NEUROLOGIC ASPECTS OF SYSTEMIC DISEASE

PART II

HANDBOOK OF CLINICAL NEUROLOGY

Series Editors

MICHAEL J. AMINOFF, FRANÇOIS BOLLER, AND DICK F. SWAAB

VOLUME 120

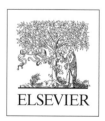

ELSEVIER

EDINBURGH LONDON NEW YORK OXFORD PHILADELPHIA
ST LOUIS SYDNEY TORONTO 2014

NEUROLOGIC ASPECTS OF SYSTEMIC DISEASE

PART II

Series Editors

MICHAEL J. AMINOFF, FRANÇOIS BOLLER, AND DICK F. SWAAB

Volume Editors

JOSÉ BILLER AND JOSÉ M. FERRO

VOLUME 120

3rd Series

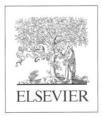

ELSEVIER

EDINBURGH LONDON NEW YORK OXFORD PHILADELPHIA
ST LOUIS SYDNEY TORONTO 2014

ELSEVIER B.V.
Radarweg 29, 1043 NX, Amsterdam, The Netherlands

ISBN: 9780702040870

British Library Cataloguing in Publication Data
A catalogue record for this book is available from the British Library

Library of Congress Cataloging in Publication Data
A catalog record for this book is available from the Library of Congress

Notice

Knowledge and best practice in this field are constantly changing. As new research and experience broaden our understanding, changes in research methods, professional practices, or medical treatment may become necessary.

Practitioners and researchers must always rely on their own experience and knowledge in evaluating and using any information, methods, compounds, or experiments described herein. In using such information or methods they should be mindful of their own safety and the safety of others, including parties for whom they have a professional responsibility.

With respect to any drug or pharmaceutical products identified, readers are advised to check the most current information provided (i) on procedures featured or (ii) by the manufacturer of each product to be administered, to verify the recommended dose or formula, the method and duration of administration, and contraindications. It is the responsibility of practitioners, relying on their own experience and knowledge of their patients, to make diagnoses, to determine dosages and the best treatment for each individual patient, and to take all appropriate safety precautions.

To the fullest extent of the law, neither the Publisher nor the contributors or editors, assume any liability for any injury and/or damage to persons or property as a matter of products liability, negligence or otherwise, or from any use or operation of any methods, products, instructions, or ideas contained in the material herein.

The Publisher

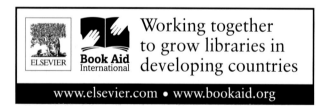

www.elsevier.com • www.bookaid.org

 your source for books, journals and multimedia in the health sciences
www.elsevierhealth.com

Printed in China

The Publisher's policy is to use **paper manufactured from sustainable forests**

Commissioning Editor: Thomas E. Stone
Development Editor: Michael Parkinson
Project Manager: Anitha Kittusamy Ramasamy
Designer/Design Direction: Alan Studholme

Handbook of Clinical Neurology 3rd Series

Available titles

Vol. 79, The human hypothalamus: basic and clinical aspects, Part I, D.F. Swaab ISBN 9780444513571
Vol. 80, The human hypothalamus: basic and clinical aspects, Part II, D.F. Swaab ISBN 9780444514905
Vol. 81, Pain, F. Cervero and T.S. Jensen, eds. ISBN 9780444519016
Vol. 82, Motor neurone disorders and related diseases, A.A. Eisen and P.J. Shaw, eds. ISBN 9780444518941
Vol. 83, Parkinson's disease and related disorders, Part I, W.C. Koller and E. Melamed, eds. ISBN 9780444519009
Vol. 84, Parkinson's disease and related disorders, Part II, W.C. Koller and E. Melamed, eds. ISBN 9780444528933
Vol. 85, HIV/AIDS and the nervous system, P. Portegies and J. Berger, eds. ISBN 9780444520104
Vol. 86, Myopathies, F.L. Mastaglia and D. Hilton Jones, eds. ISBN 9780444518996
Vol. 87, Malformations of the nervous system, H.B. Sarnat and P. Curatolo, eds. ISBN 9780444518965
Vol. 88, Neuropsychology and behavioural neurology, G. Goldenberg and B.C. Miller, eds. ISBN 9780444518972
Vol. 89, Dementias, C. Duyckaerts and I. Litvan, eds. ISBN 9780444518989
Vol. 90, Disorders of consciousness, G.B. Young and E.F.M. Wijdicks, eds. ISBN 9780444518958
Vol. 91, Neuromuscular junction disorders, A.G. Engel, ed. ISBN 9780444520081
Vol. 92, Stroke – Part I: Basic and epidemiological aspects, M. Fisher, ed. ISBN 9780444520036
Vol. 93, Stroke – Part II: clinical manifestations and pathogenesis, M. Fisher, ed. ISBN 9780444520043
Vol. 94, Stroke – Part III: Investigations and management, M. Fisher, ed. ISBN 9780444520050
Vol. 95, History of neurology, S. Finger, F. Boller and K.L. Tyler, eds. ISBN 9780444520081
Vol. 96, Bacterial infections of the central nervous system, K.L. Roos and A.R. Tunkel, eds. ISBN 9780444520159
Vol. 97, Headache, G. Nappi and M.A. Moskowitz, eds. ISBN 9780444521392
Vol. 98, Sleep disorders Part I, P. Montagna and S. Chokroverty, eds. ISBN 9780444520067
Vol. 99, Sleep disorders Part II, P. Montagna and S. Chokroverty, eds. ISBN 9780444520074
Vol. 100, Hyperkinetic movement disorders, W.J. Weiner and E. Tolosa, eds. ISBN 9780444520142
Vol. 101, Muscular dystrophies, A. Amato and R.C. Griggs, eds. ISBN 9780080450315
Vol. 102, Neuro-ophthalmology, C. Kennard and R.J. Leigh, eds. ISBN 9780444529039
Vol. 103, Ataxic disorders, S.H. Subramony and A. Durr, eds. ISBN 9780444518927
Vol. 104, Neuro-oncology Part I, W. Grisold and R. Sofietti, eds. ISBN 9780444521385
Vol. 105, Neuro-oncology Part II, W. Grisold and R. Sofietti, eds. ISBN 9780444535023
Vol. 106, Neurobiology of psychiatric disorders, T. Schlaepfer and C.B. Nemeroff, eds. ISBN 9780444520029
Vol. 107, Epilepsy Part I, H. Stefan and W.H. Theodore, eds. ISBN 9780444528988
Vol. 108, Epilepsy Part II, H. Stefan and W.H. Theodore, eds. ISBN 9780444528995
Vol. 109, Spinal cord injury, J. Verhaagen and J.W. McDonald III, eds. ISBN 9780444521378
Vol. 110, Neurological rehabilitation, M. Barnes and D.C. Good, eds. ISBN 9780444529015
Vol. 111, Pediatric neurology Part I, O. Dulac, M. Lassonde and H.B. Sarnat, eds. ISBN 9780444528919
Vol. 112, Pediatric neurology Part II, O. Dulac, M. Lassonde and H.B. Sarnat, eds. ISBN 9780444529107
Vol. 113, Pediatric neurology Part III, O. Dulac, M. Lassonde and H.B. Sarnat, eds. ISBN 9780444595652
Vol. 114, Neuroparasitology and tropical neurology, H.H. Garcia, H.B. Tanowitz and O.H. Del Brutto, eds. ISBN 9780444534903
Vol. 115, Peripheral nerve disorders, G. Said and C. Krarup, eds. ISBN 9780444529022
Vol. 116, Brain stimulation, A.M. Lozano and M. Hallett, eds. ISBN 9780444534972
Vol. 117, Autonomic nervous system, R.M. Buijs and D.F. Swaab, eds. ISBN 9780444534910
Vol. 118, Ethical and legal issues in neurology, J.L. Bernat and H.R. Beresford, eds. ISBN 9780444535016
Vol. 119, Neurologic Aspects of Systemic Disease, J. Biller and J.M. Ferro, eds. ISBN 9780702040863

Foreword

Although neurology and psychiatry are closely linked specialties, many neurologists see their specialty as part of internal medicine. Indeed, neurology departments in the United States often began as divisions within departments of internal medicine, attesting to their special relationship. With the evolution of neurology as an independent discipline, it has become particularly important for its practitioners to remain familiar with the neurologic aspects of systemic diseases as well as with the systemic aspects of neurologic disorders. This has been recognized since the *Handbook of Clinical Neurology* was founded by Pierre Vinken and George Bruyn, with volume 1 appearing in December 1968. That first series concluded in 1982 and was followed by a second series, edited by them, that concluded—in turn—in 2002. We then took over as editors of the current third series, with volume 79 appearing in late 2003 and several volumes appearing annually since then.

Two volumes (38 and 39) were published in the first series of the *Handbook,* focusing on the neurologic manifestations of systemic diseases. The second series included a further three volumes (63, 70, and 71) on the same topic, published in 1993 and 1998, with one of us (MJA) serving as an editor of those volumes. Advances in the field, but especially in immunology, genetics, imaging, pharmacotherapeutics, and intensive care, since that time have necessitated a reappraisal of the field and the publication of three new volumes on the topic. We are therefore particularly delighted at the publication of this scholarly contribution to the medical and neurologic literature and welcome it as part of the *Handbook.* We believe that it will appeal not only to neurologists but to physicians in all specialties, helping in their interactions with each other and with their patients.

Professors José Biller and José M. Ferro have together produced an authoritative, comprehensive, and up to date account of the topic and have assembled a truly international group of authors with acknowledged expertise to contribute to these important multifaceted volumes. We are grateful to them and to all the contributors for their efforts in creating such an invaluable resource. We are confident that clinicians in many different disciplines will find much in these volumes to appeal to them.

It is a pleasure, also, to thank Elsevier, our publishers – and in particular Tom Stone, Michael Parkinson, and Kristi Anderson – for unfailing and expert assistance in the development and production of these volumes.

Michael J. Aminoff
François Boller
Dick F. Swaab

Preface

Medicine has always been in a state of evolution and today, more than ever, with the accelerated growth of scientific knowledge, patients are evaluated and treated by teams of physicians. The extensive body of knowledge and the major scientific and clinical advances in neurology and internal medicine are again drawing both specialties closer together. Whatever the subspecialty area of interest, the nature of modern clinical medicine calls for multidisciplinary collaborative efforts to better meet the needs of individual patients. The aim of these three volumes of the third series of the *Handbook of Clinical Neurology* is to integrate and provide a thorough framework of the core neurologic manifestations of a wide array of systemic disorders. Each chapter provides a critical appraisal and extensive background information regarding the variety of presentations of each disorder, the characteristic clinical course, the typical neurologic manifestations of each disease, and current therapeutic strategies. Comprehensive and updated references also bring forth valuable resources for further topical reading and research. Our intended audience includes experienced practitioners and residents in neurology, neurosurgery, and internal medicine, as well as other health care professionals in different subspecialties caring for these challenging patients.

We have purposely divided these three volumes into chapters uniformly organized by organ system, which are further divided by specific conditions and disease categories. Volume I is dedicated to the neurologic aspects of cardiopulmonary diseases, renal disorders, and selective rheumatologic and musculoskeletal disorders. Volume II encompasses core neurologic aspects of gastrointestinal and hepatobiliary disorders, endocrinologic diseases, and a gamut of metabolic, nutritional and environmental conditions. Volume III concentrates on the neurologic aspects of hematologic and oncologic disorders, organ transplantation, infectious diseases, and tropical neurology. It also includes a miscellaneous group of disorders including neurodermatology, neurological complications of pregnancy, iatrogenic neurology, neuromuscular disorders in the intensive care setting, posterior reversible leukoencephalopathy and reversible cerebral vasoconstriction syndromes, neuro-Behcet's, complications of neuroimaging, neurotraumatology, and observations pertaining to neurology in the developing world. These volumes go beyond the scope of classic neurology and examine the neurologic manifestations of a wide range of medical conditions, spanning most areas of medicine, that neurologists, neurosurgeons, internists, and other specialists must diagnose and treat in everyday practice.

We are hopeful that these three volumes will contribute to the best possible care of patients with these disorders, and that the readership will find the material informative, authoritative, reliable, and stimulating

We are extremely grateful to all the contributors from across the globe, who by sharing their knowledge and expertise made these volumes possible. To bring to fruition a work of this magnitude requires a highly professional editorial effort, and for this we thank Linda Turner for her wonderful organizational skills and administrative expertise, and Mike Parkinson and the editorial staff at Elsevier for their unfailing dedication, professionalism, and expert assistance in the development and production of these three volumes.

José Biller, MD
José M. Ferro, MD

Contributors

R.J. Adams
South Carolina Stroke Center of Economic Excellence and Medical University of South Carolina Stroke Center, Charleston, SC, USA

C.L. Ahrens
Neurological Intensive Care Unit, Cleveland Clinic Cleveland, OH, USA

A. Aggarwal
Center for Brain and Nervous System, Kokilaben Dhirubhai Ambani Hospital and Medical Research Institute, Mumbai, India

L. Agrawal
Division of Endocrinology and Metabolism, Loyola University Medical Center, Maywood, IL, USA

C. Amin
Indiana Hemophilia and Thrombosis Centre, Indianapolis, IN, USA

E. Anderes
Division of Hematology and Oncology, Department of Medicine, Loyola University Chicago, Stritch School of Medicine, Maywood, IL, USA

H.C. Andersson
Hayward Genetics Center, Tulane University School of Medicine, New Orleans, LA, USA

N. Azad
Edward Hines Jr. VA Hospital, Hines, IL, USA

J.R. Berger
Department of Neurology, University of Kentucky College of Medicine, Lexington, KY, USA

M.D. Bérubé
Department of Neurology, Centre Hospitalier de l'Université de Montréal, and Faculty of Medicine, Université de Montréal, Montreal, QC, Canada

T.E. Bertorini
Department of of Neurology, Methodist University Hospital and Department of Neurology, University of Tennessee Health Science Center, Memphis, TN, USA

K. Betterman
Department of Neurology, Penn State College of Medicine, Hershey, PA, USA

M. Bhatt
Center for Brain and Nervous System, Kokilaben Dhirubhai Ambani Hospital and Medical Research Institute, Mumbai, India

N. Blais
Department of Haematology, Centre Hospitalier de l'Université de Montréal, and Faculty of Medicine, Université de Montréal, Montreal, QC, Canada

P. Bucciarelli
A. Bianchi Bonomi Hemophilia and Thrombosis Center, Department of Internal Medicine and Medical Specialties, Fondazione IRCCS Ca' Granda, Ospedale Maggiore Policlinico, University of Milan, Milan, Italy

P. Camacho
Loyola University Osteoporosis and Metabolic Bone Disease Center, Loyola University Medical Center, Maywood, IL, USA

G. Charnogursky
Division of Endocrinology and Metabolism, Loyola University Chicago, Stritch School of Medicine, Maywood, IL, USA

J. Chawla
Department of Neurology, Hines VA Hospital, Hines and Department of Neurology, Loyola University Medical Center, Maywood, IL, USA

L. Correia
Department of Gastroenterology and Hepatology,
Hospital de Santa Maria, University of Lisbon,
Lisbon, Portugal

S. Datar
Division of Critical Care Neurology, Mayo Clinic,
Rochester, MN, USA

J.F. de Lacerda
Department of Hematology and Bone Marrow
Transplantation, Hospital de Santa Maria,
Lisbon, Portugal

T. Dias
Endocrinology, Diabetes and Metabolism Unit, Hospital
de Santa Maria, Lisbon, Portugal

S. Dublis
Division of Hematology and Oncology, Department of
Medicine, Loyola University Chicago, Stritch School of
Medicine, Maywood, IL, USA

A.P. Duker
Department of Gastroenterology, Royal Hallamshire
Hospital, Sheffield, UK

P.J.B. Dyck
Mayo Clinic, Department of Neurology, Rochester,
MN, USA

M.A. Emanuele
Division of Endocrinology and Metabolism, Loyola
University Chicago, Stritch School of Medicine,
Maywood, IL, USA

N.V. Emanuele
Division of Endocrinology and Metabolism, Loyola
University Medical Center, Maywood, and
Endocrinology Section, Edward Hines Jr. VA Hospital,
Hines, IL, USA

J.M. Ferro
Neurology Service, Department of Neurosciences,
Hospital de Santa Maria, University of Lisbon,
Lisbon, Portugal

P. Foy
Department of Hematology, Medical College of
Wisconsin, Milwaukee, WI, USA

R.L. Gamelli
Department of Surgery, Loyola University Medical
Center, Maywood, IL, USA

C.R. Gomez
Neurological Institute of Alabama, Birmingham,
AL, USA

A. Griest
Indiana Hemophilia and Thrombosis Centre and
Department of Medicine, Indiana University School of
Medicine, Indianapolis, IN, USA

G. Gruener
Department of Neurology and Leischner Institute for
Medical Education, Loyola University Medical Center,
Maywood, IL, USA

Z. Habib
Division of Endocrinology and Metabolism, Loyola
University Medical Center, Maywood, IL, USA

M. Hadjivassiliou
Department of Neurology, Royal Hallamshire Hospital,
Sheffield, UK

J.C. Kattah
Department of Neurology, University of Illinois College
of Medicine, Peoria, IL, USA

W.C. Kattah
Endocrinology Department, University of the Andes,
Bogota, Colombia

R.E. Kelley
Department of Neurology, Tulane University School of
Medicine, New Orleans, LA, USA

M. Komoroski
Loyola University Osteoporosis and Metabolic Bone
Disease Center, Loyola University Medical Center,
Maywood, IL, USA

S.A.M. Kularatne
Department of Medicine, Faculty of Medicine,
University of Peradeniya, Kandy, Sri Lanka

N. Kumar
Department of Neurology, Mayo Clinic, Rochester,
MN, USA

D. Kvarnberg
Department of Neurology, Loyola University Medical
Center, Maywood, IL, USA

S. Lanthier
Department of Neurology, Centre Hospitalier de
l'Université de Montréal, and Faculty of Medicine,
Université de Montréal, Montreal, QC, Canada

H. Lee
Division of Endocrinology and Metabolism, Loyola
University Stritch School of Medicine, Maywood,
IL, USA

N. Lopez
Division of Endocrinology and Metabolism, Loyola
University Chicago, Stritch School of Medicine,
Maywood, IL, USA

I. Martinelli
A. Bianchi Bonomi Hemophilia and Thrombosis Center,
Department of Internal Medicine and Medical
Specialties, Fondazione IRCCS Ca' Granda, Ospedale
Maggiore Policlinico, University of Milan, Milan, Italy

E.W. Massey
Department of Neurology, Duke University Medical
Center, Durham, NC, USA

A. Mazhari
Division of Endocrinology and Metabolism, Loyola
University Chicago, Stritch School of Medicine,
Maywood, IL, USA

E.M. Manno
Neurological Intensive Care Unit, Cleveland Clinic,
Cleveland, OH, USA

M. McCoyd
Department of Neurology, Loyola University Medical
Center, Maywood, IL, USA

R.E. Moon
Departments of Anesthesiology and Medicine, Duke
University Medical Center, Durham, NC, USA

S. Nand
Division of Hematology and Oncology, Department of
Medicine, Loyola University Chicago, Stritch School of
Medicine, Maywood, IL, USA

S.N. Oliveira
Department of Neurology, Hospital da Luz, Lisbon,
Portugal

S.M. Passamonti
A. Bianchi Bonomi Hemophilia and Thrombosis Center,
Department of Internal Medicine and Medical
Specialties, Fondazione IRCCS Ca' Granda, Ospedale
Maggiore Policlinico, University of Milan, Milan, Italy

S. Patel
Department of Internal Medicine, Conemaugh Health
System, Jonestown, PA, USA

A. Perez
Department of Clinical Neurophysiology, University
of Tennessee Health Science Center, Memphis,
TN, USA

R.F. Pfeiffer
Department of Neurology, University of Tennessee
Health Science Center, Memphis, TN, USA

E.H. Reynolds
Department of Clinical Neurosciences, King's College,
London, UK

M.M. Rosa
Neurology Department, Hospital de Santa Maria,
Lisbon, Portugal

S. Samarasinghe
Division of Endocrinology and Metabolism, Loyola
University Chicago, Stritch School of Medicine,
Maywood, IL, USA

D.S. Sanders
Department of Neurology, University of Cincinnati,
Cincinnati, OH, USA

A. Sanford
Department of Surgery, Loyola University Medical
Center, Maywood, IL, USA

E. Schnitzler
Department of Neurology, Loyola University Medical
Center, Maywood, IL, USA

N. Senanayake
Department of Medicine, Faculty of Medicine,
University of Peradeniya, Kandy, Sri Lanka

S. Shah
Division of Hematology and Oncology, Department of
Medicine, Loyola University Chicago, Stritch School of
Medicine, Maywood, IL, USA

A. Sharathkumar
Indiana Hemophilia and Thrombosis Centre and
Department of Pediatrics, Riley Whitcomb Hospital for
Children, Indiana University School of Medicine,
Indianapolis, IN, USA

P.J. Shaw
Sheffield Institute for Translational Neuroscience,
University of Sheffield and Department of Neurology,
Royal Hallamshire Hospital,
Sheffield, UK

D. Singhal
Department of Neurology, University of Kentucky
College of Medicine, Lexington, KY, USA

U. Sobol
Department of Hematology and Oncology, Cardinal
Bernardin Cancer Center, Loyola University Medical
Center, Maywood, IL, USA

P. Stiff
Department of Hematology and Oncology, Cardinal
Bernardin Cancer Center, Loyola University Medical
Center, Maywood, IL, USA

J.A. Tracy
Mayo Clinic, Department of Neurology, Rochester, MN,
USA

J-M. Trocello
French National Wilson's Disease Centre (CNR Wilson),
Lariboisière Hospital, Paris, France

A. Venkataraman
Pediatric Neurology and Epilepsy Division, Lutheran
Medical Center, Brooklyn, NY, USA

K. Webster
Department of Pediatrics, Loyola University Medical
Center, Maywood, IL, USA

K. Weissenborn
Department of Neurology, Hanover Medical School,
Hanover, Germany

E.F.M. Wijdicks
Division of Critical Care Neurology, Mayo Clinic,
Rochester, MN, USA

F. Woimant
French National Wilson's Disease Centre (CNR Wilson),
Lariboisière Hospital, Paris, France

C.A. Wood-Allum
Sheffield Institute for Translational Neuroscience,
University of Sheffield and Department of Neurology,
Royal Hallamshire Hospital, Sheffield, UK

Contents of Part II

Contents of Part I

SECTION 2   Neurologic aspects of pulmonary diseases

SECTION 3   Neurologic aspects of renal diseases

SECTION 4   Neurologic aspects of rheumatologic/musculoskeletal diseases

Contents of Part III

SECTION 14   Miscellaneous

Section 5

Neurologic aspects of gastrointestinal/ hepatobiliary diseases

Handbook of Clinical Neurology, Vol. 120 (3rd series)
Neurologic Aspects of Systemic Disease Part II
Jose Biller and Jose M. Ferro, Editors

Chapter 39

The neurologic complications of bariatric surgery

JOSEPH R. BERGER* AND DIVYA SINGHAL
Department of Neurology, University of Kentucky College of Medicine, Lexington, KY, USA

OBESITY: AN OVERVIEW

Weight is a national obsession. In 1999, Americans spent over $300 million on prescription medications for obesity (Wilhelm, 2000) and at the end of the 20th century 2.5% of the adult population reported using such preparations (Khan et al., 2001). By some estimates, the medical costs of obesity have risen to $147 billion per year as of 2008. Obesity is now officially recognized by the US Surgeon General as a significant health risk factor. Current prevalence of obesity is estimated to be over 30% in the US (Flegal et al., 2010), and another third are overweight. Obesity increases the risk for numerous medical illnesses, among them diabetes mellitus, hypercholesterolemia, hypertension and other cardiovascular disorders, pulmonary disease, chronic diseases, including osteoarthritis, liver and kidney disease, asthma, chronic back pain, sleep apnea, and depression and some forms of cancer (Fisher and Schauer, 2002; Mokdad et al., 2003). Obesity also increases the risk of death from all causes; it is estimated that 300 000 adults in the US die from obesity-related causes annually (Allison et al., 1999). Given the increasing prevalence of obesity, it has been postulated that obesity may soon become the leading cause of death in the US (Mokdad et al., 2004). Furthermore, the average obese person costs society more than $7000 a year in lost productivity and as much as $30 000 in added medical costs over a lifetime (Freedman, 2011).

The problem of obesity is a global phenomenon consequent on the ready availability of food with high caloric content and the reduction of daily energy expenditure. While the percentage of overweight adults in most Western European countries has not surpassed that of the US, their numbers are increasing rapidly. The number of obese children in many of these countries, such as, England, is growing rapidly (Lobstein et al., 2003) and

has outstripped that in the US. In major population centers of developing countries, obesity is also seen with increasing frequency.

For medical purposes, obesity is defined by body mass index (BMI), which is derived by dividing an individual's weight in kilograms by their height in meters square. Normal weight is defined as a BMI of 18.5–24.9 (National Heart, Lung, and Blood Institute, 1998). A BMI exceeding this value is regarded as overweight. BMIs of 30 or greater are considered obese and those equal to or exceeding 40 as morbidly obese (National Heart, Lung, and Blood Institute, 1998). Prevalence data from the CDC (US Centers for Disease Control and Prevention) indicates that in 1999–2000, 64.5% of US adults were overweight, 30.5% were obese, and 4.7% were morbidly obese (Flegal et al., 2002). Despite the billions of dollars spent on diets, dietary supplements, exercise programs, and other nonsurgical modalities for weight reduction, long-term success rates have been quite variable. Increasing numbers of people are, therefore, resorting to bariatric surgery for control of their weight problem. The increasing popularity of these procedures may, in part, be attributable to media attention provided by television personalities who have undergone surgery for their own weight reduction. From 1990 to 2000, the national annual rate of bariatric surgery increased nearly sixfold, from 2.4 to 14.1 per 100 000 adults (Trus et al., 2005). Population-adjusted rates of bariatric surgery in the overall sample increased more than sevenfold in the study period, from 3.5 per 100 000 US population in 1996 to 24.0 per 100 000 in 2002 (Davis et al., 2006).

BARIATRIC SURGERY

National guidelines reserves bariatric surgery for individuals who have failed attempts of nonsurgical weight

---

*Correspondence to Dr. Joseph R. Berger, Department of Neurology, University of Kentucky College of Medicine, Kentucky Clinic L-445, 740 S. Limestone Street, Lexington, KY 40536-0284, USA. Tel: +1-859 218-5039, Fax: +1-859 323-5943, E-mail: joseph.berger@uky.edu

loss and have a BMI $\geq$ 35 with an obesity-related comorbidity or a BMI > 40 with or without a comorbidity (National Institutes of Health, 1992). A number of different surgical procedures have been employed for achieving weight reduction (Deitel and Shikora, 2002). Gastroplasties rely on the mechanical restriction of food passage through the stomach, whereas gastric bypass is considered to result in weight loss by a more physiologic mechanism (Livingston, 2002). Gastric bypass, typically the Roux-en-Y gastric bypass, is now performed more commonly than gastroplasties (Pope et al., 2002). Many of these surgical procedures can be performed laparoscopically (Azagra et al., 1999; Higa et al., 2000; Schauer et al., 2000). Average excess weight loss following laparoscopic Roux-en-Y gastric bypass has been reported to approach 70% at 12 months (Higa et al., 2000) and 83% at 24 months (Schauer et al., 2000), with excellent control of comorbidities (Buchwald et al., 2004). Although success rates have been variable, persistent, long-term weight loss of 10 or more years following these procedures has been documented (Yale, 1989; Pories et al., 1992). Studies of cost-effectiveness support the value of bariatric surgery (Clegg et al., 2003; Fang, 2003).

The complications of bariatric surgery are not insignificant, in part related to the problems inherent in operating on the obese person. In one series (Schauer et al., 2000), major complications occurred in 3.3% and the in-hospital mortality was 0.4%. Reoperation may be necessitated by bleeding, abscess, and wound dehiscence. A variety of late complications are recognized, generally the consequence of nutritional deficiency (Table 39.1). Mineral deficiencies include iron, calcium, phosphate, and magnesium, and vitamin deficiencies include thiamine (B_1), cyanocobalamin (B_{12}), folate, vitamin D, vitamin E. Iron, folate, and vitamin B_{12} deficiency have been reported to be the most common nutritional deficiencies observed following gastric bypass (Halverson, 1992; Skroubis et al., 2002; Bal et al., 2010).

Table 39.1

Micronutrient deficiencies following bariatric surgery

- Thiamine (B_1)
- Cyanocobalamin (B_{12})
- Vitamin D
- Vitamin E
- Folate
- Iron
- Calcium
- Magnesium
- Phosphate
- Copper
- Selenium

Neurologic complications of bariatric surgery

A broad spectrum of neurologic complications has been reported to occur in association with bariatric surgery (Table 39.2). No part of the neuraxis is exempt from these complications. To date, all studies addressing the neurologic complications occurring in the setting of bariatric surgery have been retrospective in nature. In 1987, Abarbanel and colleagues reported that 23 of 500 (4.6%) patients undergoing bariatric surgery experienced neurologic complications (Abarbanel et al., 1987). Of the 500 patients, 457 had a Roux-en-Y procedure and 43 had gastroplasty (Abarbanel et al., 1987). The neurologic complications became manifest 3–20 months after surgery and all affected patients experienced protracted vomiting, a symptom that may occur in up to one-third of all patients undergoing gastric bypass (Halverson, 1992; Bal et al., 2010). The constellation of neurologic complications included chronic and subacute peripheral neuropathy (52%), acute peripheral neuropathy (4%), burning feet (9%), meralgia paresthetica (9%), myotonic syndrome (4%), posterolateral myelopathy (9%), and Wernicke's encephalopathy (9%) (Abarbanel et al., 1987). In this series, individuals with burning feet and Wernicke's encephalopathy responded to thiamine administration (Abarbanel et al., 1987).

In a retrospective review of 556 patients undergoing bariatric surgery at the Mayo Clinic from 1980 through 2003, Thaisetthawatkul and colleagues observed 48 patients (8.6%) with complications affecting the peripheral nervous system (Thaisetthawatkul, 2003). Of these 48 patients, 23 (48%) developed mononeuropathies with carpal tunnel syndrome, the most common accounting for 74% of the total (Thaisetthawatkul,

Table 39.2

Neurologic complications of bariatric surgery

- Encephalopathy
- Behavioral abnormalities
- Seizures
- Cranial nerve palsies
- Ataxia
- Myelopathy
- Plexopathies
- Peripheral neuropathy
- Mononeuropathies
  - Carpal tunnel syndrome
  - Meralgia paresthetica
- Compartment syndromes
- Myopathy
- Myotonia
- Restless legs syndrome

2003). Peripheral neuropathies were observed in 20 (41.7%), plexopathies in 4 (17.4%), and myopathy in 1 (4.3%) (Thaisetthawatkul, 2003). Perhaps the most debilitating of the neurologic consequences of bariatric surgery are those occurring from vitamin deficiency, particularly vitamins B_1 and B_{12}, as these may result in permanent neurologic disability.

Thiamine deficiency (vitamin B_1)

Thiamine deficiency alters mitochondrial function, impairs oxidative metabolism, and causes selective neuronal death by diminishing thiamine-dependent enzymes (Ke et al., 2003). A deficiency of thiamine results in peripheral neuropathy, ophthalmoplegia and nystagmus, ataxia, encephalopathy and may lead to permanent impairment of recent memory. This constellation is referred to as Wernicke's encephalopathy. The diagnostic criteria of Wernicke's encephalopathy require two of the following four features: (1) dietary deficiency; (2) oculomotor abnormality; (3) cerebellar dysfunction; (4) confusion or mild memory impairment. These criteria have a very high inter-rater reliability for the diagnosis (Caine et al., 1997). This condition is most commonly described in the setting of alcohol abuse when the individual has had insufficient dietary intake of thiamine over a long period of time. However, it is important to recall one of the three cases in the initial description in 1881 by Carl Wernicke was the consequence of esophageal damage from sulfuric acid ingestion with associated refractory emesis (Wernicke, 1881). The mechanism by which bariatric surgery leads to thiamine deficiency, whether resulting in an encephalopathy or peripheral neuropathy, is almost certainly inadequate vitamin repletion attending persistent, intractable vomiting.

In 1977, Printen and Mason reported four patients who developed peripheral neuropathy and protracted emesis following gastric operations for obesity (Printen and Mason, 1977). In this and other early reports of the neurologic complications occurring with gastric bypass, the specific cause of the neurologic disorder remained uncertain. In 1981, Ayub and colleagues described confusion, slurred speech, and unsteadiness in seven of 110 patients undergoing bariatric surgery (Ayub et al., 1981). The authors listed several potential etiologies, including nutritional disturbances, metabolic abnormalities, medication side-effects, lactic acidosis, or potential "toxic" bowel product attributable to a micro-organism (Ayub et al., 1981). Some, if not all, of these cases were likely due to thiamine deficiency. Over the past three decades, several reports linked the appearance of Wernicke's encephalopathy with surgery for morbid obesity (Rothrock and Smith, 1981; Haid et al., 1982; MacLean, 1982; Milius et al., 1982; Villar and

Ranne, 1984; Oczkowski and Kertesz, 1985). Although some authors had previously considered Wernicke's encephalopathy a "very rare complication" of gastric surgery for morbid obesity (Bozbora et al., 2000), there are at least 104 cases in the world's literature and the number of cases after bariatric surgery is substantially higher than previously reported (Aasheim et al., 2009). This complication is almost always associated with severe intractable vomiting. It may be seen relatively soon after surgery, usually within 4–12 weeks (Kramer and Locke, 1987) but occasionally as late as 18 months after the procedure.

Peripheral neuropathy often, but not invariably, accompanies Wernicke's encephalopathy following surgery for morbid obesity. Peripheral neuropathy with or without Wernicke's encephalopathy that is attributable to thiamine deficiency and has occurred following surgery for morbid obesity has been referred to as "bariatric beriberi" (Gollobin and Marcus, 2002). It appears to be more common than encephalopathy and may also occur within 6 weeks of surgery (Chaves et al., 2002), although intervals exceeding 3 years have been reported (Koike et al., 2001). The neuropathy predominantly affects the lower limbs and is both sensory and motor, with variable involvement of each. While it may progress over years when untreated, rapid progression over intervals as short as 3 days may mimic Guillain–Barré syndrome (Koike et al., 2001; Chang et al., 2002). Electrophysiologic studies reveal that this neuropathy is axonal in nature with markedly reduced amplitudes of compound motor action potential and sensory nerve action potentials, especially in the lower extremities (Koike et al., 2001).

Thiamine deficiency can be confirmed by assessing the thiamine pyrophosphate effect in erythrocyte transketolase studies (Boni et al., 1980). The clinical constellation coupled with the response to parenteral thiamine, especially with the features of the encephalopathy, may prove sufficiently diagnostic. Additionally, magnetic resonance imaging (MRI) of the brain may show characteristic abnormalities, in particular, hyperintense signal abnormalities on T2-weighted images in the dorsomedial thalamic nuclei, periaqueductal gray matter, and mammillary bodies (Cirignotta et al., 2000; Toth and Voll, 2001). Both the encephalopathy and peripheral neuropathy of thiamine deficiency may occur despite oral supplementation with thiamine as emesis may preclude effective absorption. Substantial functional recovery typically occurs within 3–6 months of the initiation of therapy (Koike et al., 2001); however, neurologic recovery may be incomplete (Salas-Salvado et al., 2000), particularly if the nature of the disorder is not recognized promptly. Physical therapy for the peripheral neuropathy is also recommended (Chaves et al., 2002).

Copper deficiency myelopathy

Copper deficiency myelopathy (CDM) was first reported in 2001 and over the last decade, it has become an increasingly recognized myelopathy that most commonly occurs as a consequence of prior gastrointestinal surgery. The clinical and radiologic picture is usually indistinguishable from subacute combined degeneration (SCD) (Kumar et al., 2004) due to vitamin B_{12} (cobalamin) deficiency, and the two may coexist (Juhasz-Pocsine et al., 2007). Other, less frequently reported and less clearly causally related neurologic associations of acquired copper deficiency include isolated peripheral neuropathy, motor neuron disease, myopathy, cerebral demyelination, cognitive dysfunction, and optic neuropathy.

Jaiser and Winston (2010) reviewed 55 cases in the literature – previous upper gastrointestinal surgery was the commonest reported cause, being implicated in almost half the cases. Of these, nine cases were attributable to bariatric surgery. The interval between upper gastrointestinal surgery and symptom onset ranged from 5 to 26 years in the bariatric group (mean 11.4 years). Likely cause for copper deficiency is greater reduction in the effective absorption area for copper (postoperatively, food bypasses most of the stomach and the entire duodenum).

Copper is a component of numerous metalloenzymes and proteins that have a key role in maintaining the structure and function of the nervous system. It is a constituent of cytochrome oxidase (oxidative phosphorylation), superoxide dismutase (antioxidant defense), ceruloplasmin (iron metabolism), tyrosinase (melanin synthesis), and dopamine β-monooxygenase (catecholamine synthesis) (Kumar et al., 2004a). Based on similarities to SCD due to vitamin B_{12} deficiency and copper deficiency myelopathy, it has been hypothesized that methionine synthase and S-adenosylhomocysteine hydrolase (another enzyme involved in the cycle) may depend on copper. Dysfunction in the methylation cycle and associated failure of myelin maintenance could therefore explain the clinical and radiologic congruence between CDM and SCD, but it remains to be proven with direct biochemical evidence (Kumar et al., 2006; Kumar and Weimar, 2010).

Most common neurologic manifestation in adults is a myeloneuropathy with gait difficulties (primarily due to sensory ataxia due to dorsal column dysfunction), spastic gait and lower limb paresthesias; urinary symptoms are infrequent. Examination usually shows a spastic paraparesis or tetraparesis with a truncal sensory level for dorsal column modalities. A sensory/motor neuropathy frequently coexists and manifests as depression of distal reflexes and superimposed sensory impairment in a glove and stocking distribution. Although the hematologic hallmark of copper deficiency is anemia and neutropenia, it is being increasingly recognized that hematologic manifestations may not accompany the neurologic syndrome (Kumar et al., 2003, 2004b).

Serum copper and serum ceruloplasmin levels have consistently been found to be low and of statistical significance. Urinary copper level excretion is frequently low (when dietary copper is low). For assessment of metabolically active copper stores, activity of copper enzymes such as erythrocyte superoxide dismutase and platelet or leukocyte cytochrome c oxidase may be utilized (Kumar and Weimar, 2010). Electrophysiologic tests reveal an axonal sensorimotor peripheral neuropathy (to varying degrees). Somatosensory potentials are abnormal with impaired central conduction being a key finding (Jaiser and Winston, 2010). Spinal MRI shows an augmented T2 signal involving the dorsal column in posterior cervical or thoracic cord in nearly half of the cases with no contrast enhancement (22 cases) (Kumar, 2006); rarely, signal changes involving the lateral column may be seen (Kumar et al., 2003).

Although there have been no studies that address the most appropriate dose and duration of copper supplementation, based on a review of all articles addressing this subject, oral copper supplementation is the preferred route of supplementation. Oral supplementation equivalent to doses ranging from 2 to 8 mg of elemental copper per day have been recommended by different authors (Kumar, 2006; Jaiser and Winston, 2010). Practice at Mayo Clinic involves 6 mg/day of elemental copper orally for a week, 4 mg/day for the second week, and 2 mg/day thereafter. Periodic assessment of serum copper is essential to determine adequacy of replacement and the most appropriate long-term administration strategy is recommended (Winston and Jaiser, 2008). Since zinc can interfere with copper absorption, care must be taken to avoid copper preparations containing significant quantities of zinc, such as multivitamin tablets. As the underlying risk factor of decreased copper absorption cannot be eliminated in cases of bariatric surgery, a short 5 day course of parenteral therapy (to facilitate rapid normalization of body copper stores) followed by indefinite oral copper supplementation has been recommended. Whilst treatment causes prompt and full resolution of hematologic abnormalities, the neurologic deficits merely stabilize (51% of cases) or partially improve (49% cases). Hence, it is crucial to avoid delays in diagnosis and treatment to avert potentially irreversible neurologic deterioration (Jaiser and Winston, 2010).

Improvement when present is often subjective and preferentially involves sensory symptoms. There are some reports of definite improvement in the neurologic deficits, nerve conduction studies, evoked potential studies, and MRI T2 cord signal changes with normalization of serum copper (Kumar, 2006).

Other nutritional and metabolic disorders

Absorption of *vitamin B12* is complex and requires the presence of intrinsic factor derived from gastric parietal cells, acid gastric pH, and absorption in the ileum. Bariatric surgery may interfere with several of these mechanisms. As liver stores of cyanocobalamin are sufficient to allow for years of dietary insufficiency, these features may not appear for long periods of time. A low serum vitamin B_{12} level has been observed in as many as 70% patients undergoing gastric bypass, and vitamin B_{12} deficiency in more than 30% (Amaral et al., 1985).

The prototypical neurologic disorder occurring with cyanocobalamin deficiency is subacute combined degeneration in which the peripheral nerves and posterior columns of the spinal cord are chiefly affected. A large number of neurologic symptoms and signs have been associated with cyanocobalamin deficiency, including, paresthesias, loss of cutaneous sensation, weakness, decreased reflexes, spasticity, ataxia, incontinence, loss of vision, dementia, psychoses, and altered mood (Healton et al., 1991). Subacute combined degeneration has been reported after partial gastrectomy (Weir and Gatenby, 1963; Williams et al., 1969). The infrequency of disorders related to vitamin B_{12} has suggested to some investigators that vitamin B_{12} deficiency is seldom clinically relevant in the postgastric bypass patient (Brolin et al., 1998); however, Bloomberg and colleagues (2005) reviewed the literature and reflected on the need for further studies to evaluate the clinical significance of nutritional deficiencies and establish guidelines for supplementation.

Low plasma folate is seen in up to 42% of persons undergoing gastric bypass followed for 3 years (Halverson, 1986). Folate deficiency with an attendant peripheral neuropathy would not be unexpected. However, the literature does not suggest that it is a common problem and some investigators argue that it is not clinically relevant (Brolin et al., 1998). As with vitamin B_{12}, oral folate supplementation appears effective in maintaining levels within the normal range (Brolin et al., 1991).

Niacin deficiency and pellagra has occurred after gastroplasty (Lopez et al., 2000). This syndrome is characterized by a symmetrical rash on sun-exposed areas with hyperkeratosis, hyperpigmentation, and desquamation. Glossitis, diarrhea, fatigue, hallucinations, and encephalopathy are also features of the disorder.

Symptomatic hypocalcemia secondary to *vitamin D* deficiency after gastric bypass has been described (Marinella, 1999). Marinella reported a patient who developed carpopedal spasms, intermittent facial twitching and ophthalmoplegia in association with hypocalcemia years after gastric bypass who responded to calcium repletion (Marinella, 1999). Interestingly, Aasheim and colleagues (2009) have reported that the risk of vitamin deficiencies differs significantly based on the type of bariatric surgery – compared with gastric bypass, duodenal switch may be associated with a greater risk of thiamine, vitamin A and D deficiencies in the first year after the procedure. Hence, patients who undergo these two surgical interventions may require different monitoring and supplementation regimens in the first year after surgery. In addition to vitamin D, patients undergoing gastric bypass may also be at risk of depletion of another fat-soluble vitamin, vitamin E (Provenzale et al., 1992), which is also associated with neurologic manifestations (Satya-Murti et al., 1986).

Boldery and colleagues have reported two cases implicating selenium deficiency as a cause of heart failure in patients after gastric bypass surgery; selenium deficiency is recognized as a cause of Keshan disease, also known as nutritional cardiomyopathy. However, in postbypass surgery patients with heart failure, obstructive sleep apnea and thiamine deficiency must also be considered as potential explanations (Boldery et al., 2007).

Neurologic disorders consequent to rapid *fat metabolism* or the result of multiple nutritional and metabolic factors have been reported, but remain unproven. Feit and colleagues reported two patients who developed a severe polyneuropathy chiefly affecting position sense associated with ataxia and pseudochorea within 3 months of gastric partitioning for morbid obesity (Feit et al., 1982). In one patient who died, autopsy revealed extensive demyelination associated with extensive accumulation of lipofuscin in anterior horn cells and dorsal root ganglia and lipid in Schwann cells (Feit et al., 1982). The authors suggested that a toxin from rapid fat catabolism or loss of carnitine were responsible rather than thiamine or another vitamin deficiency (Feit et al., 1982). Similarly, Paulson and colleagues reported six patients with a clinical picture characterized by confusion, abnormal behavior, profound leg weakness, diminished or absent muscle stretch reflexes, and in three, ophthalmoplegia, or nystagmus (Paulson et al., 1985). While thiamine deficiency was considered in the differential diagnosis, the authors believed that this disorder was likely the consequence of rapid metabolism of fat in obesity (Paulson et al., 1985). Other investigators have proposed that some of the neurologic complications which follow bariatric surgery, such as the peripheral neuropathy or psychosis, arise from multifactorial causes (Seehra et al., 1996; Thaisetthawatkul et al., 2004).

Recurrent spells of encephalopathy characterized by confusion, behavioral abnormalities, weakness, lethargy, ataxia, and dysarthria occurring with *lactic acidosis* may occur after jejunoileostomy for morbid obesity (Dahlquist et al., 1984). This same disorder has been described in individuals with short bowel syndrome (Stolberg et al., 1982). It is precipitated by high carbohydrate diets. The neurologic symptoms occur in association with elevated concentrations of D-lactate in blood, urine, and stool (Dahlquist et al., 1984). The elevated levels of D-lactate are believed to result from fermentation of carbohydrates in the colon or bypassed segment of the small bowel (Dahlquist et al., 1984).

Minerals (calcium, phosphorus, and magnesium) and trace elements (zinc, iodine, copper, manganese, fluoride, chromium, molybdenum, selenium, and iron) have seldom been studied in patients following gastric bypass (Bal et al., 2010).

Miscellaneous disorders

Some of neurologic complications of bariatric surgery that are not ascribable to micronutrient insufficiency, although not exclusive to this setting, remain relatively unique. Unilateral lower compartment syndrome occurring in the immediate postoperative period may be observed (Gorecki et al., 2002). This syndrome arises from ischemic injury to tissues in the anterior compartment with progressive increase in pressure and ultimately nerve injury. Prompt recognition and fasciotomy are essential for a favorable outcome (Gorecki et al., 2002).

Lumbosacral plexopathy with an asymmetric peripheral neuropathy has been reported following gastric partitioning (Harwood et al., 1987). The specific pathogenesis of this disorder have not been addressed (Harwood et al., 1987) and whether it is due to a micronutrient deficiency or other cause remains uncertain. Similarly, Thaisetthawatkul noted plexopathy in five of his 435 patients (Thaisetthawatkul, 2003).

A wide variety of musculoskeletal symptoms have been reported to occur in association with gastric bypass (Ginsberg et al., 1979). Ginsberg and colleagues reported 13 patients who developed a constellation of arthritis, polyarthralgias, myalgias, and morning stiffness 3 weeks to 48 months after undergoing jejunoileal shunt surgery (Ginsberg et al., 1979). These symptoms tended to be transient in nature and the demonstration of circulating immune complexes suggested an autoimmune process (Ginsberg et al., 1979).

CONCLUSIONS

In summary, neurologic complications occurring in the setting of bariatric surgery are not uncommon. These complications have been reported in as many as 5–10% of patients undergoing surgery for obesity (Berger, 2004). Any part of the neuraxis, including brain, cerebellum, spinal cord, peripheral nerve, and muscle, may be involved by these complications. Most of these neurologic complications are the consequence of micronutrient deficiency. Following bariatric surgery, at 6 month intervals during the first 3 years, then once yearly ferritin, zinc, copper, magnesium, total 25-hydroxyvitamin D, folate, whole blood thiamine, vitamin B$_{12}$ and 24 h urinary calcium levels should be checked (Bal et al., 2010). Physicians need to be particularly alert to Wernicke's encephalopathy developing after bariatric surgery as it is a medical emergency and demands rapid diagnosis and intervention. Copper deficiency is an increasingly recognized complication (Jaiser and Winston, 2010) (and expected to become even more frequent with increase in number of bariatric surgeries) – early recognition and treatment is of utmost importance because it can prevent neurologic deterioration (Videt-Gibou et al., 2010). Physicians caring for patients who have undergone bariatric surgery should be familiar with the constellation of neurologic disorders that may occur.

REFERENCES

Aasheim ET, Bjorkman S, Sevik TT et al. (2009). Vitamin status after bariatric surgery: a randomized study of gastric bypass and duodenal switch. Am J Clin Nutr 90: 15–22.

Abarbanel JM, Berginer VM, Osimani A et al. (1987). Neurologic complications after gastric restriction surgery for morbid obesity. Neurology 37: 196–200.

Allison DB, Fontaine KR, Manson JE et al. (1999). Annual deaths attributable to obesity in the United States. JAMA 282: 1530–1538.

Amaral JF, Thompson WR, Caldwell MD et al. (1985). Prospective hematologic evaluation of gastric exclusion surgery for morbid obesity. Ann Surg 201: 186–193.

Ayub A, Faloon WW, Heinig RE (1981). Encephalopathy following jejunoileostomy. JAMA 246: 970–973.

Azagra JS, Goergen M, Ansay J et al. (1999). Laparoscopic gastric reduction surgery. Preliminary results of a randomized prospective trial of laparoscopic vs open vertical banded gastroplasty. Surg Endosc 13: 555–558.

Bal B, Koch TR, Finelli FC et al. (2010). Managing medical and surgical disorders after divided Roux-en-Y gastric bypass surgery. Nat Rev Gastroenterol Hepatol 7: 320–334.

Berger JR (2004). The neurological complications of bariatric surgery. Arch Neurol 61: 1185–1189.

Bloomberg RD, Fleishman A, Nalle JE et al. (2005). Nutritional deficiencies following bariatric surgery: what have we learned? Obes Surg 15: 145–154.

Boldery R, Fielding G, Rafter T et al. (2007). Nutritional deficiency of selenium secondary to weight loss (bariatric) surgery associated with life-threatening cardiomyopathy. Heart Lung Circ 16: 123–126.

Boni L, Kieckens L, Hendrikx A (1980). An evaluation of a modified erythrocyte transketolase assay for assessing thiamine nutritional adequacy. J Nutr Sci Vitaminol (Tokyo) 26: 507–514.

Bozbora A, Coskun H, Ozarmagan S et al. (2000). A rare complication of adjustable gastric banding: Wernicke's encephalopathy. Obes Surg 10: 274–275.

Brolin RE, Gorman RC, Milgrim LM et al. (1991). Multivitamin prophylaxis in prevention of post-gastric bypass vitamin and mineral deficiencies. Int J Obes 15: 661–667.

Brolin RE, Gorman JH, Gorman RC et al. (1998). Are vitamin B12 and folate deficiency clinically important after Roux-en-Y gastric bypass? J Gastrointest Surg 2: 436–442.

Buchwald H, Avidor Y, Braunwald E et al. (2004). Bariatric surgery: a systematic review and meta-analysis. JAMA 292: 1724–1737.

Caine D, Halliday GM, Kril JJ et al. (1997). Operational criteria for the classification of chronic alcoholics: identification of Wernicke's encephalopathy. J Neurol Neurosurg Psychiatry 62: 51–60.

Chang CG, Helling TS, Black WE et al. (2002). Weakness after gastric bypass. Obes Surg 12: 592–597.

Chaves LC, Faintuch J, Kahwage S et al. (2002). A cluster of polyneuropathy and Wernicke–Korsakoff syndrome in a bariatric unit. Obes Surg 12: 328–334.

Cirignotta F, Manconi M, Mondini S et al. (2000). Wernicke–Korsakoff encephalopathy and polyneuropathy after gastroplasty for morbid obesity: report of a case. Arch Neurol 57: 1356–1359.

Clegg AJ, Colquitt J, Sidhu MK et al. (2003). Clinical and cost effectiveness of surgery for morbid obesity: a systematic review and economic evaluation. Int J Obes Relat Metab Disord 27: 1167–1177.

Dahlquist NR, Perrault J, Callaway CW et al. (1984). D-Lactic acidosis and encephalopathy after jejunoileostomy: response to overfeeding and to fasting in humans. Mayo Clin Proc 59: 141–145.

Davis MM, Slish K, Chao C et al. (2006). National trends in bariatric surgery 1996–2002. Arch Surg 141: 71–74, discussion 75.

Deitel M, Shikora SA (2002). The development of the surgical treatment of morbid obesity. J Am Coll Nutr 21: 365–371.

Fang J (2003). The cost-effectiveness of bariatric surgery. Am J Gastroenterol 98: 2097–2098.

Feit H, Glasberg M, Ireton C et al. (1982). Peripheral neuropathy and starvation after gastric partitioning for morbid obesity. Ann Intern Med 96: 453–455.

Fisher BL, Schauer P (2002). Medical and surgical options in the treatment of severe obesity. Am J Surg 184: 9S–16S.

Flegal KM, Carroll MD, Ogden CL et al. (2002). Prevalence and trends in obesity among US adults 1999–2000. JAMA 288: 1723–1727.

Flegal KM, Carroll MD, Ogden CL et al. (2010). Prevalence and trends in obesity among US adults 1999–2008. JAMA 303: 235–241.

Freedman DH (2011). How to fix the obesity crisis. Sci Am 304: 40–47.

Ginsberg J, Quismorio FP Jr, DeWind LT et al. (1979). Musculoskeletal symptoms after jejunoileal shunt surgery for intractable obesity. Clinical and immunologic studies. Am J Med 67: 443–448.

Gollobin C, Marcus WY (2002). Bariatric beriberi. Obes Surg 12: 309–311.

Gorecki PJ, Cottam D, Ger R et al. (2002). Lower extremity compartment syndrome following a laparoscopic Roux-en-Y gastric bypass. Obes Surg 12: 289–291.

Haid RW, Gutmann L, Crosby TW (1982). Wernicke–Korsakoff encephalopathy after gastric plication. JAMA 247: 2566–2567.

Halverson J (1986). Micronutrient deficiencies after gastric bypass for morbid obesity. Am Surg 52: 594–598.

Halverson JD (1992). Metabolic risk of obesity surgery and long-term follow-up. Am J Clin Nutr 55 (2 Suppl): 602S–605S.

Harwood SC, Chodoroff G, Ellenberg MR (1987). Gastric partitioning complicated by peripheral neuropathy with lumbosacral plexopathy. Arch Phys Med Rehabil 68: 310–312.

Healton EB, Savage DG, Brust JC et al. (1991). Neurologic aspects of cobalamin deficiency. Medicine (Baltimore) 70: 229–245.

Higa KD, Boone KB, Ho T et al. (2000). Laparoscopic Roux-en-Y gastric bypass for morbid obesity: technique and preliminary results of our first 400 patients. Arch Surg 135: 1029–1033, discussion 1033–1034.

Jaiser SR, Winston GP (2010). Copper deficiency myelopathy. J Neurol 257: 869–881.

Juhasz-Pocsine K, Rudnicki SA, Archer RL et al. (2007). Neurologic complications of gastric bypass surgery for morbid obesity. Neurology 68: 1843–1850.

Ke ZJ, DeGiorgio LA, Volpe BT et al. (2003). Reversal of thiamine deficiency-induced neurodegeneration. J Neuropathol Exp Neurol 62: 195–207.

Khan LK, Serdula MK, Bowman BA et al. (2001). Use of prescription weight loss pills among US adults in 1996–1998. Ann Intern Med 134: 282–286.

Koike H, Misu K, Hattori N et al. (2001). Postgastrectomy polyneuropathy with thiamine deficiency. J Neurol Neurosurg Psychiatry 71: 357–362.

Kramer LD, Locke GE (1987). Wernicke's encephalopathy. Complication of gastric plication. J Clin Gastroenterol 9: 549–552.

Kumar N (2006). Copper deficiency myelopathy (human swayback). Mayo Clin Proc 81: 1371–1384.

Kumar N, Weimar LH (2013). Copper deficiency myeloneuropathy. S. Gilman (Ed.). Neurology Medlink, www.medlink.com/medlinkcontent.asp. Accessed August 10, 2013.

Kumar N, Gross Jr JB, Ahlskog JE (2003). Myelopathy due to copper deficiency. Neurology 61: 273–274.

Kumar N, Crum B, Petersen RC et al. (2004a). Copper deficiency myelopathy. Arch Neurol 61: 762–766.

Kumar N, Gross Jr JB, Ahlskog JE (2004b). Copper deficiency myelopathy produces a clinical picture like subacute combined degeneration. Neurology 63: 33–39.

Kumar N, Ahlskog JE, Klein CJ et al. (2006). Imaging features of copper deficiency myelopathy: a study of 25 cases. Neuroradiology 48: 78–83.

Livingston EH (2002). Obesity and its surgical management. Am J Surg 184: 103–113.

Lobstein TJ, James WP, Cole TJ (2003). Increasing levels of excess weight among children in England. Int J Obes Relat Metab Disord 27: 1136–1138.

Lopez JF, Halimi S, Perillat Y (2000). Pellagra-like erythema following vertical banded gastroplasty for morbid obesity. Ann Chir 125: 297–298.

MacLean JB (1982). Wernicke's encephalopathy after gastric plication. JAMA 248: 1311.

Marinella MA (1999). Ophthalmoplegia: an unusual manifestation of hypocalcemia. Am J Emerg Med 17: 105–106.

Milius G, Rose S, Owen DR et al. (1982). Probable acute thiamine deficiency secondary to gastric partition for morbid obesity. Nebr Med J 67: 147–150.

Mokdad AH, Ford ES, Bowman BA et al. (2003). Prevalence of obesity diabetes and obesity-related health risk factors 2001. JAMA 289: 76–79.

Mokdad AH, Marks JS, Stroup DF et al. (2004). Actual causes of death in the United States 2000. JAMA 291: 1238–1245.

National Heart, Lung, and Blood Institute (1998). Clinical Guidelines on the Identification Evaluation and Treatment of Overweight and Obesity in Adults: The Evidence Report. National Heart Lung and Blood Institute, Rockville, MD.

National Institutes of Health [no authors listed] (1992). Gastrointestinal surgery for severe obesity: National Institutes of Health Consensus Development Conference Statement. Am J Clin Nutr 55 (Suppl 2): S615–S619.

Oczkowski WJ, Kertesz A (1985). Wernicke's encephalopathy after gastroplasty for morbid obesity. Neurology 35: 99–101.

Paulson GW, Martin EW, Mojzisik C et al. (1985). Neurologic complications of gastric partitioning. Arch Neurol 42: 675–677.

Pope GD, Birkmeyer JD, Finlayson SR (2002). National trends in utilization and in-hospital outcomes of bariatric surgery. J Gastrointest Surg 6: 855–860, discussion 861.

Pories WJ, MacDonald Jr KG, Morgan EJ et al. (1992). Surgical treatment of obesity and its effect on diabetes: 10-y follow-up. Am J Clin Nutr 55: 582S–585S.

Printen KJ, Mason EE (1977). Gastric bypass for morbid obesity in patients more than fifty years of age. Surg Gynecol Obstet 144: 192–194.

Provenzale D, Reinhold RB, Golner B et al. (1992). Evidence for diminished B12 absorption after gastric bypass: oral supplementation does not prevent low plasma B12 levels in bypass patients. J Am Coll Nutr 11: 29–35.

Rothrock JF, Smith MS (1981). Wernicke's disease complicating surgical therapy for morbid obesity. J Clin Neuroophthalmol 1: 195–199.

Salas-Salvado J, Garcia-Lorda P, Cuatrecasas G et al. (2000). Wernicke's syndrome after bariatric surgery. Clin Nutr 19: 371–373.

Satya-Murti S, Howard L, Krohel G et al. (1986). The spectrum of neurologic disorder from vitamin E deficiency. Neurology 36: 917–921.

Schauer PR, Ikramuddin S, Gourash W et al. (2000). Outcomes after laparoscopic Roux-en-Y gastric bypass for morbid obesity. Ann Surg 232: 515–529.

Seehra H, MacDermott N, Lascelles RG et al. (1996). Wernicke's encephalopathy after vertical banded gastroplasty for morbid obesity. BMJ 312: 434.

Skroubis G, Sakellaropoulos G, Pouggouras K et al. (2002). Comparison of nutritional deficiencies after Roux-en-Y gastric bypass and after biliopancreatic diversion with Roux-en-Y gastric bypass. Obes Surg 12: 551–558.

Stolberg L, Rolfe R, Gitlin N et al. (1982). d-Lactic acidosis due to abnormal gut flora: diagnosis and treatment of two cases. N Engl J Med 306: 1344–1348.

Thaisetthawatkul P (2003). Peripheral neuropathy following gastric bypass surgery. In: 55th Annual Meeting of the American Academy of Neurology, Honolulu, Hawaii.

Thaisetthawatkul P, Collazo-Clavell ML, Sarr MG et al. (2004). A controlled study of peripheral neuropathy after bariatric surgery. Neurology 63: 1462–1470.

Toth C, Voll C (2001). Wernicke's encephalopathy following gastroplasty for morbid obesity. Can J Neurol Sci 28: 89–92.

Trus TL, Pope GD, Finlayson SR (2005). National trends in utilization and outcomes of bariatric surgery. Surg Endosc 19: 616–620.

Videt-Gibou D, Belliard S, Rivalan J et al. (2010). Acquired copper deficiency myelopathy. Rev Neurol (Paris) 166: 639–643.

Villar HV, Ranne RD (1984). Neurologic deficit following gastric partitioning: possible role of thiamine. JPEN J Parenter Enteral Nutr 8: 575–578.

Weir D, Gatenby P (1963). Subacute combined degeneration of cord after partial gastrectomy. Br Med J 2: 1175–1176.

Wernicke C (1881). Lehrbuch der Gehirnkrankheiten fur Aerzte und Studirende. Theodor Fischer, Kassel.

Wilhelm C (2000). Growing the market for anti-obesity drugs. Chem Market Rep, FR23–FR24.

Williams JA, Hall GS, Thompson AG et al. (1969). Neurological disease after partial gastrectomy. Br Med J 3: 210–212.

Winston GP, Jaiser SR (2008). Copper deficiency myelopathy and subacute combined degeneration of the cord – why is the phenotype so similar? Med Hypotheses 71: 229–236.

Yale C (1989). Gastric surgery for morbid obesity. Complications and long-term weight control. Arch Surg 124: 941–946.

Handbook of Clinical Neurology, Vol. 120 (3rd series)
Neurologic Aspects of Systemic Disease Part II
Jose Biller and Jose M. Ferro, Editors
© 2014 Elsevier B.V. All rights reserved

Chapter 40

Neurologic manifestations of inflammatory bowel diseases

JOSÉ M. FERRO[1]*, SOFIA N. OLIVEIRA[2], AND LUIS CORREIA[3]

[1]*Neurology Service, Department of Neurosciences, Hospital de Santa Maria, University of Lisbon, Lisbon, Portugal*

[2]*Department of Neurology, Hospital da Luz, Lisbon, Portugal*

[3]*Department of Gastroenterology and Hepatology, Hospital de Santa Maria, University of Lisbon, Lisbon, Portugal*

INTRODUCTION

Inflammatory bowel diseases (IBD) are chronic, relapsing and remitting inflammatory conditions affecting the digestive system, idiopathic in their etiology, comprising two main distinctive diseases, ulcerative colitis (UC) and Crohn's disease (CD).

In UC the inflammation is restricted to the mucosa of the colon, with an almost invariable involvement of the rectum and a variable continuous proximal extension.

CD is a condition that involves transmurally any segment of the digestive tract, from mouth to anus, with spared segments and skip lesions. In CD aphthoid ulcers become transmural fissures and, after a variable time interval, inflammation evolves to cause destruction and disability settles in, with fistula or fibrotic stenosis formation, as well as the potential for abscess formation or secondary occlusion (Cosnes et al., 2002). About one-third of CD patients develop perianal disease (Schwartz et al., 2002), from anal fissures to simple or complex perianal fistulae or secondary abscesses.

Both diseases can be phenotypically classified according to age, location, extension, behavior, and activity, by several clinical and endoscopic classifications. The most important of them is the Montreal classification, which allows for prognostic validation (Silverberg et al., 2005). Between 10% and 15% of colitis patients resist classification after applying strict clinical, endoscopic, radiologic, and histologic criteria, defining an intermediate condition known as unclassified colitis, or, as named by the pathologist in possession of a colectomy specimen, indeterminate colitis (Lennard-Jones, 1989).

The incidence of IBD varies between different areas of the globe, though with a north–south gradient, well documented in Europe and North America. In general,

it is recognized that there is a stable incidence of UC and a rising incidence of CD, with the former maintaining a higher incidence. In a systematic review (Molodecky et al., 2012), the highest reported incidence of UC was 24 and 19.2 per 100 000 person-years and 12.7 and 20.2 per 100 000 patient-years in CD, in Europe and the US, respectively.

The pathogenesis of IBD remains unclear. It is generally accepted that the disease appears in non-Mendelian genetically susceptible persons (Satsangi et al., 1997). The genetic predisposition can be demonstrated by an elevated concordance in twins (Orholm et al., 2000) and first-degree relatives (Lahari et al., 2001), mutations in the *NOD2/CARD15* gene (Kugathasan et al., 2004), or association with certain characteristic major histocompatibility complex elements (Bouma et al., 1997). Exposure to environmental risk factors such as infections (acute gastroenteritis, dysbiosis) (Porter et al., 2008), antibiotics, food antigens (breastfeeding, sugar or fat excess, fiber deficits, milk proteins, etc.) or nonsteroidal anti-inflammatory drugs, particularly in infancy, produces pathologic changes in the innate and adaptive immune system; these include changes in the mucosal barrier function, against luminal bacteria or antigens, eliciting an inappropriate immune response against microorganisms that generally would not generate that kind of response.

Besides the classic gastrointestinal manifestations, namely bloody diarrhea in UC or abdominal pain, fever, bowel habit change, or perianal disease in CD, a variable number of IBD patients present with complaints located outside the gastrointestinal tract, such as joints, mouth, eyes, skin, and liver, with some more rare manifestations. These are called the IBD extraintestinal manifestations (EIM) (Peyrin-Biroulet et al., 2011).

---

*Correspondence to: José M. Ferro, Department of Neurosciences, Hospital de Santa Maria, Av. Prof. Egas Moniz, 1649-035 Lisbo, Portugal. Tel: +351-21-795-7474, Fax: +351-21-795-7474, E-mail: jmferro@fm.ul.pt

EIM can have multiple mechanisms, such as metabolic complications of the disease (e.g., osteoporosis, nephrolithiasis in ileal CD), adverse effects of the medications (e.g., corticosteroid myopathy or anti-TNF demyelination), but mainly immune-mediated mechanisms. This group, classic EIM, has a phenotypic preference for colonic disease (UC and colonic CD) and can be divided in two subgroups: EIM related to intestinal activity (aphthous ulcers, peripheral arthritis or erythema nodosum) or EIM independent of the activity of the intestinal disease (axial arthritis, pyoderma gangrenosum, primary sclerosing cholangitis). Finally, it is necessary to recognize that there is an IBD-independent group of immune-mediated diseases that can coexist with greater prevalence in IBD, such as celiac or thyroid disease, vitiligo, diabetes, or, more rarely, lupus.

In general, as represented by a cohort of 950 prospectively studied Swiss patients (Vavricka et al., 2011), EIM occur more frequently in CD, both globally (43%, versus 31% in UC) and specific to the different manifestations (arthritis 33% versus 21%; aphthous stomatitis 10% versus 4%; uveitis 6% versus 4%; erythema nodosum 6% versus 3%; ankylosing spondyloarthropathy 6% versus 2%) with the exception of primary sclerosing cholangitis (CD 1% versus UC 4%).

NEUROLOGIC MANIFESTATIONS IN INFLAMMATORY BOWEL DISEASE

(Tables 40.1 and 40.2)

Table 40.1

Peripheral nervous system manifestations of inflammatory bowel disease

Peripheral neuropathy
  Axonal, large fibers
  Axonal, small fibers
  Demyelinating, acute
  Demyelinating, chronic
  Mononeuropathy
  Multifocal motor
Myopathy
  Dermatomyositis
  Polymyositis
  Rimmed vascular myopathy
  Granulomatosis myositis
Myasthenia
Cranial neuropathy
  Melkersson Rosenthal syndrome
  Optic neuritis
  Hearing loss
  Sixth nerve palsy

Table 40.2

Central nervous system manifestations of inflammatory bowel diseases

Cerebrovascular
  Ischemic arterial stroke
    Large artery disease
    Small vessel disease
    Cardioembolism, patent foramen ovale
    Cardioembolism, endocarditis
    Vasculitis
    Associated with anti-TNF-α therapy
Cerebral venous thrombosis
Demyelinating
  Multiple sclerosis
  Asymptomatic white matter lesions
  Related to anti-TNF-α therapy
Spinal cord
  Myelopathy
  Spinal empyema
Other
  Seizures
  Headache
  Encephalopathy

Prevalence

Neurologic and psychiatric involvement in inflammatory bowel disease (IBD) is rare though probably underreported. The true incidence is unknown, with values varying from 0.25% to 47.5% (Lossos et al., 1995; Elsehety and Bertorini, 1997; Oliveira et al., 2008; Sassi et al., 2009).

In a series of 638 patients with IBD, Lossos et al. (1995) reported 19 patients (3%) with neurolgic involvement that preceded the onset of intestinal symptoms by up to 10 years in 26% and started up to 12 years after IBD presentation in the remaining patients. In 10% it was associated with IBD exacerbation and most patients (53%) exhibited other extraintestinal manifestations and complications. Elsehety and Bertorini (1997) reported a 33.2% incidence of neurologic and neuropsychiatric complications in 253 patients with pathologically confirmed Crohn's disease, a much higher prevalence than that reported in other series. Two prospective cohort studies (Oliveira et al., 2008; Sassi et al., 2009) looked at the prevalence of peripheral neuropathy and found 13.4% and 8.8% respectively.

Asymptomatic focal brain white matter lesions have also been found in MRI studies of patients with IBD as compared to healthy age-matched controls (43.1% versus 16.0%; RR 2.6, 95% CI 1.3–5.3) but their clinical significance is unclear (Geissler et al., 1995).

Pathophysiology

Both the central and peripheral nervous systems can be affected in IBD. Several mechanisms are possibly involved: malabsorption and nutritional deficiencies, metabolic agents, infections induced by immunosuppresion, side-effects of medication and iatrogenic complications of surgery, thromboembolism, immunologic abnormalities, and disturbances of the so-called "brain–gut axis," referring to the neuronal influence on enteric disease and vice versa (Derbyshire, 2003; Konturek et al., 2004) via neuroendocrine pathways such as the hypothalamic–pituitary–adrenal axis, release of corticotropin and adrenal corticoid secretion, the autonomic nervous system and its effects on immune functions (Zois et al., 2010).

It is important to separate immune- and nonimmune-mediated mechanisms directly related to the disease itself from other causes, such as side-effects of medication and nutritional deficiencies.

PERIPHERAL NERVOUS SYSTEM

The peripheral nervous system (PNS) is frequently affected in IBD and peripheral neuropathy is one of the most common complications (Lossos et al., 1995; Elsehety and Bertorini, 1997; Oliveira et al., 2008), reported in up to 31.5% of patients. However, well-known causes of peripheral neuropathy such as vitamin deficiencies and secondary effects of medication should be differentiated from a primary involvement of the PNS in IBD, and prospective data are notably absent. Oliveira et al. (2008) identified peripheral neuropathy as the most common neurolgic complication in their cohort of IBD patients (36.6%), probably immune-mediated and therefore directly disease-related in 13.4%, the remainder being related to vitamin deficiency or metronidazole toxicity.

Peripheral neuropathy appeared to be more frequent in UC (Lossos et al., 1995; Gondim et al., 2005) but recent studies have shown comparable incidence in UC and CD patients (Gondim et al., 2005; Oliveira et al., 2008). Several different phenotypes have been described including sensory, motor, autonomic, and mixed, both axonal and demyelinating, acute and chronic (Gondim et al., 2005). In the largest retrospective series (Gondim et al., 2005), demyelinating chronic inflammatory polyneuropathy, small and large-fiber axonal neuropathies were found in UC patients. An acute inflammatory demyelinating polyradiculopathy has also been described in UC (Lossos et al., 1995). Axonal polyneuropathy presents with sensory loss and dysesthesias in glove and stocking distribution with decreased or absent ankle jerks. Small fiber sensory neuropathy presents with subjective numbness in the absence of objective abnormalities on electromyography and nerve conduction studies. Patients with IBD have also been found to have mononeuropathies or multifocal motor neuropathies (Gondim et al., 2005).

Patients with demyelinating neuropathies (particularly chronic inflammatory demyelinating polyneuropathy) respond better to immunomodulatory therapy that those with axonal neuropathy (Lossos et al., 1995; Gondim et al., 2005). Peripheral neuropathies are not related to disease activity and do not respond to treatment of the underlying IBD.

An inflammatory myopathy has also been found in association with IBD (Gendelman et al., 1982; Bhigjee et al., 1987; Sowa, 1991). It is probably more frequent in CD than in UC, and in the series by Lossos et al. (1995) was responsible for 16% of cases of neurolgic dysfunction. Dermatomyositis, polymyositis, rimmed vacuole myopathy, and granulomatous myositis have all been described and may also be completely asymptomatic (Hayashi et al., 1991). Myositis in CD is probably an immune-mediated disease (Shimoyama et al., 2009) as the same CD68+ macrophages that are found in the diseased colon are also present in the muscle.

Involvement of the neuromuscular junction has only rarely been described in the context of IBD (Martin and Shah, 1991; Finnie et al., 1994). It is important to report that at least one patient with CD and myasthenia had significant improvement of gastrointestinal symptoms following thymectomy (Finnie et al., 1994).

CRANIAL NEUROPATHIES

Melkersson–Rosenthal syndrome (recurrent facial nerve palsy with facial edema, tongue fissuring, and granulomas) has been described by several authors in IBD (Lloyd et al., 1994; Lossos et al., 1995).

Other cranial neuropathies, such as optic neuritis (Sedwick et al., 1984; Lossos et al., 1995), can also be found in single case reports.

Sensorineural hearing loss has also been described (Kumar et al., 2000; Akbayir et al., 2005), and is probably an under-recognized, immunologic manifestation of IBD. Of relevance also is the possibility of recovery with early treatment with steroids and immunosuppressive agents (Bachmeyer et al., 1998).

CEREBROVASCULAR COMPLICATIONS

Patients with inflammatory bowel disease (IBD) have a remarkable thromboembolic tendency and are at increased risk of both venous and arterial thrombotic complications.

In hospital series of IBD, the prevalence of arterial and venous thrombosis is around 4%, while in autopsy studies, this percentage may be more than 30%. The incidence of thrombotic complications ranges from 0.5% to 6.7% per year (Bernstein et al., 2001; Papa et al., 2003). IBD is also a risk factor for recurrent venous thromboembolism (Novacek et al., 2010).

In a cohort of 49 799 Danish patients with IBD compared with 477 504 members of the general population, patients with IBD had twice the incidence of deep venous thrombosis and pulmonary embolism. Relative risks were higher at young ages (hazard ratio 6.0 below age 20), though actual incidence increased with age (Kappelman et al., 2011). In a retrospective case control study including 17 487 IBD patients and 69 948 controls had an increased risk of arterial thrombotic events. In particular, women under the age of 40 exhibited a two-fold higher risk for stroke (Ha et al., 2009). Thromboembolism is more frequent in IBD than in other chronic inflammatory or chronic bowel diseases (Miehsler et al., 2004).

Strokes in patients with IBD were already reported in the 1930s. In 1986, Talbot and colleagues (1986) described a 1.3% prevalence of thromboembolic complications among 7199 patients with IBD observed during a 10 year period in a single institution. Among the 92 patients with thromboembolic complications, 61 had deep vein thrombosis or pulmonary embolism. Nine patients had cerebrovascular thrombotic events. There were no subarachnoid or intracerebral hemorrhages. Several other case series (Lossos et al., 1995; Elsehety and Bertorini, 1997; Barclay et al., 2010; Benavente and Morís, 2011; Cognat et al., 2011) and case reports of arterial ischemic or cerebral venous thrombosis have been published since then, with a frequency ranging from 0.6% to 4.7%.

Cerebrovascular complications are somewhat more frequent in Crohn's disease than in ulcerative colitis. They are not related to the duration or the severity of IBD, but cerebrovascular events are more frequent during bouts of inflammation. Rarely, they can antedate other manifestations of IBD.

Pathophysiology

The prothrombotic state in IBD has multiple contributors, namely blood coagulation, platelets, endothelium, prothrombotic mutations, vitamin deficiencies, inflammation, and other immune mechanisms (Santos et al., 2001; Bermejo and Burgos, 2008.

The hypercoagulation state is related to raised levels of factor V and VIII, fibrinogen, fibrinopeptide A and PAI-1, and decreased levels of protein S and antithrombin. Thrombocytosis is common in IDB, secondary both to anemia and inflammation. Platelet function is disturbed and Von Willebrand factor, a potent mediator of platelet adhesion and aggregation, is increased. In some patients endothelial dysfunction was reported. Prothrombotic mutations such as factor V Leiden and methylenetetrahydrofolate reductase (MTHFR) were identified in some IBD patients with cerebrovascular

complications. Vitamin deficiencies due to malabsorption, namely B_{12} and folate, cause hyperhomocysteinemia, in particular when combined with a MTHFR deficit. Cytokines, such as interleukin 1 and 6 and TNF-α can activate the coagulation cascade during periods of active inflammation. Other immune mechanisms include the coexistence of prothrombotic antibodies such as lupus anticoagulant, anticardiolipin antibodies, and atypical (non-MPO, non-PR3) ANCA antibodies, the latter in ulcerative colitis.

Arterial ischemic stroke

Ischemic events can be both cerebral and ocular. Ischemic stroke occurs through several mechanisms: (1) large artery disease, including even a case of common carotid occlusion; (2) small vessel disease, e.g., corona radiata (Ogawa et al., 2011) or pontine lacunar infarcts; (3) cardioembolism, related to (a) paradoxical embolism though a patent foramen ovale in patients with lower limb, pelvic, or mesenteric venous thrombosis, either symptomatic or not, (b) endocarditis (Kreuzpaintner et al., 1992); (4) vasculitis.

Stroke and anti-TNF-α therapy

A few cases of arterial ischemic complications have been reported as a complication of anti-TNF-α therapy (Vannucchi et al., 2011; Cohen et al., 2012). One of the authors (JMF) has observed two cases of deep intracerebral hemorrhage in young, nonhypertensive males with IBD treated with anti-TNF drugs. No underlying arteriovenous malformation, venous thrombosis, or other lesion was identified (Fig. 40.1).

Vasculitis

Systemic and organ-specific vasculitis, namely cerebral, has been reported in association with IBD, especially with ulcerative colitis (Scheid and Teich, 2007). However, cerebral vasculitis is very rare and only a handful of cases, small case series, and a few nonsystematic reviews have been published (Martín de Carpi et al., 2007; Scheid and Teich, 2007). Vasculitis in IBD is immune-mediated, via genetic susceptibility and HLA status, T lymphocyte-mediated cytoxicity, or immune complex deposition (Scheid and Teich, 2007). In other cases IBD is associated with primary vasculitides (giant cell arteritis, Wegener, pANCA vasculitis) (Jacob et al., 1990; Ronchetto and Pistono, 1993; Gobron et al., 2010) or with other immune diseases (Cogan syndrome, thrombotic thrombocytopenic purpura, and lupus) (Chebli et al., 2000; Baron et al., 2002; Hisada et al., 2006; Ullrich et al., 2009).

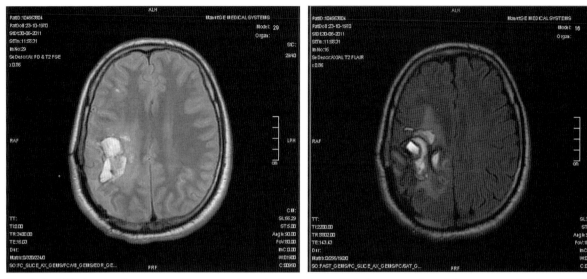

Fig. 40.1. MRI showing frontoparietal hemorrhagic stroke in a patient with inflammatory bowel disease, treated with anti-TNF-α agents.

The clinical manifestations of cerebral vasculities in IBD are protean and include headache (Holzer et al., 2009), cranial nerve palsies, focal deficits such as hemiparesis, sensory disturbances, aphasia and visual defects, multifocal signs and vigilance or cognitive troubles, isolated or in combination (Scheid and Teich, 2007). The onset can be acute or subacute. Presentation as a single stroke syndrome is infrequent. Levels of nonspecific inflammatory markers such as ESR or CRP may be elevated. Cerebrospinal fluid examination may reveal increased proteins or a mild pleiocytosis. Magnetic resonance imaging of the brain rarely shows large territorial infarcts. Acute lesions may be detected on diffusion-weighted imaging (DWI). The most common findings are deep white matter or periventricular white matter lesions, detectable in FLAIR or T2 sequences (Scheid and Teich, 2007). These lesions are not specific and *per se* do not allow a definite diagnosis of vasculitis, which relies on the demonstration of inflammation on a vessel wall. In several cases reported in the literature no imaging or biopsy of the vessels was obtained and therefore the diagnosis of vasculitis is only probable. Intra-arterial, MR (Schluter et al., 2004), or CT angiography can reveal multiple arterial stenoses or other aspects suggestive of vasculitis, but many of them can also be seen in noninflammatory vasculopathies and in the reversible cerebral vasoconstriction syndrome, in which the arterial stenoses usually regress in a follow-up angiography performed 6–8 weeks later. Moreover, angiography can be normal in vasculitis affecting only small arteries. In large artery vasculitis (Takayasu and giant cell arteritis), the temporal superficial, the carotid, and the axillary arteries are accessible to ultrasound which may demonstrate inflammatory "halos." Recently, appropriate MR sequences were reported to depict wall inflammation in medium-size intracerebral vessels, such as the proximal segments of the middle cerebral artery (Mandell et al., 2012).

In a few cases of vasculitis associated with IBD, namely UC, necropsy of brain biopsy was obtained. In three cases necrotizing vasculitis was found (Glotzer et al., 1964; Nelson et al., 1986; Carmona et al., 2000), although in one of them hemorrhagic acute disseminated encephalomyelitis could not be ruled out (Glotzer et al., 1964). In other cases only a lymphocyte infiltrate was found (Kraus et al., 1996).

Although the outcome is general favorable, a few cases were rapidly fatal. The majority improved with steroids, but in some patients symptoms developed while they were already on steroids. In these patients ciclosporin, plasma exchange, and more recently biologic anti-TNF agents (Ullrich et al., 2009) were used with variable success.

CEREBRAL VENOUS THROMBOSIS

Thrombosis of the dural sinus and cerebral veins is at least as frequent as arterial stroke in IBD. Thrombosis appears to be more common in ulcerative colitis than in Crohn's disease, but in some series the opposite was found (Cognat et al., 2011). Cognat and coworkers (2011) recently published eight cases from two centers in Paris and reviewed 49 other cases of cerebral venous thrombosis associated with IBD confirmed by MR. Other cases not included in this review have been published (Milandre et al., 1992; Lossos et al., 1995;

Papi et al., 1995; Barclay et al., 2010; Nudelman et al., 2010; Casella et al., 2011; Kothur et al., 2012). The publications of Milandre et al. (1992), Nudelman et al. (2010), and Casella et al. (2011) also provide a review of previous reports. When compared to patients with cerebral venous thrombosis with other causes, patients with IBD-related cerebral venous thrombosis are younger and more often male. A more recent review of 65 cases published in English was performed by Katsanos and coworkers (2013).

The clinical presentation, consisting of headaches, focal signs, seizures, or encephalopathy, and the sites of the venous occlusions are similar to the usual cerebral venous thromboses. They can occur from 2 months to 17 years after the first attack of IBD. Occasionally, the diagnosis of IBD is established only when cerebral venous thrombosis occurs (Cognat et al., 2011; Katsanos et al., 2013). Although IBD may be asymptomatic when the venous thrombosis occurs, almost all patients had biologic markers of inflammation such as elevated leukocyte count, CRP, or ESR.

When concomitant causes of cerebral venous thrombosis are systematically searched for, the majority had other risk factors, such as oral contraceptives, severe iron deficiency anemia, anti-TNF-α treatment, thrombocytosis, hyperhomocystenemia, folate and B$_{12}$ deficiencies, infection, lupus anticoagulant, and inherited thrombophilia (Milandre et al., 1992; Papi et al., 1995; Nudelman et al., 2010; Casella et al., 2011; Cognat et al., 2011).

Despite the potential risk of intestinal bleeding, treatment of acute cerebral venous thrombosis with full dose intravenous heparin or low molecular weight heparin is effective and safe (Tsujikawa et al., 2000; Cognat et al., 2011; Katsanos et al., 2013). Endovascular thrombolysis was tried in a few cases, with favorable and safe outcomes (Philips et al., 1999; Kothur et al., 2012). This limited evidence supports the use of approved guidelines for cerebral venous thrombosis management (Einhäupl et al., 2006; Saposnik et al., 2011) also when associated with IBD. The prognosis is usually good, but a few cases were fatal (Cognat et al., 2011; Katsanos et al., 2013).

DEMYELINATING DISEASE

Multiple sclerosis (MS) has been frequently associated with IBD, particularly with UC (Rang et al., 1982; Sadovnick et al., 1989; Purrmann et al., 1992; Buccino et al., 1994; Kimura et al., 2000; Pandian et al., 2004; Bernstein et al., 2005; Gupta et al., 2005), although evolving diagnostic criteria for MS could mean that some patients actually have an MS-like disease instead of true MS. Both patients with IBD who later developed MS and patients with MS who developed IBD have been described. Kimura et al. (2000) found a 1% prevalence of

clinically definite MS among 400 patients with IBD. Gupta et al. (2005) estimated a relative risk for MS and optic neuritis in CD of 1.54 and of 1.74 in UC when compared with the general population. Between 40% and 50% of IBD presented asymptomatic white matter lesions in a study by Perkin and Murray-Lyon (1998).

MS and IBD share similar epidemiology, age of presentation, clinical course, and geographic distribution. However, despite all evidence, the physiopathology of this relationship between diseases is still unknown, although some animal studies may shed some light on the issue. Extensive perivenular demyelination and astrocytosis has been found in monkeys suffering from IBD and cerebral venous thrombosis, possibly due to perivenular edema (Sheffield et al., 1981). Also, IBD may be viewed as a chronic variant of a predemyelinating state that can trigger demyelinating episodes. IBD has also been associated with other chronic inflammatory diseases suggesting a common immunologic etiology (Bernstein et al., 2005).

Antitumor necrosis factor-α therapy is contraindicated in the treatment of patients with IBS and multiple sclerosis and there is evidence of onset of a demyelinating process with institution of this therapy (Thomas et al., 2004; Freeman and Flak, 2005).

OTHER CENTRAL NERVOUS SYSTEM COMPLICATIONS

A slowly progressive spastic paraparesis due to myelopathy has been reported in association with IBD (Gibb et al., 1987; Ray et al., 1993; Suzuki et al., 1994; Lossos et al., 1995) and in the series by Lossos et al. was present in 26% of patients. An immune-mediated inflammatory origin has been suggested but vitamin B$_{12}$ deficiency with resulting subacute combined degeneration of the spinal cord may also be responsible in patients with CD following terminal ileum resection.

Epidural and subdural spinal empyemas secondary to fistulous extension from the rectum are rare complications of CD and can result in pain and progressive leg weakness (Sacher et al., 1989; Hershkowitz et al., 1990; Heidemann et al., 2003; Gelfenbeyn et al., 2006).

In CD patients, Elsehety and Bertorini (1997) reported seizures (5.9%), headaches (4.3%), major depression (4.3%), anxiety disorder (2%), and other less frequent complications (less than 1%) such as Parkinson-like syndrome, cerebellar syndrome, ischemic optic neuritis, orbital pseudotumor, sixth nerve palsy, organic brain syndrome, and chronic fatigue syndrome. A single case of inflammatory pseudotumor of the cerebellum in a patient with CD was reported by Derrey et al. (2012).

An association of epilepsy and IBD appears to be preferentially with CD (Elsehety and Bertorini, 1997) but secondary seizures related to metabolic and structural causes have been described in UC (Schneidermann et al., 1979; Johns, 1991; Lossos et al., 1995).

Diffuse encephalopathy may also develop in patients with CD, possibly related to vitamin deficiency including Wernicke encephalopathy, selenium toxicity due to parenteral nutrition, or precipitated by treatment with sulfasalazine (Schoonjans et al., 1993; Kawakubo et al., 1994; Hahn et al., 1998; Eggspühler et al., 2003).

PSYCHIATRIC SYNDROMES

The most frequent psychiatric syndromes associated with IBD are depression and anxiety. In two Canadian national surveys with 3076 and 1438 respondents with IBD, 16.3% and 14.7%, respectively, reported depressive symptoms (Fuller-Thomson and Sulman, 2006). Depression was more frequent in women and younger respondents and in patients with pain or functional limitations.

MEDICATION-INDUCED NEUROLGIC COMPLICATIONS

Steroids

In the 1950s, Bunim et al. (1955) described glucocorticoid-related myopathy, a well known side-effect of this therapy due to direct catabolic effects on the skeletal muscle. It can occur with any of the glucocorticoid preparations, in both initiation of treatment and chronic use. Patients typically present with painless proximal muscle wasting and weakness, normal muscle enzymes (Askari et al., 1976), and improve after decrease in drug dosage.

Metronidazole

Metronidazole is an antimicrobial agent with bactericidal effects against anaerobic agents used in the treatment of IBD. Patients treated with metronidazole, particularly with high doses, have presented seizures, dizziness and vertigo, ataxia, confusion, irritability, insomnia, headache, tremors and peripheral neuropathy (Frytak et al., 1978; Kusumi et al., 1980; Halloran, 1982). Peripheral neuropathy is usually pure sensory or autonomic with occasional ataxia; it is mostly transient and resolves completely with discontinuation.

Ciclosporin

Mild tremor, but also headache, visual abnormalities, and seizures in the context of a syndrome resembling posterior leukoencephalopathy have been described in patients treated with ciclosporin (Schwartz et al., 1995; Wijdicks et al., 1995; Hinchey et al., 1996).

Anti-TNF-α agents (infliximab, adalimumab, certolizumab)

A possible link between TNF-α and demyelinating disease has been suggested although a causal relationship has not been established. In 2001, Mohan et al. described 19 patients with brain and spinal cord demyelination on magnetic resonance imaging, presenting with confusion, ataxia, dysesthesia, and paresthesia, who improved after discontinuation of therapy (Mohan et al., 2001). In postmarketing reports both optic neuritis and demyelinating polyneuropathy have also been reported with infliximab and adalimumab (Shin et al., 2006; Simsek et al., 2007; Eguren et al., 2009).

Progressive multifocal leukoencephalopathy (PML), a severe demyelinating disease of the central nervous system caused by reactivation of the polyomavirus JC (JC virus) has been reported in patients treated with infliximab (Kumar et al., 2010) and glucocorticoids (Newton et al., 1986), alone or in combination with immune suppressive agents. The risk of PML is associated with duration of treatment, prior use of immune suppressant medication, and JC virus antibody status, being minimal in JC virus antibody-negative patients (Biogen Idec). PML typically presents with cognitive impairment and behavioral changes and can progress to cause motor weakness, visual and language disturbances, and seizures. Diagnosis can be confirmed by quantitative detection of JC virus DNA in the cerebrospinal fluid (Aksamit, 2008).

Anti-α4 integrin (natalizumab)

Natalizumab is a humanized monoclonal antibody to α4 integrin recently approved for treatment of CD (Sandborn et al., 2005) outside Europe. PML has been described in association with natalizumab in CD patients (Van Assche et al., 2005).

REFERENCES

Akbayir N, Calis AB, Alkim C et al. (2005). Sensorineural hearing loss in patients with inflammatory bowel: a subclinical extraintestinal manifestation. Dig Dis Sci 50: 1938–1945.

Aksamit AJ (2008). Progressive multifocal leukoencephalopathy. Curr Treat Options Neurol 10: 178–185.

Askari A, Vignos PJ Jr, Moskowitz RW (1976). Steroid myopathy in connective tissue disease. Am J Med 61: 485–492.

Bachmeyer C, Leclerc-Landgraf N, Laurette F et al. (1998). Acute autoimmune sensorineural hearing loss associated with Crohn's disease. Am J Gastroenterol 93: 2565–2567.

Barclay AR, Keightley JM, Horrocks I et al. (2010). Cerebral thromboembolic events in pediatric patients with inflammatory bowel disease. Inflamm Bowel Dis 16: 677–683.

Baron BW, Jeon HR, Glunz C et al. (2002). First two patients with ulcerative colitis who developed classic thrombotic thrombocytopenic purpura successfully treated with medical therapy and plasma exchange. J Clin Apher 17: 204–206.

Benavente L, Morís G (2011). Neurologic disorders associated with inflammatory bowel disease. Eur J Neurol 18: 138–143.

Bermejo PE, Burgos A (2008). Neurological complications of inflammatory bowel disease. Med Clin (Barc) 130: 666–675.

Bernstein CN, Blanchard JF, Houston DS et al. (2001). The incidence of deep venous thrombosis and pulmonary embolism among patients with inflammatory bowel disease: a population-based cohort study. Thromb Haemost 85: 430–434.

Bernstein CN, Wajda A, Blanchard JF (2005). The clustering of other chronic inflammatory diseases in inflammatory bowel disease: a population-based study. Gastroenterology 129: 827–836.

Bhigjee AI, Bill PL, Cosnett JE (1987). Ulcerative colitis and interstitial myositis. Clin Neurol Neurosurg 89: 261–263.

Biogen Idec Medical Information website. https://medinfo.biogenidec.com/medinfo/registration/reguser.do.

Bouma G, Oudkerk Pool M, Crusius JB et al. (1997). Evidence for genetic heterogeneity in inflammatory bowel disease (IBD); HLA genes in the predisposition to suffer from ulcerative colitis (UC) and Crohn's disease (CD). Clin Exp Immunol 109: 175–179.

Buccino GP, Corrente G, Visintini D (1994). Crohn's disease and multiple sclerosis: a single case report. Ital J Neurol Sci 15: 303–306.

Bunim JJ, Ziff M, McEwen C (1955). Evaluation of prolonged cortisone therapy in rheumatoid arthritis: a four-year study. Am J Med 18: 27–40.

Carmona MA, Jaume Anselmi F, Ramírez Rivera J (2000). Cerebral thrombosis and vasculitis: an uncommon complication of ulcerative colitis. Bol Asoc Med P R 92: 9–11.

Casella G, Spreafico C, Costantini M et al. (2011). Cerebral sinus thrombosis in ulcerative colitis. Inflamm Bowel Dis 17: 2214–2216.

Chebli JM, Gaburri PD, de Souza AF et al. (2000). Fatal evolution of systemic lupus erythematosus associated with Crohn's disease. Arq Gastroenterol 37: 224–226.

Cognat E, Crassard I, Denier C et al. (2011). Cerebral venous thrombosis in inflammatory bowel diseases: eight cases and literature review. Int J Stroke 6: 487–492.

Cohen M, Baldin B, Thomas P et al. (2012). Neurological adverse events under anti-TNF alpha therapy. Rev Neurol (Paris) 168: 33–39.

Cosnes J, Blain A, Cattan et al. (2002). Long-term evolution of disease behavior of Crohn's disease. Inflamm Bowel Dis 8: 244–250.

Derbyshire SWG (2003). A systematic review of neuroimaging data during visceral stimulation. Am J Gastroenterol 98: 12–20.

Derrey S, Charpentier C, Gérardin E et al. (2012). Inflammatory pseudotumor of the cerebellum in a patient with Crohn's disease. World Neurosurg 77: 201.e13–201.e16.

Eggspühler AW, Bauerfeind P, Dorn T et al. (2003). Wernicke encephalopathy – a severe neurological complication in a clinically inactive Crohn's disease. Eur Neurol 50: 184–185.

Eguren C, Díaz Ley B, Daudén E et al. (2009). Peripheral neuropathy in two patients with psoriasis in treatment with infliximab. Muscle Nerve 40: 488–489.

Einhäupl K, Bousser MG, de Bruijn SF et al. (2006). EFNS guideline on the treatment of cerebral venous and sinus thrombosis. Eur J Neurol 13: 553–559.

Elsehety A, Bertorini TE (1997). Neurologic and neuropsychiatric complications of Crohn's disease. South Med J 90: 606–610.

Finnie IA, Shields R, Sutton R et al. (1994). Crohn's disease and myasthenia gravis: a possible role for thymectomy. Gut 35: 278–279.

Freeman HJ, Flak B (2005). Demyelination-like syndrome in Crohn's disease after infliximab therapy. Can J Gastroenterol 19: 313–316.

Frytak S, Moertel CH, Childs DS (1978). Neurologic toxicity associated with high-dose metronidazole therapy. Ann Intern Med 88: 361–362.

Fuller-Thomson E, Sulman J (2006). Depression and inflammatory bowel disease: findings from two nationally representative Canadian surveys. Inflamm Bowel Dis 12: 697–707.

Geissler A, Andus T, Roth M et al. (1995). Focal white-matter lesions in brain of patients with inflammatory bowel disease. Lancet 345: 897–898.

Gelfenbeyn M, Goodkin R, Kliot M (2006). Sterile recurrent spinal epidural abscess in a patient with Crohn's disease: a case report. Surg Neurol 65: 178–184.

Gendelman S, Present D, Janowitz HD (1982). Neurological complications of inflammatory bowel disease. Gastroenterology 82: 1065.

Gibb WRG, Dhillon DP, Zilkha KJ et al. (1987). Bronchiectasis with ulcerative colitis and myelopathy. Thorax 42: 155–156.

Glotzer DJ, Yuan RH, Patterson JF (1964). Ulcerative colitis complicated by toxic megacolon, polyserositis and hemorrhagic leukoencephalitis with recovery. Ann Surg 159: 445–450.

Gobron C, Kaci R, Sokol H et al. (2010). Unilateral carotid granulomatous arteritis and Crohn's disease. Rev Neurol (Paris) 166: 542–546.

Gondim FA, Brannagan TH, Sander HW et al. (2005). Peripheral neuropathy in patients with inflammatory bowel disease. Brain 128: 867–879.

Gupta G, Gelfand JM, Lewis JD (2005). Increased risk for demyelinating diseases in patients with inflammatory bowel disease. Gastroenterology 129: 819–826.

Ha C, Magowan S, Accortt NA et al. (2009). Risk of arterial thrombotic events in inflammatory bowel disease. Am J Gastroenterol 104: 1445–1451.

Hahn JS, Berquist W, Alcorn DM et al. (1998). Wernicke encephalopathy and beriberi during total parenteral nutrition attributable to multivitamin infusion shortage. Pediatrics 101: E10.

Halloran TJ (1982). Convulsions associated with high cumulative doses of metronidazole. Drug Intell Clin Pharm 16: 409.

Hayashi K, Kurisu Y, Ohshiba J et al. (1991). Report of a case of Crohn's disease associated with hyper-creatine phosphokinasemia. Jpn J Med 30: 441–445.

Heidemann J, Spinelli KS, Otterson MF et al. (2003). Case report: magnetic resonance imaging in the diagnosis of epidural abscess perirectal fistulizing Crohn's disease. Inflamm Bowel Dis 9: 122–124.

Hershkowitz S, Link R, Ravden M et al. (1990). Spinal empyema in Crohn's disease. J Clin Gastroenterol 12: 67–69.

Hinchey J, Chaves C, Appignani B et al. (1996). A reversible posterior leukoencephalopathy syndrome. N Eng J Med 334: 494–500.

Hisada T, Miyamae Y, Mizuide M et al. (2006). Acute thrombocytopenia associated with preexisting ulcerative colitis successfully treated with colectomy. Intern Med 45: 87–91.

Holzer K, Esposito L, Stimmer H et al. (2009). Cerebral vasculitis mimicking migraine with aura in a patient with Crohn's disease. Acta Neurol Belg 109: 44–48.

Jacob A, Ledingham JG, Kerr AI et al. (1990). Ulcerative colitis and giant cell arteritis associated with sensorineural deafness. J Laryngol Otol 104: 889–890.

Johns DR (1991). Cerebrovascular complications of inflammatory bowel disease. Am J Gastroenterol 86: 367–370.

Kappelman MD, Horvath-Puho E, Sandler RS et al. (2011). Thromboembolic risk among Danish children and adults with inflammatory bowel diseases: a population-based nationwide study. Gut 60: 937–943.

Katsanos AH, Katsanos KH, Kosmidou M et al. (2013). Cerebral sinus venous thrombosis in inflammatory bowel diseases. QJM 106: 401–413.

Kawakubo K, Iida M, Matsumoto T et al. (1994). Progressive encephalopathy in a Crohn's disease patient on long-term total parenteral nutrition: possible relationship to selenium deficiency. Postgrad Med J 70: 215–219.

Kimura K, Hunter SF, Thollander MS et al. (2000). Concurrence of inflammatory bowel disease and multiple sclerosis. Mayo Clin Proc 75: 802–806.

Konturek SJ, Konturek JW, Pawlik T et al. (2004). Brain-gut axis and its role in the control of food intake. J Physiol Pharmacol 55: 137–154.

Kothur K, Kaul S, Rammurthi S et al. (2012). Use of thrombolytic therapy in cerebral venous sinus thrombosis with ulcerative colitis. Ann Indian Acad Neurol 15: 35–38.

Kraus JA, Nahser HC, Berlit P (1996). Lymphocytic encephalomyeloneuritis as a neurologic complication of ulcerative colitis. J Neurol Sci 141: 117–119.

Kreuzpaintner G, Horstkotte D, Heyll A et al. (1992). Increased risk of bacterial endocarditis in inflammatory bowel disease. Am J Med 92: 391–395.

Kugathasan S, Collins N, Maresso K et al. (2004). CARD15 gene mutations and risk for early surgery in pediatric-onset Crohn's disease. Clin Gastroenterol Hepatol 2: 1003–1009.

Kumar BN, Smith MSH, Walsh RM et al. (2000). Sensorineural hearing loss in ulcerative colitis. Clin Otolaryngol 25: 143–145.

Kumar D, Bouldin TW, Berger RG (2010). A case of progressive multifocal leukoencephalopathy in a patient treated with infliximab. Arthritis Rheum 62: 3191–3195.

Kusumi RK, Plouffe JF, Wyatt RH et al. (1980). Central nervous system toxicity associated with metronidazole therapy. Ann Intern Med 93: 59–60.

Lahari D, Debeugny S, Peeters M et al. (2001). Inflammatory bowel disease in spouses and their offspring. Gastroenterology 120: 816–819.

Lennard-Jones JE (1989). Classification of inflammatory bowel disease. Scand J Gastroenterol 170 (Suppl): 2–6.

Lloyd DA, Payton KB, Guenther L et al. (1994). Melkersson–Rosenthal syndrome and Crohn's disease: one disease or two? Report of a case and discussion of the literature. J Clin Gastroenterol 18: 213–217.

Lossos A, River Y, Eliakim A et al. (1995). Neurologic aspects of inflammatory bowel disease. Neurology 45: 416–421.

Mandell DM, Matouk CC, Farb RI et al. (2012). Vessel wall MRI to differentiate between reversible cerebral vasoconstriction syndrome and central nervous system vasculitis: preliminary results. Stroke 43: 860–862.

Martín de Carpi J, Ribó Cruz JM, Antón López J et al. (2007). Cerebral vasculitis associated with ulcerative colitis. An Pediatr (Barc) 67: 177–178.

Martin RW, Shah A (1991). Myasthenia gravis coexistent with Crohn's disease. J Clin Gastroenterol 13: 112–113.

Miehsler W, Reinisch W, Valic E et al. (2004). Is inflammatory bowel disease an independent and disease specific risk factor for thromboembolism? Gut 53: 542–548.

Milandre L, Monges D, Dor V et al. (1992). Cerebral phlebitis and Crohn disease. Rev Neurol (Paris) 148: 139–144.

Mohan N, Edwards ET, Cupps TR et al. (2001). Demyelination occurring during anti-tumor necrosis factor alpha therapy for inflammatory arthritides. Arthritis Rheum 44: 2862–2869.

Molodecky NA, Soon IS, Rabi DM et al. (2012). Increasing incidence and prevalence of the inflammatory bowel diseases with time, based on systematic review. Gastroenterology 142: 46–54.

Nelson J, Barron MM, Riggs JE et al. (1986). Cerebral vasculitis and ulcerative colitis. Neurology 36: 719–721.

Newton P, Aldridge RD, Lesseells AM et al. (1986). Progressive multifocal leukoencephalopathy complicating systemic lupus erythematous. Arthritis Rheum 29: 337–343.

Novacek G, Weltermann A, Sobala A et al. (2010). Inflammatory bowel disease is a risk factor for recurrent venous thromboembolism. Gastroenterology 139: 779–787.

Nudelman RJ, Rosen DG, Rouah E et al. (2010). Cerebral sinus thrombosis: a fatal neurological complication of ulcerative colitis. Pathol Res Int 2010: 132754.

Ogawa E, Sakakibara R, Yoshimatsu Y et al. (2011). Crohn's disease and stroke in a young adult. Intern Med 50: 2407–2408.

Oliveira GR, Teles BC, Brasil EF et al. (2008). Peripheral neuropathy and neurological disorders in an unselected Brazilian population-based cohort of IBD patients. Inflamm Bowel Dis 14: 389–395.

Orholm M, Binder V, Sørensen TI et al. (2000). Concordance of inflammatory bowel disease among Danish twins. Results of a nationwide study. Scand J Gastroenterol 35: 1075–1081.

Pandian JD, Pawar G, Singh GS et al. (2004). Multiple sclerosis in a patient with chronic ulcerative colitis. Neurol India 52: 282–283.

Papa A, Danese S, Grillo A et al. (2003). Review article: inherited thrombophilia in inflammatory bowel disease. Am J Gastroenterol 98: 1247–1251.

Papi C, Ciaco A, Acierno G et al. (1995). Severe ulcerative colitis, dural sinus thrombosis, and the lupus anticoagulant. Am J Gastroenterol 90: 1514–1517.

Perkin GD, Murray-Lyon I (1998). Neurology and the gastrointestinal system. J Neurol Neurosurg Psychiatry 65: 291–300.

Peyrin-Biroulet L, Loftus EV Jr, Colombel JF et al. (2011). Long-term complications, extraintestinal manifestations, and mortality in adult Crohn's disease in population-based cohorts. Inflamm Bowel Dis 17: 471–478.

Philips MF, Bagley LJ, Sinson GP et al. (1999). Endovascular thrombolysis for symptomatic cerebral venous thrombosis. J Neurosurg 90: 65–71.

Porter CK, Tribble DR, Aliaga PA et al. (2008). Infectious gastroenteritis and risk of developing inflammatory bowel disease. Gastroenterology 135: 781–786.

Purrmann J, Arendt G, Cleveland S et al. (1992). Association of Crohn's disease and multiple sclerosis. Is there a common background? J Clin Gastroenterol 14: 43–46.

Rang EH, Brooke BN, Hermon-Taylor J (1982). Association of ulcerative colitis with multiple sclerosis. Lancet 2: 555.

Ray DW, Bridger J, Hawnaur J et al. (1993). Transverse myelitis as the presentation of Jo-1 antibody syndrome (myositis and fibrosing alveolitis) in long-standing ulcerative colitis. Br J Rheumatol 32: 1105–1108.

Ronchetto F, Pistono PG (1993). Temporal arteritis in a patient with ulcerative colitis. Coincidental association or (immuno) pathogenetic link? Recenti Prog Med 84: 54–56.

Sacher M, Göpfrich H, Hochberger O (1989). Crohn's disease penetrating into the spinal canal. Acta Paediatr Scand 78: 647–649.

Sadovnick AD, Paty DW, Yannakoulias G (1989). Concurrence of multiple sclerosis and inflammatory bowel disease. N Eng J Med 321: 762–763.

Sandborn WJ, Colombel JF, Enns R et al. (2005). Natalizumab induction and maintenance therapy for Crohn's disease. N Eng J Med 353: 1912–1925.

Santos S, Casadevall T, Pascual LF et al. (2001). Neurological alterations related to Crohn's disease. Rev Neurol 32: 1158–1162.

Saposnik G, Barinagarrementeria F, Brown RD Jr et al. (2011). Diagnosis and management of cerebral venous thrombosis: a statement for healthcare professionals from the American Heart Association/American Stroke Association. Stroke 42: 1158–1192.

Sassi SB, Kallel L, Ben Romdhane S et al. (2009). Peripheral neuropathy in inflammatory bowel disease patients: a prospective cohort study. Scand J Gastroenterol 44: 1268–1269.

Satsangi J, Jewell DP, Bell JL (1997). The genetics of inflammatory bowel disease. Gut 40: 572.

Scheid R, Teich N (2007). Neurologic manifestations of ulcerative colitis. Eur J Neurol 14: 483–493.

Schluter A, Krasnianski M, Krivokuca M et al. (2004). Magnetic resonance angiography in a patient with Crohn's disease associated cerebral vasculitis. Clin Neurol Neurosurg 106: 110–113.

Schneidermann JH, Sharpe JA, Sutton DM (1979). Cerebral and retinal vascular complications of inflammatory bowel disease. Ann Neurol 5: 331–337.

Schoonjans R, Mast A, Van Den Abeele G et al. (1993). Sulfasalazine-associated encephalopathy in a patient with Crohn's disease. Am J Gastroenterol 88: 1416–1420.

Schwartz RB, Bravo SM, Klufas RA et al. (1995). Cyclosporine neurotoxicity and its relationship to hypertensive encephalopathy: CT and MR findings in 16 cases. AJR Am J Roentgenol 165: 627–631.

Schwartz DA, Loftus EV Jr, Tremaine WJ et al. (2002). The natural history of fistulizing Crohn's disease in Olmsted County, Minnesota. Gastroenterology 122: 875–880.

Sedwick LA, Klingele TG, Burde RM et al. (1984). Optic neuritis in inflammatory bowel disease. J Clin Neuroophthalmol 4: 3–6.

Sheffield WD, Squire RA, Strandberg JD (1981). Cerebral venous thrombosis in the rhesus monkey. Vet Pathol 18: 326–334.

Shimoyama T, Tamura Y, Sakamoto T et al. (2009). Immune-mediated myositis in Crohn's disease. Muscle Nerve 39: 101–105.

Shin IS, Baer AN, Kwon HJ et al. (2006). Guillain–Barré and Miller Fisher syndromes occurring with tumor necrosis factor alpha antagonist therapy. Arthritis Rheum 54: 1429–1434.

Silverberg MS, Satsangi J, Ahmad T et al. (2005). Toward an integrated clinical, molecular, and serological classification of inflammatory bowel disease: report of a working party of the 2005 Montreal World Congress of Gastrenterology. Can J Gastroenterol 19 (Suppl A): 5–36.

Simsek I, Erdem H, Pay S et al. (2007). Optic neuritis occurring with anti-tumour necrosis factor alpha therapy. Ann Rheum Dis 66: 1255–1258.

Sowa JM (1991). Overlapping polymyositis and ulcerative colitis: HTLV-1 infection as an alternative explanation. J Rheumatol 18: 1939.

Suzuki I, Watanabe N, Suzuki J et al. (1994). A case of bronchiectasis accompanied by ulcerative colitis and HTLV-1 associated myelopathy (HAM). Jpn J Thorac Dis 32: 358–363.

Talbot RW, Heppell J, Dozois RR et al. (1986). Vascular complications of inflammatory bowel disease. Mayo Clin Proc 61: 140–145.

Thomas CW Jr, Weinshenker BG, Sandborn WJ (2004). Demyelination during anti-tumor necrosis factor therapy with infliximab for Crohn's disease. Inflamm Bowel Dis 10: 28–31.

Tsujikawa T, Urabe M, Bamba H et al. (2000). Haemorrhagic cerebral sinus thrombosis associated with ulcerative colitis: a case report of successful treatment by anticoagulant therapy. J Gastroenterol Hepatol 15: 688–692.

Ullrich S, Schinke S, Both M et al. (2009). Refractory central nervous system vasculitis and gastrocnemius myalgia syndrome in Crohn's disease successfully treated with anti-tumor necrosis factor-alpha antibody. Semin Arthritis Rheum 38: 337–347.

Van Assche G, Van Ranst M, Sciot R et al. (2005). Progressive multifocal leukoencephalopathy after natalizumab therapy for Crohn's disease. N Eng J Med 353: 362–368.

Vannucchi V, Grazzini M, Pieralli F et al. (2011). Adalimumab-induced lupus erythematosus with central nervous system involvement in a patient with Crohn's disease. J Gastrointestin Liver Dis 20: 201–203.

Vavricka SR, Brun L, Ballabini P et al. (2011). Frequency and risk factors of extraintestinal manifestations in the Swiss inflammatory bowel disease cohort. Am J Gastroenterol 106: 110–119.

Wijdicks EF, Wiesner RH, Krom RA (1995). Neurotoxicity in liver transplant recipients with cyclosporine immunosuppression. Neurology 45: 1962–1964.

Zois CD, Katsanos K, Kosmidou M et al. (2010). Neurological manifestation of inflammatory bowel diseases: current knowledge and novel insights. J Crohns Colitis 4: 115–124.

Handbook of Clinical Neurology, Vol. 120 (3rd series)
Neurologic Aspects of Systemic Disease Part II
Jose Biller and Jose M. Ferro, Editors
© 2014 Elsevier B.V. All rights reserved

Chapter 41

Gluten-related neurologic dysfunction

MARIOS HADJIVASSILIOU[1]*, ANDREW P. DUKER[2], AND DAVID S. SANDERS[3]

[1]*Department of Neurology, Royal Hallamshire Hospital, Sheffield, UK*

[2]*Department of Gastroenterology, Royal Hallamshire Hospital, Sheffield, UK*

[3]*Department of Neurology, University of Cincinnati, Cincinnati, OH, USA*

HISTORICAL PERSPECTIVE

Celiac disease (CD) was first described by the Greek doctor Aretaeus the Cappadocian, in AD 100, only to be forgotten and then rediscovered by Samuel Gee in 1888 (Gee, 1888). In a lecture on "the coeliac affection," Gee described the classic pediatric presentation of the disease. Whilst clinicians began to recognize this disease entity, the etiologic agent remained obscure until the observations of Willem Dicke, a Dutch pediatrician, in 1953 of "the presence in wheat, of a factor having a deleterious effect in cases of celiac disease" (Dicke et al., 1953). As gastrointestinal symptoms (diarrhea, abdominal pain, bloating, weight loss) were dominant in patients with this disease, it was not surprising that CD was thought to be a disease of the gut. Indeed the introduction of endoscopy and small bowel biopsy in the 1950s confirmed the presence of an enteropathy (Paulley, 1954).

In 1963 a group of dermatologists made the interesting observation that dermatitis herpetiformis (DH), an itchy vesicular rash, was a form of gluten-related dermatopathy sharing the same small bowel pathology, but not the gastrointestinal symptoms seen in patients with CD (Marks et al., 1966). This was the first evidence of extraintestinal manifestations.

Only a small number of case reports of patients with CD and neurologic manifestations (Elders, 1925; Reed and Ash, 1927; Woltman and Heck, 1937) were published prior to the discovery of the etiologic agent and the introduction of small bowel biopsy, demonstrating the typical histologic features that define CD. Such reports need to be treated with caution given that a diagnosis of CD in those patients was speculative.

The first comprehensive case series of neurologic manifestations in the context of histologically confirmed CD was published in 1966 (Cooke and Thomas-Smith, 1966). This detailed work described the range of neurologic manifestations seen in 16 patients with established CD. Of interest was the fact that all patients had gait ataxia and some had severe peripheral neuropathy as well. The assumption was that such manifestations were nutritional as a result of malabsorption. Indeed all of these patients were grossly malnourished and cachectic. Postmortem data from the same report, however, demonstrated an inflammatory process primarily affecting the cerebellum, but also involving other parts of the central and peripheral nervous systems, a finding that was in favor of an immune-mediated pathogenesis.

Single and multiple case reports of patients with established CD who then developed neurologic dysfunction continued to be published (Binder et al., 1967; Bundey, 1967; Morris et al., 1970; Coers et al., 1971; Kepes et al., 1975; Finelli et al., 1980; Kinney et al., 1982; Ward et al., 1985; Lu et al., 1986; Kristoferitsch and Pointer, 1987; Kaplan et al., 1988; Tison et al., 1989; Collin et al., 1991; Hermaszewski et al., 1991; Bhatia et al., 1995; Dick et al., 1995; Muller et al., 1996).

The key findings from these reports were as follows:

- Ataxia (with and without myoclonus) and neuropathy were the commonest manifestations.
- Neurologic manifestations were usually reported in the context of established CD and almost always attributed to nutritional deficiencies.
- In those reports where the effect of the dietary restriction was reported, the results were mixed. None of these reports, however, documented any attempts to monitor adherence to the diet with repeat serologic testing.

*Correspondence to: Marios Hadjivassiliou, Department of Neurology, Royal Hallamshire Hospital, Glossop Road, Sheffield, S10 2JF, UK. E-mail: m.hadjivassiliou@sheffffield.ac.uk

Thirty years after the first comprehensive case series on neurologic manifestations of CD saw the publication of an original study (Hadjivassiliou et al., 1996) approaching the issue from a neurologic perspective by investigating the prevalence of serologic markers of gluten-related dysfunction (GRD) in patients presenting with neurologic dysfunction of unknown etiology. The results demonstrated that there was a high prevalence of IgG and/or IgA antigliadin antibodies (AGA) in this group of patients compared to controls. Based on duodenal biopsies the same study showed that the prevalence of CD in this group of patients with neurologic dysfunction was 16 times higher than the prevalence of CD in the healthy population. This study rekindled the interest of neurologists in a possible link between GRD and neurologic disease.

EPIDEMIOLOGY OF NEUROLOGIC MANIFESTATIONS

The prevalence of CD in the healthy population has been shown to be at least 1% in both European and North American studies (Sanders et al., 2003). There are no accurate figures of the prevalence of the neurologic manifestations of gluten sensitivity in the general population. Figures of between 10% and 22.5% have been reported amongst patients with established CD attending gastrointestinal clinics (Holmes, 1997; Briani et al., 2008). These are unlikely to be accurate because such figures are usually retrospective, derived solely from gastrointestinal clinics, concentrating exclusively on patients with classic CD presentation, and often include neurologic dysfunctions that are unlikely to be gluten related (e.g., carpal tunnel syndrome, idiopathic Parkinson's disease, etc.). Some estimates of prevalence can be made from patient populations attending specialist clinics although caution must be exercised in extrapolating these as they are inevitably affected by referral bias. Data collected from the Sheffield dedicated CD and gluten sensitivity/neurology clinics suggest that for every seven patients presenting to the gastroenterologists who are then diagnosed with CD, there are two patients presenting to the neurologists who will then be diagnosed as having CD (Hadjivassiliou et al., 2010a). This is likely to be an underestimate because this ratio does not take into account those patients with neurologic manifestations due to GRD that do not have an enteropathy (approximately two-thirds of the whole number of patients presenting with neurologic dysfunction). The authors believe that the prevalence of neurologic dysfunction even within patients with CD presenting to gastroenterologists is likely to be much higher than what has been published if such patients undergo rigorous neurologic workup including magnetic resonance (MR) spectroscopy of the cerebellum. Preliminary work on patients with CD presenting to gastroenterologists with minor neurologic complaints demonstrates that up to 80% have abnormal MR spectroscopy (low NAA/Cr ratios) of the cerebellum (Hadjivassiliou et al., 2011).

THE DIAGNOSIS OF GLUTEN-RELATED DISEASES

CD is characterized by the presence of an enteropathy, a reliable gold standard. It is now accepted, however, that an enteropathy is not a prerequisite for the diagnosis of GRD with predominantly neurologic or other extraintestinal manifestations. Furthermore, the small bowel mucosal changes in the context of GRD represent a spectrum, from histologically normal mucosa to full-blown enteropathy to a pre-lymphomatous state also referred to as the Marsh classification (Marsh, 1992). Most pathology departments have now adopted the Marsh classification when reporting the histologic findings of small bowel biopsies. Given that the histology can be normal, a definition of GRD based solely on histology becomes problematic. Furthermore the diagnosis currently has to rely on serologic tests that are not 100% specific or sensitive. For example, endomysial antibody (EMA) and antitransglutaminase-2 (TG2) IgA antibody detection are specific for the presence of an enteropathy. However, these markers are frequently not detectable in patients with neurologic manifestations, particularly in those who do not have an enteropathy (Table 41.1).

Table 41.1

Type of neurologic presentation in gluten sensitivity*

Neurologic presentation	No
Total number of patients	500
Ataxia (4 patients with myoclonus, 2 with palatal tremor)	233 (93)
Peripheral neuropathy	182 (48)
Sensorimotor axonal neuropathy	135
Mononeuropathy multiplex	19
Sensory neuronopathy	14
Small fiber neuropathy	8
Motor neuropathy	8
Encephalopathy	77 (45)
Myopathy	18 (10)
Myelopathy	9 (4)
Stiff man syndrome	7 (2)
Chorea (often with ataxia)	3 (2)
Neuromyotonia	1 (1)
Epilepsy and occipital calcifications	1 (0)

*Based on 500 patients with gluten sensitivity, presenting with neurologic dysfunction and seen in the gluten sensitivity/neurology clinic, Sheffield, UK, from 1994 to 2011. The number of patients from each group who had enteropathy on biopsy is shown in parentheses. Some patients had more than one type of neurologic presentation.

GRD cannot be diagnosed on clinical grounds alone. The majority of patients presenting with neurologic manifestations have no gastrointestinal symptoms. Patients with CD can also have no gastrointestinal symptoms. In patients without overt gastrointestinal involvement, serum antibodies to TG2 may be absent. Such patients typically have antibodies primarily reacting with different TG isozymes, TG3 in DH and TG6 in patients with gluten ataxia (Hadjivassiliou et al., 2008a). Reaction of such antibodies with TG2 in the intestinal mucosa occurs prior to overt changes in small intestinal morphology and sometimes even before the antibodies are detectable in serum (Korponay-Szabó et al., 2003). Such antibody deposits seem to be present in patients with neurologic manifestations as well, and may therefore be diagnostically useful (Hadjivassiliou et al., 2006a). However, this test is not readily available and requires experience in its interpretation. In practice, for suspected neurologic manifestations of GRD, it is best to perform serologic tests for both IgA and IgG antibodies to TG2 (and if available anti-TG6 and anti-TG3) as well as IgG and IgA antibodies to gliadin. Endomysium antibodies are very specific for the detection of enteropathy, but they detect the same antigen (transglutaminase 2) and have thus largely been replaced by TG2 antibody testing. Any differences between the two tests, however, are likely to be related to the different methodologies used (ELISA for TG2 versus immunofluorescence for the detection of EMA).

GRD have a strong genetic predisposition whereby ~40% of the genetic load comes from MHC class II association (Hunt, 2008). In Caucasian populations more than 90% of CD patients carry the HLA DQ2, with the remaining having the HLA DQ8. A small number of CD patients do not belong into either of these groups but these have been shown to carry just one chain of the DQ2 heterodimer. HLA genetic testing is therefore another useful diagnostic tool, particularly as, unlike other serologic tests, it is not dependent on an immunologic trigger. However, the HLA DQ genotype can be used only as a test of exclusion as the risk genotype DQ2 is common in Caucasian and Asian populations and many carriers will never develop GRD.

THE SPECTRUM OF GLUTEN-RELATED NEUROLOGIC MANIFESTATIONS

Gluten ataxia

Gluten ataxia (GA) was originally defined as otherwise idiopathic sporadic ataxia with positive AGA (Hadjivassiliou et al., 2003a). This original definition was based on the serologic tests available at the time. In a series of 853 patients with progressive ataxia evaluated over a period of 15 years in Sheffield, UK, there were 152 patients out of 681 with sporadic ataxia who

had serologic evidence of GRD. Therefore gluten ataxia had a prevalence of 22% amongst sporadic ataxias but as high as 45% amongst idiopathic sporadic ataxias. Using the same AGA assay the prevalence of positive AGA in genetically confirmed ataxias was 8/82 (10%), in familial ataxias (not genetically confirmed) 8/49 (16%), and in healthy volunteers 149/1200 (12%). A number of studies looking at the prevalence of antigliadin antibodies in ataxias have been published: The original publication by the authors (Hadjivassiliou et al., 2003a) reported the incidence of IgG and/or IgA AGA in a large cohort of 224 patients seen in Sheffield, UK, with idiopathic and hereditary ataxia. Antibodies were present in 41% of patients with sporadic ataxia (54/132), compared to 12% (149/1200) of normal controls from the same population. Positive antibodies were also found in 14% of patients with familial ataxia (8/59) and 15% of patients with clinically probable multiple system atrophy (MSA)-C (5/33). Among AGA-positive individuals with sporadic ataxia, evidence of celiac disease was present in 24% (12/51) of those patients who underwent duodenal biopsy. In this same study, a separate group of patients from a second center in London with sporadic ataxia showed positive antibodies in 32% (14/44). Another study (Bürk et al., 2001a) found positive antibodies in 11.5% (12/104) of patients with idiopathic ataxia and negative genetic testing, compared to 5% of 600 blood donors from the same country. An Italian study (Pellecchia et al., 1999a) confirmed a higher incidence of positive antigliadin antibodies and celiac disease on intestinal biopsy in idiopathic ataxia (3/24, 12.5%) compared to patients with known hereditary ataxia (0/23, 0%). Further confirmatory studies with smaller numbers from Finland, Japan, and France have also been published (Luostarinen et al., 2001; Anheim et al., 2006; Ihara et al., 2006). However, other studies have not shown as clear a distinction in antibody prevalence between idiopathic and other causes of ataxia. Abele et al. (2002) found positive antibodies in 15% (10/65) of patients with idiopathic ataxia compared to 9% (3/32) of patients with MSA and 7% (1/15) with genetic ataxia. In a separate study, Abele et al. (2003) found no statistically significant difference between the prevalence of positive IgG and/or IgA AGA in sporadic ataxia (19% of 32 patients), recessive ataxia (8% of 24 patients), dominant ataxia (15% of 39 patients), and controls (8% of 73 patients). Analyzing IgG and IgA subtypes separately also did not show significant differences between groups. Bushara et al. (2001) noted similar rates of positive IgG and/or IgA AGA in sporadic ataxia (27%, 7/26) and autosomal dominant ataxia (37%, 9/24). Some authors believe the elevated incidence of AGA in hereditary ataxia may be driven in part by spinocerebellar ataxia type 2 (SCA2). In one study, 23% of SCA2 patients had positive AGA, significantly higher compared to 9% of controls (Almaguer-Mederos et al., 2008). The variations in prevalence may relate to geographical differences in the prevalence of CD, referral bias, variability in the AGA assays used, patient selection (some studies included as idiopathic sporadic ataxia patients with cerebellar variant of multisystem atrophy (Combarros et al., 2000)), the small number of patients studied, and no controls. The common theme in most of these studies is the consistently high prevalence of AGA antibodies in sporadic ataxias when compared to healthy controls.

GA usually presents with pure cerebellar ataxia or rarely ataxia in combination with myoclonus, palatal tremor (Hadjivassiliou et al., 2008b), opsoclonus (Deconinck et al., 2006), or rarely, chorea (Pereira et al., 2004). GA is usually of insidious onset with a mean age at onset of 53 years. Rarely the ataxia can be rapidly progressive mimicking paraneoplastic cerebellar degeneration. Gaze-evoked nystagmus and other ocular signs of cerebellar dysfunction are seen in up to 80% of cases. All patients have gait ataxia and the majority have limb ataxia. Less than 10% of patients with GA will have any gastrointestinal symptoms but a third will have evidence of enteropathy on biopsy. Up to 60% of patients have neurophysiologic evidence of sensorimotor, length-dependent axonal neuropathy. This is usually mild and does not contribute to the ataxia. Anti-TG2 IgA antibodies are present in up to 38% of patients, but often at lower titers than those seen in patients with CD. However, unlike CD, IgG class antibodies to TG2 are more frequent than IgA. Antibodies against TG2 and TG6 combined can be found in 85% of patients with ataxia who are positive for AGA antibodies (Hadjivassiliou et al., 2009). Some patients also test positive for anti-TG3 antibodies although the prevalence of such antibodies in patients with gluten ataxia is low when compared to DH. It is unclear at present whether combined detection of TG2 and TG6 IgA/IgG without the use of antigliadin antibodies identifies all patients with gluten ataxia.

Up to 60% of patients with gluten ataxia have evidence of cerebellar atrophy on MR imaging (Fig. 41.1). Investigation of the metabolic status of the cerebellum in 15 patients with gluten ataxia and 10 controls using proton MR spectroscopy demonstrated significant differences in mean N-acetylaspartate/creatine levels between patients with GA and healthy controls, suggesting that cerebellar neuronal physiology in these patients is abnormal (Wilkinson et al., 2005). Even in those patients without cerebellar atrophy, proton MR spectroscopy of the cerebellum was abnormal. There is emerging evidence that MR spectroscopy is often abnormal in patients with newly diagnosed CD with minimal or

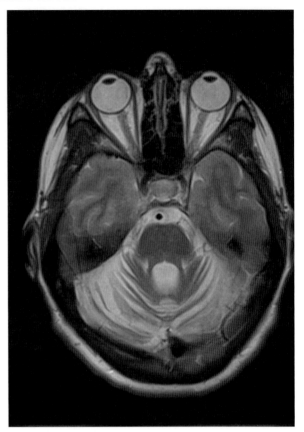

Fig. 41.1. Severe cerebellar atrophy on axial MR imaging in a 40-year-old woman with a 10 year history of progressive ataxia diagnosed eventually with gluten sensitivity. She remains stable on a gluten-free diet but the ataxia is still present as a result of permanent damage to the cerebellum.

no neurologic complaints and that such abnormalities improve with the introduction of a gluten-free diet. The clinical improvement manifests after 1 year on the diet but continues for at least 2 years. The response to treatment with a gluten-free diet depends on the duration of the ataxia prior to the diagnosis of GRD. Loss of Purkinje cells in the cerebellum, the end result of prolonged gluten exposure in patients with GA, is irreversible, and prompt treatment is more likely to result in improvement or stabilization of the ataxia. Whilst the benefits of a gluten-free diet in the treatment of patients with CD and DH have long been established, there are very few studies, mainly case reports, of the effect of a gluten-free diet on the neurologic manifestations. Most of these reports primarily concern patients with established CD who then develop neurologic symptoms (Beversdorf et al., 1996; Hahn et al., 1998; Pellecchia et al., 1999). These studies suggest variable but overall favorable responsiveness to a gluten-free diet. A small, uncontrolled study looked at the use of intravenous immunoglobulins in the treatment of four patients with

GA without enteropathy (Bürk et al., 2001b; Sander et al., 2003). All patients improved. In all of these reports, strict adherence to the gluten-free diet was assumed and no serologic evidence was provided. The best marker of strict adherence to a gluten-free diet is serologic evidence of elimination of circulating GRD-related antibodies. Only one systematic study of the effect of a gluten-free diet on a cohort of patients presenting with ataxia, with or without an enteropathy, has been published (Hadjivassiliou et al., 2003b). This study also reported serologic evidence of elimination of the antigliadin antibodies as a confirmation of strict adherence to the diet. A total of 43 patients with gluten ataxia were enrolled. Of these, 26 adhered strictly to the gluten-free diet, had serologic evidence of elimination of antibodies, and comprised the treatment group; 14 patients refused the diet and comprised the control group and 3 patients were excluded as despite the diet their antibodies were still positive. Patient and control groups were matched at baseline for all variables (age, duration of ataxia, etc.). There was no significant difference in the baseline performance for each ataxia test between the two groups. There was significant improvement in performance in test scores and in the subjective global clinical impression scale in the treatment group when compared to the control group. The improvement was apparent even after excluding patients with an enteropathy. The study concluded that gluten-free diet can be an effective treatment for GA.

There are no published randomized, placebo-controlled studies on the subject, perhaps reflecting the difficulties associated with such a study when the intervention is dietary elimination of gluten and the ethical considerations of randomizing patients with GA who have enteropathy. The current recommendation is that patients presenting with progressive cerebellar ataxia should be screened for gluten sensitivity using antigliadin IgG and IgA, anti-TG2 antibodies and if available anti-TG6 antibodies. Patients positive for any of these antibodies with no alternative cause for their ataxia should be offered a strict gluten-free diet with regular follow-up to ensure that the antibodies are eliminated (usually takes 6–12 months). Stabilization or even improvement of the ataxia at 1 year would be a strong indicator that the patient suffers from gluten ataxia. The commonest reason for lack of response is lack of compliance with the diet. If patients on strict gluten-free diet continue to progress, with or without elimination of antibodies, the use of immunosuppressive medication (mycophenolate) should be considered. Such cases are rare.

Gluten neuropathy

Up to 23% of patients with established CD on gluten-free diet have neurophysiologic evidence of a peripheral neuropathy (Luostarinen et al., 2003). A large population-based study of over 84 000 subjects in Sweden examined the risk of neurologic disease in patients with CD and found that polyneuropathy had a significant association with CD (Ludvigsson et al., 2007). In our own UK-based study, 34% of patients with idiopathic sporadic sensorimotor axonal neuropathy were found to have circulating AGA (Hadjivassiliou et al., 2006b). Using anti-TG2 antibody detection an Italian study also showed a significantly number of patients (21%) with peripheral neuropathy to be positive (Mata et al., 2006). Finally, in a tertiary referral centre in the US, retrospective evaluation of patients with neuropathy showed the prevalence of CD to be between 2.5% and 8% as compared to 1% in the healthy population (Chin et al., 2003).

Gluten neuropathy is defined as otherwise idiopathic sporadic neuropathy with serologic evidence of GRD. The commonest types are symmetric sensorimotor axonal peripheral neuropathy and sensory ganglionopathy (Hadjivassiliou et al., 2010b). Other types of neuropathies have also been reported including asymmetric neuropathy (Kelkar et al., 1996; Hadjivassiliou et al., 1997; Chin et al., 2006), small fiber neuropathy (Brannagan et al., 2005), and rarely, pure motor neuropathy (Hadjivassiliou et al., 1997) or autonomic neuropathy (Gibbons and Freeman, 2005). Gluten neuropathy is a slowly progressive disease with a mean age at onset of the neuropathy of 55 years (range 24–77 years) and a mean duration of 9 years (range 1–33 years). A third of the patients will have evidence of enteropathy on biopsy but the presence or absence of an enteropathy does not predetermine the effect of a gluten-free diet (Hadjivassiliou et al., 2006b).

Limited pathologic data available from postmortems and nerve biopsies are consistent with an inflammatory etiology (perivascular lymphocytic infiltration). The evidence of effectiveness of gluten-free diet has largely been derived from single or multiple case reports most of which suggest improvement of the neuropathy. The only systematic, controlled study of the effect of a gluten-free diet on 35 patients with gluten neuropathy, with close serologic monitoring of the adherence to the gluten-free diet, found significant improvement in the treated compared with the control group after 1 year on the diet (Hadjivassiliou et al., 2006b). The improvement took the form of an increase in the sural sensory action potential, the predefined primary endpoint, and subjective improvement of the neuropathic symptoms. Subgroup analysis suggested that the capacity for recovery of the peripheral nerves may be less when the neuropathy is severe or that more time may be needed for such recovery to manifest. As there was a correlation between disease severity and longer duration, gluten neuropathy may be considered a progressive disease if untreated. In the context of sensory ganglionopathy

GRD has been shown to be as common a cause as Sjögren's syndrome. Dorsal root ganglia demonstrate evidence of inflammatory infiltrates. The disease progresses slowly if untreated. Strict adherence to a gluten-free diet may result in stabilization or even improvement of the neuropathy irrespective of the presence of enteropathy (Hadjivassiliou et al., 2010b).

Gluten encephalopathy (headache and white matter abnormalities)

Headache is a common feature in patients with GRD. In 2001 we reported a series of 10 patients with GRD and headache who in addition had CNS white matter abnormalities on MRI scan suggesting the term "gluten encephalopathy" to describe them (Hadjivassiliou et al., 2001). The headaches are usually episodic, similar to migraines, may be associated with focal neurologic deficits, and characteristically resolve with the introduction of a gluten-free diet. The white matter abnormalities can be diffuse or focal and do not resolve following a gluten-free diet, which simply arrests progression of these changes (Fig. 41.2). Their distribution is more suggestive of a vascular rather than demyelinating etiology. Multiple sclerosis does not seem to be associated with GRD on the basis

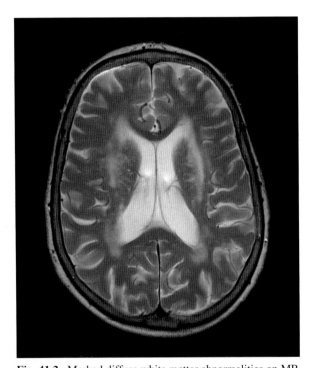

Fig. 41.2. Marked diffuse white matter abnormalities on MR imaging in a 55-year-old man with celiac disease presenting with headaches and mild ataxia. There was complete resolution of the headaches following the introduction of a gluten-free diet. Neurologically he remains stable.

of numerous studies (Pengiran Tengah et al., 2004; Hadjivassiliou et al., 2005; Borhani Haghighi et al, 2007; Nicoletti et al, 2008).

In patients with migraine there is an over-representation of CD with a prevalence of 4.4% versus 0.4% in the control population (Gabrielli et al., 2003). Using positron emission tomography (PET) brain imaging, a study on regional cerebral perfusion demonstrated that 73% of patients with CD not on a gluten-free diet, had at least one hypoperfused brain region as compared to 7% in healthy controls and in patients with CD on a gluten-free diet (Addolorato et al., 2004). Another study investigated the prevalence of white matter abnormalities in children with CD and found that 20% of patients had such abnormalities (Kieslich et al., 2001).

Over the last 14 years we have encountered 70 patients with gluten encephalopathy, a figure that includes the initial 10 patients reported in the 2001 series. Gluten encephalopathy does not always occur in isolation and such patients will often have additional neurologic features such as ataxia, neuropathy, and cognitive deficits. A study from the Mayo Clinic emphasized the significant cognitive deficits encountered in 13 such patients (Hu et al., 2006). In comparison to gluten ataxia and gluten neuropathy there is a higher prevalence of enteropathy in patients with gluten encephalopathy (40/70), but the age at onset is the same. The observed improvement of the headaches and arrest of progression in the MRI brain abnormalities, suggest a causal link with gluten ingestion. Gluten encephalopathy represents a spectrum of clinical presentations, from episodic headaches responsive to a gluten-free diet at one end to severe debilitating headaches associated with focal neurologic deficits and abnormal white matter on MRI at the other.

Myoclonic ataxia

This form of ataxia is much less common in comparison to gluten ataxia. It was first described in 1986 (Lu et al., 1986). It has been shown that the myoclonus is of cortical origin despite the presence of cerebellar atrophy (Bhatia et al., 1995). Some myoclonus can be seen in a number of such patients but it is not usually troublesome. In our series of patients (over 500) with neurologic manifestations of GRD we have encountered four patients with what appears to be focal disabling myoclonus. All patients had evidence of enteropathy on biopsy. In two patients, despite a strict gluten-free diet, their condition progressed. Both have been treated with mycophenolate resulting in some stabilization. In the remaining patients the ataxia responded to the gluten-free diet but the myoclonus persists. In some of these patients the apparent focal myoclonus resembles epilepsia partialis continua in neurophysiologic terms. The apparent refractoriness of this neurologic manifestation is mirrored by evidence of ongoing enteropathy despite a strict adherence to the gluten-free diet. The treatment of such patients remains problematic but the limited evidence from these small series suggests that mycophenolate may be a useful therapeutic intervention for those patients who appear to progress neurologically despite strict gluten-free diet.

Epilepsy

A number of reports have suggested a link between epilepsy and CD (Chapman et al., 1978; Fois et al., 1994; Cronin et al., 1998). There is a particular type of focal epilepsy associated with occipital calcifications that appears to have a strong link with CD (Gobbi et al., 1992). This entity is common in Italy but rare in other countries (Fig. 41.3). It tends to affect young patients (mean age 16 years) and in the majority the seizures are resistant to antiepileptic drugs. The pathogenesis of the cerebral calcifications remains unclear. An autopsy study showed the depositions consisted of both calcium and silica, and microscopically were found in three main types: psammoma-like bodies without any identifiable relationship to cells, vessels, or other structures; small granular deposition along small vessels; and

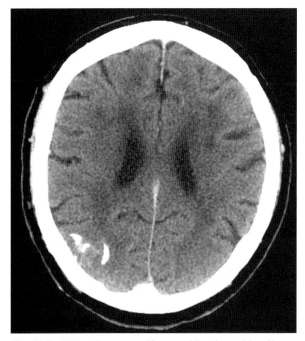

Fig. 41.3. CT head scan on a 52-year-old patient with epilepsy and gluten sensitivity demonstrating occipital calcifications. This condition is rare outside Italy and it primarily affects children. This patient presented with loss of consciousness ataxia and cognitive decline.

focal scanty areas of calcium within neurons (Toti et al., 1996). As most of the reported cases are from Italy, Spain, and Argentina, it has been hypothesized that the syndrome of celiac disease, epilepsy, and cerebral calcifications is "a genetic, non-inherited, ethnically and geographically restricted syndrome associated with environmental factors" (Gobbi, 2005).

Whilst studies examining the prevalence of CD amongst patients with epilepsy have suggested a prevalence of 1.2–2.3%, larger more recent studies failed to demonstrate such an increased prevalence (Ranua et al., 2005). However, most studies on the subject suffer from the same methodologic problem of treating epilepsy as a homogeneous disorder. The only study that attempted to look at the prevalence of GRD in well characterized subgroups of patients with epilepsy found a significant association between AGA and temporal lobe epilepsy with hippocampal sclerosis (Paltola et al., 2009). Of interest are some case reports on patients with CD and epilepsy whose epilepsy improves following the introduction of gluten-free diet (Mavroudi et al., 2005; Harper et al., 2007).

Myopathy

This is a relatively rare neurologic manifestation of GRD, first described by Henriksson et al. (1982). This study from Sweden reported that out of 76 patients with suspected polymyositis investigated at a neuromuscular unit, 17 had a history of gastrointestinal symptoms with evidence of malabsorption. Fourteen of these fulfilled the diagnostic criteria for polymyositis and of those, five were diagnosed with CD. A more recent study from Spain (Selva-O'Callaghan et al., 2007) demonstrated the prevalence of AGA antibodies amongst patients with inflammatory myopathies to be 31%. This was accompanied by a higher prevalence of CD within the same population when compared to healthy controls.

The clinical data from our series of patients are based on 18 cases encountered over the last 14 years, 13 of which have been reported previously (Hadjivassiliou et al., 2007). Enteropathy was identified following duodenal biopsy in 10 of these patients. The mean age at onset of the myopathic symptoms was 54 years. Ten patients had predominantly proximal weakness, five patients had both proximal and distal weakness, and four patients had primarily distal weakness. Two patients had ataxia and neuropathy, and one patient had just neuropathy in addition to the myopathy. Serum creatine kinase (CK) level ranged from normal (25–190 IU/L) to 4380 IU/L at presentation. Inflammatory myopathy was the most common finding on neuropathologic examination (Fig. 41.4). Six patients received immunosuppressive treatment in addition to starting a gluten-free diet whereas the others went on a gluten-free diet

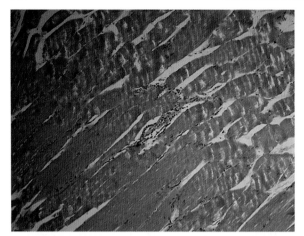

Fig. 41.4. Muscle biopsy demonstrating focal inflammatory infiltration in a 60-year-old man with celiac disease who became profoundly weak after inadvertently eating a cake made out of rye flour. His weakness was profound and necessitated admission. He made a full recovery just with reintroduction of a strict gluten-free diet.

only. In the majority of those patients who did not receive immunosuppressive treatment there was clinical improvement of the myopathy with gluten-free diet, suggesting that the myopathy was etiologically linked to the GRD. One patient developed a profound myopathy after inadvertently eating rye flour. He made a full recovery by re-establishing a strict gluten-free diet. Two patients had histologic evidence of inclusion body myositis. It is interesting to note that inclusion body myositis shares the same HLA genetic predisposition with CD.

Myelopathy

Clinical evidence of a myelopathy in the absence of vitamin and other deficiencies (particularly copper) can be a rare manifestation of CD (Fig. 41.5). It is usually associated with normal imaging of the spinal cord. However, there have been some recent reports of patients with neuromyelitis optica (Devic's disease) and GRD who have antibodies to aquaporin-4 (Jacob et al., 2005; Jarius et al., 2008). Such patients clearly had abnormal MRI of the spinal cord but the diagnosis of CD was only made at the time of their neurologic presentation. Neuromyelitis optica and CD share the same HLA genetic susceptibility (HLA DQ2). There are very limited data on the effect of the diet on the likelihood of relapse of the disease, particularly given the fact that most patients with Devic's disease end up on long-term immunosuppressive medication.

Stiff man syndrome

Stiff man syndrome (SMS) is a rare autoimmune disease characterized by axial stiffness, painful spasms, and

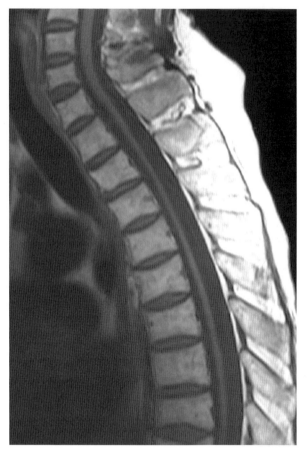

Fig. 41.5. Spinal cord atrophy on MR imaging of the thoracic cord of a 55-year-old man with celiac disease and sensory ataxia. Whilst the patient had celiac disease for many years, he never adhered to the diet strictly and went on to develop neurologic manifestations.

positivity for anti-GAD or anti-amphiphysin antibodies. It has a strong association with other autoimmune diseases (e.g., insulin-dependent diabetes mellitus (IDDM), hypothyroidism, etc.). We have found a high prevalence of gluten-related antibodies in patients with this condition over and above that expected from an association of two autoimmune diseases. The relapsing remitting nature of the condition makes a study of any responsiveness to gluten-free diet difficult. There is, however, evidence of reduction of the anti-GAD antibody titer following the introduction of a gluten-free diet suggesting that the diet may be beneficial in treating the condition (Hadjivassiliou et al., 2010c). This finding also supports the concept of prevention of autoimmunity in patients with GRD if the gluten-free diet is introduced early enough.

PATHOGENESIS

Current evidence suggests that neurologic manifestations are immune mediated. Postmortem examination from patients with gluten ataxia demonstrate patchy loss of Purkinje cells throughout the cerebellar cortex, a non-specific finding in many cerebellar disorders. However, additional findings supporting an immune-mediated pathogenesis include diffuse infiltration mainly of T lymphocytes within the cerebellar white matter as well as marked perivascular cuffing with inflammatory cells (Hadjivassiliou et al., 1998). The peripheral nervous system also shows sparse lymphocytic infiltrates with perivascular cuffing being observed in sural nerve biopsy of patients with gluten neuropathy (Hadjivassiliou et al., 2006a), in dorsal root ganglia in patients with sensory neuronopathy (Hadjivassiliou et al., 2010a) and in patients with gluten myopathy due to GRD (Hadjivassiliou et al., 2007). There is evidence to suggest that there is antibody cross-reactivity between antigenic epitopes on Purkinje cells and gluten proteins. Serum from patients with GA and from patients with CD but no neurologic symptoms, display cross-reactivity with epitopes on Purkinje cells of both human and rat cerebellum (Hadjivassiliou et al., 2002). This reactivity can also be seen using polyclonal AGA and the reactivity eliminated by absorption with crude gliadin. When using sera from patients with GA there is evidence of additional antibodies targeting Purkinje cell epitopes since elimination of AGA alone is not sufficient to eliminate such reactivity (Fig. 41.6). There is some evidence that additional antibodies that may be causing such reactivity, including antibodies against one or more transglutaminase isoenzymes.

TG2 belongs to a family of enzymes that covalently crosslink or modify proteins by formation of an isopeptide bond between a peptide-bound glutamine residue and a primary amine. However, in some instances TG2 may react with water in preference over an amine leading to the deamidation of glutamine residues. Gluten proteins (from wheat, barley, and rye), the immunologic trigger of GRD, are glutamine-rich donor substrates amenable to deamidation. Activation of TG2 and deamidation of gluten peptides appears to be central to disease development and is now well understood at a molecular level. However, events leading to the formation of autoantibodies against TG2 are still unclear. Questions also remain as to the contribution of these autoantibodies to organ-specific deficits. Anti-TG2 antibodies have been shown to be deposited in the small bowel mucosa of patients with GRD even in the absence of enteropathy. Furthermore such deposits have been found in extraintestinal sites, such as muscle and liver (Korponay-Szabó et al., 2004). Widespread deposition of transglutaminase antibodies has also been found around brain vessels in GA (Hadjivassiliou et al., 2006a). The deposition was most pronounced in the cerebellum, pons, and medulla. This finding suggests that such autoantibodies could play a role in the pathogenesis of the whole spectrum of manifestations seen in GRD. However, it is not clear whether these antibodies are derived from the circulation or if their production is mediated within target organs after stimulation of gut-primed gliadin-reactive CD4[+] T cells.

Variations in the specificity of antibodies produced in individual patients could explain the wide spectrum of manifestations. Whilst TG2 has been shown to be the autoantigen in CD (Dietrich et al., 1997), the epidermal transglutaminase TG3 has been shown to be the autoantigen in DH (Sárdy et al., 2002). More recently, antibodies against TG6, a primarily brain expressed transglutaminase, have been shown to be present in patients with GA (Hadjivassiliou et al., 2008a). In GA and DH, IgA deposits of TG6 and TG3 respectively seem to accumulate in the periphery of blood vessels. This could indicate that either the deposits originate from immune complexes formed elsewhere, and are accumulating as a consequence of enhanced vascular leaking, or that TG6/TG3 are derived from perivascular infiltrating inflammatory cells preceding deposit formation. Indeed perivascular cuffing with lymphocytes is a common finding in brain tissue from patients with GA but is also seen in peripheral nerve and muscle in patients with gluten neuropathy or myopathy. In most sera reactive

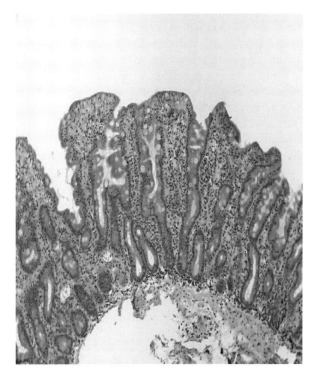

Fig. 41.6. Duodenal biopsy from a patient presenting with progressive ataxia and positive antigliadin antibodies. The biopsy demonstrates the triad of crypt hyperplasia, villous atrophy, and increase in the intraepithelial lymphocytes. Only a third of patients with gluten ataxia will have enteropathy.

with more than one TG isoenzyme, distinct antibody populations are responsible for such reactivity rather than this being a result of cross-reactivity with different TG isozymes. This makes shared epitopes less likely to be the cause for immune responses to other TGs and points to the possibility that TG isozymes other than TG2 can be the primary antigen in GRD.

IgA deposition in brain vessels and the pathologic finding of perivascular cuffing with inflammatory cells, may indicate that vasculature-centered inflammation may compromise the blood–brain barrier, allowing exposure of the CNS to pathogenic antibodies, and therefore be the trigger of nervous system involvement. Indeed, TG2 is expressed by smooth muscle and endothelial cells in noninflamed brain, is an abundant component of the blood–brain barrier and autoantibody binding could initiate an inflammatory response. Anti-TG2 and other autoantibodies (e.g., AGA) may directly cause selective neuronal degeneration. It is possible that neuronal degeneration is a consequence of the anti-TG antibody spectrum, i.e., occurs in those patients with antibodies reactive with a neuronal TG. IgG class antibodies have been shown to be present in only 60% of CD patients whereas in GA patients positive for anti-TG, the prevalence was 90%. This shift from IgA to IgG may reflect the target organ involved (central nervous system rather than the small bowel).

It could be argued that development and deposition of antibodies is an epiphenomenon rather than being pathogenic. One method to demonstrate the pathologic effect of an antibody is the passive transfer of the disease through antibody injection into a naïve animal. While such experimental evidence exists for only very few antibody-mediated diseases, IgG fractions of patients with anti-GAD ataxia and stiff man syndrome have been shown to compromise motor function and impair learning in rodents, an effect possibly ascribed to antibodies against GAD (Manto et al., 2007). A common problem in such studies is to be able to demonstrate whether it is these specific antibodies or other autoantibodies in the IgG-fraction of patient sera that cause neuronal damage. Using a mouse model we have recently shown that serum from GA patients, as well as clonal monovalent anti-TG immunoglobulins derived using phage display, cause ataxia when injected intraventricularly in mice (Boscolo et al., 2010). The fact that not only Ig fractions but also monospecific scFvs mediate functional deficits shows that there is no requirement for complement activation or for the engagement of Fc receptors on Fc receptor-bearing cells in the brain. These data therefore provide evidence that anti-TG immunoglobulins (derived from patients) compromise neuronal function in selected areas of the brain once exposed to the CNS and suggest that this involves an immune system independent mode of action. While these data implicate anti-TG antibodies in ataxia they do not explain the spectrum of distinct neurologic deficits currently ascribed to gluten sensitivity, nor why only a fraction of patients with circulating anti-TG antibodies are affected.

CONCLUSIONS

GRD include immune-mediated diseases triggered by ingestion of gluten proteins. While celiac disease has been the most comprehensively studied of all GRD, dermatitis herpetiformis and neurologic manifestations are the commonest extraintestinal manifestations. To fully understand the immunologic insults resulting from gluten ingestion, the emphasis should perhaps shift toward the study of extraintestinal manifestations. In addition there is a need for the early identification of those patients that are specifically at risk of irreversible complications (e.g., gluten ataxia). To that effect, new diagnostic tools are now becoming available (e.g., antibodies against TG6) which may make a more reliable identification of those patients with neurologic manifestations a reality. Up to 40% of patients presenting to the gastroenterologist who are ultimately diagnosed with CD also have antibodies against TG6 in addition to antibodies against TG2. This subgroup of patients with classic CD presentation may well be the ones susceptible to the development of neurologic dysfunction if they continue to consume gluten, although this remains to be shown in longitudinal studies. The presence of gastrointestinal symptoms, however, offers a major potential advantage to this group, as it substantially increases their chances of being diagnosed with, and treated for, CD, whereas the diagnosis of those patients presenting purely with extraintestinal manifestations may be more difficult. The only way that this can be improved upon is by changing the perception of physicians that gluten-related diseases are solely diseases of the gut.

REFERENCES

Abele M, Bürk K, Schöls L et al. (2002). The aetiology of sporadic adult-onset ataxia. Brain 125: 961–968.

Abele M, Schols L, Schwartz S et al. (2003). Prevalence of antigliadin antibodies in ataxia patients. Neurology 60: 1674–1675.

Addolorato G, Di Giuda D, De Rossi G et al. (2004). Regional cerebral hypoperfusion in patients with celiac disease. Am J Med 116: 312–317.

Almaguer-Mederos LE, Almira YR, Gongora EM et al. (2008). Antigliadin antibodies in Cuban patients with spinocerebellar ataxia type 2. J Neurol Neurosurg Psychiatry 79: 315–317.

Anheim M, Degos B, Echaniz-Laguna A et al. (2006). Ataxia associated with gluten sensitivity, myth or reality? Rev Neurol 162: 214–221.

Beversdorf D, Moses P, Reeves A et al. (1996). A man with weight loss, ataxia, and confusion for 3 months. Lancet 347: 448.

Bhatia KP, Brown P, Gregory R et al. (1995). Progressive myoclonic ataxia associated with celiac disease. Brain 18: 1087–1093.

Binder H, Solitaire G, Spiro H (1967). Neuromuscular disease in patients with steatorrhoea. Gut 8: 605–611.

Borhani Haghighi A, Ansari N, Mokhtari M et al. (2007). Multiple sclerosis and gluten sensitivity. Clin Neurol Neurosurg 109: 651–653.

Boscolo S, Lorenzon A, Sblattero D et al. (2010). Anti trans-glutaminase antibodies cause ataxia in mice. PLoS One 5: e9698.

Brannagan TH, Hays AP, Chin SS et al. (2005). Small-fiber neuropathy/neuronopathy associated with celiac disease: skin biopsy findings. Arch Neurol 62: 1574–1578.

Briani C, Zara G, Alaedini A et al. (2008). Neurological complications of coeliac disease and autoimmune mechanisms: a prospective study. J Neuroimmunol 195: 171–175.

Bundey S (1967). Adult coeliac disease and neuropathy. Lancet 1: 851–852.

Bürk K, Bösch S, Müller CA et al. (2001a). Sporadic cerebellar ataxia associated with gluten sensitivity. Brain 124: 1013–1019.

Bürk K, Melms A, Schulz JB et al. (2001b). Effectiveness of intravenous immunoglobulin therapy in cerebellar ataxia associated with gluten sensitivity. Ann Neurol 50: 827–828.

Bushara KO, Goebel SU, Shill H et al. (2001). Gluten sensitivity in sporadic and hereditary ataxia. Ann Neurol 49: 540–543.

Chapman RWG, Laidlow JM, Colin-Jones D et al. (1978). Increased prevalence of epilepsy in coeliac disease. BMJ 2: 250–251.

Chin RL, Sander HW, Brannagan TH et al. (2003). Celiac neuropathy. Neurology 60: 1581–1585.

Chin RL, Tseng VG, Green PHR et al. (2006). Multifocal axonal polyneuropathy in celiac disease. Neurology 66: 1923–1925.

Coers C, Telerman-Toppet N, Cremer M (1971). Regressive vacuolar myopathy in steatorrhea. Arch Neurol 24: 217–227.

Collin P, Pirttila T, Nurmikko T et al. (1991). Celiac disease, brain atrophy and dementia. Neurology 41: 372–375.

Combarros O, Infante J, López-Hoyos M et al. (2000). Celiac disease and idiopathic cerebellar ataxia. Neurology 54: 2346.

Cooke WT, Thomas-Smith W (1966). Neurological disorders associated with adult coeliac disease. Brain 89: 683–722.

Cronin CC, Jackson LM, Feighery C et al. (1998). Coeliac disease and epilepsy. QJM 91: 303–308.

Deconinck N, Scaillon M, Segers V et al. (2006). Opsoclonus-myoclonus associated with celiac disease. Pediatr Neurol 34: 312–314.

Dick DJ, Abraham D, Falkous G et al. (1995). Cerebellar ataxia in coeliac disease – no evidence of a humoral aetiology. Postgrad Med J 71: 186.

Dicke WK, Weijers HA, Van De Kamer JH (1953). Coeliac disease II The presence in wheat of a factor having a deleterious effect in cases of coeliac disease. Acta Paediatr 42: 34–42.

Dietrich W, Ehnis T, Bauer M et al. (1997). Identification of tissue transglutaminase as the autoantigen of celiac disease. Nat Med 3: 797–801.

Elders C (1925). Tropical sprue and pernicious anaemia, aetiology and treatment. Lancet 1: 75–77.

Finelli P, McEntee W, Ambler M et al. (1980). Adult celiac disease presenting as cerebellar syndrome. Neurology 30: 245–249.

Fois A, Vascotto M, Di Bartolo RM et al. (1994). Celiac disease and epilepsy in pediatric patients. Childs Nerv Syst 10: 450–454.

Gabrielli M, Cremonini F, Fiore G et al. (2003). Association between migraine and celiac disease: results from a preliminary case-control and therapeutic study. Am J Gastroenterol 98: 625–629.

Gee S (1888). On the coeliac affection. St Bartholomew's Hospital Reports 24: 17–20.

Gibbons CH, Freeman R (2005). Autonomic neuropathy and celiac disease. J Neurol Neurosurg Psychiatry 76: 579–581.

Gobbi G (2005). Coeliac disease, epilepsy and cerebral calcifications. Brain Dev 27: 189–200.

Gobbi G, Bouquet F, Greco L et al. (1992). Coeliac disease, epilepsy and cerebral calcifications. Lancet 340: 439–443.

Hadjivassiliou M, Gibson A, Davies-Jones GAB et al. (1996). Is cryptic gluten sensitivity an important cause of neurological illness? Lancet 347: 369–371.

Hadjivassiliou M, Chattopadhyay AK, Davies-Jones GAB et al. (1997). Neuromuscular disorder as a presenting feature of celiac disease. J Neurol Neurosurg Psychiatry 63: 770–775.

Hadjivassiliou M, Grunewald RA, Chattopadhyay AK et al. (1998). Clinical, radiological, neurophysiological and neuropathological characteristics of gluten ataxia. Lancet 352: 1582–1585.

Hadjivassiliou M, Grünewald RAG, Lawden M et al. (2001). Headache and CNS white matter abnormalities associated with gluten sensitivity. Neurology 56: 385–388.

Hadjivassiliou M, Boscolo S, Davies-Jones GAB et al. (2002). The humoral response in the pathogenesis of gluten ataxia. Neurology 58: 1221–1226.

Hadjivassiliou M, Grünewald RA, Sharrack B et al. (2003a). Gluten ataxia in perspective: epidemiology, genetic susceptibility and clinical characteristics. Brain 126: 685–691.

Hadjivassiliou M, Davies-Jones GAB, Sanders DS et al. (2003b). Dietary treatment of gluten ataxia. J Neurol Neurosurg Psychiatry 74: 1221–1224.

Hadjivassiliou M, Sanders DS, Grunewald RAG (2005). Multiple sclerosis and occult gluten sensitivity. Neurology 64: 933–934.

Hadjivassiliou M, Maki M, Sanders DS et al. (2006a). Autoantibody targeting of brain and intestinal transglutaminase in gluten ataxia. Neurology 66: 373–377.

Hadjivassiliou M, Grunewald RA, Kandler RH et al. (2006b). Neuropathy associated with gluten sensitivity. J Neurol Neurosurg Psychiatry 77: 1262–1266.

Hadjivassiliou M, Chattopadhyay AK, Grünewald RA et al. (2007). Myopathy associated with gluten sensitivity. Muscle Nerve 35: 443–450.

Hadjivassiliou M, Aeschlimann P, Strigun A et al. (2008a). Autoantibodies in gluten ataxia recognise a novel neuronal transglutaminase. Ann Neurol 64: 332–343.

Hadjivassiliou M, Sanders DS, Woodroofe N et al. (2008b). Gluten ataxia. Cerebellum 7: 494–498.

Hadjivassiliou M, Aeschlimann P, Sanders DS et al. (2009). Antibodies against TG6 as the only serological marker of gluten ataxia. Proceedings of the 13th International Coeliac Disease Symposium, p. 75, Amsterdam, April 09.1.

Hadjivassiliou M, Sanders DS, Grunewald RA et al. (2010a). Gluten sensitivity: from gut to brain. Lancet Neurol 9: 318–330.

Hadjivassiliou M, Rao DS, Wharton SB et al. (2010b). Sensory ganglionopathy due to gluten sensitivity. Neurology 75: 1003–1008.

Hadjivassiliou M, Aeschlimann D, Grunewald RA et al. (2010c). GAD antibody associated neurological illness and its relationship to gluten sensitivity. Acta Neurol Scand 123: 175–180. http://dx.doi.org/10.1111/J.1600-0404.2010.01356.x.

Hadjivassiliou M, Sanders DS, Hoggard N (2011). Magnetic resonance imaging and spectroscopy of the cerebellum in patients with celiac disease and minor neurological complains. Proceedings of the 14th International Coeliac Disease Symposium 2011, p. 30, Oslo, Norway, June 2011.

Hahn JS, Sum JM, Bass D et al. (1998). Celiac disease presenting as gait disturbance and ataxia in infancy. J Child Neurol 13: 351–353.

Harper E, Moses H, Lagrange A (2007). Occult celiac disease presenting as epilepsy and MRI changes that responded to gluten-free diet. Neurology 68: 533.

Henriksson KG, Hallert C, Norrby K et al. (1982). Polymyositis and adult celiac disease. Acta Neurol Scand 65: 301–319.

Hermaszewski RA, Rigby S, Dalgleish AG (1991). Coeliac disease presenting with cerebellar degeneration. Postgrad Med J 67: 1023–1024.

Holmes GKT (1997). Neurological and psychiatric complications in coeliac disease. In: G Gobbi, F Anderman, S Naccarato et al. (Eds.), Epilepsy and Other Neurological Disorders in Coeliac Disease. John Libbey, London, pp. 251–264.

Hu WT, Murray JA, Greenway MC et al. (2006). Cognitive impairment and celiac disease. Arch Neurol 63: 1440–1446.

Hunt KA (2008). Newly identified genetic risk variants for coeliac disease related immune response. Nat Genet 40: 395–402.

Ihara M, Makino F, Sawada H et al. (2006). Gluten sensitivity in Japanese patients with adult-onset cerebellar ataxia. Intern Med 45: 135–140.

Jacob S, Zarei M, Kenton A et al. (2005). Gluten sensitivity and neuromyelitis optica: two case reports. J Neurol Neurosurg Psychiatry 76: 1028–1030.

Jarius S, Jacob S, Waters P et al. (2008). Neuromyelitis optica in patients with gluten sensitivity associated with antibodies to aquaporin-4. J Neurol Neurosurg Psychiatry 79: 1084.

Kaplan JG, Pack D, Horoupian D et al. (1988). Distal axonopathy associated with chronic gluten enteropathy: a treatable disorder. Neurology 38: 642–645.

Kelkar P, Ross M, Murray J (1996). Mononeuropathy multiplex associated with celiac disease. Muscle Nerve 19: 234–236.

Kepes JJ, Chou SM, Price LW (1975). Progressive multifocal leukoencephalopathy with 10-year survival in a patient with nontropical sprue. Neurology 25: 1006–1012.

Kieslich M, Errazuriz G, Rosselt HG et al. (2001). Brain white matter lesions in celiac disease: a prospective study in diet treated patients. Paediatrics 108: E21.

Kinney HC, Burger PC, Hurwitz BJ et al. (1982). Degeneration of the central nervous system associated with celiac disease. J Neurol Sci 53: 9–22.

Korponay-Szabó IR, Laurila K, Szondy Z et al. (2003). Missing endomysial and reticulin binding of celiac antibodies in transglutaminase 2 knockout tissues. Gut 52: 199–204.

Korponay-Szabó IR, Halttunen T, Szalai Z et al. (2004). In vivo targeting of intestinal and extraintestinal transglutaminase 2 by coeliac autoantibodies. Gut 53: 641–648.

Kristoferitsch W, Pointer H (1987). Progressive cerebellar syndrome in adult coeliac disease. J Neurol 234: 116–118.

Lu CS, Thompson PD, Quin NP et al. (1986). Ramsay Hunt syndrome and coeliac disease: a new association. Mov Disord 1: 209–219.

Ludvigsson JF, Olsson T, Ekbom A et al. (2007). A population based study of celiac disease, neurodegenerative and neuroinflammatory diseases. Aliment Pharmacol Ther 25: 1317–1327.

Luostarinen LK, Collin PO, Paraaho MJ et al. (2001). Coeliac disease in patients with cerebellar ataxia of unknown origin. Ann Med 33: 445–449.

Luostarinen L, Himanen SL, Luostarinen M et al. (2003). Neuromuscular and sensory disturbances in patients with well treated celiac disease. J Neurol Neurosurg Psychiatry 74: 490–494.

Manto MU, Laute MA, Aguera M et al. (2007). Effects of anti-glutamic acid decarboxylase antibodies associated with neurological diseases. Ann Neurol 61: 544–551.

Marks J, Shuster S, Watson AJ (1966). Small bowel changes in dermatitis herpetiformis. Lancet ii: 1280–1282.

Marsh M (1992). Gluten, major histocompatibility complex and the small intestine. Gastroenterology 102: 330–354.

Mata S, Renzi D, Pinto F et al. (2006). Anti-tissue transglutaminase IgA antibodies in peripheral neuropathy and motor neuronopathy. Acta Neurol Scand 114: 54–58.

Mavroudi A, Karatza E, Papastavrou T et al. (2005). Succesful treatment of epilepsy and celiac disease with a gluten-free diet. Pediatr Neurol 33: 292–295.

Morris JS, Ajdukiewicz AB, Read AE (1970). Neurological disorders and adult celiac disease. Gut 11: 549–554.

Muller AF, Donnelly MT, Smith CML et al. (1996). Neurological complications of coeliac disease – a rare but continuing problem. Am J Gastroenterol 91: 1430–1435.

Nicoletti A, Patti F, Lo Fermo S et al. (2008). Frequency of celiac disease is not increased among multiple sclerosis patients. Mult Scler 14: 698–700.

Paltola M, Kaukinen K, Dastidar P et al. (2009). Hippocampal sclerosis in refractory temporal lobe epilepsy is associated with gluten sensitivity. J Neurol Neurosurg Psychiatry 80: 626–630.

Paulley JW (1954). Observation on the aetiology of idiopathic steatorrhoea, jejunal and lymph node biopsies. Br Med J 2: 1318–1321.

Pellecchia MT, Scala R, Filla A et al. (1999a). Idiopathic cerebellar ataxia associated with celiac disease: lack of distinctive neurological features. J Neurol Neurosurg Psychiatry 66: 32–35.

Pengiran Tengah CD, Lock RJ, Unsworth DJ et al. (2004). Multiple sclerosis and occult gluten sensitivity. Neurology 62: 2326–2327.

Pereira AC, Edwards MJ, Buttery PC et al. (2004). Choreic syndrome and coeliac disease: a hitherto unrecognised association. Mov Disord 19: 478–482.

Ranua J, Luoma K, Auvinen A et al. (2005). Celiac disease-related antibodies in an epilepsy cohort and matched reference population. Epilepsy Behav 6: 388–392.

Reed AC, Ash JE (1927). Atypical sprue. Arch Intern Med 40: 786–799.

Sander HW, Magda P, Chin RL et al. (2003). Cerebellar ataxia and celiac disease. Lancet 362: 1548.

Sanders DS, Patel D, Stephenson TJ et al. (2003). A primary care cross-sectional study of undiagnosed adult celiac disease. Eur J Gastroenterol Hepatol 15: 407–413.

Sárdy M, Kárpáti S, Merkl B et al. (2002). Epidermal transglutaminase (TGase3) is the autoantigen of dermatitis herpetiformis. J Exp Med 195: 747–757.

Selva-O'Callaghan A, Casellas F, De Torres I et al. (2007). Celiac disease and antibodies associated with celiac disease in patients with inflammatory myopathy. Muscle Nerve 35: 49.

Tison F, Arne P, Henry P (1989). Myoclonus and adult celiac disease. J Neurol 236: 307–308.

Toti P, Balestri P, Cano M et al. (1996). Celiac disease with cerebral calcium and silica deposits: X-ray spectroscopic findings, an autopsy study. Neurology 46: 1088–1092.

Ward ME, Murphy JT, Greenberg GR (1985). Celiac disease and spinocerebellar degeneration with normal vitamin E status. Neurology 35: 1199–1201.

Wilkinson ID, Hadjivassiliou M, Dickson JM et al. (2005). Cerebellar abnormalities on proton MR spectroscopy in gluten ataxia. J Neurol Neurosurg Psychiatry 76: 1011–1013.

Woltman HW, Heck FJ (1937). Funicular degeneration of the spinal cord without pernicious anemia. Arch Intern Med 60: 272–300.

Handbook of Clinical Neurology, Vol. 120 (3rd series)
Neurologic Aspects of Systemic Disease Part II
Jose Biller and Jose M. Ferro, Editors

Chapter 42

Neurologic manifestations of malabsorption syndromes

RONALD F. PFEIFFER*

Department of Neurology, University of Tennessee Health Science Center, Memphis, TN, USA

INTRODUCTION

Any engine requires fuel to run and the human body is no different. However, fueling the body is not quite as simple as placing the nozzle from the gas pump into the automobile gas tank and pumping in the gasoline. For the human body, the required fuel is complex, and multiple steps are required to ensure that the fuel is converted into usable form and actually is taken into the body. Impaired function at any of these steps can result in failure to properly absorb the fuel. The fuel itself consists of three basic types of nutrients: carbohydrates, fats, and proteins. Intermixed with these three elements are other substances or additives – vitamins and minerals – that are also required by the body to function properly and must be absorbed along with the essential nutrients.

Digestion actually begins in the mouth, where food is chewed and intermixed with salivary enzymes such as amylase. After transfer to the stomach, further mechanical disruption of the food into smaller and smaller particles takes place until the now semi-liquid chyme is ready to be disgorged from the stomach into the duodenum in an orderly fashion, which is controlled by the pyloric sphincter. Particles generally must be smaller than 0.5 mm to be allowed egress from the stomach into the duodenum through the pyloric sphincter (Meyer, 1980). Once in the small intestine, the chyme is exposed to additional enzymes secreted from the pancreas, to bile salts released from the gall bladder, and to still more enzymes found on the brush border membrane and within the mucosal surface of the small intestine itself, all of which promote digestion and ready the nutrients for absorption (Farrell, 2002). The small intestine then continues to mix and propel its contents, with the mixing ensuring maximum exposure of its contents to the intestinal mucosa, where actual absorption occurs. Although

the small intestine appears to be tucked into a relatively small compartment of the body, it is actually 22–23 feet long in adults and has an absorptive surface of approximately 300 square yards (250 square meters), which is the approximate size of a tennis court (Insel et al., 2010). This is possible because of the huge number of folds, villi, and microvilli that constitute and markedly expand the absorptive surface.

ABSORPTION AND MALABSORPTION

Absorption of nutrients

A full description of the intricacies of gastrointestinal absorption is beyond the scope of this chapter (and the expertise of this neurologist), but a very brief summary of the mechanisms of absorption of fat, carbohydrate, protein, vitamins, minerals, and trace elements will be undertaken.

Approximately 35% of adult food energy intake consists of lipids, predominantly triglyceride (Pot et al., 2012). Most dietary lipid is absorbed in the jejunum (Borel et al., 1989). Because fat is insoluble in water, intricate mechanisms exist to assist in its absorption. Dietary fat is first broken down into emulsified droplets that are stabilized by coating with phospholipid and then acted upon by lipases, initially in the stomach and then more extensively in the duodenum, which break down triglyceride into fatty acids and monoglyceride. These products of lipolysis then are formed into micelles by bile salts, which then travel to the enterocyte bush border membrane for absorption (Maldonado-Valderrama et al., 2011). Other dietary lipids, such as phospholipids and cholesterol esters, are handled in a slightly different fashion but are also transported to the enterocyte brush membrane in micelles (Farrell, 2002). Within the enterocyte, triglyceride is resynthesized and

---

*Correspondence to: Ronald F. Pfeiffer, M.D., Professor and Vice Chair, Department of Neurology, University of Tennessee Health Science Center, 855 Monroe Avenue, Memphis, TN 38163, USA. Tel: +1-901-448-5209, Fax: +1-901-448-7440, E-mail: rpfeiffer@uthsc.edu

packaged, along with cholesterol and phospholipids, into chylomicrons and very low-density lipoproteins for export into the lymphatic circulation (Thomson et al., 1993). An important component of the surface of chylomicrons is apolipoprotein, which is necessary for both their formation within and secretion from the enterocyte (Ros, 2000).

Carbohydrate accounts for approximately 48% of food energy intake in adults (Whitton et al., 2011). Digestable dietary carbohydrate consists primarily of starch in the form of the polysaccharides amylose and amylopectin, which are made up of long chains of glucose molecules, or of sugars in the form of disaccharides such as lactose and sucrose, or monosaccharides such as fructose and glucose. First salivary amylase and then pancreatic amylase break starch down into short oligosaccharides, such as maltose and maltriose. These oligosaccharides and the dietary disaccharides cannot themselves be absorbed, but are further hydrolyzed to monosaccharides (glucose, fructose, galactose) by hydrolases (e.g., maltase, lactase, sucrase) within the brush border membrane of the enterocytes, where they are then absorbed via saturable carrier-mediated transport systems.

Protein provides approximately 10–15% of energy intake in the average Western diet (Farrell, 2002) and is the primary source of amino acids. It can be derived both from animal and plant sources. Protein digestion is initiated within the stomach by the actions of proteolytic enzymes called pepsins, which break protein down into smaller peptides that are then released into the small intestine. There the peptides encounter pancreatic proteases such as trypsin, chymotrypsin, elastin, and carboxypeptidase A and B, which work together to reduce the peptides further into oligopeptides and individual amino acids. At the brush border membrane there are still more peptidases. Within the brush border there are separate systems for absorbing neutral, basic, and acidic amino acids.

Vitamins can be divided into those that are water-soluble and those that are fat-soluble. Water-soluble vitamins include ascorbic acid (vitamin C), thiamine (vitamin B_1), riboflavin (vitamin B_2), niacin (vitamin B_3), pyridoxine (vitamin B_6), cobalamin (vitamin B_{12}), folic acid, pantothenic acid, and biotin. Although in the past it was assumed that most of these substances were absorbed by passive diffusion, it is now recognized that active, carrier-mediated processes are responsible (Said, 2011). Vitamins A, D, E, and K are all polar lipids and thus, are fat-soluble rather than water-soluble. Therefore the initial steps in their digestion probably consist of their transfer from the food matrix in which they are embedded to micelles or perhaps to smaller lipid vesicles (Borel et al., 2001). They are then absorbed in the small intestine, either by passive diffusion (vitamins A, D, E) or by a carrier-mediated process (vitamin K_1)

(Farrell, 2002). Intricate systems are present to control and regulate the absorption of minerals and trace elements, which takes place primarily in the small intestine.

Malabsorption

If the stomach is unable to properly carry out its mixing function, either because prior disease has impaired its muscular function or prior surgery, such as gastric resection or bariatric surgery, has diminished its holding capacity, inadequately mixed and osmotically active material may be dumped rapidly into the duodenum. This, in turn, may result in inadequate mixing of bile salts and pancreatic enzymes with the chyme while at the same time the increased osmotic pressure draws additional fluid into the intestine, which increases the bulk of the ingested material and causes it to move rapidly through the intestine, limiting both time and extent of contact of the ingested material with the intestinal mucosa, where absorption would normally occur. The net result of this mad dash of partially digested food through the intestine can be reduced absorption of nutrients and associated diarrhea, the hallmarks of malabsorption.

Malabsorption may also occur via other mechanisms. Impaired micelle formation due to reduced luminal concentrations of bile salts, as a consequence of hepatic or gall bladder dysfunction, can result in fat malabsorption (Van Deest et al., 1968). Pancreatic insufficiency from a variety of causes can result in decreased lipase secretion with consequent fat malabsorption and decreased secretion of trypsin and chymotrypsin with resultant protein malabsorption (Owens and Greenson, 2007). Disease processes affecting the enterocytes can impair both fat absorption and chylomicron formation, with subsequent malabsorption of fat. Poor mixing of gastric and intestinal contents and mucosal disease processes also can impair protein and carbohydrate absorption. Loss or reduction of the absorptive surface, whether due to disease processes or to surgical removal, may also result in malabsorption.

The clinical signs and symptoms of malabsorption classically involve the gastrointestinal system, with abdominal distension, abdominal pain, flatulence, diarrhea, weight loss, and even ascites. However, systemic signs also may appear. Abnormalities of the skin and mucous membranes can become evident, as can musculoskeletal, renal, and hematologic dysfunction.

Neurologic involvement may develop in some malabsorptive disorders and can assume a variety of appearances. It is not possible in this chapter to fully detail all disorders of gastrointestinal absorption that may result in neurologic dysfunction. Some of these disorders are discussed in detail in their own chapters in this compendium and will be treated lightly here. Others will be discussed more fully, but the disease processes discussed in the following paragraphs might best be considered a sampling of disorders that may be of most interest to the adult neurologist.

NEUROLOGIC DYSFUNCTION IN MALABSORPTION SYNDROMES

The list of congenital disorders of the gastric and intestinal mucosa that result in malabsorption is very long and includes disorders that are characterized by malabsorption of amino acids (e.g., Hartnup disorder, cystinuria, blue diaper syndrome, Lowe's syndrome, oasthouse syndrome, and others), carbohydrates (e.g., lactase deficiency, trehalase deficiency, glucose galactose malabsorption, and others), fat (see below), and also various vitamins and minerals (Högenauer and Hammer, 2002). Many of these present during infancy and not all produce neurologic dysfunction. All cannot be covered here. The following paragraphs will focus on disorders that do produce neurologic dysfunction; both acquired and inherited disorders will be addressed and those that may appear in adult life will be preferentially described.

Vitamin E deficiency

Neurologic dysfunction in the setting of vitamin E deficiency can be genetic in origin, with an autosomal recessive inheritance pattern and a clinical presentation that can mimic Friedreich's ataxia, due to a mutation in the α-tocopherol transfer protein gene (Ben Hamida et al., 1993; Ouahchi et al., 1995; Fogel and Perlman, 2007; Di Donato et al., 2010). In most instances, however, it is the consequence of fat malabsorption (Laplante et al., 1984; Ayuso Blanco et al., 1994). This can occur following both partial and complete gastrectomy (Rino et al., 2007; Ueda et al., 2009), in the setting of primary biliary cirrhosis (Sokol et al., 1989) or other biliary diseases (Ayuso Blanco et al., 1994), in individuals with pancreatic dysfunction (Yokota et al., 1990), in patients with common variable immunodeficiency with associated enteropathy (Aslam et al., 2004; Malamut et al., 2010), in persons with inflammatory bowel disease (Howard et al., 1982; Vorgerd et al., 1996), or with cystic fibrosis (Bye et al., 1985; Willison et al., 1985).

The neurologic symptoms and signs in individuals with vitamin E deficiency can be quite varied. Ataxia is frequently present. Dysarthria and nystagmus may occur. Symptoms and signs of peripheral neuropathy, including paresthesias, impaired proprioception, impaired vibratory perception, and hyporeflexia are also common. Proximal muscle weakness, myopathy, hyperreflexia, extensor plantar responses, pigmentary retinopathy, action tremor,

limb dysmetria, and even myoclonic dystonia have also been described (Angelini et al., 2002; Aslam et al., 2004; Hammond and Wang, 2008).

Abnormalities consistent with peripheral neuropathy may be evident on electromyography and nerve conduction studies (EMG/NCV) but are not universally present (Ko and Park-Ko, 1999; Hammond and Wang, 2008). Somatosensory evoked potentials may demonstrate abnormalities indicative of posterior column dysfunction (Puri et al., 2005). Diffuse white matter changes have also been described in individuals with vitamin E deficiency, both in the cerebrum (Aslam et al., 2004) and in the spinal cord (Vorgerd et al., 1996).

The appearance of symptoms of vitamin E deficiency can be strikingly delayed. In patients post gastrectomy, it may take up to 50 months for evidence of vitamin E deficiency to appear (Ueda et al., 2009). The same investigators reported that replacement doses of vitamin E needed to be 300 mg/day or more.

Familial hypocholesterolemia

Three distinct genetic disorders, familial hypobetalipoproteinemia (FHBL), abetalipoproteinemia (ABL), and chylomicron retention disease (CRD), have been identified as causes of chronic diarrhea, malabsorption, malnutrition, growth retardation, and vitamin E deficiency. Of the three, neurologists are most familiar with ABL, previously known as the Bassen–Kornzweig syndrome (Bassen and Kornzweig, 1950; Sturman, 1968), but awareness of the other two is of value.

ABL is an autosomal recessive disorder due to a mutation in the microsomal triglyceride transfer protein (*MTP*) gene on chromosome 4 (Shoulders et al., 1993). MTP acts as a chaperone that transfers lipids such as triglycerides, cholesterol esters and phospholipids onto apolipoprotein B (APOB), thus promoting the secretion of chylomicrons from the enterocytes and very low-density lipoproteins (VLDLs) from hepatocytes (Zamel et al., 2008; Zeissig et al., 2010). Mutations lead to a nonfunctional MTP, with resultant impaired biogenesis of chylomicrons and VLDL and inability to absorb fats and fat-soluble vitamins, perhaps most importantly vitamin E. The clinical features of ABL include steatorrhea, diarrhea, retinitis pigmentosa, acanthocytosis, and a variety of neurologic features; hepatic manifestations due to hepatic steatosis, occasionally leading to cirrhosis, may also be present (Braegger et al., 1998). Blood lipid analysis demonstrates extremely low plasma levels of total cholesterol, VLDL, and low-density lipoproteins (LDL); APOB, triglycerides, and chylomicrons are virtually absent (Stevenson and Hardie, 2001; Palau and Espinós, 2006; Tarugi et al., 2007). Gastrointestinal symptoms are usually evident during infancy, but neurologic dysfunction may not appear until individuals are in their teens or even later (Fogel and Perlman, 2007). Neurologic dysfunction typically consists of progressive cerebellar ataxia. Peripheral neuropathy may also develop. The neuropathy is sensorimotor (but predominantly sensory) in character and primarily associated with impairment of position and vibratory sensation, along with reduced or absent muscle stretch reflexes; both demyelinating (Wichman et al., 1985) and axonal (Iannaccone and Sokol, 1986) pathology have been described. Both the ataxia and the peripheral neuropathy have most often been attributed to vitamin E deficiency, but investigators describing the demyelinating features of the neuropathy have questioned its relationship to vitamin E deficiency. Additional neurologic abnormalities have been described in individuals with ABL. Upper motor neuron signs, such as hyperreflexia and Babinski signs, have been reported (Zamel et al., 2008), as have resting and postural tremor (Soejima et al., 2006). Treatment of neurologic dysfunction with both vitamin E and vitamin A has been advocated, but results have been mixed (Grant and Berson, 2001; Zamel et al., 2008).

In contrast to ABL, FHBL is an autosomal codominant disorder in which heterozygotes may have mild symptoms or be asymptomatic except for low plasma cholesterol, whereas homozygotes may be clinically indistinguishable from individuals with ABL (Noto et al., 2009; Peretti et al., 2010). In approximately 50% of individuals, FHBL is due to a mutation in the *APOB* gene, which is on chromosome 2 (Whitfield et al., 2003; Tarugi et al., 2007). This results in the formation of a truncated APOB protein. The lipid profile of individuals with homozygous FHBL is similar to that of individuals with ABL; in contrast, heterozygotes have reduced but not absent total cholesterol, triglyceride, LDL, and APOB levels and high-density lipoproteins (HDL) may actually be elevated (Linton et al., 1993; Peretti et al., 2010). Homozygous individuals frequently develop retinitis pigmentosa and virtually always have acanthocytosis; neurologic dysfunction is similar to that present in ABL, but may be somewhat less severe (Linton et al., 1993). Neurologic dysfunction is unusual in heterozygotes.

CRD (also called Anderson's disease) is a very rare autosomal recessive disorder due to mutation in the *SAR1B* gene on chromosome 5, which encodes the SAR1B protein (Georges et al., 2011). SAR1B is involved with the transport of prechylomicron transport vesicles from the endoplasmic reticulum to the Golgi apparatus in enterocytes; impaired function of the protein results in failure to release chylomicrons following a fat-containing meal and the accumulation of lipids within the enterocytes (Shoulders et al., 2004; Tarugi et al.,

2007; Peretti et al., 2010). In CRD, total cholesterol, LDL, HDL, and APOB are all reduced, but triglycerides are normal. Gastrointestinal dysfunction is evident during infancy, but neurologic dysfunction typically does not appear until the teenage years or adulthood (Peretti et al., 2010). Symptoms suggestive of a peripheral polyneuropathy are the most common neurologic presentation (Peretti et al., 2009), but in adults ataxia, myopathy, and action tremor have all been described (Gauthier and Sniderman, 1983; Peretti et al., 2010). Vitamin E deficiency is the presumed etiology for the neurologic deficits; Peretti et al. (2010) noted that individuals with the more pronounced abnormalities had the lowest vitamin E levels at the time of diagnosis. Treatment with vitamins E, A, and D are recommended to prevent neurologic, ophthalmologic, and osteopenic complications of CRD (Gauthier and Sniderman, 1983; Peretti et al., 2010).

Celiac disease

The topic of gluten sensitivity is covered extensively in another chapter in this volume. Celiac disease (CD) will be covered briefly here to emphasize that patients with the classic gastrointestinal symptoms and pathology of CD may also develop neurologic dysfunction. However, it is not at all certain that the neurologic abnormalities of classic CD are the result of malabsorption; immunologic mechanisms may be a more probable explanation (Bürk et al., 2009).

The prevalence of CD, at least in American and European populations, has been estimated to be approximately 1% (Green and Cellier, 2007; Tjon et al., 2010), but recent studies suggest that the number of undiagnosed patients may be considerable and the prevalence much higher than previously proposed (Vilppula et al., 2008). The classic gastrointestinal symptoms of CD primarily are due to fat malabsorption and consist of diarrhea, weight loss, and gassy distension that develop as a consequence of damage to the mucosa of the small intestine, triggered by an immune-mediated response to gluten, the protein fraction of wheat. Malabsorption develops as a consequence of the mucosal injury, which results in blunting and atrophy of the villi, along with crypt hyperplasia. Individuals with classic CD display the presence antigliadin antibodies, both IgG and IgA. They also display the presence of additional gliadin-related antibodies, such as antiendomysial and antitransglutaminase antibodies.

Neurologic dysfunction has been reported to develop in 6–12% of individuals with CD (Pellecchia et al., 1999; Lagerqvist et al., 2001; Vaknin et al., 2004). A broad array of neurologic manifestations has been described, including peripheral neuropathy (Chin et al., 2003;

Briani et al., 2005; Bushara, 2005), myopathy (Uygur-Bayramicli and Ozel, 2011), epilepsy (Bushara, 2005), myelopathy (Cooke and Smith, 1966), neuromyelitis optica (Jacob et al., 2005), headache (Cicarelli et al., 2003; Morello et al., 2003; Bushara, 2005), restless legs (Manchanda et al., 2009; Weinstock et al., 2010; Uygur-Bayramicli and Ozel, 2011), acute inflammatory demyelinating neuropathy (Midha et al., 2007; Gupta and Kohli, 2010), chorea (Pereira et al., 2004), paroxysmal nonkinesigenic dystonia (Hall et al., 2007), autonomic imbalance (Barbato et al., 2010), and others. Some of the reports may simply reflect coincidence and in most of the others no clear connection to malabsorption has been suggested. The two neurologic disorders described most often in the setting of celiac disease are ataxia and peripheral neuropathy. With regard to peripheral neuropathy, one review of the existing literature prompted a conclusion that an association of celiac disease and peripheral neuropathy is unlikely and that celiac disease should not be considered in the workup of patients with chronic peripheral neuropathy (Rosenberg and Vermeulen, 2005).

Tropical sprue

Tropical malabsorption is a syndrome that may affect both indigenous residents of tropical countries and travelers visiting or residing in the tropics (Ramakrishna et al., 2006). Both secondary forms, in which an etiology has been identified, and primary (idiopathic) forms have been described. Small intestine mucosal damage inflicted by protozoa (e.g., *Giardia intestinalis*, *Cryptosporidium parvum*, *Isospora belli*, *Cyclospora cayetanensis*), helminths (e.g., *Strongyloides stercoralis*, *Capillaria philippinensis*), bacteria (e.g., *Mycobacterium tuberculosis*) and viruses (possibly human immunodeficiency virus) may all produce a malabsorption syndrome, as can a variety of other disease processes of inflammatory, autoimmune, neoplastic, or pancreatic origin (Ramakrishna et al., 2006).

It is in individuals in whom no etiology can be ascertained that the name tropical sprue (TS) has been applied. Although currently infrequently encountered in North America, TS has been reported to account for approximately 40% of malabsorption in children and adults in some portions of South Asia (Ranjan et al., 2004), although others have found it to be a rare cause of small bowel diarrhea (Thakur et al., 2006). Gastrointestinal symptoms of TS include chronic nonbloody diarrhea, bloating, weight loss, and abdominal cramping (Batheja et al., 2010). The mucosal changes in tropical sprue are sometimes indistinguishable from those of CD, although TS typically involves the entire length of the small intestine, whereas CD typically

spares the terminal ileum (Batheja et al., 2010). The mucosal damage in TS results in malabsorption of fat, carbohydrates, and multiple vitamins, including folate and vitamins A, E, and B_{12} (Ramirez et al., 1973; Glynn, 1986; Ramakrishna et al., 2006).

Neurologic dysfunction may develop in the setting of TS. In one study, neurologic symptoms were documented in 67% (16/24) of individuals with TS (Iyer et al., 1973). In this study, proximal muscle weakness was present in 15 of the 16 individuals with neurologic symptoms, but on electrophysiologic testing only 10 had evidence of myopathy; peripheral neuropathy was noted in eight. Night blindness, presumably due to vitamin A deficiency, and combined system degeneration, presumably the result of vitamin B_{12} deficiency, have been described in TS (Ramakrishna et al., 2006). Peripheral neuropathy in patients with TS has been attributed to vitamin E deficiency (Ghalaut et al., 1995). Periodic paralysis has been reported in an individual with TS (Ghosh et al., 1994).

Antibiotic therapy, typically with tetracycline or doxycycline for several months, and vitamin replacement therapy are the standard treatments for TS, but abnormal small intestine permeability may remain evident following treatment and some stool frequency and weight loss may persist (Kumar et al., 2011).

Wernicke's encephalopathy

Neurologists are well acquainted with Wernicke's encephalopathy (WE) in the setting of chronic alcoholism with nutritional thiamine deficiency, but it can also be the result of malabsorption of thiamine. Considering the possibility of WE in patients who are not alcoholics can be especially problematic since the full classic triad of neurologic features of WE, mental status changes, ophthalmoplegia (nystagmus is actually more common than ophthalmoplegia), and gait ataxia, develops in only 10–16% of affected individuals (Harper et al., 1986; Weathers and Lewis, 2009).

Thiamine is primarily absorbed in the duodenum, but the stomach may also play a role (Uruha et al., 2011). In keeping with this, the development of WE in a patient with peptic ulcer disease was attributed to gastric malabsorption of thiamine due to severe gastric mucosal lesions (Uruha et al., 2011). WE has also been documented following bariatric surgery, including techniques such as Roux-en-Y gastric bypass, vertical banded gastroplasty, and gastric partitioning (Rothrock and Smith, 1981; Seehra et al., 1996; Cirignotta et al., 2000; Salas-Salvadó et al., 2000; Toth and Voll, 2001; Koffman et al., 2006; Singh and Kumar, 2007). It may develop anywhere between 2 and 78 weeks following surgery, although 4–12 weeks postoperatively is the most frequent timeframe (Singh and Kumar, 2007). In a recent review, Aasheim (2008) catalogued 84 cases of WE following bariatric surgery; in 95%, gastric bypass or a restrictive procedure had been performed. The appearance of WE is more frequent in individuals who experience repeated vomiting, presumably with decreased thiamine absorption because of the vomiting (Cirignotta et al., 2000; Aasheim, 2008). However, individuals undergoing Roux-en-Y gastric bypass have an additional risk with regard to thiamine, since thiamine is predominantly absorbed in the duodenum, which is bypassed in the Roux-en-Y procedure (Escalona et al., 2004; Al-Fahad et al., 2006; Iannelli et al., 2010).

We has also been described in individuals with other causes for malabsorption. In one woman with a history of premature birth and neonatal necrotizing enterocolitis with subsequent bowel resection, WE developed during pregnancy and was attributed to longstanding chronic malabsorption exacerbated by her pregnancy (Williams et al., 2009). Another individual with colon cancer and an enterocutaneous fistula developed WE following administration of 5-fluorouracil; the role of malabsorption in this patient is uncertain (Papila et al., 2010). Either malabsorption or consumption by the tumor was considered to be responsible for the development of WE in a terminally ill cancer patient who was maintaining a reasonable caloric intake (Yae et al., 2005). WE has also been reported in the setting of pancreatic encephalopathy, but in these cases prolonged fasting and inadequate thiamine supplementation were deemed responsible (Zhang and Tian, 2007).

Pellagra

Pellagra is a disease that is often considered to have died out in the US and other developed countries; however, although rare, it still occurs (Ishii and Nishihara, 1981; Weathers and Lewis, 2009). Pellagra is due to niacin deficiency, although it can also develop in the setting of deficiency of the essential amino acid tryptophan, which is a precursor of niacin (Lanska, 2010). As with WE, pellagra is most often diagnosed in individuals with chronic alcoholism and inadequate nutritional intake, but it can also develop in other conditions, including malabsorption syndromes.

The classic clinical features of pellagra consist of the triad of dermatitis, diarrhea, and dementia. All three are not present in every individual; in one study the entire triad was present in only 22% (Spivak and Jackson, 1977). In addition to dementia, neurologic abnormalities that have been described in pellagra include headache, vertigo, myoclonus, tremor, rigidity, weakness, dysphagia, seizures, and still others; a variety of psychiatric

symptoms may also be evident (Serdaru et al., 1988; Weathers and Lewis, 2009).

Pellagra has been documented in individuals with malabsorption due to a variety of causes. Several case reports describe the development of pellagra in people with Crohn's disease, in which both niacin deficiency due to malabsorption and tryptophan wastage with increased urinary excretion of 5-hydroxyindoleacetic acid have been suggested to occur (Pollack et al., 1982; Zaki and Millard, 1995; Abu-Qurshin et al., 1997). Pellagra has been reported in an immunocompromised patient with colitis due to cytomegalovirus (Lu et al., 2001). Small intestinal bacterial overgrowth with consequent malabsorption and development of pellagra has also been described (Wierzbicka et al., 2005). Malabsorption secondary to amyloidosis in an individual with multiple myeloma is yet another reported cause of pellagra (Itami et al., 1997).

Copper deficiency myelopathy

Copper is an essential trace metal and micronutrient that is important for many biological functions (Stern, 2010; de Romaña et al., 2011). It is incorporated into at least 30 metalloenzymes and involved with catecholamine synthesis, brain peptide synthesis, oxidative defenses, and numerous other metabolic processes (Tapiero et al., 2003; Zara et al., 2009). Neurologists are most familiar with the damage that can be caused by excessive copper, as in Wilson's disease, but copper deficiency also produces neurologic dysfunction. This is, perhaps, best recognized in Menkes disease, in which there is a genetically based inability to transport copper across the intestinal barrier due to a mutation in the *ATP7A* gene (de Bie et al., 2007; Tümer and Møller, 2010; Kodama et al., 2011). However, impairment of intestinal copper absorption may also occur in the setting of other malabsorptive processes.

Copper, along with zinc, is absorbed in the proximal small intestine, primarily in the duodenum but also to a lesser extent in the stomach and more distal small intestine (Mason, 1979; Tan et al., 2006). Processes that remove these sites or otherwise impair absorption from them result in eventual copper deficiency. However, it is only within the past decade that neurologic dysfunction as a consequence of copper deficiency due to copper malabsorption has been identified in individuals who had previously undergone gastric and/or intestinal surgery (Schleper and Stuerenburg, 2001; Kumar et al., 2003b; Kumar, 2006; Tan et al., 2006; Bellance et al., 2010; Jaiser and Winston, 2010; Pineles et al., 2010).

Schleper and Stuerenburg (2001) described a 46-year-old woman who developed progressive spastic tetraparesis, sensory impairment, and sensory gait ataxia and was subsequently diagnosed with copper deficiency-associated myelopathy. She had undergone partial gastrectomy approximately 20 years earlier for treatment of gastric ulcers and a second gastric resection procedure along with resection of the transverse colon approximately 5 years earlier because of complications from the original procedure. Serum copper and ceruloplasmin levels were markedly diminished; cerebrospinal fluid copper was also diminished, excluding a diagnosis of Wilson's disease (24 hour urinary copper was not reported). Kumar et al. (2003b) subsequently described two individuals, again both women, who also developed progressive myelopathy and sensory gait ataxia following gastrointestinal surgical procedures. The first woman had undergone an intestinal bypass procedure for obesity 24 years previously; the second woman had undergone two procedures, partial small bowel resection for Crohn's disease 30 years previously and partial gastrectomy and vagotomy for refractory ulcers 15 years previously. In both individuals, serum copper and ceruloplasmin levels were markedly reduced and 24 hour urinary copper excretion was normal. Kumar (2006) subsequently reviewed the case records of 25 persons who were diagnosed with copper deficiency myelopathy (CDM); 10 of them had a history of prior gastric surgery. More recently, Jaiser and Winston (2010) reviewed 55 case reports of copper deficiency myelopathy collected from the literature and confirmed prior upper gastrointestinal surgery as an important (though not the only) risk factor. They noted a striking female predominance (F:M = 3.6:1) and attributed the copper deficiency to impaired absorption in the upper gastrointestinal tract.

Although prior gastric or intestinal surgery may be the most frequent cause of CDM, it has also been reported in individuals with excessive zinc ingestion (Kumar et al., 2003a) and in individuals with other reasons for malabsorption, such as celiac disease (Kumar and Low, 2004; Kumar, 2006; Jung and Marziniak, 2008; Jaiser and Winston, 2010).

The clinical features of CDM closely mimic those of subacute combined degeneration due to vitamin B_{12} deficiency (Kumar et al., 2004). The combination of posterior column dysfunction with sensory ataxia and associated corticospinal tract dysfunction are common to both; peripheral neuropathy may also be present in both, although it is not a predominant feature of CDM. Hematologic manifestations are frequently, though not invariably, present in both; anemia and neutropenia are characteristic in CDM and the anemia may be microcytic, macrocytic, or normocytic (Kumar, 2006). Although myelopathy, often with associated peripheral neuropathy, is the most frequent clinical presentation of CDM, optic neuropathy may also be part of the clinical picture (Spinazzi et al., 2007; Pineles et al., 2010).

Neuroradiologic changes, most typically in the form of increased T2 signal activity within the dorsal columns in the cervical cord, are often present in both CDM and subacute combined degeneration (Kumar et al., 2006).

The response to copper replacement therapy in CDM is inconsistent. Although the hematologic abnormalities typically respond promptly, neurologic dysfunction does not always do so. Progression of dysfunction is often halted, but resolution of neurologic dysfunction is often incomplete (Kumar, 2006).

Whipple's disease

Whipple's disease (WhD) is an example of a disease process in which, although characterized by both gastrointestinal malabsorption and neurologic dysfunction, the neurologic dysfunction is not the result of malabsorption but rather due to central nervous system involvement of the primary disease process itself. Nevertheless, it will be briefly detailed here because of the presence of both malabsorption and neurologic dysfunction.

Although originally described as a gastrointestinal disease, it has become abundantly clear that WhD is a multisystem disorder that may also demonstrate joint, dermatologic, lymphatic, cardiac, pulmonary, ocular, and neurologic dysfunction (Dutly and Altwegg, 2001). Thus, in addition to diarrhea, weight loss, and abdominal pain, individuals with WhD may display migratory polyarthritis, generalized lymphadenopathy, anemia, fever, generalized malaise, chronic cough, pseudo-addisonian skin pigmentation, congestive heart failure, hypotension, pericardial friction rub, splenomegaly, focal glomerulitis, visual changes, uveitis, retinitis, and a variety of neurologic manifestations (Weiner and Utsinger, 1986; Dutly and Altwegg, 2001; Ojeda et al., 2010).

The average age of symptom onset in WhD is approximately 50 years. Males are affected much more frequently than females; in the past the male-to-female ratio was 8:1 but in recent years this may have dropped to 4–5:1 (Dutly and Altwegg, 2001). Farmers have an increased risk for developing WhD (Weiner and Utsinger, 1986). The organism responsible for WhD, *Tropheryma whipplei*, has been identified and characterized as a member of the actinomycete family; it has been suggested that *Tropheryma whipplei* may be a soil-dwelling organism, which might explain the increased incidence of infection in farmers (Dutly and Altwegg, 2001). It has also been found in the influxes to sewage plants, particularly those from agricultural communities (Schöniger-Hekele et al., 2007; Schneider et al., 2008).

Neurologic dysfunction may be the presenting feature in approximately 5% of persons with WhD (Peters et al., 2002). Clinical central nervous system involvement eventually develops in 10–43% of patients with WhD; postmortem examinations demonstrate central nervous system lesions in over 90% of both symptomatic and asymptomatic individuals (Dutly and Altwegg, 2001; Peters et al., 2002). Cognitive changes appear in 71% of individuals; and may be accompanied by psychiatric symptoms such as depression and personality or behavioral changes (Louis et al., 1996; Franca et al., 2004). Insomnia, hypersomnia, hyperphagia, polyuria, and polydipsia are uncommon, but do occur (Louis et al., 1996; Perkin and Murray-Lyon, 1998; Dutly and Altwegg, 2001). Cerebellar dysfunction with gait and balance impairment and pyramidal tract abnormalities may also develop (Louis et al., 1996; Franca et al., 2004). A variety of ocular and extraocular abnormalities, such as vertical gaze impairment, extraocular muscle dysfunction, internuclear ophthalmoplegia, ptosis, and pupillary abnormalities may also occur (Chan et al., 2001; Franca et al., 2004). Oculomasticatory myorhythmia, consisting of the combination of pendular convergence nystagmus and concurrent slow, rhythmic synchronous contractions of the masticatory muscles, invariably accompanied by a supranuclear vertical gaze paresis, develops in approximately 20% of individuals with central nervous system involvement (Schwartz et al., 1986; Louis et al., 1996). Peripheral neuropathy is a neurologic feature of WhD that actually may be the direct result of nutritional deficiency due to malabsorption (Topper et al., 2002; Franca et al., 2004).

PCR analysis appears to be a more sensitive method of diagnosis than identification of PAS-positive inclusions in macrophages present in duodenal biopsy specimens, but there is some evidence that *Tropheryma whipplei* DNA may be present in healthy individuals without WhD (Dutly and Altwegg, 2001; Peters et al., 2002). In individuals with central nervous system symptomatology, brain biopsy is positive over 80% of the time; cerebrospinal fluid analysis, including PCR, may also be useful (Louis et al., 1996; Perkin and Murray-Lyon, 1998; Schijf et al., 2008).

Prompt diagnosis of WhD is important because effective treatment is available. An initial 2 week course of parenteral therapy with either a combination of penicillin G and streptomycin or with a third generation cephalosporin (e.g., ceftriaxone), followed by a 1 year course of oral trimethoprim-sulfamethoxazole has been recommended as an effective treatment approach (Dutly and Altwegg, 2001). The prolonged course of trimethoprim-sulfamethoxazole is considered by some to be important to prevent central nervous system relapses, which have a poor prognosis and high mortality rate, but not all investigators agree that this is the optimum treatment approach and instead recommend a combination of doxycycline and hydroxychloroquine, supplemented by sulfadiazine in patients with neurologic involvement (Lagier et al., 2010).

CONCLUSION

Gastrointestinal diseases resulting in malabsorption and consequent nutritional deficiencies can be accompanied by neurologic dysfunction that can manifest itself in a broad and confusing array of symptoms and signs. It is important for internists and gastroenterologists to be aware of this possibility and equally important for neurologists to think about the possibility of underlying nutritional deficiency due to malabsorption when evaluating patients for neurologic dysfunction. Prompt and appropriate testing can lead to diagnosis and treatment, which may, at a minimum, forestall further neurologic progression and, in the best of circumstances, result in complete neurologic recovery.

REFERENCES

Aasheim ET (2008). Wernicke encephalopathy after bariatric surgery: a systematic review. Ann Surg 248: 714–720.

Abu-Qurshin R, Naschitz JE, Zuckermann E et al. (1997). Crohn's disease associated with pellagra and increased excretion of 5-hydroxyindolacetic acid. Am J Med Sci 313: 111–113.

Al-Fahad T, Ismael A, Soliman MO et al. (2006). Very early onset of Wernicke's encephalopathy after gastric bypass. Obes Surg 16: 671–672.

Angelini L, Erba A, Mariotti C et al. (2002). Myoclonic dystonia as unique presentation of isolated vitamin E deficiency in a young patient. Mov Disord 17: 612–614.

Aslam A, Misbah SA, Talbot K et al. (2004). Vitamin E deficiency induced neurological disease in common variable immunodeficiency: two cases and a review of the literature of vitamin E deficiency. Clin Immunol 112: 24–29.

Ayuso Blanco T, Martin Martinez J, Figueras P et al. (1994). Chronic polyneuropathy due to vitamin E deficiency. Neurologia 9: 300–302 (Article in Spanish).

Barbato M, Curione M, Amato S et al. (2010). Autonomic imbalance in celiac disease. Minerva Pediatr 62: 333–338.

Bassen FA, Kornzweig AL (1950). Malformation of the erythrocytes in a case of atypical retinitis pigmentosa. Blood 5: 381–387.

Batheja MJ, Leighton J, Azueta A et al. (2010). The face of tropical sprue in 2010. Case Rep Gastroenterol 4: 168–172.

Bellance R, Edimo Nana M, Kone M et al. (2010). Sensory ataxic neuromyelopathy in acquired copper deficiency. Rev Neurol (Paris) 166: 734–736 (Article in French).

Ben Hamida C, Doerflinger N, Belal S et al. (1993). Localization of Friedreich ataxia phenotype with selective vitamin E deficiency to chromosome 8q by homozygosity mapping. Nat Genet 5: 195–200.

Borel P, Lairon D, Senft M et al. (1989). Wheat bran and wheat germ: effect on digestion and intestinal absorption of dietary lipids in the rat. Am J Clin Nutr 49: 1192–1202.

Borel P, Pasquier B, Armand M et al. (2001). Processing of vitamin A and E in the human gastrointestinal tract. Am J Physiol Gastrointest Liver Physiol 280: G95–G103.

Braegger CP, Belli DC, Mentha G et al. (1998). Persistence of the intestinal defect in abetalipoproteinemia after liver transplantation. Eur J Pediatr 157: 576–578.

Briani C, Zara G, Toffanin E et al. (2005). Neurological complications of celiac disease and autoimmune mechanisms: preliminary data of a prospective study in adult patients. Ann N Y Acad Sci 1051: 148–155.

Bürk K, Farecki ML, Lamprecht G et al. (2009). Neurological symptoms in patients with biopsy proven celiac disease. Mov Disord 24: 2358–2362.

Bushara KO (2005). Neurologic presentation of celiac disease. Gastroenterology 128 (4 Suppl 1): S92–S97.

Bye AM, Muller DP, Wilson J et al. (1985). Symptomatic vitamin E deficiency in cystic fibrosis. Arch Dis Child 60: 162–164.

Chan RY, Yannuzzi LA, Foster CS (2001). Ocular Whipple's disease: earlier definitive diagnosis. Ophthalmology 108: 2225–2231.

Chin RL, Sander HW, Brannagan TH et al. (2003). Celiac neuropathy. Neurology 60: 1581–1585.

Cicarelli G, Della Rocca G, Amboni M et al. (2003). Clinical and neurological abnormalities in adult celiac disease. Neurol Sci 24: 311–317.

Cirignotta F, Manconi M, Mondini S et al. (2000). Wernicke–Korsakoff encephalopathy and polyneuropathy after gastroplasty for morbid obesity: report of a case. Arch Neurol 57: 1356–1359.

Cooke WT, Smith WT (1966). Neurological disorders associated with adult coeliac disease. Brain 89: 683–722.

de Bie P, Muller P, Wijmenga C et al. (2007). Molecular pathogenesis of Wilson and Menkes disease: correlation of mutations with molecular defects and disease phenotypes. J Med Genet 44: 673–688.

de Romaña DL, Olivares M, Uauy R et al. (2011). Risks and benefits of copper in light of new insights of copper homeostasis. J Trace Elem Med Biol 25: 3–13.

Di Donato I, Bianchi S, Federico A (2010). Ataxia with vitamin E deficiency: update of molecular diagnosis. Neurol Sci 31: 511–515.

Dutly F, Altwegg M (2001). Whipple's disease and "Tropheryma whippelii". Clin Microbiol Rev 14: 561–583.

Escalona A, Pérez G, León F et al. (2004). Wernicke's encephalopathy after Roux-en-Y gastric bypass. Obes Surg 14: 1135–1137.

Farrell JJ (2002). Digestion and absorption of nutrients and vitamins. In: M Feldman, LS Friedman, MH Sleisenger (Eds.), Gastrointestinal and Liver Disease, 7th edn. Saunders, Philadelphia, pp. 1715–1750.

Fogel BL, Perlman S (2007). Clinical features and molecular genetics of autosomal recessive cerebellar ataxias. Lancet Neurol 6: 245–257.

Franca MC Jr, de Castro R, Balthazar MLF et al. (2004). Whipple's disease with neurological manifestations. Arq Neuropsiquiatr 62: 342–346.

Gauthier S, Sniderman A (1983). Action tremor as a manifestation of chylomicron retention disease. Ann Neurol 14: 591.

Georges A, Bonneau J, Bonnefont-Rousselot D et al. (2011). Molecular analysis and intestinal expression of *SAR1* genes and proteins in Anderson's disease (chylomicron retention disease). Orphanet J Rare Dis 6: 1.

Ghalaut VS, Ghalaut PS, Kharb S et al. (1995). Vitamin E in intestinal fat malabsorption. Ann Nutr Metab 39: 296–301.

Ghosh D, Dhiman RK, Kohli A et al. (1994). Hypokalemic periodic paralysis in association with tropical sprue: a case report. Acta Neurol Scand 90: 371–373.

Glynn J (1986). Tropical sprue – its aetiology and pathogenesis. J R Soc Med 79: 599–606.

Grant CA, Berson EL (2001). Treatable forms of retinitis pigmentosa associated with systemic neurological disorders. Int Ophthalmol Clin 41: 103–110.

Green PHR, Cellier C (2007). Celiac disease. N Engl J Med 357: 1731–1743.

Gupta V, Kohli A (2010). Celiac disease associated with recurrent Guillain Barre syndrome. Indian Pediatr 47: 797–798.

Hall DA, Parsons J, Benke T (2007). Paroxysmal nonkinesigenic dystonia and celiac disease. Mov Disord 22: 708–710.

Hammond N, Wang Y (2008). Fat soluble vitamins. In: J Biller (Ed.), The Interface of Neurology and Internal Medicine. Lippincott Williams and Wilkins, Philadelphia, pp. 449–452.

Harper CG, Giles M, Finlay-Jones R (1986). Clinical signs in the Wernicke–Korsakoff complex: a retrospective analysis of 131 cases diagnosed at necropsy. J Neurol Neurosurg Psychiatry 49: 341–345.

Högenauer C, Hammer HF (2002). Maldigestion and malabsorption. In: M Feldman, LS Friedman, MH Sleisenger (Eds.), Gastrointestinal and Liver Disease, 7th edn. Saunders, Philadelphia, pp. 1751–1782.

Howard L, Ovesen L, Satya-Murti S et al. (1982). Reversible neurological symptoms caused by vitamin E deficiency in a patient with short bowel syndrome. Am J Clin Nutr 36: 1243–1249.

Iannaccone ST, Sokol RJ (1986). Vitamin E deficiency in neuropathy of abetalipoproteinemia. Neurology 36: 1009.

Iannelli A, Addeo P, Novellas S et al. (2010). Wernicke's encephalopathy after laparoscopic Roux-en-Y gastric bypass: a misdiagnosed complication. Obes Surg 20: 1594–1596.

Insel P, Ross D, McMahon K et al. (2010). Nutrition. Jones and Bartlett, Burlington, VA, pp. 121–124.

Ishii N, Nishihara Y (1981). Pellagra among chronic alcoholics: clinical and pathological study of 20 necropsy cases. J Neurol Neurosurg Psychiatry 44: 209–215.

Itami A, Ando I, Kukita A et al. (1997). Pellagra associated with amyloidosis secondary to multiple myeloma. Br J Dermatol 137: 829.

Iyer GV, Taori GM, Kapadia CR et al. (1973). Neurologic manifestations in tropical sprue A clinical and electrodiagnostic study. Neurology 23: 959–966.

Jacob S, Zarei M, Kenton A et al. (2005). Gluten sensitivity and neuromyelitis optica: two case reports. J Neurol Neurosurg Psychiatry 76: 1028–1030.

Jaiser SR, Winston GP (2010). Copper deficiency myelopathy. J Neurol 257: 869–881.

Jung A, Marziniak M (2008). Copper deficiency as a treatable cause of myelopathy. Nervenarzt 79: 421–425, (Article in German).

Ko HY, Park-Ko I (1999). Electrophysiologic recovery after vitamin E-deficient neuropathy. Arch Phys Med Rehabil 80: 964–967.

Kodama H, Fujusawa C, Bhadhprasit W (2011). Pathology, clinical features and treatments of congenital copper metabolic disorders – focus on neurologic aspects. Brain Dev 33: 243–251.

Koffman BM, Greenfield LJ, Ali II et al. (2006). Neurologic complications after surgery for obesity. Muscle Nerve 33: 166–176.

Kumar N (2006). Copper deficiency myelopathy (human swayback). Mayo Clin Proc 81: 1371–1384.

Kumar N, Low PA (2004). Myeloneuropathy and anemia due to copper malabsorption. J Neurol 251: 747–749.

Kumar N, Gross JB Jr, Ahlskog JE (2003a). Myelopathy due to copper deficiency. Neurology 61: 273–274.

Kumar N, McEvoy KM, Ahlskog JE (2003b). Myelopathy due to copper deficiency following gastrointestinal surgery. Arch Neurol 60: 1782–1785.

Kumar N, Gross JB Jr, Ahlskog JE (2004). Copper deficiency myelopathy produces a clinical picture like subacute combined degeneration. Neurology 63: 33–39.

Kumar N, Ahlskog JE, Klein CJ et al. (2006). Imaging features of copper deficiency myelopathy: a study of 25 cases. Neuroradiology 48: 78–83.

Kumar S, Ghoshal UC, Jayalakshmi K et al. (2011). Abnormal small intestinal permeability in patients with idiopathic malabsorption in tropics (tropical sprue) does not change even after successful treatment. Dig Dis Sci 56: 161–169.

Lagerqvist C, Ivarsson A, Juto P et al. (2001). Screening for adult coeliac disease – which serological marker(s) to use? J Intern Med 250: 241–248.

Lagier J-C, Fenollar F, Lepidi H et al. (2010). Failure and relapse after treatment with trimethoprim/sulfamethoxazole in classic Whipple's disease. J Antimicrob Chemother 65: 2005–2012.

Lanska DJ (2010). Chapter 30: Historical aspects of the major neurological vitamin deficiency disorders: the water-soluble B vitamins. Handb Clin Neurol 95: 445–476.

Laplante P, Vanasse M, Michaud J et al. (1984). A progressive neurological syndrome associated with an isolated vitamin E deficiency. Can J Neurol Sci 11 (4 Suppl): 561–564.

Linton MF, Farese RV Jr, Young SG (1993). Familial hypobetalipoproteinemia. J Lipid Res 34: 521–541.

Louis ED, Lynch T, Kaufmann P et al. (1996). Diagnostic guidelines in central nervous system Whipple's disease. Ann Neurol 40: 561–568.

Lu JY, Yu CL, Wu MZ (2001). Pellagra in an immunocompetent patient with cytomegalovirus colitis. Am J Gastroenterol 96: 932–934.

Malamut G, Verkarre V, Suarez F et al. (2010). The enteropathy associated with common variable immunodeficiency: the delineated frontiers with celiac disease. Am J Gastroenterol 105: 2262–2275.

Maldonado-Valderrama J, Wilde P, Macierzanka A et al. (2011). The role of bile salts in digestion. Adv Colloid Interface Sci 165: 36–46.

Manchanda S, Davies CR, Picchietti D (2009). Celiac disease as a possible cause for low serum ferritin in patients with restless legs syndrome. Sleep Med 10: 763–765.

Mason KE (1979). A conspectus of research on copper metabolism and requirements of man. J Nutr 109: 1979–2066.

Meyer JH (1980). Gastric emptying of ordinary food: effect of antrum on particle size. Am J Physiol 239: G133–G135.

Midha V, Jain NP, Sood A et al. (2007). Landry–Guillaine–Barré syndrome as presentation of celiac disease. Indian J Gastroenterol 26: 42–43.

Morello F, Ronzani G, Cappellari F (2003). Migraine, cortical blindness, multiple cerebral infarctions and hypocoagulopathy in celiac disease. Neurol Sci 24: 85–89.

Noto D, Cefalù AB, Cannizzaro A et al. (2009). Familial hypobetalipoproteinemia due to apolipoprotein B R463W mutation causes intestinal fat accumulation and low postprandial lipemia. Atherosclerosis 206: 193–198.

Ojeda E, Cosme A, Lapaza J et al. (2010). Whipple's disease in Spain: a clinical review of 91 patients diagnosed between 1947 and 2001. Rev Esp Enferm Dig 102: 108–123.

Ouahchi K, Arita M, Kayden H et al. (1995). Ataxia with isolated vitamin E deficiency is caused by mutations in the alpha-tocopherol transfer protein. Nat Genet 9: 141–145.

Owens SR, Greenson JK (2007). The pathology of malabsorption: current concepts. Histopathology 50: 64–82.

Palau F, Espinós C (2006). Autosomal recessive cerebellar ataxias. Orphanet J Rare Dis 1: 47.

Papila B, Yildiz O, Tural D et al. (2010). Wernicke's encephalopathy in colon cancer. Case Rep Oncol 3: 362–367.

Pellecchia MT, Scala R, Filla A et al. (1999). Idiopathic cerebellar ataxia associated with celiac disease: lack of distinctive neurological features. J Neurol Neurosurg Psychiatry 66: 32–35.

Pereira AC, Edwards MJ, Buttery PC et al. (2004). Choreic syndrome and coeliac disease: a hitherto unrecognised association. Mov Disord 19: 478–482.

Peretti N, Roy CC, Sassolas A et al. (2009). Chylomicron retention disease: a long term study of two cohorts. Mol Genet Metab 97: 136–142.

Peretti N, Sassolas A, Roy CC et al. (2010). Guidelines for the diagnosis and management of chylomicron retention disease based on a review of the literature and the experiences of two centers. Orphanet J Rare Dis 5: 24.

Perkin GD, Murray-Lyon I (1998). Neurology and the gastrointestinal system. J Neurol Neurosurg Psychiatry 65: 291–300.

Peters G, du Plessis DG, Humphrey PR (2002). Cerebral Whipple's disease with a stroke-like presentation and cerebrovascular pathology. J Neurol Neurosurg Psychiatry 73: 336–339.

Pineles SL, Wilson CA, Balcer LJ et al. (2010). Combined optic neuropathy and myelopathy secondary to copper deficiency. Surv Ophthalmol 55: 386–392.

Pollack S, Enat R, Haim S et al. (1982). Pellagra as the presenting manifestation of Crohn's disease. Gastroenterology 82: 948–952.

Pot GK, Prynne CJ, Roberts C et al. (2012). National Diet and Nutrition Survey: fat and fatty acid intake from the first year of the rolling programme and comparison with previous surveys. Br J Nutr 107: 405–415.

Puri V, Chaudhry N, Tatke M et al. (2005). Isolated vitamin E deficiency with demyelinating neuropathy. Muscle Nerve 32: 230–235.

Ramakrishna BS, Venkataraman S, Mukhopadhya A (2006). Tropical malabsorption. Postgrad Med J 82: 779–787.

Ramirez I, Santini R, Corcino J et al. (1973). Serum vitamin E levels in children and adults with tropical sprue in Puerto Rico. Am J Clin Nutr 26: 1045.

Ranjan P, Ghoshal UC, Aggarwal R et al. (2004). Etiological spectrum of sporadic malabsorption syndrome in northern Indian adults at a tertiary hospital. Indian J Gastroenterol 23: 94–98.

Rino Y, Suzuki Y, Kuroiwa Y et al. (2007). Vitamin E malabsorption and neurological consequences after gastrectomy for gastric cancer. Hepatogastroenterology 54: 1858–1861.

Ros E (2000). Intestinal absorption of triglyceride and cholesterol Dietary and pharmacological inhibition to reduce cardiovascular risk. Atherosclerosis 151: 357–379.

Rosenberg NR, Vermeulen M (2005). Should coeliac disease be considered in the work up of patients with chronic peripheral neuropathy? J Neurol Neurosurg Psychiatry 76: 1415–1419.

Rothrock JF, Smith MS (1981). Wernicke's disease complicating surgical therapy for morbid obesity. J Clin Neuroophthalmol 1: 195–199.

Said HM (2011). Intestinal absorption of water-soluble vitamins in health and disease. Biochem J 437: 357–372.

Salas-Salvadó J, Garcia-Lorda P, Cuatrecasas G et al. (2000). Wernicke's syndrome after bariatric surgery. Clin Nutr 19: 371–373.

Schijf LJ, Becx MC, de Bruin PC et al. (2008). Whipple's disease: easily diagnosed, if considered. Neth J Med 66: 392–395.

Schleper B, Stuerenburg HJ (2001). Copper deficiency-associated myelopathy in a 46-year-old woman. J Neurol 248: 705–706.

Schneider T, Moos V, Loddenkemper C et al. (2008). Whipple's disease: new aspects of pathogenesis and treatment. Lancet Infect Dis 8: 179–190.

Schöniger-Hekele M, Petermann D, Weber B et al. (2007). *Tropheryma whipplei* in the environment: survey of sewage plant influxes and sewage plant workers. Appl Environ Microbiol 73: 2033–2035.

Schwartz MA, Selhorst JB, Ochs AL et al. (1986). Oculomasticatory myorhythmia: a unique movement disorder occurring in Whipple's disease. Ann Neurol 20: 677–683.

Seehra H, MacDermott N, Lascelles RG et al. (1996). Wernicke's encephalopathy after vertical banded gastroplasty for morbid obesity. BMJ 312: 434.

Serdaru M, Hausser-Hauw C, Laplane D et al. (1988). The clinical spectrum of alcoholic pellagra encephalopathy: a retrospective analysis of 22 cases studied pathologically. Brain 111: 829–842.

Shoulders CC, Brett DJ, Bayliss JD et al. (1993). Abetalipoproteinemia is caused by defects of the gene encoding the 97kDa subunit of a microsomal triglyceride transfer protein. Hum Mol Genet 2: 2109–2116.

Shoulders CC, Stephens DJ, Jones B (2004). The intracellular transport of chylomicrons requires the small GTPase, Sar1b. Curr Opin Lipidol 15: 191–197.

Singh S, Kumar A (2007). Wernicke encephalopathy after obesity surgery: a systematic review. Neurology 68: 807–811.

Soejima N, Ohyagi Y, Kikuchi H et al. (2006). An adult case of probable Bassen–Kornzweig syndrome, presenting resting tremor. Rinsho Shinkeigaku 46: 702–706, (Article in Japanese).

Sokol RJ, Kim YS, Hoofnagle JH et al. (1989). Intestinal malabsorption of vitamin E in primary biliary cirrhosis. Gastroenterology 96: 479–486.

Spinazzi M, De Lazzari F, Tavolato B et al. (2007). Myelo-optico-neuropathy in copper deficiency occurring after partial gastrectomy Do small bowel bacterial overgrowth syndrome and occult zinc ingestion tip the balance? J Neurol 254: 1012–1017.

Spivak JL, Jackson DL (1977). Pellagra: an analysis of 18 patients and a review of the literature. Johns Hopkins Med J 140: 295–309.

Stern BR (2010). Essentiality and toxicity in copper health risk assessment: overview, update and regulatory considerations. J Toxicol Environ Health A 73: 114–127.

Stevenson VL, Hardie RJ (2001). Acanthocytosis and neurological disorders. J Neurol 248: 87–94.

Sturman RM (1968). The Bassen–Kornzweig syndrome: 18 years in evolution. J Mt Sinai Hosp N Y 35: 489–517.

Tan JC, Burns DL, Jones HR (2006). Severe ataxia, myelopathy, and peripheral neuropathy due to acquired copper deficiency in a patient with history of gastrectomy. J Parenter Enteral Nutr 30: 446–450.

Tapiero H, Townsend DM, Tew KD (2003). Trace elements in human physiology and pathology Copper. Biomed Pharmacother 57: 386–398.

Tarugi P, Averna M, Di Leo E et al. (2007). Molecular diagnosis of hypobetalipoproteinemia: an ENID review. Atherosclerosis 195: e19–e27.

Thakur B, Mishra P, Desai N et al. (2006). Profile of chronic small-bowel diarrhea in adults in western India: a hospital-based study. Trop Gastroenterol 27: 84–86.

Thomson AB, Schoeller C, Keelan M et al. (1993). Lipid absorption: passing through the unstirred layers, brush-border membrane, and beyond. Can J Physiol Pharmacol 71: 531–555.

Tjon JM, van Bergen J, Koning F (2010). Celiac disease: how complicated can it get? Immunogenetics 62: 641–651.

Topper R, Gartung C, Block F (2002). Neurologic complications in inflammatory bowel diseases. Nervenarzt 73: 489–499, (Article in German).

Toth C, Voll C (2001). Wernicke's encephalopathy following gastroplasty for morbid obesity. Can J Neurol Sci 28: 89–92.

Tümer Z, Møller LB (2010). Menkes disease. Eur J Hum Genet 18: 511–518.

Ueda N, Suzuki Y, Rino Y et al. (2009). Correlation between neurological dysfunction with vitamin E deficiency and gastrectomy. J Neurol Sci 287: 216–220.

Uruha A, Shimizu T, Katoh T et al. (2011). Wernicke's encephalopathy in a patient with peptic ulcer disease. Case Rep Med, http://dx.doi.org/10.1155/2011/156104.

Uygur-Bayramicli O, Ozel AM (2011). Celiac disease is associated with neurological syndromes. Dig Dis Sci 56: 1587–1588.

Vaknin A, Eliakim R, Ackerman Z et al. (2004). Neurological abnormalities associated with celiac disease. J Neurol 251: 1393–1397.

Van Deest BW, Fordtran JS, Morawski SG et al. (1968). Bile salt and micellar fat concentration in proximal small bowel contents of ileectomy patients. J Clin Invest 47: 1314–1324.

Vilppula A, Collin P, Mäki M et al. (2008). Undetected celiac disease in the elderly: a biopsy-proven population-based study. Dig Liver Dis 40: 809–813.

Vorgerd M, Tegenthoff M, Kühne D et al. (1996). Spinal MRI in progressive myeloneuropathy associated with vitamin E deficiency. Neuroradiology 38 (Suppl 1): S111–S113.

Weathers AL, Lewis SL (2009). Rare and unusual . . . or are they? Less commonly diagnosed encephalopathies associated with systemic disease. Semin Neurol 29: 136–153.

Weiner SR, Utsinger P (1986). Whipple disease. Semin Arthritis Rheum 15: 157–167.

Weinstock LB, Walters AS, Mullin GE et al. (2010). Celiac disease is associated with restless legs syndrome. Dig Dis Sci 55: 1667–1673.

Whitfield AJ, Marais AD, Robertson K et al. (2003). Four novel mutations in APOB causing heterozygous and homozygous familial hypobetalipoproteinemia. Hum Mutat 22: 178.

Whitton C, Nicholson SK, Roberts G et al. (2011). National Diet and Nutrition Survey: UK food consumption and nutrient intakes from the first year of the rolling programme and comparisons with previous surveys. Br J Nutr 106: 1899–1914.

Wichman A, Buchthal F, Pezeshkpour GH et al. (1985). Peripheral neuropathy in abetalipoproteinemia. Neurology 35: 1279–1289.

Wierzbicka E, Machet L, Karsenti D et al. (2005). Pellagra and panniculitis induced by chronic bacterial colonisation of the small intestine. Ann Dermatol Venereol 132: 140–142, (Article in French).

Williams NL, Wiegand S, McKenna DS (2009). Wernicke's encephalopathy complicating pregnancy in a woman with neonatal necrotizing enterocolitis and resultant chronic malabsorption. Am J Perinatol 26: 519–521.

Willison HJ, Muller DP, Matthews S et al. (1985). A study of the relationship between neurological function and serum vitamin E concentrations in patients with cystic fibrosis. J Neurol Neurosurg Psychiatry 48: 1097–1102.

Yae S, Okuno S, Onishi H et al. (2005). Development of Wernicke encephalopathy in a terminally ill cancer patient consuming an adequate diet: a case report and review of the literature. Palliat Support Care 3: 333–335.

Yokota T, Tsuchiya K, Furukawa T et al. (1990). Vitamin E deficiency in acquired fat malabsorption. J Neurol 237: 103–106.

Zaki I, Millard L (1995). Pellagra complicating Crohn's disease. Postgrad Med J 71: 496–497.

Zamel R, Khan R, Pollex RL et al. (2008). Abetalipoproteinemia: two case reports and literature review. Orphanet J Rare Dis 3: 19.

Zara G, Grassivaro F, Brocadello F et al. (2009). Case of sensory ataxic ganglionopathy–myelopathy in copper deficiency. J Neurol Sci 277: 184–186.

Zeissig S, Dougan SK, Barral DC et al. (2010). Primary deficiency of microsomal triglyceride transfer protein in human abetalipoproteinemia is associated with loss of CD1 function. J Clin Invest 120: 2889–2899.

Zhang XP, Tian H (2007). Pathogenesis of pancreatic encephalopathy in severe acute pancreatitis. Hepatobiliary Pancreat Dis Int 6: 134–140.

Handbook of Clinical Neurology, Vol. 120 (3rd series)
Neurologic Aspects of Systemic Disease Part II
Jose Biller and Jose M. Ferro, Editors

Chapter 43

Commonly used gastrointestinal drugs

ANNU AGGARWAL AND MOHIT BHATT*

*Center for Brain and Nervous System, Kokilaben Dhirubhai Ambani Hospital
and Medical Research Institute, Mumbai, India*

INTRODUCTION

Commonly used gastrointestinal drugs, including antiemetics, motility modifying drugs, and drugs for acid-related disorders (Table 43.1), are extensively prescribed in various outpatient clinics, emergency departments, and intensive care units (Karamanolis and Tack, 2006; Herbert and Holzer, 2008). While, as a group, these drugs are generally considered safe across all age groups and many are available as over-the-counter preparations (Parikh and Howden, 2010), some of these drugs can occasionally lead to serious cardiovascular and neurologic complications (Pasricha et al., 2006). Table 43.2 lists a range of neurologic complications that have been reported following use of these gastrointestinal drugs. For instance, acute neurotoxicities including transient akathisias, oculogyric crises, delirium, seizures, strokes can develop after use of certain gastrointestinal medications (described in more detail below), while disabling and pervasive tardive syndromes are described following long-term, and often unsupervised, use of phenothiazines, metoclopramide, and other drugs. In rare instances, some of the antiemetics can precipitate life-threatening extrapyramidal reactions, neuroleptic malignant syndrome, or serotonin syndrome. At the extreme, concerns over the cardiovascular toxicity of drugs such as cisapride or tegaserod have been grave enough to lead to their withdrawal from many world markets.

However, most often the symptoms of neurotoxicity are innocuous (as in akathisias and various tardive dyskinesias), not readily reported by patients or attributed to a gastrointestinal medication, and the offending drug is continued (Miller and Jankovic, 1989).

In this chapter we review the mode of action of the commonly used gastrointestinal drugs as well as the spectrum and mechanism of their neurotoxicity, (Tables 43.1 and 43.2). This information should help a clinician weigh the benefits of prescribing the particular gastrointestinal drug against the associated risk of adverse effects, and recognise symptoms of neurotoxicity if they occur.

ANTIEMETICS

Nausea and vomiting are triggered by stimulation of the medullary chemoreceptor trigger zone located outside the blood–brain barrier, the medullary central pattern generator, and the limbic forebrain regions (Hesketh, 2008). Development of antiemetics has paralleled understanding of neurotransmitters and neuroreceptors responsible for emesis. Early research on antiemetics focused on dopamine 2 (D_2) receptor antagonists (phenothiazines, substituted benzamides, and butyrophenones). A recent advance in antiemetic therapy has been the elucidation of the key role of serotonin and tachykinins in stimulating emesis through central and peripheral receptors and development of selective serotonin 3 (5-HT_3) receptor antagonists and selective neurokinin 1 (NK_1) receptor antagonists (Roila and Fatigoni, 2006; Herrstedt and Dombernowsky, 2007; Hesketh, 2008; Feyer and Jordan, 2011).

Since the introduction of cisplatin, a highly emetogenic chemotherapeutic agent, in the late 1970s, the main clinical drive to develop potent antiemetics has been to help prevent or abolish chemotherapy-induced nausea and vomiting (CINV) (Herrstedt, 2008). Currently, the therapeutic usefulness of an antiemetic is classified as high or low (Hesketh, 2008) based on their ability to prevent CINV (Roila and Fatigoni, 2006; Herrstedt and Dombernowsky, 2007; Hesketh, 2008; Feyer and Jordan, 2011).

*Correspondence to: Dr. Mohit Bhatt, Center for Brain and Nervous System, Kokilaben Dhirubhai Ambani Hospital and Medical Research Institute, Four Bungalows, Andheri West, Mumbai 400053, India. Tel: +91-986-704-0404, E-mail: drmbhatt@gmail.com

Table 43.1

Commonly used gastrointestinal drugs

Antiemetics	Phenothiazines, e.g., chlorpromazine, prochlorperazine, promethazine
	Substituted benzamides – metoclopramide
	Butyrophenones – domperidone, droperidol
	Sertons, e.g., ondansetron, granisetron, tropisetron, dolasetron, palonosetron
	Neurokinin (NK1) receptor antagonists, e.g., aprepitant and fosaprepitant
Promotility drugs	Substituted benzamides – metoclopramide
	Butyrophenones – domperidone, droperidol
	Cisapride
	Mosapride
	Renzapride
	Tegaserod
	Levosulpiride
Laxatives	Stimulant laxatives, e.g., bisacodyl, sodium picosulfate
	Osmotic laxatives, e.g. (magnesium salts)
Antimotility agents	Bismuth salts
	Dronobinol
Drugs for acid-related disorders	Selective H_2 blockers, e.g., cimetidine, ranitidine, famotidine, nizatidine
	Proton pump inhibitors (PPI), e.g., omeprazole, esomeprazole, lansoprazole, pantoprazole, tenatoprazole, rabeprazole

Table 43.2

Potential neurologic adverse effects associated with various commonly used gastrointestinal drugs[#]

Headache	
Dizziness	
Extrapyramidal syndromes	
Acute	Akathisias
	Dystonia including oculogyric crisis, oromandibular dystonia, retrocollis, opisthotonus posturing, dysphagia,[*] respiratory spasm,[*] status dystonicus[*]
	Tremor
	Myoclonus
	Drug induced parkinsonism
Chronic	Akathisias
	Tardive dyskinesias[*]
	Tardive dystonia
	Myoclonus
Mood disorders	Anxiety
	Psychosis
	Depression
Encephalopathy	
Seizures	
Cataplexy	
Syncopy	
Strokes	
Hyperthermic syndromes	Neuroleptic malignant syndrome[*]
	Serotonin syndrome[*]

[#]Neurologic adverse effects associated with a particular gastrointestinal drug are detailed in the text.
[*]Potentially life-threatening neurotoxicities.

Phenothiazines

Antipsychotics, phenothiazines (for example, chlorpromazine, prochlorperazine, promethazine) were the first effective antiemetics. They acted by blocking central D_2 receptors. Their antiemetic doses were limited by hypotension, restlessness, and sedation. At tolerable doses phenothiazines had a low therapeutic usefulness as antiemetics and extrapyramidal reactions and depression were a serious concern (Bateman et al., 1989; Weiden et al., 1987; Burke et al., 1989). Over the last three decades the availability of newer antiemetics with safer adverse effect profile (like selective serotonin 3 (5-HT$_3$) receptor antagonists and selective neurokinin 1 (NK$_1$) receptor antagonists) has helped curtail the use of phenothiazines as antiemetics.

Metoclopramide

Metoclopramide is a benzamide derivative of procaine that was developed in 1964 to equal the antiemetic properties of phenothiazines. Like phenothiazines, metoclopramide is a selective D_2 receptor blocker, but unlike phenothiazines it has only a weak antipsychotic effect (Schulze-Delrieu, 1981). Additionally, metoclopramide has a partial 5-HT$_4$ receptor agonist activity that enhances release of acetylcholine in the myenteric plexus and is responsible for its gastrointestinal prokinetic action. Metoclopramide is equipotent to chlorpromazine in preventing vomiting, at one-tenth of chlorpromazine doses (Harrington et al., 1983; Ganzini et al., 1993). In high doses, metoclopramide can prevent cisplatin-induced vomiting from antagonism of 5-HT$_3$ receptors (Gralla et al., 1981; Schulze-Delrieu, 1981; Karamanolis and Tack, 2006).

Metoclopramide was initially approved for use in diagnostic radiology to facilitate duodenal intubation and barium studies of upper gastrointestinal tract in patients with delayed gastric emptying. Later its use was extended to treat nausea and vomiting, diabetic gastroparesis, refractory gastroesophageal reflux and postoperative ileus. Over time, metoclopramide found application in a range of disorders including nonmigrainous headaches,

Tourette's syndrome, hiccups, neurogenic bladder, orthostatic hypotension, anorexia nervosa, and select cases of amenorrhea (Schulze-Delrieu, 1981; Tisdale, 1981; Harrington et al., 1983; Miller and Jankovic, 1989; Ellis et al., 1993). Currently, metoclopramide is used extensively as a prokinetic and to lesser extent as an antiemetic agent.

Metoclopramide use can lead to extrapyramidal symptoms (movement disorders or parkinsonism) that develop acutely (within minutes or days) to more pervasive disorders that develop after high doses or long-term use. The extrapyramidal symptoms comprise acute akathisia, dystonia, oculogyric crisis, tremor, and parkinsonism, to tardive syndromes such as tardive dyskinesias, dystonia, tremor or myoclonus, and rarely catalepsy (Costall and Naylor, 1973; Miller and Jankovic, 1989; Sethi, 2004). Mixed movement disorders may occur and may be accompanied by behavioral changes such as restlessness, anxiety, or frank psychosis. The manufacturer's package inserts (http://dailymed.nlm.nih.gov/dailymed) warn of extrapyramidal reactions in 1:500 patients treated with metoclopramide, but reviews of case series suggest a higher figure (1–15%) (Miller and Jancovic, 1989; Parkman et al., 2004; Pasricha et al., 2006). A prospective study of physician-reported drug-induced dyskinesias-dystonia estimated the incidence of metoclopramide-induced dyskinesias-dystonia to be 1/213 new prescriptions (Bateman et al., 1989). Miller and Jankovic (1989) identified 131 patients with drug-induced movement disorders (DIMD) from a database of 3000 patients seen over 12 years, of whom 16 (12.2%) had metoclopramide-induced DIMD. The average duration of metoclopramide use prior to DIMD onset was 12 months (range 1 day to 4 years). Interestingly, the drug was continued for 6 months after developing DIMD, indicating either failure to diagnose DIMD or failure to attribute the DIMD to metoclopramide.

Tardive dyskinesias (TD) are persistent and often irreversible involuntary movements that occur following prolonged neuroleptic therapy (Sethi, 2004). TD is the commonest of the metoclopramide-induced movement disorders. In an epidemiologic study in the UK a review of 15.9 million metoclopramide prescriptions from 1967 to 1982 identified 455 patients with TD (Bateman et al., 1985). Ganzini et al. (1993) examined 51 patients prescribed metoclopramide over a 4 month period at a veterans hospital medical outpatient clinic with an age- and gender-matched control population for DIMD. The authors found relative risk of TD to be 1.67 in the metoclopramide group. A retrospective analysis of 434 patients followed up for TD at a movement disorder clinic revealed that metoclopramide was responsible for 39.4% of cases, and was the second most common medicine to induce TD following haloperidol (Kenney et al., 2008). Withdrawal of cisapride from the US

markets in 2000, following reports of its cardiotoxicity, led to a surge of metoclopramide use as a prokinetic and an increase in the incidence of metoclopramide-induced TD (Shaffer et al., 2004; Kenney et al., 2008). Currently, metoclopramide accounts for a third of all reported DIMDs (Pasricha et al., 2006).

TD are characterized by involuntary, repetitive movements typically involving the oromandibular muscles and axial muscles, including lip puckering, pursing and smacking, facial grimacing, tongue protrusion, rapid eye movements or blinking, and choreiform movements of the limbs. The movements may be accompanied by tremor, dystonia, or parkinsonism. Metoclopramide-induced TD have been reported to lead to life-threatening dyspnea and dysphagia (Samie et al., 1987). High cumulative doses and long duration of treatment are the major risk factors for metoclopramide-induced TD. Elderly women and those with a family history of DIMD and diabetes (Miller and Jankovic, 1989; Sewell and Jeste, 1992; Ganzini et al., 1993) are vulnerable to metoclopramide-induced TD. In 2009, the US Food and Drug Administration (FDA) issued a black box warning for metoclopramide, advising that the drug use be restricted to recommended doses and for not more than 12 weeks. It warned that chronic use of metoclopramide therapy should be avoided in all but rare cases where the benefits were believed to outweigh the risks (http://dailymed.nlm.nih.gov/dailymed). In a minority of patients TD can abate or resolve after discontinuing metoclopramide but in 71% of patients or more TD are persistent despite drug withdrawal (Grimes, 1981; Grimes et al., 1982a, b; Sewell and Jeste, 1992; Tarsy and Indorf, 2002). Currently there is no known treatment for TD (Samie et al., 1987; Miller and Jancovic, 1989; Sethi, 2004). TD developing after discontinuation of long-term metoclopramide is also described (Lavy et al., 1978).

Acute dystonic reactions including retrocollis, oculogyric crisis, trismus, facial grimacing, dysarthria, dysphagia, and opisthotonus spasms are observed in approximately 1% of patients receiving metoclopramide (Robinson, 1973). Dystonic spasms are often painful and frightening. The resultant disability may vary from a slight neck discomfort from cervical dystonia to potentially life-threatening status dystonicus, dysphagia, respiratory distress, or respiratory arrest. Acute rhabdomyolysis and myoglobinuria are known to occur (Mark and Newton-John, 1988; Mastaglia and Argov, 2007). The dystonic reactions commence within minutes to hours of drug administration and are often self-remitting, or resolve within minutes of anticholinergic or dopamine agonist treatment (Bhatt et al., 2004). Dystonia may be accompanied by acute parkinsonism, dyskinesia, asterixis, and myoclonus (Grimes et al., 1982b; Lu and Chu, 1988; Miller and Jankovic, 1989).

Children, young adults, and men are susceptible to developing acute dystonia following normal recommended doses of metoclopramide (Casteels-Van Daele et al., 1970; Robinson, 1973; Reid, 1977; Grimes et al., 1982b; Ganzini et al., 1993; Sethi, 2004). Acute dystonic reactions are also reported following metoclopramide overdose or accidental injection (Sills and Glass, 1978; Kerr, 1996). Metoclopramide doses need to be reduced in patients with renal failure (Bateman and Gokal, 1980; Grimes et al., 1982b). A familial tendency towards metoclopramide-induced dystonia is described (Gatrad and Gatrad, 1979; Miller and Jankovic, 1989; Guala et al., 1992). Poorly functioning or nonfunctioning CYP2D6 alleles, which slow metoclopramide metabolism, are reported in some familial cases of metoclopramide-induced dystonia (Van der Padt et al., 2006). Re-exposure to metoclopramide can cause recurrent dystonic reactions and the drug is best avoided if an extrapyramidal reaction has occurred. Rarely, recurrent dystonic reactions such as oculogyric crisis develop despite complete withdrawal of metoclopramide (Sethi, 2004; Schneider et al., 2009).

Metoclopramide-induced parkinsonism or worsening of idiopathic Parkinson disease usually develops in the first 3 months of therapy and resolves within months of discontinuation of the drug. Symptoms persisting for a year after drug withdrawal are described (Miller and Jankovic, 1989). Compared to idiopathic Parkinson disease, patients with drug-induced parkinsonism are younger and have a symmetrical tremor (Indo and Ando, 1982; Yamamoto et al., 1987; Miller and Jankovic, 1989; Bondon-Guitton et al., 2011). People at the extremes of the age spectrum, children and the elderly, are at risk of metoclopramide-induced parkinsonism (Andrejak et al., 1990; Perez-Lloret et al., 2010).

Akathisia, or motor restlessness, relieved by movements such as pacing, body rocking, crossing and uncrossing of legs, foot tapping, folding and unfolding of arms, or hand rubbing, is observed in association with metoclopramide use. Acute-onset akathisia is reported following intravenous metoclopramide use. Rapid infusions are associated with earlier onset and more severe akathisia (Parlak et al., 2005). Oral metoclopramide use reaching high peak plasma concentrations (over 100 ng/dL) can also lead to akathisia (Bateman et al., 1978), lasting for days after drug cessation (Poortinga et al., 2001). Acute akathisia was observed generally within the first 3 months of metoclopramide therapy (Lang, 1988). Acute onset akathisia is often self-remitting but may be associated with considerable anxiety, feelings of impending doom, and agitation, leading to refusal of treatment or surgery, violence, and even attempted suicide (Drake and Ehrlich, 1985; Caldwell et al., 1987; Sachdev and Kruk, 1994; Chow et al., 1997;

LaGorio et al., 1998). Tardive akathisia has been observed years after metoclopramide exposure (Burke et al., 1989).

High-amplitude resting and postural tremor following chronic metoclopramide use has been reported (Stacy and Jankovic, 1992; Tarsy and Indorf, 2002). Reversible palatopharyngeal tremor with parkinsonism was observed in a woman following oral metoclopramide for 3 weeks (Nampiaparampil and Oruc, 2006).

Metoclopramide-induced depression can develop after a few doses or after more protracted use (Anfinson, 2002).

Domperidone

Domperidone is a peripheral D_2 receptor antagonist and is used as a prokinetic and antiemetic of low therapeutic efficacy. It is the preferred drug to counteract levodopa-induced vomiting and constipation in patients with Parkinson disease as in recommended doses domperidone does not block central dopamine receptors (Critchley et al., 1985). There are isolated reports of domperidone-induced akathisia, parkinsonism, depression, and tardive dyskinesias (Franckx and Noel, 1984; Biasini and Alberti, 1985; Leeser and Bateman, 1985; Steinherz et al., 1986; Bondon-Guitton et al., 2011), usually in the context of high doses. Psychosis following domperidone withdrawal after chronic use is described (Roy-Desruisseaux et al., 2011). Overdosage can lead to seizures (Weaving et al., 1984).

Setrons (5-hydroxytryptamine 3 (5-HT$_3$) receptor antagonists, serotonin 3 receptor antagonist)

Setrons are antiemetics that selectively block peripheral and central 5-HT$_3$ receptors. Ondansetron and granisetron were the first setrons marketed in 1990s, followed by introduction of tropisetron, dolasetron, and finally the second generation setron, palonosetron, in 2003. Ramosetron and azasetron are currently available only in Japan. The available setrons have high therapeutic usefulness, and can prevent cisplatin-induced nausea and vomiting. The first generation setrons are interchangeable at equivalent doses. The drugs are safe, with the commonest adverse effects being constipation, transient elevation of hepatic aminotransferases, mild headache, and lightheadedness. Extrapyramidal reactions are rare (Kovac, 2003; Feyer and Jordan, 2011).

Dramatic acute extrapyramidal syndromes have been observed following intravenous ondansetron. These complex involuntary movements variably include multi-focal myoclonus, jerky "seizure-like" movements, tremor, involuntary eye blinking, eye deviation, facial grimacing, tongue protrusion, oromandibular dystonia, generalized dystonia, or opisthotonus spasms (Dobrow et al., 1991; Tolan et al., 1999; Duncan et al., 2001; Ritter et al., 2003; Sprung et al., 2003; Spiegel et al., 2005; Kumar and Hu, 2009). The movements are focal or generalized, and occasionally voluntarily suppressible for short periods of time. Associated confusion, agitation, pyramidal signs, and hemodynamic instability are described (Ritter et al., 2003). Involuntary movements have also been described following use of oral ondansetron for several days (Lee et al., 2010) or overdosage (Sprung et al., 2003). Dose reduction has been shown to prevent the extrapyramidal reaction (Sprung et al., 2003). Benzodiazepines, diphenhydramine, or procyclidine (Stonell, 1998; Ritter et al., 2003; Sprung et al., 2003; Kumar and Hu, 2009) have helped ameliorate these extrapyramidal symptoms.

Ondansetron has no direct effect on dopamine receptors. It is postulated that an overlap of central serotonergic and central dopaminergic systems is responsible for the observed extrapyramidal reaction to ondansetron. This hypothesis is supported by animal studies and benefit of ondansetron in levodopa-induced psychosis and dyskinesias in patients with Parkinson's disease (Ritter et al., 2003; Sprung et al., 2003; Kumar and Hu, 2009).

In a 2 year retrospective analysis of 1521 inpatients who received ondansetron for nausea and vomiting, Singh et al. (2009) identified three patients who developed brief generalized tonic-clonic seizures after intravenous ondansetron. Clinical seizures have also been reported following intravenous ondansetron use with other epileptogenic drugs (Sargent et al., 1993; Sharma and Raina, 2001). However, in the absence of electroencephalographic evidence of seizure, some authors have suggested that the "seizure-like" movements may be involuntary movements of extrapyramidal origin (Kanarek et al., 1992; Sprung et al., 2003; Singh et al., 2009).

As yet no extrapyramidal reaction has been reported following granisetron or dolasetron, though cross-reactivity with ondansetron is described (Lee et al., 1993; Sorbe et al., 1994). There are isolated reports of palonosetron-induced seizures (Zambelli et al., 2009).

Neurokinin receptor antagonists

Aprepitant and its prodrug fosaprepitant are nonpeptide molecules that cross the blood–brain barrier and inhibit both peripheral and central receptors of substance P (neurokinin 1 (NK$_1$) receptors). The drugs were initially developed as potential analgesics and antidepressants and later found to have a beneficial antiemetic effect. Both aprepitant and fosaprepitant are highly efficacious antiemetics and have emerged as the first-line antiemetics for controlling CINV. They are well tolerated and are not known to have any serious neurologic adverse effects (Feyer and Jordan, 2011). Aprepitant is metabolized by P450 (CYP) 3A4 and when coadministered with ifosfamide may aggravate ifosfamide-induced encephalopathy (Aapro and Walko, 2010).

DRUGS AFFECTING GASTROINTESTINAL MOTILITY

Gastrointestinal motility is regulated by a complex interaction of the enteric nervous system, interstitial cells of Cajal (gastrointestinal pacemakers), smooth muscle cells (effectors of gastrointestinal motility), mucosal neuroendocrine cells, and the autonomic nervous system. Various neuroendocrine mediators including serotonin, dopamine, acetylcholine, motilin, cholecystokinin, and catecholamines help regulate gastrointestinal motility (Grundy et al., 2006; Herbert and Holzer, 2008).

Promotility drugs

These accelerate gastric emptying and colonic transit and are used for treating symptoms associated with gastroparesis, functional dyspepsia, or constipation. Currently, metoclopramide is the most widely used gastrointestinal prokinetic. Development of newer prokinetics has been modeled to stimulate the prokinetic properties of metoclopramide without its extrapyramidal adverse effects.

Cisapride is a serotonin 5-HT$_4$ receptor agonist and 5-HT$_3$ receptor antagonist that increases gastrointestinal motility by augmenting cholinergic transmission through the myenteric plexus. In 2000, cisapride was withdrawn from the North American and most European markets because of concerns about its potential to induce serious cardiac arrhythmias. Cisapride interferes with the pore-forming subunits of hERG (human Ether-a-go-go-Related Gene) K+ channels, delaying the ventricular repolarization and prolonging the QTc interval on ECG. Cisapride associated cardiotoxicity is enhanced when cisapride coadministered with drugs that inhibit the CYP3A4 enzyme and slow its metabolism (Karamanolis and Tack, 2006; Toga et al., 2007). Cisapride is available in some markets as a prokinetic for infants and young children (Raschetti et al., 2001; Vandenplas et al., 2001).

Neurotoxicity from cisapride use is rare. Cisapride-induced chorea in an 8-month-old boy (Lucena et al., 1998) and torticollis, dystonia, and myoclonus during infancy (Dieckmann et al., 1996) are described. Cisapride has been associated with persistent akathisia in a 3-year-old child from neonatal life. The movements resolved 2 months after discontinuation of the drug. The authors postulated that children are prone to neurotoxicity because of poorly developed blood–brain barrier and CYP3A4 enzymes (Elzinga-Huttenga et al., 2006). Dystonia, orofacial dyskinesias, and aggravation of parkinsonism following cisapride use in adults is reported (Naito and Kuzuhara, 1994).

Renzapride and mosapride are benzapride derivatives, partial 5-HT$_4$ receptor agonists, and 5-HT$_3$ receptor antagonists. They are less efficacious than cisapride but have a good cardiac safety profile (with little or no action on hERG K + channels). Renzapride has application in constipation-dominant irritable bowel syndrome while mosapride is used for upper gastrointestinal motility disorders (Karamanolis and Tack, 2006; Toga et al., 2007). Neurotoxicity has not been described as yet.

Tegaserod is a partial 5-HT$_4$ receptor agonist and 5-HT$_{2b}$ receptor antagonist. Antagonism of the 5-HT$_{2b}$ receptor results in decreased prokinetic efficacy. Post-marketing surveys have shown an increased risk of cardiovascular events (unstable angina, myocardial infarction, and stroke) and death with tegaserod use compared to placebo, leading to tegaserod withdrawal from the US and other markets. However, tegaserod is used in some regions for chronic constipation and constipation-dominant irritable bowel syndrome in women (Pasricha, 2007; Herbert and Holzer, 2008).

Levosulpiride is a benzamide derivative, a selective D$_2$ receptor inhibitor, 5-HT$_4$ and partial 5-HT$_3$ receptor stimulator. It is as effective as cisapride, but more effective than metoclopramide and domperidone, in increasing gastric and small intestinal motility (Rossi and Forgione, 1995; Karamanolis and Tack, 2006). Over the past decade there has been a considerable increase in levosulpiride prescriptions, especially in Asia and Europe. In South Korea, levosulpiride prescriptions were almost double of metoclopramide prescriptions (Shin et al., 2009). Extrapyramidal reactions have been reported following levosulpiride use and may be related to its ability to cross the blood–brain barrier (Rossi and Forgione, 1995; Kim et al., 2003; Karamanolis and Tack, 2006; Baik et al., 2008). In a movement disorder clinic in South Korea, 91 of 132 patients diagnosed with DIMD between 2002 and 2008 developed DIMD secondary to levosulpiride use. A majority of patients were elderly. Parkinsonism (n = 85) was the commonest DIMD followed by TD (restricted to the orolingual region) (n = 9) and isolated tremor (n = 3). Levosulpiride was administered for period ranging from a few days to a few weeks (up to 3 years) prior to development of DIMD. Parkinsonism was reversible in 51.9% of patients within months of drug withdrawal. Three of the nine patients with TD and all three patients with isolated tremor recovered after levosulpiride withdrawal (Shin et al., 2009).

Antimotility and antidiarrheal agents

Bismuth salts have been used for dyspepsia, peptic ulcer disease, colitis, and parasitic infections for many centuries. In 1970s, there was a series of reports of a potentially fatal myoclonic encephalopathy following use of bismuth salts (Ford et al., 2008). In France, 1000 cases of encephalopathy with 72 deaths were reported within a short period leading to the withdrawal of bismuth. The encephalopathy was characterized by a subacute confusional state, visual and auditory hallucinations, generalized tremulousness, myoclonic jerks, and gait problems. The encephalopathy was associated with high serum and CSF levels of bismuth and periodic complexes on EEG (Morrow, 1973; Burns et al., 1974; Escourelle et al., 1977; Supino-Viterbo et al., 1977; Tillman et al., 1996). Autopsy showed bismuth deposits in the brain, primarily in the gray matter, perivenular lymphocytic infiltration, and intracytoplasmic lipofuscin accumulation. Bismuth withdrawal led to remission. Recently there has been a renewed interest in using bismuth salts in smaller doses and for short periods for *Helicobacter pylori* eradication (Tillman et al., 1996; Ford et al., 2008).

Dronabinol is a nonselective cannabinoid receptor agonist and is used to delay gastric emptying. Neurologic adverse events are uncommon and include headaches, dry mouth, lightheadedness and vasovagal syncopes, and poor concentration (Herbert and Holzer, 2008).

LAXATIVES

Stimulant (bisacodyl, sodium picosulfate) and osmotic (magnesium salts) laxatives are safe and free from major adverse effects but can cause electrolyte disturbances (Herbert and Holzer, 2008).

DRUGS FOR ACID-RELATED DISORDERS

Selective histamine 2 (H$_2$) blockers (cimetidine, ranitidine, famotidine, nizatidine) and proton pump inhibitors (omeprazole, esomeprazole, lansoprazole, pantoprazole, tenatoprazole, rabeprazole) are widely used to treat acid-related diseases and functional gastrointestinal disorders (Lewis, 1991; Howden and Tytgat, 1996). As a class, both H$_2$ blockers and proton pump inhibitors are safe with very few adverse effects other than diarrhea, headache, and dizziness, even on long-term use (Parikh and Howden, 2010). In fact, pooled data analysis suggested that incidence of adverse effects following ranitidine and famotidine use was no more than seen following placebo use (Lewis, 1991; Howden and Tytgat, 1996). A concern with the use of H$_2$ blockers and proton pump inhibitors is inhibition of cytochrome 450 and the prolongation of the half-life of drugs with low therapeutic index (such as warfarin, phenytoin, tacrolimus, ciclosporin, theophylline, and others). However, clinically relevant drug-to-drug interactions are not observed on chronic outpatient use of H_2 blockers or proton pump inhibitors and these drugs are freely available as over-the-counter medications (Parikh and Howden, 2010).

Long-term proton pump inhibitor treatment can lead to hypomagnesemia-induced seizure (Cundy and Dissnayake, 2008). Cimetidine (Edmonds et al., 1979; Flind and Rowley-Jones, 1979; Sharpe and Burland, 1980; Cerra et al., 1982; Handler et al., 1982), ranitidine (Bories et al., 1980; Hughes et al., 1983; Davis, 1984; Silverstone, 1984), famotidine (Henann et al., 1988; Catalano et al., 1996; Rodgers and Brengel, 1998; Yuan et al., 2001) and nizatidine (Galynker and Tendler, 1997; Bhanji and Margolese, 2004) induced mental confusion is described in elderly inpatients with coexistent liver or renal failure, or drug overdose. The confusion may be variable, associated with seizures, and visual hallucinations, cerebellar signs, and mild extrapyramidal features are reported. Symptoms remit with dose reduction or drug withdrawal.

Dystonia is reported following acute use of cimetidine (Peiris and Peckler, 2001), acute and long-term use of ranitidine (Wilson et al., 1997), and overdosage of nizatidine (Bhanji and Margolese, 2004). Ranitidine-induced acute hemiballismus and dyskinesias are described (Fouddah et al., 2001; Elzinga-Huttenga et al., 2006). There are isolated reports of cimetidine-induced parkinsonism (Leo et al., 1995), myopathy, and motor neuropathy (Feest and Read, 1980; Walls et al., 1980). Further, both H_2 blockers and proton pump inhibitors can theoretically impair neuromuscular transmission (Kounenis et al., 1994).

CENTRAL HYPERTHERMIA SYNDROMES AND GASTROINTESTINAL DRUGS

Antiemetic use is associated with two life-threatening hyperthermic syndromes; the neuroleptic malignant syndrome (NMS) and the serotonin syndrome.

NMS is characterized by hyperthermia, muscle rigidity, fluctuating sensorium, and autonomic instability. It is caused by abrupt central dopamine blockade and has been associated with prochlorperazine, promethazine, metoclopramide, and droperidol use. Dehydration and concomitant lithium therapy are risk factors. The syndrome can be rapidly fatal from rhabdomyolysis and multiorgan failure. Treatment involves withdrawal of the offending drug, hydration, benzodiazepines, dantrolene (muscle relaxants), dopamine agonists and supportive care (Guzé and Baxter, 1985; Fisher and Davis, 2002).

Serotonin syndrome results from a hyperserotonergic state following therapeutic drug use or inadvertent drug-to-drug interactions. Manifestations of the serotonin syndrome range from mild akathisia and tachycardia to severe tremulousness, myoclonus, rigidity, sustained clonus, delirium, autonomic instability, hyperthermia, and cardiovascular shock. Metoclopramide and the setrons have been implicated in causing serotonin syndrome. Their use with serotonin reuptake inhibitors, antidepressants, lithium, triptans, opioid analgesics, valproate, linezolid, and other proserotonergic drugs can heighten the symptoms. Treatment involves withdrawal of the offending drug(s), hydration, benzodiazepines, HT_{2a} antagonists, control of hyperthermia and autonomic dysfunction, and supportive care (Fisher and Davis, 2002; Boyer and Shannon, 2005; George et al., 2008; Patel et al., 2011).

CONCLUSION

Antiemetic therapy has evolved from the use of dopamine blockers like the phenothiazines with the potential for serious extrapyramidal reactions to selective serotonin and neurokinin receptor inhibitors that are more potent than the phenothiazines (D_2 blockers) and have a better safety profile. While metoclopramide remains the most extensively used prokinetic in most parts of the world, newer prokinetic agents with better adverse effect profiles are under development and review.

Postmarketing surveys have been critical in identifying serious adverse effects such as the cardiotoxicity of cisapride, cardiovascular events following tegaserod use, and risk of tardive dyskinesias following long-term use of metoclopramide or levosulpiride. Epidemiologic studies have also helped in defining the spectrum of drug-induced neurotoxicity and at-risk populations. For instance, young men are susceptible to metoclopramide-induced acute dystonic reactions while the elderly are more vulnerable to suffering tardive dyskinesias (Bhatt et al., 2004).

The commonly used gastrointestinal drugs, comprising antiemetics, promotility drugs and drugs to treat acid-related disorders, are used to treat disorders that can lead to morbidity but are not fatal (Parikh and Howden, 2010). Therefore, the benefits of their use should be evaluated taking into account possible adverse effects, even if these are uncommon. As far as possible, drugs such as metoclopramide and others that can lead to tardive dyskinesias should be used for as short a time as possible, with close clinical monitoring and patient education.

ACKNOWLEDGEMENT

The authors would like to thank Dr. Amruta Ravan for help with manuscript assembly and proofreading.

References

Aapro MS, Walko CM (2010). Aprepitant: drug-drug interactions in perspective. Ann Oncol 21: 2316–2323.

Andrejak M, Masmoudi K, Mizon JP (1990). Acute dyskinesia after the ingestion of antiemetics leading to emergency hospitalization. Therapie 45: 33–35.

Anfinson TJ (2002). Akathisia, panic, agoraphobia, and major depression following brief exposure to metoclopramide. Psychopharmacol Bull 36: 82–93.

Baik JS, Lyoo CH, Lee JH et al. (2008). Drug-induced and psychogenic resting suprahyoid neck and tongue tremors. Mov Disord 23: 746–748.

Bateman DN, Gokal R (1980). Metoclopramide in renal failure. Lancet 1: 982.

Bateman DN, Kahn C, Mashiter K et al. (1978). Pharmacokinetic and concentration-effect studies with intravenous metoclopramide. Br J Clin Pharmacol 6: 401–407.

Bateman DN, Rawlins MD, Simpson JM (1985). Extrapyramidal reactions with metoclopramide. Br Med J (Clin Res Ed) 291: 930–932.

Bateman DN, Darling WM, Boys R et al. (1989). Extrapyramidal reactions to metoclopramide and prochlorperazine. Q J Med 71: 307–311.

Bhanji NH, Margolese HC (2004). Extrapyramidal symptoms related to adjunctive nizatidine therapy in an adolescent receiving quetiapine and paroxetine. Pharmacotherapy 24: 923–925.

Bhatt M, Sethi K, Bhatia K (2004). Acute and tardive dystonia. In: K Sethi (Ed.), Drug-Induced Movement Disorders. Marcel Dekker, New York, pp. 111–128.

Biasini A, Alberti A (1985). Extrapyramidal dysfunction after domperidone. Helv Paediatr Acta 40: 93–94.

Bondon-Guitton E, Perez-Lloret S, Bagheri H et al. (2011). Drug-induced parkinsonism: a review of 17 years' experience in a regional pharmacovigilance center in France. Mov Disord 26: 2226–2231.

Bories P, Michel H, Brigitte D et al. (1980). Use of ranitidine, without mental confusion, in patient with renal failure. Lancet 2: 755.

Boyer EW, Shannon M (2005). The serotonin syndrome. N Engl J Med 352: 1112–1120.

Burke RE, Kang UJ, Jankovic J et al. (1989). Tardive akathisia: an analysis of clinical features and response to open therapeutic trials. Mov Disord 4: 157–175.

Burns R, Thomas DW, Barron VJ (1974). Reversible encephalopathy possibly associated with bismuth subgallate ingestion. Br Med J 1: 220–223.

Caldwell C, Rains G, McKiterick K (1987). An unusual reaction to preoperative metoclopramide. Anesthesiology 67: 854–855.

Casteels-Van Daele M, Jaeken J, Van der Schueren P et al. (1970). Dystonic reactions in children caused by metoclopramide. Arch Dis Child 45: 130–133.

Catalano G, Catalano MC, Alberts VA (1996). Famotidine-associated delirium. A series of six cases. Psychosomatics 37: 349–355.

Cerra BF, Schentag JJ, Mcmillen M et al. (1982). Mental status, the intensive care unit and cimetidine. Ann Surg 196: 565–570.

Chow LY, Chung D, Leung V et al. (1997). Suicide attempt due to metoclopramide-induced akathisia. Int J Clin Pract 51: 330–331.

Costall B, Naylor RJ (1973). Is there a relationship between the involvement of extrapyramidal and mesolimbic brain areas with the cataleptic action of neuroleptic agents and their clinical antipsychotic effect? Psychopharmacologia 32: 161–170.

Critchley P, Langdon N, Parkes JD et al. (1985). Domperidone. Br Med J (Clin Res Ed) 290: 788.

Cundy T, Dissanayake A (2008). Severe hypomagnesaemia in long-term users of proton-pump inhibitors. Clin Endocrinol (Oxf) 69: 338–341.

Davis WA (1984). Mental confusion associated with ranitidine. Med J Aust 140: 478.

Dieckmann K, Maurage C, Rolland JC et al. (1996). Torticollis as a side effect of cisapride treatment in an infant. J Pediatr Gastroenterol Nutr 22: 336.

Dobrow RB, Coppock MA, Hosenpud JR (1991). Extrapyramidal reaction caused by ondansetron. J Clin Oncol 9: 1921.

Drake RE, Ehrlich J (1985). Suicide attempts associated with akathisia. Am J Psychiatry 142: 499–501.

Duncan MA, Nikolov NM, O'Kelly B (2001). Acute chorea due to ondansetron in an obstetric patient. Int J Obstet Anesth 10: 309–311.

Edmonds ME, Ashford RF, Brenner MK et al. (1979). Cimetidine: does neurotoxicity occur? J R Soc Med 72: 172.

Ellis GL, Delaney J, DeHart DA et al. (1993). The efficacy of metoclopramide in the treatment of migraine headache. Ann Emerg Med 22: 191–195.

Elzinga-Huttenga J, Hekster Y, Bijl A et al. (2006). Movement disorders induced by gastrointestinal drugs: two paediatric cases. Neuropediatrics 37: 102–106.

Escourelle R, Bourdon R, Galli A et al. (1977). Neuropathologic and toxicologic study of 12 cases of bismuth encephalopathy. Rev Neurol 133: 153–163.

Feest TG, Read DJ (1980). Myopathy associated with cimetidine? Br Med J 281: 1284–1285.

Feyer P, Jordan K (2011). Update and new trends in antiemetic therapy: the continuing need for novel therapies. Ann Oncol 22: 30–38.

Fisher AA, Davis MW (2002). Serotonin syndrome caused by selective serotonin reuptake-inhibitors-metoclopramide interaction. Ann Pharmacother 36: 67–71.

Flind AC, Rowley-Jones D (1979). Mental confusion and cimetidine. Lancet 1: 379.

Ford AC, Malfertheiner P, Giguere M et al. (2008). Adverse events with bismuth salts for *Helicobacter pylori* eradication: systematic review and meta-analysis. World J Gastroenterol 14: 7361–7370.

Fouddah A, Canivet JL, Damas P (2001). Clinical case of the month. Severe dyskinetic syndrome induced by ranitidine. Rev Med Liege 56: 548–551.

Franckx J, Noel P (1984). Acute extrapyramidal dysfunction after domperidone administration. Report of a case. Helv Paediatr Acta 39: 285–288.

Galynker II, Tendler DS (1997). Nizatidine-induced delirium in a nonagenarian. J Clin Psychiatry 58: 327.

Ganzini L, Casey DE, Hoffman WF et al. (1993). The prevalence of metoclopramide-induced tardive dyskinesia and acute extrapyramidal movement disorders. Arch Intern Med 153: 1469–1475.

Gatrad AR, Gatrad AH (1979). Familial incidence of dystonic reactions to metoclopramide (Maxolon). Br J Clin Pract 33: 111–115.

George M, Al-Duaij N, O'Donnell KA et al. (2008). Obtundation and seizure following ondansetron overdose in an infant. Clin Toxicol 46: 1064–1066.

Gralla RJ, Itri LM, Pisko SE et al. (1981). Antiemetic efficacy of high-dose metoclopramide: randomized trials with placebo and prochlorperazine in patients with chemotherapy-induced nausea and vomiting. N Engl J Med 305: 905–909.

Grimes JD (1981). Parkinsonism and tardive dyskinesia associated with long-term metoclopramide therapy. N Engl J Med 305: 1417.

Grimes JD, Hassan MN, Krelina M (1982a). Long-term follow-up of tardive dyskinesia due to metoclopramide. Lancet 4: 563.

Grimes JD, Hassan MN, Preston DN (1982b). Adverse neurologic effects of metoclopramide. Can Med Assoc J 126: 23–25.

Grundy D, Al-Chaer ED, Aziz Q et al. (2006). Fundamentals of neurogastroenterology: basic science. Gastroenterology 130: 1391–1411.

Guala A, Mittino D, Fabbrocini P et al. (1992). Familial metoclopramide-induced dystonic reactions. Mov Disord 7: 385–386.

Guzé BH, Baxter LR Jr (1985). Current concepts. Neuroleptic malignant syndrome. N Engl J Med 313: 163–166.

Handler CE, Besse CP, Wilson AO (1982). Extrapyramidal and cerebellar syndrome with encephalopathy associated with cimetidine. Postgrad Med J 58: 527–528.

Harrington RA, Hamilton CW, Brogden RN et al. (1983). Metoclopramide. An updated review of its pharmacological properties and clinical use. Drugs 25: 451–494.

Henann NE, Carpenter DU, Janda SM (1988). Famotidine-associated mental confusion in elderly patients. Drug Intell Clin Pharm 22: 976–978.

Herbert MK, Holzer P (2008). Standardized concept for the treatment of gastrointestinal dysmotility in critically ill patients – current status and future options. Clin Nutr 27: 25–41.

Herrstedt J (2008). Antiemetics: an update and the MASCC guidelines applied in clinical practice. Nat Clin Pract Oncol 5: 32–43.

Herrstedt J, Dombernowsky P (2007). Anti-emetic therapy in cancer chemotherapy: current status. Basic Clin Pharmacol Toxicol 101: 143–150.

Hesketh PJ (2008). Chemotherapy-induced nausea and vomiting. N Engl J Med 358: 2482–2494.

Howden CW, Tytgat GN (1996). The tolerability and safety profile of famotidine. Clin Ther 18: 36–54.

Hughes JD, Reed WD, Serjeant CS (1983). Mental confusion associated with ranitidine. Med J Aust 2: 12–13.

Indo T, Ando K (1982). Metoclopramide-induced Parkinsonism. Clinical characteristics of ten cases. Arch Neurol 39: 494–496.

Kanarek BB, Curnow R, Palmer J et al. (1992). Ondansetron: confusing documentation surrounding an extrapyramidal reaction. J Clin Oncol 10: 506–507.

Karamanolis G, Tack J (2006). Promotility medications – now and in the future. Dig Dis 24: 297–307.

Kenney C, Hunter C, Davidson A et al. (2008). Metoclopramide, an increasingly recognized cause of tardive dyskinesia. J Clin Pharmacol 48: 379–384.

Kerr GW (1996). Dystonic reactions: two case reports. J Accid Emerg Med 13: 221–222.

Kim JS, Ko SB, Han SR et al. (2003). Levosulpiride-induced Parkinsonism. J Korean Neurol Assoc 21: 418–421.

Kounenis G, Koutsoviti-Papadopoulou, Elezoglou V (1994). Effect of nizatidine and ranitidine on the D-tubocurarine neuromuscular blockade in the toad rectus abdominis muscle. Pharmacol Res 29: 155–161.

Kovac AL (2003). Benefits and risks of newer treatments for chemotherapy-induced and postoperative nausea and vomiting. Drug Saf 26: 227–259.

Kumar N, Hu WT (2009). Extrapyramidal reaction to ondansetron and propofol. Mov Disord 24: 312–313.

LaGorio J, Thompson VA, Sternberg D et al. (1998). Akathisia and anesthesia: refusal of surgery after the administration of metoclopramide. Anesth Analg 87: 224–227.

Lang AE (1988). Akathisia and restless leg syndrome. In: J Jankovic, E Tolosa (Eds.), Parkinson's Disease and Movement Disorders. Urban and Schwarzenberg, Baltimore, pp. 349–364.

Lavy S, Melamed E, Penchas S (1978). Tardive dyskinesia associated with metoclopramide. Br Med J 1: 77–78.

Lee CR, Plosker GL, McTavish D (1993). Tropisetron. A review of its pharmacodynamic and pharmacokinetic properties, and therapeutic potential as an antiemetic. Drugs 46: 925–943.

Lee CY, Ratnapalan S, Thompson M et al. (2010). Unusual reactions to 5-HT3 receptor antagonists in a child with rhabdomyosarcoma. Can J Clin Pharmacol 17: 1–4.

Leeser J, Bateman DN (1985). Domperidone. Br Med J (Clin Res Ed) 290: 241–242.

Leo RJ, Lichter DG, Hershey LA (1995). Parkinsonism associated with fluoxetine and cimetidine: a case report. J Geriatr Psychiatry Neurol 8: 231–233.

Lewis JH (1991). Safety profile of long-term H2-antagonist therapy. Aliment Pharmacol Ther 5: 49–57.

Lu CS, Chu NS (1988). Acute dystonic reaction with asterixis and myoclonus following metoclopramide therapy. J Neurol Neurosurg Psychiatry 51: 1002–1003.

Lucena R, Monteiro L, Melo A (1998). Cisapride related movement disorders. J Pediatr 74: 416–418.

Mark R, Newton-John H (1988). Acute upper airway obstruction due to supraglottic dystonia induced by a neuroleptic. Br Med J 297: 964–965.

Mastaglia FL, Argov Z (2007). Toxic and iatrogenic myopathies. Handb Clin Neurol 86: 321–341.

Miller LG, Jankovic J (1989). Metoclopramide-induced movement disorders. Clinical findings with a review of the literature. Arch Intern Med 149: 2486–2492.

Morrow AW (1973). Requests for reports; adverse reactions with bismuth subgallate. Med J Aust 1: 912.

Naito Y, Kuzuhara S (1994). Parkinsonism induced or worsened by cisapride. Nihon Ronen Igakkai Zasshi 31: 899–902.

Nampiaparampil D, Oruc NE (2006). Metodopramide-induced palatopharyngeal myoclonus. Mov Disord 21: 2028–2029.

Parikh N, Howden CW (2010). The safety of drugs used in acid-related disorders and functional gastrointestinal disorders. Gastroenterol Clin North Am 39: 529–542.

Parkman HP, Hasler WL, Fisher RS et al. (2004). American Gastroenterology Association review on the diagnosis and treatment of gastroparesis. Gastroenterology 127: 1592–1622.

Parlak I, Atilla R, Cicek M et al. (2005). Rate of metoclopramide infusion affects the severity and incidence of akathisia. Emerg Med J 22: 621–624.

Pasricha PJ (2007). Desperately seeking serotonin. A commentary on the withdrawal of tegaserod and the state of drug development for functional and motility disorders. Gastroenterology 132: 2287–2290.

Pasricha PJ, Pehlivanov N, Sugumar A et al. (2006). Drug insight: from disturbed motility to disordered movement – a review of the clinical benefits and medicolegal risks of metoclopramide. Nat Clin Pract Gastroenterol Hepatol 3: 138–148.

Patel A, Mittal S, Manchanda S et al. (2011). Ondansetron-induced dystonia, hypoglycemia, and seizures in a child. Ann Pharmacother 45: 7.

Peiris RS, Peckler BF (2001). Cimetidine-induced dystonic reaction. J Emerg Med 21: 27–29.

Perez-Lloret S, Bondon-Guitton E, Rascol O et al. (2010). Adverse drug reactions to dopamine agonists: a comparative study in the French Pharmacovigilance Database; French Association of Regional Pharmacovigilance Centers. Mov Disord 25: 1876–1880.

Poortinga E, Rosenthal D, Bagri S (2001). Metoclopramide-induced akathisia during the second trimester of a 37-year-old woman's first pregnancy. Psychosomatics 42: 153–156.

Raschetti R, Maggini M, Da Cas R et al. (2001). Time trends in the coprescribing of cisapride and contraindicated drugs in Umbria, Italy. JAMA 285: 1840–1841.

Reid M (1977). Dystonic reactions to metoclopramide (Maxolon). Ulster Med J 46: 38–40.

Ritter MJ, Goodman BP, Sprung J et al. (2003). Ondansetron-induced multifocal encephalopathy. Mayo Clin Proc 78: 1150–1152.

Robinson OP (1973). Metoclopramide – side effects and safety. Postgrad Med J 49: 77–80.

Rodgers PT, Brengel GR (1998). Famotidine-associated mental status changes. Pharmacotherapy 18: 404–407.

Roila F, Fatigoni S (2006). New antiemetic drugs. Ann Oncol 2: ii96–ii100.

Rossi F, Forgione A (1995). Pharmacotoxicological aspects of levosulpiride. Pharmacol Res 31: 81–94.

Roy-Desruisseaux J, Landry J, Bocti C et al. (2011). Domperidone-induced tardive dyskinesia and withdrawal psychosis in an elderly woman with dementia. Ann Pharmacother 45: 51.

Sachdev P, Kruk J (1994). Clinical characteristics and predisposing factors in acute drug-induced akathisia. Arch Gen Psychiatry 51: 963–974.

Samie MR, Dannenhoffer MA, Rozek S (1987). Life-threatening tardive dyskinesia caused by metoclopramide. Mov Disord 2: 125–129.

Sargent AI, Deppe SA, Chan FA (1993). Seizure associated with ondansetron. Clin Pharmacol 12: 613–615.

Schneider SA, Udani V, Sankhla CS et al. (2009). Recurrent acute dystonic reaction and oculogyric crisis despite withdrawal of dopamine receptor blocking drugs. Mov Disord 24: 1226–1229.

Schulze-Delrieu K (1981). Drug therapy. Metoclopramide. N Engl J Med 305: 28–33.

Sethi KD (2004). Drug-Induced Movement Disorders, Marcel Dekker, New York.

Sewell DD, Jeste DV (1992). Metoclopramide-associated tardive dyskinesia. An analysis of 67 cases. Arch Fam Med 1: 271–278.

Shaffer D, Butterfield M, Pamer C et al. (2004). Tardive dyskinesia risks and metoclopramide use before and after U.S. market withdrawal of cisapride. J Am Pharm Assoc 44: 661–665.

Sharma A, Raina V (2001). Generalized seizures following ondansetron. Ann Oncol 12: 131–132.

Sharpe PC, Burland WL (1980). Mental confusion and H2-receptor blockers. Lancet 2: 924.

Shin HW, Kim MJ, Kim JS et al. (2009). Levosulpiride-induced movement disorders. Mov Disord 24: 2249–2253.

Sills JA, Glass EJ (1978). Metoclopramide in young children. Br Med J 2: 431.

Silverstone PH (1984). Ranitidine and confusion. Lancet 1: 1071.

Singh NN, Rai A, Selhorst JB et al. (2009). Ondansetron and seizures. Epilepsia 50: 2663–2666.

Sorbe B, Hallén C, Frankendal B (1994). An open, randomized study to compare the efficacy and tolerability of tropisetron with that of a metoclopramide-containing antiemetic cocktail in the prevention of cisplatin-induced emesis. Cancer Chemother Pharmacol 33: 298–302.

Spiegel JE, Kang V, Kunze L et al. (2005). Ondansetron-induced extrapyramidal symptoms during cesarean section. Int J Obstet Anesth 14: 368–369.

Sprung J, Choudhry FM, Hall BA (2003). Extrapyramidal reactions to ondansetron: cross-reactivity between ondansetron and prochlorperazine? Anesth Analg 96: 1374–1376.

Stacy M, Jankovic J (1992). Tardive tremor. Mov Disord 7: 53–57.

Steinherz R, Levy Y, Ban-Amiti D et al. (1986). Extrapyramidal reactions to domperidone. J Pediatr 108: 630–631.

Stonell C (1998). An extrapyramidal reaction to ondansetron. Br J Anaesth 81: 658.

Supino-Viterbo V, Sicard C, Risvegliato M et al. (1977). Toxic encephalopathy due to ingestion of bismuth salts: clinical and EEG studies of 45 patients. J Neurol Neurosurg Psychiatry 40: 748–752.

Tarsy D, Indorf G (2002). Tardive tremor due to metoclopramide. Mov Disord 17: 620–621.

Tillman LA, Drake FM, Dixon JS et al. (1996). Review article: safety of bismuth in the treatment of gastrointestinal diseases. Aliment Pharmacol Ther 10: 459–467.

Tisdale SA (1981). Metoclopramide. N Engl J Med 305: 1093.

Toga T, Kohmura Y, Kawatsu R (2007). The 5-HT(4) agonists cisapride, mosapride, and CJ-033466, a novel potent compound, exhibit different human ether-a-go-go-related gene (hERG)-blocking activities. J Pharmacol Sci 105: 207–210.

Tolan MM, Fuhrman TM, Tsueda K et al. (1999). Perioperative extrapyramidal reactions associated with ondansetron. Anesthesiology 90: 340–341.

Van der Padt A, Van Schaik RH, Sonneveld P (2006). Acute dystonic reaction to metoclopramide in patients carrying homozygous cytochrome P450 2D6 genetic polymorphisms. Neth J Med 64: 160–162.

Vandenplas Y, Benatar A, Cools F et al. (2001). Efficacy and tolerability of cisapride in children. Paediatr Drugs 3: 559–573.

Walls TJ, Pearce SJ, Venables GS (1980). Motor neuropathy associated with cimetidine. Br Med J 281: 974–975.

Weaving A, Bezwoda WR, Derman DP (1984). Seizures after antiemetic treatment with high dose domperidone: report of four cases. Br Med J (Clin Res Ed) 288: 1728.

Weiden PJ, Mann JJ, Haas G et al. (1987). Clinical nonrecognition of neuroleptic-induced movement disorders: a cautionary study. Am J Psychiatry 144: 1148–1153.

Wilson LB, Woodward AM, Ferrara JJ (1997). An acute dystonic reaction with long-term use of ranitidine in an intensive care unit patient. J La State Med Soc 149: 36–38.

Yamamoto M, Ujike H, Ogawa N (1987). Metoclopramide-induced parkinsonism. Clin Neuropharmacol 10: 287–289.

Yuan RY, Kao CR, Sheu JJ et al. (2001). Delirium following a switch from cimetidine to famotidine. Ann Pharmacother 35: 1045–1048.

Zambelli A, Sagrada P, Pavesi L (2009). Seizure associated with palonosetron. Support Care Cancer 17: 217.

Handbook of Clinical Neurology, Vol. 120 (3rd series)
Neurologic Aspects of Systemic Disease Part II
Jose Biller and Jose M. Ferro, Editors

Chapter 44

Neurologic manifestations of acute liver failure

SUDHIR DATAR AND EELCO F.M. WIJDICKS*

Division of Critical Care Neurology, Mayo Clinic, Rochester, MN, USA

INTRODUCTION

Neurologists have been familiar with the manifestations of chronic liver disease for more than a century but in acute liver failure most have been on less sure ground. Acute liver failure (ALF) (Trey and Davidson, 1970; Lee et al., 2008), best known as fulminant hepatic failure, is a clinical syndrome of acute onset of encephalopathy and coagulopathy (international normalized ratio (INR) ≥ 1.5) resulting from massive loss of hepatocyte function in a patient without any pre-existing liver disease, with an illness duration of < 26 weeks (Trey and Davidson, 1970; Lee et al., 2012). Suicide attempt with acetaminophen (paracetamol) remains a common cause. Fortunately, such a catastrophic event is rare and in the US, about 2000 cases are reported annually (Lee et al., 2008). In the pre-transplant era, morbidity and mortality was high and autopsies would show brain edema, but these manifestations were viewed as terminal events in a critically ill mechanically ventilated patient.

There has been a paradigm shift in our understanding of acute liver failure over the last 20 years and, as a result of the discovery that cerebral edema is treatable, it has become partly a neurologic disease. Emergency liver transplantation (Bismuth et al., 1987; Emond et al., 1989; Brandsaeter et al., 2002; Fujiwara and Mochida, 2002; Russo et al., 2004; Montalti et al., 2005; Detry et al., 2007; O'Grady, 2007) and management in modern intensive care units (ICUs) equipped to handle the complications have increased survival rates to 65%, far better than the miserable earlier survival rates of $< 15\%$ (Ostapowicz et al., 2002; Khashab et al., 2007).

It has become apparent that one of the major causes of death in these patients is cerebral edema and intracranial hypertension, eventually leading to brain death if untreated. Technology is now available to monitor intracranial pressure (ICP), which, combined with mean arterial pressure (MAP), provides an estimation of cerebral perfusion. However, these techniques are invasive, needing burr holes and placement of intracranial monitoring devices in a patient with very poor coagulation.

The roles that a neurologist can play when evaluating a patient with ALF are: (1) to rapidly identify patients who are at risk of cerebral edema and intracranial hypertension; (2) to carefully select the patient population who will benefit from invasive monitoring; (3) to select the correct time to start monitoring; (4) to suggest to the neurosurgeon the appropriate tissue compartment (subdural, epidural, or parenchymal) for the placement of ICP monitors; (5) to participate in treatment of cerebral edema and increased ICP; (6) to manage complications such as intracranial hemorrhage or seizures; (7) to assist in selection of candidates for liver transplantation and referral to transplant center.

This chapter illustrates the clinical presentation and overall management of ALF, with a focus on the management of cerebral edema.

HISTORICAL PERSPECTIVE

The liver plays an indispensable role in homeostasis, playing a major role in synthesis of proteins and removal of waste products of metabolism. With acute liver failure, these mechanisms are compromised with the major consequences being coagulopathy and encephalopathy with or without cerebral edema. Cerebral edema in ALF was described as early as the 1960s. Williams and colleagues examined 92 cases of fulminant hepatic failure over a 7 year period and found the presence of cerebral edema in 31% of the cases (Record et al., 1975). Mortality seems to be associated with brain herniation, which was found in 20 patients.

The causes of acute injury to the hepatocytes have changed over the last few decades. In the 1980s, acute

---

*Correspondence to: Eelco F.M. Wijdicks, M.D., Ph.D., Department of Neurology, Mayo Clinic, 200 First Street SW, 55905, Rochester, MN, USA. E-mail: wijde@mayo.edu

viral hepatitis played a major role. However, with time, paracetamol (acetaminophen) toxicity started emerging as a major cause and today about half of all cases of ALF are due to paracetamol (acetaminophen) overdose. Other causes of acute loss of hepatocyte function are idiosyncratic drug reaction, hepatic venous thrombosis (Budd–Chiari syndrome), acute fatty liver of pregnancy/HELLP (hemolysis, elevated liver enzymes, low platelet count) syndrome, ingestion of certain types of mushrooms, Wilson's disease, autoimmune hepatitis, cardiac arrest, or any other severe episode of sufficiently prolonged hypotension leading to "shock liver," infiltration of the liver by malignancy, etc. Reye's syndrome (Meythaler and Varma, 1987) associated with the use of aspirin or viral infections (influenza-like illness or varicella) is now extraordinarily rare and any child presenting with a similar clinical picture should undergo extensive investigations to rule out inborn errors of metabolism which can mimic Reye's syndrome (Belay et al., 1999).

Attempts at using artificial livers go back to the 1970s. Williams and colleagues, from King's College Hospital, London, described the use of temporary liver support using isolated but functioning pig's liver in an extracorporeal perfusion circuit. Attempts were also made at using human liver or the liver of a baboon. Perfusion could be continued for only up to 48 hours with human or baboon's liver and for up to 6–8 hours with pig's liver. This was followed by only temporary improvement in laboratory abnormalities or level of consciousness. However, overall, long-term results were discouraging (Williams, 1975).

The main conceptional change has been to connect brain edema with care of acute liver failure and to prioritize liver transplantation. A new liver may be the only effective treatment of brain edema in some patients.

CLINICAL PRESENTATION

ALF is commonly seen in critically ill patients already admitted to the hospital in the setting of multiorgan failure, shock or cardiac arrest, and a neurologist may get involved quickly. Often these patients are admitted to the ICU for several reasons which could include difficulty with airway protection and respiratory failure needing mechanical ventilation, severe hypotension, sepsis syndrome, and rapidly worsening "hepatic encephalopathy."

As expected, the initial symptoms are typical of any encephalopathy. Apathy is one of the earliest psychiatric symptoms (Wijdicks, 2009). Other symptoms are hypersomnia and impaired judgment (Rothstein and Herlong, 1989). Surprisingly, patients may present with agitated delirium or even euphoria with a transition to mania (Zacharski et al., 1970).

Spatial disorientation, impairment in thought process and content, fluctuations in attention, slowed cognitive processing and impairment of short-term and immediate memory may be present. Multifocal myoclonus and excessive startle responses can occur. In contrast to chronic liver disease, asterixis is rather uncommon (Wijdicks, 2009). Encephalopathy of any grade may signify the onset of cerebral edema, but the probability increases with worsening encephalopathy (Table 44.1).

Pupillary responses are normal initially but may become impaired when cerebral herniation develops, eventually progressing to fixed midposition pupils (4–6 mm) due to displacement and compression of the mesencephalon from the diffuse mass effect. Oculocephalic responses usually remain normal but may become brisk or transiently disappear (Heubi et al., 1984). Dysconjugate gaze occurs rarely (Caplan and Scheiner, 1980) and an equally rare but reported phenomenon is the occurrence of periodic alternating gaze deviation (PAGD) in patients with hepatic encephalopathy without any identifiable structural injury, which can resolve with the treatment of encephalopathy (Averbuch-Heller and Meiner, 1995). In general, however, oculomotor dysfunction is uncommon and its presence should raise suspicion for alternative causes other than hepatic encephalopathy.

Decerebrate and decorticate posturing, albeit very dramatic, may be completely reversible after correction of ammonia and improvement of liver function (Conomy and Swash, 1968). Other common findings are increased muscle tone, exaggerated deep tendon reflexes, and Babinski's signs (Wijdicks, 2009).

Table 44.1

Grades of encephalopathy: West Haven criteria (adapted from Ferenci et al., 2002)

Grade	Clinical characteristics
I	Trivial lack of awareness
	Euphoria or anxiety
	Shortened attention span
	Impaired performance of addition
II	Lethargy or apathy
	Minimal disorientation for time or place
	Subtle personality change
	Inappropriate behavior
	Impaired performance of subtraction
III	Somnolence to semistupor, but responsive to verbal stimuli
	Confusion
	Gross disorientation
IV	Coma (unresponsive to verbal or noxious stimulus)

As the severity of liver failure increases, consciousness becomes impaired, eventually progressing to coma. Even if these patients initially present with mild encephalopathy, they can worsen rapidly from quick development of cerebral edema and hence they need close monitoring in the hospital which may be best done in an ICU setting. Grades of hepatic encephalopathy are summarized in Table 44.1.

Generally any pathologic motor response or abnormality of mesencephalic or pontine reflexes is suspicious for diffuse cerebral edema. Classic clinical signs of increased ICP, such as Cushing's response of systemic hypertension and bradycardia, are not always present. Computed tomography (CT) scans should be repeated even if transport of the patient is far from ideal.

Both focal and generalized seizures have been reported to occur, even in the absence of radiographically identifiable focal brain injury which could account for it. In severely encephalopathic patients a low index of suspicion must be maintained for ongoing subclinical seizures. A review of electroencephalograms (EEGs) over a 10 year period identified 18 (15%) with epileptiform abnormalities (Ficker et al., 1997). In another study, by Ellis and colleagues, 13 out of 42 patients with ALF who underwent continuous EEG monitoring were found to have electrographic seizures (Ellis et al., 2000). Subclinical seizure activity is probably an under-recognized occurrence which also potentially contributes towards cerebral hypoxia and cerebral edema.

As expected, jaundice, hepatic tenderness, and ascites (in cases of acute hepatic vein thrombosis) may be present. However, signs of chronic liver failure are usually absent, as by definition, acute liver failure implies absence of any chronic liver disease.

Contrary to liver cirrhosis commonly presenting with gastrointestinal bleeding, in ALF spontaneous hemorrhage is rather uncommon and any significant hemorrhage requiring transfusion is rare (Boks et al., 1986). Acute portal hypertension can develop from ALF, but bleeding from varices seldom occurs.

LABORATORY TESTS AND IMAGING STUDIES

Laboratory tests show marked elevation of transaminases, increased INR and increased serum ammonia. Phosphorus, magnesium, and potassium are frequently low and may need supplementation. Glucose should be monitored and replaced if indicated, as severe hypoglycemia may occur and markedly confound the clinical presentation. Similarly severe hyponatremia may be present. Acute elevation of blood urea nitrogen and creatinine suggests acute renal failure, which also complicates the clinical picture. These acute metabolic abnormalities in theory could contribute toward encephalopathy; they are usually transient as they are easily correctable. However, a worsening encephalopathy should not be readily attributed to these metabolic factors as any appreciable change can signify the onset of cerebral edema with fatal consequences if untreated.

Elevation of white blood cell count could suggest the presence of an underlying infection, especially if it is associated with a left shift. Thrombocytopenia may be present. Blood gas measurement may reveal acidosis but more commonly shows alkalosis which could be respiratory or metabolic. Other pertinent laboratory studies include tests to identify a cause for the ALF. This may include testing of paracetamol (acetaminophen) levels in cases of suspected exposure, viral hepatitis panel testing for A, B, C and, if indicated, D and E viruses. If there is clinical suspicion, testing for autoimmune hepatitis may be indicated with serum antinuclear antibody, smooth muscle antibody, antibodies to liver and kidney microsomes (anti-LKM), antimitochondrial antibody and serum protein electrophoresis. Liver ultrasound with Doppler studies can identify portal vein or hepatic vein thrombosis.

Brain CT scan is usually the first neuroimaging study performed as it is quick, readily available, and can identify complications of ALF such as cerebral edema with evidence of mass effect (Wijdicks et al., 1995) or, in rare cases, acute intracranial hemorrhage. Brain edema on CT scan is demonstrated by effacement of cortical sulci, blurring of gray–white differentiation, and obliteration of basal cisterns (Fig. 44.1). However, it should be noted that brain CT scan is not a very sensitive way of excluding early cerebral edema and early abnormalities can be very subtle, such as disappearance of some sulci and sylvian fissures (Fig. 44.2) (Munoz et al., 1991). Any patient with ALF and advanced hepatic encephalopathy with a normal CT scan can still be at high risk of rapidly developing intracranial hypertension (IH) and it makes perfect sense to be proactive and consider ICP monitoring.

Magnetic resonance (MR) imaging abnormalities have been described in the periventricular white matter, thalami, posterior limb of the internal capsule, dorsal brainstem and cortex. These abnormalities are seen on both fluid attenuated inversion recovery (FLAIR) as well as diffusion-weighted imaging (DWI). Serum ammonia has been shown to correlate strongly with FLAIR and DWI severity and clinical outcome (McKinney et al., 2010). Diffusion restriction is likely explained by cytotoxic edema from astrocyte swelling (Ranjan et al., 2005). Diffuse cortical involvement has a higher potential for neurologic sequelae but these changes are reversible (Fig. 44.3).

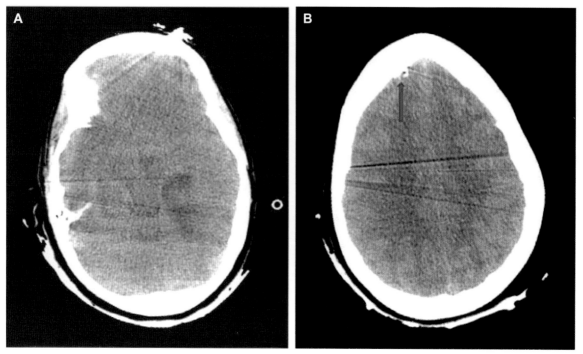

Fig. 44.1. A 30-year-old woman with acute hepatic failure due to HELLP syndrome. (**A** and **B**) CT of the brain without contrast showing cerebral edema with effacement of the sulci, blurring of gray–white differentiation and obliteration of cisterns. Bolt for ICP monitoring can be seen in image (**B**) (arrow). The patient received liver transplantation but did poorly postoperatively due to high intracranial pressure and died from cerebral herniation.

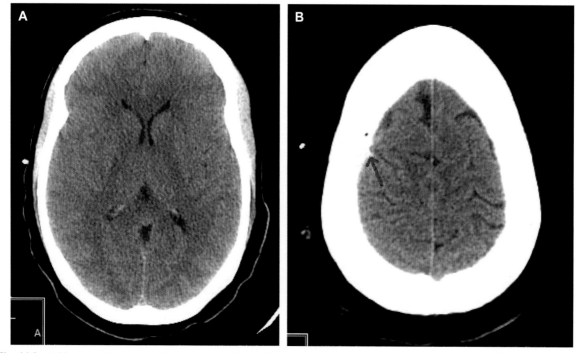

Fig. 44.2. A 32-year-old woman with acute hepatic failure from paracetamol (acetaminophen) overdose. (**A**) Normal noncontrast head CT scan without any evidence of cerebral edema but showing effacement of both sylvian fissures. Intracranial pressure (ICP) was elevated. (**B**) Placement of bolt for monitoring ICP (arrow). She went on to receive a liver transplant and did well.

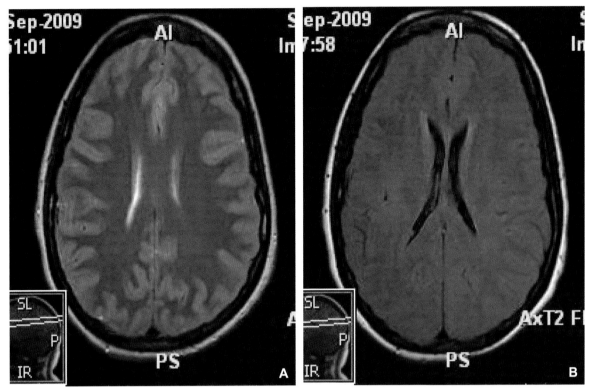

Fig. 44.3. MRI of the brain without contrast showing evidence of cerebral edema. (**A**) T2-weighted image showing diffuse efface-ment of sulci and increased cortical T2 signal suggestive of cerebral edema. (**B**) Fluid attenuated inversion recovery (FLAIR) image showing periventricular T2 signal abnormalities in addition to cortical signal changes, suggestive of cerebral edema.

Somatosensory evoked potentials (SSEP) are mark-edly different in patients with fulminant liver failure (Madl et al., 1994). A study using bilateral median nerve-stimulated short- and long-latency sensory evoked potentials found that nine patients had spontaneous recovery, eight patients underwent emergency liver transplantation, and eight patients died (Madl et al., 1994). Probability of correct outcome prediction by sen-sory evoked potentials versus that based on clinical cri-teria alone was 0.96 versus 0.72, respectively. It was concluded that serial recording of sensory evoked poten-tials may help identify a subgroup of patients who should undergo early liver transplantation even though they do not fulfill the King's College criteria (Table 44.2). How-ever, experience with SSEPs is very limited and until there are more data, SSEPs should be used cautiously for this purpose.

REFERRAL TO TRANSPLANT CENTER

Once a diagnosis of acute liver failure is established, the next step is to quickly determine if the patient is a trans-plant candidate. Urgent liver transplantation is indicated in ALF where prognostic indicators suggest a high prob-ability of poor outcome (see section on outcome). However, complete reliance on the prognostic scoring

systems is not recommended as they do not adequately predict outcome and candidacy for liver transplantation (Lee et al., 2012). Other factors that also play a role in determining the candidacy of transplantation include overall medical comorbidities. Conditions such as severe coexistent medical disease, progressive inotropic or ven-tilator support, irreversible brainstem dysfunction, mul-tiple previous episodes of self-harm (>5), especially if nondrug methods were used, refractory or resistant mental illness, incapacitating dementia or mental retar-dation, active intravenous drug use, or excessive alcohol use may be relative contraindications for transplantation (Simpson et al., 2009). Nonetheless, the threshold to pri-oritize patients for transplantation is low because the time window for effective treatment is very narrow. Timely referral to a center where liver transplantation can be done is critical. Even if the encephalopathy is mild to begin with, it can progress quickly, with development of cerebral edema.

MEDICAL MANAGEMENT OF ACUTE LIVER FAILURE

Even if not directly involved with care, it is important for neurologists to have a good understanding of this emerg-ing critical illness and in particular the degree of

Table 44.2

King's College criteria (adapted from Lee et al., 2012)

Acetaminophen-induced ALF	Strongly consider OLT listing if: • Arterial lactate > 3.5 mmol/L after early fluid resuscitation List for OLT if: • pH < 7.3 *OR* • Arterial lactate > 3.0 mmol/L after adequate fluid resuscitation List for OLT if all three occur within a 24-hour period: • Presence of grade 3 or 4 hepatic encephalopathy • INR > 6.5 • Creatinine > 3.4 mg/dL
Nonacetaminophen-induced ALF	List for OLT if: INR > 6.5 and encephalopathy present (irrespective of grade) *OR* Any three of the following (encephalopathy present; irrespective of grade): • Age < 10 or > 40 years • Jaundice for > 7 days before development of encephalopathy • INR ≥ 3.5 • Serum bilirubin ≥ 17 mg/dL • Unfavorable etiology, such as Wilson disease, idiosyncratic drug reaction, seronegative hepatitis

ALF, acute liver failure; OLT, orthotopic liver transplantation; INR, international normalized ratio.

coagulopathy in ALF. By definition, patients with ALF are coagulopathic and thrombocytopenic. Correction of INR is not indicated unless the patient is actively bleeding or an invasive procedure – which may include a lumbar puncture in selected cases – is planned. Fresh frozen plasma (FFP) has been used for decades to correct the coagulopathy before invasive procedures. However, it is associated with the drawbacks of transfusion reactions including transfusion-related acute lung injury (TRALI) and volume overload. Plasma infusion alone may not adequately correct severely elevated INR and with the risk of volume overload, plasmapheresis may be an option (Munoz et al., 1989). Recently, factor VIIa has been explored for this purpose. In one study, factor VIIa was used in patients with ALF undergoing procedures and the authors found it to be more effective over FFP in transiently controlling the parameters of coagulation (Shami et al., 2003). There remains a risk of thromboembolic complications with the use of factor VIIa (myocardial infarction and portal vein thrombosis) (Pavese et al., 2005). However, none of these concerns were found in a study of 11 patients who received factor

VIIa for placement of ICP monitors, once again in ALF, reported no hemorrhagic or thrombotic complications (Le et al., 2010). Further randomized studies are needed to prove the safety, efficacy, and cost-effectiveness of factor VIIa in this group of patients; however, it remains an available option.

Precise guidelines for safe coagulation parameters for the performance of invasive procedures in patients with ALF do not exist. A common practice is to keep the INR below 1.5. Vitamin K (10 mg intravenously) should be routinely administered since vitamin K deficiency has been reported in patients with ALF (Pereira et al., 2005).

Some investigators have used thromboelastography (TEG) and demonstrated that despite elevated INR, most patients with ALF maintain normal hemostasis, mechanisms of which include an increase in clot strength with increasing severity of liver injury, increased factor VIII levels, and a reduction in pro- and anticoagulant proteins (Stravitz et al., 2012). Therefore, the actual bleeding risk based on elevated INR may be less than expected (Lee et al., 2012).

Similar to INR, correction of platelets is not indicated unless an invasive procedure is planned or there is evidence of active bleeding. Platelet counts of > 10 000/mm³ are generally well tolerated, with a preference of > 20 000/mm³ in the setting of active infection/sepsis. Transfusion should be considered for patients with active bleeding and platelet counts < 50 000/mm³. If an invasive procedure is planned, then counts between 50 000 and 70 000/mm³ are acceptable (Munoz et al., 2009).

Lactulose has not been formally tested in a randomized controlled fashion in ALF; however, we have extensive experience with its use in chronic liver failure to treat hyperammonemia. Thus, combined with the fact that ammonia likely plays a central role in the pathogenesis of encephalopathy and cerebral edema, in theory lactulose may be beneficial in these patients. The dose should be titrated to produce 2–3 bowel movements, but not to the point of producing diarrhea. A small retrospective study showed no difference in overall outcome, but a small increase in survival time in those who received lactulose was observed (Jalan, 2005; Lee et al., 2012). One concern with its use, however, is distension of the bowel and interference with the surgical field during liver transplantation.

Fever due to infection can worsen ICP. ALF increases the risk of infection by bacterial and fungal agents. Routine surveillance cultures should be drawn in all patients and treatment with antibiotics should be instituted at the first sign of infection/systemic inflammatory response syndrome (SIRS). Studies suggest an association between infection/SIRS and progression to deeper stages of encephalopathy (Rolando et al., 2000; Vaquero et al., 2003).

Another important factor in management of ICP is maintenance of adequate mean arterial pressure (MAP). Patients are often intravascularly volume depleted, either from poor oral intake or from third spacing. In addition, they may have low peripheral vascular resistance from vasodilation. Hypotension can decrease cerebral blood flow (CBF) and increase the risk of cerebral ischemia. Hypotensive patients should be volume resuscitated initially with normal saline followed by isotonic sodium bicarbonate if acidosis develops. Patients may need norepinephrine for the support of blood pressure to maintain a MAP of at least 75 mmHg or cerebral perfusion pressure (CPP) of at least > 60 mmHg, preferably between 60 and 80 mmHg if that can be achieved.

Vasopressin, or its analog terlipressin, can be considered to reduce the need for high doses of norepinephrine, which can cause intense peripheral vasoconstriction and tissue ischemia. Although terlipressin produces systemic vasoconstriction, it produces cerebral vasodilatation and may inadvertently increase cerebral blood flow (CBF), thereby having additional benefit. One study comparing terlipressin and noradrenaline showed little effect on ICP while increasing CPP (Eefsen et al., 2007), but there was a suggestion of increase in ICP in one study (Shawcross et al., 2004). It should be used with extreme caution in patients with cerebral edema and only if ICP can be monitored.

MANAGEMENT OF CEREBRAL EDEMA

Ammonia has been implicated in the pathogenesis of hepatic encephalopathy, perhaps through an imbalance between inhibitory and excitatory neurotransmitters. The γ-aminobutyric acid (GABA) neurotransmitter system, an inhibitory system, possibly plays a prominent role (Grimm et al., 1988; Bassett et al., 1987; Jones et al., 1989; Jones et al., 1990; Lavoie et al., 1990). GABA causes hyperpolarization of neuronal membrane through opening of chloride channel and influx of chloride inside the cells. Barbiturates and benzodiazepines potentiate this action. It has been observed in animal models that hepatic encephalopathy has many similarities to encephalopathy induced by drugs that potentiate GABA action. It appears that the degree of hepatic encephalopathy is correlated with cerebrospinal fluid (CSF) levels of GABA. Furthermore, flumazenil, a benzodiazepine antagonist, has been shown to improve the encephalopathy at least in some cases, if not all (Bassett et al., 1987; Grimm et al., 1988; Jones et al., 1990). These findings have led to the suggestion that an endogenous substance with benzodiazepine-like properties contributes to the neuropsychiatric manifestations of hepatic encephalopathy (Jones et al., 1989). However, based on limited data, flumazenil cannot be recommended for all patients with hepatic encephalopathy; nevertheless, it has an important role in patients with fulminant hepatic failure who have received repeated doses of benzodiazepines. This may help correctly stage hepatic encephalopathy, which is relevant when emergency transplantation is being considered. Other potential mechanisms of hepatic encephalopathy are mercaptans, short-chain fatty acids, and depletion of neurotransmitters, such as norepinephrine and dopamine.

Cerebral edema is a well-known complication of ALF (Ware et al., 1971), mechanisms of which are partially understood (Blei and Larsen, 1999; Rao and Norenberg, 2001; Butterworth, 2003; Jalan, 2005). Ammonia must play an important role in the pathogenesis of cerebral edema although there may be downstream effects. During ALF, hyperammonemia has been shown to increase the risk of cerebral edema (Clemmesen et al., 1999). Patients rarely develop hepatic encephalopathy with arterial ammonia concentration less than 75 μmol/L (Bernal et al., 2007). A level > 100 μmol/L at admission is an independent risk factor for the development of high grade hepatic encephalopathy (Bernal et al., 2007). Conversely a level of > 200 μmol/L is strongly associated with cerebral edema.

Under normal circumstances, ammonia which is produced in the gut is metabolized by the liver to urea and glutamine. However, when the liver fails, ammonia starts building up and is then metabolized in tissues such as the brain and skeletal muscle. Ammonia crosses the blood–brain barrier by diffusion. The glutamine hypothesis proposes that astrocytes which are the sites of ammonia detoxification in the brain metabolize excess ammonia to glutamine (Blei and Larsen, 1999; Blei, 2001; Jalan, 2005). Glutamine, being osmotically active, causes the astrocytes to swell. This process takes place rapidly during ALF, thereby preventing cellular adaptation to the changes in osmolality, a process which does occur with chronic ammonia elevation as seen in liver cirrhosis. Electron microscopy has demonstrated marked swelling of the perivascular astroglial foot processes (Kato et al., 1992).

Impaired cerebral autoregulation with massive liver necrosis has been demonstrated using rat models (Dethloff et al., 2008). Patients with cerebral edema and intracranial hypertension have been shown to have higher cerebral blood flow (CBF) (Aggarwal et al., 1994; Durham et al., 1995). Alterations in cerebral hemodynamics result from locally induced cerebral hyperemia. Other mechanisms that have been implicated include production of nitric oxide (Blei and Larsen, 1999). There is increasing evidence that this increase in CBF is of importance for the development of cerebral edema and intracranial hypertension (Raghavan and Marik, 2006) (Fig. 44.4).

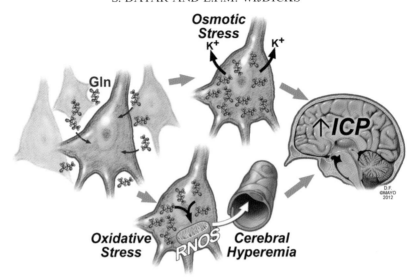

Fig. 44.4. Illustration of the pathophysiologic mechanisms of cerebral edema in acute liver failure. Gln, glutamine; RNOS, reactive nitrogen oxide species; ICP, intracranial pressure. (Reproduced by permission of the Mayo Foundation for Medical Education and Research. All rights reserved.)

Dysfunction of the sodium-potassium adenosine triphosphate (ATPase) pump also likely plays a role. Inhibition of enzyme α-ketoglutarate dehydrogenase (a key enzyme in the Krebs cycle) by ammonia impairs generation of ATP and increases anaerobic metabolism. Cerebral microdialysis studies in patients with ALF revealed elevated lactate in patients with high ICP, which further increased before surges of ICP (Tofteng et al., 2002).

Deficits in the ability of astrocytes to take up glutamate from the extracellular space may lead to excitotoxicity of neuronal and glial glutamate receptors and glial dysfunction (Norenberg, 1998).

The observation that hemodynamic status as well as IH improves after removal of native liver during transplantation raises the possibility of necrotic liver being the source of vasoactive cytokines inducing the hemodynamic changes.

Finally, aquaporin-4, a molecule which modulates brain water transport, may play a role, and inhibition of this water channel may provide a new therapeutic option for reducing brain edema (Manley et al., 2000).

The incidence of cerebral edema increases with increasing grades of encephalopathy (Wijdicks et al., 1995), reaching 75% or more with grade IV encephalopathy (Munoz, 1993). The subsequent course depends upon the volume of brain tissue in relation to the volume of the cranial vault. As alluded to earlier, almost half of the cases of ALF occur with paracetamol (acetaminophen) overdose and these patients are relatively young (in their 30s to 40s). They have less or no cerebral atrophy, which can give rise to rapid increases in ICP with small increases in the volume of intracranial contents due to cerebral edema (Monro-Kellie hypothesis) (Mokri, 2001). Untreated, this can lead to cerebral herniation, vascular compression, and cerebral infarction, which result in more edema and set up a vicious cycle. The eventual outcome can be fatal.

Treatment of cerebral edema follows traditional methods of ICP management. Any underlying factors which can worsen the ICP, such as agitation, coughing, frequent turning, endotracheal suctioning and severe hypertension, need to be eliminated.

In the emergency setting, it is important to raise the head of the bed to at least 30° and to keep the neck straight, to facilitate venous return from the brain. If the patient is intubated, then hyperventilation can be used as a temporary measure, maintaining partial pressure of carbon dioxide (pCO_2) between 28 and 35 mmHg (Wijdicks, 2009). The resulting hypocapnic alkalosis causes potent cerebral vasoconstriction, thereby reducing cerebral blood volume and consequently ICP (Laffey and Kavanagh, 2002). Intracranial pressure may decrease transiently at the expense of cerebral perfusion. In addition, vasoconstriction induced by hypocapnia can decrease regional cerebral blood flow and inflict secondary ischemic brain injury. Not all patients are pCO_2 responders and moreover the effect is short lived. Increasing evidence suggests that hypocapnia can induce substantial adverse effects, including cardiac arrhythmias, myocardial ischemia, and bronchospasm to mention a few. Thus, therapeutic hypocapnia should generally be limited to emergency management of life-threatening increases in intracranial pressure (Laffey and Kavanagh, 2002).

Seizures increase ICP (Gabor et al., 1984; Shah et al., 2007) and when they occur, they must be promptly controlled. Both focal and generalized seizures are known to occur in these patients even in the absence of radiographically detectable structural brain injury. Traditionally phenytoin has been used for the treatment of seizures. As subclinical seizures also occur and can worsen cerebral edema, there is a suggestion that prophylactic phenytoin may be of benefit. One study indeed showed benefit with prophylactic phenytoin administration (Ellis et al., 2000). However, one small trial failed to show any improvement in survival or cerebral edema with prophylactic use of phenytoin (Bhatia et al., 2004). Hence seizure prophylaxis with phenytoin is currently not recommended (Lee et al., 2012).

ICP monitoring in cases of ALF is currently controversial. Some studies have suggested that ICP monitoring is clinically useful in ALF despite the risk of hemorrhage (Lidofsky et al., 1992).

One study in 1993 reported a complication rate approaching 20% (Blei et al., 1993), but the numbers vary based on the type and location of the ICP monitoring device. Epidural location had the lowest complication rate (3.8%). Subdural and parenchymal locations have more benefit in regards to accuracy; however, they also have a higher rate of complications (20% and 22%, respectively) (Blei et al., 1993). Ventricular catheters are rarely, if ever, used. In general, epidural catheters provide a relatively safe way of monitoring ICP although they are not as accurate as subdural and parenchymal devices. One survey (Vaquero et al., 2005) evaluated 332 patients across 24 centers constituting the US ALF study group. ICP monitoring was used in 92 (28%) of the patients and was strongly associated with referral for liver transplantation. The rate of intracranial hemorrhage was 10.3% in a subset of 52 patients, with half of the complications being incidental radiologic findings. Survival at 30 days in both monitored and nonmonitored patients post-transplantation was similar. However, this study was retrospective and it is possible that monitoring was undertaken in sicker patients. To date, although proof of improved survival with ICP monitoring is lacking, many liver transplant surgeons, hepatologists, and neurointensivists consider it a useful tool and, despite some increased risk of hemorrhage, would strongly favor its use.

However, the more difficult question is to decide which patient to select for ICP monitoring. In other words, who will benefit most from aggressive treatment of elevated ICP? As pointed out earlier (Bernal et al., 2007), it was found that an ammonia level of > 200 μmol/L is strongly associated with cerebral edema. Other factors which also increase the risk of cerebral edema are grade III or IV encephalopathy, acute renal failure, and the need for vasopressors to maintain MAP. Furthermore, CT scan of the brain may not reliably demonstrate evidence of edema, especially in early stages (Munoz et al., 1991). Intracranial hypertension is of particular concern during orthotopic liver transplantation (OLT), when rapid shifts in electrolytes and hemodynamics can cause large fluctuations in ICP.

Hence, a high index of suspicion must be maintained, with a low threshold to use ICP monitoring in patients who are at increased risk of cerebral edema. According to an update released by the American Association for the Study of Liver Diseases (AASLD) in 2011, ICP monitoring is recommended in ALF patients with high grade hepatic encephalopathy, in centers with expertise in ICP monitoring, in patients awaiting and undergoing liver transplantation (Lee et al., 2012). Monitoring is usually started around the time of intubation for worsening encephalopathy and should be continued at least 1–2 days postoperatively, following liver transplantation.

Hyperosmolar therapy can be given following or simultaneous to the above measures for the treatment of ICP (Bhardwaj and Ulatowski, 2004b; Diringer and Zazulia, 2004; Suarez, 2004; Aiyagari et al., 2006; Wakai et al., 2007). These solutions increase osmolality of the serum. This facilitates osmotic movement of water out of the brain tissue according to Starling's law and thereby helps reduce cerebral edema. Mannitol in addition also results in osmotic diuresis thereby facilitating excretion of excess sodium and water out of the body. The usual first dose of mannitol is 1 g/kg. Additional doses of 0.5 g/kg can be given as needed while monitoring serum osmolality. The usual trigger for administration is ICP elevation to > 20 mmHg for > 5 min. Mannitol effectively reduces ICP within 10–20 minutes of infusion and the effect may last up to 4–6 hours. As mannitol induces diuresis, it is also important to maintain relative euvolemia as volume depletion in the setting of elevated ICP can lower CBF and increase ischemic complications.

Mannitol was used in 17 out of 34 patients with ALF and was found to resolve cerebral edema with greater frequency than in those patients who did not receive it (Canalese et al., 1982). Problems arise with its use in the presence of renal failure as mannitol can lead to volume overload which may necessitate the use of dialysis to remove three times the given volume, 15–30 minutes following infusion. Mannitol has traditionally been used cautiously when the osmolality reaches > 320 mOsm for fear of toxicity, especially in renal failure. This concern comes from a small study in which high doses of mannitol were used as continuous infusions. Crossing the 320 mOsm threshold may probably be safe (Diringer and Zazulia, 2004), but caution is advised as patients with ALF are already at risk of acute renal failure from hepatorenal syndrome.

Alternatively, hypertonic saline can be used. Induction and maintenance of hypernatremia can reduce the incidence and severity of intracranial hypertension in patients with ALF (Murphy et al., 2004). The ability of an intact blood–brain barrier (BBB) to exclude a given compound is expressed as reflection coefficient (zero = freely permeable and 1 = completely impermeable) (Schell et al., 1996; Paczynski, 1997). Compounds with reflection coefficient approaching 1 are theoretically better osmotic agents because they are completely excluded by an intact BBB and therefore are less likely to exhibit rebound cerebral edema. Sodium has a reflection coefficient of 1.0 for the BBB, hence in theory, hypertonic saline is an effective dehydrating agent (mannitol has reflection coefficient of 0.9) and reduces brain water content in humans and animal models (Suarez, 2004). Other mechanisms which may possibly play a role include enhanced microvascular blood flow and maintenance of integrity of BBB (Raghavan and Marik, 2006). In ALF patients at high risk of cerebral edema, induced hypernatremia in the range of 145–155 mEq/L with hypertonic saline is currently recommended (Lee et al., 2012). This can be achieved either by bolus doses or continuous infusion of hypertonic saline. The different available concentrations are 3%, 7.5%, 10%, and 23.4%. Potential complications with hypertonic saline include transient hypotension, pulmonary edema and heart failure, hypokalemia, hyperchloremic acidemia, coagulopathy, intravascular hemolysis, myelinolysis (only with rapid overcorrection of pre-existing hyponatremia), and encephalopathy (Worthley et al., 1988; Bhardwaj and Ulatowski, 2004a). Phlebitis can occur if peripheral venous access is used for infusion.

Serum sodium level has to be monitored when hyperosmolar therapy is used. It is generally accepted that hypertonic saline should not be used if the serum sodium level is > 160 mEq/L. In a study of 600 patients in the neurointensive care unit, there was an independent increase in mortality in patients with serum sodium > 160 mEq/L (Aiyagari et al., 2006). In the same study, the incidence of renal failure was also high in patients with hypernatremia.

Whether to choose mannitol or hypertonic saline depends upon the clinical situation. No study has proven superiority of one therapy over the other.

Propofol, a highly lipophilic agent, has been used extensively in the ICU for sedation of mechanically ventilated patients (Marik, 2004). Importantly, its rapid onset and short duration of action (Fulton and Sorkin, 1995) makes it easier to follow neurologic status of comatose patients, as wakefulness returns rapidly following discontinuation of infusion. Propofol has been reported to reduce cerebral metabolic rate, cerebral blood flow, and ICP (Vandesteene et al., 1988;

Newman et al., 1995; Ergun et al., 2002; Jalan, 2005). Its pharmacokinetic properties and protein binding remain largely unaffected even in patients with liver failure (Servin et al., 1988a, b; Veroli et al., 1992; Costela et al., 1996). Propofol may also have a neuroprotective role mediated through GABA receptors (Ito et al., 1999) and potentially through its antioxidant properties (Sagara et al., 1999). In seven patients with ALF treated with an infusion of 50 µg/kg/min, ICP remained within normal limits in six (Wijdicks and Nyberg, 2002).

Propofol has favorable pharmacokinetics and along with its potential to reduce ICP (Merlo et al., 1991; Watts et al., 1998; Wijdicks and Nyberg, 2002) in patients with elevated intracranial pressure, it should be considered as an option for this purpose, even perhaps as a first-line agent. The suggested dose is 1–3 mg/kg/hour. A major side-effect is hypotension, which is usually transient following a bolus. Another rare but potentially life-threatening complication, when used at high doses of ~5 mg/kg/hour, is propofol infusion syndrome (PRIS), a state of severe metabolic acidosis and circulatory collapse. However, this complication is rare, predominantly seen at high doses and in younger patients, and should not preclude its use. Besides, patients with ALF would only need it for short period of time.

Barbiturates are an option in cases resistant to hyperosmolar therapy. This is usually achieved with pentobarbital or pentothal infusion. Some experience has been published and in one study (Forbes et al., 1989) thiopental coma was induced in 13 cases of fulminant hepatic failure with intracranial hypertension unresponsive to other modes of therapy. All had developed acute renal failure. ICP was measured by extradural transducers. The dosage of thiopental was adjusted incrementally until intracranial pressure was normalized or hypotension developed. ICP was reduced by a median dose of 250 mg of thiopental given over 15 minutes. Eight cases needed continuing infusion. Five patients made complete recovery and there were only three deaths from IH. Side-effects included minor hypotension controlled by dose reduction. It should be recognized that barbiturate clearance is markedly reduced in patients with ALF precluding neurologic assessment for prolonged periods of time, thus making it a less attractive option to treat IH. A common dose of thiopental is 4 mg/kg loading dose followed by infusion starting at 1 mg/kg/hour with gradual upward titration until ICP control is established or hypotension develops. A common method of monitoring these patients is EEG, as patients undergoing barbiturate coma have no clinical examination. Dose can be titrated up until burst suppression is achieved on EEG.

Mild hypothermia (35°C) in rat models of acute liver failure was found to prevent the development of brain edema. A proposed mechanism of this action was inhibition of blood–brain transfer of ammonia at least in part from reduced cerebral blood flow (Butterworth, 2001; Chatauret et al., 2001). In humans, several uncontrolled studies suggest effective control of brain edema and intracranial hypertension with the induction of hypothermia (core temperature 32–35°C) (Jacob et al., 2009; Stravitz and Larsen, 2009). Potential deleterious effects of hypothermia include increased risk of infection, coagulation disturbance, and cardiac arrhythmias.

OUTCOME

Although liver transplantation may seem a necessary step in most patients, only 25% actually receive it, either because of spontaneous recovery from paracetamol (acetaminophen) toxicity or due to failure to find a suitable liver match. Usually patients are grafted within 3 days of hospitalization as the window of opportunity is small (Lee and Wijdicks, 2008).

It is important to quickly and accurately predict which patients have a good chance of recovering spontaneously and which patients will need emergency liver transplantation. This distinction is important as the patients who will eventually recover spontaneously can be spared the hazards of transplantation and lifelong immunosuppression. This will also save precious and scarce organs for those who will need them the most. In a large study in 2002, etiology of acute liver failure was one of the important predictors of outcome (Ostapowicz et al., 2002). Transplant free survival was more than 50% with paracetamol (acetaminophen), hepatitis A, shock liver, or pregnancy-related disease, whereas it was less than 25% for all other etiologies. Patients with grade III or IV hepatic encephalopathy are less likely to survive without transplantation than those with grade I or grade II. A model for end stage liver disease (MELD) score has been tested in ALF from paracetamol (acetaminophen) toxicity but was not found to be superior to INR or King's College criteria (KCC) (Schmidt and Larsen, 2007). The Clichy criteria developed in a cohort of French patients used factor V level measurements to predict outcome. Serum factor V level of less than 20% in patients younger than 30 years of age or less than 30% in any patient with grade 3–4 encephalopathy predicted mortality with a positive predictive value of 82% and a negative predictive value of 98%. At present, KCC is the most commonly used prognostic tool, with a sensitivity of 68–69% and specificity of 82–92% (Bailey et al., 2003; McPhail et al., 2010).

Auxiliary partial orthotopic liver transplantation was tested in both adults and children in a small study done in France and was found to be a feasible option. In this procedure, the native liver is left in place and a graft (auxiliary liver) is implanted to temporarily support the native liver until its function recovers. This way immunosuppression can be limited to the time period for which the auxiliary liver is in place. In this study, regeneration of the native liver occurred in 11 of 15 patients and in 8 of 10 survivors. Six of these eight patients had permanently stopped immunosuppressant therapy (Jaeck et al., 2002). Similar findings were reported in one other study (Chenard-Neu et al., 1996).

Living donor liver transplantation (LDLT) has also been attempted. Right lobe LDLT improves survival of patients with acute liver failure. In one study 7 out of 10 patients with ALF who received LDLT survived (Campsen et al., 2008). The median period of follow-up was 5 years. Five of the 10 living donors had a total of seven post-transplant complications. Currently LDLT is rarely performed. The transplant team must consider the associated complications related to the donor before proceeding.

ARTIFICIAL LIVERS

Limited experience in humans supports the use of hypothermia as a bridge to liver transplantation, cooling to a core temperature of 32–33°C, in cases of intracranial hypertension which are refractory to mannitol or hypertonic saline (Jalan et al., 2004).

Artificial liver support systems can work as a bridge for patients with severe liver disease, either to give them time to recover or to go to transplant.

Many attempts have been made to develop artificial liver support devices (ALSD). These include nonbiologic ones such as hemodialysis, charcoal hemoperfusion, selective plasma filtration, plasma exchange, hemodiadsorption, albumin dialysis, and biologic ones such as whole liver perfusion, liver cell transplantation, and bioartificial liver support.

Use of albumin-collodion microencapsulated activated charcoal (ACAC) hemoperfusion in fulminant hepatic coma showed promising results in rat models (Chirito et al., 1977). However, randomized trial using charcoal hemoperfusion in fulminant hepatic failure in humans did not show any benefit (O'Grady et al., 1988).

The molecular adsorbent recycling system (MARS) used a membrane impermeable to proteins but capable of exchanging water soluble and protein-bound toxins and a recycled protein containing dialysate (Stange et al., 1999). A meta-analysis of studies using MARS did not show significant survival benefit in patients with liver failure when compared with standard medical therapy (Khuroo and Farahat, 2004). Randomized trials are needed to define the role of MARS in the treatment of these patients.

A bioartificial liver (BAL) is a bioreactor charged with liver cells that is connected externally to the circulation. In animal models they have been shown to prolong survival significantly in comparison to the standard treatment (Flendrig et al., 1999; Hochleitner et al., 2006; Kawazoe et al., 2006). Five systems have been tested clinically. HepatAssist™ is a BAL based on porcine hepatocytes. In a prospective randomized controlled trial it demonstrated safety and improved survival in patients with fulminant/subfulminant hepatic failure (Demetriou et al., 2004).

Another bridging method is hepatocyte infusion. Using advanced femoral artery catheter, cryopreserved human hepatocytes are infused into the splenic artery. These hepatocytes appear to survive and even proliferate in the spleen, resulting in a 40–60% reduction of ammonia levels (Strom et al., 1997).

Artificial support systems have not been shown to reliably reduce mortality in the setting of ALF (Kjaergard et al., 2003; McKenzie et al., 2008). The standard of care continues to be urgent cadaveric liver transplantation. The concept of a bioengineered liver is only in a very preliminary and experimental phase (Chan et al., 2004; Diekmann et al., 2006; Linke et al., 2007; Fiegel et al., 2008; Ishii et al., 2008).

REFERENCES

Aggarwal S, Kramer D, Yonas H et al. (1994). Cerebral hemodynamic and metabolic changes in fulminant hepatic failure: a retrospective study. Hepatology 19: 80–87.

Aiyagari V, Deibert E, Diringer MN (2006). Hypernatremia in the neurologic intensive care unit: how high is too high? J Crit Care 21: 163–172.

Averbuch-Heller L, Meiner Z (1995). Reversible periodic alternating gaze deviation in hepatic encephalopathy. Neurology 45: 191–192.

Bailey B, Amre DK, Gaudreault P (2003). Fulminant hepatic failure secondary to acetaminophen poisoning: a systematic review and meta-analysis of prognostic criteria determining the need for liver transplantation. Crit Care Med 31: 299–305.

Bassett ML, Mullen KD, Skolnick P et al. (1987). Amelioration of hepatic encephalopathy by pharmacologic antagonism of the GABAA-benzodiazepine receptor complex in a rabbit model of fulminant hepatic failure. Gastroenterology 93: 1069–1077.

Belay ED, Bresee JS, Holman RC et al. (1999). Reye's syndrome in the United States from 1981 through 1997. N Engl J Med 340: 1377–1382.

Bernal W, Hall C, Karvellas CJ et al. (2007). Arterial ammonia and clinical risk factors for encephalopathy and intracranial hypertension in acute liver failure. Hepatology 46: 1844–1852.

Bhardwaj A, Ulatowski JA (2004a). Hypertonic saline solutions in brain injury. Curr Opin Crit Care 10: 126–131.

Bhardwaj A, Ulatowski JA (2004b). Hypertonic saline solutions in brain injury. Curr Opin Crit Care 10: 126–131.

Bhatia V, Batra Y, Acharya SK (2004). Prophylactic phenytoin does not improve cerebral edema or survival in acute liver failure – a controlled clinical trial. J Hepatol 41: 89–96.

Bismuth H, Samuel D, Gugenheim J et al. (1987). Emergency liver transplantation for fulminant hepatitis. Ann Intern Med 107: 337–341.

Blei AT (2001). Pathophysiology of brain edema in fulminant hepatic failure, revisited. Metab Brain Dis 16: 85–94.

Blei AT, Larsen FS (1999). Pathophysiology of cerebral edema in fulminant hepatic failure. J Hepatol 31: 771–776.

Blei AT, Olafsson S, Webster S et al. (1993). Complications of intracranial pressure monitoring in fulminant hepatic failure. Lancet 341: 157–158.

Boks AL, Brommer EJ, Schalm SW et al. (1986). Hemostasis and fibrinolysis in severe liver failure and their relation to hemorrhage. Hepatology 6: 79–86.

Brandsaeter B, Hockerstedt K, Friman S et al. (2002). Fulminant hepatic failure: outcome after listing for highly urgent liver transplantation – 12 years experience in the Nordic countries. Liver Transpl 8: 1055–1062.

Butterworth RF (2001). Mild hypothermia prevents cerebral edema in acute liver failure. J Hepatobiliary Pancreat Surg 8: 16–19.

Butterworth RF (2003). Molecular neurobiology of acute liver failure. Semin Liver Dis 23: 251–258.

Campsen J, Blei AT, Emond JC et al. (2008). Outcomes of living donor liver transplantation for acute liver failure: the adult-to-adult living donor liver transplantation cohort study. Liver Transpl 14: 1273–1280.

Canalese J, Gimson AE, Davis C et al. (1982). Controlled trial of dexamethasone and mannitol for the cerebral oedema of fulminant hepatic failure. Gut 23: 625–629.

Caplan LR, Scheiner D (1980). Dysconjugate gaze in hepatic coma. Ann Neurol 8: 328–329.

Chan C, Berthiaume F, Nath BD et al. (2004). Hepatic tissue engineering for adjunct and temporary liver support: critical technologies. Liver Transpl 10: 1331–1342.

Chatauret N, Rose C, Therrien G et al. (2001). Mild hypothermia prevents cerebral edema and CSF lactate accumulation in acute liver failure. Metab Brain Dis 16: 95–102.

Chenard-Neu MP, Boudjema K, Bernuau J et al. (1996). Auxiliary liver transplantation: regeneration of the native liver and outcome in 30 patients with fulminant hepatic failure – a multicenter European study. Hepatology 23: 1119–1127.

Chirito E, Reiter B, Lister C et al. (1977). Artificial liver: the effect of ACAC microencapsulated charcoal hemoperfusion on fulminant hepatic failure. Artif Organs 1: 76–83.

Clemmesen JO, Larsen FS, Kondrup J et al. (1999). Cerebral herniation in patients with acute liver failure is correlated with arterial ammonia concentration. Hepatology 29: 648–653.

Conomy JP, Swash M (1968). Reversible decerebrate and decorticate postures in hepatic coma. N Engl J Med 278: 876–879.

Costela JL, Jimenez R, Calvo R et al. (1996). Serum protein binding of propofol in patients with renal failure or hepatic cirrhosis. Acta Anaesthesiol Scand 40: 741–745.

Demetriou AA, Brown RS Jr, Busuttil RW et al. (2004). Prospective, randomized, multicenter, controlled trial of a bioartificial liver in treating acute liver failure. Ann Surg 239: 660–667, discussion 667–670.

Dethloff TJ, Knudsen GM, Larsen FS (2008). Cerebral blood flow autoregulation in experimental liver failure. J Cereb Blood Flow Metab 28: 916–926.

Detry O, De Roover A, Coimbra C et al. (2007). Cadaveric liver transplantation for non-acetaminophen fulminant hepatic failure: a 20-year experience. World J Gastroenterol 13: 1427–1430.

Diekmann S, Bader A, Schmitmeier S (2006). Present and future developments in hepatic tissue engineering for liver support systems: state of the art and future developments of hepatic cell culture techniques for the use in liver support systems. Cytotechnology 50: 163–179.

Diringer MN, Zazulia AR (2004). Osmotic therapy: fact and fiction. Neurocrit Care 1: 219–233.

Durham S, Yonas H, Aggarwal S et al. (1995). Regional cerebral blood flow and CO_2 reactivity in fulminant hepatic failure. J Cereb Blood Flow Metab 15: 329–335.

Eefsen M, Dethloff T, Frederiksen HJ et al. (2007). Comparison of terlipressin and noradrenalin on cerebral perfusion, intracranial pressure and cerebral extracellular concentrations of lactate and pyruvate in patients with acute liver failure in need of inotropic support. J Hepatol 47: 381–386.

Ellis AJ, Wendon JA, Williams R (2000). Subclinical seizure activity and prophylactic phenytoin infusion in acute liver failure: a controlled clinical trial. Hepatology 32: 536–541.

Emond JC, Aran PP, Whitington PF et al. (1989). Liver transplantation in the management of fulminant hepatic failure. Gastroenterology 96: 1583–1588.

Ergun R, Akdemir G, Sen S et al. (2002). Neuroprotective effects of propofol following global cerebral ischemia in rats. Neurosurg Rev 25: 95–98.

Ferenci P, Lockwood A, Mullen K et al. (2002). Hepatic encephalopathy – definition, nomenclature, diagnosis, and quantification: final report of the working party at the 11th World Congresses of Gastroenterology, Vienna, 1998. Hepatology 35: 716–721.

Ficker DM, Westmoreland BF, Sharbrough FW (1997). Epileptiform abnormalities in hepatic encephalopathy. J Clin Neurophysiol 14: 230–234.

Fiegel HC, Kaufmann PM, Bruns H et al. (2008). Hepatic tissue engineering: from transplantation to customized cell-based liver directed therapies from the laboratory. J Cell Mol Med 12: 56–66.

Flendrig LM, Calise F, Di Florio E et al. (1999). Significantly improved survival time in pigs with complete liver ischemia treated with a novel bioartificial liver. Int J Artif Organs 22: 701–709.

Forbes A, Alexander GJ, O'Grady JG et al. (1989). Thiopental infusion in the treatment of intracranial hypertension complicating fulminant hepatic failure. Hepatology 10: 306–310.

Fujiwara K, Mochida S (2002). Indications and criteria for liver transplantation for fulminant hepatic failure. J Gastroenterol 37 (Suppl 13): 74–77.

Fulton B, Sorkin EM (1995). Propofol. An overview of its pharmacology and a review of its clinical efficacy in intensive care sedation. Drugs 50: 636–657.

Gabor AJ, Brooks AG, Scobey RP et al. (1984). Intracranial pressure during epileptic seizures. Electroencephalogr Clin Neurophysiol 57: 497–506.

Grimm G, Ferenci P, Katzenschlager R et al. (1988). Improvement of hepatic encephalopathy treated with flumazenil. Lancet 2: 1392–1394.

Heubi JE, Daugherty CC, Partin JS et al. (1984). Grade I Reye's syndrome – outcome and predictors of progression to deeper coma grades. N Engl J Med 311: 1539–1542.

Hochleitner B, Hengster P, Bucher H et al. (2006). Significant survival prolongation in pigs with fulminant hepatic failure treated with a novel microgravity-based bioartificial liver. Artif Organs 30: 906–914.

Ishii Y, Saito R, Marushima H et al. (2008). Hepatic reconstruction from fetal porcine liver cells using a radial flow bioreactor. World J Gastroenterol 14: 2740–2747.

Ito H, Watanabe Y, Isshiki A et al. (1999). Neuroprotective properties of propofol and midazolam, but not pentobarbital, on neuronal damage induced by forebrain ischemia, based on the GABAA receptors. Acta Anaesthesiol Scand 43: 153–162.

Jacob S, Khan A, Jacobs ER et al. (2009). Prolonged hypothermia as a bridge to recovery for cerebral edema and intracranial hypertension associated with fulminant hepatic failure. Neurocrit Care 11: 242–246.

Jaeck D, Boudjema K, Audet M et al. (2002). Auxiliary partial orthotopic liver transplantation (APOLT) in the treatment of acute liver failure. J Gastroenterol 37 (Suppl 13): 88–91.

Jalan R (2005). Pathophysiological basis of therapy of raised intracranial pressure in acute liver failure. Neurochem Int 47: 78–83.

Jalan R, Olde Damink SW, Deutz NE et al. (2004). Moderate hypothermia in patients with acute liver failure and uncontrolled intracranial hypertension. Gastroenterology 127: 1338–1346.

Jones EA, Skolnick P, Gammal SH et al. (1989). NIH conference. The gamma-aminobutyric acid A (GABAA) receptor complex and hepatic encephalopathy. Some recent advances. Ann Intern Med 110: 532–546.

Jones EA, Basile AS, Mullen KD et al. (1990). Flumazenil: potential implications for hepatic encephalopathy. Pharmacol Ther 45: 331–343.

Kato M, Hughes RD, Keays RT et al. (1992). Electron microscopic study of brain capillaries in cerebral edema from fulminant hepatic failure. Hepatology 15: 1060–1066.

Kawazoe Y, Eguchi S, Sugiyama N et al. (2006). Comparison between bioartificial and artificial liver for the treatment of acute liver failure in pigs. World J Gastroenterol 12: 7503–7507.

Khashab M, Tector AJ, Kwo PY (2007). Epidemiology of acute liver failure. Curr Gastroenterol Rep 9: 66–73.

Khuroo MS, Farahat KL (2004). Molecular adsorbent recirculating system for acute and acute-on-chronic liver failure: a meta-analysis. Liver Transpl 10: 1099–1106.

Kjaergard LL, Liu J, Als-Nielsen B et al. (2003). Artificial and bioartificial support systems for acute and acute-on-chronic liver failure: a systematic review. JAMA 289: 217–222.

Laffey JG, Kavanagh BP (2002). Hypocapnia. N Engl J Med 347: 43–53.

Lavoie J, Layrargues GP, Butterworth RF (1990). Increased densities of peripheral-type benzodiazepine receptors in brain autopsy samples from cirrhotic patients with hepatic encephalopathy. Hepatology 11: 874–878.

Le TV, Rumbak MJ, Liu SS et al. (2010). Insertion of intracranial pressure monitors in fulminant hepatic failure patients: early experience using recombinant factor VII. Neurosurgery 66: 455–458, discussion 458.

Lee WM, Wijdicks EF (2008). Fulminant hepatic failure: when the hepatologist meets the neurointensivist. Neurocrit Care 9: 1–2.

Lee WM, Squires RH Jr, Nyberg SL et al. (2008). Acute liver failure: Summary of a workshop. Hepatology 47: 1401–1415.

Lee WM, Stravitz RT, Larson AM (2012). Introduction to the revised American Association for the Study of Liver Diseases position paper on acute liver failure 2011. Hepatology 55: 965–967.

Lidofsky SD, Bass NM, Prager MC et al. (1992). Intracranial pressure monitoring and liver transplantation for fulminant hepatic failure. Hepatology 16: 1–7.

Linke K, Schanz J, Hansmann J et al. (2007). Engineered liver-like tissue on a capillarized matrix for applied research. Tissue Eng 13: 2699–2707.

McKenzie TJ, Lillegard JB, Nyberg SL (2008). Artificial and bioartificial liver support. Semin. Liver Dis 28: 210–217.

McKinney AM, Lohman BD, Sarikaya B et al. (2010). Acute hepatic encephalopathy: diffusion-weighted and fluid-attenuated inversion recovery findings, and correlation with plasma ammonia level and clinical outcome. Am J Neuroradiol 31: 1471–1479.

McPhail MJ, Wendon JA, Bernal W (2010). Meta-analysis of performance of Kings's College Hospital Criteria in prediction of outcome in non-paracetamol-induced acute liver failure. J Hepatol 53: 492–499.

Madl C, Grimm G, Ferenci P et al. (1994). Serial recording of sensory evoked potentials: a noninvasive prognostic indicator in fulminant liver failure. Hepatology 20: 1487–1494.

Manley GT, Fujimura M, Ma T et al. (2000). Aquaporin-4 deletion in mice reduces brain edema after acute water intoxication and ischemic stroke. Nat Med 6: 159–163.

Marik PE (2004). Propofol: therapeutic indications and side-effects. Curr Pharm Des 10: 3639–3649.

Merlo F, Demo P, Lacquaniti L et al. (1991). Propofol in single bolus for treatment of elevated intracranial hypertension. Minerva Anestesiol 57: 359–363.

Meythaler JM, Varma RR (1987). Reye's syndrome in adults. Diagnostic considerations. Arch Intern Med 147: 61–64.

Mokri B (2001). The Monro-Kellie hypothesis: applications in CSF volume depletion. Neurology 56: 1746–1748.

Montalti R, Nardo B, Beltempo P et al. (2005). Liver transplantation in fulminant hepatic failure: experience with 40 adult

patients over a 17-year period. Transplant Proc 37: 1085–1087.

Munoz SJ (1993). Difficult management problems in fulminant hepatic failure. Semin Liver Dis 13: 395–413.

Munoz SJ, Ballas SK, Moritz MJ et al. (1989). Perioperative management of fulminant and subfulminant hepatic failure with therapeutic plasmapheresis. Transplant Proc 21: 3535–3536.

Munoz SJ, Robinson M, Northrup B et al. (1991). Elevated intracranial pressure and computed tomography of the brain in fulminant hepatocellular failure. Hepatology 13: 209–212.

Munoz SJ, Stravitz RT, Gabriel DA (2009). Coagulopathy of acute liver failure. Clin Liver Dis 13: 95–107.

Murphy N, Auzinger G, Bernel W et al. (2004). The effect of hypertonic sodium chloride on intracranial pressure in patients with acute liver failure. Hepatology 39: 464–470.

Newman MF, Murkin JM, Roach G et al. (1995). Cerebral physiologic effects of burst suppression doses of propofol during nonpulsatile cardiopulmonary bypass. CNS Subgroup of McSPI. Anesth Analg 81: 452–457.

Norenberg MD (1998). Astroglial dysfunction in hepatic encephalopathy. Metab Brain Dis 13: 319–335.

O'Grady J (2007). Modern management of acute liver failure. Clin Liver Dis 11: 291–303.

O'Grady JG, Gimson AE, O'Brien CJ et al. (1988). Controlled trials of charcoal hemoperfusion and prognostic factors in fulminant hepatic failure. Gastroenterology 94: 1186–1192.

Ostapowicz G, Fontana RJ, Schiodt FV et al. (2002). Results of a prospective study of acute liver failure at 17 tertiary care centers in the United States. Ann Intern Med 137: 947–954.

Paczynski RP (1997). Osmotherapy. Basic concepts and controversies. Crit Care Clin 13: 105–129.

Pavese P, Bonadona A, Beaubien J et al. (2005). FVIIa corrects the coagulopathy of fulminant hepatic failure but may be associated with thrombosis: a report of four cases. Can J Anaesth 52: 26–29.

Pereira SP, Rowbotham D, Fitt S et al. (2005). Pharmacokinetics and efficacy of oral versus intravenous mixed-micellar phylloquinone (vitamin K_1) in severe acute liver disease. J Hepatol 42: 365–370.

Raghavan M, Marik PE (2006). Therapy of intracranial hypertension in patients with fulminant hepatic failure. Neurocrit Care 4: 179–189.

Ranjan P, Mishra AM, Kale R et al. (2005). Cytotoxic edema is responsible for raised intracranial pressure in fulminant hepatic failure: in vivo demonstration using diffusion-weighted MRI in human subjects. Metab Brain Dis 20: 181–192.

Rao KV, Norenberg MD (2001). Cerebral energy metabolism in hepatic encephalopathy and hyperammonemia. Metab Brain Dis 16: 67–78.

Record CO, Chase RA, Hughes RD et al. (1975). Glycerol therapy for cerebral oedema complicating fulminant hepatic failure. Br Med J 2: 540.

Rolando N, Wade J, Davalos M et al. (2000). The systemic inflammatory response syndrome in acute liver failure. Hepatology 32: 734–739.

Rothstein JD, Herlong HF (1989). Neurologic manifestations of hepatic disease. Neurol Clin 7: 563–578.

Russo MW, Galanko JA, Shrestha R et al. (2004). Liver transplantation for acute liver failure from drug induced liver injury in the United States. Liver Transpl 10: 1018–1023.

Sagara Y, Hendler S, Khoh-Reiter S et al. (1999). Propofol hemisuccinate protects neuronal cells from oxidative injury. J Neurochem 73: 2524–2530.

Schell RM, Applegate RL 2nd, Cole DJ (1996). Salt, starch, and water on the brain. J Neurosurg Anesthesiol 8: 178–182.

Schmidt LE, Larsen FS (2007). MELD score as a predictor of liver failure and death in patients with acetaminophen-induced liver injury. Hepatology 45: 789–796.

Servin F, Desmonts JM, Farinotti R et al. (1988a). Pharmacokinetics of propofol administered by continuous infusion in patients with cirrhosis. Preliminary results. Anaesthesia 43 (Suppl): 23–24.

Servin F, Desmonts JM, Haberer JP et al. (1988b). Pharmacokinetics and protein binding of propofol in patients with cirrhosis. Anesthesiology 69: 887–891.

Shah AK, Fuerst D, Sood S et al. (2007). Seizures lead to elevation of intracranial pressure in children undergoing invasive EEG monitoring. Epilepsia 48: 1097–1103.

Shami VM, Caldwell SH, Hespenheide EE et al. (2003). Recombinant activated factor VII for coagulopathy in fulminant hepatic failure compared with conventional therapy. Liver Transpl 9: 138–143.

Shawcross DL, Davies NA, Mookerjee RP et al. (2004). Worsening of cerebral hyperemia by the administration of terlipressin in acute liver failure with severe encephalopathy. Hepatology 39: 471–475.

Simpson KJ, Bates CM, Henderson NC et al. (2009). The utilization of liver transplantation in the management of acute liver failure: comparison between acetaminophen and non-acetaminophen etiologies. Liver Transpl 15: 600–609.

Stange J, Mitzner SR, Risler T et al. (1999). Molecular adsorbent recycling system (MARS): clinical results of a new membrane-based blood purification system for bioartificial liver support. Artif Organs 23: 319–330.

Stravitz RT, Larsen FS (2009). Therapeutic hypothermia for acute liver failure. Crit Care Med 37: S258–S264.

Stravitz RT, Lisman T, Luketic VA et al. (2012). Minimal effects of acute liver injury/acute liver failure on hemostasis as assessed by thromboelastography. J Hepatol 56: 129–136.

Strom SC, Fisher RA, Thompson MT et al. (1997). Hepatocyte transplantation as a bridge to orthotopic liver transplantation in terminal liver failure. Transplantation 63: 559–569.

Suarez JI (2004). Hypertonic saline for cerebral edema and elevated intracranial pressure. Cleve Clin J Med 71 (Suppl 1): S9–S13.

Tofteng F, Jorgensen L, Hansen BA et al. (2002). Cerebral microdialysis in patients with fulminant hepatic failure. Hepatology 36: 1333–1340.

Trey C, Davidson CS (1970). The management of fulminant hepatic failure. Prog Liver Dis 3: 282–298.

Vandesteene A, Trempont V, Engelman E et al. (1988). Effect of propofol on cerebral blood flow and metabolism in man. Anaesthesia 43 (Suppl): 42–43.

Vaquero J, Polson J, Chung C et al. (2003). Infection and the progression of hepatic encephalopathy in acute liver failure. Gastroenterology 125: 755–764.

Vaquero J, Fontana RJ, Larson AM et al. (2005). Complications and use of intracranial pressure monitoring in patients with acute liver failure and severe encephalopathy. Liver Transpl 11: 1581–1589.

Veroli P, O'Kelly B, Bertrand F et al. (1992). Extrahepatic metabolism of propofol in man during the anhepatic phase of orthotopic liver transplantation. Br J Anaesth 68: 183–186.

Wakai A, Roberts I, Schierhout G (2007). Mannitol for acute traumatic brain injury. Cochrane Database Syst Rev CD001049.

Ware AJ, D'Agostino AN, Combes B (1971). Cerebral edema: a major complication of massive hepatic necrosis. Gastroenterology 61: 877–884.

Watts AD, Eliasziw M, Gelb AW (1998). Propofol and hyperventilation for the treatment of increased intracranial pressure in rabbits. Anesth Analg 87: 564–568.

Wijdicks EF (2009). Neurologic complications of acute liver failure. In: Neurologic Complications of Critical Illness, Contemporary Neurology, 3rd edn. Vol. 74. Oxford University Press, New York, pp. 204–217.

Wijdicks EF, Nyberg SL (2002). Propofol to control intracranial pressure in fulminant hepatic failure. Transplant Proc 34: 1220–1222.

Wijdicks EF, Plevak DJ, Rakela J et al. (1995). Clinical and radiologic features of cerebral edema in fulminant hepatic failure. Mayo Clin Proc 70: 119–124.

Williams R (1975). Artificial liver support in fulminant hepatic failure. Bull N Y Acad Med 51: 508–518.

Worthley LI, Cooper DJ, Jones N (1988). Treatment of resistant intracranial hypertension with hypertonic saline. Report of two cases. J Neurosurg 68: 478–481.

Zacharski LR, Litin EM, Mulder DW et al. (1970). Acute, fatal hepatic failure presenting with psychiatric symptoms. Am J Psychiatry 127: 382–386.

Handbook of Clinical Neurology, Vol. 120 (3rd series)
Neurologic Aspects of Systemic Disease Part II
Jose Biller and Jose M. Ferro, Editors

Chapter 45

Portosystemic encephalopathy

KARIN WEISSENBORN*

Department of Neurology, Hanover Medical School, Hanover, Germany

HISTORY

Scientific interest in the relationship between the liver and the brain dates back to ancient times. The basis for our current understanding of hepatic encephalopathy (HE), however, was provided at the end of the 19th century, when Nencki, Pavlov, and Zaleski observed that dogs developed a behavioral syndrome following the formation of a portocaval shunt (Eck's fistula). Symptoms worsened after a meat feed and thus the phrase "meat intoxication syndrome" was coined. Nencki and coworkers saw that the arterial ammonia levels in the dogs increased after protein ingestion, accompanied by an increase in urinary ammonia excretion. After ammonia ingestion the dogs died. Analysis of the animals' brain ammonia content showed a fourfold increase of ammonia compared to normal. Thus, it was concluded that the behavioral changes in the animals were induced by ammonia (Shawcross et al., 2005). At the beginning of the 20th century, clinical observations led to the conclusion that there is a connection between raised ammonia levels in the blood and the development of neuropsychiatric symptoms in patients with severe liver disease (Zieve, 1991). In 1952, Phillips et al. established a regular relationship between raised ammonia levels and the development of HE. Later a detailed analysis of the clinical features of HE was performed by Dame Sheila Sherlock and her coworkers (Sherlock et al., 1954; Sherlock, 1958). It was Sherlock who coined the term "portosystemic encephalopathy" for HE in patients with liver cirrhosis. In 2002, a working party on clinical research in hepatic encephalopathy recommended changes in the terminology and the differentiation of three types of HE (Ferenci et al., 2002):

1. encephalopathy associated with acute liver failure (type A)

2. encephalopathy associated with portal-systemic bypass and no intrinsic hepatocellular disease (type B)

3. encephalopathy associated with cirrhosis and portal hypertension (type C).

CLINICAL FINDINGS

Portosystemic encephalopathy, or type C hepatic encephalopathy (HE), is characterized by disturbances of cognition, motor abilities, and consciousness. Symptoms range from minimal changes in personality or altered sleep pattern to deep coma (Sherlock et al., 1954). Sleep disturbances and slight behavioral changes are usually overlooked as they are not apparent in the clinical examination, but can be detected only by a directed inquiry. HE may stay in this covert stage for a long time but may also proceed to more severe stages with clinically obvious disturbance of consciousness: mild confusion in grade I, drowsiness, lethargy and disorientation in grade II, somnolence in grade III, and coma, with or without response to painful stimuli, in grade IV (a and b) HE (Fig. 45.1). Cognitive dysfunction is the major problem in minimal HE (mHE) and grades I and II HE. While this is obvious in grades I and II HE, it remains unnoticed with clinical examination in patients with mHE, since the patients' verbal abilities are preserved (Schomerus and Hamster, 1998). Neuropsychological examinations, however, show deficits in attention and visual perception combined with a reduction in motor speed and accuracy (Weissenborn et al., 2001). The patients are especially impaired in their mechanical skills or in tasks which require sustained attention and quick reaction. Schomerus and Hamster (1998) were able to show that mHE decreases the

---

*Correspondence to: Karin Weissenborn, M.D., Department of Neurology, Hannover Medical School, Carl-Neuberg-Str. 1, 30625 Hanover, Germany. Tel: +49-511-532-2339, Fax: +49-511-532-3115, E-mail: weissenborn.karin@mh-hannover.de

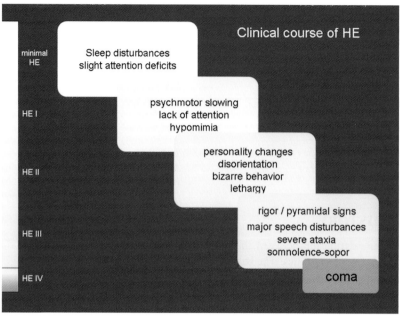

Fig. 45.1. Classification of hepatic encephalopathy according to alterations in attention and alertness (West Haven Criteria).

working ability of blue collar workers, while white collar workers are not impaired unless HE becomes clinically overt. It has repeatedly been shown that minimal HE also affects driving ability (Schomerus et al., 1981; Watanabe et al., 1995; Wein et al., 2004; Bajaj et al., 2009; Kircheis et al., 2009).

In patients with grade 1 HE lack of attention and psychomotor slowing is clinically obvious. In patients with grade 2 HE cognitive dysfunction is accompanied by a further decrease of alertness and disorientation for time and sometimes also for place and situation.

Motor symptoms such as asterixis, dysarthria, ataxia, tremor, hypokinesia, muscular rigidity, and posture abnormalities are hallmarks of hepatic encephalopathy. They are usually attributed to grade 2 HE. In practice, however, these symptoms are detectable by subtle neurologic assessment even in patients with mild HE (Krieger et al., 1996; Spahr et al., 1996). Speech disturbances and writing disabilities belong to the first symptoms of HE. Initially speech is monotonous and slow. With increasing ataxia speech becomes slurred, dysarthric. In stuporous patients dysphasia occurs combined with perseveration. Writing disabilities are traditionally used for follow-up examinations. Initially omission of single letters, reversal of order and misspellings are common. Later the patients become unable to sign their names or to move the pencil from left to right.

Hyperreflexia and ankle clonus is a characteristic finding in grade 3 HE, but can be observed also in patients with mild HE, in principle.

Personality changes are frequent. Mood fluctuates. While some of the patients appear euphoric the majority present with mild to moderate depression. Confusion, bizarre behavior, and paranoid symptoms are common in grade 2–3 HE. In addition, hallucinations may be observed (Sherlock et al., 1954; Summerskill et al., 1956).

Rare symptoms of type C HE are headaches, blurred or double vision, focal neurologic signs such as hemiparesis and epileptic seizures (Sherlock et al., 1954; Cadranel et al., 2001).

While type C HE occurs episodically in the majority of patients, some show chronic progressive symptoms. In general, these patients have extensive portosystemic shunts either developed in the course of liver cirrhosis or following shunt operation or TIPSS (transjugular intrahepatic portosystemic stent shunt). Occasionally chronic progressive HE can be observed as a complication of a congenital intrahepatic portosystemic venous shunt despite normal liver function (type B HE) (Da Rocha et al., 2004). Read et al. (1967) observed five different syndromes of chronic persistent HE in patients who had undergone shunt operations: "1. predominant psychiatric disorder, 2. paraplegia, 3. cerebellar and basal ganglia disorder, 4. paroxysmal disorders of consciousness or muscle spasms, 5. localized or generalized cortical disease." While the psychiatric disorder and paraplegia occurred within several months up to 1½ years after shunt operation in their patients, cerebellar and basal ganglia disorder was observed 7 and 8 years after the procedure.

Nowadays, paraplegia in patients with chronic liver disease is referred to as hepatic myelopathy (HM) (Campellone et al., 1996; Lewis et al., 2000). In most cases HM will develop after several episodes of HE. Upper extremities are affected minimally, if at all. Brisk tendon reflexes and increased tone of the lower extremities are the predominant findings. Plantar reflexes may be flexor, even in patients with ankle clonus. Disturbances of sensation or bladder function are uncommon. After months of progressing disability most patients either depend upon an assistive device or are confined to a wheelchair. For unknown reasons, most patients described are men.

Acquired hepatocerebral degeneration (AHD) is a further intriguing neurologic syndrome associated with extensive portosystemic shunting. While patients with AHD suffer the whole spectrum of cerebral dysfunction present in HE, cognitive dysfunction and alteration of consciousness are by far less prominent than motor dysfunction. Parkinsonism, ataxia, dystonia, chorea, and orobuccolingual dyskinesia can be observed. Parkinsonism in AHD is characterized by a rapid progression and postural instability or cognitive impairment early in the course of disease. The most characteristic motor phenotype of AHD is cranial dyskinesia, which is often intermixed with dystonic elements such as forced grimacing, jaw opening or blepharospasm (Burkhard et al., 2003; Ferrara and Jankovic, 2009).

DIFFERENTIAL DIAGNOSIS

None of the symptoms present in patients with hepatic encephalopathy proves the diagnosis of HE. Thus the exclusion of other possible causes of brain dysfunction is requested. Any patient has to undergo a thorough diagnostic workup that includes laboratory investigations and neuroimaging. Conditions that have to be considered are intracranial bleeding, especially chronic subdural haematoma, Wernicke's encephalopathy, alcohol or drug withdrawal, intoxication, hypoglycemia, electrolyte disturbances, and in rare cases encephalitis. Hyponatremia has gained special interest recently, as it could be shown that the frequency of HE increased with the reduction in serum sodium levels (15%, 24%, and 38% in patients with serum sodium > 135, 130–135, and < 130 mEq/L, respectively) (Angeli et al., 2006). Guevara et al. (2009) showed that hyponatremia is a strong predictor of the development of overt HE. Hyponatremia is considered to facilitate astrocytic swelling in patients with severe liver disease and thereby to facilitate the development of HE. Although the clinical presentation of hyponatremic and hepatic encephalopathy share only the alteration of consciousness, hyponatremia should

be addressed in every individual case before neuropsychiatric symptoms are related to HE (Cordoba et al., 2010).

Kril and Butterworth (1997) noted the high prevalence of unexpected evidence for thiamine deficiency in patients who died with HE, even in patients with nonalcoholic cirrhosis. Thus, Wernicke's encephalopathy has to be considered and thiamine should be given in case of doubt.

DIAGNOSIS OF MINIMAL HEPATIC ENCEPHALOPATHY

While the pattern of cerebral dysfunction in minimal hepatic encephalopathy (mHE) has been well known for decades (e.g., Zeegen et al., 1970; Rehnström et al., 1977; Rikkers et al., 1978; Gilberstadt et al., 1980; Tarter et al., 1984), the diagnostic approach is controversial. People working on HE seem to be evenly divided: some plead for the use of a neuropsychological test battery that is able to represent the different cognitive domains which are affected in mHE, while others aim to find a single means as surrogate marker of brain dysfunction in HE. Recently the International Society for Hepatic Encephalopathy and Nitrogen Metabolism (ISHEN) formed a commission to review the available data on the role of neuropsychological testing in HE, and to make recommendations regarding the routine assessment of patients with liver disease (Randolph et al., 2009). They recommended the use of either the Repeatable Battery for the Assessment of Neuropsychological Status (RBANS) (Randolph, 1998) or the PSE-Syndrome-Test (Schomerus et al., 1999). The choice of which battery to use should be based upon the availability of local translations and normative data. Moreover the commission recommended future systematic studies to compare approaches to diagnosing and monitoring mHE. The PSE syndrome test is a test battery consisting of five paper and pencil tests: the Number Connection Tests (NCT) A and B, the Digit Symbol Test (DST), the Serial Dotting Test (SDT), and the Line Tracing Test (LTT) (Fig. 45.2). In the NCTA the subject is asked to connect the numbers from 1 to 13 as quickly as possible. In the NCTB subjects are asked to connect numbers from 1 to 13 and letters from A to L in alternating order. In the Digit Symbol Test each of the numbers 1–9 is paired with a specific symbol in adjacent boxes. Subjects are requested to draw the missing symbol in a row of boxes filled with numbers. In the Serial Dotting Test subjects are requested to place a dot as quickly as possible in the center of 100 circles, and in the Line Tracing Test the task is to draw a continuous line between two parallel (winding) lines. The test battery is able to detect deficits in attention, visual perception, visual scanning efficiency, motor speed, and accuracy. The PSE syndrome

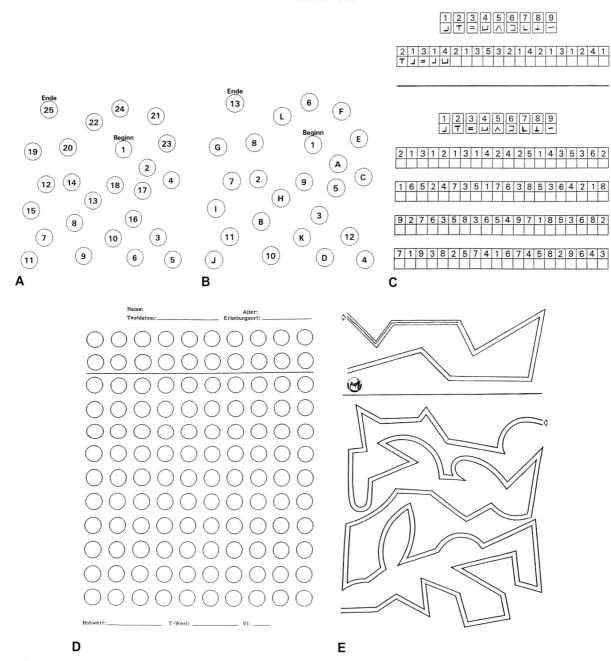

Fig. 45.2. Subtests of the PSE syndrome test (PSE-Syndrome-Test): Number Connection Test A and B, Digit Symbol Test (upper line from left to right), Serial Dotting Test, and Line Tracing Test (lower line).

test is predominantly used in Europe where normative data have been collected for the German (Schomerus et al., 1999), the Italian (Amodio et al., 2008), the Spanish (Romero-Gomez et al., 2006) and the British (Marks et al., 2008) population. Meanwhile the test has also recently been validated and standardized in Poland (Wunsch et al., 2013); and an altered test version has been standardized in India (Thumburu et al., 2008). The RBANS has been developed and standardized in the US, where it is also used predominantly (Mooney et al., 2007). This test battery contains measures of verbal and visual anterograde memory, working memory, cognitive processing speed, language (including semantic fluency), and visuospatial function (line orientation and figure copy). The results of 12 subtests are converted into age-adjusted index scores for five domains (immediate memory, visuospatial/constructional, language, attention, and delayed memory). The PSE syndrome test takes about 20 minutes for completion and evaluation, the RBANS 25–35 minutes.

Critics of the test batteries complain about the time needed to apply and evaluate the tests, the psychological expertise needed to interpret the test results, and the impact of learning effects, age, and education on test results. In addition copyright was mentioned as barrier to using the test batteries. The search for "simple" diagnostic methods has resulted so far in the recommendation of the Inhibitory Control Test (ICT), a computerized test of attention and response inhibition, which is freely available (Bajaj et al., 2007), and examination of the critical flicker frequency (CFF) (Kircheis et al., 2002). The ICT results were repeatedly shown to be worse in patients with minimal HE as diagnosed by standard psychometric tests than in patients without mHE (Bajaj et al., 2007; Amodio et al., 2010). The diagnostic use of the test, however, remains to be proven. The ICT results have been shown to depend – similar to other neuropsychological tests – upon age and education, and to some extent even upon sociocultural factors (Amodio et al., 2010), and the elaboration of normative data has still to be undertaken.

CFF was recommended for diagnosing mHE by Kircheis et al. in 2002. CFF decreases with increasing grade of HE, but there is an overlap between the normal range and the test results in patients with mHE as defined by psychometric tests. In addition, CFF in patients with alcohol-induced cirrhosis differs significantly from CFF in patients with cirrhosis from other causes. The data available at present suggest that alterations in CFF go in parallel with alterations in psychometric tests in a proportion of the patients, while a pathologic result in one of the two does not predict a pathologic result in the other (Romero-Gomez et al., 2007; Sharma et al., 2007).

Neurophysiologic methods have been used for diagnosis and follow-up of HE for decades. The majority of patients with clinically overt HE show alterations of the EEG with an increasing amount of θ and δ rhythms with increasing grade of HE, an initial increase, followed by a decrease, in EEG amplitude, a discontinuous pattern, and finally an isoelectric EEG (Fig. 45.3) (Parsons-Smith et al., 1957; Davies et al., 1991; Montagnese et al., 2004; Guerit et al., 2009). Characteristic is the appearance of triphasic waves. However, normal EEGs have been found in up to 60% of patients with distinct clinical symptoms of HE (Penin 1967; Weissenborn et al., 1990; Montagnese et al., 2007). Since EEG slowing was shown also in up to 30% of patients with liver cirrhosis but no clinical signs of encephalopathy (van der Rijt et al., 1990; Montagnese et al., 2007), EEG is used for the detection of mHE in addition to other means by several groups (Quero et al., 1996).

Visual evoked potentials (VEP), somatosensory evoked potentials (SSEP), and the P300 wave elicited in an auditory oddball paradigm have been intensively studied in patients with HE. They have been proven to be useful for follow-up examinations, as they show an increase or decrease of latency in close correlation to the clinical course of the disease. Endogenous evoked potentials in addition may provide an insight into the alteration of cognitive processes in HE. The clinical use of evoked potentials, however, is limited (Weissenborn, 1991). They are less sensitive than psychometric tests and clinical assessment. The widespread use of endogenous evoked potentials is in addition hampered by the need for sophisticated technical equipment and the need for trained personnel.

NATURAL HISTORY

The natural history of hepatic encephalopathy is not well known since long-term follow-up studies are sparse. In most cases HE is observed to occur episodically, generally related to a precipitating factor that triggers a toxin load to the brain.

Cirrhotic patients with minimal HE are more prone to develop overt HE than those without. (Romero-Gomez et al., 2001) identified altered CFF, Child–Pugh score, and mHE as diagnosed by psychometric tests to be significantly associated with lower survival and higher risk of overt HE. The percentage of patients who developed overt HE was 45% when either psychometric tests or CFF indicated abnormal scores and 3.3% in patients with normal values in both tests ($p < 0.0001$).

Dhiman et al. (2010) applied a variant of the PSE syndrome test and CFF examination to 100 patients without clinical signs of HE. Minimal HE was detected in 48% considering the PSE syndrome test sum score PHES (psychometric hepatic encephalopathy score). CFF was pathologic in 21%. The prevalence of mHE increased with increasing liver dysfunction. During follow-up of up to 2 years, 39.1% died among those who had mHE compared to 22.9% of those without HE. The probability of survival in patients with PHES ≤ -6 was 67.7% at 1 year of follow-up, and 26.4% at 2 years, compared to 88.7% at 1 year and 74.6% at 2 years in patients with PHES > -6 ($p = 0.003$). CFF was evaluated according to age-adjusted normal data in this study, and thereby did not show any predictive value.

In a recent population-based study, Jepsen et al. (2010) showed that overt HE is associated with a high mortality rate in patients with alcohol-toxic cirrhosis. Patients with HE had a median survival time of 2.4 months from its onset; 45% died within 1 month, 64% died within 1 year, and 85% died within 5 years. Of note, patients do not die *of*, but *with* hepatic encephalopathy. The presence of HE is just an indication of severe liver dysfunction.

Fichet et al. (2009) did a retrospective analysis of the case records of 71 patients who were admitted to the

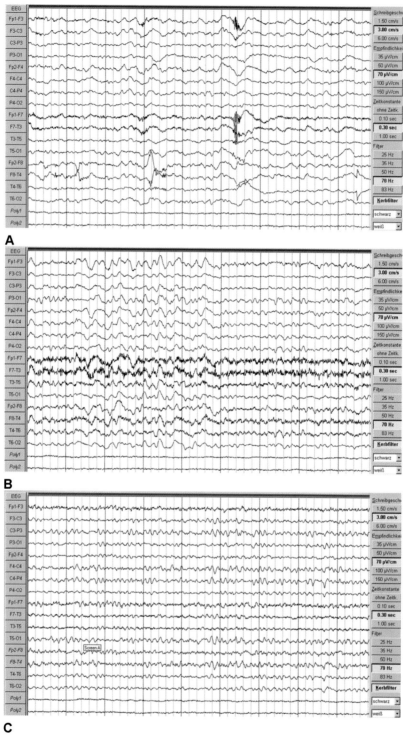

Fig. 45.3. EEG follow-up in a patient who was admitted with grade 2 hepatic encephalopathy (HE) (**A**) and swiftly improved after therapy with lactulose and antibiotics was started (**B** and **C**).

intensive care unit (ICU) of their hospital with grade III and IV HE. Mortality rate at 1 year was 54%. 35% of the patients died during ICU care. The mortality rate was 8.9% in the patients with isolated HE and 80.7% in the patients with accompanying organ dysfunction.

LABORATORY INVESTIGATIONS

Laboratory investigations and neuroimaging do not provide findings specific for HE. An elevated ammonia level hints at a potential hepatic origin of a patient's cerebral condition, but is nevertheless unspecific. Serum ammonia levels correlate broadly with stages of encephalopathy; however, there is substantial overlap between values at different stages, and ammonia levels may even be in the normal range in patients with clinical symptoms of HE.

NEUROIMAGING INVESTIGATIONS

For a while the bright pallidal hyperintensities found on T1-weighted magnetic resonance images (MRI) in about 90% of the patients with cirrhosis of the liver were considered as representative of HE (Fig. 45.4). Meanwhile it is clear that the T1 alterations are due to the deposition of manganese and depend on the presence of portosystemic shunting, while their extent relates only slightly to HE symptoms (Pujol et al., 1993; Krieger et al., 1996; Spahr et al., 1996; Pomier-Layrargues et al., 1998; Rose et al., 1999a). The MRI alterations usually disappear within 1 year after liver transplantation (Lockwood et al., 1997). Recently MRI has successfully been used to support the pathophysiologic model of a slightly increased brain water content – "a low-grade

cerebral edema" – as a milestone in the development of HE in liver cirrhosis (Häussinger et al., 2000). Methods applied were magnetization transfer ratio (MTR) imaging (Rovira et al., 2001; Balata et al., 2003), diffusion-weighted imaging (DWI) and diffusion tensor imaging (DTI) (Kale et al., 2006; Kumar et al., 2008), water content mapping (Shah et al., 2008) and T2 relaxometry (Singhal et al., 2009). While an increase of brain water content in cirrhotic patients with hepatic encephalopathy is generally agreed on, it has to be clarified by further investigations if the patient develops an intra- or extracellular edema, or both (Shah et al., 2008; Poveda et al., 2010). Proton magnetic resonance spectra (MRS) of the brain in patients with liver cirrhosis and HE shows a characteristic alteration of the metabolite pattern – a decrease in the myoinositol and choline signal intensity combined with an increase in the glutamate/glutamine (Glx) signal intensity (Fig. 45.5). These alterations rise with increasing grade of HE and MR has been shown to be a sensitive means to represent metabolic alterations in these patients, with induced hyperammonemia leading to an immediate and significant alteration of the MR spectra (Balata et al., 2003). The MRS alterations have

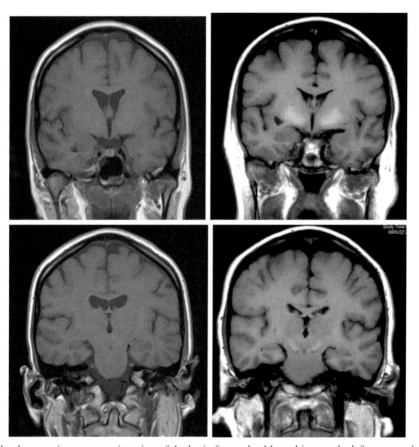

Fig. 45.4. T1-weighted magnetic resonance imaging of the brain from a healthy subject on the left compared with a patient with cirrhosis on the right. Coronal slices show bilateral hyperintensities in the pallidum and substantia nigra in the patient (due to manganese deposition).

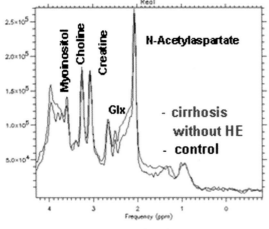

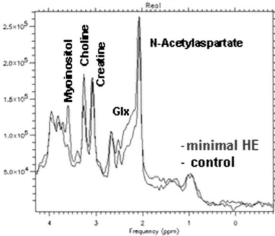

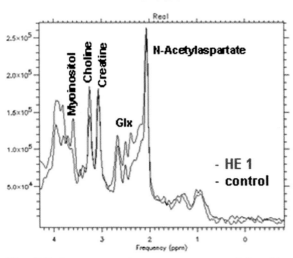

Fig. 45.5. Proton magnetic resonance spectra of the white matter in patients with liver cirrhosis but no hepatic encephalopathy) (HE) (top), minimal HE (center), and grade 1 HE (bottom) compared to a control spectrum.

also been studied for their diagnostic use but without satisfying results (Köstler, 1998; Poveda et al., 2010).

Positron emission tomography (PET) has been applied for the study of some pathophysiologic aspects of HE, such as cerebral ammonia metabolism. In 1991a, Lockwood et al. suggested a significantly increased blood–brain barrier permeability for ammonia in patients with liver cirrhosis and minimal HE compared to controls based on their findings in a 13 N-ammonia PET study. This assumption was well in line with experimental and clinical observations, and backed up the hypothesis that hyperammonemia and an increase of brain ammonia uptake were the main causes for the development of HE. Recently, their data have been contradicted by two further studies which included patients with different grades of liver disease – from mild fibrosis to cirrhosis – and different grades of HE compared to controls, and which did not find a significant difference of the blood–brain barrier permeability for ammonia between the groups (Keiding et al., 2006; Goldbecker et al., 2010). Nevertheless the metabolic flux of ammonia into glutamine was increased in the brain of cirrhotic patients compared to controls as their plasma ammonia levels were increased and in consequence also their brain ammonia levels. Ahl et al. (2004) showed significant regional differences in cerebral ammonia metabolism with an excess of ammonia supply to the basal ganglia and the cerebellum mainly due to differences in the regional cerebral blood flow (CBF).

Cagnin et al. (2006) described an increased PK 11195 binding in the basal ganglia, dorsolateral prefrontal regions, and anterior cingulate gyrus in patients with liver cirrhosis and minimal HE (Cagnin et al., 2006). PK 11195 is a specific high-affinity ligand to the "peripheral-type" benzodiazepine receptors (PTBR) (recently renamed the 18 kDa translocator protein) which in the brain are localized especially in the outer mitochondrial membrane of astrocytes and activated microglia. PTBR are considered to play a role in the pathophysiology of HE via their role in the neurosteroid synthesis (Cagnin et al., 2006). Activation of PTBR results in increased synthesis of neurosteroids – especially allopregnanolone – a potent modulator of GABA-ergic neurotransmission, which enhances GABA-elicited chloride currents and positively modulates the binding of GABA and benzodiazepines to their respective sites on the GABA-A receptor complex (Ahboucha and Butterworth, 2007).

In accordance with the clinical observation that HE especially affects the basal ganglia, the cerebellum and the "attention system," Lockwood and coworkers were able to show by [18] F-fluorodeoxyglucose PET that the glucose utilization is decreased in the cingulum and frontal and parieto-occipital cortex and increased in the basal ganglia, cerebellum, and temporomesial structures in patients with HE compared to healthy controls and patients without HE (Lockwood et al., 1993, 2002). Glucose metabolism of the cingulate gyrus and cortical areas mentioned was significantly decreased even in patients with minimal HE and was positively correlated to their neuropsychological and motor performance (Lockwood et al., 2002; Giewekemeyer et al., 2007).

PATHOLOGY/PATHOPHYSIOLOGY

The pathogenesis of HE is far from being fully understood, but there is a working hypothesis which is continuously adjusted to new findings, and which at present includes ammonia and systemic inflammation as the key players. Blood ammonia levels may be increased about two- to threefold in patients with liver cirrhosis compared to controls and brain–blood concentration ratios of ammonia increase from 2 in controls to 3–4 in patients with chronic liver failure (for comparison: the brain–blood ammonia ratio in patients with acute liver failure is 8) (Butterworth, 2002). In the brain, ammonia is detoxified by astrocytes via the synthesis of glutamine. Accordingly proton MRS studies of the brain in patients with liver cirrhosis and different grades of HE show an increase of the glutamate/glutamine signal. It is hypothesized that the brain osmolyte myoinositol is extruded from the astrocytes to avoid astrocyte swelling in spite of increasing intracellular glutamine levels and thus to maintain astrocyte function. Of note, astrocyte swelling may be induced not only by ammonia detoxification but also by other factors such as inflammatory cytokines, hyponatremia, or benzodiazepines (Häussinger et al., 2000), and in fact HE is often precipitated in patients with liver cirrhosis by concomitant disorders such as electrolyte dysbalance, sedation with benzodiazepines, or infection. The vulnerability of the brain to these factors is postulated to depend upon the extent of the myoinositol depletion. Low baseline myoinositol levels were observed to predispose for neuropsychological deterioration by an experimental amino acid load (Shawcross et al., 2004a). Comparing the response of patients with liver cirrhosis to an oral amino acid challenge in the presence of a systemic inflammation response syndrome (SIRS) and again after its solution, Shawcross et al. (2004b) were able to show that the presence of inflammation increases the effect of ammonia on brain function. Unfortunately, patients with liver cirrhosis carry an increased risk of infection, since their neutrophils and macrophages have a reduced phagocytosis capacity (Mookerjee et al., 2007). Thus the synergism between ammonia and inflammation effects can frequently be observed in these patients.

There is ample experimental evidence that astrocyte swelling induces the formation of reactive oxygen and nitrogen oxide species, including nitric oxide (NO), while on the other hand oxidative stress induces astrocyte swelling (Schliess et al., 2006; Norenberg et al., 2009). Astrocyte swelling is considered the key factor in the pathogenesis of HE as it has been shown to trigger multiple alterations of astrocyte function and gene expression in part through oxidative stress-dependent modifications of proteins and RNA. Ammonia as well as TNF-α, benzodiazepines, and hypo-osmotic swelling were shown to induce RNA oxidation in cultured astrocytes and brain slices and thereby to compromise synaptic plasticity and glutamatergic neurotransmission (Görg et al., 2008; Häussinger and Schliess, 2008). Recently, Görg et al. (2010) showed evidence for oxidative/nitrosative stress, protein tyrosine nitration, and RNA oxidation also in postmortem cortical brain tissue from patients with cirrhosis and hepatic encephalopathy.

Ammonia has also been shown to induce mitochondrial permeability transition (mPT), probably mediated by oxidative stress. Induction of the mPT leads to a collapse of the mitochondrial inner membrane potential, swelling of the mitochondrial matrix, defective oxidative phosphorylation, cessation of ATP synthesis, and finally the generation of reactive oxygen species. Thus induction of the mPT is part of the vicious circle of oxidative/nitrosative stress and astrocytic dysfunction (Norenberg et al., 2009).

The characteristic neuropathologic feature of the brain in patients who died with hepatic coma is an increase in the size and number of protoplasmatic astrocytes, the so-called Alzheimer type II astrocytes (Adams and Foley, 1952). They are characterized by large, chromatin-deficient nuclei with prominent nucleoli surrounded by a small rim of cytoplasm. The Alzheimer type II astrocytes were found in all parts of the cerebral cortex, the basal ganglia, thalamus, amygdala, midbrain, pons, and cerebellum. The number of Alzheimer type II astrocytes within the pallidum is representative for the degree of astrocytic changes in each individual case. The extent of Alzheimer type II astrocytosis is significantly correlated with blood ammonia levels and severity of encephalopathy (Martin et al., 1987). Neurons appear healthy in neuropathologic studies of the brain from patients with end stage chronic liver disease, except for those cases with "acquired hepatocerebral degeneration." Here the brain shows a patchy, spongy degeneration especially in the deep layers of cerebral cortex and subcortical white matter, particularly in the parieto-occipital cortex, basal ganglia, and cerebellum. Microscopically these regions are characterized by a diffuse increase in the size and number of protoplasmic astrocytes with glycogen inclusions and regional parenchymal degeneration with zones of pseudolaminar microcavitation, together with shrunken, pyknotic nerve cells and some swelling and fragmentation of the myelin (Victor et al., 1965; Plum and Hindfelt, 1976). Butterworth (2007) hints to the fact that neuronal cell death in brain in liver failure is considerably less than would be predicted considering the numerous cell death mechanisms present in this condition, such as NMDA receptor-mediated excitotoxicity, oxidative/nitrosative stress, and the presence of proinflammatory cytokines. Therefore he hypothesizes that the extent of neuronal damage in liver failure may be attenuated by compensatory mechanisms including downregulation of NMDA receptors or the presence of neuroprotective steroids such as allopregnanolone.

Of note, histologic alterations of the brain are most pronounced in those regions with high blood supply and thus the highest ammonia load: the basal ganglia, the cerebellum, and the cortex. The above average effect on the basal ganglia can be explained by a synergism of ammonia and manganese. Rose and coworkers (1999a) showed that the manganese concentration in postmortem brain of patients who died with HE is significantly increased compared to controls and most evident in the globus pallidus. Manganese is probably actively transported and deposited in the pallidum, thalamic nuclei, and substantia nigra (Aschner et al., 2007). Manganese deposition *per se* results in neuronal loss, Alzheimer type II astrocytosis, and alteration of dopaminergic neurotransmission (Butterworth et al., 1995). Manganese has also been shown to increase ammonia toxicity in astrocyte cultures (Jayakumar et al., 2004) and – like ammonia – to induce the expression of the "peripheral-type" benzodiazepine receptor mentioned above.

MANAGEMENT

HE episodes are frequently provoked by nutritional protein overload, gastrointestinal bleeds, infection, medication (especially sedatives or diuretics), or constipation. Therefore, identification and treatment of the precipitating factor should be the first step in its management. In addition, correction of electrolyte disturbances is essential. Considering the role of ammonia in the pathogenesis of HE, at present the main route of HE therapy aims at the reduction of ammonia production and absorption.

Nonabsorbable disaccharides – lactulose and lactitol – are an established first-line therapy in HE. The daily dose of lactulose should be titrated to result in two to four soft, acidic stools per day (30–60 g per day). In comatose patients lactulose-containing enemas (250 mL lactulose in 750 mL water) can be used instead of the oral preparation (Uribe et al., 1987). Lactitol has been shown to be as effective as lactulose (Morgan and Hawley, 1987). Lactulose is considered to be effective by several mechanisms: (1) the cathartic effect; (2) acidification of the intestinal content resulting in a reduction of ammonia absorption and net movement from ammonia from the blood into the bowel; (3) reduced bacterial production of ammonia

in the colonic lumen due to environmental changes with promotion of the growth of nonurease producing bacteria; (4) interference with the uptake of glutamine and its metabolism into NH_3 in the gut wall (Conn and Lieberthal, 1979). Lactulose therapy has been shown to reduce plasma ammonia levels (Als-Nielsen et al., 2004; Poo et al., 2006), to improve cognitive function in patients with minimal HE (Prasad et al., 2007), and to reduce interstitial brain edema in cirrhotics with mild HE with corresponding improvement in neuropsychological test scores (Kale et al., 2006). Sharma et al. (2009) showed that lactulose was effective in the secondary prevention of HE episodes. In practice, side-effects such as diarrhea, flatulence, and abdominal pain reduce patients' compliance with this therapy.

Antibiotics directed at urease-producing bacteria have similar efficacy in HE to nonabsorbable disaccharides (Als-Nielsen et al., 2004). In the past, neomycin and metronidazole have been used. Currently rifaximin, a nonabsorbed derivative of rifamycin, is recommended (Leevy and Phillips, 2007; Bass et al., 2010). It has been shown to be well tolerated, safe and efficacious in both short- and long-term use. The most recent study analyzed in a double-blind, placebo-controlled design the protective effect of rifaximin against breakthrough episodes of HE in patients with advanced liver disease, who had suffered at least two episodes of HE ≥ 2 during the previous 6 months. The study drug was added to an ongoing lactulose therapy in about 90% of the patients. Rifaximin significantly reduced the risk of an episode of HE over a 6 month period (HR 0.42, 95% CI 0.28–0.64; $p < 0.001$) and also reduced the frequency of hospitalization due to HE by half (Bass et al., 2010). The rifaximin dose applied was 550 mg twice per day.

A decrease of plasma ammonia levels can also be achieved by the application of L-ornithine-L-aspartate (LOLA). Ornithine stimulates both the urea cycle and glutamine synthesis. The major effect results from stimulation of glutamine synthesis in skeletal muscle (Rose et al., 1999b). A significant reduction of plasma ammonia levels and improvement of clinical symptoms after intravenous application of 80–120 g LOLA was shown in cirrhotic patients with grade III–IV HE as long ago as 1972 (Leonhardt and Bungert). With regard to lower grades of HE, data are contradictory (Kircheis et al., 1997; Stauch et al., 1998; Poo et al., 2006). Nevertheless LOLA (three to six sachets daily in three divided doses) is recommended in addition to or as an alternative to rifaximin if there is not complete remission of encephalopathy within 24 hours after lactulose treatment onset (Cash et al., 2010).

Studies on the use of branched-chain amino acids (BCAA) for therapy of HE date back more than 30 years. A comprehensive Cochrane review (Als-Nielsen et al., 2004) showed that compared to the control treatment,

BCAA significantly increased the number of patients improving from hepatic encephalopathy (59% versus 41%; RR 1.31; 95% confidence limits 1.04–1.66). Two recent studies of BCAA supplementation showed a significant positive effect compared to placebo with regard to mortality and the progression of liver disease (Marchesini et al., 2003; Muto et al., 2005).

Hepatic myelopathy and acquired hepatocerebral degeneration do not respond to conventional HE therapy. Here immediate liver transplantation is recommended (Weissenborn et al., 2003).

CONCLUSIONS

Hepatic encephalopathy is a frequent complication of end stage chronic liver disease indicating poor prognosis. Neuropathologic findings indicate that it is a glial disease that results in severe neuronal dysfunction. The characteristic extrapyramidal and cerebellar symptoms distinguish HE from metabolic encephalopathies due to other causes. Diagnosis has to be made with careful exclusion of other possible causes of brain dysfunction. Even mild degrees of HE should be treated, as they significantly impair quality of life and activities of daily living. Further efforts are needed to clarify the pathogenesis of HE, to identify new therapeutic targets, and to harmonize the diagnostic approach.

REFERENCES

Adams RD, Foley JM (1952). The neurological disorders associated with liver disease. Proc Assoc Res Nerv Ment Dis 32: 198–237.

Ahboucha S, Butterworth RF (2007). The neurosteroid system: implication in the pathophysiology of hepatic encephalopathy. Neurochem Int 52: 575–587.

Ahl B, Weissenborn K, van den Hoff J et al. (2004). Regional differences in cerebral blood flow and cerebral ammonia metabolism in patients with cirrhosis. Hepatology 40: 73–79.

Als-Nielsen B, Gluud LL, Gluud C (2004). Non-absorbable disaccharides for hepatic encephalopathy: systematic review of randomised trials. BMJ 328: 1046–1051.

Amodio P, Campagna F, Olianas S et al. (2008). Detection of minimal hepatic encephalopathy: normalization and optimization of the Psychometric Hepatic Encephalopathy Score. A neuropsychological and quantified EEG study. J Hepatol 49: 346–353.

Amodio P, Ridola L, Schiff S et al. (2010). Improving detection of minimal hepatic encephalopathy using the inhibitory control task. Gastroenterology 139: 510–518.

Angeli P, Wong F, Watson H et al. (2006). Hyponatremia in cirrhosis: results of a patient population survey. Hepatology 44: 1535–1542.

Aschner M, Guilarte TR, Schneider JS et al. (2007). Manganese: recent advances in understanding its transport and neurotoxicity. Toxicol Appl Pharmacol 221: 131–147.

Bajaj JS, Saeian K, Verber MD et al. (2007). Inhibitory control test is a simple method to diagnose minimal hepatic encephalopathy and predict development of overt hepatic encephalopathy. Am J Gastroenterol 102: 754–760.

Bajaj JS, Saeian K, Schubert CM et al. (2009). Minimal hepatic encephalopathy is associated with motor vehicle crashes: the reality beyond the driving test. Hepatology 50: 1175–1183.

Balata S, Olde Damink SWM, Ferguson K et al. (2003). Induced hyperammonemia alters neuropsychology, brain MR spectroscopy and magnetization transfer in cirrhosis. Hepatology 37: 931–939.

Bass NM, Mullen KD, Sanyal A et al. (2010). Rifaximin treatment in hepatic encephalopathy. N Engl J Med 362: 1071–1081.

Burkhard PR, Delavelle J, Du Pasquier R et al. (2003). Chronic parkinsonism associated with cirrhosis: a distinct subset of acquired hepatocerebral degeneration. Arch Neurol 60: 521–528.

Butterworth RF (2002). Pathophysiology of hepatic encephalopathy: a new look at ammonia. Metab Brain Dis 17: 221–227.

Butterworth RF (2007). Neuronal cell death in hepatic encephalopathy. Metab Brain Dis 22: 309–320.

Butterworth RF, Spahr L, Fontaine S et al. (1995). Manganese toxicity, dopaminergic dysfunction and hepatic encephalopathy. Metab Brain Dis 10: 259–227.

Cadranel J-F, Lebiez E, Di Martino V et al. (2001). Focal neurological signs in hepatic encephalopathy in cirrhotic patients: an underestimated entity? Am J Gastroenterol 96: 515–518.

Cagnin A, Taylor-Robinson S, Forton DM et al. (2006). In vivo imaging of cerebral "peripheral benzodiazepine binding sites" in patients with hepatic encephalopathy. Gut 55: 547–553.

Campellone JV, Lacomis D, Giuliani MJ et al. (1996). Hepatic myelopathy. Case report with review of the literature. Clin Neurol Neurosurg 98: 242–246.

Cash WJ, McConville P, McDermott E et al. (2010). Current concepts in the assessment and treatment of hepatic encephalopathy. Q J Med 103: 9–16.

Conn HO, Lieberthal MM (1979). The Hepatic Coma Syndromes and Lactulose. Williams and Wilkins, Baltimore.

Cordoba J, Garcia-Martinez R, Simon-Talero M (2010). Hyponatremic and hepatic encephalopathies: similarities, differences and coexistence. Metab Brain Dis 25: 73–80.

Davies MG, Rowan MJ, Feely J (1991). EEG and event related potentials in hepatic encephalopathy. Metab Brain Dis 6: 175–186.

Da Rocha, Braga FT, da Silva CJ et al. (2004). Reversal of parkinsonism and portosystemic encephalopathy following embolization of a congenital intrahepatic venous shunt: brain MR imaging and 1H spectroscopic findings. AJNR 25: 1247–1250.

Dhiman RK, Kurmi R, Thumburu KK et al. (2010). Diagnosis and prognostic significance of minimal hepatic encephalopathy in patients with cirrhosis of liver. Dig Dis Sci 55: 2381–2390.

Ferenci P, Lockwood A, Mullen K et al. (2002). Hepatic encephalopathy – definition, nomenclature, diagnosis, and quantification: final report of the working party at the 11th World Congresses of Gastroenterology, Vienna, 1998. Hepatology 35: 716–721.

Ferrara J, Jankovic J (2009). Acquired hepatocerebral degeneration. J Neurol 256: 320–332.

Fichet J, Mercier E, Genee O et al. (2009). Prognosis and 1-year mortality of intensive care unit patients with severe hepatic encephalopathy. J Crit Care 24: 364–370.

Giewekemeyer K, Berding G, Ahl B et al. (2007). Bradykinesia in cirrhotic patients with early hepatic encephalopathy is related to a decreased glucose uptake of frontomesial cortical areas relevant for movement initiation. J Hepatol 46: 1034–1039.

Gilberstadt SJ, Gilberstadt H, Zieve L et al. (1980). Psychomotor performance defects in cirrhotic patients without overt encephalopathy. Arch Intern Med 140: 519–521.

Goldbecker A, Buchert R, Berding G et al. (2010). Blood brain barrier permeability for ammonia in patients with different grades of liver fibrosis and normal plasma ammonia levels is not different from healthy controls. J Cereb Blood Flow Metab 30: 1384–1393.

Görg B, Qvartskhava N, Keitel V et al. (2008). Ammonia induces RNA oxidation in cultured astrocytes and brain in vivo. Hepatology 48: 567–579.

Görg B, Qvartskhava N, Bidmon H-J et al. (2010). Oxidative stress markers in the brain of patients with cirrhosis and hepatic encephalopathy. Hepatology 52: 256–265.

Guerit JM, Amantini A, Fischer C et al. (2009). Neurophysiological investigations of hepatic encephalopathy: ISHEN practice guidelines. Liver Int 29: 789–796.

Guevara M, Baccaro ME, Torre A et al. (2009). Hyponatremia is a risk factor of hepatic encephalopathy in patients with cirrhosis: a prospective study with time-dependent analysis. Am J Gastroenterol 104: 1382–1389.

Häussinger D, Schliess F (2008). Pathogenetic mechanisms of hepatic encephalopathy. Gut 57: 1156–1165.

Häussinger D, Kircheis G, Fischer R et al. (2000). Hepatic encephalopathy in chronic liver disease: a clinical manifestation of astrocyte swelling and low-grade cerebral edema? J Hepatol 32: 1035–1038.

Jayakumar AR, Rama Rao KV, Kalaiselvi P et al. (2004). Combined effects of ammonia and manganese on astrocytes in culture. Neurochem Res 29: 2051–2056.

Jepsen P, Ott P, Andersen PK et al. (2010). Clinical course of alcoholic liver cirrhosis: a Danish population-based cohort study. Hepatology 51: 1675–1682.

Kale RA, Gupta RK, Saraswat VA et al. (2006). Demonstration of interstitial cerebral edema with diffusion tensor MR imaging in type C hepatic encephalopathy. Hepatology 43: 698–706.

Keiding S, Sørensen M, Bender D et al. (2006). Brain metabolism of 13 N-ammonia during acute hepatic encephalopathy in cirrhosis measured by positron emission tomography. Hepatology 43: 42–50.

Kircheis G, Nilius R, Held C et al. (1997). Therapeutic efficacy of L-ornithine-L-aspartate infusions in patients with cirrhosis and hepatic encephalopathy: results of a placebo-controlled, double-blind study. Hepatology 25: 1351–1360.

Kircheis G, Wettstein M, Timmermann L et al. (2002). Critical flicker frequency for quantification of low-grade hepatic encephalopathy. Hepatology 35: 357–366.

Kircheis G, Knoche A, Hilger N et al. (2009). Hepatic encephalopathy and fitness to drive. Gastroenterology 137: 1706–1715.

Krieger S, Jauß M, Jansen O et al. (1996). Neuropsychiatric profile and hyperintense globus pallidus on T1-weighted magnetic resonance images in liver cirrhosis. Gastroenterology 111: 147–155.

Kril JJ, Butterworth RF (1997). Diencephalic and cerebellar pathology in alcoholic and nonalcoholic patients with end-stage liver disease. Hepatology 26: 837–841.

Köstler H (1998). Proton magnetic resonance spectroscopy in portal-systemic encephalopathy. Metab Brain Dis 13: 291–301.

Kumar R, Gupta RK, Elderkin-Thompson V et al. (2008). Voxel-based diffusion tensor magnetic resonance imaging evaluation of lowgrade hepatic encephalopathy. J Magn Reson Imaging 27: 1061–1068.

Leevy CB, Phillips JA (2007). Hospitalizations during the use of rifaximin versus lactulose for the treatment of hepatic encephalopathy. Dig Dis Sci 52: 737–741.

Leonhardt H, Bungert HJ (1972). Therapie der schweren Hyper ammoniamie. Med Klin 67: 1052–1056.

Lewis MB, MacQillan G, Bamford JM, Howdle PD (2000). Delayed myelopathic presentation of the acquired hepatocerebral degeneration syndrome. Neurology 54: 1011.

Lockwood AH, Yap EWH, Wong W-H (1991a). Cerebral ammonia metabolism in patients with severe liver disease and minimal hepatic encephalopathy. J Cereb Blood Flow Metab 11: 337–341.

Lockwood AH, Murphy BW, Donnelly KZ et al. (1993). Positron emission tomographic localization of abnormalities of brain metabolism in patients with minimal hepatic encephalopathy. Hepatology 18: 1061–1068.

Lockwood AH, Weissenborn K, Butterworth RF (1997). An image of the brain in patients with liver disease. Curr Opin Neurol 10: 525–533.

Lockwood AH, Weissenborn K, Bokemeyer M et al. (2002). Correlations between cerebral glucose metabolism and neuropsychological test performance in non-alcoholic cirrhotics. Metab Brain Dis 17: 29–40.

Marchesini G, Bianchi G, Merli M et al. (2003). Nutritional supplementation with branched-chain amino acids in advanced cirrhosis: a double-blind, randomized trial. Gastroenterology 124: 1792–1801.

Marks ME, Jackson CD, Montagnese S et al. (2008). Derivation of a normative UK database for the psychometric hepatic encephalopathy score (PHES): confounding effect of ethnicity and test scoring. J Hepatol 48: S119.

Martin H, Voss K, Hufnagl P et al. (1987). Morphometric and densitometric investigations of protoplasmic astrocytes and neurons in human hepatic encephalopathy. Exp Pathol 32: 241–250.

Montagnese S, Amodio P, Morgan MY (2004). Methods for diagnosing hepatic encephalopathy in patients with cirrhosis: a multidimensional approach. Metab Brain Dis 19: 281–312.

Montagnese S, Jackson C, Morgan MY (2007). Spatio-temporal decomposition of the electroencephalogram in patients with cirrhosis. J Hepatol. 46 (3): 447–458.

Mookerjee R, Stadlbauer V, Lidder S et al. (2007). Neutrophil dysfunction in alcoholic hepatitis superimposed on cirrhosis is reversible and predicts outcome. Hepatology 46: 831–840.

Mooney S, Hasssanein TI, Hilsabeck RC et al. (2007). The UCSD Hepatology Neurobehavioral Research Program. Utility of the Repeatable Battery for the Assessment of Neuropsychological Status (RBANS) in patients with end-stage liver disease awaiting liver transplant. Arch Clin Neuropsychol 22: 175–186.

Morgan MY, Hawley KE (1987). Lactitol versus lactulose in the treatment of acute hepatic encephalopathy in cirrhotic patients: a double-blind, randomized trial. Hepatology 7: 1278–1284.

Muto Y, Sato S, Watanabe A et al. (2005). Effects of oral branched-chain amino acid granules on event-free survival in patients with liver cirrhosis. Clin Gastroenterol Hepatol 3: 705–713.

Norenberg MD, Rama Rao KV, Jayakumar AR (2009). Signaling factors in the mechanism of ammonia neurotoxicity. Metab Brain Dis 24: 103–117.

Parsons-Smith BG, Summerskill WHJ, Dawson AM et al. (1957). The electroencephalograph in liver disease. Lancet ii: 867–871.

Penin H (1967). Über den diagnostischen Wert des Hirnstrombildes bei der hepato-portalen Encephalopathie. Fortschr Neurol Psychiatr 35: 174–234.

Phillips G, Schwartz R, Gabuzda G et al. (1952). The syndrome of impending hepatic coma in patients with cirrhosis of the liver given certain nitrogenous substances. N Engl J Med 247: 239–246.

Plum F, Hindfelt B (1976). The neurological complications of liver disease. In: P Vinken, DF Bruyn (Eds.), Metabolic and Deficiency Diseases of the Nervous System. Handbook of Clinical Neurology. vol. 27, Elsevier, Amsterdam, pp. 349–377.

Pomier-Layrargues G, Rose C, Spahr L et al. (1998). Role of manganese in the pathogenesis of portal-systemic encephalopathy. Metab Brain Dis 13: 311–317.

Poo JL, Gongora J, Sanchez-Avila F et al. (2006). Efficacy of oral L-ornithine-L-aspartate in cirrhotic patients with hyperammonemic hepatic encephalopathy. Results of a randomized, lactulose-controlled study. Ann Hepatol 5: 281–288.

Poveda M-J, Bernabeu A, Concepción L et al. (2010). Brain edema dynamics in patients with overt hepatic encephalopathy. A magnetic resonance imaging study. Neuroimage 52: 481–487.

Prasad S, Dhiman RK, Duseja A et al. (2007). Lactulose improves cognitive functions and health-related quality of life in patients with cirrhosis who have minimal hepatic encephalopathy. Hepatology 45: 549–559.

Pujol A, Pujol J, Graus F et al. (1993). Hyperintense globus pallidus on T1-weighted MRI in cirrhotic patients is associated with severity of liver failure. Neurology 43: 65–69.

Quero JC, Hartmann IJ, Meulstee J et al. (1996). The diagnosis of subclinical hepatic encephalopathy in patients with cirrhosis using neuropsychological tests and automated electroencephalogram analysis. Hepatology 24: 556–560.

Randolph C (1998). The Repeatable Battery for the Assessment of Neuropsychological Status (RBANS). Psychological Corporation, San Antonio.

Randolph C, Hilsabeck R, Kato A et al. (2009). Neuropsychological assessment of hepatic encephalopathy: ISHEN practice guidelines. Liver Int 29: 629–635.

Read A, Sherlock S, Laidlaw J et al. (1967). The neuropsychiatric syndromes associated with chronic liver disease and an extensive portal-systemic collateral circulation. Q J Med 36: 135–150.

Rehnström S, Simert G, Hansson JA et al. (1977). Chronic hepatic encephalopathy. A psychometric study. Scand J Gastroenterol 12: 305–311.

Rikkers L, Jenko P, Rudman D et al. (1978). Subclinical hepatic encephalopathy: detection, prevalence, and relationship to nitrogen metabolism. Gastroenterology 75: 462–469.

Romero-Gomez M, Boza F, Garcia-Valdecasas MS et al. (2001). Subclinical hepatic encephalopathy predicts the development of overt hepatic encephalopathy. Am J Gastroenterol 96: 2718–2723.

Romero Gomez M, Cordoba J, Jover R et al. (2006). Normality tables in the Spanish population for psychometric tests used in the diagnosis of minimal hepatic encephalopathy. Med Clin (Barc) 127: 246–249.

Romero Gomez M, Cordoba J, Jover R et al. (2007). Value of the critical flicker frequency in patients with minimal hepatic encephalopathy. Hepatology 45: 879–885.

Rose C, Butterworth RF, Zayed J et al. (1999a). Manganese deposition in basal ganglia structures results from both portal-systemic shunting and liver dysfunction. Gastroenterology 117: 640–644.

Rose C, Michalak A, Rao KV et al. (1999b). L-ornithine-L-aspartate lowers plasma and cerebrospinal fluid ammonia and prevents brain edema in rats with acute liver failure. Hepatology 30: 636–640.

Rovira A, Grive E, Pedraza S et al. (2001). Magnetization transfer ratio values and proton MR spectroscopy of normal appearing cerebral white matter in patients with liver cirrhosis. AJNR 22: 1137–1142.

Schliess F, Görg B, Häussinger D (2006). Pathogenetic interplay between osmotic and oxidative stress: the hepatic encephalopathy paradigm. Biol Chem 387: 1363–1370.

Schomerus H, Hamster W (1998). Neuropsychological aspects of portal-systemic encephalopathy. Metab Brain Dis 13: 361–377.

Schomerus H, Hamster W, Blunck H et al. (1981). Latent portasystemic encephalopathy: I. Nature of cerebral functional defects and their effect on fitness to drive. Dig Dis Sci 26: 622–630.

Schomerus H, Weissenborn K, Hamster W et al. (1999). PSE-Syndrom-Test. Swets Test Services. Swets and Zeitlinger B.V., Frankfurt.

Shah NJ, Neeb H, Kircheis G et al. (2008). Quantitative cerebral water content mapping in hepatic encephalopathy. Neuroimage 41: 706–717.

Sharma P, Sharma BC, Puri V et al. (2007). Critical flicker frequency: diagnostic tool for minimal hepatic encephalopathy. J Hepatol 47: 67–73.

Sharma BC, Sharma P, Agarwal A et al. (2009). Secondary prophylaxis of hepatic encephalopathy: an open label randomized controlled trial of lactulose versus placebo. Gastroenterology 137: 885–891.

Shawcross DL, Balata S, Olde-Damink SW et al. (2004a). Low myoinositol and high glutamine levels in brain are associated with neuropsychological deterioration after induced hyperammonemia. Am J Physiol 287: G503–G509.

Shawcross DL, Davies NA, Williams R et al. (2004b). Systemic inflammatory response exacerbates the neuropsychological effects of induced hyperammonemia in cirrhosis. J Hepatol 40: 247–254.

Shawcross DL, Olde Daminck SWM, Butterworth RF et al. (2005). Ammonia and hepatic encephalopathy: the more things change, the more they remain the same. Metab Brain Dis 20: 169–179.

Sherlock S (1958). Pathogenesis and management of hepatic coma. Am J Med 24: 805–813.

Sherlock S, Summerskill WHJ, White LP et al. (1954). Portal-systemic encephalopathy. neurological complications of liver disease. Lancet I: 453–457.

Singhal A, Nagarajan R, Kumar R et al. (2009). Magnetic resonance T2-relaxometry and 2D L-correlated spectroscopy in patients with minimal hepatic encephalopathy. J Magn Reson Imaging 30: 1034–1041.

Spahr L, Butterworth RF, Fontaine S et al. (1996). Increased blood manganese in cirrhotic patients: relationship to pallidal magnetic resonance signal hyperintensity and neurological symptoms. Hepatology 24: 1116–1120.

Stauch S, Kircheis G, Adler G et al. (1998). Oral L-ornithine-L-aspartate therapy of chronic hepatic encephalopathy: results of a placebo-controlled double-blind study. J Hepatol 28: 856–864.

Summerskill WHJ, Davidson EA, Sherlock S et al. (1956). The neuropsychiatric syndrome associated with hepatic cirrhosis and an extensive portal collateral circulation. Q J Med 25: 245–266.

Tarter RE, Hegedus AM, Van Thiel DH et al. (1984). Nonalcoholic cirrhosis associated with neuropsychological dysfunction in the absence of overt evidence of hepatic encephalopathy. Gastroenterology 86: 1421–1427.

Thumburu KK, Kurmi R, Dhiman RK et al. (2008). Psychometric hepatic encephalopathy score, critical flicker frequency and P300 event-related potential for the diagnosis of minimal hepatic encephalopathy: evidence that psychometric hepatic encephalopathy score is enough. 13th ISHEN, Padua, 2008 [abstract].

Uribe M, Campollo O, Vargas F et al. (1987). Acidifying enemas (lactitol and lactose) vs. nonacidifying enemas (tap water) to treat acute portal-systemic encephalopathy: a double-blind randomized clinical trial. Hepatology 7: 639–643.

Van der Rijt CDC, Schalm S, De Groot GH et al. (1990). Objective measurement of hepatic encephalopathy by means of automated EEG analysis. Electroencephalogr Clin Neurophysiol 75: 289–295.

Victor M, Adams RD, Cole M (1965). The acquired (non-Wilsonian) type of chronic hepatocerebral degeneration. Medicine (Baltimore) 44: 345–396.

Watanabe A, Tuchida T, Yata Y et al. (1995). Evaluation of neuropsychological function in patients with liver cirrhosis with special reference to their driving ability. Metab Brain Dis 10: 239–248.

Wein C, Koch H, Popp B et al. (2004). Minimal hepatic encephalopathy impairs fitness to drive. Hepatology 39: 739–745.

Weissenborn K, Scholz M, Hinrichs H, Wiltfang J, Schmidt FW, Künkel H (1990). Neurophysiological assessment of early hepatic encephalopathy. Electroencephalogr Clin Neurophysiol. 75 (4): 289–295.

Weissenborn K (1991). Neurophysiological methods in the diagnosis of early hepatic encephalopathy. In: F Bengtsson, B Jeppsson, T Almdal et al. (Eds.), Progress in Hepatic Encephalopathy and Metabolic Nitrogen Exchange. CRC Press, Boca Raton, pp. 27–39.

Weissenborn K, Ennen J, Schomerus H et al. (2001). Neuropsychological characterisation of hepatic encephalopathy. J Hepatol 34: 768–773.

Weissenborn K, Tietge UJ, Bokemeyer M et al. (2003). Liver transplantation improves hepatic myelopathy: evidence by three cases. Gastroenterology 124: 346–351.

Wunsch E, Koziarska D, Kotarska K et al. (2013). Normalization of the psychometric hepatic encephalopathy score in polish population. A prospective, quantified electroencephalography study. Liver Int 33: 1332–1340.

Zeegen R, Drinkwater JE, Dawson AM (1970). Method for measuring cerebral dysfunction in patients with liver disease. Br Med J 2: 633–636.

Zieve L (1991). Historical remarks and recent trends in hepatic encephalopathy. In: F Bengtsson, B Jeppsson, T Almdal et al. (Eds.), Progress in Hepatic Encephalopathy and Metabolic Nitrogen Exchange. CRC Press, Boca Raton, pp. 3–8.

Handbook of Clinical Neurology, Vol. 120 (3rd series)
Neurologic Aspects of Systemic Disease Part II
Jose Biller and Jose M. Ferro, Editors
© 2014 Elsevier B.V. All rights reserved

Chapter 46

Neurotoxicity of commonly used hepatic drugs

CHRISTINE L. AHRENS AND EDWARD M. MANNO*
Neurological Intensive Care Unit, Cleveland Clinic, Cleveland, OH, USA

INTRODUCTION

The increased need for and utility of organ transplantation including liver transplantation has increased the use of immunosuppressive agents to prevent rejection. Neurologic complications are common with many of these medications (Table 46.1). The neurologist, surgeon, or intensivist will often be confronted with a variety of these complications.

Similarly, the use of interferons has improved the care of patients with hepatitis C and other hepatic infections.

This chapter will review the medications used to treat hepatic infections and to prevent liver rejection post-transplantation. Neurologic complications commonly encountered will be emphasized.

CALCINEURIN INHIBITORS

Calcineurin inhibitors are a class of immunosuppressant drugs that decrease lymphocytic proliferation through the inhibition of a phophatase calcineurin. The two commonly employed drugs are ciclosporin and tacrolimus (previously referred to as FK 506). These drugs represent the mainstay of immunosuppression after orthotopic liver transplantation (OLT).

MECHANISM OF ACTION

The lymphocytic response to an antigen is mediated through antigenic binding of the T-helper membrane receptor. This results in the opening of calcium channels which facilitates calcium influx into the cell. Intracellular calcium subsequently binds to calmodulin. This complex stimulates calcineurin (a phosphatase) which activates various transcription factors (primarily IL-2). These factors lead to a clonal expansion of new lymphocytes while inhibiting the apoptosis of existing lymphocytic lines.

This process of antigen-induced clonal expansion is inhibited by ciclosporin. Ciclosporin binds to a cytosolic protein named cyclophilin. This complex inhibits calcineurin-mediated activation of several transcriptases. Tacrolimus inhibits calcineurin through binding to FK-binding protein which in turn inhibits the function of calcineurin (Rang et al., 2003).

NEUROTOXICITY

The range of neurologic signs and symptoms attributable to the use of calcineurin inhibitors is considerable. Symptoms can vary from mild headache, paresthesias, and confusion to psychosis and coma. Neurologic signs include tremor, visual disturbances, and seizures. Other reported neurologic complications include speech apraxia, cortical blindness, hemiparesis, parkinsonism, peripheral neuropathy, and ocular motor difficulties (Muellar et al., 1994; Wijdicks et al., 1994, 1995; Bechstein, 2000).

The incidence of neurologic complications reported after liver transplantation ranges between 10% and 47% with most studies limiting the range between 20% and 30% (Saner et al., 2007, 2009, 2010). The exact incidence of side-effects attributable to calcineurin inhibitors is difficult to assess. Pre-existing or post-transplant encephalopathy can complicate the evaluation of immunosuppressant medications. Drug interactions with glucocorticoids can confuse which medication is the source of the problem. Other complications can include issues attributable to electrolyte disturbances, infections, sepsis, or sedative medications. Thus, neurotoxicity attributable to calcineurin inhibitors is often a diagnosis of exclusion (Bechstein, 2000).

Neurotoxicity attributable to calcineurin inhibitors is often classified as mild, moderate, or severe. The most common side-effect is tremor, seen in up to 40% of

*Correspondence to: Edward M. Manno, M.D., Head, Neurocritical Care, Cleveland Clinic, 9500 Euclid Ave, HB-105, Cleveland, OH 44195, USA. Tel: +1-216-445-1624, E-mail: MANNOE@ccf.org

Table 46.1

Potential central nervous system adverse effects of immunosuppresent medications

Medication	Central nervous system adverse effects
Immunosuppressants	
Calcineurin inhibitors (ciclosporin, tacrolimus)	Headache, paresthesias, confusion, tremor, visual disturbances, apraxia, parkinsonism, peripheral neuropathy, ocular motor difficulties, psychosis, coma seizures, hemiparesis, cortical blindness, leukoencephalopathy
Sirolimus	Headache, arthralgias, insomnia, dizziness, neuropathy, confusion, abnormal vision, leukoencephalopathy (rare)
Mycophenolate mofetil	Headache, insomnia, dizziness, anxiety, pain, psychosis, seizure
Antihepatitis therapies	
Interferons	Depression, asthenia, myalgia, psychosis, insomnia, irritability
Ribavirin	Headache, fatigue
Lamivudine	Headache, fatigue, insomnia, neuropathy
Adefovir dipivoxil	Headache, asthenia
Entecavir	Headache, fatigue, dizziness
Telbivudine	Headache, dizziness, insomnia, peripheral neuropathy (occurs in combination with pegylated interferon (peg-IFN))

patients. This can resolve spontaneously but usually requires dose reduction. Paresthesias can respond similarly to dose adjustments. Headache, neuralgia, and peripheral neuropathies are also quite common. Severe complications such as psychosis, coma or a leukoencephalopathy occur in approximately 5% of patients and may not be amenable to dose reduction or discontinuation of the calcineurin inhibitor (Bechstein, 2000; Saner et al., 2009).

MECHANISM OF NEUROTOXICITY

The mechanism of neurologic cellular dysfunction after the initiation of calcineurin inhibitors is not completely understood. There are, however, several observations and findings that are common to both tacrolimus and ciclosporin toxicity. Both animal models and clinical studies suggest that calcineurin inhibitors increase sympathetic outflow and nerve activity (Scherrer et al., 1990; Lyson et al., 1993). The exact localization of this process is unknown but probably involves both central and peripheral mechanisms (Sander et al., 1996; Bechstein, 2000).

Increased sympathetic activity may also be modulated through both pre- and postsynaptic effects on excitatory and inhibitory amino acid receptors. Ciclosporin may decrease GABA-mediated inhibition. In rat brain slice models a ciclosporin–cyclophilin complex can desensitize GABA receptors (Martina et al., 1996). Similarly, tacrolimus has been shown to increase NMDA-induced transmitter release (Lu et al., 1996).

Calcineurin inhibition may also be selectively toxic to white matter. *In vitro* studies of cells incubated with ciclosporin suggest selective toxicity of glial cells

(Stoltenburg-Didinger and Boegner, 1992). Similarly, ciclosporin induces apoptosis in oligodendrocytes (McDonald et al., 1996). Cell lines with the highest density of calcineurin appear to be most affected. These effects increase with the length of exposure, possibly accounting for the delayed development of a leukoencephalopathy seen in some patients (Bechstein, 2000).

The white matter changes commonly seen on computed tomography (CT) and magnetic resonance imaging (MRI) may represent vascular injury. Ciclosporin and tacrolimus induced white matter changes on MRI, typically in the occipital white matter and border zone areas similar to those areas encountered during hypoperfusion (Bartynski et al., 1994). Tacrolimus can also affect the thalami and produce vascular injury in animal models (Frank et al., 1993). Patients after liver transplant will develop cortical hyperintensities involving the cingulate gyrus and the occipital lobes noted on proton density-weighted imaging (Jansen et al., 1996). This may represent ciclosporin-induced changes to the vascular basement membrane (Sloane et al., 1985).

SPECIFIC COMPLICATIONS

Mild symptoms of calcineurin inhibition include tremor, sleep disturbances, mood alterations, headaches, and confusion. These are commonly encountered and may even have a higher incidence than reported if a thorough neurologic and mental status examination is performed. Moderate and severe symptoms of cortical blindness, seizures, coma, and encephalopathy are found in a smaller percentage of patients and may be more common with tacrolimus (Muellar et al., 1994). The incidence of these complications appears to be higher for liver transplantation compared to other solid organ transplants (Muellar et al., 1994) and may be related to high plasma concentration of tacrolimus.

The leukoencephalopathy encountered with calcineurin use is difficult to predict or characterize. Clearly white matter tracts are involved as central pontine myelinolysis can occur with devastating effects (Saner et al., 2007). Calcineurin effects on MRI can occur early but also in a delayed fashion after several weeks or months (Saner et al., 2009). Interestingly, MRI changes in white matter do not necessarily correlate with neurologic symptoms (Wijdicks et al., 1995).

Seizures are seen most commonly immediately post-transplant. Early studies had suggested that calcineurin inhibition-induced seizures had a poor outcome (Adams et al., 1987; Estol et al., 1989). Wijdicks, however, in a retrospective analysis of post liver transplant patients, suggested that this may not be accurate. In the Mayo series, most seizures occurred during the time of initiation or adjustment of ciclosporin or tacrolimus. All patients had supratherapeutic levels and did not have further seizures with dose reduction (Wijdicks et al., 1996).

Hypertension has been shown to be an independent risk factor for developing seizures post-transplant (Erer et al., 1996), and seizures may be associated with hypomagnesemia (Thompson et al., 1989).

The significance of calcineurin-induced neurotoxicity post liver transplant is unclear. Mild symptoms probably have little significance; however, older literature has suggested that patients with late onset or severe neurologic complications have worse outcome (Wszolek et al., 1991; Muellar et al., 1994). It is difficult, however, to discern if late neurologic complications are due to calcineurin inhibitors or a late complication of a failing transplant (Bechstein, 2000).

There are a number of predisposing factors that can increase the risk to post-transplant patients of calcineurin inhibition toxicity. Liver failure can lead to blood–brain barrier disruption and increased access of ciclosporin and tacrolimus to the brain (Freise et al., 1993). Intravenous administration of drug, concurrent use of prednisone, and hypocholesterolemia can increase the total and unbound level of calcineurin inhibitors, thus increasing brain uptake of the drug used (Freise et al., 1991, 1993; Bechstein, 2000).

TREATMENT OF COMPLICATIONS

The correlation between neurotoxicity and calcineurin inhibitor drug levels is weak and routine monitoring of drug levels is usually not indicated. A simple dose response relationship does not exist and discontinuation of drug does not always reverse symptomatology. Severe toxicity, however, does occur with higher drug levels. Toxicity may be mediated through ciclosporin and tacrolimus metabolites which can cross the blood–brain barrier. Impaired hepatic function can also increase these metabolites. Monitoring of these metabolites to assess for neurotoxicity has been suggested but has not gained wide acceptance (Trull et al., 1989).

In some instances maneuvers designed to decrease drug levels can help with symptomatology. These can include lowering the dose, switching to oral therapy (Wijdicks et al., 1999), or treating renal failure. Lipid supplementation with soybean oil has been used in five patients post liver transplant to prevent lipophillic calcineurin inhibtors from crossing the blood–brain barrier (Ide et al., 2007). Several antibiotics can have drug interactions which can increase ciclosporin or tacrolimus levels. The use of combined immunosuppressant regimens can be used to lower the levels of any individual drug (Bechstein, 2000).

Treatment of post liver transplant hypertension is important to decrease the incidence of neurologic complications. Drug-induced blood–brain barrier and vascular membrane disruption may impair cerebral autoregulation rendering the brain susceptible to a form of malignant hypertension. This may account for the MRI changes commonly encountered which resemble the posterior reversible encephalopathy syndrome (PRES).

Seizure control post liver transplant can be difficult. Management involves dose reduction and the initiation of anticonvulsants. Phenytoin, phenobarbital, and carbamazepine will decrease ciclosporin levels. Valproate or levetiracetam may be preferred. Levetiracetam dosing will need to be adjusted based on renal function.

Early post-transplant seizures do not appear to affect long-term outcome; however, status epilepticus and epiletiform activity on EEG monitoring has an ominous prognosis (Wszolek et al., 1991; Wijdicks et al., 1996).

OTHER MEDICATIONS USED FOR IMMUNOSUPPRESION AFTER ORTHOTOPIC LIVER TRANSPLANTATION

Sirolimus

Sirolimus is the generic name for a drug also known as rapamycin. It has a similar mechanism of action to tacrolimus in that sirolimus binds to the intracelluler FK-12 protein but inhibits a regulatory kinase (mTOR) which leads to the suppression of T cell proliferation. No evidence of direct central neurotoxicity could be attributed to sirolimus use in a review of over 200 transplant patients (Maramattom and Wijdicks, 2004). A demyelinating sensorimotor polyneuropathy, however, has been described (Bilodeau et al., 2008).

Mycophenolate mofetil (CellCept)

Mycophenolate mofetil is a prodrug which is hydrolyzed to mycophenolic acid. Mycophenolic acid is a noncompetitive inhibitor of inosine monophosphate dehydrogenase, an enzyme required for B and T cell proliferation (Krensky et al., 2006). The toxicity for this drug is primarily GI and hematopoietic. Use can lead to hyperlipidemia, thrombocytopenia, and leukopenia. Levels can be increased with ingestion of grapefruit juice. A review of 191 liver transplant patients treated with mycophenolate did not report any neurologic complications (Pfitzmann et al., 2003).

Mycophenolate has been used for rescue therapy in patients that have developed neurotoxicty from calcineurin inhibitors (Klupp et al., 1997). Two studies have suggested that mycophenolate is a safe and useful adjuvant for immunosuppression in post liver transplant patients (Freise et al., 1993; Klupp et al., 1997).

INTERFERONS, RIBAVIRIN AND NUCLEOSIDE AND NUCLEOTIDE ANALOGS USED IN THE TREATMENT OF HEPATITIS B AND C VIRUS

There are a select number of medications available for the treatment of hepatitis B virus (HBV) and hepatitis C virus (HCV) (Lok and McMahon, 2009). Interferons, ribavirin, lamivudine, entecavir, tenofovir, telbivudine, and adefovir make up the armamentarium of commonly used antivirals considered in the treatment of hepatitis. Interferon monotherapy or in combination with ribavirin are the recommended medications for the treatment of chronic hepatitis C virus (HCV). Not all patients with HBV and/or HCV receive pharmacologic treatment. However, for those appropriately selected candidates who do, there exists a potential for adverse effects related to these therapies. Particular adverse events to some of these therapies are the primary reason patients discontinue therapy. Understanding the potential for these effects to occur and patient counseling may reduce discontinuation or denial of therapy (Ghany et al., 2009).

Interferons

Interferons (INF) are a class of cytokines which have antiviral, immunomodulating, and antiproliferative effects (Lok and McMahon, 2009). Three classes of human IFNs exist (α, β, and γ) with significant antiviral activity; however, only recombinant α and β IFNs are clinically utilized. Standard IFNs were first available for the treatment of HBV and HCV but have been replaced by the newer pegylated interferons (peg-IFN). Certain advantages exist with peg-IFNs compared to the standard formulations, including a reduction in the severity of side-effects. Commercially available IFNs used in the treatment of HBV are standard IFN-α2b (Intron®A) and peg-IFN-α2a (PEGASYS®) and IFN-α 2b, peg-IFN-α2a, peg-IFN-α2b (PegIntron®), and IFN alfacon-1 (Infergen®).

MECHANISM OF ACTION

IFNs activate the JAK-STAT signal-transduction pathway on the surface of target cells leading to nuclear translocation of a cellular protein complex that binds to genes containing an IFN-specific response element. This leads to synthesis of over two dozen proteins that contribute to viral resistance mediated at a different stage of viral penetration. IFN-induced proteins can inhibit protein synthesis in the presence of double-stranded RNA. IFN also induces a phosphodiesterase which cleaves a portion of transfer RNA thus preventing peptide elongation. IFNs may modify the immune response to infection as well through enhancement of the lytic effects of cytotoxic T lymphocytes (Pegasys, 2011).

NEUROTOXICITY

Pegylated interferons have several, undesirable adverse effects. Nearly every patient treated with the combination therapy (peginterferon and ribavirin) will experience one or more adverse effects, potentially resulting in discontinuation of therapy. The two most common adverse effects are influenza-like symptoms (fatigue, headache, fever, rigors), asthenia, myalgia, and psychiatric effects, specifically depression, irritability, and insomnia. The incidence of depression is approximately 30% and occurs typically in the first few months of therapy (Lok and McMahon, 2009). An exact causative mechanism for interferon-induced depression has not been fully elucidated. Risk factors linked to the development of depression include a premorbid presence of mood and anxiety symptoms. To a lesser extent, history of depression, higher doses of interferon, and female gender are also considered risk factors.

Two syndromes describe interferon-induced depression: a depression-specific syndrome characterized by mood, anxiety, and cognitive complaints and a neurovegetative syndrome characterized by fatigue, anorexia, pain, and psychomotor slowing. Preassessment for neuropsychiatric conditions should be completed prior to initiating interferon therapy. Selective serotonin reuptake inhibitors (SSRIs) have been studied in both prevention and treatment of symptoms associated with depression-specific syndromes. Some centers have a low threshold for initiating SSRIs, even prior to interferon therapy. While debatable, consideration of prophylactic antidepressants use should be given for patients with risk factors for the development of depression. Use of certain antidepressants (citalopram, fluoxetine, imipramine, nortriptyline, paroxetine, sertraline) has over an 85% success rate in treating interferon-induced depression. Consideration should be given to which antidepressant to use, based on the particular adverse effects of these agents (Lok and McMahon, 2009).

Ribavirin

Ribavirin is indicated for the treatment of chronic hepatitis C in combination with interferon α-2B (pegylated and nonpegylated) in patients with compensated liver disease. (Rebetol®, 2013) (ribavirin) monotherapy is not effective for the treatment of hepatitis C (37).

MECHANISM OF ACTION

Ribavirin is a neucleoside analog and has antiviral activity against multiple RNA viruses. However, its mechanism in the treatment of hepatitis C has not been fully elucidated. It is proposed that ribavirin has effects on the host immune response (Lau et al., 2002).

NEUROTOXICITY

The most concerning adverse effect associated with ribavirin use is hemolytic anemia. Other adverse effects include fatigue, leukopenia, pruritis, rash, and gout. Ribavirin is a well known teratogenic drug and is US Food and Drug Administration (FDA) pregnancy category X. Clear recommendations on use in women of childbearing age are outlined within the prescribing information (Epivir-HBV, 2011).

Lamivudine

Lamivudine (Epivir-HBV®) is approved for the treatment of chronic hepatitis B and may be considered as initial therapy for patients with compensated liver disease. This indication is supported by 1 year data of histologic and serologic responses in adult patients. Advantages of this therapy over IFN-α or adefovir as first line include lower cost and tolerability. Disadvantages are the potential for increased resistance and worsening of hepatic disease.

MECHANISM OF ACTION

Lamivudine is a synthetic nucleoside analog and is incorporated into viral DNA by HBV polymerase resulting in premature DNA termination (Lau et al., 2002).

NEUROTOXICITY

Lamivudine is generally well tolerated. A black box warning within the prescribing information states lactic acidosis and severe hepatomegaly with steatosis, including fatal cases, have been reported. Female gender, obesity, pregnancy, and prolonged exposure may increase the risk of these occurring. While these adverse effects are rare, there should be heightened consideration of encephalopathy related to these metabolic processes in critically ill patients presenting on lamivudine. In addition, severe acute exacerbations of hepatitis B have been reported in patients who have discontinued antihepatitis B therapy, including Epivir-HBV®. Less severe CNS effects include headache (21%), fatigue and malaise (24%), and insomnia (11%). Musculoskeletal pain (12%), neuropathy (12%), and myalgias (8–14%) also commonly occurred. In clinical trials of lamivudine for HBV, increases in creatine kinase levels were observed in 9% of patients (Lau et al., 2002; Lai et al., 2006).

Adefovir dipivoxil (Hepsera®)

Adefovir dipivoxil is a prodrug of adefovir, a nucleotide analog of adenosine monophosphate. Hepsera® is approved for the treatment of chronic hepatitis B in adults with evidence of active viral replication and either evidence of persistent elevations in serum aminotransferases or histologically active disease (Hepsera, 2009).

MECHANISM OF ACTION

Adefovir is phosphorylated to its active metabolite, adefovir diphosphate, which inhibits HBV DNA polymerase resulting in inhibition of viral replication.

NEUROTOXICITY

Adefovir has multiple black box warnings within its prescribing information, including lactic acidosis and severe hepatomegaly with steatosis; severe, acute exacerbation of hepatitis B upon discontinuation; and cautious use in patients with renal dysfunction since chronic administration may result in nephrotoxicity.

CNS toxicities associated with adefovir are minimal. In clinical studies adefovir had a similar side-effect profile to placebo. More commonly occurring central nervous system effects are headache (25%) and asthenia (13%). These adverse effects, however, have not been reported to significantly result in discontinuation of patient therapy. If patients experience headache, it is recommended they consult their healthcare provider for appropriate selection of analgesic therapy (Hadziyannis et al., 2003; Marcellin et al., 2003).

Entecavir (Baraclude®)

Entecavir is approved for the treatment of hepatitis B infection with compensated or decompensated liver disease in adults with evidence of active viral replication and either evidence of persistent transaminase elevations or histologically active disease. Entecavir can also be used for patients with lamivudine-resistant viremia. Adjustment in dosing should be considered for patients with CrCl < 50 mL/min (Baraclude, 2010).

MECHANISM OF ACTION

Entecavir is a guanosine nucleoside analog. Intracellularly it is phosphorylated to guanosine triphosphate which competes with natural substrates to inhibit HBV reverse transcriptase in three activities: (1) base priming, (2) reverse transcription of the negative strand DNA from the pregenomic messenger RNA, (3) synthesis of the positive strand of HBV DNA (Baraclude, 2010).

NEUROTOXICITY

The adverse effect profile of entecavir is similar to lamivudine, including the same black box warnings (Sherman et al., 2006; Baraclude, 2010). Common CNS effects include pyrexia (14% with decompenstated liver disease), headache (2–4%), fatigue (1–3%), and dizziness. In preclinical animal trials, there was a higher incidence of solid tumors with high-dose, prolonged administration of entecavir (Baraclude, 2010). Studies are ongoing to evaluate long-term treatment effects with entecavir.

Telbivudine (Tyzeka®)

Telbivudine is indicated for the treatment of chronic HBV in adult patients. It is well tolerated and has been shown to be more efficacious compared to lamivudine and adefovir in treating compensated chronic HBV (Chan et al., 2007; Lai et al., 2007; Liaw et al., 2009). Its use in special populations, such as patients with renal insufficiency, has not been reported.

MECHANISM OF ACTION

Telbivudine is a synthetic thymidine nucleoside analog reverse transcriptase inhibitor. Intracellularly it is phosphorylated to its active triphosphate form which competes with naturally occurring thymidine triphosphate for HBV viral DNA elongation. This incorporation into viral DNA results in DNA chain termination (Bryant et al., 2001).

NEUROTOXICITY

The same boxed warning which exists for other nucleoside analogs is included in the prescribing information for telbivudine. In clinical trials comparing telbivudine to lamivudine, side-effects were similar with the exception of increased creatinine kinase levels in the telbivudine patients (Liaw et al., 2009). During these trials, the most commonly occurring neurologic adverse effects seem with telbivudine included headache (10%), dizziness (4%), and insomnia (3%) (Baraclude, 2010). Peripheral neuropathy has been reported with telbivudine either as monotherapy (< 1%) or in combination with peg-IFNs (16%) (Marcellin et al., 2005; Baraclude, 2010). The mechanism of this adverse effect is unknown. A clinical trial was terminated early as a result of the higher incidence of peripheral neuropathy when telbivudine was used in combination with peg-IFN. Peripheral neuropathy did not reverse in some of these patients (Marcellin et al., 2005). Use of this combination should be avoided. Patients are instructed to contact their physician should they develop any numbness, tingling, and/or burning sensations in the upper or lower extremities while receiving telbivudine. If peripheral neuropathy is suspected in a patient, therapy should be held and if a diagnosis is confirmed, therapy should be permanently discontinued (Baraclude, 2010).

CONCLUSIONS

Neurologic complications do occur with the use of hepatic medications to treat hepatitis and in medications used to prevent liver rejection post-transplant. The major side-effects variably result in an encephalopathy or depression. Awareness of these effects may be useful for the recognition of early management.

REFERENCES

Adams DH, Ponsford S, Gunson B et al. (1987). Neurologic complications following liver transplantation. Lancet 1: 949–951.

Baraclude [package insert] (2010). Bristol-Myers Squibb, Princeton, NJ, December 2010.

Bartynski WS, Grabb BC, Zeiger Z et al. (1994). Watershed imaging features and clinical vascular injury in cyclosporine A neurotoxicity. J Comput Assist Tomogr 21: 872–880.

Bechstein WO (2000). Neurotoxicity of calcineurin inhibitors: impact and clinical management. Transpl Int 13: 313–326.

Bilodeau M, Hassoun Z, Brunet D (2008). Demyelinating sensorimotor polyneuropathy associated with the use of sirolimus: a case report. Transplant Proc 40: 1545–1547.

Bryant M, Bridges E, Placidi L et al. (2001). Antiviral L-nucleosides specific for hepatitis B virus infection. Antimicrob. Agents Chemother 45: 229–235.

Chan HL, Heathcote EJ, Marcellin P et al. (2007). Treatment of hepatitis B e antigen positive chronic hepatitis with telbivudine or adefovir: a randomized trial. Ann Intern Med 147: 745–754.

Epivir-HBV [package insert] (2011). GlaxoSmithKline, Research Triangle Park, NC; January 2011.

Erer B, Polchi P, Lucarelli G et al. (1996). Cyclosporine-associated neurotoxicity and ineffective prophylaxis with clonazepam in patients transplanted for thalassemia major: analysis and risk factors. Bone Marrow Transpl 18: 157–162.

Estol CJ, Lopez O, Brenner RP et al. (1989). Seizures after liver transplantation: a clinicopathologic study. Neurology 29: 1297–1301.

Frank B, Perdrizet GA, White HM et al. (1993). Neurotoxicity of FK506 in liver transplant recipients. Transpl Proc 25: 1887–1888.

Freise CE, Rowley H, Lake M et al. (1991). Similar clinical presentation of neurotoxicity following FK506 and cyclosporine in a liver transplant recipient. Transpl Proc 23: 3173–3174.

Freise CE, Hebert M, Osorio B et al. (1993). Maintenance immunosuppression with prednisone RS-61443 alone following liver transplantation. Transplant Proc 25: 1758–1759.

Ghany MG, Strader DB, Thomas DL et al. (2009). AASLD practice guideline diagnosis, management, and treatment of hepatitis C: an update. Hepatology 49: 1335–1374.

Hadziyannis SJ, Tassopoulos NC, Heathcote EJ et al. (2003). Adefovir dipivoxil for the treatment of hepatitis B e-antigen negative chronic hepatitis B. N Engl J Med 348: 800–807.

Hepsera [package insert] (2009). Gilead Sciences, Foster City, CA, October 2009.

Ide K, Ohdan H, Tahara H et al. (2007). Possible therapeutic effect of lipid supplementation on neurological complications in liver transplant recipients. Transpl Int 20: 632–635.

Jansen O, Krieger D, Krieger S et al. (1996). Cortical hyperintensity on proton density-weighted images: an MR sign of cyclosporine-related encephalopathy. Am J Neuroradiol 17: 337–344.

Klupp J, Bechstein WO, Platz KP et al. (1997). Mycophenolate mofetil added to immunosuppression after liver transplantation-first results. Transpl Int 10: 223–238.

Krensky AM, Vincenti F, Bennett WM (2006). Immunosuppresents toleragens and immunostimulants. In: LL Brunton, JS Lazo, KL Parker (Eds.), Goodman and Gilman's The Pharmacological Basis of Therapeutics. 11th edn, McGraw-Hill, New York, ch. 52, pp. 1405–1431.

Lai CL, Shouval D, Lok A (2006). Entecavir versus lamivudine for patients with HBeAg-negative chronic hepatitis B. N Engl J Med 354: 1011–1020.

Lai CL, Gane E, Liaw YF et al. (2007). Telbivudine versus lamivudine in patients with chronic hepatitis B. N Engl J Med 357: 2576–2588.

Lau JYN, Tam RC, Lian TJ et al. (2002). Mechanism of action of ribavirin in the combination treatment of chronic HCV infection. Hepatology 35: 1002–1009.

Liaw YF, Gane E, Leung N et al. (2009). 2-year GLOBE trial results: telbivudine is superior to lamivudine in patients with chronic hepatits B. Gastroenterology 136: 486–495.

Lok ASF, McMahon BJ (2009). AASLD practice guideline update chronic hepatitis B: update 2009. Hepatology 50: 1–36.

Lu YF, Tomizawa K, Moriwaki A et al. (1996). Calcineurin inhibitors, FK506 and cyclosporine A, suppress the NMDA receptor-mediated potentials and LTP, but not depotentiation in the rat hippocampus. Brain Res 729: 142–146.

Lyson T, Ermel LD, Belshaw PJ et al. (1993). Cyclosporin and FK506 induced sympathetic activation correlated with calcineurin-mediated inhibition of T-cell signaling. Circ Res 73: 596–602.

Maramattom BV, Wijdicks EFM (2004). Sirolimus may not cause neurotoxicity in kidney and liver transplant recipients. Neurology 63: 1958–1959.

Marcellin P, Chang TT, Lim SG et al. (2003). Adefovir dipivoxil for the treatment of hepatits B e antigen-positive chronic hepatitis B. N Engl J Med 348: 808–816.

Marcellin P, Asselah T, Boyer N (2005). Treatment of chronic hepatitis B. J Viral Hepat 12: 333–345.

Martina M, Mozrzymas JW, Boddeke HW et al. (1996). The calcineurin inhibitor cyclosporine A-cycolphilin A complex reduces desensitization of GABA-mediated responses in acutely disassociated rat hippocampal neurons. Neurosci Lett 215: 95–98.

McDonald JW, Goldberg MP, Gwag BJ et al. (1996). Cyclosporine induces neuronal apotosis and selective oligodendrocyte death in cortical cultures. Ann Neurol 40: 750–758.

Muellar AR, Platz KP, Bechstein WO et al. (1994). Neurotoxicity after orthotopic liver transplantation. A comparison between cyclosporine and FK506. Transplantation 58: 155–169.

Pegasys [prescribing information] (2011). Hoffman-LaRoche, Nutly, NJ; February 2011.

Pfitzmann R, Klupp J, Langrehr JM et al. (2003). Mycophenolatemofetil for immunosuppression after liver transplantation: a follow-up study of 191 patients. Transplantation 76: 130–136.

Rang HP, Dale MM, Ritter JM et al. (2003). Anti-inflammatory and immunosuppressant drugs. In: Pharmacology, 5th edn. Churchill Livingstone, Edinburgh, pp. 244–263.

Rebetol® (2013). Merck & Co., Whitehouse Station, NJ; July 2012.

Sander M, Lyson T, Thomas GD et al. (1996). Sympathetic neural mechanisms of cyclosporine induce hypertension. Am J Hypertens 9: 121S–138S.

Saner FH, Sotiropoulos GC, Gu Y et al. (2007). Severe neurological events following liver transplantation. Arch Med Res 38: 75–79.

Saner FH, Nadalin S, Radtke A et al. (2009). Liver transplant and neurological side effects. Metab Brain Dis 24: 183–187.

Saner FH, Gensicke J, Damink SWMO et al. (2010). Neurologic complications in adult living donor liver transplant patients: an underestimated factor? J Neurol 257: 243–258.

Scherrer U, Vissing SF, Morgan BJ et al. (1990). Cyclosporin induced sympathetic activation and hypertension after heart transplantation. N Engl J Med 323: 693–699.

Sherman M, Yurdayin C, Sollano J et al. (2006). AI436026 Behold Study Group Entecavir for the treatment of lamivudine-refractory HBeAg-positive chronic hepatitis B. Gastroenterology, 130. 2039–2049.

Sloane JP, Lwin KY, Gore ME et al. (1985). Disturbances in blood-brain barrier after bone marrow transplantation (letter). Lancet 2: 280–281.

Stoltenburg-Didinger G, Boegner F (1992). Glia toxicity in dissociated cell cultures induced by cyclosporine. Neurotoxicology 13: 179–184.

Thompson CB, June CH, Sullivan KM et al. (1989). Association between cyclosporine neurotoxicty and hypomagnesemia. Lancet 2: 1116–1120.

Trull AK, Tan KKC, Roberts NB et al. (1989). Cyclosporine metabolites and neurotoxicity. Lancet 2: 448.

Wijdicks EFM, Wiesner RH, Dahlke LJ et al. (1994). FK506-induced neurotoxicity in liver transplantation. Ann Neurol 35: 498–501.

Wijdicks EFM, Wiesner RH, Krom RAF (1995). Neurotoxicity in liver transplant recipients with cyclosporine immunosuppression. Neurology 45: 1962–1964.

Wijdicks EFM, Plevak DJ, Wiesner RH et al. (1996). Causes and outcome of seizures in liver transplant reipients. Neurology 47: 1523–1525.

Wijdicks EFM, Dahlke LJ, Wiesner RH (1999). Oral cyclosporine decreases severity of neurotoxicity in liver transplant recipients. Neurology 52: 1708–1710.

Wszolek ZK, Aksamit AJ, Ellingson RJ et al. (1991). Epileptiform electroencephalographic abnormalities in liver transplant recipients. Ann Neurol 130: 37–41.

Section 6

Neurologic aspects of endocrinologic diseases

Handbook of Clinical Neurology, Vol. 120 (3rd series)
Neurologic Aspects of Systemic Disease Part II
Jose Biller and Jose M. Ferro, Editors

Chapter 47

Neurology of the pituitary

SHANIKA SAMARASINGHE*, MARY ANN EMANUELE, AND ALALEH MAZHARI
Division of Endocrinology and Metabolism, Loyola University Chicago,
Stritch School of Medicine, Maywood, IL, USA

BACKGROUND

The anterior pituitary hormones are essential for reproduction, growth, metabolic homeostasis, stress response, and adaptation to the external environment. Each pituitary hormone is secreted in a distinctive pulsatile manner reflecting its regulation by the central nervous system through a complex interaction between hypothalamic neuroendocrine pathways, feedback effects from peripheral target gland hormones, and intrapituitary mechanisms (Table 47.1).

PITUITARY ADENOMAS: EPIDEMIOLOGY AND PATHOGENESIS

Pituitary adenomas can be classified based on size (<1 cm adenomas are classified as microadenomas and ≥ 1 cm as macroadenomas) or functionality (nonsecretory or secretory). The prevalence of pituitary adenomas is as high as 20–25% (Molitch, 2009). The majority of pituitary adenomas occur sporadically; however, about 5% occur in a familial setting, of which over half are due to multiple endocrine neoplasia type 1 (MEN-1). Recently non-MEN-1 familial pituitary tumors have been described, a condition named familial isolated pituitary adenomas (Tichomirowa et al., 2009). While the most common cause of a pituitary mass is an adenoma, the differential diagnosis includes pituitary hyperplasia, lymphocytic hypophysitis, granulomatous hypophysitis, sarcoidosis, pituitary abscess, craniopharyngioma, Rathke's cleft cyst, pars intermedia cyst, colloid cyst, arachnoid cyst, empty sella, germ cell tumors, hamartoma, astrocytoma, aneurysm, histiocytosis X, chordoma, melanoma, and metastatic carcinoma.

Biological behavior and tumor aggressiveness can be predicted with the use of electron microscopy, immunohistochemistry, *in situ* hybridization for measurement

of mRNA, and assessment of cell proliferation markers such as p53, a tumor suppressor gene and indicator of rapid growth. In marked contrast to other tumors, pituitary adenomas are less vascular than the normal pituitary gland, suggesting that inhibitors of angiogenesis may play an important role in their behavior (Vierimaa et al., 2006). Pituitary development and anterior pituitary cell differentiation involve the sequential expression of several transcription factors including pituitary transcription factor-1, PROP-1 (prophet of Pit-1), bone morphogenic protein-4 (Giacomini et al., 2006), and HMGA2 (Fedele et al., 2006). The pituitary tumor transforming gene (PTTG), is overexpressed in most human pituitary adenomas compared with nonadenomatous pituitary tissue (Vlotides et al., 2007). Loss of function mutations of the MEN-1 tumor suppressor gene appears to be responsible for the tumors that occur in the parathyroids, pancreatic islets, and pituitary glands of patients who have MEN-1 (Vierimaa et al., 2006). An activating mutation of the α subunit of the guanine nucleotide stimulatory protein (Gs-α) gene is found in approximately 40% of somatotroph adenomas (Melmed, 2006; Iwata et al., 2007). These mutations result in constitutive activation of adenylyl cyclase, which may play a role in both cell division and excessive growth hormone secretion. Cytokines also play an important role in maintaining pituitary physiology, affecting not only cell proliferation but also hormone secretion (Haedo et al., 2009).

NEUROLOGIC MANIFESTATIONS OF PITUITARY LESIONS

Patients with pituitary adenomas can be asymptomatic or present with symptoms due to mass effect, pituitary hormone dysfunction, or both (Molitch, 2008).

---
*Correspondence to: Shanika Samarasinghe, M.D., Division of Endocrinology and Metabolism, Department of Medicine, Loyola University Chicago, Stritch School of Medicine, 2160 S. First Avenue, Maywood, IL 60153, USA. Tel: +1-708-216-6435, E-mail: ssamarasinghe@lumc.edu

Table 47.1

Pituitary and target hormones

Pituitary hormone	Target gland	Feedback hormone
Growth hormone (GH)	Liver, bone, adipocytes, and other tissues	IGF-1
Luteinizing hormone (LH)	Gonad	Testosterone (men) Estradiol (women)
Follicle-stimulating hormone (FSH)	Gonad	Testosterone (men) Estradiol (women)
Thyrotropin (TSH)	Thyroid	T_4, T_3
Corticotropin (ACTH)	Adrenal	Cortisol
Prolactin	Breast	Unknown

Nonfunctioning intrasellar adenomas are often asymptomatic and usually diagnosed incidentally on imaging. Neurologic symptoms occur most commonly when pituitary adenomas extend beyond the sella causing compression of surrounding structures or cause pituitary hormone deficiencies (Jaffe, 2006). The magnitude and severity of the neurologic symptoms is dependent on several factors including size, location, and the rate of enlargement of the adenoma.

Pituitary hyperplasia can at times mimic pituitary adenoma and manifest in diffuse or nodular morphologic forms (Horvath et al., 1999). Pituitary hyperplasia is most commonly seen as a physiologic response in pregnancy secondary to lactotroph hyperplasia. It can also be seen when there is failure of the pituitary hormone target gland such as thyrotroph hyperplasia secondary to hypothyroidism or gonadotroph hyperplasia secondary to primary hypogonadism. (Al-Gahtany et al., 2003). In rare cases somatotroph hyperplasia has been reported secondary to ectopic secretion of growth hormone-releasing hormone (Ezzat et al., 1994).

Patients with large tumors, rapidly enlarging tumors, or those with rapid expansion of the contents of the sella have acute onset of signs and symptoms associated with neurologic and/or hormonal dysfunction. This is classically seen in pituitary apoplexy when there is acute hemorrhage or infarction of a pre-existing pituitary adenoma (usually a macroadenoma). Patients commonly present with sudden onset, severe headache which is usually located in the retro-orbital region (Randeva et al., 1999; Nawar et al., 2008). Other symptoms may include nausea, lethargy, altered consciousness, cranial nerve palsies, and visual field defects. Compression of the pituitary gland and its vasculature supply can lead to partial or complete hypopituitarism (Bills et al., 1993; Ayuk et al., 2004). If there is compromise of the hypothalamic–pituitary–adrenal axis it is crucial that it is diagnosed and glucocorticoid replacement therapy is initiated, as untreated secondary adrenal insufficiency can lead to adrenal crisis and death.

The diagnosis of pituitary apoplexy is a clinical one and needs to be distinguished from other intracranial pathology such as subarachnoid hemorrhage, meningitis/encephalitis, cervicocranial artery dissection, cerebral venous and dural sinus thrombosis, acute stroke and mass lesion. Characteristics on imaging studies such as computed tomography (CT) or magnetic resonance imaging (MRI) can help solidify the diagnosis (Fig. 47.1). The prevalence of pituitary apoplexy is estimated to be approximately 2–3% (Randeva et al., 1999; Nawar et al., 2008).

There are several theories regarding the pathophysiology of pituitary apoplexy. Some authors have theorized

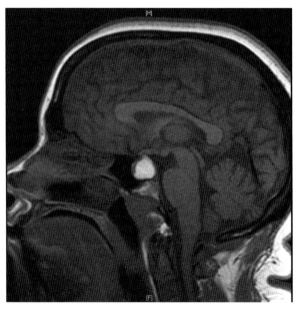

Fig. 47.1. A T1-weighted MR image showing an enlarged pituitary gland with areas of high intensity, suggesting recent hemorrhage.

that a rapidly growing adenoma can outgrow its vascular supply leading to necrosis and subsequent hemorrhage. Others propose that it is the direct compression of the pituitary infundibulum and therefore portal blood vessels that can lead to the development of pituitary apoplexy. Another proposed mechanism is that the vascular supply to the adenoma is unique and different from the vascular supply in a normal pituitary gland and therefore more susceptible to hemorrhage with changes in perfusion pressure. There is some evidence that certain inherent features of the vasculature supplying the adenoma, such as incomplete maturation of the vessels, poor fenestration, and basal membrane abnormalities predispose the adenoma to sudden hemorrhage and infarction (Biousse et al., 2001; Nawar et al., 2008).

In a majority of cases pituitary apoplexy is a spontaneous event. A precipitating factor can be identified in less than 50% of the cases. Some of the known precipitating factors or events for development of pituitary apoplexy include fluctuations in blood pressure such as hypotension, increased intracranial pressure, increased blood flow to the pituitary gland, head trauma, surgical procedures and vascular compromise as a result of changes occurring post brain irradiation. Pituitary stimulation such as in cases of high estrogen state, dynamic pituitary testing, treatment with dopamine agonists as well as stressors such as an acute systemic illness can also lead to the development of pituitary apoplexy. Anticoagulation, thrombolytic therapy or the presence of thrombocytopenia have also been identified as potential predisposing factors for pituitary apoplexy (Biousse et al., 2001).

Pituitary apoplexy is considered an endocrine emergency and untreated patients can have high morbidity and mortality. Management needs to address neurologic, endocrinologic and neuro-ophthalmologic abnormalities. Glucocorticoid treatment is commonly used not just for hormone replacement but also to control the effect of inflammation and edema on parasellar structures. Surgical intervention may be necessary to reverse or prevent further neurologic compromise (Bills et al., 1993; Ayuk et al., 2004).

There is also an entity termed subclinical pituitary apoplexy which is due to asymptomatic pituitary hemorrhage, usually diagnosed incidentally based on histopathologic findings in surgically resected or postmortem adenoma specimens, with an incidence of up to 25%. The clinical relevance of this entity is not entirely clear (Nawar et al., 2008).

The neurologic manifestation of pituitary adenomas that are small and those that are slow growing usually does not become apparent until there are signs and symptoms of hormonal dysfunction or the tumor has extended beyond the sella to cause mass effect. Visual compromise is not seen in patients with microadenomas or tumors extending just beyond the sella, given the distance between the diaphragm and the optic chiasm. Patients with macroadenomas are more likely to present with visual field defects at time of diagnosis.

The direction and extent of adenoma growth can lead to a variety of neurologic manifestations. Expansion of the adenoma superiorly can lead to compression of the optic nerve or optic chiasm resulting in visual field defects. In the majority of cases, the compression of the optic chiasm is insidious and the progression of visual loss is gradual, so that most patients are not aware of any visual changes until visual field testing is performed (Jaffe, 2006). The most common presentation is diminished or loss of vision in the temporal fields secondary to symmetric compression of the optic chiasm (bitemporal hemianopsia). At the optic chiasm there is partial decussation of the optic nerve fibers. The axons from the medial part of each retina (nasal hemiretina) cross, whereas the axons from the lateral part of the retina (temporal hemiretina) remain uncrossed (Jäger, 2005). Selective compression of the crossed and uncrossed visual fibers can result in unilateral temporal or nasal hemianopic field defect, respectively (Lee et al., 1997). Compression of the crossing inferonasal nerve fibers anterior to the chiasm can lead to bitemporal superior quadrantanopsia (Dekkers et al., 2008). Optic nerve involvement at the junction of the optic chiasm can lead to unilateral visual field loss (Lee et al., 1997).

Lateral expansion of the adenoma can lead to cranial nerve (CN) palsies (CN III, IV, V and VI) resulting in diplopia and other visual deficits. The third cranial nerve is the most commonly affected, either in isolation or in combination with other cranial nerve palsies (Yen et al., 1990). Although much less frequent, isolated CN IV and VI involvement has been reported (Lopez et al., 1981; Peterman and Newman, 1999). Involvement of the CN V is unusual and mostly seen in cases of pituitary apoplexy. In cases of very large adenomas, the tumor can compress surrounding brain tissue and manifest as partial complex seizures and hydrocephalus (secondary to compression of foramen of Monro or the aqueduct of Sylvius) (Jaffe, 2006). If there is compromise of the intracavernous portion of the carotid artery patients can present with lethargy or hemiplegia. Mass effect on the brainstem or hypothalamus can lead to altered levels of consciousness (Nawar et al., 2008).

Rare cases of prolactinomas presenting as painful postganglionic Horner syndrome responding to treatment with dopamine agonist have been reported (Talkad et al., 2004). There have also been cases of giant prolactinomas associated with bilateral scotomata (Casanueva et al., 2006).

Cerebrospinal fluid (CSF) rhinorrhea can occur due to inferior expansion of the pituitary adenoma with subsequent disruption of the arachnoid and the dura, coupled with an osseous defect secondary to the tumor erosion through the bone. CSF rhinorrhea is most commonly seen in the setting of trauma or after pituitary surgery but it can also occur after treatment of prolactinoma with dopamine agonist (due to tumor shrinkage resulting in unplugging defects in the dura and the bone resulting in CSF leakage) (Suliman et al., 2007). There have been rare case reports of untreated pituitary adenomas presenting with CSF rhinorrhea (Obana et al., 1990). If blood or necrotic tissue enters the subarachnoid space patients can present with meningitis.

Headache is the most commonly reported symptom at presentation in patients with pituitary adenomas with the majority of patients having macroadenomas. The incidence of headaches in patients with pituitary adenoma is approximately 33–72% (Fleseriu et al., 2009). In one large prospective study, 46% of the patients reported chronic migraine headaches and 30% of the patients reported episodic migraine headaches. Other patients presented with short-lasting unilateral neuralgiform headache attacks with conjunctival injection and tearing (SUNCT), cluster headaches, hemicrania continua, and primary stabbing headaches. Interestingly, SUNCT syndrome was only seen in patients with prolactin and growth hormone secreting tumors. It was not possible to classify the headache in 7% of the patients. (Levy et al., 2005).

The exact pathophysiology of headaches in this setting is not known; however, it appears that multiple factors may play a role. These include biochemical changes, compression of vessels and pain-sensitive structures (cavernous sinus, dural arteries, first branch of the trigeminal nerve), and increased intrasellar pressure (Arafah et al., 2000; Fleseriu et al., 2009). Regarding biochemical changes, growth hormone and prolactin secreting tumors in particular have been associated with headaches. Improvement in headaches has been reported with medical management of these tumors. However, it is not known if the improvement was related to the hormonal changes or changes in the tumor or tumor size. Interestingly some patients have reported exacerbation of the headache with the use of dopamine agonists for treatment of prolactin secreting tumors. This paradoxical effect may be due to central actions of dopamine agonists or the effects on the trigeminovascular system. Improvement in headaches has been reported in both microadenomas and macroadenomas following surgery (Levy et al., 2005; Fleseriu et al., 2009). The above data suggest that biochemical and structural changes may play a role in the pathophysiology of headaches in patients with pituitary adenomas.

Empty sella results from arachnoid herniation into the sella causing flattening of the pituitary gland against the floor of the sella. Empty sella can result from pituitary adenoma infarction or after pituitary surgery or radiation. Patients can also have primary empty sella due to a congenital defect. The prevalence has been reported to be 5.5–23% based on autopsy series. The clinical picture of patients with empty sella can be complex and it is not always clear if the symptoms are due to the empty sella or other etiology with incidental diagnosis of empty sella. Headache is the most commonly reported symptom and may be related to pressure on the suprasellar dural covering or due to intracranial hypertension. Patients can also have symptoms of increased intracranial pressure, rhinorrhea, dizziness, syncope, cranial nerve disorders, and other neuro-ophthalmologic disturbances. While most patients have normal pituitary function, pituitary hormone abnormalities can be present so pituitary function should be evaluated. Hyperprolactinemia is the most common pituitary hormone abnormality reported which may be secondary to pituitary stalk compression. Isolated deficiencies of growth hormone (GH), adrenocorticotropic hormone (ACTH), and thyroid-stimulating hormone (TSH) have been reported; however, panhypopituitarism is very rare (Vance, 1994; Marinis et al., 2005).

HYPOPITUITARISM

Pituitary adenomas are a common cause of pituitary hormone deficiencies. Other causes of hypopituitarism include compression of normal pituitary tissue (empty sella, suprasellar masses, metastases, internal carotid artery aneurysm), vascular (impaired blood flow to the pituitary gland secondary to infarct, trauma or Sheehan syndrome), infiltrative processes, surgery, cranial irradiation, and interference with hypothalamic production or delivery of releasing hormones to the pituitary gland. Congenital deficiencies of pituitary hormones due to genetic defects can lead to isolated or combined deficiencies of pituitary hormones and at times are associated with specific syndromes (Vance, 1994; Ascoli and Cavagnini, 2006). Traumatic brain injury (TBI) can also lead to hypopituitarism and the risk of pituitary failure has been evaluated in retrospective and prospective studies. There is now increased awareness of the need for testing of pituitary function in patients both immediately after and during long-term follow up of TBI (Tanriverdi et al., 2006).

Hypopituitarism in patients with pituitary adenomas can be partial or complete. The clinical picture will depend on the type, degree, and rapidity of onset of pituitary hormone deficiency. Most of the signs and symptoms of pituitary hormone deficiencies are similar to the hormone deficiencies associated with the target gland. In patients with pituitary macroadenomas 30%

or more can have pituitary hormone deficiencies, with the most common being growth hormone deficiency. In patients with microadenomas gonadotropin deficiency is the most common deficiency (Vance, 1994).

SECONDARY ADRENAL INSUFFICIENCY

Patients with secondary adrenal insufficiency can present with a wide range of symptoms depending on the degree and duration of glucocorticoid deficiency. The symptoms can range from subtle nonspecific symptoms to hypotension and adrenal crisis. Excluding adrenal crisis, patients with secondary adrenal insufficiency commonly report fatigue, weakness, mental dysfunction, dizziness (orthostatic hypotension may be present), anorexia, and weight loss. It is important to note that all patients with secondary adrenal insufficiency who are not on glucocorticoid therapy are at high risk for adrenal crisis if exposed to a stressor as the pituitary–adrenal axis is not able to respond to stress appropriately. Patients with adrenal crisis can present with nausea, vomiting, abdominal pain, severe hypotension, or hypovolemic shock. Biochemically patients have a low cortisol level with low or inappropriately normal ACTH level. The gold standard for diagnosing secondary adrenal insufficiency is the insulin tolerance test to evaluate the entire hypothalamic–pituitary–adrenal axis. However, in the acute setting, treatment of patients with high likelihood of secondary adrenal insufficiency based on history and clinical assessment should not be delayed in order to do further testing. Patients can be treated with glucocorticoids and further testing can be done at a later time if necessary (Ascoli and Cavagnini, 2006; Reimondo et al., 2008; Arlt, 2009).

On examination patients do not have hyperpigmentation; this is in contrast to patients with primary adrenal insufficiency who have hyperpigmentation due to elevated pro-opiomelanocortin (POMC) and ACTH levels. Patients may have hyponatremia (due to lack of negative feedback on vasopressin secretion secondary to cortisol deficiency). Serum potassium concentration is usually normal as the renin–angiotensin–aldosterone system is intact (in contrast to primary adrenal insufficiency where there is mineralocorticoid deficiency). Metabolic acidosis, hypercalcemia and/or hypoglycemia, normocytic anemia, and eosinophilia may also be present (Arlt and Allolio, 2003; Arlt, 2009).

SECONDARY HYPOTHYROIDISM

Central hypothyroidism (CH) is a rare cause of hypothyroidism characterized by deficiency of thyroid stimulating hormone (TSH). Both primary and secondary hypothyroidism can manifest with the same clinical picture. In CH symptoms of hypothyroidism tend to be milder than in primary hypothyroidism given there is some residual TSH secretion. Patients can present with fatigue, cold intolerance, constipation, weight gain or inability to lose weight, dry skin, hair loss, puffiness, nonpitting edema (myxedema), diffuse myalgias exacerbated by exercise, carpal tunnel, peripheral neuropathy, cognitive impairment, and myxedema coma. On examination, bradycardia and diastolic hypertension can be present as well as periorbital edema, proximal muscle weakness, and a slow relaxation phase of muscle stretch reflexes. Patients with secondary hypothyroidism do not present with goiter in contrast to those with primary hyperthyroidism. Biochemically patients have a low free/total triiodothyronine and thyroxine levels with inappropriately normal or low TSH. Most patients also suffer from other pituitary hormone deficiencies which can make the diagnosis difficult. (Ascoli and Cavagnini, 2006; Lania et al., 2008).

SECONDARY HYPOGONADISM

Clinical manifestation of secondary hypogonadism varies depending on the age of onset. If hypogonadism is present before puberty in men it can lead to delayed puberty, presence of small testes, phallus, scant pubic and axillary hair, as well as eunuchoid proportions with disproportionately long arms and legs secondary to delayed epiphyseal closure. There is reduced male musculature, gynecomastia, and persistent high-pitched voice. Men who develop hypogonadism after puberty can present with diminished facial and body hair, fine wrinkles, gynecomastia, soft testes, progressive decrease in muscle mass, increase in visceral fat, decreased libido, erectile dysfunction, oligo/azospermia, hot flashes (less common), and decreased bone mass (Isidori et al., 2008).

In women, hypogonadism presents prior to puberty and can lead to primary amenorrhea and absent breast development. After puberty, women with hypogonadism can present with hot flashes, vaginal dryness, dyspareunia, breast atrophy, decreased libido, low bone density. Premenopausal women can present with menstrual irregularities. Secondary hypogonadism is characterized by low or normal LH and FSH in the setting of low testosterone and low sperm count in men and low estradiol in women (Rothman and Wierman, 2008).

Secondary or hypogonadotropic hypogonadism can be congenital. An example of congenital hypogonadotropic hypogonadism is Kallman syndrome. There is failure of the gonadotropin-releasing hormone (GnRH) neurons to migrate from the olfactory placode into the hypothalamus during fetal life. Therefore GnRH is not produced by the hypothalamus and the pituitary gland is not stimulated to make LH/FSH. It can be sporadic or familial (X-linked, autosomal dominant, or recessive). Anosmia, midline facial abnormalities, urogenital abnormalities, and synkinesis can be seen in this disorder (Brioude et al., 2010). Hypogonadotropic hypogonadism can also be associated with other pituitary deficiencies as a result of impaired differentiation during fetal development due to impaired expression of transcription factors including LHX3 and PROP-1, to name a few (Rothman and Wierman, 2008).

Acquired causes of hypogonadotropic hypogonadism include acute or chronic illness, GnRH analogs which can suppress gonadotropins, and long-term use of glucocorticoids (Rothman and Wierman, 2008). Hyperprolactinemia can affect the GnRH pulse generator and therefore LH/FSH production causing hypogonadism. In women, Sheehan syndrome, which is characterized by pituitary infarct due to peri/postpartum hemorrhage, can lead to hypogonadotropic hypogonadism (Ascoli and Cavagnini, 2006).

GROWTH HORMONE DEFICIENCY

Growth hormone (GH) deficiency in childhood manifests as growth failure. In adulthood GH deficiency can present with reduced lean body mass, increased abdominal adiposity, reduced energy, higher risk of fracture, depressed mood, and increased risk of cardiovascular mortality. Exercise capacity is impaired and there is decreased muscle mass and muscle strength. The contractile properties of muscles are affected in patients with GH deficiency (Cuneo et al., 1990; Carrol et al., 1998). Since GH is secreted in a pulsatile manner, a random GH level is not helpful in the diagnosis of GH deficiency. GH stimulates hepatic production of insulin-like growth factor 1 (IGF-1, also known as somatomedin C). It is easier to interpret the age-specific IGF-1 level given its longer half-life and more steady blood level. A low age-specific IGF-1 level may be indicative of growth hormone deficiency. The best two tests for diagnosis of GH deficiency are the insulin tolerance test and the growth hormone-releasing hormone (GHRH) arginine test (Biller et al., 2002).

PROLACTIN DEFICIENCY

Prolactin is the only pituitary hormone that is under tonic inhibition (via dopamine) under normal circumstances. Prolactin level is rarely low and it tends to occur in conjunction with other pituitary hormone deficiencies. The main clinical presentation of prolactin deficiency is inability to lactate in women.

CENTRAL DIABETES INSIPIDUS

Central diabetes insipidus (DI) or neurogenic DI is characterized by an absolute or relative deficiency of

arginine vasopression (AVP) or antidiuretic hormone (ADH). More than 90% of the magnocellular AVP neurons in the supraoptic and paraventricular nuclei need to be damaged for DI to occur. DI can be due to congenital or acquired etiology. It is unusual for pituitary adenomas to present with DI due to the fact that AVP is synthesized in the supraoptic and paraventricular nuclei of the hypothalamus rather than the posterior pituitary. Even in cases of large pituitary adenomas, given the slow growth of the tumors there is adaptation of the neurohypophyseal function with the ADH release site shifting from posterior pituitary to median eminence. Central DI is most commonly seen in the postoperative setting (Adams et al., 2006; Loh and Verbalis, 2008).

Patients can present with polydipsia (craving ice cold liquids) and variable degrees of polyuria depending on the severity of ADH deficiency. In adults with intact thirst mechanism and cognitive function who have access to water, true hypernatremia usually does not occur as loss of water stimulates the thirst mechanism, resulting in an increase in intake to match the urinary losses. However, if the thirst mechanism is impaired causing hypodipsia or adipsia then patients can become hypernatremic. Biochemical data may reveal hypernatremia, elevated plasma osmolality with submaximally concentrated urine. The gold standard for diagnosis of DI is the water deprivation test (Adams et al., 2006; Loh and Verbalis, 2008).

EVALUATION OF THE HYPOTHALAMIC–PITUITARY AXIS

Proper sample collection and transport, including timing and condition (e.g., fasting, stress, sleep, posture, and drugs), are of primary importance in the evaluation of all hormone levels, and the responsible laboratory should be consulted prior to obtaining a sample. Basal evaluation should consist of trophic and target hormone levels (Table 47.1). Stimulatory tests provide insight into cases of hypofunction, whereas suppression tests are best for cases of hyperfunction.

HORMONAL HYPERFUNCTION

Hyperprolactinemia

Hyperprolactinemia is the most common neuroendocrine condition in clinical practice and the many etiologies of hyperprolactinemia are listed in Table 47.2. Prolactin is synthesized in lactotrope cells in the anterior pituitary, which account for 10–20% of pituitary cells (Molitch, 2009). In contrast to other anterior pituitary hormones, prolactin regulation is unique in that the predominant hypothalamic influence on its secretion is inhibitory rather than stimulatory. This regulation is

Table 47.2

Causes of hyperprolactinemia

Physiologic	Drugs
Pregnancy	Neuroleptics
Lactation	(e.g., haloperidol)
Pathologic	Dopamine receptor
Hypothalamic-pituitary	blockers
disorders	(e.g., metoclopramide)
Tumors	Antidepressants
Craniopharyngioma	(e.g., imipramine)
Glioma	Antihypertensives
Hamartoma	(e.g., α-methyldopa)
Microadenoma	Estrogens
Macroadenoma	Opiates
Metastatic cancer	Neurogenic
Germinoma	Spinal cord lesions
Meningioma	Chest wall lesions
Infiltrative disorders	Breast stimulation
Sarcoidosis	Miscellaneous
Giant cell granuloma	Primary hypothyroidism
Eosinophilic	Chronic renal failure
granuloma	Cirrhosis
Lymphocytic	Stress (physical,
hypophysitis	psychological)
Other	Idiopathic
Cranial radiation	
Pseudotumor cerebri	
Pituitary stalk section	
(trauma)	
Empty sella	

provided primarily by tonic inhibition by hypothalamic dopamine, which reaches the lactotropes through the hypothalamic–pituitary portal system and inhibits prolactin release, prolactin gene expression, and lactotrope proliferation. Conversely disruption of the hypothalamic–pituitary stalk leads to increased prolactin secretion (Molitch, 2008). A pituitary mass arising from any cause (neoplastic, inflammatory, vascular, or other) results in hyperprolactinemia secondary to the pressure of the mass on pituitary dopamine pathways (stalk section phenomenon). Clinically the challenge is to determine if the high prolactin levels are due to direct prolactinoma hypersecretion and require one set of therapeutic options, or if a nonfunctioning mass is causing the prolactin to rise. Chronic hyerprolactinemia causes hypogonadism through a negative effect on the secretion of GnRH, which leads to reduction of luteinizing hormone (LH) and follicle-stimulating hormone (FSH) and gonadal hormone production. This leads to amenorrhea/oligomenorrhea in women, impotence and decreased libido in men, and infertility in both genders, in addition to galactorrhea and decreased bone mineral density (Molitch, 2008). In cases of prolactinomas, mass effect such as headache,

visual field defects, decreased visual acuity, and ophthalmoplegia can be seen. The prevalence of medication-induced hyperprolactinemia varies between medications, with antipsychotics resulting in hyperprolactinemia in up to 70% of patients. If the patient is taking a medication known to cause hyperprolactinemia it is still essential to rule out a coincident prolactinoma. This can be done if the prolactin level is normalized by stopping the medication.

Prolactinomas

Prolactinomas account for 40% of pituitary tumors with 90% being microadenomas. Macroadenomas are more commonly seen in men and postmenopausal women. Prolactin levels ≥ 100 ng/mL in the face of a nonfunctioning mass implies that that patient harbors a prolactinoma and not a nonfunctioning macroadenoma (Schlechte, 2003). This well-defined cutoff value will be of great help in clinical management of patients with elevated prolactin levels and a large pituitary mass. A pituitary macroadenoma associated with only a mild elevation in prolactin level raises concern for either a nonprolactin-producing tumor causing hyperprolactinemia through pituitary stalk compression or a prolactinoma where the prolactin level, though very elevated, is artificially low due to the assay used. This artifact, called the hook effect, can be avoided by dilution of the serum.

Growth hormone excess

Growth hormone (GH) exerts a broad spectrum of effects, resulting in growth promotion and the regulation of carbohydrate, protein, lipid, and mineral metabolism. It is synthesized in and released from somatotroph cells, which constitute the most numerous cell type in the anterior pituitary. GH secretion is controlled by hypothalamic growth hormone-releasing hormone (GHRH) and somatostatin (somatotroph release-inhibiting factor, or SRIF) (Melmed, 2006). GH stimulates hepatic production of insulin-like growth factor 1 (IGF-1), which carries out the action of GH.

Acromegaly

Prolonged excessive secretion of GH and IGF-1 over years results in the clinical picture of acromegaly. A GH-secreting adenoma of the anterior pituitary is present in over 95% of cases and approximately 60% secrete exclusively GH with 25% secreting both GH and prolactin (PRL). The onset of acromegaly is insidious, and its progression is usually very slow. The interval from the onset of symptoms until diagnosis is about 12 years (Colao et al., 2004), with the mean age at diagnosis

45 years. Because of late detection, at diagnosis 75% of patients have macroadenomas which can extend to the parasellar or suprasellar region. Most patients will present with headaches and visual symptoms (Molitch, 2008), classically bitemporal hemianopsia and cranial nerve palsies. A somatotroph macroadenoma, by its mass, can cause decreased secretion of other pituitary hormones, most commonly gonadotropins (Colao et al., 2004). An activating mutation of the Gs-α gene is found in approximately 40% of somatotroph adenomas (Sam and Molitch, 2005). Neurologic manifestations include paresthesias of the hands with carpal tunnel syndrome occurring in 20% of patients. MRI studies suggest that the pathology of median neuropathy is increased edema of the median nerve (Jenkins et al., 2000). Other patients have a symmetric sensorimotor peripheral neuropathy unrelated to entrapment. Acral changes including enlarged hands and feet as well as coarsened facial features develops, along with joint cartilage and synovial tissue hypertrophy, leading to arthritis and arthralgias. Macroglossia and enlargement of the soft tissues of the pharynx and larynx lead to obstructive sleep apnea in about 50% of patients. The skin thickens and skin tags may appear. Hyperhidrosis is common. Cardiac function is frequently impaired, presenting as left ventricular hypertrophy with diastolic dysfunction. Systemic hypertension magnifies the cardiac dysfunction. GH contributes to insulin resistance, and glucose intolerance and diabetes are commonly seen. A number of studies have reported an increased risk of adenomatous colonic polyps in patients with acromegaly in addition to an increased risk of colon cancer, and colonoscopy is recommended at 3–4 year intervals in patients over age 55 (Melmed et al., 2009). In addition to an excess risk of colon polyps and cancer, acromegaly may be associated with an excess number of malignant tumors including adenocarcinomas of the stomach and esophagus, and melanoma. Patients can also have loss of other pituitary trophic hormones such as FSH, LH, TSH, and ACTH. The major diagnostic criteria are elevation of IGF-1 and nonsuppressibility of GH in response to oral glucose loads. Random GH levels are often misleading due to the pulsatile nature of GH secretion and because of its short plasma half-life. IGF-1 is a stable, integrated assessment of GH activity and IGF-1 concentrations are elevated in virtually all patients with acromegaly, providing an excellent discriminator from normal individuals. Among patients with equivocal values, serum GH levels can be measured after an oral glucose load (OGTT) (Carmichael et al., 2009). This test is the most specific dynamic test for establishing the diagnosis of acromegaly. Once GH hypersecretion has been confirmed, the next step is magnetic resonance imaging (MRI) of the pituitary.

Excess ACTH

The hypothalamic–pituitary–adrenal (HPA) axis is tightly regulated to ensure adequate glucocorticoid secretion in response to stress and to avoid excess glucocorticoid release. Corticotroph cells comprise 20% of anterior pituitary cells and are located in the central median portion of the pituitary. Pituitary ACTH release is stimulated primarily by corticotropin-releasing hormone (CRH) that is synthesized by CRH neurons located in the paraventricular hypothalamus. Levels of ACTH and glucocorticoids follow a circadian rhythm, the levels peak in the early morning and gradually decline during the day to reach a nadir at midnight. Glucocorticoid feedback action is essential for the control of this circadian rhythm.

Cushing's disease

The etiology of Cushing's syndrome can broadly be divided into two categories: ACTH-dependent and ACTH-independent. Of the ACTH-dependent forms, pituitary-dependent Cushing's syndrome, Cushing's disease, is the most common, accounting for 60–80% of all cases, usually due to a pituitary microadenoma. Overall, the onset of symptoms is usually insidious and gradually progressive over 2–10 years before the diagnosis (Kovacs et al., 2006). The clinical manifestations associated with hypercortisolemia are variable and differ widely in severity. Gross obesity of the trunk with wasting of the limbs, facial rounding and plethora, hirsutism with frontal balding, proximal muscle weakness, vertebral fractures, hypertension, and diabetes mellitus can all be seen in its most obvious form. Common symptoms also include depression, acne, easy bruising, loss of libido, and menstrual irregularity. Tests used to help confirm the diagnosis include measurement of urinary free cortisol (UFC) which produces an integrated measure of serum cortisol, smoothing out the variations in cortisol during the day. A midnight salivary cortisol measurement, which accurately reflects the plasma free cortisol concentration and can conveniently be performed at home, is highly sensitive and specific. The overnight dexamethasone suppression test can also be used as a screen. After establishing the diagnosis of Cushing's syndrome, the next step is to determine if the excess cortisol is ACTH-dependent or not and the most common test used for differentiation is the high-dose dexamethasone suppression test. It relies on the concept that high dose dexamethasone can suppress ACTH in Cushing's disease. Pituitary MRI should be done in all patients with ACTH-dependent Cushing's syndrome. A pituitary tumor larger than 6 mm with biochemical testing indicating Cushing's disease may be sufficient to confirm the diagnosis (Agha et al., 2006). However, 10% of unaffected patients may be identified as having pituitary adenoma by MRI scans and therefore, if the results are not confirmatory, bilateral inferior petrosal sinus sampling (BIPSS) should be done. This procedure requires placement of catheters in the left and right inferior petrosal sinuses and measuring ACTH simultaneously from both sinuses and peripherally before and after CRH stimulation. It is debatable whether the BIPSS should be done routinely since incidentalomas are common.

Thyroid-stimulating hormone excess

TSH is secreted from thyrotroph cells, which constitute 5% of anterior pituitary cells. The α subunit is common to TSH, follicle-stimulating hormone (FSH), and luteinizing hormone (LH) (and also chorionic gonadotropin) but the β subunit is unique to the thyrotroph and confers specificity of biologic action. The primary neuroendocrine regulation of TSH is mediated through TRH, which stimulates the transcription of both α and β subunits. Thyroid hormone inhibits the stimulatory effect of TRH on TSH release, which occurs in a pulsatile manner with secretory pulses every 2–3 hours. There is also a diurnal pattern of TSH secretion with a nocturnal surge that occurs before the onset of sleep. The feedback regulation of TSH secretion occurs principally as the result of changes in peripheral thyroid hormone levels in classic negative feedback fashion.

TSH-producing adenomas

Thyrotroph adenomas are characterized by a clinically hyperthyroid patient who has a diffuse goiter and elevations in serum free T_4 and T_3 levels, but an inappropriately normal or elevated serum TSH level. A sellar mass without excess target hormone production or without elevated prolactin, GH, ACTH, or TSH levels indicates a nonfunctional pituitary adenoma. The α subunit, which is common to FSH, LH, and TSH and has no metabolic activity, can be elevated. If initially high, this level can be followed as a marker of tumor recurrence.

Gonadotropin-producing adenomas

The gonadotrophs constitute 7–15% of the cells in the anterior pituitary gland. LH and FSH are glycoproteins with a common α subunit and distinct β subunits that confer specificity to each hormone. Both FSH and LH are synthesized and released in a pulsatile manner in response to hypothalamic GnRH. The frequency of the GnRH pulses is a critical factor that determines LH and FSH synthesis and secretion. Also important in gonadotropin synthesis and secretion are inhibins, activins, and follistatin. Sex steroids are important regulators of GnRH and gonadotropin release through classic feedback mechanisms in the hypothalamus and the pituitary. Gonadotroph adenomas can be identified by characteristic patterns and their subunits, which differ in men and women.

Gonadotropin producing adenomas are the most common clinically nonfunctioning pituitary adenomas, and usually come to clinical attention when they become large enough to cause neurologic symptoms. They may also be found on imaging for an unrelated reason. Impaired vision is the most common presenting symptom, caused by suprasellar extension of the adenoma compressing the optic chiasm. Other presenting neurologic symptoms include headache, diplopia, cerebrospinal fluid rhinorhea, and pituitary apoplexy induced by sudden hemorrhage. Importantly, apoplexy can be precipitated by administration of a drug that stimulates gonadotroph adenomas, such as GnRH analog treatment of prostate cancer (Davis et al., 2006). The least common clinical presentation is one that results from hormonal abnormalities, as gonadotroph adenomas are hormonally inefficient and the LH and FSH produced are not usually sufficient to result in hormonal derangements. Also only about 35% of these tumors secrete enough gonadotropins to raise the serum levels (Sam and Molitch, 2005), and the hormone combinations differ in men and women. In men an elevated basal serum FSH concentration with an intrasellar mass lesion usually indicates that the lesion is a gonadotroph adenoma. The diagnosis is strengthened if the patient also has a supranormal level of the free α subunit and serum LH accompanied by an elevated testosterone level. In women, recognizing the gonadotroph origin of an intrasellar mass on the basis of serum intact FSH and LH is more difficult, especially in women over 50 years of age. However, a gonadotroph adenoma is suspected if there is a markedly elevated FSH level associated with a subnormal LH concentration, as this pattern is not likely in the postmenopausal state or in premature ovarian failure (Mor et al., 2005). An elevated serum free α subunit concentration is also helpful. An elevated serum estradiol with an FSH concentration that is not suppressed, associated with endometrial hyperplasia and polycystic ovaries by ultrasound in a woman of premenopausal age who presents with amenorrhea or oligomenorrhea strongly suggests a gonadotroph adenoma secreting FSH constantly and causing ovarian hyperstimulation (Daneshdoost et al., 1991). It is important to remember that a "normal" FSH is not appropriate when the estradiol is markedly elevated and the LH suppressed. Prepubertal girls may present with breast development, vaginal bleeding, and abdominal distension (Daneshdoost et al., 1991), and young boys with premature puberty.

Hormonal deficiencies due to compression of nona-denomatous pituitary cells by the macroadenoma can also be the initial presentation. The diagnosis is established by finding abnormalities of the subunits of LH and FSH that are characteristic of a gonadotroph adenoma and by follow-up imaging. By the time a gonadotroph adenoma produces supranormal serum concentrations of intact gonadotropins or their subunits, it is sufficiently large to be seen by imaging. A pituitary adenoma of gonadotroph or thyrotroph cell origin should be suspected if the serum prolactin is less than 100 ng/mL, the patient does not appear acromegalic and the insulin-like growth factor 1 (IGF-1) is not elevated, and the patient does not have Cushing's syndrome or supranormal salivary, serum, or urine cortisol levels.

Nonfunctional adenomas

Clinically nonfunctioning pituitary adenomas range from being completely asymptomatic, and therefore being detected either at autopsy or as incidental findings on head MRI or CT scans performed for other reasons (pituitary incidentalomas), to causing significant hypothalamic/pituitary dysfunction and visual field compromise due to their large size. Patients with pituitary incidentalomas should all be screened for hypersecretion of prolactin (PRL), acromegaly (IGF-1), Cushings's disease (salivary and urine cortisol levels), and those with macroadenomas should also be screened for hypopituitarism and for visual field defects if the tumor abuts the optic chiasm. Growth of nonfunctioning pituitary adenomas without treatment occurs in about 10% of microadenomas and 24% of macroadenomas (Sam and Molitch, 2005). In the absence of hypersecretion, hypopituitarism, or visual field defects, patients may be followed up by periodic screening by MRI for enlargement. Growth of a pituitary incidentaloma is an indication for surgery.

IMAGING

The key imaging features of pituitary tumors relate to the demonstration of a mass and displacement of adjacent structures. Characterizing the type of tumor is based on location, shape and size, and on the density/intensity characteristics of the mass.

An MRI specifically focused on the sellar region is the imaging modality of choice as the more widely spaced cuts of a routine brain MRI are often inadequate to visualize small pituitary tumors. This technique delineates the pituitary gland, stalk, optic tracts and surrounding structures such as the cavernous sinus. The posterior pituitary exhibits a bright spot of high signal intensity thought to reflect the presence of vasopressin localized within neurosecretory vesicles. Lack of this feature can represent a nonspecific indicator of central diabetes insipidus. The pituitary gland can transiently enlarge during puberty, pregnancy, and in the postpartum period. The stalk should not exceed 4 mm in diameter; a thickened stalk can indicate hypophysitis, histiocytosis, lymphoma, or granulomatous disease (Morana et al., 2010).

Most microadenomas are hypointense on T1-weighted MR images in relation to adjacent pituitary tissue. This difference is accentuated after contrast enhancement with gadolinium. Macroadenomas, which tend to be more vascular tumors, show intermediate signal on unenhanced images, and can enhance after gadolinium administration. They often enlarge the sella turcica by gradual remodeling of the bony fossa and show frequent extrasellar extension (Sam and Molitch, 2005) (Fig. 47.2). Subacute hemorrhage shows high signal on T1- and T2-weighted images.

Certain lesions have specific signal characteristics which may aid in diagnosis. Rathke cleft cysts and craniopharyngiomas have a common origin from remnants of Rathke's pouch. Craniopharyngiomas are benign yet aggressive squamous epithelial tumors that are predominantly suprasellar. Prominent cystic portions with wall enhancement or varying signal intensities of mixed cystic and solid components with calcification are typical imaging features (Komotar et al., 2009) (Fig. 47.3). CT is superior to MRI in the identification of calcifications

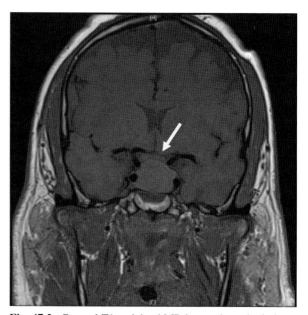

Fig. 47.2. Coronal T1-weighted MR image through pituitary fossa showing a pituitary macroadenoma elevating and compressing optic chiasm (arrow).

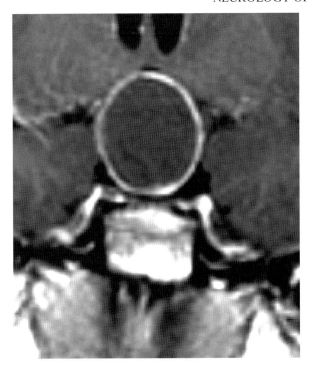

Fig. 47.3. Craniopharyngioma. Coronal T1-weighted MR image. Large well-defined cystic mass with wall enhancement. (Image courtesy of Jordan Rosenblum, M.D., Loyola University Medical Center, Chicago, IL, USA.)

which represent the hallmark of craniopharyngiomas. Rathke's cleft cysts are benign lesions containing mucoid material and usually show a sellar epicenter, smooth contour, and reduced MR signal intensity on T1-weighted and increased MR signal intensity on T2-weighted imaging (Anderson et al., 1999).

Meningiomas, primitive germ cell tumors, chordomas, and metastasis also represent neoplasms which appear in the sellar region. Meningiomas may arise from any dural site, including the diaphragma sella, turberculum, dorsum sella as well as the dura of the adjacent cavernous sinuses. Characteristic features include dense homogenous enhancement after gadolinium, dural tail enhancement and adjacent hyperosteosis (bone thickening) (Sam and Molitch, 2005). Germinomas are generally isointense on T1- and T2- weighted imaging. Chordomas, arising from the notochordal remnants of the clivus, typically produce bony destruction and can lead to cranial neuropathy and neurologic symptoms. Finally, pituitary metastases are found in 1–2% of patients, with breast and lung carcinoma being the most common primary sources. Interestingly, the posterior pituitary can be involved in 70% of these cases and patients present with diabetes insipidus. The MRI/CT features are those of an enhancing mass, but potential multiplicity of lesions,

with a history of a known primary tumor, often leads to the diagnoses.

MANAGEMENT OF PITUITARY TUMORS

Management of pituitary tumors ranges from observation of nonfunctioning microadenomas through medical, surgical, and radiotherapeutic approaches dependant on tumor type, function, size, and invasiveness. The choice of treatment modality is determined by several factors including: relief of mass effect, treatment of hormone excess or restoration of hormone deficits, prevention of tumor regrowth, and minimizing long-term morbidity and mortality.

Observation

Asymptomatic patients with nonfunctioning pituitary adenomas may be candidates for conservative management. Although studies are heterogeneous, the clinical course of microadenomas suggests a low growth propensity (3.2–12.5%), whereas tumor enlargement was reported in up to 24% of patients with macroadenomas (Greenman and Stern, 2009). Therefore, medical follow-up appears reasonable for microadenomas. In the case of macroadenomas, the higher incidence of tumor enlargement can be associated with the appearance of new pituitary dysfunction, visual field defects, or apoplexy. As a predictor of tumor growth, adenomas larger than 15 mm have been shown to increase the risk of symptom development over a mean of 5 years (Arita et al., 2006). Early surgery may increase the chance of complete tumor removal with a resultant decrease in tumoral complications and recurrence.

Surgical management

Surgery remains the first-line treatment of symptomatic pituitary tumors with the exception of prolactinomas. Indications include mass effect with visual compromise, primary correction of hormonal hypersecretion, resistance to medical therapy, pituitary hemorrhage/apoplexy, and need for tissue histology for diagnosis. The most rapid and reliable relief from optic nerve and chiasmal compression is surgery; visual deficits improve in over 85% of patients (Ausiello et al., 2008). Minimally invasive transsphenoidal microsurgery is used in the vast majority of pituitary tumors. This approach precludes invasion of the cranial cavity and manipulation of brain tissue and allows for a clearly visible operative field (Fig. 47.4). Normal pituitary can be clearly distinguished from tumor tissue, facilitating dissection. The mortality in experienced hands is excellent, between 0.2% and 1%, depending on the case mix

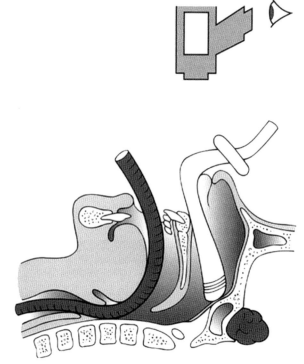

Fig. 47.4. After preparation of a mucosal tunnel a speculum is inserted which is placed right in front of the sphenoid sinus (transsphenoidal approach) The sinus has been opened so that the sellar floor can be identified using a microscopic view. (Reproduced from Buchfelder and Schlaffer, 2009, with permission.)

(Joshi and Cudlip, 2008). Exceptions to the transsphenoidal technique are tumors with significant temporal or suprasellar extension, especially those contained by a small diaphragmatic aperture (dumbbell configuration), invasion into the posterior clivus, or coexisting intrasellar vascular lesions. In such cases, a transcranial approach is undertaken.

An endoscopic approach is increasingly being utilized. Use of an endoscope allows for a superior view of the target area, an enlarged working angle with panoramic views of bony landmarks, and access to tumor extension into the cavernous sinus. Disadvantages include management of perioperative intrasellar bleeding and the requirement for a preoperative CT scan (Cappabianca et al., 2008). The long-term outcomes for this relatively new technique are not yet well defined and often a combination approach is used. Additional advances in the operating room include intraoperative MRI which allows for real-time assessment of the dimensions and extent of the pituitary mass concealed from the operating microscope (Jones and Ruge, 2007). Neuronavigation employs a 3D data set provided by preoperative imaging to gain additional anatomic orientation, identifying tumor shape and major arteries superimposed onto the surgical field (Buchfelder and Schlaffer, 2009). These techniques improve the rate of completely excised tumors, but long-term benefits await further follow-up.

In terms of surgical outcomes, the tumor size, magnitude of hormonal hypersecretion, local invasion, and experience of the neurosurgeon are critical factors in determining the likelihood of success. In hormonally active pituitary microadenomas, expert surgeons report remissions in up to 90% of patients (Buchfelder and Schlaffer, 2009). However, with macroadenomas, remission rates vary widely depending on the series and definition of cure. Craniopharyngiomas demonstrate variable tumor extension, thus total resection is more difficult to achieve and is associated with higher postoperative morbidity.

Postoperative complications

The low morbidity and mortality associated with transsphenoidal surgery is a major advantage of this approach. Anterior pituitary insufficiency and diabetes insipidus can occur in up to 20% of cases (Ciric et al., 1997). Major neurosurgical complications such as CSF leak, meningitis, stroke, intracranial hemorrhage, and visual loss are relatively rare (1.5–4%) (Dumont et al., 2005). Minor complications including sinus disease, septal perforation, epistaxis, and wound issues occur in approximately 6.5% (Dumont et al., 2005). As transcranial surgery necessitates direct dissection of the brain, vascular structures and visual pathways, the complication rate is considerably higher.

A main focus of postoperative assessment after transsphenoidal surgery is monitoring for anterior and posterior pituitary dysfunction. Disruption of the hypothalamic–pituitary–adrenal axis is covered with perioperative glucocorticoids. Monitoring for water imbalances due to deficiency or excess of AVP requires strict assessment of fluid intake, urine output and urine osmolality in conjunction with frequent electrolyte measurements. Diabetes insipidus is often transient in the postoperative period. Most patients maintain adequate fluid intake and euvolemia. Desmopressin (DDAVP) therapy should be undertaken with care and is usually only needed once or twice. If the patient is alert with intact thirst mechanisms, the degree of thirst can be used to guide water replacement. An analysis of 1571 patients undergoing transphenoidal surgery demonstrated various patterns of postoperative polyuria and hyponatremia; only 0.9% of patients at 3 months and only 0.25% of patients at 1 year still had polyuria or needed DDAVP (Hensen et al., 1999).

Syndrome of inappropriate antidiuretic hormone (SIADH) can occur up to 2 weeks postoperatively in 5–10% of patients, with peak incidence on day seven (Ausiello et al., 2008). It can present with hyponatremia that can be severe and symptomatic. Management generally consists of fluid restriction. A few weeks after surgery, the adrenal, thyroid, and gonadal axes are assessed. New persistent hypopituitarism is relatively uncommon in experienced hands. Long-term monitoring should initially include imaging every 6–12 months to detect growth of residual adenoma tissue and laboratory testing to gauge adequacy of hormonal replacement. Vision should also be periodically evaluated if affected preoperatively. If there is no tumor regrowth, the intervals between imaging can be lengthened.

Medical management

Several established and emerging medical therapies are available for the treatment of prolactinomas, acromegaly, and Cushing's disease.

PROLACTINOMAS

Dopamine agonists (DA) are the first line of management in patients with hyperprolactinoma. As dopamine is the endogenous negative regulator of prolactin release, prolactin gene expression, and lactotrope proliferation, medical treatments are based on activation of the lactotrope D_2 receptor. They normalize prolactin levels, control galactorrhea, restore reproductive function, and decrease tumor size in most patients (Klibanski, 2010). DA include bromocriptine and cabergoline (ergot derivatives), and quinagolide (nonergot derivative) available outside the US. Pergolide was withdrawn from the US market in 2007 following concerns of cardiac valvular damage (Patil et al., 2009). Cabergoline, with a high affinity for the lactotrope D_2 receptor, is often considered the initial DA of choice, although it is more expensive. In a randomized trial involving 459 women, cabergoline was associated with fewer side-effects and normalized prolactin levels in 83% of patients compared to 59% of those treated with bromocriptine (Klibanski and Greenspan, 1986). In addition, cabergoline may be effective in patients intolerant of or resistant to bromocriptine. DA decrease tumor mass in the majority of patients and are used as primary therapy as tumor shrinkage and visual field improvement may occur in weeks. Adverse effects include gastrointestinal symptoms and orthostatic hypotension which can be minimized by slow titration of medication dosage. A recent study (Schade et al., 2007) has suggested that the high doses of cabergoline used to treat Parkinson's patients may be associated with cardiac valve insufficiency. The cumulative daily dose was > 3.0 mg,

significantly higher than that routinely administered to prolactinoma patients (0.25–1.0 mg/week). Further study is necessary to determine the clinical significance of this finding in prolactinomas as many patients can be treated for decades.

Patients with DA agonist-resistant prolactinomas by definition have more aggressive tumors, thus recurrence rates after surgery tend to be higher.

ACROMEGALY

Surgical treatment remains the initial treatment of choice in acromegaly, specifically for tumors that are small, large but resectable, or large and causing visual symptoms. Surgery may also be considered for debulking of unresectable adenomas with the goal of increasing the success of subsequent adjuvant therapy. Medical therapy for acromegaly is indicated in patients who do not achieve biochemical cure after resection or have disease recurrence. The biochemical criteria for cure have become more stringent in recent years with the recognition of the considerable cardiovascular, metabolic, and respiratory comorbidities and reduction in life expectancy associated with growth hormone excess (Melmed, 2009). These include the normalization of serum IGF-1 levels and suppression of the serum GH concentration to < 1 ng/mL after a glucose load as measured by a high sensitivity immunoradiometric or chemiluminescent assay (Chanson et al., 2009).

The mainstays of medical therapy for acromegaly are the somatostatin analogs (SSA), octreotide and lanreotide. Octreotide is available in short- and long-acting forms; lanreotide is a long-acting depot. They bind to somatostatin receptor subtypes 2 and 5 to inhibit GH secretion as well as reduce tumor volume (Freda et al., 2005). These drugs achieve remission in 60–70% of patients and reduce tumor volume in 20–40% of patients (Colao et al., 2001; Freda et al., 2005; Melmed et al., 2005). The reduction in tumor volume is usually modest and more significant when the SSA is the first-line treatment (either before or as an alternative to surgery and radiotherapy). These agents can be continued indefinitely, with cost as the major obstacle. They have gastrointestinal adverse effects which are generally transient, and cause gallstones in 10–20% of patients (Lamberts et al., 1996). They have also been found to decrease fasting plasma insulin, but their clinical impact on glucose homeostasis appears minimal (Mazziotti et al., 2009).

Pegvisomant acts in the periphery, blocking the effects of GH on its target organs by binding to GH receptors and preventing their dimerization. This blocks GH activity including production of IGF-1, but does not inhibit GH secretion. Pegvisomant is a highly effective therapy for lowering IGF-1; levels normalize in more than 90% of patients (Chanson et al., 2009) with subsequent improvement in symptoms. Continued adenoma growth is possible and should be monitored by MRI, but this appears uncommon. An increase in tumor size was noted in 3.2% of 684 patients for whom MRI data were available over a mean duration of 1.7 years (Trainer, 2009). Elevations in hepatic transaminases have also been reported (Melmed, 2009). Finally, as somatotroph tumors also express D_2 receptors, DA agonists do have a limited role in the treatment of acromegaly, especially in those that cosecrete prolactin. High-dose bromocriptine (20–40 mg/day) normalizes IGF-1 in 10% of patients (Colao et al., 1997). Cabergoline appears to be more effective, with up to 40% of select patients responding (Abs et al., 1998).

CUSHING'S DISEASE

Surgery is also the primary treatment modality for Cushing's disease. Unfortunately, 10–30% of patients fail to achieve remission after initial surgery and a similar percentage may recur (Patil et al., 2009). Thus limited medical therapy, radiotherapy, and bilateral adrenalectomy are also utilized in the management of Cushing's disease. Pharmacologic treatments focus on diminishing adrenal cortisol synthesis by enzymatic inhibition and include agents such as ketoconazole, metyrapone, etomidate, and mitotane. Side-effects are common. In addition, if the pharmacologic blockade is incomplete, the rise in ACTH secretion overrides the blockade and hypercortisolemia remains. Their primary role is to temporarily control cortisol levels in patients awaiting the therapeutic effects of radiation.

Agents that specifically target the pituitary in Cushing's disease include the DA agonist cabergoline and the somatostatin analogue pasireotide. Chronic cabergoline therapy has been associated with a clinically relevant reduction in hypercortisolemia, although rare normalization. Pasireotide has a high affinity for somatostatin receptor subtype 5 which can be present in corticotroph adenomas. Activation of this subtype inhibits corticotropin secretion. In a recent study by Colao et al, pasireotide decreased urinary free cortisol by a mean of 48% and normalized it in 26% and 15% of patients receiving a 900 mcg or 600 mcg dose, respectively (Colao et al., 2012). However, hyperglycemia-related adverse events were common, occurring in 73% of patients (Colao et al., 2012). Another medical therapeutic option is mifepristone, which at high doses is a glucocorticoid receptor antagonist. It has been shown to be rapidly effective for certain symptoms of Cushing's syndrome, such as cortisol-induced psychosis and hyperglycemia (Castinetti et al., 2009). As such, mifepristone has been recently approved in the United States to control hyperglycemia in adults with endogenous Cushing's syndrome and type 2 diabetes who have failed surgery. Adverse effects include moderate to severe hypokalemia, hypertension and clinical signs of adrenal insufficiency (Castinetti et al., 2009).

Radiotherapy

Radiotherapy is reserved for patients who have failed surgical and/or medical therapies or who are unable to tolerate the risks of surgery due to medical comorbidites. This includes those with persistent or recurrent hormonal hypersecretion states. It is the rational step after failed transsphenoidal surgery in Cushing's disease as medical therapy is poor. Pituitary irradiation has also decreased the incidence of Nelson's syndrome, the development of locally aggressive ACTH-producing tumors due to loss of feedback inhibition at the corticotrope in patients who have undergone bilateral adrenalectomy.

Radiation may be indicated after resection of a recurrent or inadequately resected sellar mass. These tend to display aggressive features such as cavernous sinus invasion, compression of the carotid artery, erosion into the clivus or sphenoid sinus. Postoperative radiotherapy is favored in those with craniopharyngioma. Radiotherapy has a high therapeutic index, delivering high-energy ionizing radiation to arrest growth of tumor while minimizing exposure to the normal surrounding tissue (Minniti et al., 2009). The aim is to prevent tumor progression and normalize elevated hormone levels. It is successful in achieving tumor control in up to 95–97% of patients at 10 years and 88–92% of patients at 20 years. Hormonal control is less successful with 60–80% of patients in remission dependant on tumor type after radiotherapy (Patil et al., 2009). Conventional radiotherapy requires several years to become maximal and may require continued medical therapy in the interim. Hypopituitarism is the most common complication with up to 80% of patients demonstrating gonadotroph, somatotroph, thyrotroph, or corticotroph deficits within 10 years after radiation (Anderson et al., 1999). Additional complications of conventional radiotherapy include optic neuropathy (1.5% risk), brain necrosis (0.2%), secondary malignancies such as gliomas and astrocytomas (2%), cerebrovascular disease, and possible cognitive impairment (Brada et al., 2004; Vance, 2005). The development of modern stereotactic technologies that can deliver high dose radiation more precisely to the tumor can minimize complications and allow for more rapid reduction in hormonal hypersecretion. Stereotactic irradiation can be given as a single fraction radiosurgery (SRS) using either a cobalt unit (Gamma knife) or linear accelerator (LINAC) or as lower fractionated doses over several treatments using a linear accelerator or proton source (Castinetti et al., 2010). The precision achieved with stereotactic techniques allows for a reduction in safety margins around the tumor leading to sparing of normal brain from high radiation doses. Despite theoretical advantages, long-term outcomes and efficacy have yet to be defined.

FUTURE DIRECTIONS

Improvement in hormonal assays and imaging techniques will allow for earlier diagnosis of pituitary problems even prior to symptom development. Further development of molecular tools will help determine the aggressiveness and genetic implications of pituitary adenomas. Continued advancements in surgical and radiation techniques as well as newer medical therapies will continue to evolve.

REFERENCES

Abs R, Verhelst J, Maiter D et al. (1998). Cabergoline in the treatment of acromegaly: a study in 64 patients. J Clin Endocrinol Metab 83: 374–378.

Adams JR, Belvins LS, Allen GS et al. (2006). Disorders of water metabolism following transsphenoidal pituitary surgery: a single institutions experience. Pituitary 9: 93–99.

Agha A, Tomlinson JW, Clark PM et al. (2006). The long-term predictive accuracy of the short synacthen (corticotropin) stimulation test for assessment of the hypothalamic-pituitary-adrenal axis. J Clin Endocrinol Metab 91: 43–47.

Al-Gahtany M, Horvath E, Kovacs K (2003). Pituitary hyperplasia. Hormones 2: 149–158.

Anderson JR, Antoun N, Burnet N et al. (1999). Neurology of the pituitary gland. J Neurol Neurosurg Psychiatry 66: 703–721.

Arafah BM, Prunty D, Ybarra J et al. (2000). The dominant role of increased intrasellar pressure in the pathogenesis of hypopituitarism, hyperprolactinemia and headaches in patients with pituitary adenomas. J Clin Endocrinol Metab 85: 1789–1793.

Arita K, Tominaga A, Sugiyama K et al. (2006). Natural course of incidentally found nonfunctioning pituitary adenoma, with special reference to pituitary apoplexy during follow-up examination. J Neurosurg 104: 884–891.

Arlt W (2009). The approach to the adult with newly diagnosed adrenal insufficiency. J Clin Endocrinol Metab 94: 1059–1067.

Arlt W, Allolio B (2003). Adrenal insufficiency. Lancet 361: 1881–1893.

Ascoli P, Cavagnini F (2006). Hypopituitarism. Pituitary 9: 335–342.

Ausiello JC, Bruce JN, Freda PU (2008). Postoperative assessment of the patient after transsphenoidal pituitary surgery. Pituitary 11: 391–401.

Ayuk J, McGregor EJ, Mitchell RD et al. (2004). Acute management of pituitary apoplexy – surgery or conservative management. Clin Endocrinol 61: 747–752.

Biller MBK, Samuels MH, Zagar A et al. (2002). Sensitivity and specificity of six tests for the diagnosis of adult growth hormone deficiency. J Clin Endocrinol Metab 87: 2067–2079.

Bills DC, Meyer FB, Laws ER et al. (1993). A retrospective analysis of pituitary apoplexy. Neurology 33: 602–609.

Biousse V, Newman NJ, Oyesiku NM (2001). Precipitating factors in pituitary apoplexy. J Neurol Neurosurg Psychiatry 71: 524–525.

Brada M, Ajithkumar TV, Minniti G (2004). Radiosurgery for pituitary adenomas. Clin Endocrinol (Oxf) 61: 531–543.

Brioude F, Bouligand J, Trabado S et al. (2010). Non-syndromic congenital hypogonadotropic hypogonadism: clinical presentation and genotype-phenotype relationships. Eur J Endocrinol 162: 835–851.

Buchfelder M, Schlaffer S (2009). Surgical treatment of pituitary tumours. Best Pract Res Clin Endocrinol Metab 23: 677–692.

Cappabianca P, Cavallo LM, de Divitiis O et al. (2008). Endoscopic pituitary surgery. Pituitary 11: 385–390.

Carmichael JD, Bonert VS, Mirocha JM et al. (2009). The utility of oral glucose tolerance testing for diagnosis and assessment of treatment outcomes in 166 patients with acromegaly. J Clin Endocrinol Metab 94: 523.

Carrol PV, Christ ER, Bengtsson BA et al. (1998). Growth hormone deficiency in adulthood and the effect of growth hormone replacement: a review. J Clin Endocrinol Metab 83: 382–395.

Casanueva FF, Molitch ME, Schlechte JA et al. (2006). Guidelines of the pituitary society for the diagnosis and management of prolactinomas. Clin Endocrinol 65: 265–273.

Castinetti F, Regis J, Dufour H et al. (2010). Role of stereotactic radiosurgery in the management of pituitary adenomas. Nat Rev Endocrinol 6: 214–223.

Castinetti F, Fassnacht M, Johanssen S et al. (2009). Merits and pitfalls of mifepristone in Cushing's syndrome. Eur J Endocrinol 160 (6): 1003.

Chanson P, Salenave S, Kamenicky P et al. (2009). Pituitary tumours: acromegaly. Best Pract Res Clin Endocrinol Metab 23: 555–574.

Ciric I, Ragin A, Baumgartner C et al. (1997). Complications of transsphenoidal surgery: results of a national survey, review of the literature, and personal experience. Neurosurgery 40: 225–236, discussion 236–227.

Colao A, Di Sarno A, Sarnacchiaro F et al. (1997). Prolactinomas resistant to standard dopamine agonists respond to chronic cabergoline treatment. J Clin Endocrinol Metab 82: 876–883.

Colao A, Ferone D, Marzullo P et al. (2001). Long-term effects of depot long-acting somatostatin analog octreotide on hormone levels and tumor mass in acromegaly. J Clin Endocrinol Metab 86: 2779–2786.

Colao A, Ferone D, Marzullo P et al. (2004). Systemic complications of acromegaly: epidemiology, pathogenesis, and management. Endocr Rev 25: 102.

Colao A, Petersenn S, Newell-Price J et al. (2012). A 12-month phase 3 study of pasireotide in Cushing's disease. N Engl J Med. 366 (10): 914–924.

Cuneo RC, Salomon F, Wiles CM et al. (1990). Skeletal muscle performance in adults with growth hormone deficiency. Horm Res 33: 55–60.

Daneshdoost L, Gennarelli TA, Bashey HM et al. (1991). Recognition of gonadotroph adenomas in women. N Engl J Med 324: 589–594.

Davis A, Goel S, Picolos M et al. (2006). Pituitary apoplexy after leuprolide. Pituitary 9: 263–265.

Dekkers OM, Pereira AM, Romjin JA (2008). Treatment and follow up of clinically nonfunctioning pituitary macroadenomas. J Clin Endocrinol Metab 93: 3717–3726.

Dumont AS, Nemergut EC 2nd, Jane JA Jr et al. (2005). Postoperative care following pituitary surgery. J Intensive Care Med 20: 127–140.

Ezzat S, Asa SL, Stefaneanu L et al. (1994). Somatotroph hyperplasia without pituitary adenoma associated with a long standing growth hormone-releasing hormone producing bronchial carcinoid. J Clin Endocrinol Metab 78: 555–560.

Fedele M, Pierantoni GM, Visone R et al. (2006). Critical role of the HMGA2 gene in pituitary adenomas. Cell Cycle 5: 2045–2048.

Fleseriu M, Yedinak C, Campbell C et al. (2009). Significant headache improvement after transsphenoidal surgery in patients with small sellar lesions. J Neurosurg 110: 354–358.

Freda PU, Katznelson L, van der Lely AJ et al. (2005). Long-acting somatostatin analog therapy of acromegaly: a meta-analysis. J Clin Endocrinol Metab 90: 4465–4473.

Giacomini D, Paez-Pereda M, Theodoropoulou M et al. (2006). Bone morphogenetic protein-4 inhibits corticotroph tumor cells: involvement in the retinoic acid inhibitory action. Endocrinology 147: 247–256.

Greenman Y, Stern N (2009). Non-functioning pituitary adenomas. Best Pract Res Clin Endocrinol Metab 23: 625–638.

Haedo MR, Gerez J, Fuertes M et al. (2009). Regulation of pituitary function by cytokines. Horm Res 72: 266–274.

Hensen J, Henig A, Fahlbusch R et al. (1999). Prevalence, predictors and patterns of postoperative polyuria and hyponatraemia in the immediate course after transsphenoidal surgery for pituitary adenomas. Clin Endocrinol (Oxf) 50: 431–439.

Horvath E, Kovacs K, Scheithauer BW (1999). Pituitary hyperplasia. Pituitary 1: 169–180.

Isidori AM, Giannetta E, Lenzi A (2008). Male hypogonadism. Pituitary 11: 171–180.

Iwata T, Yamada S, Mizusawa N et al. (2007). The aryl hydrocarbon receptor-interacting protein gene is rarely mutated in sporadic GH-secreting adenomas. Clin Endocrinol (Oxf) 66: 499–502.

Jaffe CA (2006). Clinically non-functioning pituitary adenoma. Pituitary 9: 317–321.

Jäger HR (2005). Loss of vision: imaging the visual pathways. Eur Radiol 15: 501–510.

Jenkins PJ, Sohaib SA, Akker S et al. (2000). The pathology of median neuropathy in acromegaly. Ann Intern Med 133: 197.

Jones J, Ruge J (2007). Intraoperative magnetic resonance imaging in pituitary macroadenoma surgery: an assessment of visual outcome. Neurosurg Focus 23: E12.

Joshi SM, Cudlip S (2008). Transsphenoidal surgery. Pituitary 11: 353–360.

Klibanski A (2010). Clinical practice Prolactinomas. N Engl J Med 362: 1219–1226.

Klibanski A, Greenspan SL (1986). Increase in bone mass after treatment of hyperprolactinemic amenorrhea. N Engl J Med 315: 542–546.

Komotar RJ, Roguski M, Bruce JN (2009). Surgical management of craniopharyngiomas. J Neurooncol 92: 283–296.

Kovacs K, Horvath E, Coire C et al. (2006). Pituitary corticotroph hyperplasia preceding adenoma in a patient with Nelson's syndrome. Clin Neuropathol 25: 74–80.

Lamberts SW, van der Lely AJ, de Herder WW et al. (1996). Octreotide. N Engl J Med 334: 246–254.

Lania A, Persani L, Beck-Peccoz P (2008). Central hypothyroidism. Pituitary 11: 181–186.

Lee AG, Siebert KJ, Sanan A (1997). Radiologic-clinical correlation junctional visual field loss. AJNR Am J Neuroradiol 18: 1171–1174.

Levy MJ, Matharu MS, Meeran K et al. (2005). The clinical characteristics of headache in patients with pituitary tumours. Brain 128: 1921–1930.

Loh JA, Verbalis JG (2008). Disorders of water and salt metabolism associated with pituitary disease. Endocrinol Metab Clin North Am 37: 213–234.

Lopez R, David NJ, Gargano F et al. (1981). Bilateral sixth nerve palsies in a patient with massive pituitary adenoma. Neurology 31: 1137–1138.

Marinis LD, Bonadonna S, Bianchi A et al. (2005). Primary empty sella. J Clin Endocrinol Metab 90: 5471–5477.

Mazziotti G, Floriani I, Bonadonna S et al. (2009). Effects of somatostatin analogs on glucose homeostasis: a metaanalysis of acromegaly studies. J Clin Endocrinol Metab 94: 1500–1508.

Melmed S (2006). Medical progress: acromegaly. N Engl J Med 355: 2558.

Melmed S (2009). Acromegaly pathogenesis and treatment. J Clin Invest 119: 3189–3202.

Melmed S, Sternberg R, Cook D et al. (2005). A critical analysis of pituitary tumor shrinkage during primary medical therapy in acromegaly. J Clin Endocrinol Metab 90: 4405–4410.

Melmed S, Colao A, Barkan A et al. Acromegaly Consensus Group (2009). Guidelines for acromegaly management: an update. J Clin Endocrinol Metab 94: 1509–1517.

Minniti G, Gilbert DC, Brada M (2009). Modern techniques for pituitary radiotherapy. Rev Endocr Metab Disord 10: 135–144.

Molitch ME (2008). Nonfunctioning pituitary tumors and pituitary incidentalomas. Endocrinol Metab Clin North Am 37: 151–171.

Molitch ME (2009). Pituitary tumours: pituitary incidentalomas. Best Pract Res Clin Endocrinol Metab 23: 667–675.

Mor E, Rodi IA, Bayrak A et al. (2005). Diagnosis of pituitary gonadotroph adenomas in reproductive-aged women. Fertil Steril 84: 757.

Morana G, Maghnie M, Rossi A (2010). Pituitary tumors: advances in neuroimaging. Endocr Dev 17: 160–174.

Nawar RN, AbdelMannan D, Selman WR et al. (2008). Analytic review Pituitary tumor apoplexy: a review. J Intensive Care Med 23: 75–90.

Obana WG, Hodes JE, Weinstein PR et al. (1990). Cerebrospinal fluid rhinorrhea in patients with untreated pituitary adenoma: report of two cases. Surg Neurol 33: 336–340.

Patil CG, Hayden M, Katznelson L et al. (2009). Non-surgical management of hormone-secreting pituitary tumors. J Clin Neurosci 16: 985–993.

Peterman SH, Newman NJ (1999). Pituitary macroadenoma manifesting as isolated fourth nerve palsy. Am J Ophthalmol 127: 235–236.

Randeva HS, Schoebel J, Byrne J et al. (1999). Classical pituitary apoplexy: clinical features, management and outcome. Clin Endocrinol 51: 181–188.

Reimondo G, Bovio S, Allasino B et al. (2008). Secondary hypoadrenalism. Pituitary 11: 147–154.

Rothman MS, Wierman ME (2008). Female hypogonadism, evaluation of the hypothalamic pituitary ovarian axis. Pituitary 11: 163–169.

Sam S, Molitch ME (2005). The pituitary mass: diagnosis and management. Rev Endocr Metab Disord 6: 55–62.

Schade R, Andersohn F, Suissa S et al. (2007). Dopamine agonists and the risk of cardiac-valve regurgitation. N Engl J Med 356: 29–38.

Schlechte JA (2003). Clinical practice Prolactinoma Review. N Engl J Med 349: 2035–2041.

Suliman SGI, Gurlek A, Byrne JV et al. (2007). Neurosurgical cerebrospinal fluid rhinorrhea in invasive macroprolactinoma: incidence, radiological and clinicopathological features. J Clin Endocrinol Metab 92: 3829–3835.

Talkad AV, Kattah JC, Xu MY (2004). Prolactinoma presenting as painful postganglionic Horner syndrome. Neurology 62: 1400–1401.

Tanriverdi F, Senyurek H, Unluhizarci K et al. (2006). High risk of hypopituitarism after traumatic brain injury: a prospective investigation of anterior pituitary function in the acute phase and 12 months after trauma. J Clin Endocrinol Metab 91: 2105–2111.

Tichomirowa MA, Daly AF, Beckers A (2009). Familial pituitary adenomas. J Intern Med 266: 5–18.

Trainer PJ (2009). ACROSTUDY: the first 5 years. Eur J Endocrinol 161 (Suppl 1): S19–S24.

Vance ML (1994). Hypopituitarism. N Engl J Med 330: 1651–1662.

Vance ML (2005). Pituitary radiotherapy. Endocrinol Metab Clin North Am 34: 479–487, xi.

Vierimaa O, Georgitsi M, Lehtonen R et al. (2006). Pituitary adenoma predisposition caused by germline mutations in the AIP gene. Science 312: 1228–1230.

Vlotides G, Eigler T, Melmed S (2007). Pituitary tumor-transforming gene: physiology and implications for tumorigenesis. Endocr Rev 28: 165–186.

Yen MY, Liu JH, Jaw SJ (1990). Ptosis as the early manifestation of pituitary tumour. Br J Ophthalmol 74: 188–191.

Handbook of Clinical Neurology, Vol. 120 (3rd series)
Neurologic Aspects of Systemic Disease Part II
Jose Biller and Jose M. Ferro, Editors

Chapter 48

Thyroid disease and the nervous system

CLARE A. WOOD-ALLUM AND PAMELA J. SHAW*
*Sheffield Institute for Translational Neuroscience, University of Sheffield and Department of Neurology,
Royal Hallamshire Hospital, Sheffield, UK*

INTRODUCTION

Disorders of the thyroid gland are common and frequently accompanied by neurologic complications. A recent study of unselected general medical, geriatric, and psychiatric inpatients showed that 1–2% of patients had some form of thyroid disease (Attia et al., 1999). A 2008 population-based study carried out in Tayside, Scotland, revealed a prevalence of ever having had hyperthyroidism of 1.26% in women, 0.24% in men and a prevalence of hypothyroidism of 5.14% in women and 0.88% in men (Leese et al., 2008). It is important for the neurologist to be aware of the neurologic complications of thyroid disease because thyroid disorders may present first to the neurologist but, more important still, most may be readily corrected with appropriate treatment.

The neurologic complications of thyroid disease may be the direct result of changes in the levels of thyroid hormones, may arise from immune-mediated mechanisms, or else may be the result of mechanical compression of neural structures. Alteration in the levels of circulating thyroid hormones may produce a new neurologic complication, exacerbate a pre-existing neurologic problem, or unmask a subclinical neurologic problem. Antibodies raised against targets in the thyroid gland may have effects on neural tissue with antigens in common. Autoimmune disease of the thyroid may be associated with other autoimmune diseases affecting the nervous system such as myasthenia gravis. Compression of adjacent neural structures by an enlarging thyroid gland, an enlarging pituitary gland, or infiltrated ocular muscles and fat may result in neurologic complications. Patients with thyroid carcinoma may develop intracranial metastases. Whilst research in this area continues apace, it is clear that the cellular and molecular mechanisms underlying many neurologic complications of thyroid disease remain incompletely understood.

NEUROLOGIC COMPLICATIONS OF HYPOTHYROIDISM

The neurology of congenital hypothyroidism

Congenital hypothyroidism (CH), historically termed cretinism, is the commonest treatable cause of mental retardation, with a prevalence of 1/2000 to 1/4000 (Fisher, 1983). It is due to a deficiency in thyroid hormone present at birth. Congenital hypothyroidism may be subdivided into primary (due to agenesis of the thyroid or dyshormonogenesis), secondary (due to deficient TSH signal transduction or else as part of congenital hypopituitarism), or peripheral (due to deficits in the transport or metabolism of thyroid hormone) (Rastogi and LaFranchi, 2010). It may be permanent or transient. Endemic cretinism is the commonest form of transient CH although its effects on the fetus, if maternal iodine supplementation is not instituted in the first trimester of pregnancy, are permanent (Bunevicius and Prange, 2010). It occurs in neonates born to mothers whose diet is deficient in iodine and in consequence cannot make adequate thyroid hormone. Maternal thyroid hormone deficiency early in gestation results in devastating irreversible neurodevelopmental deficits regardless of treatment after birth. In these cases both mother and baby have thyroid glands capable of generating and responding to thyroid hormone normally although common polymorphisms in the gene coding a thyroid hormone deiodinase may modulate the severity of the phenotype resulting from a lack of maternal dietary iodine (Guo et al., 2004).

Neonates with CH not born in areas where diets are deficient in iodine may be clinically normal or present only

*Correspondence to: Pamela J. Shaw, Academic Neurology Unit, Department of Neuroscience, Sheffield Institute of Translational Neuroscience, University of Sheffield, 385a Glossop Road, Sheffield S10 2HQ, UK. Tel: +44-114-222-2260, E-mail: pamela.shaw@sheffield.ac.uk

subtle clinical signs at birth as thyroid hormone made by their mother may partially compensate the deficit *in utero*. If diagnosis and the institution of treatment is delayed postpartum, however, they too may go on to manifest irreversible neurodevelopmental deficits. Due to the widespread introduction of neonatal screening programs, manifest CH is now extremely rare in the developed world. It is a sobering fact that ~75% of the world's neonates are not screened for CH and because of this and the resultant delayed diagnosis and treatment, preventable permanent learning disability still occurs due to CH.

ETIOLOGY OF PERMANENT CONGENITAL HYPOTHYROIDISM

A detailed consideration of inborn errors of thyroid gland development and thyroid hormone synthesis responsible for permanent congenital hypothyroidism lies beyond the scope of this chapter. A summary is provided but the topic has been recently reviewed (Djemli et al., 2006; Rastogi and LaFranchi, 2010). Some 85% of permanent primary CH is due to abnormal development of the thyroid gland (Clifton-Bligh et al., 1998; Macchia et al., 1998; Krude et al., 2002). As an example, a group of patients with congenital hypothyroidism poorly responsive to treatment and featuring additional choreoathetosis, muscular hypotonia, and pulmonary problems were found to be due to mutations in thyroid transcription factor 1 (Krude et al., 2002). Mutations in genes coding proteins required for thyroid hormone synthesis cause 10–15% of permanent primary CH. These include thyroid peroxidase, the most commonly affected protein (Bakker et al., 2000), thyroglobulin (Vono-Toniolo and Kopp, 2004), the sodium/iodide symporter (Dohan and Carrasco, 2003; Dohan et al., 2003), and nicotinamide adenine dinucleotide phosphate (NADP) oxidases (Moreno et al., 2002). Mutations in the thyrotropin receptor are responsible for permanent secondary CH (Abramowicz et al., 1997; Jordan et al., 2003), whilst mutations to a transmembrane thyroid hormone transporter, MCT-8, cause permanent peripheral CH (Dumitrescu et al., 2004). MCT-8 mutations cause abnormal levels of circulating iodothyronines as well as global developmental delay, central hypotonia, spastic quadriplegia, dystonic movements, rotatory nystagmus and impaired gaze and hearing in affected males. Heterozygous females have a milder thyroid phenotype and no neurologic abnormalities.

CLINICAL AND RADIOLOGIC FEATURES

A study of endemic foci of CH in western China and central Java described mental retardation, proximal pyramidal signs, and extrapyramidal signs as the commonest features of CH (Halpern et al., 1991). Many patients had a characteristic gait, reflecting dysfunction of both the pyramidal and the extrapyramidal motor systems, in combination with laxity and deformity of the joints. Other clinical features commonly seen in patients with congenital hypothyroidism included strabismus, deafness, ataxia, and persistent primitive reflexes. Adult patients with CH have a characteristic motor phenotype: rigidity and spasticity affecting the trunk and proximal limb girdle musculature, and relative sparing of the distal extremities. In this study computed tomography (CT) imaging of the brain showed basal ganglia calcification in one-third of patients. Magnetic resonance imaging (MRI) of the head in three CH patients showed abnormalities in the globus pallidus and substantia nigra. There was only modest cerebral atrophy, and the cerebral cortical gyral pattern and thickness appeared normal. The corpus callosum and cerebral white matter were well myelinated, and there was no significant atrophy of the brainstem and cerebellum (Ma et al., 1993).

PATHOGENESIS

Recent studies have shown that, in the developing brain, thyroid hormone has important effects on the regulation of neurofilament gene expression (Ghosh et al., 1999) and on the expression of genes encoding mitochondrial proteins (Vega-Nunez et al., 1995). Hypothyroidism increases adenosine monophosphate (AMP) hydrolysis in the hippocampal and cortical synaptosomes of rats and influences synaptic function control throughout cortical development (Bruno et al., 2005). Thyroid hormone also regulates the timing of appearance and regional distribution of laminin, an extracellular matrix protein that provides key guidance signals to migrating neurons within the central nervous system (CNS). It has been suggested that disruption in the expression of laminin may play a role in the derangement of neuronal migration observed in the brain of patients with congenital hypothyroidism (Farwell and Dubord-Tomasetti, 1999).

TREATMENT AND PROGNOSIS

Prompt initiation of treatment is essential in CH; indeed there is an inverse relationship between ultimate IQ score and time to treatment (Boileau et al., 2004). A recent review of outcomes in the postneonatal screening era indicated that in 18 of 51 reviewed studies the ultimate attained IQs of children with CH were as high as those of unaffected controls. In the other 33 studies, however, children with CH had ultimate IQs 5–25 points lower than unaffected controls (LaFranchi and Austin, 2007). A recent Dutch study found worsened motor performance in young adults diagnosed on neonatal screening with CH, the degree of impairment correlating with the severity of hypothyroidism (Kempers et al., 2006). If CH is permanent, lifelong treatment is required. In transient CH euthyroidism is gradually regained over the first few months or years of life, therefore treatment is only required until then. It should be emphasized that the cause of many cases of primary CH may not be clear – for the overwhelming majority of cases treatment does not depend upon this but upon the closely monitored replacement of thyroxine and the restoration of euthyroidism.

Encephalopathy, coma, and seizures

MYXEDEMA COMA

Clinical features

Slowness, impairment of attention and concentration, somnolence, and lethargy are common symptoms in hypothyroidism. Occasionally, a life-threatening encephalopathy known as myxedema coma develops in patients with chronic, untreated hypothyroidism. Whilst diminution of mentation and sleepiness are invariable in myxedema coma, patients do not usually, despite the name, present in coma. Myxedema coma may result from a variety of precipitating factors (see below) causing decompensation of the physiologic adaptations to the hypothyroid state (Wall, 2000). In the compensated hypothyroid state, physiologic adaptations include a shift of the vascular pool away from the periphery to the central core, to sustain normal body temperature (Nicoloff and LoPresti, 1993). In chronic hypothyroidism, these adaptations tend to produce a degree of diastolic hypertension, as well as a decrease in blood volume of up to 20%. Many other organ systems and metabolic pathways are profoundly altered by chronic deficiency of thyroid hormone. Alterations in myocardial biochemistry produce impairment of cardiac contractility; the ventilatory response to hypercapnia is abnormal; hyponatremia may result from a reduction in free water clearance; and there may be a degree of suppression of bone marrow function resulting in normochromic normocytic anemia and an impaired white blood cell response to infection. Reduction in insulin clearance and decreased gluconeogenesis may produce a tendency to hypoglycemia, and patients are predisposed to toxic side-effects of medication due to reduced plasma clearance of all drugs. The corticosteroid response to stress is likely to be impaired, even when basal serum cortisol levels are normal (Nicoloff and LoPresti, 1993).

The majority of patients who develop myxedema coma are elderly, yet a high index of suspicion is required to diagnose myxedema coma in this group in whom features of hypothyroidism may be difficult to distinguish from the effects of aging. It is not uncommon for myxedema coma to be the presenting complaint of previously undiagnosed hypothyroidism. In more than 50% of cases, coma develops after the patient has been admitted to the hospital, often following a history of gradual deterioration (Nicoloff and LoPresti, 1993).

Three key clinical features are universally present in myxedema coma: altered mentation which may include depression of level of consciousness, defective temperature control, and a precipitant (Beynon et al., 2008). Precipitants include infection, trauma or surgery, exposure to the cold, and the administration of certain medications. There is even a case report of myxedema coma precipitated in an elderly Japanese lady by several months' excessive intake of raw Bok Choy, a form of cabbage that when raw contains a goitrogen that inhibits the uptake of iodine by the thyroid (Chu and Seltzer, 2010). Body temperature is lower than normal in the majority of cases, but there may also be relative hypothermia – that is a normal body temperature in the presence of sepsis, which may complicate diagnosis. Most patients have clinical signs in keeping with long-standing hypothyroidism which can help with diagnosis – dry skin, sparse hair, periorbital edema, hoarse voice, macroglossia and nonpitting peripheral edema. Seizures occur in approximately 20% of cases. Focal neurologic signs are not usually observed unless there has been a concomitant cerebrovascular event.

The pathophysiology of myxedema coma is not fully understood, but is likely to be multifactorial. Contributory factors may include derangement of blood gas levels, hyponatremia, hypopituitarism, hypotension, sepsis, and seizure activity (Myers and Hays, 1991). Neuropathologic studies of patients with myxedema coma have been few and have usually shown only the presence of cerebral edema with or without diffuse neuronal changes.

Laboratory investigations

Laboratory investigations are often abnormal, but are not pathognomonic (Wall, 2000). In critically ill patients, distinguishing between severe hypothyroidism (low T_4, low T_3, and, unless due to secondary hypothyroidism, a high TSH) and the euthyroid sick syndrome may be difficult and it may be necessary to measure levels of free circulating thyroid hormone. The electrocardiogram typically shows sinus bradycardia, with low voltage and prolongation of the QT interval. Chest radiography may reveal pleural effusion or enlargement of the cardiac silhouette due to pericardial effusion. The patient may be mildly anemic, usually with normochromic normocytic indices. Hyponatremia may be present, and serum cholesterol level may be elevated. Serum creatine kinase and lactate dehydrogenase are often raised, sometimes in a pattern suggestive of myocardial damage. Arterial blood gases may be abnormal, with carbon dioxide retention and/or hypoxia. Lumbar puncture may reveal a high cerebrospinal fluid (CSF) opening pressure often with a high CSF protein. The electroencephalogram (EEG) is likely to be abnormal (Cadilhac, 1976). Initially, there is a decrease in the frequency of the α rhythm, a reduction of photic responses, and an overall decrease in the amplitude and slowing of the dominant rhythm, often with low-range θ activity. Triphasic waves have also been described in some individuals.

Management of myxedema coma

The key to the successful treatment of myxedema coma is early diagnosis and the rapid institution of appropriate therapeutic measures in an intensive care unit setting (Myers and Hays, 1991; Nicoloff and LoPresti, 1993; Wall, 2000). The main principles of management include correction of electrolyte and blood sugar abnormalities; passive rewarming; treatment of associated infections; control of seizures; respiratory and circulatory support; administration of stress doses of glucocorticoids; and thyroid hormone replacement. Myxedema coma has a high mortality rate (20–40%) (Beynon et al., 2008), and treatment should not be deferred pending confirmatory laboratory results. Empiric initial treatment should comprise intravenous thyroxine, broad-spectrum antibiotics to cover any underlying infection, and hydrocortisone. When thyroxine is replaced in these patients the metabolism of cortisol is increased. If this is not anticipated and hydrocortisone given, a secondary adrenal crisis may be precipitated. Patients may not develop a fever or raise their leukocyte count even in the presence of severe infection – the absence of these features should not be interpreted as an absence of sepsis. Intravenous thyroxine (200–500 μg initially, followed by 50–100 μg daily) has been recommended (Myers and Hays, 1991; Rodriguez et al., 2004). Whether optimal replacement therapy should be with thyroxine (T_4), triiodothyronine (T_3), or a combination of the two is unclear from the evidence, as is whether oral T_4 is as efficacious as intravenous T_4. Studies in this area are limited by the small numbers of patients and the large numbers of variables in the initial presentation (Beynon et al., 2008). A recent study from Japan examined factors associated with mortality in eight cases of myxedema coma of their own and reviewed 87 cases reported in the literature (Yamamoto et al., 1999). Increased age, cardiac complications, and high-dose thyroid hormone replacement (thyroxine, ≥ 500 μg/day, or triiodothyronine, ≥ 75 μg/day) were significantly associated with a fatal outcome within 4 weeks of the development of myxedema coma. Reduced conscious level on admission to hospital was shown to predict poor outcome in another study (Rodriguez et al., 2004).

SEIZURES

There is a relatively high incidence of seizures in hypothyroidism (Evans, 1960). Approximately 20% of patients with untreated hypothyroidism will develop seizures or syncopal episodes. Drop attacks (sudden repeated falls without warning symptoms and without loss of consciousness) have also been reported as a complication of hypothyroidism that resolves with therapy (Kramer and Achiron, 1993). There have also been reports of patients with severe hypothyroidism presenting in status epilepticus (Jansen et al., 2006). Clinicians should be alert to the possibility of underlying hypothyroidism when the recovery time of the patient following a seizure is unusually prolonged.

Mental changes

Hypothyroidism may be associated with mood disorder, in particular depression (Bunevicius and Prange, 2010). Treatment of the hypothyroidism usually resolves this although interestingly it seems likely that the response of individuals to treatment may be modulated by common polymorphisms of thyroid hormone transporters and deiodinases (Panicker et al., 2009; Bunevicius and Prange, 2010). Severe psychiatric features also occur in untreated hypothyroidism and may be florid. Asher coined the colorful term *myxedematous madness* to describe the mental state changes that can occur in some hypothyroid patients, including irritability, paranoia, hallucinations, delirium, and psychosis (Asher, 1949). This problem resolves rapidly following the administration of thyroid hormone replacement therapy (Cook and Boyle, 1986). Evidence for mental changes in subclinical hypothyroidism is conflicting. A recent study in 164 elderly Korean people found no evidence of what they called neuropsychiatric derangements in subclinical hypothyroidism (Park et al., 2010).

An increased incidence of hypothyroidism has been reported in various groups of patients with major psychiatric illnesses. An association between hypothyroidism and bipolar affective disorder has been proposed (Szabadi, 1991). Even higher rates of hypothyroidism have been reported in manic-depressive patients with the "rapid cycling" form of the illness of whom up to 50% have positive antithyroid antibody titers (Kilzieh and Akiskal, 1999). Clinical and subclinical hypothyroidism in depression and bipolar disorder may adversely affect or delay the response to treatment (Cole et al., 2002). Many patients with depression, when by usual definitions biochemically euthyroid, have subtle alterations in their thyroid function, including slight elevation of serum thyroxine, blunting of the thyroid-stimulating hormone (TSH) response to thyrotropin-releasing hormone (TRH), detectable antithyroid antibody titers (Heinrich and Grahm, 2003) and loss of the normal nocturnal TSH rise (Jackson, 1998). These changes are generally reversed following alleviation of the depression.

Hypothyroidism is an important cause of reversible dementia, most commonly manifesting as psychomotor slowing, memory impairment, visuoperceptual problems, and reduced constructional dexterity (Dugbartey, 1998). One study reported reversible cerebral hypoperfusion, determined by single-photon emission computed tomography (SPECT) brain imaging, in a patient with hypothyroid dementia caused by excessive treatment of a hyperthyroid state (Kinuya et al., 1999). Both the mental changes and the SPECT abnormalities reversed following return of the patient to euthyroidism. Interestingly, recent work in rats suggested that hypothyroidism may increase the vulnerability of cortical neurons to the deposition of amyloid protein (Ghenimi et al., 2010).

More subtle neuropsychological abnormalities have also been documented in hypothyroidism. In one study, 54 nondemented hypothyroid patients were compared with 30 controls (Osterweil et al., 1992). Hypothyroid patients had lower Mini-Mental Status Test scores and performed worse in five of 14 neuropsychological tests applied. The aspects of cognitive function most affected included learning, word fluency, visuospatial abilities, and some aspects of attention, visual scanning, and motor speed. Treatment of the hypothyroidism resulted in improvement in three of the most sensitive neuropsychological measures employed.

A review of the literature suggests that thyroid replacement does not always lead to complete resolution of cognitive impairment (Clarnette and Patterson, 1994). Lai et al. investigated the potential for recovery of CNS complications of hypothyroidism by serially measuring central conduction in rats (Lai et al., 2000). Before thyroxine treatment, there was a consistent prolongation of central conduction. After treatment, central conduction usually returned to normal if the animals had been hypothyroid for less than 5 months. However, if they had been hypothyroid for 7 months or more, there was incomplete recovery. The authors suggested that there may be a "therapeutic window" for reversal of the CNS effects of hypothyroidism. Recent evidence suggested that mood and neuropsychological function may improve more in hypothyroid patients treated with both thyroxine and triiodothyronine, rather than with thyroxine alone (Bunevicius et al., 1999).

Peripheral neuropathy

Hypothyroidism may be complicated by the development of entrapment mononeuropathies or a more diffuse peripheral neuropathy.

ENTRAPMENT NEUROPATHY

Evidence of entrapment neuropathy is found in around 35% of patients with hypothyroidism (Khedr et al., 2000). The most common mononeuropathy is carpal tunnel syndrome (CTS), which may occur in as many as 29% of patients (Purnell et al., 1961; Bastron, 1984). Compression of the median nerve results from deposition of acid mucopolysaccharides in the nerve and surrounding tissues (Purnell et al., 1961). Tarsal tunnel syndrome frequently coexists in patients with hypothyroidism who develop carpal tunnel syndrome (Schwartz et al., 1983). Surgical decompression for median nerve entrapment is not usually required in patients with underlying hypothyroidism, as symptoms gradually resolve once euthyroidism is achieved (Kececi and Degirmenci, 2006). De Rijk et al. recently reported the results of thyroid function tests performed in 516 consecutive patients diagnosed on electrophysiology with CTS and without known hypothyroidism or other underlying cause. Only two cases of hypothyroidism were detected suggesting that thyroid function testing, even in confirmed CTS, is probably not worthwhile if there are no other clinical pointers to the hypothyroid state (de Rijk et al., 2007).

DIFFUSE PERIPHERAL NEUROPATHY

The peripheral neuropathy of hypothyroidism is usually relatively mild and predominantly sensory. Knee and ankle reflexes are reduced, distal vibration and joint position sense are mildly impaired. The patient may describe episodes of lancinating pain (Pollard et al., 1982). The reported incidence of peripheral neuropathy in hypothyroidism has varied widely, ranging from 9% to 60% (Nickel et al., 1961; Watanakunakorn et al., 1965). In a study of 39 consecutive patients with hypothyroidism, Beghi et al. found subjective sensory symptoms in 64% of cases, objective clinical findings supporting a diagnosis of polyneuropathy in 33%, and neurophysiologic evidence of polyneuropathy in 72% (Beghi et al., 1989). More recently, Duyff et al. studied 24 patients newly diagnosed with hypothyroidism. Of this group 42% had clinical signs of a predominantly sensory peripheral neuropathy (Duyff et al., 2000). Guieu et al. studied the nociceptive threshold in 12 hypothyroid patients and found values significantly higher than those of normal control subjects; values returned to normal 6 weeks after starting thyroxine replacement therapy (Guieu et al., 1993).

Pollard reported absent sensory action potentials and significant slowing of motor conduction velocities in hypothyroid patients, suggesting segmental demyelination (Pollard et al., 1982). Other studies have shown decreased motor and sensory action potential amplitudes and mild slowing of sensory and motor conduction velocities consistent with axonal pathology (Nemni et al., 1987).

The pathologic changes described in hypothyroid neuropathy include segmental demyelination, axonal degeneration, increased numbers of mitochondria, and deposition of mucopolysaccharides in the endoneurial interstitium and perineurial sheath. Opinions differ as to whether axonal degeneration (Pollard et al., 1982; Nemni et al., 1987; Shinoda et al., 1987) or demyelination (Dyck and Lambert, 1970) is the primary pathologic process.

Toscano et al. report a single case of multifocal motor neuropathy with elevated titers of IgM antibodies against GM1 in association with Hashimoto's thyroiditis (Toscano et al., 2002). The patient in this case responded to intravenous immunoglobulin therapy.

Disorders of sleep

Both obstructive and central sleep apnea may occur in patients with hypothyroidism. Depression of the respiratory center, an altered bellows action of the thorax, and physical obstruction of the airway by an enlarged tongue and pharyngeal muscles have all been described. In one recent study of 50 newly diagnosed, untreated hypothyroid patients, 30% had sleep disordered breathing (defined as an apnea–hypopnea index ≥ 5) (Jha et al., 2006). Of these patients, 10 of 12 returned to normal once euthyroidism was achieved with treatment of the hypothyroidism. Factors contributing to the development of obstructive sleep apnea are likely to include narrowing of the upper airway due to deposition of mucopolysaccharides and extravasation of protein into the tissues of the tongue and nasopharynx, as well as hypertrophy of the genioglossus muscle. Zwillich et al. showed that decreased hypoxic ventilatory drive in hypothyroidism can be corrected with thyroid hormone replacement therapy (Zwillich et al., 1975). The mechanism of central apnea in hypothyroidism may involve a disturbance in serotonin (5-HT) neurotransmission (Vaccari, 1982). Thyroid hormone replacement usually results in rapid improvement in ventilatory drive. Improvement in airway dimensions may require a longer period of euthyroidism (up to 12 months), and only at this stage will nocturnal snoring decrease (Lin et al., 1992). In some patients, sleep apnea does not satisfactorily remit with adequate treatment of the hypothyroidism, and additional measures such as overnight continuous positive airway pressure ventilation (CPAP) may be required.

Cerebellar ataxia

Reference to unsteadiness of gait may be found in the earliest clinical descriptions of hypothyroidism. Further interest in this neurologic complication was generated in a paper published in 1960 (Jellinek and Kelly, 1960). Studies indicate that 5–10% of hypothyroid patients develop significant gait ataxia (Jellinek and Kelly, 1960; Cremer et al., 1969; Swanson et al., 1981; Harayama et al., 1983). A detailed assessment of 24 patients with hypothyroidism and ataxia was reported by Cremer et al. (1969). All complained of poor balance, a tendency to fall, or poor limb coordination, and in many cases ataxia was the presenting complaint. Ten patients had poor limb coordination, one had cerebellar dysarthria, but none had nystagmus. The cause of the hypothyroidism varied in these patients. Near complete or complete resolution of the cerebellar features rapidly followed achievement of euthyroidism.

The pathophysiologic basis of cerebellar dysfunction in hypothyroidism remains unknown. The rapid resolution of ataxia with thyroid replacement therapy suggests that the problem may be caused by a reversible metabolic factor. Some authors have suggested that ataxia only becomes apparent when hypothyroidism is superimposed upon a pre-existing, subclinical cerebellar deficit (Barnard et al., 1971). Selim and Drachman reported six patients with Hashimoto's thyroiditis who developed ataxia while euthyroid (three were on oral replacement with L-thyroxine) (Selim and Drachman, 2001). All had midline cerebellar atrophy on MRI and alternative causes were excluded. The authors postulated an immune-mediated mechanism of cerebellar degeneration in a subset of patients and suggest that immune suppression may be a therapeutic option for this group. Pathologic reports are few, and those cases that have been described had complicating coexisting medical problems. Depletion of Purkinje cells was reported in one patient, novel "myxedema bodies" were recorded in the brain of another, and cerebellar atrophy most markedly affecting the anterosuperior vermis in a third (Barnard et al., 1971).

Developmental studies in young rats have shown that hypothyroidism interferes with the development of Purkinje cell dendrites and the normal inward migration of cells from the external granular layer (Nicholson and Altman, 1972; Koibuchi and Iwasaki, 2006). Cerebellar ataxia has been less frequently reported in children with CH or childhood hypothyroidism. A small number of cases are now present in the literature, many featuring ataxia as only one of several features of a hypothyroid syndrome. Tajima et al. reported a case of promptly diagnosed and treated CH who nevertheless suffered mental and growth retardation along with ataxia. MRI imaging revealed dramatic cerebellar atrophy in this case (Tajima et al., 2007).

Cranial nerve disorders

Primary thyroid failure may be associated with pituitary enlargement resulting from hyperplasia due to lack of negative feedback from circulating thyroid hormones. In one recent study pituitary enlargement on MRI was found in 37 of 53 (70%) of patients with primary hypothyroidism (Khawaja et al., 2006). Subtle visual field defects resulting from pressure on the optic chiasm have been reported in the majority of patients with primary hypothyroidism (Yamamoto et al., 1983). Visual evoked potentials may be abnormal in hypothyroid patients (Ladenson et al., 1984) but severe visual field loss and blindness are rare. Thyroid hormone replacement therapy may lead to a reduction in pituitary size and an improvement in vision along with development of an empty sella in some (LaFranchi et al., 1986; Lecky et al., 1987). If the association between pituitary gland enlargement and primary hypothyroidism is remembered, unnecessary invasive interventions can be avoided when pituitary hyperplasia is detected on neuroimaging. Occasionally patients with hypothyroidism develop headache and papilledema secondary to benign intracranial hypertension after the initiation of thyroxine replacement therapy (Van Dop et al., 1983).

Hearing impairment and tinnitus commonly occur in hypothyroid patients (Anand et al., 1989). Pure-tone audiometry reveals hearing loss in as many as 85% of cases. Brainstem auditory evoked potentials in hypothyroidism are "slow and low" compared with those in normal subjects. Hearing loss in this group of patients may be due to pathology at several sites. Abnormalities in the middle ear and inner ear have been described, and the resultant hearing loss may have conductive, neural, and central components. Hearing loss may improve when the hypothyroidism is treated. Dysphonia in patients with hypothyroidism appears to arise from local myxedematous changes in the larynx, rather than from lower cranial nerve dysfunction. An atypical facial pain syndrome has also been described in hypothyroidism (Watts, 1951).

Hypothyroid myopathy

CLINICAL FEATURES

Muscle involvement is common in both clinical and subclinical hypothyroidism. More than 60% of patients have an elevated creatine kinase level (Hekimsoy and Oktem, 2005). Creatine kinase levels correlate with the severity of hypothyroidism and correct when thyroid function normalizes with treatment. Symptomatic muscle disease, however, is less common. Clinically evident hypothyroid myopathy occurs in 30–80% of hypothyroid patients (Duyff et al., 2000). Myopathy may preface biochemical hypothyroidism or else develop concurrently (Kung et al., 1987). Kliachko and Prikhozhan studied 81 patients 4 weeks after thyroxine treatment was stopped (Kliachko and Prikhozhan, 1970). Half

developed muscle pain, 82% had prolonged ankle reflexes, 14% had objective muscle weakness, 6% had muscle cramps, and 6% had myopathic features on electromyography.

The clinical features of hypothyroid myopathy include weakness, cramps, aching or painful muscles, sluggish movements and reflexes, and myoedema (mounding up of the muscle on percussion). There may also be an increase in muscle bulk. Affected patients typically have a slow and clumsy gait most apparent on initiation of walking and in cold ambient temperatures. Muscle weakness is usually relatively mild and tends to involve the pelvic and shoulder girdle muscles (Swanson et al., 1981). Patients may be more severely affected by muscle weakness although this is less common. Several reports of rhabdomyolysis associated with hypothyroidism, in some cases leading to renal failure, are to be found in the literature, although this too does not occur often (Kisakol et al., 2003; Kuo and Jeng, 2010). Case reports of atypical presentations with head-drop (Furutani et al., 2007) or camptocormia (Kim et al., 2009) indicate that, rarely, non-limb girdle muscle groups may also be predominantly affected. Infrequently the diaphragm and other muscles of respiration may be affected causing neuromuscular respiratory insufficiency occasionally requiring long-term ventilatory support (Pandya et al., 1989). Martinez and colleagues described several patients who developed diaphragmatic dysfunction. The severity varied from mild weakness predominantly affecting exercise tolerance to severe compromise mimicking diaphragmatic paralysis (Martinez et al., 1989).

Muscle pain, particularly during and after exertion, is a prominent feature of hypothyroid myopathy (Lochmuller et al., 1993). Patients may also experience widespread, painful muscle cramps (Nickel et al., 1961). For this reason it is important to consider hypothyroidism in patients presenting with musculoskeletal pains of uncertain cause. The differential diagnosis of hypothyroid myopathy includes other causes of painful stiff muscles, such as polymyalgia rheumatica and polymyositis. Interestingly, a polymyositis-like condition has been reported in the literature in association with hypothyroidism (Madariaga, 2002).

The muscles in hypothyroid myopathy often have a feeling of increased volume and firmness. This muscle enlargement is most obvious in the tongue, arms, and legs (Fig. 48.1). There have even been occasional reports of patients with hypothyroidism developing an acute compartment syndrome (Hsu et al., 1995; Ramdass et al., 2007) or presenting with acute muscle edema (Bhansali et al., 2000). Frank muscle pseudohypertrophy associated with muscle stiffness and cramps in adults with hypothyroidism is sometimes known as Hoffman's

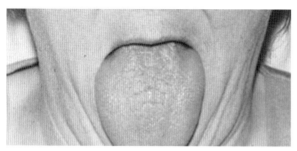

Fig. 48.1. Patient with hypothyroid myopathy in whom there was an increase in muscle bulk including macroglossia.

syndrome (Deepak et al., 2004; Tuncel et al., 2008; Turker et al., 2008). Kocher–Debré–Semelaigne syndrome is the rarer equivalent found in childhood hypothyroidism. These children may display the typical features of cretinism, including delayed development, constipation, bradycardia, the characteristic facies (large tongue, coarse hair and skin), hypotonia, and prolonged tendon reflexes but also have generalized muscular hypertrophy which gives the child an athletic, almost herculean appearance (Spiro et al., 1970; Salaria and Parmar, 2004).

A delay in the relaxation of muscle (pseudomyotonia) is commonly observed on eliciting the tendon reflexes in hypothyroid patients. Lambert et al. showed that all phases of the tendon reflex are delayed, although only slowing of the relaxation phase is clinically apparent (Lambert et al., 1951). Pseudomyotonia differs from true myotonia in that in pseudomyotonia there is reduction in the speed of both contraction and relaxation, and slowing is not increased after rest nor relieved by repeated muscle contractions. The characteristic "dive-bomber" effect seen in true myotonia on electromyography is not a feature of the pseudomyotonia of hypothyroidism. Instead, there is a continuous burst of action potentials that begin abruptly, fire at a constant rate, and then terminate abruptly (Pearce and Aziz, 1969). Percussion of the muscle commonly causes a slow prolonged mounding effect, called myoedema. Myoedema, unlike myotonia, is electrically silent. It is believed that myoedema results from derangement of intracellular calcium homeostasis. Occasionally, hypothyroidism may precipitate true myotonia in patients who have underlying myotonic dystrophy or myotonia congenita (Venables et al., 1978).

Increasing evidence suggests that the use of statins in hypothyroidism may increase the risk of myopathy (Hung and Yeung, 2000) and case reports exist of severe myopathy sometimes with rhabdomyolysis (Kursat et al., 2005; Qari, 2009) when statins are used in patients with hypothyroidism. The use of statins and the subsequent development of a myopathy may serve to unmask previously undetected hypothyroidism (Bar et al., 2007; Krieger and Knopp, 2009). Whether the resultant muscle symptoms are due to an exacerbation of a previously unnoticed hypothyroid myopathy or due to a true statin-induced myopathy is less clear (Herwig, 2008). As hypothyroidism predisposes patients to dyslipidemia (Morris et al., 2001) and subclinical hypothyroidism is common, some argue that baseline CK and thyroid function testing should be performed prior to starting a statin. Those with dyslipidemia due to hypothyroidism are frequently resistant to antilipid drug treatment. Should a patient with raised cholesterol fail to respond to treatment it is even more important to check thyroid function. Fortunately, treatment of the underlying hypothyroidism returns the lipid profile back to normal (Monzani et al., 2004).

INVESTIGATIONS

The majority of patients with hypothyroidism have an elevated serum creatine kinase (CK), even when myopathic features are not clinically obvious. In symptomatic patients, the serum CK level may rise to more than 10 times the upper limit of normal (Hekimsoy and Oktem, 2005). Neurophysiologic assessment may show no significant abnormalities. However, in approximately 30% of patients with hypothyroidism, significant abnormalities are observed on electromyography (EMG). These include abnormal insertional activity or hyperirritability, an increase in polyphasic motor unit potentials, and a reduction in duration and amplitude of motor unit potentials (Kendall-Taylor and Turnbull, 1983; Duyff et al., 2000). The EMG features of pseudomyotonia and myoedema have been discussed above.

PATHOLOGY

There is no pathognomonic histologic feature of hypothyroid myopathy and in most cases pathologic changes in muscle are subtle. Changes seen on light microscopy include fiber atrophy, necrosis or hypertrophy, increased numbers of nuclei, and an accumulation of interstitial connective tissue and glycogen (McKeran et al., 1980). There may be vacuolation in many large fibers (Pearce and Aziz, 1969), and crescents of material containing acid mucopolysaccharides may be found beneath the sarcolemmal sheath. Selective atrophy of type II fibers, with hypertrophy of type I fibers has been reported (McKeran et al., 1975). The neuromuscular junction appears normal, but there may be loss of the myelin sheath of intramuscular nerves. On electron microscopy there may be mitochondrial swelling and inclusions, fragmentation and disorganization of myofibrils, accumulation of glycogen or lipoid granules, T-tubule proliferation, dilatation of the sarcoplasmic reticulum, and autophagic vacuoles (Ruff and Weissmann, 1988). Pathologic changes resolve with thyroxine replacement therapy.

PATHOPHYSIOLOGY

Thyroid hormone is intimately linked to carbohydrate metabolism and mitochondrial function and, possibly, to the function of the sarcoplasmic reticulum and intrinsic contractile properties of muscle (McKeran et al., 1980). A deficit of thyroid hormone, regardless of cause, would therefore be expected to impact on these intracellular processes. The pathology of hypothyroid myopathy suggests that excessive glycogen storage and mitochondrial dysfunction are likely to be important factors in the pathogenesis of muscle dysfunction in hypothyroidism (McKeran et al., 1980). Magnetic resonance spectroscopy of hypothyroid muscle shows a low intracellular pH in resting muscle and delayed glycogen breakdown in exercising muscle (Taylor et al., 1992). Hurwitz and associates undertook detailed analysis of muscle enzymes in hypothyroidism and found a reduction in activity of the glycolytic enzyme α-glucosidase (acid maltase) in hypothyroid myopathy, which may contribute to glycogen accumulation (Hurwitz et al., 1970). Mitochondrial oxidative capacity is reduced in hypothyroidism (Zoll et al., 2001) and there is decreased responsiveness of β-adrenergic receptors to the enzymes of glycogen metabolism (Chu et al., 1985). Low levels of the mitochondrial transcription factor A (h-mtTFA), a proposed thyroid hormone target, occur in hypothyroid myopathy and it has been suggested that abnormal h-mtTFA turnover may be implicated in mitochondrial alterations in the condition (Siciliano et al., 2002). Decreased responsiveness to adrenergic stimulation and alterations in muscle carbohydrate metabolism may contribute to the impaired ischemic lactate production, weakness, exertional pain, and fatigue occurring in hypothyroidism. Alterations in myosin, lactate dehydrogenase, and myofibrillar ATPase activity occur in hypothyroidism such that muscle fibers switch from a pattern characteristic of fast-twitch fibers to one characteristic of slow-twitch fibers (Salviati et al., 1985). These changes may underlie the observed slowing of muscle contraction and relaxation. Both protein synthesis and breakdown are reduced in hypothyroidism but the result is net protein catabolism (Schwartz and Oppenheimer, 1978). Na$^+$-K$^+$ pump activity in skeletal muscle is also reduced in the hypothyroid state (Kjeldsen et al., 1984).

TREATMENT AND PROGNOSIS

The only effective therapy for hypothyroid myopathy is to restore the patient to the euthyroid state. Most patients respond to thyroxine therapy with complete clinical and biochemical recovery, although in some individuals this may take some time. Khaleeli and Edwards reported that 7 of 19 patients with hypothyroid myopathy still had myopathic weakness 12 months after euthyroidism had been restored (Khaleeli and Edwards, 1984). Torres and Moxley described persistent weakness and wasting 6 years after restoration of euthyroidism in another case (Torres and Moxley, 1990). Serum CK levels correct very rapidly with thyroxine replacement, normalizing even before the TSH level (Ruff and Weissmann, 1988). Some patients may develop increased muscle pain and weakness after starting thyroxine replacement, and the short-term addition of corticosteroid therapy may be helpful if this problem arises. Recent attention has been given to the frequency of neuromuscular symptoms in patients with subclinical hypothyroidism, and the suggestion has been made that such patients should be treated early not only to prevent progression to frank hypothyroidism, but also to improve their neuromuscular dysfunction (Monzani et al., 1999).

MISCELLANEOUS NEUROLOGIC CONDITIONS AND HYPOTHYROIDISM

Myasthenia gravis

An association between myasthenia gravis and hypothyroidism has been reported, although this is less common than its association with hyperthyroidism (Sahay et al., 1965). The myasthenic symptoms may precede or present with the hypothyroidism or else develop subsequently. The severity of the myasthenia may or may not improve following treatment of the hypothyroidism.

Giant cell arteritis and polymyalgia rheumatica

In 1977, How and coworkers described a patient in whom both giant cell arteritis and hypothyroidism were present, and suggested a common cause (How et al., 1977). Subsequently, Wiseman and associates reviewed 36 elderly patients presenting with giant cell arteritis or polymyalgia rheumatica during a 6 year period (Wiseman et al., 1989). A total of 15 of the 36 (42%) patients had hypothyroidism before or at the time of presentation or else developed it during subsequent follow-up. The authors stressed the importance of recognizing this association lest the musculoskeletal symptoms of hypothyroidism misinterpreted as an exacerbation of polymyalgia rheumatica and the steroid dose escalated unnecessarily.

Hypothyroidism related to anticonvulsant therapy

The problem of subclinical hypothyroidism in children with epilepsy treated with valproate or carbamazepine therapy has been highlighted (Eiris-Punal et al., 1999).

Elevation of TSH was found in 8.2% of children on carbamazepine therapy and 26% of those on valproate therapy, compared with only 3.6% of healthy controls. It was suggested that thyroid function should be monitored at intervals in children on long-term therapy with these antiepileptic agents. More recently, Miller reported three cases of central hypothyroidism believed to be secondary to treatment with oxcarbazepine (Miller and Carney, 2006). A steadily increasing number of case reports document the complex interaction of phenytoin and thyroid function (Aanderud and Strandjord, 1980; Kushnir et al., 1985; Horii et al., 1991; Betteridge and Fink, 2009). It appears that phenytoin may bring about hypothyroidism or else worsen pre-existing hypothyroidism, whilst hypothyroidism in turn increases the risk of phenytoin toxicity.

Neuroleptic malignant syndrome

There have been occasional reports of neuroleptic malignant syndrome developing in patients with hypothyroidism (Moore et al., 1990; Taskapan et al., 2005). Moore et al. described two patients with primary hypothyroidism who developed neuroleptic malignant syndrome while taking a neuroleptic drug (Moore et al., 1990). They suggested that thyroid disease may predispose to the development of neuroleptic malignant syndrome by altering brain dopamine metabolism.

NEUROLOGIC COMPLICATIONS OF HYPERTHYROIDISM AND GRAVES' DISEASE

There are several potential underlying causes of hyperthyroidism, including (1) Graves' disease; (2) excess release of stored hormone during subacute thyroiditis or following thyroid irradiation; (3) uncontrolled hormone formation in single or multinodular goiters (Plummer's disease); (4) ingestion of excess thyroid hormone; (5) rare TSH-secreting pituitary tumors; (6) drug-induced disease. Graves' disease is the commonest cause of thyrotoxicosis and occurs with a female-to-male preponderance of 7:1. The neurologic complications of hyperthyroidism are diverse, as will be evident from following discussion.

Hyperthyroid myopathy

CLINICAL FEATURES

Predominantly proximal muscle weakness occurs in the majority of hyperthyroid patients and may be accompanied by muscle wasting. In a carefully assessed cohort of 54 patients with thyrotoxicosis, Ramsay reported that 82% had evidence of muscle weakness (Ramsay, 1966). Weakness was confined to the proximal muscles in 63% and involved both proximal and distal muscles in

18.5%. More recently, Duyff et al. carried out a prospective cohort study of patients with newly diagnosed thyroid dysfunction. A total of 67% of 21 hyperthyroid patients had neuromuscular complaints whilst 62% had objective muscle weakness (Duyff et al., 2000). In his series of 50 hyperthyroid cases, Havard reported that wasting of the pectoral or pelvic girdle musculature was evident in 46% of hyperthyroid patients with atrophy most often affecting the deltoid, supraspinatus, and quadriceps muscles (Havard et al., 1963). Patients may further complain of muscle pain, stiffness, cramping and fatigability (Araki et al., 1968). Superimposed thyrotoxic tremor may suggest fasciculation, but once the muscle is completely relaxed this usually disappears. Tendon reflexes are normal or brisk with shortening of the relaxation phase.

Symptomatic weakness of the bulbar musculature resulting in dysphagia and dysarthria is very uncommon in hyperthyroidism, but there is a limited literature based on case reports, well reviewed by Chiu (Chiu et al., 2004). In the vast majority of cases bulbar involvement follows the development of limb weakness although there are case reports of isolated bulbar dysfunction, sometimes of acute onset, attributed to hyperthyroid myopathy (Kammer and Hamilton, 1974; Marks et al., 1980; Lleo et al., 1999). It is important to realize that bulbar symptoms in hyperthyroid patients may not be due to bulbar myopathy but may have another cause. A large goiter or thymic hyperplasia may physically compress the esophagus leading to mechanical dysphagia or else compress the recurrent laryngeal nerve leading to dysphonia. Coincident myasthenia gravis may cause dysphagia due to neuromuscular junction dysfunction rather than muscle dysfunction *per se*. As treatment of these causative conditions differs, establishing a clear diagnosis is important. In hyperthyroid bulbar myopathy, dysphagia may be the result of esophageal dysfunction as well as bulbar muscle weakness. Of the 13 cases reviewed by Chiu et al., six developed aspiration pneumonia. This seemed to be more of a risk in those affected by oropharyngeal weakness rather than esophageal dysmotility. Very rarely, involvement of the respiratory muscles occurs in hyperthyroid myopathy and patients may need ventilatory support.

Some authors distinguish acute and chronic forms of thyrotoxic myopathy. In chronic thyrotoxic myopathy, the patient is said to present with insidiously progressive generalized weakness and wasting, worse in proximal muscles, and weight loss. Other features of thyrotoxicosis may not be obvious or may be masked by β-blocker therapy. This combination of features may be mistaken for progressive muscular atrophy (PMA), the lower motor neuron variant of motor neuron disease. The severity of the muscle weakness may be marked, but most patients retain the ability to walk. Acute thyrotoxic myopathy was first described by Laurent in 1944, in this first instance presenting as a bulbar palsy (Laurent, 1944). Acute onset of weakness due to hyperthyroidism is very uncommon and some authors have even suggested that in these cases the weakness is due not to thyroid myopathy but to unrecognized concomitant myasthenia gravis. This said, there are reports of patients in whom myasthenia gravis was carefully excluded who presented with an acute onset myopathy. These patients presented with muscle weakness progressing rapidly over a few days. The weakness may be profound, bulbar muscles are often affected, and the patient may develop respiratory failure. The tendon reflexes may be reduced or absent. Some of these patients have developed an associated encephalopathic state.

INVESTIGATIONS

In contrast to hypothyroid myopathy, the serum CK level in hyperthyroid myopathy is usually normal or reduced. There are a small number of case reports of rhabdomyolysis and elevation of CK in hyperthyroidism (Bennett and Huston, 1984; Hosojima et al., 1992; Lichtstein and Arteaga, 2006).

Havard reported electromyographic changes in a cohort of 50 consecutive patients with hyperthyroidism in 1963. Only two cases showed fasciculation and there were no cases with fibrillations. Cases where motor unit potentials were polyphasic and were judged to be of shorter duration were described as myopathic and ascribed to three categories, severe, moderate and mild. Based on these subjective criteria, eight patients were judged to be severely myopathic, 16 moderately myopathic and 20 mildly myopathic. Six patients had normal electromyography (Havard et al., 1963). More recently, Duyff et al. performed extensive electrophysiology on their cohort of 21 hyperthyroid patients of whom 67% had neuromuscular complaints. Only 10% of their hyperthyroid patients had myopathic changes, while 24% had neuropathic changes. These categories are not, however, further defined. Subclinical sensory carpal tunnel syndrome was identified in two patients and central motor conduction times were normal in all patients (Duyff et al., 2000). The fact that these two studies were carried out almost 40 years apart makes comparison difficult. Given this and the paucity of other literature on the subject, it is reasonable only to say that electrophysiology is commonly abnormal in hyperthyroid myopathy and that there is no pathognomonic electrophysiologic feature of hyperthyroid myopathy. Despite this, electrophysiologic examination looking for evidence of concomitant myasthenia gravis should be considered in these patients, particularly if there is prominent fatigability or other pointers such as ptosis and ophthalmoplegia.

There is no published modern study of muscle pathology in hyperthyroid myopathy. There are, however, earlier studies done using both light (Havard et al., 1963) and electron microscopy (Engel, 1966). As is the case with electrophysiology, there is no diagnostically useful pathognomonic pathologic finding in hyperthyroid myopathy. Biopsy may be needed on occasion, however, to rule out other muscle pathologies.

PHYSIOLOGIC AND BIOCHEMICAL CHANGES IN SKELETAL MUSCLE

Significant research effort has been directed at elucidating how skeletal muscle is affected by the hyperthyroid state. Skeletal muscle is a major target organ of the thyroid hormones so it is unsurprising that this work has shown that the biochemistry, electrophysiology and even structure of skeletal muscle is profoundly affected by an excess of thyroid hormone. A detailed review of this literature lies beyond the scope of this review, but a summary is provided here and the reader is directed to Brennan et al. for a more detailed consideration of the subject (Brennan et al., 2006b).

Hyperthyroidism affects both the physiologic and the biochemical properties of skeletal muscle with a preferential effect on type 1 (slow) muscle fibers used during prolonged effort (Sickles et al., 1987). This preferential effect may relate to the greater density of cytoplasmic thyroid hormone receptors and the greater capillary density and blood supply in slow-twitch fibers. Hyperthyroidism moreover shifts the characteristics of slow muscle fibers towards those resembling fast muscle fibers (Levine et al., 2003). The speed of muscle contraction is enhanced and its duration is reduced. This effect underlies the clinical observation that the duration of muscle contraction after a deep tendon is struck with a tendon hammer is briefer than normal in the hyperthyroid state and prolonged in the hypothyroid state. The expression of isotypes of the myosin heavy chain is altered in hyperthyroidism to favor expression of MHC type IIx associated with fast fiber characteristics, with this isoform replacing MHC type I associated with slow fiber characteristics. These changes reverse on treatment (Brennan et al., 2006a).

The pattern of glycogen utilization and lactate production in muscle is altered in hyperthyroidism. Using *in vivo* phosphorus-31 magnetic resonance spectroscopy, Erkintalo et al. found that skeletal muscle was less efficient in hyperthyroidism (Erkintolo et al., 1998). At rest, the concentration of phosphocreatine was reduced in thyrotoxic patients compared with that in control subjects. At the onset of exercise, the magnitude of glycolysis activation was significantly larger in the thyrotoxic group, and this resulted in a marked decrease in pH. The energy cost of exercise was significantly higher in thyrotoxic patients, with greater activation of both anaerobic and aerobic pathways throughout 3 minutes of exercise. The authors concluded that muscle requires more energy to function in the hyperthyroid state when compared with the euthyroid state. Evidence that in hyperthyroidism the mitochondrial transport chain is uncoupled backs up this finding (Martin et al., 1991; Lebon et al., 2001). There is also good evidence that in hyperthyroidism there is muscle catabolism and a net breakdown of muscle protein (Morrison et al., 1988; Riis et al., 2005). It seems reasonable to assume that this effect underlies the muscle atrophy that so frequently accompanies muscle weakness in hyperthyroid myopathy.

Whilst more and more is being discovered about various aspects of muscle structure and function in the hyperthyroid state, a coherent picture of the primary mechanisms underlying the clinical features of hyperthyroid myopathy is yet to emerge. That the symptoms and signs of hyperthyroid myopathy typically resolve quickly with restoration of euthyroidism suggests that the changes described above should be reversible with treatment. Brennan et al. studied muscle protein metabolism in eight patients with hyperthyroid myopathy before and after treatment and demonstrated that, at least for the parameters studied, this was the case (Brennan et al., 2006a).

TREATMENT AND PROGNOSIS

The muscle weakness and EMG changes of hyperthyroid myopathy typically resolve as euthyroidism is achieved, generally doing so faster than is the case in hypothyroid myopathy. In Duyff's series mean resolution of muscle weakness in the hyperthyroid group was 3.6 months compared to 6.9 months in the hypothyroid group. Where there is dysphagia and dysarthria due to hyperthyroid myopathy, symptoms also typically resolve on treatment of the hyperthyroidism. Resolution in Chiu's cases took around 3 weeks.

MYOPATHY WITH RAISED CREATINE KINASE ON COMMENCEMENT OF TREATMENT FOR HYPERTHYROIDISM

Shaheen and Kim describe a case of Graves' disease initially presenting with no neuromuscular features who developed myalgia and a raised CK on starting propylthiouracil (Shaheen and Kim, 2009). The drug was discontinued and total thyroidectomy performed but despite cessation of the drug the myalgia and CK elevation worsened. The myalgia and CK both responded to treatment with triiodothyronine and relapsed with its discontinuation, despite higher than normal thyroid hormone levels. These authors made reference to two other similar cases (Suzuki et al., 1997; Mizuno et al., 2006) and suggest that some patients with hyperthyroidism may be particularly sensitive to a fall in their thyroid hormone levels such that relative muscle hypothyroidism develops leading to muscular symptoms and a raised CK more typical of a hypothyroid myopathy. As Shaheen and Kim state, the nature of this phenomenon requires further clarification.

INFLAMMATORY MYOPATHY IN HYPERTHYROIDISM

Hardiman reports a case in which a patient presented with biochemically proven hyperthyroidism and symptoms and signs in keeping with hyperthyroid myopathy (Hardiman et al., 1997). Concomitant myasthenia gravis was excluded. A modestly raised CK prompted a muscle biopsy which showed features of an inflammatory myositis with a marked endomysial mononuclear cell infiltrate. There are two further case reports of a polymyositis-like picture in the setting of hyperthyroidism (Araki et al., 1990; Stevanato et al., 1991).

Peripheral neuropathy

Peripheral neuropathy occurs much less commonly in hyperthyroidism than it does in hypothyroidism and was thought to occur only rarely. More recent studies suggest that although peripheral nerve involvement in hyperthyroidism is much less common than myopathy, it does occur (Ludin et al., 1969; Caparros-Lefebvre et al., 2003). In Duyff's cohort of 21 hyperthyroid cases three patients complained of distal sensory abnormalities and electrophysiology revealed a "neuropathic" pattern in 24% (Duyff et al., 2000). A recent report described a severe subacute motor axonal neuropathy induced by T_3 hyperthyroidism which reversed on treatment of the hyperthyroidism (Caparros-Lefebvre et al., 2003).

Mononeuropathies associated with hyperthyroidism are relatively uncommon. A prospective study of 60 patients with untreated hyperthyroidism showed that 5% had clinical and neurophysiologic features of carpal tunnel syndrome and an additional 8% had subclinical neurophysiologic abnormalities (Roquer and Cano, 1993). Two of Duyff's 21 hyperthyroid patients had evidence of a subclinical sensory carpal tunnel syndrome on electrophysiology. The symptoms of median nerve compression typically resolve once the hyperthyroidism has been treated and surgery is not usually necessary. Ijichi reported two hyperthyroid patients, one with a common peroneal neuropathy and one with meralgia paresthetica (Ijichi et al., 1990). Mononeuropathies occur in other patient groups and in the normal population – the sparse literature on their occurrence in hyperthyroidism makes it difficult to assess whether the two are associated or simply occurring together by chance.

A rare Guillain–Barré-like acute peripheral neuropathy causing paraplegia was first described by Charcot and termed Basedow's paraplegia by Joffroy (Charcot, 1889; Joffroy, 1894). The subsequent literature contains a scattering of case reports (Feibel and Campa, 1976). In 1998, Pandit et al. reported a more recent case and were the first to include details of a sural nerve biopsy including ultrastructural studies (Pandit et al., 1998). As originally described by Charcot, the syndrome is acute in onset, and presents as a flaccid paraplegia with upper limbs much less affected than the lower limbs. Tendon reflexes are absent. There is sensory involvement in some cases. Sphincters are typically intact. Electrophysiology in Pandit's case showed evidence of a mixed sensorimotor peripheral neuropathy with evidence both of demyelination and of axonal loss. Neuropathology in this case identified loss of myelinated fibers, thinly myelinated large nerve fibers and evidence of mitochondrial degeneration and cytoskeletal abnormalities in affected axons.

A possible association between hyperthyroidism and Guillain–Barré syndrome was reported by Bronsky and colleagues (Bronsky et al., 1964).

Corticospinal tract disorders

In 1988 one of us (PJS) reported the case of a 60-year-old man with a progressive spastic paraparesis and hyperthyroidism (Shaw et al., 1988). Extensive testing to identify another cause of his symptoms and signs revealed no other cause. Resolution of his upper motor neuron symptoms and signs followed treatment of his hyperthyroidism with carbimazole and, tellingly, temporary cessation of treatment pending radioiodide treatment provoked their relapse. A review of the literature performed at that time identified only nine other cases in which hyperthyroidism and an upper motor neuron syndrome were convincingly documented together (Bulens, 1981; Newcomer et al., 1983; Fisher et al., 1985; Shaw et al., 1988). Clinical features emphasized in these reports included spasticity and weakness, particularly affecting the lower limbs, as well as hyperreflexia, clonus at the ankles and knees, and extensor plantar responses. Only a subset of these reported cases represent a pure upper motor neuron syndrome. In others there were additional features such as sensory dysfunction including impaired vibration sensation and proprioception, upper motor neuron bladder disturbance, and urinary incontinence, or alteration in conscious level (Bulens, 1981; Newcomer et al., 1983). Some patients had both upper and lower motor neuron signs, a combination mimicking amyotrophic lateral sclerosis (ALS)

(Fisher et al., 1985; Shaw et al., 1988; Patial et al., 1995). Treatment of the hyperthyroid state in these cases resulted in complete or nearly complete recovery of their motor symptoms. These cases provide a strong argument in favor of routine thyroid function testing in patients in whom ALS is being considered.

An electrical correlate of upper motor neuron features in hyperthyroidism has been documented by Ozata et al. (1996). This group studied central motor conduction following transcranial magnetic stimulation of the motor cortex in 19 patients with hyperthyroidism. The mean central motor conduction time (CMCT) was significantly prolonged in the hyperthyroid group compared with a control group. Two of the nineteen patients (10.5%) had abnormal CMCT values that exceeded the mean + 2.5 SD of the normal control subjects. There have been no histopathologic studies of corticospinal tract dysfunction in hyperthyroidism and the underlying cause remains unclear. Experimental work in animal models makes it clear that thyroid hormones can have important effects on CNS neurotransmitter systems (Savarad et al., 1983; Atterwill et al., 1984; Carageprgiou et al., 2005) and enzyme function (Murthy and Baquer, 1982; Carageprgiou et al., 2005) but further histopathologic and neurochemical studies in animal models are needed to define the pathophysiologic basis of corticospinal tract dysfunction in thyrotoxicosis.

Movement disorders

TREMOR

Tremor is almost invariably seen in hyperthyroidism, so is best considered a feature of the hyperthyroid state rather than a neurologic complication. The tremor seen in thyrotoxicosis can be considered an exaggerated physiologic tremor (Milanov and Sheinkova, 2000). It is postural, persists on movement, but is not present at rest and has a frequency of 8–12 Hz. The tremor affects outstretched hands and tongue most commonly, but the lips and facial muscles may also be affected. Therapy with β-blockers alleviates tremor in hyperthyroidism suggesting that increased β-adrenergic activity is likely to be responsible (Feely and Peden, 1984).

CHOREA AND OTHER MOVEMENT DISORDERS

Chorea is an unusual complication of hyperthyroidism. The literature on the subject comprises individual case reports or reviews of small numbers of case reports (Shahar et al., 1988) and perhaps for this reason the association of chorea with hyperthyroidism is not universally accepted. Some authors suggest that it is simply an exaggeration of the fidgetiness seen in many thyrotoxic patients. Others suggest that hyperthyroidism unmasks pre-existing and subclinical basal ganglia dysfunction. The problem appears to be more common in women and the underlying cause of the hyperthyroidism is most commonly Graves' disease. Choreiform movements typically involved the limbs with the face, neck, or tongue affected in some cases. There are case reports of hemichorea (Baba et al., 1992; Nagaoka et al., 1998; Miao et al., 2010), bilateral ballism (Ristic et al., 2004), and paroxysmal choreoathetosis (Drake, 1987) associated with thyrotoxicosis. The chorea usually resolves once hyperthyroidism has been controlled, but there are reports of chorea persisting long after euthyroidism has been achieved (Baba et al., 1992).

The pathophysiologic basis of hyperthyroid chorea is unknown. Given that most cases occur in autoimmune hyperthyroidism many have assumed that the associated chorea also has an autoimmune basis. It has been suggested that chorea may be mediated by the sympathetic nervous system, because β-blockers have been reported to be helpful in controlling symptoms. Klawans and Shenker suggested that thyrotoxicosis induces increased responsiveness of striatal dopamine receptors, resulting in reduced dopamine turnover within the brain and decreased levels of homovanillic acid, a dopamine metabolite, in CSF (Klawans and Shenker, 1972). Indeed, dopamine receptor antagonists, such as haloperidol and sulpiride, have been effective in the treatment of hyperthyroid chorea (Yu and Weng, 2009). Cases in which chorea develops when a patient is hyperthyroid, resolves on treatment, then, due to poor compliance with medication, recurs again when the patient once more becomes hyperthyroid lend support to the idea that the chorea is a direct effect of high levels of thyroid hormone on the function of the basal ganglia. This contention is supported by a single case report of chorea associated with iatrogenic hyperthyroidism due to overtreatment of hypothyroidism in an elderly woman (Isaacs et al., 2005).

There are also case reports of hyperthyroidism and associated spasmodic truncal flexion (Loh et al., 2005), platysmal myoclonus (Teoh and Lim, 2005), and paroxysmal kinesogenic dyskinesia (Puri and Chaudhry, 2004).

Thyroid-associated ophthalmopathy (Graves' ophthalmopathy)

Graves' disease is an autoimmune condition in which antibodies to thyrotropin receptors are generated and bind to their antigen on follicular cells in the thyroid gland, inducing them to make and release excess thyroid hormone which causes hyperthyroidism. This condition is associated with two main extrathyroid complications – thyroid dermopathy (also known as pretibial myxedema), in which the skin of the lower

limbs, especially that over the shins, becomes thickened, and thyroid-associated ophthalmopathy. Thyroid-associated ophthalmopathy, sometimes called Graves' ophthalmopathy or Graves' orbitopathy, is a potentially disfiguring and sight-threatening complication most commonly occurring in patients with hyperthyroidism due to Graves' disease or else a past history of hyperthyroid Graves' disease. Approximately 50% of patients with Graves' hyperthyroidism report symptoms of Graves' ophthalmopathy whilst subclinical disease is evident on orbital imaging in nearly 70% (Enzmann et al., 1979). Thyroid-associated ophthalmopathy may less commonly occur in euthyroid or hypothyroid Graves' patients, making up approximately 5% of all Graves' ophthalmopathy (Eckstein et al., 2009) and in Hashimoto's (autoimmune) thyroiditis regardless of levels of thyroid hormone. Fortunately only 3–5% of patients with Graves' disease have severe, sight-threatening ophthalmopathy requiring aggressive therapeutic intervention (Wiersinga and Bartalena, 2002). Graves' ophthalmopathy is generally managed by ophthalmologists. For this reason a detailed review of the pathogenesis and management of the disease is not given here, but interested readers are referred to two good recent reviews that address the current state of knowledge and controversies in the field (Bahn, 2010; Smith, 2010). Patients do, however, present to neurology with complaints of visual loss or diplopia, therefore a summary focusing on these neurologic presentations and diagnosis follows.

CLINICAL FEATURES

Symptoms and signs of Graves' ophthalmopathy are usually bilateral and begin within 18 months of the onset of Graves' hyperthyroidism. Ophthalmopathy in Graves' disease may uncommonly appear to be unilateral (5–14%) although in these cases orbital imaging usually identifies subclinical involvement of the clinically unaffected eye. The onset of ophthalmopathy may precede the development of hyperthyroidism and may also develop some years after Graves' disease has been diagnosed and treated (Bartley et al., 1996a). Whether or not Graves' ophthalmopathy may be induced or existing eye disease worsened by radioiodine treatment for hyperthyroidism remains contentious – most authorities suspect this does happen although evidence in the literature is contradictory (Tallstedt et al., 1992; Bartalena et al., 1998). What is clear is that smoking is an independent and modifiable risk factor for Graves' ophthalmopathy and that the more cigarettes smoked, the greater the risk (Prummel and Wiersinga, 1993). Patients with Graves' hyperthyroidism who smoke carry a 7.7-fold increased risk for development of ophthalmopathy and those who continue to smoke having developed eye problems are more likely to progress than those who manage to quit. The group at most risk appears to be patients treated with radioiodine who also smoke (Traisk et al., 2009).

The majority of eye symptoms and signs in Graves' ophthalmopathy are the result of the expansion of orbital contents. This expansion is due to an increase in both the amount of cushioning fat within the orbit and to enlargement of the extraocular muscles. Patients complain of a sensation of grittiness in the eyes, photophobia, and pressure or pain behind the eyes. The commonest features of Graves' ophthalmopathy are periorbital and conjunctival edema and erythema (secondary to compression of orbital veins and resultant venous stasis), retraction of the upper eyelid (due to overactive sympathetic activity), and proptosis due to the increased volume of orbital contents (Fig. 48.2). If proptosis is severe ptosis may occur. Proptosis is defined as measured exophthalmos greater than 2 mm above the upper normal limit. It is found in approximately 20–30% of patients with Graves' disease and results from increased volume of the orbital contents. Proptosis serves to decompress the orbit – visual loss due to compressive optic neuropathy occurs more often in those with no, or little, compensatory proptosis. Apart from the cosmetic problems that come with proptosis, failure of the eyelids to completely close the eyes may result in sight-threatening exposure keratopathy (Wiersinga et al., 1989). Although Graves' ophthalmopathy is the commonest cause of unilateral proptosis, being responsible for 15–30% of the total (Wiersinga et al., 1989), where proptosis is on one side only it is important rapidly to exclude other causes, for example orbital infiltration by malignancy or granulomatous disease.

Extraocular muscle involvement leading to ophthalmoparesis is clinically apparent in 10–15% of patients with Graves' hyperthyroidism (Fig. 48.2). Orbital imaging demonstrates enlargement of the extraocular muscles in 60–98% of these patients (Fig. 48.3). Patients may complain of blurred vision with binocular gaze, diplopia that may be continuous or intermittent, or a pulling

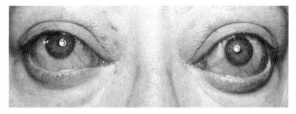

Fig. 48.2. Clinical appearance of moderately severe dysthyroid eye disease. The patient has bilateral proptosis, injection and edema of the eyelids and conjunctiva as well as strabismus.

sensation on attempted upgaze. For reasons that are not understood, there is preferential involvement of the inferior and medial rectus muscles in Graves' ophthalmopathy. Upward gaze is the most commonly restricted eye movement although other eye movements may also be affected (Rundle, 1964).

Optic nerve compression occurs in fewer than 5% of patients with Graves' disease (Trobe, 1981). It occurs as a result of apical crowding of the orbit due to enlargement of the extraocular muscles and excess orbital connective tissue. Early recognition of the problem is very important as up to 21% of untreated patients experience permanent loss of vision (Trobe, 1981). Patients may present with loss of visual acuity of rapid or gradual onset, impairment of color vision, or with a visual field defect. On fundoscopy optic disc swelling is seen in 25–33% of patients whilst optic disc pallor is seen in 10–20%. In occasional patients, choroidal folds are observed (Trobe, 1981). A recent review highlighted the fact that dysthyroid optic neuropathy may not be accompanied by proptosis and orbital inflammation and that the most useful diagnostic criteria are optic disc swelling, impaired color vision, and radiologic evidence of optic nerve compression (McKeag et al., 2007).

Other ocular symptoms may also occur. Episodic extraocular muscle spasm and ocular neuromyotonia have been described (Chung et al., 1997). There have also been reports of patients complaining of flashing lights (photopsia) in the superior visual field on upgaze. These are probably due to compression of the globe by a tight inferior rectus or traction on the insertion of the inferior rectus (Danks and Harrad, 1998).

DIAGNOSTIC TOOLS

Diagnosis is largely clinical based on the features outlined above with orbital imaging used to confirm the diagnosis and exclude differentials in apparently unilateral cases. As levels of antithyrotropin antibody correlate with disease severity, these should be measured, as should thyroid function tests. Advances have occurred in investigative techniques. STIR (short tau inversion recovery) MRI gives an indication of muscle water content, and a high signal is seen in patients with active ophthalmopathy (Bailey et al., 1996). Cine-MRI undertaken in the burned-out phase of the disease is useful in demonstrating reduced elasticity of the extraocular muscles, with failure of the normal stretching on eye movement (Bailey et al., 1996). The value of amplitude reduction on pattern electroretinography as a sensitive measure for demonstrating early impairment of optic nerve function has been reported (Genovesi-Ebert et al., 1998). Measurement of visual evoked potentials

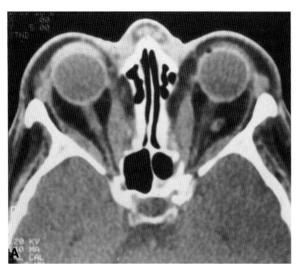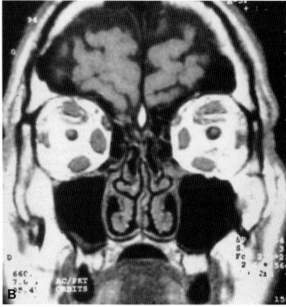

Fig. 48.3. Transverse (**A**) and coronal (**B**) orbital CT scans showing enlargement of the extraocular muscles, particularly inferior rectus and medial rectus, in dysthyroid eye disease.

is also useful in the detection of subclinical optic nerve involvement (Genovesi-Ebert et al., 1998).

PATHOGENESIS

Whilst there has been significant recent progress in the understanding of the pathogenesis of Graves' ophthalmopathy, there remain a number of contentious issues and unanswered questions (Bahn, 2010; Smith, 2010). Environmental and immunogenetic factors are both likely to play a part. Any schema of disease pathogenesis needs to explain the following features of the disease: (1) the occurrence of markedly asymmetric disease in some patients, (2) the exacerbation of the disease by smoking, (3) the improvement in ophthalmopathy that occurs when euthyroidism is regained, (4) its occurrence years after Graves' hyperthyroidism has been diagnosed and treated, and (5) its apparent exacerbation by radioiodine therapy. It is widely accepted that antithyrotropin antibodies are pathogenic in Graves' ophthalmopathy and that their target within the eye is orbital fibroblasts which express the thyrotropin receptor to a greater extent than do orbital fibroblasts in unaffected subjects (Bahn et al., 1998; Wakelkamp et al., 2003). Interaction of these pathogenic antibodies with the thyrotropin receptor on orbital fibroblasts triggers an inflammatory cascade within the orbit resulting in the expansion of orbital adipose tissue due first to generation of orbital adipocytes from a subgroup of orbital fibroblasts called preadipocytes and second, to the laying down of hydrophilic hyaluronan. This substance is also laid down between extraocular muscle fibers causing their enlargement. Antithyrotropin antibodies are not the only pathogenic antibodies in Graves' ophthalmopathy. The best supported of several additional candidates are antibodies to IGF-1. It seems likely that many of the other antibodies detected in Graves' ophthalmopathy will turn out to be secondary markers of the orbital immune-mediated reaction, rather than pathogenic effectors.

TREATMENT

A consensus statement on the management of thyroid-associated ophthalmopathy was released by the European Group on Graves' Orbitopathy in 2008 (Bartalena et al., 2008), whilst Bahn and Bartalena provide additional reviews (Bartalena et al., 1998; Bahn, 2010). In summary, there is currently no recommended preventive therapy and the condition is usually only treated when symptoms are severe or vision is threatened. In ophthalmopathy where there is evidence of active inflammation, corticosteroids and orbital radiotherapy may be used. Sight-threatening keratopathy due to proptosis and optic neuropathy due to apical crowding are treated surgically with orbital decompression. A variety of techniques are used to achieve this, including endoscopic approaches (Kasperbauer and Hinkley, 2005; Metson and Pletcher, 2006). Some authorities use a 3 month course of corticosteroids starting immediately after radioiodine treatment to prevent exacerbation of existing Graves' ophthalmopathy or its *de novo* development. Whether such treatment is effective remains unclear as the literature is contradictory (Vannucchi et al., 2009; Lai et al., 2010). Treatment of dysthroid strabismus once Graves' disease has burnt out and the ophthalmoparesis is stable is surgical. Prism glasses are an alternative in those preferring not to undergo surgery. During the active phase of the disease botulinum toxin may also be used to improve strabismus. A number of new, immunomodulatory therapies have been suggested as of potential use in Graves' ophthalmopathy, usefully summarized in a recent review (Bahn, 2010). These include rituximab directed against B cells, currently being assessed in clinical trials, and anti-TNF agents such as etanercept (Paridaens et al., 2005).

PROGNOSIS

Thyroid-associated ophthalmopathy tends to follow a fairly rapidly progressive course, reaching a peak after 6–24 months, followed by a prolonged plateau phase, and then a gradual but often incomplete regression of the eye changes. Lid retraction is the feature most likely to remit, and orbital soft tissue changes resolve over 1–5 years in most patients. Ophthalmoparesis is less likely to resolve rapidly, but one-third of patients show some improvement without specific therapy. Proptosis is the feature least likely to improve or resolve (Rundle, 1964). Bartley and colleagues undertook a long-term follow-up study of Graves' ophthalmopathy in an incidence cohort of 120 patients, following more than 80% for over 5 years (Bartley et al., 1996b). Persistent visual loss from optic neuropathy occurred in only two eyes, and only two patients had persistent diplopia, this being readily corrected with prism glasses. One-third of patients had some persistent ocular discomfort, usually dryness of the eyes. Some 60% of patients reported that the appearance of their eyes had not returned to normal, and one-third of patients were dissatisfied with the appearance of their eyes. The authors concluded that few patients have significant long-term functional impairment from Graves' ophthalmopathy, but that there are nevertheless important psychological, esthetic, and social sequelae for many.

Thyrotoxic hypokalemic periodic paralysis

Thyrotoxic hypokalemic periodic paralysis (TPP) is a condition in which a small proportion of hyperthyroid patients develop recurrent episodes of often profound muscular weakness associated with hypokalemia in response to recognized precipitants. Once the cause of the underlying hyperthyroidism is identified and patients are rendered euthyroid, the episodes of weakness stop completely. TPP can be caused by all forms of hyperthyroidism. Commonest is Graves' disease, but TPP is also seen in toxic goiter, autoimmune thyroiditis, and toxic thyroid adenomas. TPP has also been reported in overtreated hypothyroidism and in Jod-Basedow hyperthyroidism secondary to the use of iodinated contrast agents (Kane and Busch, 2006).

CLINICAL FEATURES

TPP typically affects young, hyperthyroid Asian or Hispanic men. Although hyperthyroidism is commoner in women, men with TPP outnumber women by ∼20:1. In Asian populations ∼2% of hyperthyroid men have TPP whereas only ∼0.1% of hyperthyroid Caucasians develop the condition (Kelley et al., 1989). TPP was rarely recognized outside Asia until recently but increasing geographic mobility and with it improved clinical awareness is changing this. The first attack of weakness usually occurs at 20–40 years of age, lower than that in familial hypokalemic periodic paralysis (FHPP). The mean age of onset in a recent Korean cohort was ∼30 years (16–54) (Hsieh et al., 2008). Attacks of weakness typically occur in the early hours of the morning, hence the name "nocturnal palsy." Exercise and/or a meal with a high salt or carbohydrate content the evening before typically precede an attack. Attacks are commonest in summer in temperate areas, most likely due to a combination of increased physical activity and the consumption of sugary drinks. Other recognized precipitants include trauma, infection, alcohol, cold, stress, menstruation, and certain prescription drugs such as amiodarone and steroids (Wongraoprasert et al., 2007).

Neurologic features

Patients report muscle stiffness, ache, and cramping before an attack. Weakness usually affects proximal limb muscles first, but this is not invariable. Weakness may be asymmetric or affect only exercised muscles. Respiratory, bulbar, and ocular muscles are not usually affected, nor is smooth muscle. Reflexes are most often reduced but hyperreflexia may also be seen. Sensory symptoms and signs are not a feature. Attacks of weakness are usually short. In one retrospective study most patients recovered either sporadically or with treatment within 24 hours. The longest time to recovery was 96 hours (Hsieh et al., 2008). Patients with TPP have no neuromuscular symptoms between bouts and do not develop the fixed weakness and muscle pathology seen in FHPP patients after multiple bouts of weakness.

Non-neurologic features

Patients with TPP may have no clinical evidence of hyperthyroidism at the time of their first attack of weakness. Patients may have a goiter or palpable thyroid nodule, but most will not. During attacks patients may be hypertensive and tachycardic. Patients may develop atrial or less often ventricular tachyarrythmias. Cardiac arrest secondary to ventricular tachycardia is uncommon but has been reported (Fisher, 1982; Tassone et al., 2004).

DIAGNOSIS

Diagnosis relies on consideration of the condition in a young man presenting with otherwise unexplained rapid-onset weakness in the presence of a low serum potassium with no family history of periodic paralysis. Although serum potassium is typically low, it may lie within the normal range. Urinary excretion of potassium is reduced with a low potassium-creatinine ratio. Serum phosphate and magnesium are low during an attack (Manoukian et al., 1999). Spot testing of urine in the emergency department for urinary calcium (high) and phosphate (low) has been advocated as a quick and useful diagnostic test. Acid–base balance is typically normal. In addition to the electrocardiographic findings typical of hypokalemia, TPP patients may have high voltage QRS complexes and first degree A-V block. Electromyography performed during an attack typically shows low amplitude compound muscle action potentials. Motor nerve conduction studies are normal confirming that TPP is a disease of muscle not nerve. In severe attacks there may be rhabdomyolysis.

PATHOPHYSIOLOGY

Clinical attacks of weakness in TPP are clinically similar to those of FHPP, a channelopathy caused by inherited defects to genes encoding sodium and calcium channels in skeletal muscle. This phenotypic similarity led investigators to postulate that TPP too might be a channelopathy, albeit one that manifests only in the presence of excess thyroid hormone. In the past TPP was considered to be a sporadic condition. It is now thought that TPP patients have a genetic predisposition to the disease unmasked by independently occurring hyperthyroidism.

Gene sequencing in cohorts of largely Asian TPP patients have revealed no mutations in FHPP-causing genes or in components of the $Na^+K^+ATPase$ pump (Kung et al., 2006). Recently six different mutations to an inwardly rectifying potassium channel, Kir2.6, expressed strongly in skeletal muscle were found in 33% of an unrelated cohort of TPP patients from the US, Brazil, and France, 25% of a Singaporean cohort, but none of 31 tested Thai patients (Ryan et al., 2010). The mutations discovered all had effects upon the stability of the muscle cell membrane, altering its excitability. The gene for Kir2.6 is transcriptionally regulated by thyroid hormone. Levels of the channel are increased in hyperthyroidism explaining why it is only in this circumstance that the mutation becomes manifest. It seems

likely that in future further TPP genes will be discovered and that their prevalence will vary between populations.

The hypokalemia seen in attacks of weakness in TPP is not due to loss of potassium, but to shift of extracellular potassium into cells driven by the $Na^+K^+ATPase$ pump (Chan et al., 1991). TPP patients do not have a potassium deficit and this has implications for treatment (see below). TPP patient platelets and muscle cells have increased $Na^+K^+ATPase$ activity compared to those of non-TPP hyperthyroid patients (Chan et al., 1991). Clinical observations of the epidemiology of TPP and the precipitants of weakness have provided further insights into the molecular mechanisms of TPP. $Na^+K^+ATPase$ pump activity is increased by β-adrenergic stimulation – this is potentiated by hyperthyroidism. Insulin also drives the pump providing an explanation for the precipitation of attacks by carbohydrate meals and exercise. A small study of hyperthyroid patients showed that those with TPP were more obese than those without and demonstrated higher basal levels of insulin (Soonthornpun et al., 2009). Insulin levels are moreover elevated in TPP patients during attacks of weakness. Animal studies suggest that testosterone may stimulate the $Na^+K^+ATPase$ pump, perhaps explaining the overwhelming male preponderance in TPP (Magsino and Ryan, 2000).

MANAGEMENT

Management of TPP is in three phases as summarized in Table 48.1. First, there is the emergency treatment of the attack of weakness and hypokalemia and any complications. Next, efforts must be made to reduce the likelihood of recurrent attacks of weakness pending

Table 48.1

Management of thyrotoxic hypokalemic periodic paralysis

Emergency treatment
    Oral or intravenous potassium chloride
    Oral or intravenous propranolol
    Supportive therapy if cardiac arrhythmia or respiratory
      muscle involvement
Prevention of further attacks whilst still hyperthyroid
    Avoidance of precipitants
      High carbohydrate meals
      High salt intake
      Alcohol
      Exercise
      Provocative drugs
        Steroids
        Amiodarone
    Regular propranolol
    Antithyroid medication
Definitive treatment of hyperthyroidism

investigation and treatment of the underlying hyperthyroidism. Finally, definitive treatment of the hyperthyroidism and return of the patient to the euthyroid state stops further attacks of weakness altogether. TPP patients are most at risk during their first attack of weakness when no diagnosis has been made. This is especially the case in non-Asian countries where the condition is seen only rarely. The often scant history suggestive of underlying hyperthyroidism complicates the situation. Diagnosis of hyperthyroidism at first presentation of TPP is important if patients are not to be discharged home only to have recurrent episodes of weakness.

Emergency treatment

TPP patients presenting with severe weakness are treated with potassium chloride to speed recovery. Urgent assessment of cardiac and respiratory involvement must be carried out and appropriate supportive management and monitoring instituted pending recovery. Potassium chloride may be administered orally or intravenously (10 mEq/hour) until weakness resolves. Mid-attack, TPP patients do not have a potassium deficit but rather an intracellular shift of their potassium. There is therefore a risk of rebound hyperkalemia on recovery as the potassium shift reverses. In one study patients given potassium recovered twice as fast as untreated patients, but 70% experienced rebound hyperkalemia (Lu et al., 2004). In practice this is rarely of clinical importance but most authorities recommend giving lower doses of potassium (<50 mEq total) which are effective at shortening an attack but are less likely to cause rebound. Hypophosphatemia and hypomagnesemia do not need treatment. Potassium chloride does not always abort an attack of weakness in TPP. In cases of refractory weakness propranolol can be effective. In one study, intravenous propranolol rapidly resolved weakness but was associated with rebound hyperkalemia and cardiac arrhythmia. Oral propranolol (3–4 mg/kg) was also effective but was not associated with rebound. Some clinicians favor the use of propranolol as first-line treatment but there are no data currently available to support this approach.

Prevention of further attacks pending resolution of hyperthyroidism

On recovery from their first attack of weakness patients should be educated about TPP and its precipitants in order that further attacks can be avoided. Patients should avoid food and drink with high salt or carbohydrate content. Alcohol should likewise be avoided. Formal exercise is best halted until the patient is euthyroid. Patients who live alone should be encouraged to call for help as soon as an attack starts. Propranolol 40 mg four times a day has been shown to reduce the likelihood of further attacks until the euthyroid state is regained. Likewise antithyroid drugs may have a role in reducing levels of thyroid hormones pending definitive treatment of the hyperthyroidism. Depending upon the underlying cause it may take months for the euthyroid state to be achieved. In the meantime the patient remains at risk of further attacks and the importance of compliance with antithyroid medication and avoidance of known precipitants must be emphasized.

Definitive treatment of the underlying hyperthyroidism

Euthyroid TPP patients do not have attacks of weakness – therefore definitive treatment of the hyperthyroidism brings to an end the risk of further attacks. The treatment deployed obviously depends upon the underlying cause, but may include surgery, radioiodine and/or antithyroid medication.

Thyroid storm

Florid thyrotoxic encephalopathy, sometimes referred to as "thyroid storm," is seen less often now that active monitoring and treatment of hyperthyroidism is the norm. Its clinical features and treatment have been well reviewed (Sarlis and Gourgiotis, 2003). Thyrotoxic storm is thought to make up 1–2% of thyroid-related admissions. Precipitating factors include radioactive iodine therapy, surgery (either thyroid or nonthyroid), trauma, pregnancy, and intercurrent illness. Thyroid storm is best seen as an exaggerated form of hyperthyroidism. No consensus definition of what comprises thyroid storm exists but four groups of symptoms dominate the clinical picture: fever, tachycardia, CNS dysfunction, and gastrointestinal symptoms. Fever is high and associated with profound sweating. Patients may develop supraventricular tachyarrythmias including atrial fibrillation (AF), with consequent cardiac failure or embolic cerebral infarction. Diarrhea and vomiting are common and patients may develop jaundice. Biochemically thyroid storm may be indistinguishable from uncomplicated thyrotoxicosis making its diagnosis a clinical one.

CNS symptoms may be prominent. Affected individuals are commonly confused or agitated and may present with frank pyschosis (Snabboon et al., 2009). The patient's conscious level may deteriorate, with the development of coma sometimes associated with seizures, bulbar weakness, and corticospinal tract signs (Newcomer et al., 1983). An increased risk of cerebral infarction has been identified in thyroid storm – whether this is attributable in its entirety to the risk associated with new-onset AF is not clear but if the patient does develop AF prompt anticoagulation is recommended

(Haynes and Kageler, 1989; Page and Scott, 1993). Patients with hyperthyroidism are more sensitive to warfarin than are euthyroid patients due to the increased clearance of vitamin K-dependent clotting factors (Kellett et al., 1986) and most require less warfarin to achieve therapeutic anticoagulation.

The mortality of thyroid storm is between 20% and 50% (Burch and Wartofsky, 1993; Tietgens and Leinung, 1995) so patients should be nursed on an intensive care unit. Successful treatment depends on early recognition and aggressive intervention. Treatment is aimed at: (1) reducing production and secretion of thyroid hormones by the thyroid gland, for which antithyroid medication ± iodine is used; (2) reduction of the effects of the excess thyroid hormone on target organs in the periphery, for which β-blockade is used; (3) reversing systemic problems such as fever and cardiovascular compromise; (4) treatment of any treatable precipitating factor such as systemic infection. Management of systemic disturbances in thyroid storm is likely to involve active cooling and close attention to fluid balance, treatment of arrhythmia and cardiac failure, and the administration of steroids in recognition of the risk of functional adrenal insufficiency due to a combination of increased cortisol clearance and markedly increased demand (Burger and Philippe, 1992; Migneco et al., 2005). Plasmapheresis has been employed for occasional patients to reduce levels of thyroid hormone (Newcomer et al., 1983). The pathogenesis of thyroid storm has not been established, and at postmortem examination few changes are found in organs other than the thyroid gland.

Seizures

Seizures are a relatively frequent complication of metabolic encephalopathies, but they are not a common complication of thyrotoxicosis. The literature mostly comprises cases reports or small groups of cases but two studies reported generalized or focal seizures in 9% (Salviati et al., 1985) and 10% (Jabbari and Huott, 1980) of thyrotoxic patients requiring admission to hospital. Seizures may be the first clinical manifestation of thyrotoxicosis but this is rare. Case reports of seizures in thyrotoxicosis typically occur in the setting of a thyroid encephalopathy in untreated hyperthyroidism. In most of these cases glucose, electrolytes, and osmolarity are normal and with treatment of the hyperthyroidism seizures cease. Several reports document recurrence of encephalopathy and seizures when compliance with antithyroid treatment is poor or treatment ceases, seizure control being regained when thyroid hormone levels are returned to normal. These cases suggest that thyroxine may act directly to lower seizure threshold as has been shown in animal models of epilepsy and hyperthyroidism. The cause of the hyperthyroidism appears not to be important – seizures have been reported in patients with Graves' disease (Jabbari and Huott, 1980) and in those with iatrogenic hypothyroidism overtreated with thyroxine (Aydin et al., 2004). As well as the provocation of *de novo* seizures, hyperthyroidism may also exacerbate a pre-existing seizure disorder (Su et al., 1993). β-Blockers used in the treatment of thyroid storm have also been implicated as a potential contributory factor in the development of seizures in thyrotoxicosis (Smith and Looney, 1983).

EEG abnormalities are more common in hyperthyroidism than are seizures. Skanse and Nyman found definite abnormalities in 43% of their patients and borderline abnormalities in a further 25% (Skanse and Nyman, 1956). In one series of 20 patients with hyperthyroidism, 17 had mild to moderate abnormalities before treatment and 16 showed reactivity to photic stimulation. After 4 weeks of treatment, all patients were clinically euthyroid but 12 continued to have some milder degree of EEG changes (Leubuscher et al., 1988). The commonest changes are generalized slow activity, but focal slowing and excess fast activity have been documented. The EEG sometimes shows definite epileptiform activity, as well as increased voltage of the photic response (Wilson and Johnson, 1964; Leubuscher et al., 1988). These EEG changes can also be found in normal subjects following the administration of thyroxine (Wilson and Johnson, 1964). In patients with florid thyrotoxic encephalopathy or thyroid storm, the EEG may show triphasic δ waves (Primavera et al., 1990). EEG changes usually improve once the thyrotoxic state is controlled.

Mental and psychiatric disorders

Minor mental disturbances are almost uniformly found in patients presenting with untreated hyperthyroidism. Complaints of insomnia and impairment of concentration and attention span are common. Patients' relatives frequently describe irritability, emotional lability, and capricious behavior. More serious neuropsychological disturbances reported include pyschosis (Bursten, 1961), affective disorders (Larisch et al., 2004), agitated delirium, with confusion, restlessness, and hyperkinesia (Brownlie et al., 2000), and an apathetic state with lethargy and depression (Thomas et al., 1970). These problems typically resolve on treatment of the hyperthyroidism. Evidence from case series regarding the occurrence of psychiatric disorders in thyroid disease, however, is conflicting. Demet et al. reviewed 32 hyperthyroid patients and 30 euthyroid controls. They found an excess of depression-anxiety symptoms in hyperthyroidism (Demet et al., 2002). In contrast, when Engum et al. assessed thyroid function and self-rating of depression and anxiety of 589 adults they found no significant association between thyroid dysfunction and depression or anxiety (Engum et al., 2002). Recent FDG-PET (positron emission tomography) studies of hyperthyroid patients suffering from severe anxiety showed increased glucose metabolism in limbic areas of the brain (Schreckenberger et al., 2006).

Several studies have examined the incidence of subclinical thyroid disorders in patients with psychiatric diseases. These studies have produced conflicting results, with some showing no clear association and others showing surprisingly high rates of thyroid disorder (Spratt et al., 1982; Tappy et al., 1987). No systematic study has been undertaken of the effect of correcting these subclinical thyroid problems on the course or prognosis of the psychiatric disorder.

Miscellaneous conditions associated with hyperthyroidism

HEADACHE

The evidence base underlying an association between hyperthyroidism and headache is weak. Iwasaki et al. reported six cases of hyperthyroidism (and none of hypothyroidism) of 30 cases of chronic headache assessed (Iwasaki et al., 1991). Larner et al. collated the thyroid function tests of 13 of 119 patients referred to a headache clinic and found that in no case could the headache be attributed to thyroid dysfunction. Stone et al. recently reported three patients referred from primary care with new-onset unremitting headache who on subsequent assessment were found to have Graves' disease. The headache in each of these cases resolved when the hyperthyroidism was successfully treated (Stone et al., 2007). One of the three cases had previously suffered from migraine and another's headache had previously been diagnosed as migraine. Another report, albeit in abstract form, exists of a further four patients known to suffer from migraine whose headache was exacerbated when they became hyperthyroid due to Graves' disease (three cases) and iatrogenic hyperthyroidism (one case) (Thomas et al., 1996). The authors suggest that in these patients hyperthyroidism may have lowered their migraine threshold. It has also been suggested that intracranial pressure may be reversibly increased in patients with thyrotoxicosis (Stern et al., 1984; Herwig and Sturzenegger, 1999) but this possibility has not been investigated systematically.

CEREBRAL VENOUS SINUS THROMBOSIS

Several case reports have now been published suggesting an association between hyperthyroidism, in most cases thyroid storm, and cerebral venous sinus thrombosis (Schutta et al., 1991; Siegert et al., 1995; Dulli et al., 1996; Silburn et al., 1996; De Schryver et al., 1999; Verberne et al., 2000; Ra et al., 2001; Maes et al., 2002; Molloy et al., 2003; Karouache et al., 2004; Madroñero-Vuelta et al., 2004; Nagumo et al., 2007; Kim et al., 2008; Pekdemir et al., 2008; Usami et al., 2009). Details of several of these cases are provided by Squizzato et al. (2005), whilst a recent systematic review of hyperthyroidism and venous thromboembolism has been undertaken by Franchini et al. (2010). It is already known that hyperthyroidism due to any cause results in a significant increase in levels of factor VIII and von Willebrand's factor that reverse with treatment of hyperthyroidism (Simone et al., 1965; Burggraaf et al., 2001). It has also been demonstrated that increased factor VIII levels increase the risk of venous thromboembolism (Koster et al., 1995; Kyrle et al., 2000). Most of the reported cases of venous sinus thrombosis and hyperthyroidism were found to have another, independent, risk factor for venous thromboembolism, e.g., use of the oral contraceptive pill (Maes et al., 2002; Kim et al., 2008), protein C deficiency (De Schryver et al., 1999; Ra et al., 2001; Nagumo et al., 2007), factor V Leiden (Molloy et al., 2003), prothrombin G20210A heterozygous mutation (Madroñero-Vuelta et al., 2004). This suggests that in most cases the vascular effects of hyperthyroidism are not alone sufficient to induce venous sinus thrombosis. The increasing number of cases, however, suggests that the dehydration, stasis of venous blood flow due to goiter and other hemodynamic factors attributable to thyroid disease may well contribute to the development of cerebral venous sinus thrombosis in those already predisposed. Finally, Peralta reports two cases of concomitantly diagnosed *hypo*thyroidism due to autoimmune thyroiditis (one mild, one subclinical) and cerebral venous sinus thrombosis (Peralta and Canhao, 2008). As far as we are aware there has been only one subsequent case report of concomitant hypothyroidism and cerebral venous sinus thrombosis (Chen et al., 2008).

STROKE

The association between disease of the thyroid and cerebrovascular disease has been thoroughly reviewed elsewhere (Squizzato et al., 2005). Atrial fibrillation develops in 10–15% of patients with hyperthyroidism (Presti and Hart, 1989) and it has been suggested that 10–40% of patients with thyrotoxic AF have embolic events, the majority of which are cerebral (Parmar, 2005). Whether thyrotoxic patients in AF have a higher embolic risk than euthyroid patients with chronic atrial fibrillation is unclear as the literature is contradictory. A very recent study by Sheu et al. followed over 3000 young hyperthyroid patients (18–44 years) for 5 years and compared their incidence of ischemic stroke with a large cohort of euthyroid controls (Sheu et al., 2010). Although the absolute risk of stroke in both groups was small (1.0% of hyperthyroid patients versus 0.6% of controls) once confounders such as AF, age, hypertension and diabetes were taken into account, there was an increased risk of ischemic stroke in the hyperthyroid patients (hazard ratio = 1.44). Little previous evidence existed to suggest an increased risk of ischemic stroke in hyperthyroidism in the absence of cardiac arrhythmia.

Evidence for associations between hyperthyroidism and rarer causes of stroke, is sparser still. Case reports of patients with concomitant moyamoya and Graves' disease suggest that cerebral infarcts tended to occur while patients were thyrotoxic, but no causative relationship between the thyroid and underlying vascular malformation is suggested (Tendler et al., 1997; Kim et al., 2001; Nakamura et al., 2003). A sixfold overrepresentation of hyperthyroid patients has been reported in two case series of giant cell arteritis (Thomas and Croft, 1974; Nicholson et al., 1984). This association, however, was refuted by a third (Duhaut et al., 1999). Whether or not the two conditions are truly associated remains unclear. Finally, there is at least one documented case where physical compression of a carotid artery in the neck by a thyroid nodule associated with a large goiter caused a right temporoparietal infarct (Silvestri et al., 1990).

Hashimoto's encephalopathy

Hashimoto's encephalopathy (HE) is a relatively rare condition arising as a complication of Hashimoto's thyroiditis, an autoimmune thyroid disorder. In Hashimoto's thyroiditis (HT) an antibody-mediated attack on the thyroid gland eventually brings about hypothyroidism although there may be an initial, transient hyperthyroidism and a period of intervening euthyroidism. Most HE occurs in patients with HT who are hypothyroid or euthyroid but it can, less often, occur in hyperthyroid patients. For this reason HE is not believed to be a consequence of the patient's thyroid status. Numerous variably well-defined case studies of Hashimoto's encephalopathy exist as well as a few small case series (Shaw et al., 1991; Castillo et al., 2006). The largest of these (Chong et al., 2003), describes only 85 patients.

The rarity of the disorder and the absence of consensus diagnostic criteria mean that qualifying clinical features and even the existence of HE as an entity are an ongoing subject of debate.

CLINICAL FEATURES

Clinical features of HE include relapsing episodes of encephalopathy, seizures, and often superimposed stroke-like neurologic deficits. The encephalopathy ranges from confusion to coma with an acute or subacute onset but it may also present insidiously as gradual cognitive decline in adults often confused with dementia (Spiegel et al., 2004) or a falling-off of school performance in children (Vasconcellos et al., 1999). Seizures in HE may be focal or generalized and patients with HE may present recurrently in status epilepticus (Ferlazzo et al., 2006; Tsai et al., 2007). Patients have high levels of antithyroid antibodies and the episodes are characteristically responsive to treatment with steroids. The first case termed Hashimoto's encephalopathy was described in 1966 (Brain et al., 1966). The authors presented a man with biopsy-proven Hashimoto's thyroiditis and antithyroid antibodies who developed progressive aphasia, hemiplegia and blindness eventually leading to coma. Ironically this patient failed to respond to steroids, improving only with return to a euthyroid state with thyroxine treatment. Two alternative names for HE have been proposed, steroid-responsive encephalopathy associated with autoimmune thyroiditis (SREAT) (Castillo et al., 2006) and nonvasculitic autoimmune inflammatory meningoencephalitis (NAIM) (Caselli et al., 1999). Neither of these terms is in widespread use.

Patients with Hashimoto's encephalopathy are usually euthyroid but may be hypothyroid. Cases of encephalopathy with antithyroid antibodies, an abnormal EEG, and hyperthyroidism have also been reported and are termed thyrotoxic Hashimoto's thyroiditis (Barker et al., 1996). Women are affected by HE more than men – 81% in Chong's series of 85 adult patients (Chong et al., 2003). The mean age of onset is reported to be 41 but the condition has been reported in children as young as 9 years of age (Alink and de Vries, 2008). Few would argue that encephalopathy must feature for a diagnosis of HE to be contemplated but there is less agreement about associated features. Cases of HE featuring encephalopathy with additional aphasia, ataxia, myoclonus, tremor, headache, psychosis, and visual hallucinations have all been reported.

PATHOPHYSIOLOGY

The presence of antithyroid antibodies is a prerequisite for the diagnosis of HE but it remains far from clear whether these antibodies are pathogenetic effectors or simply proxy markers of the disease. The fact that antithyroid antibodies are associated with diverse and unrelated conditions and are found in a small proportion of the healthy population argues against a direct role. Few reports have found HE-specific CNS epitopes to which antithyroid antibodies bind. Antithyroid peroxidase (Anti-TPO) antibodies were found to bind to cerebellar astrocytes in HE but not HT, although the significance of this finding is unclear (Blanchin et al., 2007). The presence of lymphocytic infiltration of CNS vessels in some cases of HE has been used by some to suggest that the disorder is a vasculitis. Excess TSH-releasing hormone has also been suggested to underlie the encephalopathy in HE.

NEUROPATHOLOGY

The small number of reports of the neuropathology of HE that have been published have recently been summarized (Schiess and Pardo, 2008). Of these papers some (Duffey et al., 2003), but not all (Striano et al., 2006), report lymphocytic infiltration of vessels implying vasculitis. It is clear that further studies are needed before any conclusion can be drawn – the largely favorable outcome in this anyway rare condition inevitably means that few cases come to autopsy when the condition is active.

DIAGNOSIS

Differential diagnosis

The lack of clear diagnostic criteria and the variety of neurologic symptoms and signs reported in addition to encephalopathy in HE mean that it should be considered in the differential of all cases of encephalopathy in which an alternative explanation is not quickly evident. Although HE is rare it is treatable which makes it even more important that thyroid antibodies are sent as part of the encephalopathy workup. In the Mayo Clinic series (Castillo et al., 2006), of 20 patients with a final diagnosis of HE all were initially given another diagnosis, including dementia, encephalitis, stroke, Creutzfeldt–Jakob disease and even migraine. The case described in Jacob (Jacob and Rajabally, 2005) presented with multiple episodes of encephalopathy over many years and was variously diagnosed with viral meningoencephalitis, anxiety, and mania. Fourteen years after her first presentation a diagnosis of HE was made, underlying the multiple (more common) mimics of HE.

Antithyroid antibodies

Antibodies directed against thyroid antigens are a defining feature of HE. Despite this there is little consensus about what antithyroid antibodies are associated with HE and whether those that are have a role in pathogenesis. Antithyroid peroxidase antibodies are raised in almost all cases of HE. They are also, however, raised in other nonthyroid autoimmune disorders and in some healthy controls, and reference ranges and sensitivity vary depending upon the laboratory test used. Antibodies against thyroglobulin (Anti-TG) are often found in cases of HE but less commonly than are anti-TPO. Anti-TG antibodies are also found in a proportion of healthy subjects without thyroid disease. Anti-α-enolase antibodies have recently been found in the serum of patients with HE (Yoneda et al., 2007). These antibodies too have been found associated with nonthyroid autoimmune disorders. The issues around antibody testing in HE have recently been reviewed (Sinclair, 2008).

Other diagnostic tests

Cerebrospinal fluid. The most common finding in HE is a raised protein in the absence of a raised white cell count although a mild pleocytosis and, independently, oligoclonal bands have also been reported.

Imaging. CT scanning in HE is typically normal. MRI scanning has shown diffuse white matter abnormalities in up to half of patients in some series, these abnormalities sometimes resolving on treatment. Although a variety of other abnormalities have been reported in individual cases (Castillo et al., 2006), no HE-defining abnormality has been identified using MRI. The few reports of SPECT in HE document focal hypoperfusion, generalized hypoperfusion, or no abnormalities at all. The few reports of cerebral angiography in HE are generally normal, showing no evidence of large vessel vasculitis.

Electrical encephalography. Reviews of EEG findings in HE (Chong et al., 2003; Schauble et al., 2003) indicate that the vast majority of HE patients have an abnormal EEG. Generalized slowing is the commonest abnormality, whilst triphasic sharp waves and periodic complexes have been reported. Again no HE-specific EEG features have been identified.

TREATMENT

There is reasonable evidence that the vast majority of episodes of Hashimoto's encephalopathy respond to treatment with steroids. Of the 85 cases reviewed by Chong et al. (2003), 98% responded to steroids alone whereas of those treated with levothyroxine alone only 67% improved. Other immunosuppressants have also been used with success. Plasmapheresis has been effective including in cases resistant to steroids (Nieuwenhuis et al., 2004). Treated, the prognosis of HE is on the whole good. Consideration of a trial of steroids in an encephalopathic patient with antithyroid antibodies and no other obvious underlying cause is therefore sensible provided that intracerebral infection has been excluded.

MISCELLANEOUS NEUROLOGIC DISORDERS AND THYROID DISEASE

Myasthenia gravis

A long-recognized association exists between thyroid disease and myasthenia gravis. There is no evidence that thyroid dysfunction causes myasthenia gravis, or vice versa, and their coexistence is likely to be due to an underlying genetic predisposition to autoimmune disease. Myasthenia gravis may be associated with both hyperthyroidism and hypothyroidism (Sahay et al., 1965). Hyperthyroidism occurs in 2–17.5% of patients with myasthenia gravis (Trabelsi et al., 2006). In one study of 104 myasthenic patients, 6% had thyrotoxicosis, 10% had subclinical hyperthyroidism, 2% had hypothyroidism, 3.4% had subclinical hypothyroidism, and 11.5% had autoantibodies directed against thyroid antigens (Kiessling et al., 1981). The incidence of myasthenia gravis in patients with hyperthyroidism is less than 1%. In general, when hyperthyroidism and myasthenia occur in the same patient, their coexistence confers few unusual features upon either condition. Marino et al., however, studied 129 patients with myasthenia gravis, of whom 56 had autoimmune thyroid disease (25 with autoimmune thyroiditis and three with Graves' disease). They concluded that myasthenia associated with autoimmune thyroid disease has a mild clinical expression, with preferential ocular involvement, a lower frequency of thymic disease, and less likelihood of detectable acetylcholine receptor antibodies in serum (Marino et al., 1997). The control of myasthenia gravis may deteriorate with departure from the euthyroid state (Engel, 1992); however, treatment of the thyroid disorder does not have a predictable effect on myasthenia. Dramatic deteriorations in myasthenia have been reported following treatment of thyroid disease, although this is uncommon (Sahay et al., 1965). In some patients, an improvement in myasthenic weakness occurs after treatment of hyperthyroidism, perhaps because of the decreased magnitude of miniature end-plate potentials in untreated hyperthyroidism (Herwig and Denys, 1972). There have been reports of thyrotoxic myasthenic patients in whom repetitive nerve stimulation suggested the presence of either a disorder such as the Lambert–Eaton myasthenic syndrome or both presynaptic and postsynaptic disturbances of neuromuscular transmission (Mori and Takamori, 1976).

Differentiating between ophthalmoplegia due to myasthenia gravis and dysthyroid eye disease may be difficult, and the two may coexist (Vargas et al., 1993). Signs of orbital congestion or abnormal forced ductions suggest the presence of ophthalmopathy. Ptosis, exotropia, or weakness of the orbicularis oculi should alert the physician to the possibility of myasthenia gravis.

Multiple sclerosis and thyroid disease

Karni and Abramsky undertook a controlled prospective study to evaluate the prevalence of thyroid disease in patients with multiple sclerosis and found that thyroid disorders were at least three times more common in women with multiple sclerosis than in female control subjects (Karni and Abramsky, 1999). This was predominantly due to an increase in the prevalence of hypothyroidism. The authors suggested that this association may support the concept of an autoimmune pathogenesis for multiple sclerosis. Another interesting report documented thyroid-related complications in a group of 27 patients with multiple sclerosis treated with pulsed monoclonal antibody therapy (humanized anti-CD52 monoclonal antibody Campath-1H) to deplete circulating lymphocytes (Coles et al., 1999). Although radiologic and clinical markers of disease activity related to multiple sclerosis were significantly decreased for at least 18 months following therapy, one-third of treated patients developed antibodies against the thyrotropin receptor and autoimmune hyperthyroidism. The authors concluded that Campath-1H changed the immune response away from the Th1 phenotype, suppressing disease activity in multiple sclerosis, but permitting the generation of antibody-mediated thyroid disease.

Endocrine dysfunction in long-term survivors of primary brain tumors

Endocrine dysfunction, including hypothyroidism, has been highlighted as a frequent and frequently overlooked long-term complication of radiotherapy for primary brain tumors, with a significant impact on patient well-being (Araki et al., 1997). In one series of 31 patients examined 1.5–11 years after radiotherapy, 26% showed evidence of hypothalamic hypothyroidism. Hypothalamic hypogonadism in males and hyperprolactinemia and oligomenorrhea in female patients were also frequently found. It was suggested that endocrine function should be evaluated periodically in long-term survivors of primary brain tumors treated with radiotherapy.

Recurrent laryngeal nerve palsy

Both malignant disease of the thyroid gland (Takashima et al., 2003; Okuda et al., 2004) and thyroidectomy (Chiang et al., 2005) may be associated with hoarseness and other bulbar symptoms due to damage to the recurrent laryngeal nerve. Invasion of the recurrent laryngeal nerve by thyroid carcinoma can be accurately predicted by the finding of effaced fatty tissue on MR imaging (Takashima et al., 2003).

References

Aanderud S, Strandjord RE (1980). Hypothyroidism induced by anti-epileptic therapy. Acta Neurol Scand 61: 330–332.

Abramowicz MJ, Duprez L, Parma J et al. (1997). Familial congenital hypothyroidism due to inactivating mutation of the thyrotropin receptor causing profound hypoplasia of the thyroid gland. J Clin Invest 99: 3018–3024.

Alink J, de Vries TW (2008). Unexplained seizures, confusion or hallucinations: think Hashimoto encephalopathy. Acta Paediatr 97: 451–453.

Anand VT, Mann SB, Dash RJ et al. (1989). Auditory investigations in hypothyroidism. Acta Otolaryngol 108: 83–87.

Araki S, Terao A, Matsumoto I et al. (1968). Muscle cramps in chronic thyrotoxic myopathy Report of a case. Arch Neurol 19: 315–320.

Araki K, Minami Y, Ueda Y et al. (1990). A case of polymyositis associated with chronic thyroiditis presenting as hyperthyroidism. Jpn J Med 29: 46–51.

Araki W, Hove U, Muller B et al. (1997). Frequent and frequently overlooked: treatment-induced endocrine dysfunction in adult long-term survivors of primary brain tumors. Neurology 49: 498–506.

Asher R (1949). Myxoedematous madness. Br Med J 2: 555–562.

Atterwill CK, Bunn SJ, Atkinson DJ et al. (1984). Effects of thyroid status on presynaptic alpha 2-adrenoceptor function and beta-adrenoceptor binding in the rat brain. J Neural Transm 59: 43–55.

Attia J, Margetts P, Guyatt G (1999). Diagnosis of thyroid disease in hospitalized patients: a systematic review. Arch Intern Med 159: 658–665.

Aydin A, Cemeroglu AP, Baklan B (2004). Thyroxine-induced hypermotor seizure. Seizure 13: 61–65.

Baba M, Terada A, Hishida R et al. (1992). Persistent hemichorea associated with thyrotoxicosis. Intern Med 31: 1144–1146.

Bahn RS (2010). Graves' ophthalmopathy. N Engl J Med 362: 726–738.

Bahn RS, Dutton CM, Natt N et al. (1998). Thyrotropin receptor expression in Graves' orbital adipose/connective tissues: potential autoantigen in Graves' ophthalmopathy. J Clin Endocrinol Metab 83: 998–1002.

Bailey CC, Kabala J, Laitt R et al. (1996). Magnetic resonance imaging in thyroid eye disease. Eye (Lond) 10: 617–619.

Bakker B, Bikker H, Vulsma T et al. (2000). Two decades of screening for congenital hypothyroidism in the Netherlands: TPO gene mutations in total iodide organification defects (an update). J Clin Endocrinol Metab 85: 3708–3712.

Bar SL, Holmes DT, Frohlich J (2007). Asymptomatic hypothyroidism and statin-induced myopathy. Can Fam Physician 53: 428–431.

Barker R, Zajicek J, Wilkinson I (1996). Thyrotoxic Hashimoto's encephalopathy. J Neurol Neurosurg Psychiatry 60: 234.

Barnard RO, Campbell MJ, McDonald WI (1971). Pathological findings in a case of hypothyroidism with ataxia. J Neurol Neurosurg Psychiatry 34: 755–760.

Bartalena L, Marcocci C, Bogazzi F et al. (1998). Relation between therapy for hyperthyroidism and the course of Graves' ophthalmopathy. N Engl J Med 338: 73–78.

Bartalena L, Baldeschi L, Dickinson AJ et al. (2008). Consensus statement of the European Group On Graves' Orbitopathy (EUGOGO) on management of Graves' orbitopathy. Thyroid 18: 333–346.

Bartley GB, Fatourechi V, Kadrmas EF et al. (1996a). Clinical features of Graves' ophthalmopathy in an incidence cohort. Am J Ophthalmol 121: 284–290.

Bartley GB, Fatourechi V, Kadrmas EF et al. (1996b). Long-term follow-up of Graves ophthalmopathy in an incidence cohort. Ophthalmology 103: 958–962.

Bastron JA (1984). Neuropathy in disease of the thyroid. In: PJ Dyck (Ed.), Peripheral Neuropathy. WB Saunders, Philadelphia.

Beghi E, Delodovici ML, Bogliun G et al. (1989). Hypothyroidism and polyneuropathy. J Neurol Neurosurg Psychiatry 52: 1420–1423.

Bennett WR, Huston DP (1984). Rhabdomyolysis in thyroid storm. Am J Med 77: 733–735.

Betteridge T, Fink J (2009). Phenytoin toxicity and thyroid dysfunction. N Z Med J 122: 102–104.

Beynon J, Akhtar S, Kearney T (2008). Predictors of outcome in myxoedema coma. Crit Care 12: 111.

Bhansali A, Chandran V, Ramesh J et al. (2000). Acute myoedema: an unusual presenting manifestation of hypothyroid myopathy. Postgrad Med J 76: 99–100.

Blanchin S, Coffin C, Viader F et al. (2007). Antithyroperoxidase antibodies from patients with Hashimoto's encephalopathy bind to cerebellar astrocytes. J Neuroimmunol 192: 13–20.

Boileau P, Bain P, Rives S et al. (2004). Earlier onset of treatment or increment in LT4 dose in screened congenital hypothyroidism: which as the more important factor for IQ at 7 years? Horm Res 61: 228–233.

Brain L, Jellinek EH, Ball K (1966). Hashimoto's disease and encephalopathy. Lancet 2: 512–514.

Brennan MD, Coenen-Schimke JM, Bigelow ML et al. (2006a). Changes in skeletal muscle protein metabolism and myosin heavy chain isoform messenger ribonucleic acid abundance after treatment of hyperthyroidism. J Clin Endocrinol Metab 91: 4650–4656.

Brennan MD, Powell C, Kaufman KR et al. (2006b). The impact of overt and subclinical hyperthyroidism on skeletal muscle. Thyroid 16: 375–380.

Bronsky D, Kaganiec GI, Waldstein SS (1964). An association between the Guillain–Barré syndrome and hyperthyroidism. Am J Med Sci 247: 196–200.

Brownlie BE, Rae AM, Walshe JW et al. (2000). Psychoses associated with thyrotoxicosis – "thyrotoxic psychosis" A report of 18 cases, with statistical analysis of incidence. Eur J Endocrinol 142: 438–444.

Bruno AN, Ricachenevsky FK, Pochmann D et al. (2005). Hypothyroidism changes adenine nucleotide hydrolysis in synaptosomes from hippocampus and cerebral cortex of rats in different phases of development. Int J Dev Neurosci 23: 37–44.

Bulens C (1981). Neurologic complications of hyperthyroidism: remission of spastic paraplegia, dementia, and optic neuropathy. Arch Neurol 38: 669–670.

Bunevicius R, Prange AJ Jr (2010). Thyroid disease and mental disorders: cause and effect or only comorbidity? Curr Opin Psychiatry 23: 363–368.

Bunevicius R, Kazanavicius G, Zalinkevicius R et al. (1999). Effects of thyroxine as compared with thyroxine plus triiodothyronine in patients with hypothyroidism. N Engl J Med 340: 424–429.

Burch HB, Wartofsky L (1993). Life-threatening thyrotoxicosis Thyroid storm. Endocrinol Metab Clin North Am 22: 263–277.

Burger AG, Philippe J (1992). Thyroid emergencies. Baillieres Clin Endocrinol Metab 6: 77–93.

Burggraaf J, Lalezari S, Emeis JJ et al. (2001). Endothelial function in patients with hyperthyroidism before and after treatment with propranolol and thiamazol. Thyroid 11: 153–160.

Bursten B (1961). Psychoses associated with thyrotoxicosis. Arch Gen Psychiatry 4: 267–273.

Cadilhac J (1976). EEG in thyroid function. In: A Remond (Ed.), Handbook of Electroencephalopathy and Clinical Neurophysiology, vol. 15C. Elsevier, Amsterdam.

Caparros-Lefebvre D, Benabdallah S, Bertagna X et al. (2003). Subacute motor neuropathy induced by T3 hyperthyroidism. Ann Med Interne (Paris) 154: 475–478.

Carageprgiou H, Pantos C, Zarros A et al. (2005). Changes in antioxidant status, protein concentration, acetylcholinesterase, (Na+, K+)-, and Mg2+ -ATPase activities in the brain of hyper- and hypothyroid adult rats. Metab Brain Dis 20: 129–139.

Caselli RJ, Boeve BF, Scheithauer BW et al. (1999). Nonvasculitic autoimmune inflammatory meningoencephalitis (NAIM): a reversible form of encephalopathy. Neurology 53: 1579–1581.

Castillo P, Woodruff B, Caselli R et al. (2006). Steroid-responsive encephalopathy associated with autoimmune thyroiditis. Arch Neurol 63: 197–202.

Chan A, Shinde R, Chow CC et al. (1991). In vivo and in vitro sodium pump activity in subjects with thyrotoxic periodic paralysis. BMJ 303: 1096–1099.

Charcot J (1889). Nouveaux signes de la maladie de Basedow. Bull Med 3: 147–149.

Chen Q, Yao ZP, Zhou D et al. (2008). Lateral sinus thrombosis and intracranial hypertension associated with primary hypothyroidism: case report. Neuro Endocrinol Lett 29: 41–43.

Chiang FY, Wang LF, Huang YF et al. (2005). Recurrent laryngeal nerve palsy after thyroidectomy with routine identification of the recurrent laryngeal nerve. Surgery 137: 342–347.

Chiu WY, Yang CC, Huang IC et al. (2004). Dysphagia as a manifestation of thyrotoxicosis: report of three cases and literature review. Dysphagia 19: 120–124.

Chong JY, Rowland LP, Utiger RD (2003). Hashimoto encephalopathy: syndrome or myth? Arch Neurol 60: 164–171.

Chu M, Seltzer TF (2010). Myxedema coma induced by ingestion of raw bok choy. N Engl J Med 362: 1945–1946.

Chu DT, Shikama H, Khatra BS et al. (1985). Effects of altered thyroid status on beta-adrenergic actions on skeletal muscle glycogen metabolism. J Biol Chem 260: 9994–10000.

Chung SM, Lee AG, Holds JB et al. (1997). Ocular neuromyotonia in Graves dysthyroid orbitopathy. Arch Ophthalmol 115: 365–370.

Clarnette RM, Patterson CJ (1994). Hypothyroidism: does treatment cure dementia? J Geriatr Psychiatry Neurol 7: 23–27.

Clifton-Bligh RJ, Wentworth JM, Heinz P et al. (1998). Mutation of the gene encoding human TTF-2 associated with thyroid agenesis, cleft palate and choanal atresia. Nat Genet 19: 399–401.

Cole DP, Thase ME, Mallinger AG et al. (2002). Slower treatment response in bipolar depression predicted by lower pretreatment thyroid function. Am J Psychiatry 159: 116–121.

Coles AJ, Wing M, Smith S et al. (1999). Pulsed monoclonal antibody treatment and autoimmune thyroid disease in multiple sclerosis. Lancet 354: 1691–1695.

Cook DM, Boyle PJ (1986). Rapid reversal of myxedema madness with triiodothyronine. Ann Intern Med 104: 893–894.

Cremer GM, Goldstein NP, Paris J (1969). Myxedema and ataxia. Neurology 19: 37–46.

Danks JJ, Harrad RA (1998). Flashing lights in thyroid eye disease: a new symptom described and (possibly) explained. Br J Ophthalmol 82: 1309–1311.

de Rijk MC, Vermeij FH, Suntjens M et al. (2007). Does a carpal tunnel syndrome predict an underlying disease? J Neurol Neurosurg Psychiatry 78: 635–637.

De Schryver EL, Hoogenraad TU, Banga JD et al. (1999). Thyrotoxicosis, protein C deficiency and lupus anticoagulant in a case of cerebral sinus thrombosis. Neth J Med 55: 201–202.

Deepak S, Harikrishnan, Jayakumar B (2004). Hypothyroidism presenting as Hoffman's syndrome. J Indian Med Assoc 102: 41–42.

Demet MM, Ozmen B, Deveci A et al. (2002). Depression and anxiety in hyperthyroidism. Arch Med Res 33: 552–556.

Djemli A, Van Vliet G, Delvin EE (2006). Congenital hypothyroidism: from paracelsus to molecular diagnosis. Clin Biochem 39: 511–518.

Dohan O, Carrasco N (2003). Advances in Na(+)/I(-) symporter (NIS) research in the thyroid and beyond. Mol Cell Endocrinol 213: 59–70.

Dohan O, De la Vieja A, Paroder V et al. (2003). The sodium/iodide symporter (NIS): characterization, regulation, and medical significance. Endocr Rev 24: 48–77.

Drake ME Jr (1987). Paroxysmal kinesigenic choreoathetosis in hyperthyroidism. Postgrad Med J 63: 1089–1090.

Duffey P, Yee S, Reid IN et al. (2003). Hashimoto's encephalopathy: postmortem findings after fatal status epilepticus. Neurology 61: 1124–1126.

Dugbartey AT (1998). Neurocognitive aspects of hypothyroidism. Arch Intern Med 158: 1413–1418.

Duhaut P, Bornet H, Pinede L et al. (1999). Giant cell arteritis and thyroid dysfunction: multicentre case-control study

The Groupe de Recherche sur l'Artéritéa Cellules Géantes. BMJ 318: 434–435.

Dulli DA, Luzzio CC, Williams EC et al. (1996). Cerebral venous thrombosis and activated protein C resistance. Stroke 27: 1731–1733.

Dumitrescu AM, Liao XH, Best TB et al. (2004). A novel syndrome combining thyroid and neurological abnormalities is associated with mutations in a monocarboxylate transporter gene. Am J Hum Genet 74: 168–175.

Duyff RF, Van den Bosch J, Laman DM et al. (2000). Neuromuscular findings in thyroid dysfunction: a prospective clinical and electrodiagnostic study. J Neurol Neurosurg Psychiatry 68: 750–755.

Dyck PJ, Lambert EH (1970). Polyneuropathy associated with hypothyroidism. J Neuropathol Exp Neurol 29: 631–658.

Eckstein AK, Losch C, Glowacka D et al. (2009). Euthyroid and primarily hypothyroid patients develop milder and significantly more asymmetrical Graves ophthalmopathy. Br J Ophthalmol 93: 1052–1056.

Eiris-Punal J, Del Rio-Garma M, Del Rio-Garma MC et al. (1999). Long-term treatment of children with epilepsy with valproate or carbamazepine may cause subclinical hypothyroidism. Epilepsia 40: 1761–1766.

Engel AG (1966). Electron microscopic observations in thyrotoxic and corticosteroid-induced myopathies. Mayo Clin Proc 41: 785–796.

Engel AG (1992). Myasthenia gravis and myasthenic syndromes. In: PJ Vinken, GW Bruyn, HL Klawans (Eds.), Handbook of Clinical Neurology, vol. 62, Myopathies, Elsevier Science, Amsterdam, Chapter 14, pp. 391–456.

Engum A, Bjoro T, Mykletun A et al. (2002). An association between depression, anxiety and thyroid function – a clinical fact or an artefact? Acta Psychiatr Scand 106: 27–34.

Enzmann DR, Donaldson SS, Kriss JP (1979). Appearance of Graves' disease on orbital computed tomography. J Comput Assist Tomogr 3: 815–819.

Erkintolo M, Bendahan D, Mattei JP et al. (1998). Reduced metabolic efficiency of skeletal muscle energetics in hyperthyroid patients evidenced quantitatively by in vivo phosphorus-31 magnetic resonance spectroscopy. Metabolism 47: 769–776.

Evans EC (1960). Neurologic complications of myxedema: convulsions. Ann Intern Med 52: 434–444.

Farwell AP, Dubord-Tomasetti SA (1999). Thyroid hormone regulates the expression of laminin in the developing rat cerebellum. Endocrinology 140: 4221–4227.

Feely J, Peden N (1984). Use of beta-adrenoceptor blocking drugs in hyperthyroidism. Drugs 27: 425–446.

Feibel JH, Campa JF (1976). Thyrotoxic neuropathy (Basedow's paraplegia). J Neurol Neurosurg Psychiatry 39: 491–497.

Ferlazzo E, Raffaele M, Mazzu I et al. (2006). Recurrent status epilepticus as the main feature of Hashimoto's encephalopathy. Epilepsy Behav 8: 328–330.

Fisher J (1982). Thyrotoxic periodic paralysis with ventricular fibrillation. Arch Intern Med 142: 1362–1364.

Fisher DA (1983). Second International Conference on Neonatal Thyroid Screening: progress report. J Pediatr 102: 653–654.

Fisher M, Mateer JE, Ullrich I et al. (1985). Pyramidal tract deficits and polyneuropathy in hyperthyroidism, combination clinically mimicking amyotrophic lateral sclerosis. Am J Med 78: 1041–1044.

Franchini M, Lippi G, Targher G (2010). Hyperthyroidism and venous thrombosis: a casual or causal association? A systematic literature review. Clin Appl Thromb Hemost 17: 387–392.

Furutani R, Ishihara K, Miyazawa Y et al. (2007). A case of hypothyroidism displaying "dropped head" syndrome. Rinsho Shinkeigaku 47: 32–36.

Genovesi-Ebert F, Di Bartolo E, Lepri A et al. (1998). Standardized echography, pattern electroretinography and visual-evoked potential and automated perimetry in the early diagnosis of Graves' neuropathy. Ophthalmologica 212 (Suppl 1): 101–103.

Ghenimi N, Alfos S, Redonnet A et al. (2010). Adult-onset hypothyroidism induces the amyloidogenic pathway of amyloid precursor protein processing in the rat hippocampus. J Neuroendocrinol 22: 951–959.

Ghosh S, Rahaman SO, Sarkar PK (1999). Regulation of neurofilament gene expression by thyroid hormone in the developing rat brain. Neuroreport 10: 2361–2365.

Guieu R, Harley JR, Blin O et al. (1993). Nociceptive threshold in hypothyroid patients. Acta Neurol (Napoli) 15: 183–188.

Guo TW, Zhang FC, Yang MS et al. (2004). Positive association of the DIO2 (deiodinase type 2) gene with mental retardation in the iodine-deficient areas of China. J Med Genet 41: 585–590.

Halpern JP, Boyages SC, Maberly GF et al. (1991). The neurology of endemic cretinism A study of two endemias. Brain 114: 825–841.

Harayama H, Ohno T, Miyatake T (1983). Quantitative analysis of stance in ataxic myxoedema. J Neurol Neurosurg Psychiatry 46: 579–581.

Hardiman O, Molloy F, Brett F et al. (1997). Inflammatory myopathy in thyrotoxicosis. Neurology 48: 339–341.

Havard CW, Campbell ED, Ross HB et al. (1963). Electromyographic and histological findings in the muscles of patients with thyrotoxicosis. Q J Med 32: 145–163.

Haynes JH 3rd, Kageler WV (1989). Thyrocardiotoxic embolic syndrome. South Med J 82: 1292–1293.

Heinrich TW, Grahm G (2003). Hypothyroidism presenting as psychosis: myxedema madness revisited. Prim Care Companion J Clin Psychiatry 5: 260–266.

Hekimsoy Z, Oktem IK (2005). Serum creatine kinase levels in overt and subclinical hypothyroidism. Endocr Res 31: 171–175.

Herwig D (2008). Myopathy associated with statin therapy. Neuromuscul Disord 18: 97–98.

Herwig WW, Denys EH (1972). Effects of thyroid hormone at the neuromuscular junction. Am J Physiol 223: 283–287.

Herwig U, Sturzenegger M (1999). Hyperthyroidism mimicking increased intracranial pressure. Headache 39: 228–230.

Horii K, Fujitake J, Tatsuoka Y et al. (1991). A case of phenytoin intoxication induced by hypothyroidism. Rinsho Shinkeigaku 31: 528–533.

Hosojima H, Iwasaki R, Miyauchi E et al. (1992). Rhabdomyolysis accompanying thyroid crisis: an autopsy case report. Intern Med 31: 1233–1235.

How J, Bewsher PD, Walker W (1977). Giant-cell arteritis and hypothyroidism. Br Med J 2: 99.

Hsieh MJ, Lyu RK, Chang WN et al. (2008). Hypokalemic thyrotoxic periodic paralysis: clinical characteristics and predictors of recurrent paralytic attacks. Eur J Neurol 15: 559–564.

Hsu SI, Thadhani RI, Daniels GH (1995). Acute compartment syndrome in a hypothyroid patient. Thyroid 5: 305–308.

Hung YT, Yeung VT (2000). Hypothyroidism presenting as hypercholesterolaemia and simvastatin-induced myositis. Hong Kong Med J 6: 423–424.

Hurwitz LJ, McCormick D, Allen IV (1970). Reduced muscle alpha-glucosidase (acid-maltase) activity in hypothyroid myopathy. Lancet 1: 67–69.

Ijichi S, Niina K, Tara M et al. (1990). Mononeuropathy associated with hyperthyroidism. J Neurol Neurosurg Psychiatry 53: 1109–1110.

Isaacs JD, Rakshi J, Baker R et al. (2005). Chorea associated with thyroxine replacement therapy. Mov Disord 20: 1656–1657.

Iwasaki Y, Kinoshita M, Ikeda K et al. (1991). Thyroid function in patients with chronic headache. Int J Neurosci 57: 263–267.

Jabbari B, Huott AD (1980). Seizures in thyrotoxicosis. Epilepsia 21: 91–96.

Jackson IM (1998). The thyroid axis and depression. Thyroid 8: 951–956.

Jacob S, Rajabally YA (2005). Hashimoto's encephalopathy: steroid resistance and response to intravenous immunoglobulins. J Neurol Neurosurg Psychiatry 76: 455–456.

Jansen HJ, Doebe SR, Louwerse ES et al. (2006). Status epilepticus caused by a myxoedema coma. Neth J Med 64: 202–205.

Jellinek EH, Kelly RE (1960). Cerebellar syndrome in myxoedema. Lancet 2: 225–227.

Jha A, Sharma SK, Tandon N et al. (2006). Thyroxine replacement therapy reverses sleep-disordered breathing in patients with primary hypothyroidism. Sleep Med 7: 55–61.

Joffroy M (1894). Hospice de la Salpêtrière, Clinique Nerveuse, Leçons faite en Decembre 1891. Prog Med 22: 61–62.

Jordan N, Williams N, Gregory JW et al. (2003). The W546X mutation of the thyrotropin receptor gene: potential major contributor to thyroid dysfunction in a Caucasian population. J Clin Endocrinol Metab 88: 1002–1005.

Kammer GM, Hamilton CR Jr (1974). Acute bulbar muscle dysfunction and hyperthyroidism A study of four cases and review of the literature. Am J Med 56: 464–470.

Kane MP, Busch RS (2006). Drug-induced thyrotoxic periodic paralysis. Ann Pharmacother 40: 778–781.

Karni A, Abramsky O (1999). Association of MS with thyroid disorders. Neurology 53: 883–885.

Karouache A, Mounach J, Bouraza A et al. (2004). Cerebral thrombophlebitis revealing hyperthyroidism: two cases report and literature review. Rev Med Interne 25: 920–923.

Kasperbauer JL, Hinkley L (2005). Endoscopic orbital decompression for Graves' ophthalmopathy. Am J Rhinol 19: 603–606.

Kececi H, Degirmenci Y (2006). Hormone replacement therapy in hypothyroidism and nerve conduction study. Neurophysiol Clin 36: 79–83.

Kellett HA, Sawers JS, Boulton FE et al. (1986). Problems of anticoagulation with warfarin in hyperthyroidism. Q J Med 58: 43–51.

Kelley DE, Gharib H, Kennedy FP et al. (1989). Thyrotoxic periodic paralysis Report of 10 cases and review of electromyographic findings. Arch Intern Med 149: 2597–2600.

Kempers MJ, van der Sluijs Veer L, Nijhuis-van der Sanden MW et al. (2006). Intellectual and motor development of young adults with congenital hypothyroidism diagnosed by neonatal screening. J Clin Endocrinol Metab 91: 418–424.

Kendall-Taylor P, Turnbull DM (1983). Endocrine myopathies. Br Med J (Clin Res Ed) 287: 705–708.

Khaleeli AA, Edwards RH (1984). Effect of treatment on skeletal muscle dysfunction in hypothyroidism. Clin Sci (Lond) 66: 63–68.

Khawaja NM, Taher BM, Barham ME et al. (2006). Pituitary enlargement in patients with primary hypothyroidism. Endocr Pract 12: 29–34.

Khedr EM, El Toony LF, Tarkhan MN et al. (2000). Peripheral and central nervous system alterations in hypothyroidism: electrophysiological findings. Neuropsychobiology 41: 88–94.

Kiessling WR, Pflughaupt KW, Ricker K et al. (1981). Thyroid function and circulating antithyroid antibodies in myasthenia gravis. Neurology 31: 771–774.

Kilzieh N, Akiskal HS (1999). Rapid-cycling bipolar disorder An overview of research and clinical experience. Psychiatr Clin North Am 22: 585–607.

Kim JY, Kim BS, Kang JH (2001). Dilated cardiomyopathy in thyrotoxicosis and moyamoya disease. Int J Cardiol 80: 101–103.

Kim DD, Young S, Chunilal S et al. (2008). Possible association of venous thromboembolism and hyperthyroidism: 4 case reports and literature review. N Z Med J 121: 53–57.

Kim JM, Song EJ, Seo JS et al. (2009). Polymyositis-like syndrome caused by hypothyroidism, presenting as camptocormia. Rheumatol Int 29: 339–342.

Kinuya S, Michigishi T, Tonami N et al. (1999). Reversible cerebral hypoperfusion observed with Tc-99m HMPAO SPECT in reversible dementia caused by hypothyroidism. Clin Nucl Med 24: 666–668.

Kisakol G, Tunc R, Kaya A (2003). Rhabdomyolysis in a patient with hypothyroidism. Endocr J 50: 221–223.

Kjeldsen K, Norgaard A, Gotzsche CO et al. (1984). Effect of thyroid function on number of Na-K pumps in human skeletal muscle. Lancet 2: 8–10.

Klawans HL Jr, Shenker DM (1972). Observations on the dopaminergic nature of hyperthyroid chorea. J Neural Transm 33: 73–81.

Kliachko VR, Prikhozhan VM (1970). Neurologic disorders in primary hypothyroidism. Probl Endokrinol (Mosk) 16: 24–29.

Koibuchi N, Iwasaki T (2006). Regulation of brain development by thyroid hormone and its modulation by environmental chemicals. Endocr J 53: 295–303.

Koster T, Blann AD, Briet E et al. (1995). Role of clotting factor VIII in effect of von Willebrand factor on occurrence of deep-vein thrombosis. Lancet 345: 152–155.

Kramer U, Achiron A (1993). Drop attacks induced by hypothyroidism. Acta Neurol Scand 88: 410–411.

Krieger EV, Knopp RH (2009). Hypothyroidism misdiagnosed as statin intolerance. Ann Intern Med 151: 72.

Krude H, Schutz B, Biebermann H et al. (2002). Choreoathetosis, hypothyroidism, and pulmonary alterations due to human NKX2-1 haploinsufficiency. J Clin Invest 109: 475–480.

Kung AW, Ma JT, Yu YL et al. (1987). Myopathy in acute hypothyroidism. Postgrad Med J 63: 661–663.

Kung AW, Lau KS, Cheung WM et al. (2006). Thyrotoxic periodic paralysis and polymorphisms of sodium-potassium ATPase genes. Clin Endocrinol (Oxf) 64: 158–161.

Kuo HT, Jeng CY (2010). Overt hypothyroidism with rhabdomyolysis and myopathy: a case report. Chin Med J (Engl) 123: 633–637.

Kursat S, Alici T, Colak HB (2005). A case of rhabdomyolysis induced acute renal failure secondary to statin-fibrate-derivative combination and occult hypothyroidism. Clin Nephrol 64: 391–393.

Kushnir M, Weinstein R, Landau B et al. (1985). Hypothyroidism and phenytoin intoxication. Ann Intern Med 102: 341–342.

Kyrle PA, Minar E, Hirschl M et al. (2000). High plasma levels of factor VIII and the risk of recurrent venous thromboembolism. N Engl J Med 343: 457–462.

Ladenson PW, Stakes JW, Ridgway EC (1984). Reversible alteration of the visual evoked potential in hypothyroidism. Am J Med 77: 1010–1014.

LaFranchi SH, Austin J (2007). How should we be treating children with congenital hypothyroidism? J Pediatr Endocrinol Metab 20: 559–578.

LaFranchi SH, Hanna CE, Krainz PL (1986). Primary hypothyroidism, empty sella, and hypopituitarism. J Pediatr 108: 571–573.

Lai CL, Lin RT, Tai CT et al. (2000). The recovery potential of central conduction disorder in hypothyroid rats. J Neurol Sci 173: 113–119.

Lai A, Sassi L, Compri E et al. (2010). Lower dose prednisone prevents radioiodine-associated exacerbation of initially mild or absent Graves' orbitopathy: a retrospective cohort study. J Clin Endocrinol Metab 95: 1333–1337.

Lambert EH, Underdahl LO, Beckett S et al. (1951). A study of the ankle jerk in myxedema. J Clin Endocrinol Metab 11: 1186–1205.

Larisch R, Kley K, Nikolaus S et al. (2004). Depression and anxiety in different thyroid function states. Horm Metab Res 36: 650–653.

Laurent L (1944). Acute thyrotoxic bulbar palsy. Lancet 1: 87.

Lebon V, Dufour S, Petersen KF et al. (2001). Effect of triiodothyronine on mitochondrial energy coupling in human skeletal muscle. J Clin Invest 108: 733–737.

Lecky BR, Williams TD, Lightman SL et al. (1987). Myxoedema presenting with chiasmal compression: resolution after thyroxine replacement. Lancet 1: 1347–1350.

Leese GP, Flynn RV, Jung RT et al. (2008). Increasing prevalence and incidence of thyroid disease in Tayside, Scotland The thyroid epidemiology and audit and research study (TEARS). Clin Endocrinol 68: 311–316.

Leubuscher HJ, Herrmann F, Hambsch K et al. (1988). EEG changes in untreated hyperthyroidism and under the conditions of thyreostatic treatment. Exp Clin Endocrinol 92: 85–90.

Levine JA, Nygren J, Short KR et al. (2003). Effect of hyperthyroidism on spontaneous physical activity and energy expenditure in rats. J Appl Physiol 94: 165–170.

Lichtstein DM, Arteaga RB (2006). Rhabdomyolysis associated with hyperthyroidism. Am J Med Sci 332: 103–105.

Lin CC, Tsan KW, Chen PJ (1992). The relationship between sleep apnea syndrome and hypothyroidism. Chest 102: 1663–1667.

Lleo A, Sanahuja J, Serrano C et al. (1999). Acute bulbar weakness: thyrotoxicosis or myasthenia gravis? Ann Neurol 46: 434–435.

Lochmuller H, Reimers CD, Fischer P et al. (1993). Exercise-induced myalgia in hypothyroidism. Clin Investig 71: 999–1001.

Loh LM, Hum AY, Teoh HL et al. (2005). Graves' disease associated with spasmodic truncal flexion. Parkinsonism Relat Disord 11: 117–119.

Lu KC, Hsu YJ, Chiu JS et al. (2004). Effects of potassium supplementation on the recovery of thyrotoxic periodic paralysis. Am J Emerg Med 22: 544–547.

Ludin HP, Spiess H, Koenig MP (1969). Neuromuscular dysfunction associated with thyrotoxicosis. Eur Neurol 2: 269–278.

Ma T, Lian ZC, Qi SP et al. (1993). Magnetic resonance imaging of brain and the neuromotor disorder in endemic cretinism. Ann Neurol 34: 91–94.

Macchia PE, Lapi P, Krude H et al. (1998). PAX8 mutations associated with congenital hypothyroidism caused by thyroid dysgenesis. Nat Genet 19: 83–86.

Madariaga MG (2002). Polymyositis-like syndrome in hypothyroidism: review of cases reported over the past twenty-five years. Thyroid 12: 331–336.

Madroñero-Vuelta A, Sanahuja-Montesinos J, Bergua-Llop M et al. (2004). Cerebral venous thrombosis associated to subacute De Quervain's thyroiditis in a carrier for the G20210A mutation of the prothrombin gene. Rev Neurol 39: 533–535.

Maes J, Michotte A, Velkeniers B et al. (2002). Hyperthyroidism with increased factor VIII procoagulant protein as a predisposing factor for cerebral venous thrombosis. J Neurol Neurosurg Psychiatry 73: 458.

Magsino CH Jr, Ryan AJ Jr (2000). Thyrotoxic periodic paralysis. South Med J 93: 996–1003.

Manoukian MA, Foote JA, Crapo LM (1999). Clinical and metabolic features of thyrotoxic periodic paralysis in 24 episodes. Arch Intern Med 159: 601–606.

Marino M, Ricciardi R, Pinchera A et al. (1997). Mild clinical expression of myasthenia gravis associated with autoimmune thyroid diseases. J Clin Endocrinol Metab 82: 438–443.

Marks P, Anderson J, Vincent R (1980). Thyrotoxic myopathy presenting as dysphagia. Postgrad Med J 56: 669–670.

Martin WH 3rd, Spina RJ, Korte E et al. (1991). Mechanisms of impaired exercise capacity in short duration experimental hyperthyroidism. J Clin Invest 88: 2047–2053.

Martinez FJ, Bermudez-Gomez M, Celli BR (1989). Hypothyroidism: a reversible cause of diaphragmatic dysfunction. Chest 96: 1059–1063.

McKeag D, Lane C, Lazarus JH et al. (2007). Clinical features of dysthyroid optic neuropathy: a European Group On Graves' Orbitopathy (EUGOGO) survey. Br J Ophthalmol 91: 455–458.

McKeran RO, Slavin G, Andrews TM et al. (1975). Muscle fibre type changes in hypothyroid myopathy. J Clin Pathol 28: 659–663.

McKeran RO, Slavin G, Ward P et al. (1980). Hypothyroid myopathy A clinical and pathologaical study. J Pathol 132: 35–54.

Metson R, Pletcher SD (2006). Endoscopic orbital and optic nerve decompression. Otolaryngol Clin North Am 39: 551–561, ix.

Miao J, Liu R, Li J et al. (2010). Meige's syndrome and hemichorea associated with hyperthyroidism. J Neurol Sci 288: 175–177.

Migneco A, Ojetti V, Testa A et al. (2005). Management of thyrotoxic crisis. Eur Rev Med Pharmacol Sci 9: 69–74.

Milanov I, Sheinkova G (2000). Clinical and electromyographic examination of tremor in patients with thyrotoxicosis. Int J Clin Pract 54: 364–367.

Miller J, Carney P (2006). Central hypothyroidism with oxcarbazepine therapy. Pediatr Neurol 34: 242–244.

Mizuno H, Sugiyama Y, Nishi Y et al. (2006). Elevation of serum creatine kinase in response to medical treatment of Graves' disease in children. Acta Paediatr 95: 243–245.

Molloy E, Cahill M, O'Hare JA (2003). Cerebral venous sinus thrombosis precipitated by Graves' disease and factor V Leiden mutation. Ir Med J 96: 46–47.

Monzani F, Caraccio N, Del Guerra P et al. (1999). Neuromuscular symptoms and dysfunction in subclinical hypothyroid patients: beneficial effect of L-T4 replacement therapy. Clin Endocrinol (Oxf) 51: 237–242.

Monzani F, Caraccio N, Kozakowa M et al. (2004). Effect of levothyroxine replacement on lipid profile and intima-media thickness in subclinical hypothyroidism: a double-blind, placebo- controlled study. J Clin Endocrinol Metab 89: 2099–2106.

Moore AP, Macfarlane IA, Blumhardt LD (1990). Neuroleptic malignant syndrome and hypothyroidism. J Neurol Neurosurg Psychiatry 53: 517–518.

Moreno JC, Bikker H, Kempers MJ et al. (2002). Inactivating mutations in the gene for thyroid oxidase 2 (THOX2) and congenital hypothyroidism. N Engl J Med 347: 95–102.

Mori M, Takamori M (1976). Hyperthyroidism and myasthenia gravis with features of Eaton–Lambert syndrome. Neurology 26: 882–887.

Morris MS, Bostom AG, Jacques PF et al. (2001). Hyperhomocysteinemia and hypercholesterolemia associated with hypothyroidism in the third US National Health and Nutrition Examination Survey. Atherosclerosis 155: 195–200.

Morrison WL, Gibson JN, Jung RT et al. (1988). Skeletal muscle and whole body protein turnover in thyroid disease. Eur J Clin Invest 18: 62–68.

Murthy AS, Baquer NZ (1982). Changes of pyruvate dehydrogenase in rat brain with thyroid hormones. Enzyme 28: 48–53.

Myers L, Hays J (1991). Myxedema coma. Crit Care Clin 7: 43–56.

Nagaoka T, Matsushita S, Nagai Y et al. (1998). A woman who trembled, then had chorea. Lancet 351: 1326.

Nagumo K, Fukushima T, Takahashi H et al. (2007). Thyroid crisis and protein C deficiency in a case of superior sagittal sinus thrombosis. Brain Nerve 59: 271–276.

Nakamura K, Yanaka K, Ihara S et al. (2003). Multiple intracranial arterial stenoses around the circle of Willis in association with Graves' disease: report of two cases. Neurosurgery 53: 1210–1214, discussion 1214–1215.

Nemni R, Bottacchi E, Fazio R et al. (1987). Polyneuropathy in hypothyroidism: clinical, electrophysiological and morphological findings in four cases. J Neurol Neurosurg Psychiatry 50: 1454–1460.

Newcomer J, Haire W, Hartman CR (1983). Coma and thyrotoxicosis. Ann Neurol 14: 689–690.

Nicholson JL, Altman J (1972). The effects of early hypo- and hyperthyroidism on the development of rat cerebellar cortex I Cell proliferation and differentiation. Brain Res 44: 13–23.

Nicholson GC, Gutteridge DH, Carroll WM et al. (1984). Autoimmune thyroid disease and giant cell arteritis: a review, case report and epidemiological study. Aust N Z J Med 14: 487–490.

Nickel SN, Frame B, Bebin J et al. (1961). Myxedema neuropathy and myopathy A clinical and pathologic study. Neurology 11: 125–137.

Nicoloff JT, LoPresti JS (1993). Myxedema coma A form of decompensated hypothyroidism. Endocrinol Metab Clin North Am 22: 279–290.

Nieuwenhuis L, Santens P, Vanwalleghem P et al. (2004). Subacute Hashimoto's encephalopathy, treated with plasmapheresis. Acta Neurol Belg 104: 80–83.

Okuda S, Kanda F, Kawamoto K et al. (2004). Subacute bulbar palsy as the initial sign of follicular thyroid cancer. Intern Med 43: 997–999.

Osterweil D, Syndulko K, Cohen SN et al. (1992). Cognitive function in non-demented older adults with hypothyroidism. J Am Geriatr Soc 40: 325–335.

Ozata M, Ozkardes A, Dolu H et al. (1996). Evaluation of central motor conduction in hypothyroid and hyperthyroid patients. J Endocrinol Invest 19: 670–677.

Page SR, Scott AR (1993). Thyroid storm in a young woman resulting in bilateral basal ganglia infarction. Postgrad Med J 69: 813–815.

Pandit L, Shankar SK, Gayathri N et al. (1998). Acute thyrotoxic neuropathy – Basedow's paraplegia revisited. J Neurol Sci 155: 211–214.

Pandya K, Lal C, Scheinhorn D et al. (1989). Hypothyroidism and ventilator dependency. Arch Intern Med 149: 2115–2116.

Panicker V, Saravanan P, Vaidya B et al. (2009). Common variation in the DIO2 gene predicts baseline psychological well-being and response to combination thyroxine plus triiodothyronine therapy in hypothyroid patients. J Clin Endocrinol Metab 94: 1623–1629.

Paridaens D, van den Bosch WA, van der Loos TL et al. (2005). The effect of etanercept on Graves' ophthalmopathy: a pilot study. Eye (Lond) 19: 1286–1289.

Park YJ, Lee EJ, Lee YJ et al. (2010). Subclinical hypothyroidism (SCH) is not associated with metabolic derangement, cognitive impairment, depression or poor quality of life (QoL) in elderly subjects. Arch Gerontol Geriatr 50: e68–e73.

Parmar MS (2005). Thyrotoxic atrial fibrillation. MedGenMed 7: 74.

Patial RK, Kumar V, Kumari R (1995). Motor neurone disease like picture in hyperthyroidism. Indian J Med Sci 49: 114–116.

Pearce J, Aziz H (1969). The neuromyopathy of hypothyroidism Some new observations. J Neurol Sci 9: 243–253.

Pekdemir M, Yilmaz S, Ersel M et al. (2008). A rare cause of headache: cerebral venous sinus thrombosis due to hyperthyroidism. Am J Emerg Med 26: 383.e1–383.e2.

Peralta AR, Canhao P (2008). Hypothyroidism and cerebral vein thrombosis – a possible association. J Neurol 255: 962–966.

Pollard JD, McLeod JG, Honnibal TG et al. (1982). Hypothyroid polyneuropathy Clinical, electrophysiological and nerve biopsy findings in two cases. J Neurol Sci 53: 461–471.

Presti CF, Hart RG (1989). Thyrotoxicosis, atrial fibrillation, and embolism, revisited. Am Heart J 117: 976–977.

Primavera A, Brusa G, Novello P (1990). Thyrotoxic encephalopathy and recurrent seizures. Eur Neurol 30: 186–188.

Prummel MF, Wiersinga WM (1993). Smoking and risk of Graves' disease. JAMA 269: 479–482.

Puri V, Chaudhry N (2004). Paroxysmal kinesigenic dyskinesia manifestation of hyperthyroidism. Neurol India 52: 102–103.

Purnell DC, Daly DD, Lipscomb PR (1961). Carpal-tunnel syndrome associated with myxedema. Arch Intern Med 108: 751–756.

Qari FA (2009). Severe rhabdomyolysis and acute renal failure secondary to use of simvastatin in undiagnosed hypothyroidism. Saudi J Kidney Dis Transpl 20: 127–129.

Ra CS, Lui CC, Liang CL et al. (2001). Superior sagittal sinus thrombosis induced by thyrotoxicosis Case report. J Neurosurg 94: 130–132.

Ramdass MJ, Singh G, Andrews B (2007). Simvastatin-induced bilateral leg compartment syndrome and myonecrosis associated with hypothyroidism. Postgrad Med J 83: 152–153.

Ramsay ID (1966). Muscle dysfunction in hyperthyroidism. Lancet 2: 931–934.

Rastogi MV, LaFranchi SH (2010). Congenital hypothyroidism. Orphanet J Rare Dis 5: 17.

Riis AL, Jorgensen JO, Gjedde S et al. (2005). Whole body and forearm substrate metabolism in hyperthyroidism: evidence of increased basal muscle protein breakdown. Am J Physiol Endocrinol Metab 288: E1067–E1073.

Ristic AJ, Svetel M, Dragasevic N et al. (2004). Bilateral chorea-ballism associated with hyperthyroidism. Mov Disord 19: 982–983.

Rodriguez I, Fluiters E, Perez-Mendez LF et al. (2004). Factors associated with mortality of patients with myxoedema coma: prospective study in 11 cases treated in a single institution. J Endocrinol 180: 347–350.

Roquer J, Cano JF (1993). Carpal tunnel syndrome and hyperthyroidism A prospective study. Acta Neurol Scand 88: 149–152.

Ruff RL, Weissmann J (1988). Endocrine myopathies. Neurol Clin 6: 575–592.

Rundle F (1964). Eye signs of Graves' disease. In: R Pitt-Rivers, WR Trotter (Eds.), The Thyroid. Butterworth, Washington DC, p. 171.

Ryan DP, da Silva MR, Soong TW et al. (2010). Mutations in potassium channel Kir26 cause susceptibility to thyrotoxic hypokalemic periodic paralysis. Cell 140: 88–98.

Sahay BM, Blendis LM, Greene R (1965). Relation between myasthenia gravis and thyroid disease. Br Med J 1: 762–765.

Salaria M, Parmar VR (2004). Kocher Debre Semelaigne syndrome – a case report and review of literature. J Indian Med Assoc 102: 645–646.

Salviati G, Zeviani M, Betto R et al. (1985). Effects of thyroid hormones on the biochemical specialization of human muscle fibers. Muscle Nerve 8: 363–371.

Sarlis NJ, Gourgiotis L (2003). Thyroid emergencies. Rev Endocr Metab Disord 4: 129–136.

Savarad P, Merand Y, Di Paolo T et al. (1983). Effects of thyroid state on serotonin, 5-hydroxyindoleacetic acid and substance P contents in discrete brain nuclei of adult rats. Neuroscience 10: 1399–1404.

Schauble B, Castillo PR, Boeve BF et al. (2003). EEG findings in steroid-responsive encephalopathy associated with autoimmune thyroiditis. Clin Neurophysiol 114: 32–37.

Schiess N, Pardo CA (2008). Hashimoto's encephalopathy. Ann N Y Acad Sci 1142: 254–265.

Schreckenberger MF, Egle UT, Drecker S et al. (2006). Positron emission tomography reveals correlations between brain metabolism and mood changes in hyperthyroidism. J Clin Endocrinol Metab 91: 4786–4791.

Schutta HS, Williams EC, Baranski BG et al. (1991). Cerebral venous thrombosis with plasminogen deficiency. Stroke 22: 401–405.

Schwartz HL, Oppenheimer JH (1978). Physiologic and biochemical actions of thyroid hormone. Pharmacol Ther B 3: 349–376.

Schwartz MS, Mackworth-Young CG, McKeran RO (1983). The tarsal tunnel syndrome in hypothyroidism. J Neurol Neurosurg Psychiatry 46: 440–442.

Selim M, Drachman DA (2001). Ataxia associated with Hashimoto's disease: progressive non-familial adult onset cerebellar degeneration with autoimmune thyroiditis. J Neurol Neurosurg Psychiatry 71: 81–87.

Shahar E, Shapiro MS, Shenkman L (1988). Hyperthyroid-induced chorea Case report and review of the literature. Isr J Med Sci 24: 264–266.

Shaheen D, Kim CS (2009). Myositis associated with the decline of thyroid hormone levels in thyrotoxicosis: a syndrome? Thyroid 19: 1413–1417.

Shaw PJ, Bates D, Kendall-Taylor P (1988). Hyperthyroidism presenting as pyramidal tract disease. BMJ 297: 1395–1396.

Shaw PJ, Walls TJ, Newman PK et al. (1991). Hashimoto's encephalopathy: a steroid-responsive disorder associated with high anti-thyroid antibody titers – report of 5 cases. Neurology 41: 228–233.

Sheu JJ, Kang JH, Lin HC (2010). Hyperthyroidism and risk of ischemic stroke in young adults: a 5-year follow-up study. Stroke 41: 961–966.

Shinoda K, Hosokawa S, Mozai T (1987). Peripheral neuropathy in hypothyroidism II Morphometrical and electron microscopical studies on sural nerve in hypothyroidism and axonal atrophy in hypothyroid polyneuropathy. Bull Osaka Med Sch 33: 149–163.

Siciliano G, Monzani F, Manca ML et al. (2002). Human mitochondrial transcription factor A reduction and mitochondrial dysfunction in Hashimoto's hypothyroid myopathy. Mol Med 8: 326–333.

Sickles DW, Oblak TG, Scholer J (1987). Hyperthyroidism selectively increases oxidative metabolism of slow-oxidative motor units. Exp Neurol 97: 90–105.

Siegert CE, Smelt AH, de Bruin TW (1995). Superior sagittal sinus thrombosis and thyrotoxicosis Possible association in two cases. Stroke 26: 496–497.

Silburn PA, Sandstrom PA, Staples C et al. (1996). Deep cerebral venous thrombosis presenting as an encephalitic illness. Postgrad Med J 72: 355–357.

Silvestri R, De Domenico P, Raffaele M et al. (1990). Vascular compression from goiter as an unusual cause of cerebrovascular accident. Ital J Neurol Sci 11: 307–308.

Simone JV, Abildgaard CF, Schulman I (1965). Blood coagulation in thyroid dysfunction. N Engl J Med 273: 1057–1061.

Sinclair D (2008). Analytical aspects of thyroid antibodies estimation. Autoimmunity 41: 46–54.

Skanse B, Nyman GE (1956). Thyrotoxicosis as a cause of cerebral dysrhythmia and convulsive seizures. Acta Endocrinol (Copenh) 22: 246–263.

Smith TJ (2010). Pathogenesis of Graves' orbitopathy: a 2010 update. J Endocrinol Invest 33: 414–421.

Smith DL, Looney TJ (1983). Seizures secondary to thyrotoxicosis and high-dosage propranolol therapy. Arch Neurol 40: 457–458.

Snabboon T, Khemkha A, Chaiyaumporn C et al. (2009). Psychosis as the first presentation of hyperthyroidism. Intern Emerg Med 4: 359–360.

Soonthornpun S, Setasuban W, Thamprasit A (2009). Insulin resistance in subjects with a history of thyrotoxic periodic paralysis (TPP). Clin Endocrinol (Oxf) 70: 794–797.

Spiegel J, Hellwig D, Becker G et al. (2004). Progressive dementia caused by Hashimoto's encephalopathy – report of two cases. Eur J Neurol 11: 711–713.

Spiro AJ, Hirano A, Beilin RL et al. (1970). Cretinism with muscular hypertrophy (Kocher–Debre–Semelaigne syndrome) Histochemical and ultrastructural study of skeletal muscle. Arch Neurol 23: 340–349.

Spratt DI, Pont A, Miller MB et al. (1982). Hyperthyroxinemia in patients with acute psychiatric disorders. Am J Med 73: 41–48.

Squizzato A, Gerdes VE, Brandjes DP et al. (2005). Thyroid diseases and cerebrovascular disease. Stroke 36: 2302–2310.

Stern BJ, Gruen R, Koeppel J et al. (1984). Recurrent thyrotoxicosis and papilledema in a patient with communicating hydrocephalus. Arch Neurol 41: 65–67.

Stevanato F, Martinello F, Pesce R et al. (1991). A case of polymyositis in autoimmune thyroiditis with hyperthyroidism. Riv Neurol 61: 17–19.

Stone J, Foulkes A, Adamson K et al. (2007). Thyrotoxicosis presenting with headache. Cephalalgia 27: 561–562.

Striano P, Pagliuca M, Andreone V et al. (2006). Unfavourable outcome of Hashimoto encephalopathy due to status epilepticus One autopsy case. J Neurol 253: 248–249.

Su YH, Izumi T, Kitsu M et al. (1993). Seizure threshold in juvenile myoclonic epilepsy with Graves disease. Epilepsia 34: 488–492.

Suzuki S, Ichikawa K, Nagai M et al. (1997). Elevation of serum creatine kinase during treatment with antithyroid drugs in patients with hyperthyroidism due to Graves disease A novel side effect of antithyroid drugs. Arch Intern Med 157: 693–696.

Swanson JW, Kelly JJ Jr, McConahey WM (1981). Neurologic aspects of thyroid dysfunction. Mayo Clin Proc 56: 504–512.

Szabadi E (1991). Thyroid dysfunction and affective illness. BMJ 302: 923–924.

Tajima T, Fujiwara F, Sudo A et al. (2007). A Japanese patient of congenital hypothyroidism with cerebellar atrophy. Endocr J 54: 941–944.

Takashima S, Takayama F, Wang J et al. (2003). Using MR imaging to predict invasion of the recurrent laryngeal nerve by thyroid carcinoma. AJR Am J Roentgenol 180: 837–842.

Tallstedt L, Lundell G, Torring O et al. (1992). Occurrence of ophthalmopathy after treatment for Graves' hyperthyroidism The Thyroid Study Group. N Engl J Med 326: 1733–1738.

Tappy L, Randin JP, Schwed P et al. (1987). Prevalence of thyroid disorders in psychogeriatric inpatients A possible relationship of hypothyroidism with neurotic depression but not with dementia. J Am Geriatr Soc 35: 526–531.

Taskapan C, Sahin I, Taskapan H et al. (2005). Possible malignant neuroleptic syndrome that associated with hypothyroidism. Prog Neuropsychopharmacol Biol Psychiatry 29: 745–748.

Tassone H, Moulin A, Henderson SO (2004). The pitfalls of potassium replacement in thyrotoxic periodic paralysis: a case report and review of the literature. J Emerg Med 26: 157–161.

Taylor DJ, Rajagopalan B, Radda GK (1992). Cellular energetics in hypothyroid muscle. Eur J Clin Invest 22: 358–365.

Tendler BE, Shoukri K, Malchoff C et al. (1997). Concurrence of Graves' disease and dysplastic cerebral blood vessels of the moyamoya variety. Thyroid 7: 625–629.

Teoh HL, Lim EC (2005). Platysmal myoclonus in subclinical hyperthyroidism. Mov Disord 20: 1064–1065.

Thomas RD, Croft DN (1974). Thyrotoxicosis and giant-cell arteritis. Br Med J 2: 408–409.

Thomas FB, Mazzaferri EL, Skillman TG (1970). Apathetic thyrotoxicosis: a distinctive clinical and laboratory entity. Ann Intern Med 72: 679–685.

Thomas DJ, Robinson S, Robinson A et al. (1996). An association between migraine and hyperthyroidism. JNNP 61: 213–226.

Tietgens ST, Leinung MC (1995). Thyroid storm. Med Clin North Am 79: 169–184.

Torres CF, Moxley RT (1990). Hypothyroid neuropathy and myopathy: clinical and electrodiagnostic longitudinal findings. J Neurol 237: 271–274.

Toscano A, Rodolico C, Benvenga S et al. (2002). Multifocal motor neuropathy and asymptomatic Hashimoto's thyroiditis: first report of an association. Neuromuscul Disord 12: 566–568.

Trabelsi L, Charfi N, Triki C et al. (2006). Myasthenia gravis and hyperthyroidism: two cases. Ann Endocrinol (Paris) 67: 265–269.

Traisk F, Tallstedt L, Abraham-Nordling M et al. (2009). Thyroid-associated ophthalmopathy after treatment for Graves' hyperthyroidism with antithyroid drugs or iodine-131. J Clin Endocrinol Metab 94: 3700–3707.

Trobe JD (1981). Optic nerve involvement in dysthyroidism. Ophthalmology 88: 488–492.

Tsai MH, Lee LH, Chen SD et al. (2007). Complex partial status epilepticus as a manifestation of Hashimoto's encephalopathy. Seizure 16: 713–716.

Tuncel D, Cetinkaya A, Kaya B et al. (2008). Hoffmann's syndrome: a case report. Med Princ Pract 17: 346–348.

Turker H, Bayrak O, Gungor L et al. (2008). Hypothyroid myopathy with manifestations of Hoffman's syndrome and myasthenia gravis. Thyroid 18: 259–262.

Usami K, Kinoshita T, Tokumoto K et al. (2009). Successful treatment of plasma exchange for severe cerebral venous thrombosis with thyrotoxicosis. J Stroke Cerebrovasc Dis 18: 239–243.

Vaccari A (1982). Decreased central serotonin function in hypothyroidism. Eur J Pharmacol 82: 93–95.

Van Dop C, Conte FA, Koch TK et al. (1983). Pseudotumor cerebri associated with initiation of levothyroxine therapy for juvenile hypothyroidism. N Engl J Med 308: 1076–1080.

Vannucchi G, Campi I, Covelli D et al. (2009). Graves' orbitopathy activation after radioactive iodine therapy with and without steroid prophylaxis. J Clin Endocrinol Metab 94: 3381–3386.

Vargas ME, Warren FA, Kupersmith MJ (1993). Exotropia as a sign of myasthenia gravis in dysthyroid ophthalmopathy. Br J Ophthalmol 77: 822–823.

Vasconcellos E, Pina-Garza JE, Fakhoury T et al. (1999). Pediatric manifestations of Hashimoto's encephalopathy. Pediatr Neurol 20: 394–398.

Vega-Nunez E, Menendez-Hurtado A, Garesse R et al. (1995). Thyroid hormone-regulated brain mitochondrial genes revealed by differential cDNA cloning. J Clin Invest 96: 893–899.

Venables GS, Bates D, Shaw DA (1978). Hypothyroidism with true myotonia. J Neurol Neurosurg Psychiatry 41: 1013–1015.

Verberne HJ, Fliers E, Prummel MF et al. (2000). Thyrotoxicosis as a predisposing factor for cerebral venous thrombosis. Thyroid 10: 607–610.

Vono-Toniolo J, Kopp P (2004). Thyroglobulin gene mutations and other genetic defects associated with congenital hypothyroidism. Arq Bras Endocrinol Metabol 48: 70–82.

Wakelkamp IM, Bakker O, Baldeschi L et al. (2003). TSH-R expression and cytokine profile in orbital tissue of active vs inactive Graves' ophthalmopathy patients. Clin Endocrinol (Oxf) 58: 280–287.

Wall CR (2000). Myxedema coma: diagnosis and treatment. Am Fam Physician 62: 2485–2490.

Watanakunakorn C, Hodges RE, Evans TC (1965). Myxedema; a study of 400 cases. Arch Intern Med 116: 183–190.

Watts FB (1951). Atypical facial neuralgia in the hypothyroid state. Ann Intern Med 35: 186–193.

Wiersinga WM, Bartalena L (2002). Epidemiology and prevention of Graves' ophthalmopathy. Thyroid 12: 855–860.

Wiersinga WM, Smit T, van der Gaag R et al. (1989). Clinical presentation of Graves' ophthalmopathy. Ophthalmic Res 21: 73–82.

Wilson WP, Johnson JE (1964). Thyroid hormone and brain function I The EEG in hyperthyroidism with observations on the effect of age, sex, and reserpine in the production of abnormalities. Electroencephalogr Clin Neurophysiol 16: 321–328.

Wiseman P, Stewart K, Rai GS (1989). Hypothyroidism in polymyalgia rheumatica and giant cell arteritis. BMJ 298: 647–648.

Wongraoprasert S, Buranasupkajorn P, Sridama V et al. (2007). Thyrotoxic periodic paralysis induced by pulse methylprednisolone. Intern Med 46: 1431–1433.

Yamamoto K, Saito K, Takai T et al. (1983). Visual field defects and pituitary enlargement in primary hypothyroidism. J Clin Endocrinol Metab 57: 283–287.

Yamamoto T, Fukuyama J, Fujiyoshi A (1999). Factors associated with mortality of myxedema coma: report of eight cases and literature survey. Thyroid 9: 1167–1174.

Yoneda M, Fujii A, Ito A et al. (2007). High prevalence of serum autoantibodies against the amino terminal of alpha-enolase in Hashimoto's encephalopathy. J Neuroimmunol 185: 195–200.

Yu JH, Weng YM (2009). Acute chorea as a presentation of Graves disease: case report and review. Am J Emerg Med 27: 369.e1–369.e3.

Zoll J, Ventura-Clapier R, Serrurier B et al. (2001). Response of mitochondrial function to hypothyroidism in normal and regenerated rat skeletal muscle. J Muscle Res Cell Motil 22: 141–147.

Zwillich CW, Pierson DJ, Hofeldt FD et al. (1975). Ventilatory control in myxedema and hypothyroidism. N Engl J Med 292: 662–665.

Handbook of Clinical Neurology, Vol. 120 (3rd series)
Neurologic Aspects of Systemic Disease Part II
Jose Biller and Jose M. Ferro, Editors

Chapter 49

Neurologic disorders of mineral metabolism and parathyroid disease

LILY AGRAWAL[1]*, ZEINA HABIB[1], AND NICHOLAS V. EMANUELE[1,2]

[1]*Division of Endocrinology and Metabolism, Loyola University Medical Center, Maywood, IL, USA*

[2]*Endocrinology Section, Edward Hines Jr. VA Hospital, Hines, IL, USA*

CALCIUM, PHOSPHORUS, AND MAGNESIUM HOMEOSTASIS

Calcium participates in many biological functions of the body including cell signaling, neural transmission, muscle function, blood coagulation, enzymatic cofactor activity, membrane and cytoskeletal functions, secretion and biomineralization (Fig. 49.1) (Endotext.org, Ch. 2). The major regulating organ systems of calcium, magnesium, and phosphorus are the parathyroid gland, kidney, bone, and gastrointestinal tract. The four parathyroid glands, located on the posterior aspect of the thyroid gland, secrete parathyroid hormone (PTH), an important calcium and phosphorus regulatory hormone. The three calcitropic hormones, PTH, calcitonin (CT), and vitamin D metabolites maintain serum and extracellular fluid calcium within a normal range.

Calcium is absorbed from the diet primarily in the duodenum. In the intestine, vitamin D enhances the movement of calcium into the cell. PTH plays a role in intestinal absorption of calcium by activation of vitamin D (Favus, 1992). PTH further modulates serum calcium levels by activating osteoclasts leading to bone resorption and release of calcium into the circulation. Calcium enters the extracellular fluid space and becomes incorporated into the skeleton through mineralization of the osteoid matrix of bone. Some 99% of total body calcium is found in the skeleton and only 1% in blood and body fluids, intracellular structures, etc. (Brown, 2001). Approximately 50% of this calcium in serum is bound to albumin or forms complexes with other ions, including phosphate, citrate, bicarbonate, and lactate. The rest is ionized, and is maintained within a narrow range for the optimal activity of extracellular and intracellular

processes. About 10 g is filtered through the kidneys each day, of which 99% is reabsorbed by active and passive mechanisms. PTH increases the reabsorption of calcium, predominantly in the distal convoluted tubule, and inhibits the reabsorption of phosphate in the renal proximal tubule. The parathyroid gland senses the concentration of extracellular ionized calcium through a cell-surface calcium-sensing receptor (CaSR) and this regulates serum level of PTH. An increase in ionized calcium inhibits PTH secretion.

The endogenous form of vitamin D, cholecalciferol (vitamin D_3), is synthesized in the skin from the cholesterol metabolite 7-dehydrocholesterol under the influence of ultraviolet radiation. In the liver, vitamin D is converted to 25-hydroxyvitamin D (25-D). PTH stimulates the conversion of 25-hydroxyvitamin D to 1,25-dihydroxyvitamin D, the most active form of the hormone, in the kidney. In the bone, PTH and calcitonin are the major regulators of cellular calcium and phosphate transport, and vitamin D provides appropriate concentrations of these minerals through its actions on the renal and GI tract (Bruder, 2001).

Calcitonin is secreted by parafollicular C cells of the thyroid and other neuroendocrine cells, and it inhibits osteoclast-mediated bone resorption (Konrad et al., 2004). In contrast to PTH, hypercalcemia increases secretion of calcitonin while hypocalcemia inhibits secretion. Calcitonin secretion is controlled by serum calcium through the same CaSR that regulates PTH secretion, but in an inverse manner and at higher concentrations of calcium.

Phosphorus is absorbed from the GI tract distal to duodenum. Active metabolites of vitamin D, through

---

*Correspondence to: Lily Agrawal, M.D., FACE, Endocrinology Section, Edward Hines Jr. VA Hospital, 5000 S. Fifth Avenue, Hines, IL 60141, USA. Tel: +1-708-202-2701, Fax: +1-708-202-2195, E-mail: lily.agrawal@va.gov

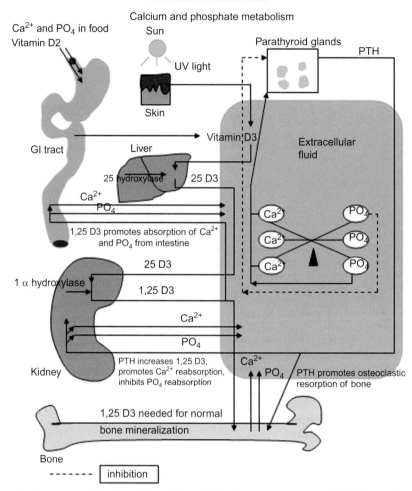

Fig. 49.1. Calcium and phosphate metabolism (adapted from Netterimages.com, image 8094, Elsevier Inc by R Agrawal).

the action of PTH, increase its absorption while calcitonin and phosphate binders (calcium, aluminum) decrease its absorption. Some 85% of phosphorus is found in the skeleton as hydroxyapatite and 15% is distributed among extraskeletal sites such as phosphoproteins, phospholipids, and nucleic acids. PTH, calcitonin, and acidosis increase renal phosphorus excretion, and vitamin D decreases its excretion (Drezner, 2002). Hypermagnesemia can inhibit PTH secretion and hypomagnesemia can stimulate PTH secretion. However, prolonged depletion of magnesium will inhibit PTH biosynthesis and secretion. Hypomagnesemia also attenuates the biological effect of PTH (Konrad et al., 2004).

DISORDERS ASSOCIATED WITH HYPERCALCEMIA

These disorders can be classified into two groups: PTH-mediated hypercalcemia, and non-PTH-mediated hypercalcemia; they are listed in Table 49.1.

Hyperparathyroidism and malignancy-associated hypercalcemia are the most common causes of hypercalcemia. Since the neurologic symptoms reviewed for primary hyperparathyroidism (PHPT) are in part those of hypercalcemia, they can appear in patients with hypercalcemia of any cause if the calcium elevation is severe enough.

Primary hyperparathyroidism

PATHOPHYSIOLOGY

Primary hyperparathyroidism (PHPT) results from autonomous PTH secretion from one or more parathyroid glands, without a clearly identifiable cause. Inappropriate secretion of PTH in the absence of external stimuli results in an unwarranted increase in bone resorption, renal calcium reabsorption, renal phosphate excretion, and intestinal calcium absorption, leading to hypercalcemia and hypophosphatemia (DeLellis et al., 2008). Elevated PTH also promotes further formation of 1,25-D, which increases intestinal calcium absorption

Table 49.1

Causes of hypercalcemia

PTH-mediated
  Primary hyperparathyroidism
  Familial hypocalciuric hypercalcemia
  Tertiary hyperparathyroidism
  Lithium-associated hypercalcemia
  Calcium-sensing receptor antibodies
Non-PTH-mediated
  Hypercalcemia of malignancy
    PTH-related protein
    Other humoral factors
    Bone metastases
  Vitamin D intoxication
  Vitamin A intoxication
  Milk-alkali syndrome
  Granulomatous diseases
  Hyperthyroidism
  Adrenal insufficiency
  Immobilization
Medications
    Thiazide diuretics
    Theophylline

PTH, parathyroid hormone.

and bone resorption (Sitges-Serra and Bergenfelz, 2007). Primary hyperparathyroidism is due to a single parathyroid adenoma in 75–85% of cases, to parathyroid hyperplasia in about 15% of cases, and rarely to parathyroid carcinoma in less than 1% of cases (Fraser, 2009). Possible etiologies of PHPT include exposure to ionizing radiation, and genetic mutations such as those seen in multiple endocrine neoplasia and other inherited forms of hyperparathyroidism (Sitges-Serra and Bergenfelz, 2007; DeLellis et al., 2008; Fraser, 2009).

OVERVIEW OF THE CLINICAL AND BIOCHEMICAL FEATURES OF PRIMARY HYPERPARATHYROIDISM

The clinical picture of PHPT, classically a disease of hypercalcemia, bone disease and kidney stones, has changed significantly in the past few decades. Since the introduction of routine calcium screening in the mid-1970s, PHPT has become a primarily asymptomatic, incidentally discovered disease (Khan et al., 2009a). Primary hyperparathyroidism in its current clinical phenotype is asymptomatic in up to 80% of cases (Fraser, 2009).

Among the traditional symptoms of PHPT, nephrolithiasis is the most common (Bilezikian and Potts, 2002; Mollerup et al., 2002). Additional manifestations involve: the neurologic system, e.g., difficulty concentrating, confusion, depression, dementia, anxiety and fatigue (Coker et al., 2005; Dotzenrath et al., 2006; Benge et al., 2009); the cardiovascular system, e.g., hypertension, left ventricular hypertrophy, QT prolongation, bradycardia, valvular calcifications, and arrhythmias (Niederle et al., 1990; Piovesan et al., 1999; Kiewiet et al., 2004; Vázquez-Díaz et al., 2009); the gastrointestinal system, e.g., anorexia, nausea, vomiting, abdominal pain, constipation, pancreatitis, and peptic ulcer disease (Chan et al., 1995; Carnaille et al., 1998); the kidney, e.g., renal insufficiency, polyuria, polydipsia, and nephrocalcinosis (Peacock, 2002); and the musculoskeletal system, e.g., osteopenia, osteoporosis, osteitis fibrosa cystica, proximal muscle weakness, gout, pseudogout, bone or joint pains, and chondrocalcinosis (Rubin and Silverberg, 2002; Farford et al., 2007; Rubin et al., 2008; Fraser, 2009).

Primary hyperparathyroidism is characterized by an elevated or inappropriately normal PTH level in the presence of hypercalcemia, due to autonomous PTH secretion. Patients with PHPT can also have hypophosphatemia, hypomagnesemia, and hypercalciuria. Despite the hypocalciuric effect of PTH, it is common to find hypercalciuria among patients with PHPT. This is due to several factors, including a high filtered load of calcium due to hypercalcemia, as well as the activation by hypercalcemia of the calcium-sensing receptor, which indirectly inhibits calcium reabsorption (Bringhurst et al., 2008). Mineral abnormalities in primary hyperparathyroidism include:

1. Hypercalcemia. Parathyroid hormone, through an increase in bone resorption, intestinal calcium reabsorption, and tubular calcium reabsorption, results in an elevated calcium level. Normocalcemic PHPT has been described but it is unclear at this point whether the normocalcemic variant is associated with complications similar to those seen with the hypercalcemic form of PHPT. It is important in those normocalcemic cases to rule out any causes of secondary hyperparathyroidism, particularly vitamin D deficiency and renal dysfunction (Bringhurst et al., 2008; Silverberg et al., 2009).
2. Hypophosphatemia. Elevated PTH results in decreased tubular phosphate reabsorption and therefore hypophosphatemia (Bringhurst et al., 2008).
3. Hypomagnesemia. Although PTH stimulates tubular reabsorption of magnesium, patients with PHPT are usually normomagnesemic or mildly hypomagnesemic, due to a direct effect of hypercalcemia and hypophosphatemia on the renal tubules limiting magnesium reabsorption (Bringhurst et al., 2008).

Neurologic and muscular manifestations of symptomatic primary hyperparathyroidism

It appears that neurologic symtpoms seen in PHPT are largely due to hypercalcemia and other mineral abnormalities in phosphorus and magnesium which occur in tandem in PHPT. These manefestations become more prominent with increasing degrees of hypercalcemia. However, it is important to note that they can be seen in any condition in which there is hypercalcemia, hypophosphatemia, and/or hypomagnesemia. For clarity of presentation, these neurologic manifestations are reviewed in this section on PHPT and other causes of these mineral abnormalities are listed in Tables 49.2, 49.3, and 49.4.

Depending on the severity and rate of development of hypercalcemia, neuropsychiatric manifestations of PHPT can range from subtle personality changes to stupor and coma which can be seen in severe hypercalcemia. Memory problems, dementia, confusion, delirium, and obtundation have been reported with severe PHPT, mostly in elderly patients (Mannix et al., 1980; Tonner and Schlechte, 1993). Psychotic behavior, catatonia, and mania have also been described as manifestations of PHPT (Tonner and Schlechte, 1993; Brown et al., 2007). In addition, patients with PHPT may present with focal neurologic deficits due to mass effects from brown tumors (Tonner and Schlechte, 1993). In one case report, the inital presentation of PHPT was spastic paraparesis, urinary incontinence, and confusion, which improved with bisphosphonate therapy and normalization of serum calcium (Thomas and Lebrun, 1994). Primary hyperparathyroidism has also been associated with a neuropsychiatric illness with clinical manifestations and electroencephalographic changes similar to those seen with Creutzfeldt–Jakob disease. This syndrome may resolve with treatment of the hyperparathyroidism (Bertolucci and Malheiros, 1990; Goto et al., 2000; Karatas et al., 2007; Chadenat et al., 2009).

Neurologic and muscular manifestations of asymptomatic primary hyperparathyroidism

In recent years, more data have emerged about the presence of nontraditional manifestations of PHPT, specifically cardiovascular and neuropsychiatric manifestations, in patients who appear to have asymptomatic disease (Silverberg et al., 2009). The nature, degree, and reversibility of cognitive and psychological impairment associated with mild, asymptomatic PHPT are currently areas of active investigation. Neurologic symptoms such as lethargy, confusion, and memory impairment, and psychiatric disorders such as depression, paranoia, and hallucinations are part of the classic presentation of symptomatic PHPT (Coker et al., 2005). Patients with mild, asymptomatic PHPT display some vague, nonspecific symptoms such as generalized fatigue, bone and joint pains, weakness, anxiety, irritability, depressed mood, sleep disturbances, difficulty in completing daily tasks, loss of initiative, decreased social interaction, cognitive impairment, and

somatization. These symptoms may be due to elevated serum calcium, elevated PTH levels, or coexisting vitamin D deficiency (Coker et al., 2005; Walker and Silverberg, 2007; Silverberg et al., 2009).

Muscle disorders described with PHPT include generalized fatigue, muscle weakness, particularly in proximal muscles, and myopathy with characteristic electromyographic changes and muscle fiber atrophy seen on biopsy.

Parathyroidectomy led to improvement in muscular symptoms, memory, and anxiety in a cohort of patients who underwent surgery for PHPT (Tonner and Schlechte, 1993; Walker et al., 2004). In a case-control study that examined neuropsychological manifestations in patients with PHPT, cognitive impairment did not correlate with serum calcium or PTH levels. In this study, extensive cognitive and neuropsychological testing was used to compare patients with PHPT to normal controls. PHPT was associated with more depression and anxiety symptoms, delayed recall of contextually related materials, delayed immediate word list recall, and abnormalities in nonverbal abstraction. There were no differences between PHPT patients and controls with regards to delayed word list recall, visual memory, visual concentration, and visual and auditory attention. Only depressive symptoms, contextual recall and nonverbal abstraction improved after parathyroidectomy (Walker et al., 2009a). Two randomized controlled trials demonstrated no difference in baseline general health status between patients with PHPT and controls, but did show an improvement in social functioning, emotional functioning, pain, general health, vitality, or mental health after parathyroidectomy (Rao et al., 2004; Ambrogini et al., 2007). In a larger randomized controlled trial, there were significant baseline differences in quality of life and neuropsychiatric symptoms between patients with PHPT and normal controls, but no improvement was seen in patients with PHPT after parathyroidectomy (Bollerslev et al., 2007). In a recent study, improvement in neuropsychological symptoms after parathyroidectomy was more prominent in younger patients (Benge et al., 2009).

The potential vascular dysfunction of PHPT may adversely affect the cerebral vasculature. There are numerous studies linking PHPT (hypercalcemia and/or high PTH levels) to cardiovascular mortality (Nilsson et al., 2004; Hagstrom et al., 2009; Silverberg et al., 2009), coronary atherosclerosis, myocardial and valvular calcifications, conduction abnormalities, arrhythmias, left ventricular hypertrophy, and increased aortic stiffness (Piovesan et al., 1999; Rubin et al., 2005; Silverberg et al., 2009; Vázquez-Díaz et al., 2009), as well as increased carotid intima media thickness (Walker et al., 2009b). Patients with mild asymptomatic disease, however, did not have a higher risk of coronary atherosclerosis based on tomographic coronary calcium scores (Streeten et al., 2008; Kepez et al., 2009). In addition, some recent data have shown that patients with PHPT have impaired nitric oxide-induced vasodilatation and flow-mediated vasodilatation compared to controls. These abnormalities resolved after successful parathyroidectomy (Ekmekci et al., 2009; Virdis et al., 2010). Patients with PHPT were also found to have alterations in tissue plasminogen activator and other important factors in the coagulation and fibrinolytic pathways, resulting in a possible hypercoagulable and hypofibrinolytic state (Erem et al., 2009). There are fewer data on the cerebral vasculature. In one study, PHPT was shown to be associated with regional cerebral hypoperfusion. The degree of hypoperfusion was positively correlated with serum calcium and PTH levels (Cermik et al., 2007). The implications of PHPT on cerebrovascular function remain to be investigated.

Neurologic manifestations of hypophosphatemia.
Hypophosphatemia can occur in PHPT. Mild hypophosphatemia is generally asymtomatic. In severe cases of hypophosphatemia, a number of neurologic abnormalities have been described, including mental status changes such as disorientation, confusion, hallucinations, lethargy, encephalopathy, and coma; cerebellar or extrapyramidal signs such as ataxia, nystagmus, tremor, and ballismus; peripheral sensory neuropathies; and Guillain–Barré-like paralysis. Severe hypophosphatemia may lead to seizures, coma, and death. Muscular manifestations include rhabdomyolysis and muscle weakness, which can potentially affect the cardiac and respiratory muscles leading to cardiorespiratory failure (Berkelhammer and Bear, 1984; Bringhurst et al., 2008).

Other etiologies of hypophosphatemia.
There is a wide array of disorders that can cause hypophosphatemia besides PHPT (Table 49.2), and these can be classified into three categories based on the mechanism of hypophosphatemia: decreased tubular reabsorption, transcellular phosphorus shifts, and phosphorus malabsorption. Since the neurologic symptoms reviewed for PHPT are in part those of hypophosphatemia, they can appear in patients with hypophosphatemia of any cause if the phosphorus disturbance is severe enough.

Neurologic manifestations of hypomagnesemia.
Hypopmagnesemia can occur in PHPT. Several neurologic abnormalities have been reported with hypomagnesemia, and those include tremor, seizures, ataxia, nystagmus, movement disorders, and vertigo. Changes in mental status and mood perturbations associated with hypomagnesemia include apathy, depression, irritability, agitation, confusion, delirium, and psychosis. In addition, hypomagnesemia is associated with muscular manifestations such as muscle weakness,

Table 49.2

Causes of hypophosphatemia

Decreased tubular reabsorption
Elevated PTH or PTHrp vitamin D deficiency
Excess FGF-23
Hypophosphatemic rickets
Tumor-induced osteomalacia
Fanconi syndrome and other renal tubular disorders
Transcellular shifts
Intravenous glucose, insulin, or catecholamines
Acute respiratory alkalosis
Acute gout
Salicylate toxicity
Sepsis or toxic shock syndrome
Recovery from acidosis, starvation, anorexia nervosa, or hepatic failure
States of rapid cellular proliferation
Postparathyroidectomy
Decreased intestinal absorption
Aluminum containing antacids

PTH, parathyroid hormone; PTHrp, Parathyroid Hormone related protein; FGF-23, Fibroblast Growth Factor 23.

twitching, cramps, and tetany, as well as positive Chvostek's and Trousseau's signs (Berkelhammer and Bear, 1985; Bringhurst et al., 2008).

Other etiologies of hypomagnesemia.
Magnesium depletion can occur in cases of decreased magnesium absorption, increased gastrointestinal magnesium loss, renal magnesium wasting, and acute magnesium shifts. These etiologies are listed in Table 49.3. Since the neurologic symptoms reviewed for PHPT are in part those of hypomagnesemia, they can appear in patients with hypomagnesemia of any cause if the magnesium disturbance is severe enough.

MANAGEMENT OF HYPERCALCEMIA, INCLUDING PRIMARY HYPERPARATHYROIDISM

An acute rise in serum calcium to 12–14 mg/dL or a serum calcium > 14 mg/dL requires administration of isotonic saline with careful monitoring of fluid status. A loop diuretic may need to be added to further increase urinary calcium excretion. Calcitonin can be added in severe hypercalcemia with bisphosphonates for a more sustained effect. Glucocorticoids are effective in patients with hypercalcemia due to excess vitamin D, chronic granulomatous disease, or lymphoma. Parathyroidectomy is the treatement of choice for patients with PHPT who develop complications of the disease such as bone disease, nephrolithiasis, or life-theatening hypercalcemia (Phitayakorn and McHenry, 2008; Bilezikian et al., 2009). For patients who have

Table 49.3

Causes of hypomagnesemia

Decreased absorption
    Malabsorption syndromes
    Vitamin D deficiency
Increased gastrointestinal losses
    Vomiting
    Diarrhea
    Bowel preparation for procedures
Renal wasting
  Genetic
    Bartter syndrome
    Gitelman syndrome
  Acquired renal diseases
    Renal transplantation
    Diuretic phase of acute tubular necrosis
    Tubulointerstitial nephritis
  Drugs
    Diuretic
    Ethanol
    Digoxin, and aminoglycosides
  Endocrinopathies
    Diabetes mellitus
    Hypercalcemia,
    Hypophosphatemia,
    Hyperthyroidism
    Hyperaldosteronism
    Syndrome of inappropriate
      antidiuretic hormone secretion
Transcellular shifts
    Catecholamines
    Recovery from respiratory acidosis or diabetic
    ketoacidosis
    Refeeding syndrome
    Correction of vitamin D deficiency
    After parathyroidectomy

---

asymptomatic PHPT, recommendations from the Third International Workshop on the Management of Asymptomatic Primary Hyperparathyroidism include surgical referral for patients with any of the following: serum calcium more than 1.0 mg/dL above the upper limit of normal; creatinine clearance less than 60 mL/min, age less than 50 years, and bone mineral density (BMD) T-score less than −2.5 at any site and/or history of low-trauma fracture (Bilezikian et al., 2009). Surgery should also be considered in patients for whom medical surveillance is difficult or not feasible (Bilezikian et al., 2002).

Bisphosphonates and calcimimetics can be considered in patients with PHPT requiring therapy if they are not good candidates for surgery because of high surgical risk or inoperable disease, if they decline surgery, or if they have persistent disease. In a meta-analysis comparing the effects of parathyroidectomy, bisphosphonate therapy, and no intervention on BMD in patients with mild PHPT, BMD increased to a similar extent in patients treated with bisphosphonates or with surgery, and slowly decreased in patients with no intervention (Sankaran et al., 2010). This suggests that bisphosphonate therapy may be a reasonable alternative to surgery in patients with asymptomatic PHPT and bone loss, especially those who cannot or are not willing to go for surgery (Khan et al., 2009b). Cinacalcet, a calcimimetic, targets an allosteric site of the calcium sensing receptor (CaSR) on the parathyroid cells to inhibit PTH secretion and has been shown to normalize serum calcium levels and reduce PTH levels though it may not have a significant effect in improving BMD (Khan et al., 2009b; Marcocci et al., 2009; Peacock et al., 2009).

Patients who are asymptomatic and do not have indications for surgical intervention can be observed, with annual calcium and creatinine checks, and BMD evaluation every 1–2 years (Bilezikian et al., 2009).

DISORDERS ASSOCIATED WITH HYPOCALCEMIA

Pathophysiology

Low serum calcium concentrations are most often caused by disorders of parathyroid hormone (PTH) or vitamin D. Other causes may include conditions in which serum protein is reduced, e.g., volume overload, chronic illness, malnutrition, or nephrotic syndrome (Table 49.4). Serum concentration of calcium falls ~0.8 mg/dL for every 1 g/dL reduction in serum albumin. Binding of calcium within the vascular space or by its deposition in tissues, such as with hyperphosphatemia, can also result in a reduction in total serum calcium. In these situations, an ionized serum calcium may more accurately reflect the true calcium concentration. However, serum ionized calcium may be reduced by citrate (used to inhibit coagulation in banked blood or plasma), lactate, foscarnet, and acute respiratory alkalosis. Medicines that have been known to cause hypocalcemia include antiepileptic drugs, some chemotherapeutic drugs, bisphosphonates, cinacalcet, foscarnet, paromomycin, and excess fluoride (Fitzpatrick, 2002).

SECONDARY AND TERTIARY HYPERPARATHYROIDISM

Secondary hyperparathyroidism is evoked in response to changes in renal function or situations where there is a deficiency of calcium and/or vitamin D. Renal insufficiency, whatever the cause, leads to secondary hyperparathyroidism in several ways. First, a decline in glomerular filtration results in increased serum phosphorus. Phosphorus complexes with calcium producing a fall in ionized calcium, a signal to the parathyroid gland, which then increases its secretion of PTH to restore calcium to baseline levels. Over time, as the renal

Table 49.4

Causes of hypocalcemia

Associated with low parathyroid hormone
 Surgical hypoparathyroidism after thyroid, parathyroid,
  or radical neck surgery for head and neck cancer
 Autoimmune hypoparathyroidism with or without
  polyendocrine syndrome type I (other features are chronic
  mucocutaneous candidiasis, adrenal insufficiency,
  hypothyroidism, hypogonadism, vitiligo)
 Parathyroid destruction
  Radiation
  Infiltrative and storage diseases (hemochromatosis,
   Wilson's disease, sarcoidosis, amyloidosis, metastasis)
 Postparathyroidectomy hungry bone syndrome
 Familial syndromes
  DiGeorge syndrome (aplasia or hyperplasia of the
   thymus, immunodeficiency, aplasia or hypoplasia of
   the parathyroid glands, abnormal facies and congenital
   heart defects)
  Kearns–Sayre syndrome (heart block, retinitis
   pigmentosa, ophthalmoplegia)
  Kenny–Caffey syndrome (medullary stenosis of the long
   bones and growth retardation)
 Activating mutations of the calcium sensing receptor gene
  (PTH is not released at serum concentrations of calcium
  that normally trigger PTH release)
 Hypomagnesemia (inhibits PTH release and produces end
  organ resistance depending on magnesium level)
 Severe hypermagnesemia (by suppressing the secretion
  of PTH)
Associated with high parathyroid hormone
 Secondary or tertiary hyperparathyroidism (vitamin D
  deficiency or resistance, anticonvulsant drugs, renal
  disease, hyperphosphatemia)
 Extravascular deposition (acute pancreatitis)
 Parathyroid resistance syndromes
  Pseudohypoparathyroidism (PHP)
  Hypomagnesemia
 Osteoblastic metastases of breast and prostate cancer
 Hypomagnesemia (produces end organ resistance
  depending on magnesium level)
Pseudohypocalcemia
 Hypoalbuminemia
 Acid–base disturbances
 Gadolinium-based contrast agents

disease worsens, PTH increases more but, ultimately, serum calcium falls to below normal levels. Secondly, the fall in renal mass leads to a fall in activated vitamin D, since the kidney is a prime location for l-α-hydroxylation of 25-hydroxy-vitamin D. The reduction in active vitamin D causes reduced absorption of calcium from the gut, further worsening the falling serum calcium and this, in turn, acts as a signal to provoke more PTH secretion. Activated vitamin D itself acts in a negative feedback loop, along with calcium, to restrain PTH secretion, so that low calcium and low vitamin D together create a situation where restraints on PTH release are markedly reduced. Over time, the lack of inhibitory signals not only allows for hypersecretion of PTH but also for hyperplasia of the glandular tissue itself. In some instances, this will progress to totally unrestrained PTH release from excessive glandular mass and the production of hypercalcemia, a condition referred to as tertiary hyperparathyroidism. Thus, the calcium levels can be anywhere from normal (in early, compensated secondary hyperparathyroidism), to low (in advanced secondary hyperparathyroidism), to high (in tertiary hyperparathyroidism). Outside the clinical context of renal disease, secondary hyperparathyroidism can also be caused by states where there is a deficiency of calcium and/or vitamin D such as a variety of malabsorptive states or simply poor nutritional intake or, in the case of vitamin D, inadequate exposure to the sun.

Laboratory tests that may be helpful in establishing the etiology of hypocalcemia include measurement of serum intact parathyroid hormone (iPTH), serum magnesium, creatinine, phosphate, 25-hydroxyvitamin D, 1,25-D, and alkaline phosphatase. Amylase, urinary calcium and magnesium may be useful in selected patients.

Clinical features of hypocalcemia

Acute hypocalcemia is associated with neuromuscular irritability manifesting as circumoral numbness, paresthesias of the fingertips, muscle cramps, carpopedal spasm, tetany, laryngospasm, bronchospasm, or seizures. This can be demonstrated by eliciting Chvostek's or Trousseau's signs. For the Chvostek's sign, the skin over the facial nerve anterior to the external auditory meatus is tapped sharply. In a patient with acute hypocalcemia, ipsilateral contraction of the facial muscles will occur. Trousseau's sign is the carpal spasm induced by inflation of the blood pressure cuff to 20 mmHg above the patient's systolic blood pressure for 3–5 minutes. The nerves are more irritable under ischemic conditions induced by the blood pressure cuff. Paresthesias are followed by flexion of the wrist and metacarpal phalangeal joints, extension of the intraphalangeal joints, and adduction of thumb (Endotext.org, Ch. 7). Mental status changes such as confusion, disorientation, psychosis, and psychoneurosis may occur. Severe hypocalcemia may be associated with a prolonged Q-T_c interval on electrocardiography. Smooth muscle involvement due to irritability of autonomic ganglia can result in dysphagia, abdominal pain, biliary colic, wheezing, and dyspnea.

Patients with chronic hypocalcemia, such as seen in idiopathic hypoparathyroidism or pseudohypoparathyroidism, may have calcification of the basal ganglia or more widespread intracranial calcification which can be seen with a skull X-ray or CT scan. Calcification of the basal ganglia suggests long-standing hypocalcaemia (Danowski et al., 1960). Extrapyramidal neurologic symptoms such as Parkinsonism, choreoathetosis, dystonic spasms, focal, grand mal or petit mal seizures have been described (Basser et al., 1969). Increased intracranial pressure and papilledema may be present. Electroencephalographic changes may be seen with or without symptoms of hypocalcemia. Other manifestations include fatigue, impaired intellectual ability, irritability, personality disturbance, psychoses, psychoneuroses, organic brain syndrome, and subnormal intelligence. In some cases, treatment of the hypocalcemia may improve intelligence and personality, but amelioration of psychiatric symptoms is inconsistent.

Epidermal changes include dry skin, coarse hair, brittle nails, dental abnormalities, alopecia, atopic eczema, exfoliative dermatitis, impetigo herpetiformis, and psoriasis. Restoration of normocalcemia has improved these skin disorders (Endotext.org, Ch. 7). Subcapsular cataracts, band keratopathy, and sensorineural deafness has also been observed.

Because patients with secondary and tertiary hyperparathyroidism may have serum calcium concentrations varying from low to high, the clinical presentation of these disorders is, in part at least, the clinical presentation of any patient with hypo- or hypercalcemia. In addition, there are some unique clinical presentations mediated by other mechanisms.

Patients with secondary or tertiary hyperparathyroidism due to renal disease have renal osteodystrophy. This is a spectrum of bone disorders including osteitis fibrosa cystica, osteomalacia, and adynamic bone disease. Rarely, as part of the hyperparathyroid process, brown tumors may appear. These are focal areas of intense osteoclast-mediated bone resorption, fibrous tissue, and blood. Their high hemosiderin content imparts the characteristic brown color for which they are named. Though the differential diagnosis of these lesions includes malignancy, they are benign. They can undergo central necrosis and cyst formation. They are typically located in the hands, but can be seen in other sites such as the facial bones, pelvis, ribs, and femoral bones. Complications are rare but, if they are located in critical areas, they may result in several neurologic syndromes. Spinal cord compression secondary to expansion of the tumor as well as to vertebral body collapse or pathologic fracture has been reported. The clinical presentation depends on the location of the lesion (Mourad et al., 1996; Fuster et al., 2006; Mak et al., 2009). There is an interesting case report of a young man with chronic renal failure on dialysis who presented with painful proptosis, opthalmoplegia, and a palpable frontotemporal mass which turned out to be a brown tumor (Zwick et al., 2006).

The treatment is surgical removal of the brown tumor which has usually resulted in cure of the neurologic symptoms. In addition to brown tumors, extraskeletal tumoral calcification can occur. Rare instances of cord compression have been reported by this entity (Jackson et al., 2007). Secondary hyperparathyroidism can cause calvarial hypertrophy (sometimes referred to as uremic leontiasis ossea or bighead disease) and dense calcification of the dura. These result in compression of cranial nerves. Deafness, recurrent facial nerve palsy, and optic neuropathy have been reported (Schmidt et al., 2001; Abid et al., 2007; Shenoy and Oghalai, 2008). Another compressive neuropathic syndrome seen in secondary hyperparathyroidism and rarely reported is carpal tunnel syndrome due to soft tissue calcium hydroxyapatite deposition in the carpal tunnel (Firooznia et al., 1981). Each of these clinical situations is amenable to surgical decompression, acutely. Ultimately, medical and/or surgical treatment of the underlying hyperparathyroidism is warranted.

Systemic calciphylaxis is a rare complication of secondary hyperparathyroidism and this has been associated with stroke. The usual presentation of systemic calciphylaxis is a diffuse calcification of the medial layer of the smaller arteries which leads to ischemic skin lesions. Soft tissue calcification may occur in a variety of organs and mitral valve annular calcification can be seen. Multiple calcified cerebral emboli presumably emanating from such valves have been described and associated with clinical strokes (Katsamakis et al., 1998).

Analogous to the well known clinical syndrome of pituitary apoplexy wherein there is hemorrhage into the pituitary gland causing symptoms locally from rapid pituitary expansion and systemically from sudden alteration of pituitary hormones, there is the less well recognized phenomenon of parathyroid apoplexy. There is an interesting case report of a patient with sudden onset of dysphonia and pain on the right side of her neck (Terada et al., 2007). She had severe tertiary hyperparathyroidism from renal failure. At surgery, she was found to have a hyperplastic parathyroid gland with hemorrhage which abutted the recurrent laryngeal nerve. The gland could not easily be removed from the nerve and though surgery cured the hypercalcemia, the dysphonia persisted.

Muscle weakness and myalgia have been frequently reported in secondary and tertiary hyperparathyroidism (Chou et al., 1999; Drakopoulos et al., 2009). This has been attributed to multiple causes including the hyperparathyroidism itself, abnormalities of vitamin D metabolism, and peripheral neuropathy. The response to parathyroidectomy is often dramatic.

Improvement in frequently seen sleep disturbances and reduction in use of sleeping pills has been observed after parathyroid removal (Chou et al., 2005). The mechanism for this is not clear, but the improvement has been attributed, at least in part, to relief of troublesome symptoms which could impair sleep, such as skin itching and bone pain.

There is some information, such as that in the Tromso study, that suggests that secondary hyperparathyroidism may be associated with impaired cognitive and emotional function (Jorde et al., 2006). However, the conclusions from this study, by the authors' own admission, are flawed by the relatively small number of subjects (84), not large enough for statistical significance to be achieved if adjusted for multiple testing. Previously, (Driessen et al., 1995) had reported a relationship between high depression scores and elevated PTH levels in another small study of 75 patients, 59 of whom had chronic renal failure and secondary or tertiary hyperparathyroidism.

PSEUDOPSEUDOHYPOPARATHYROIDISM

This is a group of disorders characterized by end organ resistance to PTH (Endotext.org, Ch. 9). In addition to physical findings described as Albright hereditary osteodystrophy, patients may have thickened calvaria, mental deficit, and basal ganglia calcification (Wilson and Trembath, 1994). They are associated with hypocalcemia, hyperphosphatemia, and increased iPTH, but target tissue unresponsiveness to the hormone manifests as a lack of increased cAMP excretion in response to PTH administration.

Management of hypocalcemia

Treatment of hypocalcemia depends on its severity and underlying cause. Acute symptomatic hypocalcemia can be a life-threatening situation and requires aggressive treatment with intravenous calcium administration. Calcium gluconate (containing 90 mg of elemental calcium per 10 mL ampoule) diluted in 50–100 mL of 5% dextrose is infused slowly over 10 minutes to avoid arrhythmias and local vein irritation. This can be repeated until the patient's symptoms have cleared. The goal should be to raise serum calcium by 2–3 mg/dL with the administration of 15 mg/kg of elemental calcium over 4–6 hours so that calcium is maintained in the low-normal range. Oral calcium supplementation should be initiated concurrently. For seizures due to hypocalcemia, correction of the hypocalcemia, rather than the use of anticonvulsants, is effective treatment. For patients with milder symptoms, or if the corrected calcium concentration is greater than 7.5 mg/dL, oral calcium supplementation can be used. In patients with impaired renal function, correction of hyperphosphatemia and/or low 1,25-dihyroxyvitamin D is indicated instead of intravenous calcium. One must measure serum magnesium in any patient who is hypocalcemic, since correction of hypomagnesemia must occur to overcome PTH resistance before serum calcium will return to normal.

Chronic hypocalcemia in patients who are asymptomatic or mildly symptomatic can be treated with oral calcium and vitamin D. Oral calcium carbonate with 1–3 g of elemental calcium in three to four divided doses with meals is most commonly given. Calcium carbonate contains 40% elemental calcium and is relatively inexpensive. Lower amounts of elemental calcium are present in other types of calcium such as calcium citrate (21%), calcium lactate (13%), and calcium gluconate (9%), requiring a larger number of tablets. The goal of therapy is to maintain serum calcium in the low-normal range. Serum calcium should be tested every 3–6 months. One potential side-effect is hypercalciuria with nephrocalcinosis and/or nephrolithiasis, therefore a 24 hour urine calcium should be determined and should be < 4 mg/kg/24 h. Thiazide diuretics can increase renal calcium absorption in patients with hypoparathyroidism and may be useful to titrate urinary calcium to < 4 mg/kg/day. Furosemide and other loop diuretics can depress serum calcium levels and should be avoided. In patients with hypoparathyroidism, calcitriol, the active form of vitamin D, is preferably used at 0.25 μg twice daily up to 0.5 μg four times a day. A long-acting and less expensive vitamin D preparation, ergocalciferol, can also be used in doses of 50 000–100 000 IU weekly to daily. In postsurgical hypoparathyroidism, autotransplantation of parathyroid tissue at the time of parathyroidectomy can be done to preserve parathyroid function.

The treatment for secondary hyperparathyroidism associated with renal disease is phosphorus reduction and supplementation with vitamin D and calcium. If this does not reduce PTH to desired levels, the oral agent cinacalcet can be added. As stated above, this is a drug which reduces PTH by increasing the sensitivity of the parathyroid cell calcium sensing receptor to ambient circulating calcium concentrations. Finally, parathyroid surgery with or without parathyroid autotransplantation is an option for those who fail medical therapy.

CONCLUSION

Abnormalities in calcium, phosphorus and magnesium metabolism can result in behavioral abnormalities, symptoms of neuromuscular irritability, and cardiac and smooth muscle changes, and knowledge of these conditions is essential for appropriate diagnosis and treatment.

REFERENCES

Abid F, Lalani I, Zakaria A et al. (2007). Cranial nerve palsies in renal osteodystrophy. Pediatr Neurol 36: 64–65.

Ambrogini E, Cetani F, Cianferotti L et al. (2007). Surgery or surveillance for mild asymptomatic primary hyperparathyroidism: a prospective, randomized clinical trial. J Clin Endocrinol Metab 92: 3114–3121.

Basser LS, Neale FC, Ireland AW et al. (1969). Epilepsy and electroencephalographic abnormalities in chronic surgical hypoparathyroidism. Ann Intern Med 71: 507–515.

Benge JF, Perrier ND, Massman PJ et al. (2009). Cognitive and affective sequelae of primary hyperparathyroidism and early response to parathyroidectomy. J Int Neuropsychol Soc 15: 1002–1011.

Berkelhammer C, Bear RA (1984). A clinical approach to common electrolyte problems: 3. Hypophosphatemia. Can Med Assoc J 130: 17–23.

Berkelhammer C, Bear RA (1985). A clinical approach to common electrolyte problems: 4. Hypomagnesemia. Can Med Assoc J 132: 360–368.

Bertolucci PH, Malheiros SF (1990). Hyperparathyroidism simulating Creutzfeldt–Jakob disease. Arq Neuropsiquiatr 48: 245–249.

Bilezikian JP, Potts JT (2002). Asymptomatic primary hyperparathyroidism: new issues and new questions – bridging the past with the future. J Bone Miner Res 17 (Suppl. 2): N57–N67.

Bilezikian JP, Potts JT Jr, Fuleihan Gel H et al. (2002). Summary statement from a workshop on asymptomatic primary hyperparathyroidism: a perspective for the 21st century. J Clin Endocrinol Metab 87: 5353–5361.

Bilezikian JP, Khan AA, Potts JT Jr (2009). Guidelines for the management of asymptomatic primary hyperparathyroidism: summary statement from the third international workshop. J Clin Endocrinol Metab 94: 335–339.

Bollerslev J, Jansson S, Mollerup CL et al. (2007). Medical observation, compared with parathyroidectomy, for asymptomatic primary hyperparathyroidism: a prospective, randomized trial. J Clin Endocrinol Metab 92: 1687–1692.

Bringhurst FR, Demay MB, Kronenberg HM (2008). Disorders of mineral metabolism. In: Kronenberg HM, Schlomo M, Polansky KS, Larsen PR, (Eds.), *Williams Textbook of Endocrinology*. 11th edn. WB Saunders, St. Louis, Mo, chap. 27.

Brown EM (2001). Physiology of calcium homeostasis. In: JP Bilezikian, R Marcus, A Levine (Eds.), The Parathyroids. 2nd edn. Academic Press ch. 10, pp. 167–182.

Brown SW, Vyas BV, Spiegel DR (2007). Mania in a case of hyperparathyroidism. Psychosomatics 48: 265–268.

Carnaille B, Oudar C, Pattou F et al. (1998). Pancreatitis and primary hyperparathyroidism: forty cases. Aust N Z J Surg 68: 117–119.

Cermik TF, Kaya M, Ugur-Altun B et al. (2007). Regional cerebral blood flow abnormalities in patients with primary hyperparathyroidism. Neuroradiology 49: 379–385.

Chadenat ML, Dalloz MA, D'Anglejean J et al. (2009). Primary hyperparathyroidism as a differential diagnosis of Creutzfeldt–Jakob disease. Rev Neurol (Paris) 165: 185–188.

Chan AK, Duh Q-Y, Katz MH et al. (1995). Clinical manifestations of primary hyperparathyroidism before and after parathyroidectomy. A case control study. Ann Surg 222: 402–412.

Chou F, Lee C, Chen J (1999). General weakness as an indication for parathyroid surgery in patients with secondary hyperparathyroidism. Arch Surg 134: 1108–1111.

Chou F, Lee C, Chen J et al. (2005). Sleep disturbances before and after parathyroidectomy for secondary hyperparathyroidism. Surgery 137: 426–430.

Coker LH, Rorie K, Cantley L et al. (2005). Primary hyperparathyroidism, cognition, and health-related quality of life. Ann Surg 245: 642–650.

Danowski TS, Lasser EC, Wechsler RL (1960). Calcification of basal ganglia in post-thyroidectomy hypoparathyroidism. Metabolism 9: 1064–1065.

DeLellis RA, Mazzaglia P, Mangray S (2008). Primary hyperparathyroidism: a current perspective. Arch Pathol Lab Med 132: 1251–1262.

Dotzenrath CM, Kaetsch AK, Pfingsten H et al. (2006). Neuropsychiatric and cognitive changes after surgery for primary hyperparathyroidism. World J Surg 30: 680–685.

Drakopoulos S, Koukoulaki M, Phil M et al. (2009). Total parathyroidectomy without autotransplantation in dialysis patients and renal transplant recipients, long-term follow-up evaluation. Am J Surg 198: 178–183.

Drezner MK (2002). Phosphorus homeostasis and related disorders. In: JP Bilezikian, LG Raisz, GA Rodan (Eds.), Principles of Bone Biology. 2nd edn. Academic Press Ch. 22, pp. 321–338.

Driessen M, Wetterling T, Wedel R et al. (1995). Secondary hyperparathyroidism and depression in chronic renal failure. Nephron 70: 334–339.

Ekmekci A, Abaci N, Colak Ozbey A et al. (2009). Endothelial function and endothelial nitric oxide synthase intron 4a/b polymorphism in primary hyperparathyroidism. J Endocrinol Invest 32: 611–616.

Endotext.org/ Deftos L Calcium and phosphate homeostasis. Ch. 2 In: F Singer (Ed.), Diseases of Bone and Mineral Metabolism.

Endotext.org/ Schafer AL MD, Fitzpatrick LA MD, Shoback DM MD. Hypocalcemia: diagnosis and treatment. Ch. 7 In: F Singer (Ed.), Diseases of Bone and Mineral Metabolism.

Endotext.org/ Cole DEC MD, Hendy GN PhD, Bastepe M MD PhD. Hypoparathyroidism and pseudohypoparathyroidism. Ch. 9 In: F Singer (Ed.), Diseases of Bone and Mineral Metabolism.

Erem C, Kocak M, Nuhoglu I et al. (2009). Increased plasminogen activator inhibitor-1, decreased tissue factor pathway inhibitor, and unchanged thrombin-activatable fibrinolysis inhibitor levels in patients with primary hyperparathyroidism. Eur J Endocrinol 160: 863–868.

Farford B, Presutti RJ, Moraghan TJ (2007). Nonsurgical management of primary hyperparathyroidism. Mayo Clin Proc 82: 351–355.

Favus MJ (1992). Intestinal Absorption of Calcium, Magnesium, and Phosphorus. In: FL Coe, MJ Favus (Eds.), Disorder of Bone and Mineral Metabolism, pp. 57–82. Chapter 3.

Firooznia H, Golimbu C, Rafii M (1981). Carpal tunnel syndrome as manifestation of secondary hyperparathyroidism. Arch Intern Med 141: 959.

Fitzpatrick LA (2002). The hypocalcemic states. In: M Favus (Ed.), Disorders of Bone and Mineral Metabolism.

Lippincott Williams and Wilkins, Philadelphia, pp. 568–588.

Fraser WD (2009). Hyperparathyroidism. Lancet 374: 145–158.

Fuster D, Monegal A, Torregrosa J (2006). Progressive paraplegia in a renal transplant patient with normal allograft function. Kidney Int 70: 1533.

Goto F, Kano S, Ogawa K (2000). Creutzfelt–Jakob disease presenting hyperparathyroidism. Auris Nasus Larynx 27: 281–283.

Hagstrom E, Hellman P, Larsson TE et al. (2009). Plasma parathyroid hormone and the risk of cardiovascular mortality in the community. Circulation 119: 2765–2771.

Jackson W, Sethi A, Carp J et al. (2007). Unusual spinal manifestation in secondary hyperparathyroidism. Spine 32: E557–E560.

Jorde R, Waterloo K, Saleh F et al. (2006). Neuropsychological function in relation to serum parathyroid hormone and serum 25-hydroxyvitamin D levels. J Neurol 253: 464–470.

Karatas H, Dericioglu N, Kursun O et al. (2007). Creutzfeldt–Jakob disease presenting as hyperparathyroidism and generalized tonic status epilepticus. Clin EEG Neurosci 38: 203–206.

Katsamakis G, Lukovits T, Gorelick P (1998). Calcific cerebral embolism in systemic calciphylaxis. Neurology 51: 295–297.

Kepez A, Harmanci A, Hazirolan T et al. (2009). Evaluation of subclinical coronary atherosclerosis in mild asymptomatic primary hyperparathyroidism patients. Int J Cardiovasc Imaging 25: 187–193.

Khan AA, Bilezikian JP, Potts JT (2009a). The diagnosis and management of asymptomatic primary hyperparathyroidism revisited. J Clin Endocrinol Metab 94: 333–334.

Khan A, Grey A, Shoback D (2009b). Medical management of asymptomatic primary hyperparathyroidism: proceedings of the third international workshop. J Clin Endocrinol Metab 94: 373–381.

Kiewiet RM, Ponssen HH, Janssens ENW et al. (2004). Ventricular fibrillation in hypercalcemic crisis due to primary hyperparathyroidism. Neth J Med 62: 94–96.

Konrad M, Schlingmann KP, Gudermann T (2004). Insights into the molecular nature of magnesium homeostasis. Am J Physiol Renal Physiol 286: F599–F605.

Mak K, Wong Y, Luk K (2009). Spinal cord compression secondary to brown tumour in a patient on long-term haemodialysis: a case report. J Orthop Surg 17: 90–95.

Mannix H Jr, Pyrtek LJ, Crombie HD Jr et al. (1980). Hyperparathyroidism in the elderly. Am J Surg 139: 581–585.

Marcocci C, Chanson P, Shoback D et al. (2009). Cinacalcet reduces serum calcium concentrations in patients with intractable primary hyperparathyroidism. J Clin Endocrinol Metab 94: 2766–2772.

Mollerup CL, Vestergaard P, Frøkjær VG et al. (2002). Risk of renal stone events in primary hyperparathyroidism before and after parathyroid surgery: controlled retrospective follow-up study. BMJ 325: 807.

Mourad G, Deschodt G, Turc-Baron C et al. (1996). The dialysis patient with cystic bone defects and spinal cord symptoms. Nephrol Dial Transplant 11: 1870–1873.

Niederle B, Stefenelli T, Glogar D et al. (1990). Cardiac calcific deposits in patients with primary hyperparathyroidism: preliminary results of a prospective echocardiographic study. Surgery 108: 1052–1056.

Nilsson I-L, Wadsten C, Brandt L et al. (2004). Mortality in sporadic primary hyperparathyroidism: nationwide cohort study of multiple parathyroid gland disease. Surgery 136: 981–987.

Peacock M (2002). Primary hyperparathyroidism and the kidney: biochemical and clinical spectrum. J Bone Miner Res 17 (Suppl. 2): N87–N94.

Peacock M, Bolognese MA, Borofsky M et al. (2009). Cinacalcet treatment of primary hyperparathyroidism: biochemical and bone densitometric outcomes in a five-year study. J Clin Endocrinol Metab 94: 4860–4867.

Phitayakorn R, McHenry CR (2008). Hyperparathyroid crisis: use of bisphosphonates as a bridge to parathyroidectomy. J Am Coll Surg 206: 1106–1115.

Piovesan A, Molineri N, Casasso F et al. (1999). Left ventricular hypertrophy in primary hyperparathyroidism. Effects of successful parathyroidectomy. Clin Endocrinol 50: 321–328.

Rao DS, Phillips ER, Divine GW et al. (2004). Randomized controlled clinical trial of surgery versus no surgery in patients with mild asymptomatic primary hyperparathyroidism. J Clin Endocrinol Metab 89: 5415–5422.

Rubin MR, Silverberg SJ (2002). Rheumatic manifestations of primary hyperparathyroidism and parathyroid hormone therapy. Curr Rheumatol Rep 4: 179–185.

Rubin MR, Maurer MS, McMahon DJ et al. (2005). Arterial stiffness in mild primary hyperparathyroidism. J Clin Endocrinol Metab 90: 3326–3330.

Rubin MR, Bilezikian JP, McMahon DJ et al. (2008). The natural history of primary hyperparathyroidism with or without parathyroid surgery after 15 years. J Clin Endocrinol Metab 93: 3462–3470.

Sankaran S, Gamble G, Bolland M et al. (2010). Skeletal effects of interventions in mild primary hyperparathyroidism: a meta-analysis. J Clin Endocrinol Metab 95: 1653–1662.

Schmidt R, Rietz L, Bhupendra C et al. (2001). Compressive optic neuropathy caused by renal osteodystrophy. J Neurosurg 95: 704–709.

Shenoy V, Oghalai J (2008). Chronic pachymeningitis and bilateral facial paralysis secondary to renal osteodystrophy. Arch Otolaryngol Head Neck Surg 134: 324–326.

Silverberg SJ, Lewiecki EM, Mosekilde L et al. (2009). Presentation of asymptomatic primary hyperparathyroidism: proceedings of the third international workshop. J Clin Endocrinol Metab 94: 351–365.

Sitges-Serra A, Bergenfelz A (2007). Clinical update: sporadic primary hyperparathyroidism. Lancet 370: 468–470.

Streeten EA, Munir K, Hines S et al. (2008). Coronary artery calcification in patients with primary hyperparathyroidism in comparison with control subjects from the multi-ethnic study of atherosclerosis. Endocr Pract 14: 155–161.

Terada T, Kawata R, Higashino M et al. (2007). Sudden dysphonia due to spontaneous bleeding in secondary parathyroid hyperplasia. Arch Otolaryngol Head Neck Surg 133: 608–609.

Thomas P, Lebrun C (1994). Progressive spastic paraparesis revealing primary hyperparathyroidism. Neurology 44: 178–179.

Tonner DR, Schlechte JA (1993). Neurologic complications of thyroid and parathyroid disease. Med Clin North Am 77: 251–263.

Vázquez-Díaz O, Castillo-Martínez L, Orea-Tejeda A et al. (2009). Reversible changes of electrocardiographic abnormalities after parathyroidectomy in patients with primary hyperparathyroidism. Cardiol J 16: 241–245.

Virdis A, Cetani F, Giannarelli C et al. (2010). The sulfaphenazole-sensitive pathway acts as a compensatory mechanism for impaired nitric oxide availability in patients with primary hyperparathyroidism. Effect of surgical treatment. J Clin Endocrinol Metab 95: 920–927.

Walker MD, Silverberg SJ (2007). Parathyroidectomy in asymptomatic primary hyperparathyroidism: improves "bones" but not "psychic moans. J Clin Endocrinol Metab 92: 1613–1615.

Walker RP, Paloyan E, Gopalsami C (2004). Symptoms in patients with primary hyperparathyroidism: muscle weakness or sleepiness. Endocr Pract 10: 404–408.

Walker MD, McMahon DJ, Inabnet WB et al. (2009a). Neuropsychological features in primary hyperparathyroidism: a prospective study. J Clin Endocrinol Metab 94: 1951–1958.

Walker MD, Fleischer J, Rundek T et al. (2009b). Carotid vascular abnormalities in primary hyperparathyroidism. J Clin Endocrinol Metab 94: 3849–3856.

Wilson LC, Trembath RC (1994). Albright's hereditary osteodystrophy. J Med Genet 31: 779–784.

Zwick O, Vagefi M, Cockerham K et al. (2006). Brown tumor of secondary hyperparathyroidism involving the superior orbit and frontal calvarium. Ophthal Plast Reconstr Surg 22: 304–306.

Handbook of Clinical Neurology, Vol. 120 (3rd series)
Neurologic Aspects of Systemic Disease Part II
Jose Biller and Jose M. Ferro, Editors

Chapter 50

Neurologic complications of disorders of the adrenal glands

TULIO E. BERTORINI[1]* AND ANGEL PEREZ[2]

[1]*Department of Neurology, Methodist University Hospital and Department of Neurology,
University of Tennessee Health Science Center, Memphis, TN, USA*

[2]*Department of Clinical Neurophysiology, University of Tennessee Health Science Center, Memphis, TN, USA*

INTRODUCTION

In order to understand the neurologic manifestations of diseases of the adrenal glands, their anatomy and physiology must first be understood. Each adrenal gland has two distinct areas, the medulla and the cortex. The adrenal medulla derives from the neuroectoderm, and its chromaffin cells secrete catecholamines in a process controlled by preganglionic sympathetic neurons. The adrenal cortex derives from the mesoderm and has three defined functional zones. The zona reticularis adjacent to the medulla secretes sex hormones, and the middle zone secretes corticosteroids. The secretion from both of these zones is under the control of the hypothalamus–pituitary axis. The outer area or zona glomerulosa secretes mineralocorticoids and is controlled by the renin–angiotensin system.

A spectrum of diseases can cause adrenal hormonal dysfunction. In this chapter, their clinical and physiopathological aspects are discussed with emphasis on their neurologic manifestations, their diagnosis, and their management.

HISTORICAL ASPECTS

The anatomy of the adrenal glands was initially described by Bartholomeo Eustachius (Eustachius, 1774). Their function was defined by Thomas Addison, who in 1855 reported the disease that was named after him (Addison, 1855). That same year, Charles Brown-Séquard demonstrated the necessity of the glands for survival by performing adrenalectomies in animals. (Brown-Séquard, 1856).

William Osler, in 1896, was the first physician to treat a patient with Addison's disease with adrenal extracts

(Osler, 1896). In 1901, Takamine and Aldrich isolated adrenaline (Bishop, 1949), and in 1917, Rogoff and Stewart began more detailed research in totally adrenalectomized animals, establishing that cortical adrenal extracts have life-preserving properties (Bishop, 1949). In 1912, Harvey Cushing reported a polyglandular syndrome caused by pituitary basophilism, and later in 1932, he associated this with adrenal hyperactivity (Cushing, 1932).

The control of adrenocortical function by a "pituitary factor" was demonstrated in the 1920s, leading to the isolation of the adrenocorticotrophic hormone (ACTH) by Li, Evans and Simpson in 1943 (Li et al., 1943). In 1937, Reischestein prepared deoxycorticosterone acetate synthetically, while Philip Hench of the Mayo Clinic demonstrated that cortisone relieved symptoms of rheumatoid arthritis (Bishop, 1949). Harris et al. described the neural control of ACTH by the corticotrophin-releasing hormone (CRH) in 1940 (Harris, 1948), and Wylie Vale synthesized this hormone in 1981 (Raux-Demay and Girard, 1985).

FUNCTION OF THE ADRENAL GLANDS

All steroid hormones secreted by the adrenal cortex derive from a cyclopentanoperhydrophenanthrene structure. Cholesterol, which is the precursor of all adrenal steroidogenesis. This is released in the circulation in the form of low-density lipoproteins (LDL) that enter into the adrenal cells by endocytosis. The first rate-limiting step in steroidogenesis is the transport of cholesterol intracellularly from the outer to the inner mitochondrial membrane for conversion to pregnenolone by the cytochrome P450 system. Pregnenolone is then converted to progesterone by the type II isozyme 3β-hydroxysteroid dehydrogenase.

*Correspondence to: Tulio E. Bertorini, M.D., FAAN, FACP, Chief of Neurology, Methodist University Hospital, Professor of Neurology and Pathology, acting Chairman of Neurology, University of Tennessee Health Science Center, 116 Johnson Building, Memphis, TN 38163, USA. Tel: +1-901-448-8353, E-mail: tbertorini@aol.com

The 21-hydroxylation of progesterone and 17-OH-progesterone by 21-hydroxilase produces deoxycortisol and deoxycorticosterone (DOC), respectively. In the final step of cortisol biosynthesis, deoxycortisol is converted to cortisol, which is subsequently converted to cortisone in the peripheral tissues. Most of the secreted cortisol is bound to corticosteroid-binding globulin (CBG). Only 5–10% accounts for the biological active hormone (Larsen et al., 2003). Increased levels of cortisol occur in physiological states such as stress, excessive exercise, hypoglycemia, fever, or surgery (Larsen et al., 2003).

The corticotrophin-releasing hormone is synthesized in neurons of the paraventricular nucleus of the hypothalamus. Its secretion triggers the pituitary production of ACTH which promotes glucocorticoid secretion by the adrenal cortex. CRH binds to specific type I CRH receptors to stimulate pro-opiomelanocortin (POMC) gene transcription (Larsen et al., 2003). POMC is an ACTH precursor containing 241 amino acids. Its secretion is controlled by numerous factors such as CRH, arginine vasopressin (AVP), the endogenous circadian rhythm, stress, and the feedback inhibition by cortisol itself. The circadian rhythm controls CRH and ACTH secretion, which peaks at 3:00–4:00 a.m. and bottoms at about 10:00–11:00 p.m.

CUSHING SYNDROME

Cushing syndrome (CS) is a metabolic disorder caused by chronic high levels of endogenous cortisol or by exogenous exposure to corticosteroids that impairs carbohydrate, protein, and lipid metabolism. Cushing syndrome includes all causes of hypercortisolism, while Cushing disease is reserved for cases of pituitary-dependent CS.

Historical aspects

In 1912 Harvey Cushing described a young woman with obesity, hirsutism, and amenorrhea. Later, he reported 12 additional patients with this syndrome, and in 1932 postulated that this "polyglandular syndrome" was caused by a primary pituitary abnormality that resulted in adrenal hyperplasia (Cushing, 1932). Adrenal tumors or ectopic ACTH production as a cause of CS were not recognized until 1962 (Medvei, 1991).

Etiology

Endogenous CS can be ACTH dependent or independent. ACTH-dependent CS occurs in approximately 80–85% of patients (Fig. 50.1A) (Bertorini et al., 2008), and is most often caused by hyperplasia of the adrenal glands secondary to ACTH secretion from pituitary adenomas. Less frequently it is caused by ectopic production of ACTH by small cell carcinomas of the

lung, medullary thyroid carcinoma, or even more rarely by prostate, pancreatic, adrenal, or thyroid carcinomas. Very infrequently, ectopic production of CRH can also cause CS. The ACTH-independent syndrome is caused by adenomas, carcinomas or macronodular hyperplasia of the adrenal glands (Fig. 50.1B–D).

The most common etiology of CS, however, is the exogenous administration of corticosteroids or ACTH for therapeutic purposes. Because medroxyprogesterone and progesterone also have some intrinsic glucocorticoid activity, their administration might also cause the syndrome.

Clinical manifestations

CS is most frequent in adults between 20 and 50 years of age. It affects all body systems. Patients may have abnormal fat distribution with a "buffalo hump," temporal wasting, central obesity, moon face, weight gain, acne, purple striae, hirsutism (Fig. 50.2), cataracts, menstrual irregularities, arterial hypertension, and hyperglycemia (Nieman, 2013a).

Thinning of the skin with easy bruising and poor wound healing are common, and there is an increased tendency to infections, hypercholesterolemia, and hypertriglyceridemia. Diabetes or glucose intolerance may be accompanied by decreased libido and impotence. Osteoporosis may result in pathological fractures. Patients may complain of back pain caused by osteoporotic vertebral compressions fractures (Fig. 50.3A). Aseptic necrosis of the femoral head is a dreaded complication (Fig. 50.3B). Visual abnormalities may result from optic chiasm compression by the surrounding tumor. Symptom severity varies according to several factors, including the cause of hypercortisolism, its duration, and the presence or absence of androgen excess.

Psychiatric manifestations develop in more than half of patients with CS (Bertorini et al., 2008). Presenting symptoms may include emotional lability, irritability, anxiety, panic attacks, and paranoia. Depression with weight gain and increased appetite also occurs, and severely depressed patients might be suicidal. Some have anorexia and weight loss. Mania may develop in some patients. Insomnia is mostly related to high serum cortisol concentrations during sleep from the absence of normal diurnal variations of its secretion. Learning, cognition, and memory, especially short-term memory, can be impaired in CS (Mauri et al., 1993); this appears to be related to cortical cerebral atrophy and reduction in hippocampal volumes (Momose et al., 1971; Starkman et al., 1992).

Proximal muscle weakness and wasting occur in about 60% of patients (Nieman, 2013a). This "steroid myopathy" is more prominent in the legs, with sparing

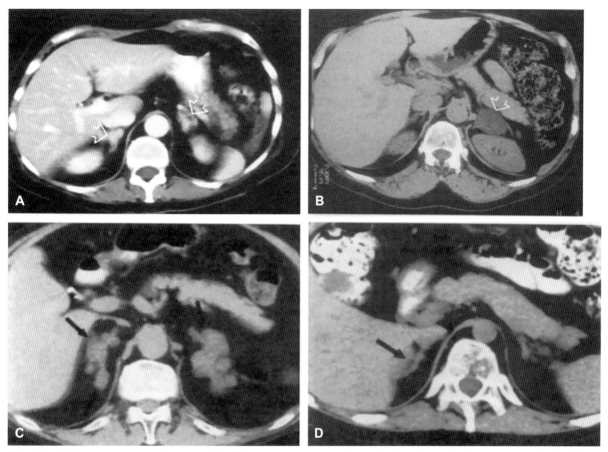

Fig. 50.1. (**A**) Adrenal computed tomographic (CT) scan demonstrating bilateral adrenal hyperplasia in a patient with Cushing's diease. (**B**) CT scan of a typical solitary left adrenal adenoma causing Cushing's syndrome. (**C**) Cushing's syndrome caused by massive macronodular hyperplasia. (**D**) Cushing's syndrome caused by surgically proven primary pigmented nodular adrenal disease. Notice the multiple small nodules with the relatively atrophic internodular adrenocortical tissue inviolving the medial limb of the right adrenal gland (arrow). (**A** and **B** reproduced with permission from Stewart, 2003; **C** and **D** reproduced with permission from Findling and Doppman, 1994.)

of the sphincter muscles. Serum muscle enzymes are usually normal, and nerve conduction tests are unremarkable. Needle examination demonstrates a lack of spontaneous potentials, while the motor unit action potentials may be normal in mild cases or have low amplitude and are polyphasic. The characteristic histological finding is selective type II muscle fiber atrophy, particularly of type IIB subtype fibers (Fig. 50.4). Electron microscopy may show some aggregations of mitochondria and vacuolization (Ferguson et al., 1990; Ubogu et al., 1994).

A number of mechanisms have been proposed to account for the pathogenesis of steroid myopathy. These putative mechanisms are related to abnormalities of carbohydrate metabolism and negative protein balance, because high levels of corticosteroids stimulate dose-related protein degradation. Protein synthesis is also inhibited, affecting type II fibers predominantly. High levels of mineralocorticoids can cause hypokalemia that

can increase muscle weakness. Decreased physical activity might also be a contributing factor. The muscle damage caused by steroids is usually reversible (Bertorini et al., 2008).

Critical illness myopathy (CIM) is a paralytic disorder that occurs predominantly in patients in intensive care units who have received high doses of corticosteroids and neuromuscular blocking agents (Danon and Carpenter, 1991; Danon and Edinger, 1999; Bolton, 2005). Characteristically, weakness is diffuse, affecting predominantly proximal muscles. Muscle stretch reflexes are decreased, and afflicted subjects might also have an associated "neuropathy of the gravely ill." Serum CK is normal or mildly elevated. Muscle biopsy shows characteristic features with muscle atrophy particularly of type II muscle fibers, basophilic stippling, necrosis, and reduction of adenosine triphosphatase (ATPase) activity electron microscopy shows a diffuse loss of thick filaments (Fig. 50.5)

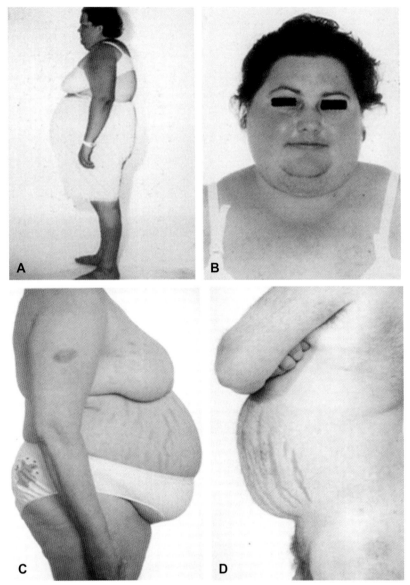

Fig. 50.2. Clinical features of Cushing's syndrome. (**A**) Centripetal and some generalized obesity and dorsal kyphosis in a 30-year-old woman with Cushing's disease. (**B**) Same woman as in (**A**), showing moon facies, plethora, hirsutism and enlarged supraclavicular fat pads. (**C** and **D**) Typical centripetal obesity with livid abdominal striae. (Reproduced from Stewart, 2003, with permission.)

(Bertorini et al., 2008). The etiology of CIM and the role of corticosteroids in its development are uncertain, but several hypotheses have been proposed. CIM seems to be related to a systemic inflammatory response with cytokine-induced muscle injury and activation of proteases (Lacomis et al., 1996; Danon and Edinger, 1999; Di Giovanni et al., 2004).

Diagnosing Cushing syndrome

The first step in the diagnosis of CS is the demonstration of an elevated urinary free cortisol in a 24 hour sample.

Once an elevated urinary cortisol is observed, a dexamethasone suppression test should be ordered to confirm the diagnosis. The final step is to determine the cause of hypercortisolism and to determine if this is ACTH-dependent or independent.

The low-dose dexamethasone suppression test is based on the fact that dexamethasone suppresses ACTH release from the pituitary gland, leading to reduction of serum cortisol levels and, therefore, decreased urinary excretion of cortisol and its metabolites (Nieman, 2013b). Dexamethasone is usually given at 11 p.m. and serum cortisol is measured at 8 a.m. the next morning.

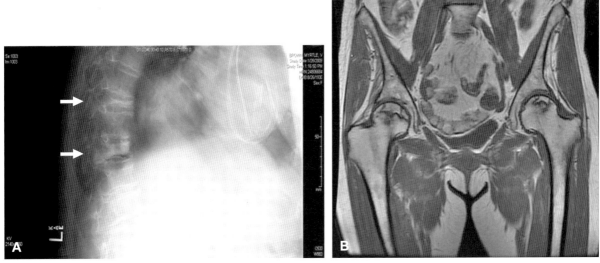

Fig. 50.3. (**A**) Vertebral compression at T8 and T10 levels (arrows), and diffuse osteoporosis of an 80-year-old woman with iatrogenic Cushing's syndrome. (**B**) MRI demonstrating bilateral aseptic necrosis of the femoral head in a patient with Cushing's syndrome.

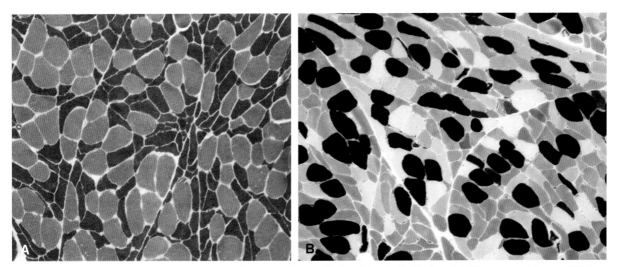

Fig. 50.4. (**A**) Selective atrophy of type II muscle fibers. (ATPase stain, PH 9.4 × 100). (**B**) Atrophic fibers are mainly type IIB that stain intermediate with ATPase at PH 4.6 (×100). (Reproduced from Bertorini et al., 2008, with permission.)

A cortisol level over 3 µg/dL suggests hypercortisolism (David, 1995; Findling et al., 2004). Some drugs, such as phenytoin and rifampicin, can cause false-positive results by increasing the clearance of dexamethasone.

Measurement of serum or salivary cortisol is also of great diagnostic value. Patients collect samples on three consecutive evenings, and CS is considered if the cortisol serum level is above 5 µg/dL (Nieman, 2013b) or if the cortisol salivary level is above 1.3 ng/mL.

Diagnosing the cause of Cushing syndrome

Once CS is diagnosed, the determination of whether cortisol secretion is ACTH dependent or independent is made by measuring plasma ACTH levels. Concentration below 5 pg/mL is diagnostic of ACTH independent CS. A concentration over 15 pg/mL indicates ACTH-dependent CS (Nieman, 2013c).

A standard high-dose dexamethasone suppression test can also be done in patients with suspected

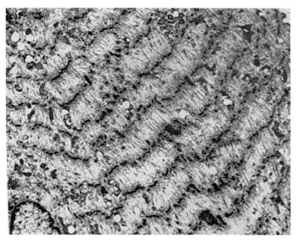

Fig. 50.5. Electron microscopy of a muscle biopsy from a patient with critical illness myopathy showing loss of thick filaments (×7500). (Reproduced from Bertorini et al., 2008, with permission.)

ACTH-dependent CS from a pituitary cause. If cortisol secretion is suppressed by high doses of dexamethasone, Cushing disease (CD) should be considered. If cortisol is not suppressed by low or high doses of dexamethasone, an adrenal tumor or an ectopic ATCH-secreting tumor should be suspected. In patients diagnosed with CD a head computed tomography (CT) scan, or preferably brain MRI, is done to search for a pituitary adenoma. In patients with inadequate suppression of cortisol after dexamethasone administration, an octreotide scan and chest and abdominal CT or MRI are done to rule out possible tumors causing ectopic ACTH production.

Treatment

The treatment of choice for patients with CD consists of transphenoidal microadenalectomy or partial resection of the anterior pituitary gland. Patients are considered cured if their morning plasma cortisol levels are undetectable and ACTH levels are below 5 pg/mL 24 hours after the last dose of hydrocortisone 4–7 days postsurgery. Patients require daily glucocorticoid replacement therapy from the time of surgery until their adrenal function recovers, which might take up to 6–12 months (Larsen et al., 2003; Bertorini et al., 2008).

Most cases of primary adrenal hyperplasia respond to bilateral adrenalectomy. Unilateral adrenalectomy should be performed in those with an adrenal adenoma or carcinoma (David, 1995). Adrenal enzyme inhibitors such as aminoglutethimide, metyrapone, and etomidate should also be considered to control hypercortisolism in patients with carcinoma. Ketoconazole is also effective for long-term control of hypercortisolism (Larsen et al., 2003).

The treatment of steroid myopathy consists of removal of the primary cause. A high protein diet may be helpful. CIM is treated with a reduction of corticosteroid dosage and discontinuation of paralyzing agents. Patients should have increased mobility and receive adequate physical therapy.

ADRENAL INSUFFICIENCY

Adrenal insufficiency (AI) refers to inadequate adrenocortical function that causes reduction of corticoid secretion. Two distinct types of AI are distinguished: primary or Addison disease (AD), in which the glucocorticoid deficiency is caused by disorders of the adrenal glands, and a secondary form resulting from pituitary or hypothalamic disorders causing ACTH deficiency.

Historical aspects

On March 15, 1849, Thomas Addison, described at the South London Medical Society: "a remarkable form of anemia in adult males, ages 20 to 60, which lasts a period of several weeks, or even months. Its approach is indicated by a certain amount of languor and restlessness, paleness, loss of muscular strength, general relaxation or feebleness of the whole frame, and indisposition to, or incapacity for, bodily and mental exertion" (Bishop, 1949).

Addison also described progressive and severe paleness, tachycardia, dyspnea, edema, and generalized weakness. Only three of his patients were autopsied, and all demonstrated a disease of the suprarenal capsules. When Addison's monograph was published, the functions of the glands were almost unknown, and in common with the spleen, thymus, and thyroid, they were believed to be in charge of the elaboration of blood (Bishop, 1949).

In 1856, Charles E. Brown-Séquard performed his classic experiments involving the removal of the adrenal glands from animals and concluded that all had died of Addison disease. Later, in 1899, Kippel introduced the concept of "encephalopathy addisonienne," noting that neuropsychiatric symptoms are common in adrenal insufficiency (Bishop, 1949).

Etiology and pathogenesis

Primary AI is caused by different disorders categorized as:

* destructive lesions of the adrenal glands
* developmental defects of the glands manifested with several phenotypes associated with different grades of psychomotor retardation
* impaired steroidogenesis secondary to defects in cholesterol metabolism or mitochondrial DNA abnormalities (Arlt and Allolio, 1881, Ten et al., 2001).

DISORDERS CAUSING DESTRUCTIVE LESIONS

Most cases of AD are autoimmune. These disorders occur either in isolation or as part of an autoimmune polyglandular syndrome. Around 50% of patients with AD have other autoimmune disorders (Myhre et al., 2002; Falorni et al., 2004), such as thyroid disease (Hashimoto thyroiditis or Graves' disease), type 1 diabetes mellitus, premature ovarian failure, celiac disease, and autoimmune gastritis (Myhre et al., 2003; Falorni et al., 2004).

In the rare autoimmune polyendocrine syndrome type I (APS-I), AI is associated with hypoparathyroidism and chronic mucocutaneous candidiasis. APS-II describes AD in combination with autoimmune thyroid disease and/or type-1 diabetes. APS-IV is characterized by AD without thyroid involvement or type-1 diabetes, but in combination with other autoimmune disorders such as autoimmune gonadal insufficiency and celiac disease. APS-III describes cases without involvement of the adrenal glands (Larsen et al., 2003).

Other destructive causes of AI include infections such as tuberculosis, often in combination with human immunodeficiency virus (HIV) infection (Piedrola et al., 1996). Mycobacterium tuberculosis causes a gradual destruction of the adrenal glands that initially appear enlarged. Later, the tissue is replaced by caseous nodules and fibrosis. Calcifications are usually seen on some radiographic studies (Larsen et al., 2003). Other pathogens such as *Mycobacterium avium*, toxoplasma, pneumocystis species, and cytomegalovirus may also result in AI in AIDS patients. Histoplasmosis, cryptococcosis, and paracoccidioidomycosis have a predilection for infecting the adrenal glands and should be included in the differential diagnosis in endemic areas.

Destruction of the adrenal glands from hemorrhages is a rare cause of AI. A classic cause is meningococcal septicemia (Waterhouse–Friderichsen syndrome). This has also been reported as a complication of heparin treatment (Fig. 50.6) (Bakaeen et al., 2005) and in the antiphospholipid syndrome (Presotto et al., 2005). Infrequent destructive causes include metastasis (mostly from lung or breast tumors), amyloidosis, sarcoidosis, hemorrhagic infarction, hemochromatosis, surgical removal of the glands, adrenoleukodystrophy, congenital hypoplasia, and other rare hereditary disorders (Carey, 1997; Ten et al., 2001).

Pathophysiology of autoimmune Addison disease

The immunology of AD was unknown until 1992, when Winqvist et al. identified the steroidogenic enzyme 21-hydroxylase as the main target of pathogenic autoantibodies (Winqvist and Karlsson, 1992). About 95% of AD patients have elevated anti-21-hydroxylase

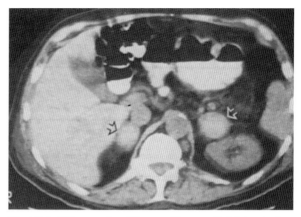

Fig. 50.6. CT scan of an 80-year-old man with bilateral adrenal hemorrhage resulting from anticoagulation for pulmonary emboli. (Reproduced from Stewart, 2003, with permission).

antibodies at diagnosis, but this typically declines to about 50% after 20 years of disease duration (Laureti et al., 1998; Myhre et al., 2002). The presence of these antibodies is predictive of the development of adrenal failure (Yu, 1999).

At autopsy, there is lymphocytic infiltration of the atrophic glands (al Sabri et al., 1997), but this finding is not specific and can also can be observed in some healthy older people without adrenal insufficiency (Hayashi et al., 1989; al Sabri et al., 1997). Nerup demonstrated that patients with AD had T lymphocytes reactive to fetal adrenal glands or to mitochondrial fractions from the glands (Nerup et al., 1969, 1970). Recently, patients with APS-II, but not those with isolated AD, were found to have CD4+CD25+ regulatory T cells with defective suppressive capacity (Kriegel et al., 2004), suggesting that a break of peripheral tolerance could activate pathogenic T cells with an ability to target adrenocortical cells. Reduced expression of caspase-3, a mediator in activation-induced cell death, may also contribute to the break of tolerance in patients with APS-II and thyroid autoimmunity (Vendrame et al., 2006).

AD has been associated with certain MHC haplotypes, in particular DR3-DQ2 and DR4-DQ8 (Nejentsev and Howson, 2007). Also, MHC class I chain-related gene A has been found to be related to the disease (Gambelunghe et al., 1999). Some specific genotypes increase the risk for the disease, while others confer protection (Myhre et al., 2002).

Cytotoxic T lymphocyte antigen 4 inhibits T cell activation, and this seems to be involved with disease susceptibility in autoimmune AD (Husebye and Lovas, 2009). An association with the gene protein tyrosine phosphatase nonreceptor type 22 occurs in some cases (Skinningsrud et al., 2008), while an association with polymorphisms of the vitamin D receptors has also been reported (Pani et al., 2002). Associations with polymorphisms in the la-hydroxylase promoter region have been found in some patients (Lopez et al., 2004; Jennings et al., 2005).

DISORDERS CAUSED BY DEVELOPMENTAL DEFECTS

Developmental defects from genetic disorders causing AD are very rare. In adrenal dysgenesis there are mutations of the dosage-sensitive sex reversal-adrenal hypoplasia gene 1 on Xp21 (DAX-1), and mutations of steroidogenic factor-1 gene (SF-1) have also been reported (Guo et al., 1995). In *congenital adrenal hypoplasia*, due to DAX-1 mutations, development of the adrenal cortex is arrested. The X-linked form associated with primary AI manifests at birth, and patients develop hypogonadotrophic hypogonadism (Reutens et al., 1999). Another X-linked form of adrenal insufficiency has also been described in association with glycerol kinase deficiency (Reutens et al., 1999). In this disorder, the onset of symptoms varies from birth to childhood, and the clinical presentation includes psychomotor retardation, muscular dystrophy, hypertelorism, strabismus, drooping mouth, anorchia or cryptochidism, short stature, and osteoporosis (Sjarif et al., 2000). SF-1 mutations were found in 46 XY female patients with severe gonadal dysgenesis and primary adrenal insufficiency (Guo et al., 1995; Köhler et al., 2008).

Familial glucocorticoid deficiency (FGD), a rare autosomal recessive disorder, is characterized by deficient cortisol and androgen secretions. In this disorder the adrenal glands do not respond to ACTH; aldosterone secretion is normal or partially deficient (Ten et al., 2001).

The *Allgrove or triple A syndrome* is an autosomal recessive disorder that maps to 12q13 and consists of the triad of ACTH resistance, alacrima, and achalasia. Patients have gradual neurologic dysfunction, polyneuropathy, deafness, mental retardation, and hyperkeratosis of palms and soles. Aldosterone deficiency may be seen (Huebner et al., 1999).

DISORDERS CAUSING IMPAIRED STEROIDOGENESIS

Smith–Lemli–Opitz syndrome, congenital adrenal hyperplasias, lipoid congenital adrenal hyperplasia, abetalipoproteinemia and homozygous familial hypercholesterolemia are included in this group of disorders characterized by adrenal insufficiency because of impaired steroidogenesis, but these are not usually associated with neurologic manifestations (Ten et al., 2001; Larsen et al., 2003).

Congenital adrenal hyperplasia, however, is particularly important because patients with this disorder frequently have neurologic and particularly behavioral manifestations. This is an autosomal recessive condition caused by mutation of the CYP21 gene that encodes 21-hydroxylase, a deficiency that affects cortisol biosynthesis and is associated with corticotrophin hypersecretion and increased androgen production. Patients with this disorder may have temporal lobe atrophy and may show white matter abnormalities on MRI (Nass et al., 1997), while functional MRI shows that females, but not males, may activate the amygdalae more than healthy controls during visual tasks (Ernst et al., 2007). There also is evidence of abnormalities of brain development affecting behavior (Berenbaum and Snyder, 1995; Meyer-Bahlburg, 2011). Females may display masculine-like behavior and boy-like activities and may have genital abnormalities such as an enlarged clitoris (Dittman et al., 1990; Zucker et al., 1996; Speiser and White, 2003).

Mitochondrial diseases can also manifest with endocrine disturbances; for example, the Kearns–Sayre syndrome, an unusual disorder characterized by myopathy with ptosis and opthalmoplegia, deafness, and endocrine dysfunction (short stature, hypogonadism, hypoparathyroidism, hypothyroidism, cardiac arrhythmia and adrenal deficiency) (Sanaker et al., 2007).

Finally, several drugs can affect cortisol biosynthesis and cause adrenal failure. Examples include aminoglutethimide, metyrapone, and etomidate, which are used to treat hypercortisolism in CS. Other drugs such as phenytoin and barbiturates accelerate cortisol metabolism. Anti-infective medications such as ketoconazole, rifampicin, and trimethoprim might precipitate adrenal insufficiency (Ten et al., 2001; Larsen et al., 2003).

Secondary AI is commonly caused by the sudden cessation of chronic exogenous glucocorticoid therapy. Secondary AI may also occur following surgical removal of pituitary adenomas or infections. Preserved mineralocorticoid secretion and decreased CRH or ACTH synthesis and secretion are typical.

Isolated ACTH deficiency is a rare disorder of possible autoimmune etiology in which there is no ACTH-secretory response to CRH (Sauter et al., 1990). A defect in conversion of POMC to ACTH by the prohormone convertase enzymes has been described. Other causes of secondary AI include pituitary apoplexy, Sheehan syndrome, lymphocytic hypophysitis, radiation, and surgical resection of parts of the hypothalamus.

Pituitary apoplexy is characterized by an acute onset of headache, visual disturbances, altered mental status, and hormonal dysfunction caused by hemorrhage or infarction of the hypophysis. Usually a pre-existing pituitary adenoma is found (Larsen et al., 2003). *Sheehan syndrome* is a caused by a severe vascular insufficiency of the pituitary gland caused by massive postpartum hemorrhage. The clinical picture varies from nonspecific symptoms to coma. Decreased or absent postpartum lactation and failure to resume menses after delivery are the most common presenting symptoms. All patients have hypogonadism and growth hormone and prolactin deficiencies. Approximately 90% of patients have secondary hypothyroidism, and 55% have adrenal failure (Dökmetas et al., 2006). Because most patients have a mild disease, this disorder is often undiagnosed and remains untreated for a long time. Brain MRI demonstrates a totally or partially empty sella in all patients. Treatment consists of hormone replacement with corticosteroids, levothyroxine, estrogen, and growth hormone (Kelestimur, 2003; Dökmetas et al., 2006).

Clinical manifestations

The clinical presentation of AI depends on the rate and degree of the hormonal deficiency. AD is associated with glucocorticoiod and mineralocorticoid deficiencies, while secondary AI has an intact renin–angiotensin–adosterone system. The onset of AI is usually insidious and is characterized by nonspecific symptoms of corticosteroid deficiency, such as chronic weakness, fatigue, general malaise, dizziness, weight loss, fever, anorexia, and orthostatic hypotension, which is more prominent in AD (Nieman, 2013). Other symptoms include headaches, visual disturbances, craving for salt, abdominal cramps, nausea, vomiting, or diarrhea alternating with constipation. Patients with AD also have increased daytime fatigue without excessive sleepiness (Lovas et al., 2003). Hyponatremia, hyperkalemia, acidosis, elevated serum creatinine, hypoglycemia, hypercalcemia, mild normocytic anemia, lymphocytosis, and mild eosinophilia have been described (Wolfgang, 1996).

The most significant finding differentiating the types of AI is the presence of hyperpigmentation of the skin and mucous surfaces present in the primary form (Fig. 50.7). This hyperpigmentation is caused by high plasma corticotrophin concentrations resulting from decreased cortisol feedback, which increase melanocyte-stimulating hormone (MSH) levels (Piedrola et al., 1996; Larsen et al., 2003).

Because secondary AI is also associated with hypopituitarism, the clinical presentation may be related to other hormonal deficiencies, especially luteinizing hormone (LH), follicle-stimulating hormone (FSH), or thyroid-stimulating hormone (TSH) (Larsen et al., 2003). Symptoms usually are not as severe as in AD and the lassitude, weakness and lack of energy might resemble a myopathy; this is usually caused by dehydration and hypoglycemia.

Acute adrenal crisis, or "Addisonian crisis," is a medical emergency. Patients become hypotensive and may develop acute circulatory failure, hypoglycemia, severe abdominal pain, confusion, convulsions, lethargy, coma, and death. The crisis may result from an acute process affecting adrenal function (e.g., adrenal hemorrhage) or an intercurrent illness or stress (e.g., infection, trauma, surgery, and burns) in patients with known Addison disease. The most common cause is the abrupt withdrawal of steroids in patients on long-term of oral glucocorticoids (Ten et al., 2001; Larsen et al., 2003).

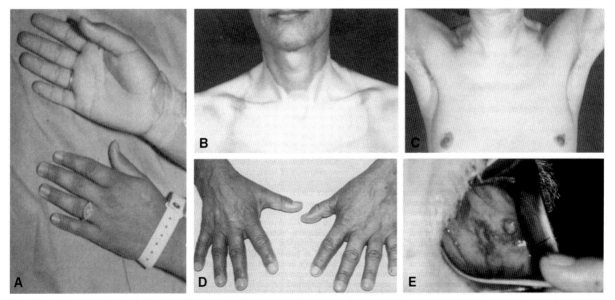

Fig. 50.7. Pigmentation in Addison's disease. (**A**) Hands of an 18-year-old woman with autoimmune polyendocrine syndrome and Addison's disease. Pigmentation in a patient with Addison's disease before (**B**) and after (**C**) treatment with hydrocortisone and fludrocortisone. (**D**) Similar changes also seen in a 60-year-old man with tuberculous Addison's disease before and after corticosteroid therapy. (**E**) Buccal pigmentation in the same patient. (**B** and **C**, courtesy of Professor C.R.W. Edwards.) (Reproduced from Stewart, 2003, with permission.)

The neurologic manifestations of AI include neuro-psychiatric symptoms, myopathy, flexion contractures of the legs, and rarely seizures (Nieman, 2013d). Muscle pain and generalized weakness can occur, affecting mostly the lower extremities, when associated with a metabolic abnormality. Muscle biopsy and electromyographic studies are usually normal or nonspecific without consistent and reproducible abnormalities. Factors contributing to muscle weakness include circulatory insufficiency, fluid imbalance, electrolyte abnormalities, impaired carbohydrate metabolism, and starvation (Benvenga et al., 2001).

Flexion contractures syndrome is a rare disorder associated with AD or hypopituitarism and rarely with isolated ACTH deficiency (Nakamagoe et al., 1994; Odagaki et al., 2003; Syriou et al., 2008). This has also been reported as a paraneoplastic manifestation (Eekhoff et al., 1998). The syndrome is characterized by progressive painful flexion contractures of the pelvic girdle, hips, and knees without involvement of the extensor muscles. Normal conduction tests and nonspecific EMG findings without myopathic changes or spontaneous discharges have been described (Nishikawa, 2003; Odagaki et al., 2003). Two cases of isolated adrenal insufficiency associated with "frozen shoulders" have been reported as a focal flexion contractures syndrome (Choy et al., 1991; Romney and Chik, 2001). The exact mechanism involved in this disorder is unknown, although an autoimmune basis cannot be excluded.

The neuropsychiatric manifestations of AI were initially described by Addison in 1855. Addison reported that patients could develop "attacks of giddiness," "anxiety in the face" and "delirium." Mood and behavioral symptoms are common. Psychosis and marked cognitive changes, including delirium, appear to occur more rarely and are associated with severe disease (Lever and Stansfeld, 1983; Varadaraj and Cooper, 1986; Anglin et al., 2006). Rare cases of catatonia and self-mutilation have been reported (Thompson, 1973; Rajathurai et al., 1983; Varadaraj and Cooper, 1986). These neuropsychiatric symptoms may be a presenting feature of an Addisonian crisis (Anglin et al., 2006) or may be present in patients with adrenoleukodystrophy or Hashimoto encephalopathy, disorders that are associated with primary AI.

In patients with neuropsychiatric symptoms, EEG studies are frequently abnormal with diffuse slowing (Cohen and Marks, 1961; McFarland, 1963) or bursts of 1–3 or 3–6 seconds of high voltage waves (Smith, 1958).

The pathophysiology of the neuropsychiatric manifestations of AD remains unclear. Several theories have been proposed, including:

- Metabolic abnormalities: hyponatremia in most patients may produce cognitive changes and encephalopathy (Moritz, and Ayus, 2003). Severe hypoglycemia can precipitate cognitive changes and coma. Hypoxia secondary to severe hypotension may be responsible for mental status changes, but this is less likely because of cerebral vascular autoregulation (Michiels, 2004).

- Glucocorticoid receptors are distributed throughout the brain and are particularly abundant in the hippocampus. It has been demonstrated that adrenalectomy produces massive granular cell death in the dentate gyrus of the hippocampus (McNeill et al., 1991; Gould et al., 1992; Sloviter et al., 1993), and it is conceivable that this could interrupt the hippocampal trisynaptic circuit, producing memory impairment and cognitive changes (Sloviter et al., 1993; Mizoguchi et al., 2004).

- Glucocorticoids are essential for maintaining prefrontal cortical cognitive function (Mizoguchi et al., 2004). Henkin proposed that a reduction of glucocorticoids results in an enhanced ability to detect sensory inputs (Henkin et al., 1963, 1970, 1973). There is a loss of perceptual ability and decreased integration of sensory inputs; for example, the ability to recognize the four qualities of taste, understand speech, recognize changes in tone, and localize auditory stimuli is impaired with decreased glucocorticoids levels. Therefore, it is possible that if patients receive abnormally high sensory signals but are unable to process and integrate these signals appropriately, there may be a tendency to develop hallucinations.

- An increase in endorphin levels has been proposed in AD (Anglin et al., 2006), which might cause psychosis. In response to decreased glucocorticoid production by the adrenal cortex, the anterior pituitary synthesizes proopiomelanocortin (POMC) which is cleaved to release ACTH and β-endorphin. The association of increased endorphins with psychosis has been suggested based on the findings of elevated CSF endorphins in schizophrenic patients (Lindstrom et al., 1978), the ability of phencyclidine to act on opiate receptors and cause psychosis (Steinpresis, 1996), and the amelioration of auditory hallucinations with the opioid antagonist naloxone (Lehmann et al., 1979).

Diagnosis

Several methods are used to diagnose adrenal insufficiency. A useful screening test is measurement of serum cortisol. An intact adrenocortical reserve is confirmed with basal morning cortisol levels of over 500 nmol/L

(Grinspoon and Biller, 1994; Arlt and Allolio, 2003; Dorin et al., 2003).

After screening, the most widely used test in the assessment of adrenal insufficiency is the Synacthen or Cortrosyn test (synthetic ACTH). Baseline cortisol concentrations are obtained before and 30 or 60 minutes after 250 μg of Synacthen is administered. Levels above 500–600 nmol/L are considered to indicate a normal adrenal reserve (Dickstein et al., 1991; Gonzalbez et al., 2000; Dorin et al., 2003). Many patients with pituitary disease have marginal responses, and should be tested further with the insulin tolerance or the overnight metyrapone test (Mayenknecht et al., 1998; Salvatori, 2005).

The insulin tolerance test (ITT) is considered the goldstandard for assessment of HPA reserve and is particularly useful in the detection of early secondary AI and growth hormone deficiency. This test is based on the stress response to hypoglycemia following insulin administration. Hypoglycemia causes release of ACTH and growth hormone, and ACTH elevation produces secretion of cortisol from the adrenal glands. The ITT is contraindicated in patients with epilepsy, cardiovascular or cerebrovascular disease, or basal cortisol concentrations < 100 nmol/L (Finucane et al., 2008). Also, this test may precipitate an acute hypoadrenal crisis. The ITT is particularly useful in patients whose Synacthen test is borderline or patients who have had recent pituitary surgery (Dorin et al., 2003; Reynolds et al., 2006; Finucane et al., 2008).

Metyrapone inhibits the adrenal cortex enzyme 11β-hydroxylase, thus inhibiting the conversion of 11-deoxycortisol to cortisol. Metyrapone is administered at midnight, and cortisol and 11-deoxycortisol levels are measured at 8:00 a.m. (Fiad et al., 1994). In normal individuals, postmetyrapone cortisol concentrations are low, but 11-deoxycortisol concentrations rise significantly, while this does not occur in patients with AI (Grinspoon and Biller, 1994; Berneis et al., 2002; Arlt and Allolio, 2003).

ACTH concentrations above 100 ng/L are usually observed in primary AI (Dorin et al., 2003), while elevated ACTH concentrations accompanied by normal cortisol concentrations represent a state of subclinical AI that could progress to overt clinical AI (Dorin et al., 2003). In patients with secondary adrenal insufficiency, plasma ACTH concentrations are usually undetectable (Grinspoon and Biller, 1994; Salvatori, 2005).

In secondary AI, the CRH test can be used to differentiate pituitary from hypothalamic etiologies (Salvatori, 2005). The test consists of the administration of human or ovine CRH and measurement of serum cortisol at baseline and at 15, 30, and 60 minutes.

In primary AI aldosterone concentrations typically are low and are associated with elevated renin concentrations.

In secondary AI the renin–angiotensin system can function normally and aldosterone concentrations usually fall within the normal range (Salvatori, 2005).

In clinically apparent autoimmune AI, adrenocortical autoantibodies (ACA) are detected in more than 90% of patients with AD (Betterle et al., 2002); these antibodies destroy adrenal tissue, interfering with hormone production. The 21-hydroxylase antibodies are ACA, which are considered more sensitive indicators of autoimmune adrenal insufficiency, and their presence together with other ACA makes a diagnosis of autoimmune primary AI with up to 99% probability (Falorni et al., 1997; Betterle et al., 2002; Coco et al., 2006).

Radiologic tests are usually not necessary in patients with autoimmune adrenalitis (Arlt and Allolio, 2003), but for other forms of AI either CT or MR imaging may be used. With infiltrative causes, such as infection, hemorrhage, neoplasm, hemochromatosis, and sarcoidosis, the radiological findings are characteristic (Salvatori, 2005). In late stages of tuberculous adrenalitis, calcifications are more readily identified on CT than on MRI (Sawczuk et al., 1986). In suspected secondary adrenal insufficiency, MRI of the pituitary gland is indicated (Salvatori, 2005).

CT-guided adrenal biopsy can be used in patients with suspected metastases and in whom a known primary tumor remains unidentified and a pheochromocytoma has been excluded (Arlt and Allolio, 2003). Adrenal biopsy may also have some additional diagnostic utility in patients with other infiltrative etiologies.

Treatment

Treatment of AI consists of replacement of glucocorticoids and mineralocorticoids, in conjunction with fluid and electrolyte replacement. Patients should receive hydrocortisone or cortisone. The oral dose of hydrocortisone is 25 mg/day (15 mg in the morning and 10 mg at night), while cortisone could be given in dosages of 25 mg in the morning and 12.5 mg in the evening. In primary AI, oral fludrocortisone is added in doses of 0.05–2 mg daily for mineralocorticoid replacement (Larsen et al., 2003; Salvatori, 2005). Physical therapy and gait training are important.

Patients should be advised regarding the risk of an Addisonian crisis, particularly during times of stress or surgery, and the dosage of hydrocortisone should be doubled or tripled during these situations (Arlt and Allolio, 2003). During a crisis, patients should receive hydrocortisone intravenously in a dosage of 100 mg every 8 hours.

ADRENOLEUKODYSTROPHY AND ADRENOMYELONEUROPATHY

Adrenoleukodystrophy (ALD) and adrenomyeloneuropathy (AMN) are allelic X-linked genetic diseases with different clinical presentation. Both are associated with accumulations of saturated very long chain fatty acids (VLCFA) in the brain and adrenal cortex, and are caused by a mutated gene known as *ABCD1*, which codes a protein that transfers VLCFA into the peroxisome to undergo β-oxidation. Their exact pathogenesis, however, is unclear.

Historical aspects

Adrenoleukodystrophy, first described by Siemerling and Creutzfeld in 1923 (Aubourg, 1996), was originally called Schilder–Addison disease because of the presence of features of Addison disease, such as "bronze" skin changes, along with findings of Schilder disease. Schilder disease is a rare condition that affects children and is characterized by a severe and acute demyelinating diffuse cerebral sclerosis; deafness and cortical blindness are common findings, and the prognosis is poor (Barbieri et al., 1982). The X-linked inheritance in adrenoleukodystrophy was proposed by Fanconi et al. in 1963. Blaw coined the name adrenoleukodystrophy in 1970 based on the association of a leukodystrophy with adrenal insufficiency (Aubourg, 1996).

In 1975, Schaumburg et al. performed extensive neuropathological analyses of ALD patients. One year later, Budka and Griffin recognized that a form of this disease occurred in young adults with progressive spastic paraplegia and neoplasty and adrenal insufficiency. They named this form of the disorder adrenomyeloneuropathy (Budka et al., 1976; Griffin et al., 1977). In 1973, Powers and Schaumburg demonstrated the presence of trilamellar inclusions in the adrenocortical cells (Powers and Schaumburg, 1973), and in 1976 Igarashi et al. showed that the cholesterol ester lipid fraction from the ALD brain and adrenal cortex contained high levels of saturated very long chain fatty acids, concluding that the disease was a lipid storage disease (Igarashi et al., 1976).

Moser et al. identified heterozygous women as an at-risk group for ALD, and made prenatal diagnoses in children of affected families in 1982 and 1983 (Moser et al., 1982, 1983). An impaired capacity to β-oxidase VLCFA was found. Later studies demonstrated that ALD fibroblasts normally transport VLCFA across the peroxisomal membrane and oxidize the coenzyme A ester of VLCFA at a normal rate. This suggested that accumulation of VLCFA was caused by a deficiency of the first enzyme of the peroxisomal β-oxidation pathway, VLCFA-CoA synthetase or ligase. Recently, the gene for the disease was demonstrated by positional cloning (Mosser et al., 1993).

Clinical manifestations

Adrenoleukodystrophy has a variable age of onset in childhood and different phenotypes. Neurologic symptoms usually precede adrenal insufficiency, and about 90% of these patients show melanodermia and increased ACTH levels (Aubourg, 1996). The clinical characteristics correspond to demyelinating lesions involving primarily the white matter of the parieto-occipital lobes of the brain (Aubourg, 1996) (Fig. 50.8). Patients may have moderate dystonia and pyramidal signs. Also, marked behavioral changes occur between the ages of 4 and 8 years, with signs of withdrawal or hyperactivitiy. Some patients have attention deficit disorder and may be diagnosed as having a psychiatric disease. In 2009, Kaga et al. demonstrated that abnormal neuropsychological findings can precede the onset of clinical and MRI alterations (Kaga et al., 2009). Patients may lose the ability to read and to understand the oral language, and some also develop seizures. Visual impairment and "word deafness," as well as apraxia, asterognosia, and agraphesthesia, are frequently described. Gait disturbances with features of cerebellar and pyramidal tract involvement are often seen (Aubourg, 1996). Psychomotor development is normal until the onset of the first demyelinating lesion. On rare occasions, the disease may have a remitting course, which is not seen in adrenomyeloneuropathy (AMN) (Aubourg, 1996).

Adrenomyeloneuropathy usually manifests around the age of 20–30 years with an abnormal gait, paraparesis, and spasticity, as well as proprioceptive deficits and mild signs of neuropathy (Aubourg, 1996). Other symptoms include urinary difficulties and impotence. Cognitive function is usually normal, and there are no cerebellar or extrapyramidal signs. AI may be manifested clinically before the diagnosis of the disease or may be evident biochemically at the time of neurologic diagnosis (Aubourg, 1996). Clinically, patients may also show early balding and appear older than their chronological age. Other features include hypogonadism and testicular atrophy in males. Heterozygote females may also manifest the disease (Brian et al., 1984). ALD and AMN can be observed in the same family, and they clearly represent variants of the same disease (Aubourg, 1996).

Diagnosis

The first laboratory diagnosis of ALD and AMN is based on measurement of plasma VLCFA. All affected and asymptomatic males have markedly elevated C26:0 levels with an increased ratio of C24:0/C22:0 and C26:0/C22:0. Very rarely, patients may have normal levels of C26, but all have abnormal ratios (Spurek et al., 2004). These assays should be performed in all males with idiopathic AD and in patients with undiagnosed progressive paraparesis. No correlation exists between absolute levels of VLCFA and the degree of neurologic involvement. Heterozygous female carriers may also have elevated VLCFA, but false-negative tests

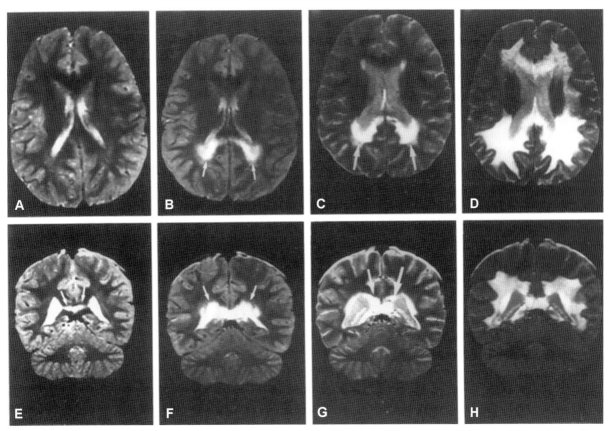

Fig. 50.8. T2-weighted MRI scans showing the progression of demyelinating lesions in an occipital cerebral form of adrenoleukodystrophy (ALD) over the course of 4 years in a 6-year-old boy with ALD. Demyelination initially struck the splenium of the corpus callosum (**E**, arrows). The patient developed neuropsychological deficits associated with the progress of the demyelinating lesions. (Reproduced from Aubourg, 1996, with permission.)

occur in 20%, and DNA sequencing analysis is recommended for diagnosis (Moser et al., 2005a). Once a mutation is identified, other family members can be rapidly tested for the presence of the same mutation. Prenatal diagnosis can be made by measuring VLCFA levels in cultured amniocytes and chorionic villus cells, but this should be confirmed by DNA analysis (Moser and Moser, 1999).

The cerebrospinal fluid (CSF) in patients with ALD shows marked elevation of protein content and may demostrate increased immunoglobulin secretion, with the presence of oligoclonal bands similar to MS. The CSF, however, is usually normal in AMN.

MRI in ALD characteristically shows involvement of the occipital lobes and the splenium and genu of the corpus callosum. The lesions may also involve the corticospinal tracts (Fig. 50.9A) and frontal lobes. Later, there is evidence of hydrocephalus (Fig. 50.10). In AMN, the brain MRI can be normal. The spinal cord shows mainly atrophy (Fig. 50.9B), although in some patients central demyelination is also observed (Spurek et al., 2004; Moser et al., 2005b).

Visual evoked potentials (VER) may be normal initially in ALD, but then become abnormal when the occipital and parietal white matter is severely affected. Brainstem auditory evoked reponse (BAER) abnormalities may be present after 10 years of disease without demyelinating lesions being seen on MRI. Severely delayed wave V bilaterally, as well as delayed III–V and I–V interpeak latencies, can be found (Bhuwan et al., 1983; Aubourg, 1996). Somatosensory evoked potentials may show large parietal waves with delayed N11–P14 and P14–N20 interpeak latencies bilaterally (Bhuwan et al., 1983). The EEG shows slowing of posterior waves, particularly when there is a clinical manifestation of occipital lobe involvement (Mamoli et al., 1979).

In AMN, the VERs are usually normal. BAER abnormalities are found more frequently than in ADL, with delayed I–V interpeak latency. Somatosensory evoked potential abnormalities may be similar to those with ALD (Aubourg, 1996). Motor nerve conduction velocities are slow in the legs. Low amplitude and slow velocities are detected in sensory conduction studies.

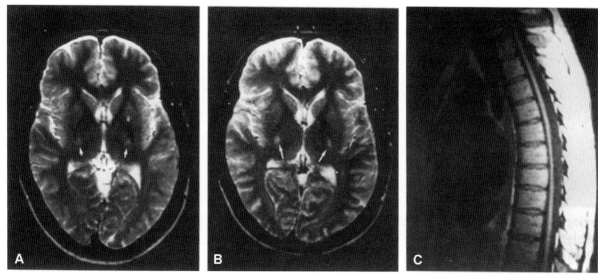

Fig. 50.9. Weight MRI scans showing intensity of the posterior internal capsules (**A**, arrows) and abnormal intensity of pyramidal tracts in posterior internal capsules of a case of adrenomyeloneuropathy (**B**, arrows). Spinal cord atrophy is shown in (**C**). (Reproduced from Aubourg, 1996, with permission.)

Pathological findings in ALD consist of demyelination, with loss of oligodendrocytes and reactive glyosis, and PAS-positive macrophage and mononuclear cells, some in the perivascular areas. Inflammation is usually found around demyelination foci.

Pathological findings in AMN affect mainly the spinal cord. There is loss of myelin in axons with a distal axonopathy pattern involving mainly the corticospinal tracts. In some patients, cerebral demyelination may be similar to ALD (Aubourg, 1996). Sural nerve biopsies in AMN show loss of small and large myelinated fibers with endoneural fibrosis, and sometimes trilamellar bodies are seen in Schwann cells (Powers and Schaumburg, 1974).

After diagnosis, patients should be evaluated regularly and monitored for adrenal insufficiency. Testing is done by measuring serum ACTH levels and, if necessary, the ACTH stimulation test.

Treatment

Because most patients with ALD and AMN develop adrenal insufficiency, corticosteroid replacement is critical. Hydrocortisone, 10–40 mg a day in divided doses, is usually given. Testosterone replacement may also be helpful. Treatment of spasticity, physical therapy, and mobilization are beneficial.

Lorenzo's oil has proven to be effective in preventing or delaying the onset in asymptomatic boys with ALD and may be beneficial in patients with AMN. The oil is a 4:1 mixture of two long chain fatty acids, glyceryl tioleate and glyceryl trierucate. These fatty acids inhibit endogenous VLCFA synthesis. When patients take this medication orally in a dosage of 1 mL/kg per day along with a low VLCFA diet, the level of VLCFA normalizes (Aubourg, 1996). Because of this, it was thought that this form of treatment might slow the progression of the disease and decrease MRI abnormalities. Unfortunately, different trials concluded that Lorenzo's oil did not benefit symptomatic ALD patients (Aubourg et al., 1993; Korenke et al., 1995; van Geel et al., 1999). However, Moser et al. (2005b) found that 74% of asymptomatic ALD boys had normal neurologic and MRI examinations after 7 years of treatment with Lorenzo's oil; 24% had abnormal MRI, and 11% developed clinical and radiological abnormalities. For this reason, it is recommended that this form of treatment be used early in asymptomatic ALD patients.

The only treatment shown to produce clear benefit in early symptomatic X-ALD is hematopoetic stem cell therapy. With this approach, 50–75% of boys show improvement or stabilization in clinical and/or radiological findings (Loes et al., 1994; Shapiro et al., 2000; Aubourg, 2007). This is a risky procedure with a mortality of about 10–20%, and risk versus benefit assessment should be carefully considered, particularly in patients with severe cerebral inflammation on MRI. Bone marrow transplantation may also be a good optional therapy in AMN patients (Lloyd and Chaudhry, 2011).

Other drugs that have been tried for patients with ALD and AMN include lovastatin, 4-phenylbutyrate, and compounds that upregulate the expression of ABCD2 protein, which potentially compensates for the loss of ABCD1 (Lloyd and Chaudhry, 2011).

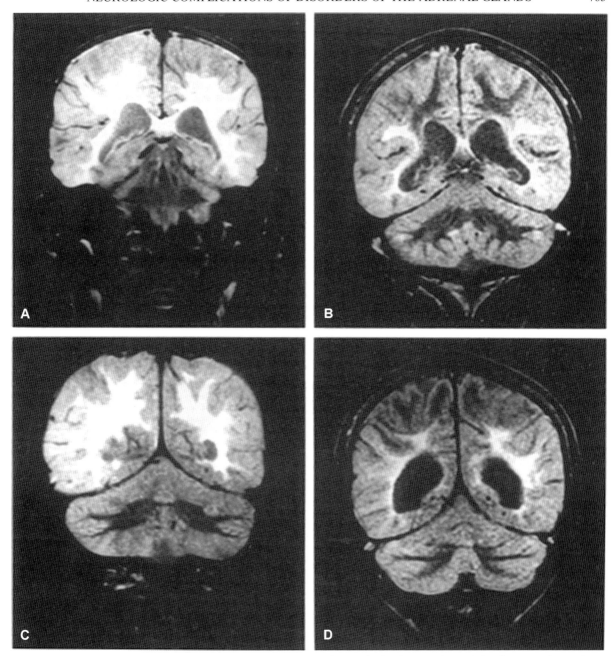

Fig. 50.10. T2-weighted MRI scans showing the progression of ventricular dilation in "chronic" occipital form over 4 years in an 11-year old boy with adrenoleukodystrophy. Although the demyelinating lesions made little progress from figures (**A**) and (**B**) to figures (**C**) and (**D**), the patient developed significant neuropsychological deterioration. (Reproduced from Aubourg, 1996, with permission.)

HYPERALDOSTERONISM

Hyperaldosteronism is defined as a state of selective increase of mineralocorticoid secretion by a primary disorder of the zona glomerulosa of the adrenal glands. Hyperaldosteronism is relatively uncommon and may be caused by adrenal hyperplasia, or less commonly by an adenoma or carcinoma.

Historical aspects

In 1943, during World War II, because acclimatization to tropical heat was a major military concern in the South Pacific, Dr. Jerome W. Conn investigated the regulation of salt loss among people exposed to elevated heat and humidity. He established that the acclimatization response involved diminished renal, sweat, and salivary excretion of sodium and water, and suggested that this was due to increased adrenocortical function with excessive production of salt-retaining steroids (Loriaux, 2008).

In 1954, Conn described a patient with a 7 year history of muscle spasms, tetany, weakness, arterial hypertension, severe hypokalemia, mild hypernatremia, and alkalosis, with no findings of an excess of glucocorticoids or androgens. Elevated urinary excretion of mineralocorticoids confirmed his suspicions that this patient had an excess secretion of the adrenal salt-retaining corticoid. Conn called this new clinical syndrome primary aldosteronism (Conn et al., 1964).

Etiology

Primary hyperaldosteronism is caused by aldosterone-secreting adenomas or carcinomas, bilateral adrenal hyperplasia (idiopathic hyperaldosteronism), or primary unilateral adrenal hyperplasia (Larsen et al., 2003). Familial hyperaldosteronism (FH) is a rare autosomal dominant disorder with two typical presentations. Type I is associated with different degrees of hyperaldosteronism and high levels of hybrid steroids (e.g., 18-hydroxycortisol and 18-oxocortisol) and responds to exogenous glucocorticoid administration. Clinical features of type I hyperaldosteronism include hypertension, weakness, failure to thrive, and increased incidence of intracranial aneurysms (Spoto et al., 2004). Type II hyperaldosteronism is not suppressed by glucocorticoids; patients have an aldosterone-producing adenoma, bilateral idiophatic hyperaldosteronism, or both (Spoto et al., 2004).

Secondary hyperaldosteronism results from overactivation of the renin–angiotensin system, and occurs in patients with severe accelerated hypertension, renovascular hypertension, estrogen administration, renin-secreting tumors, and Bartter syndrome. The latter is a rare disorder causing hypokalemia, metabolic alkalosis, hyperrenininemia, hyperaldosteronism, and hyperplasia of the juxtaglomerular apparatus (Bertorini et al., 2008). Kearns–Sayre syndrome may also cause hyperaldosteronism, hypokalemic alkalosis, and symptoms similar to Bartter syndrome (Emma et al., 2006). Other causes of hyperaldosteronism include potassium sodium-wasting nephropathy, renal tubular acidosis, diuretic or laxative abuse, and chronic edematous state. Congenital absence of adrenal enzymes such as 11β-hydroxylase, 17α-hydroxylase, and 11β-hydroxysteroid dehydrogenase, as well as administration of licorice, carbenoxolone, fludrocortisone or other steroids, are other unusual causes of hyperaldosteronism (Larsen et al., 2003).

Clinical manifestations

Hyperaldosteronism manifests as hypertension, hypokalemia, and metabolic alkalosis. Mild hypokalemia causes fatigue, nocturia, and headaches. Severe hypokalemia results in polyuria, polydipsia, paresthesias, and sometimes temporary muscle weakness or a persistent myopathy (Bautista et al., 1979; Talib et al., 2004). Thus, hyperaldosteronism should be considered in patients presenting with muscle weakness associated with low potassium regardless of the degree of arterial hypertension. Patients may also complain of leg pain and develop tetany secondary to metabolic alkalosis manifesting with Trousseau or Chvostek signs (Fujihara et al., 1990). Other neurologic manifestations include a static tremor, encephalopathy, and syncope. Rarely, idiopathic intracranial hypertension may be associated with primary hyperaldosteronism (Weber et al., 2002). Ischemic optic neuropathy is an unusual association. Patients also may present with depression (Bertorini et al., 2008).

Diagnosis

The diagnosis of hyperaldosteronism is suspected in patients with arterial hypertension associated with hypokalemia and muscle weakness; particularly if not receiving diuretics. Diagnosis requires measurement of aldosterone and plasma renin activity (PRA) in the early morning hours. A serum aldosterone to PRA ratio > 20 ng/dL and a serum aldosterone level of over 15 ng/dL suggest the diagnosis of primary hyperaldosteronism (Larsen et al., 2003).

The second step in diagnosis consists of determining if the cause is an adrenal adenoma or bilateral adrenal hyperplasia. The postural challenge test is useful in this regard (Larsen et al., 2003). A baseline plasma aldosterone of < 20 ng/dL that increases upon standing suggests bilateral hyperplasia. With adenomas, baseline levels are over 20 ng/dL and decrease upon standing as a result of decreased stimulation of ACTH. After this test is performed, an abdominal CT scan or other imaging helps to localize the tumor (Larsen et al., 2003).

Treatment

The treatment of hyperaldosteronism consists of removal of the adenoma by laparoscopic adrenalectomy (Duncan et al., 2000). Ablative procedures using percutaneous acetic acid injection may also be effective for unilateral adenomas (Minowada et al., 2003). This approach may cause marked reduction of aldosterone secretion with orthostatic hypotension (Milsom et al., 1986). Hypertension may persist after treatment in as many as 40–65% of patients, likely caused by nephrosclerosis after a prolonged period of uncontrolled hypertension (Milsom et al., 1986; Horito et al., 2001; Larsen et al., 2003).

Mineralocorticoid receptor antagonists, such as spironolactone and eplerenone, may be used to normalize blood pressure and serum potassium levels, especially in patients with idiopathic hyperaldosteronism (Brown et al., 1972; Lim et al., 2001). If patients fail to tolerate any of these treatments, the potassium-sparing diuretic amiloride can be used. Amiloride has been shown to reduce the systolic and diastolic blood pressure values and increase plasma potassium levels (Griffing et al., 1982). Hydrochlorothiazide can be added for better control of arterial hypertension.

DISORDERS OF THE ADRENAL MEDULLA

The adrenal medulla is the area of the adrenal gland that produces catecholamines from secreting cells called chromaffin cells or pheochromocytes because they stain brown with chromium salts. Tumors affecting the adrenal medulla cause increased secretion of norepinephrine and epinephrine, and are called pheochromocytomas. Pheochromocytomas are rare tumors that can be single or multiple, benign or malignant.

Historical aspects

The association between adrenal medullary tumors and their symptom spectrum was first noticed by Fränkel in 1886, when he described a patient who had intermittent attacks of palpitations, anxiety, vertigo, headaches, and chest pain, as well as cold sweats and vomiting. When this patient died, her autopsy showed bilateral adrenal tumors (Frankel, 1984).

The name pheochromocytoma was proposed by Pick in 1912 (Larsen et al., 2003). This term comes from the Greek words *phaios* ("dusky") and *chroma* ("color"). In 1926, Roux in Switzerland and Charles Mayo in Rochester performed successful surgical removal of adrenal pheochromocytomas (Larsen et al., 2003). In 1929, it was discovered that pheochromocytomas contained an excess of a pressor substance (Manger and Gifford, 1996); subsequently, catecholamines were isolated from these tumors (Manger and Gifford, 1996).

Etiology

Catecholamine-secreting tumors arising from the adrenal medulla are called pheocromocytomas. Those tumors arising in the sympathetic ganglia are called extra-adrenal paragangliomas (Lloyd et al., 2004). Both have similar clinical presentations and are treated similarly.

A number of genetic conditions associated with pheochromocytomas have been described:

- *Multiple endocrine neoplasia type 2A* (MEN 2A), or *Sipple syndrome*, is an autosomal dominant disease characterized by primary hyperparathyroidism, medullary carcinoma of the thyroid, and bilateral pheochromocytomas (Marx, 2005; Peczkowska and Januszewic, 2005).

- *Multiple endocrine neoplasia type 2B* (MEN 2B) is also an autosomal dominant disorder and is phenotypically characterized by the association of pheochromocytomas, mucosal neuromas, and thickening of the optic nerves. Patients may also have intestinal ganglioneuromas. These tumors produce predominantly epinephrine and metanephrine (Carling, 2005; Marx, 2005; Peczkowska and Januszewicz, 2005).

- Many patients with MEN 2A or 2B have mutations of the *RET* proto-oncogene, and genetic testing for this mutation is now commercially available (Larsen et al., 2003).

- *Von Hippel–Lindau* disease is another autosomal dominant disorder. Which is characterized by the presence of paragangliomas, pheochromocytomas, retinal angiomas, cerebellar hemangioblastomas, renal and pancreatic cysts, and renal cell carcinomas. Most of these tumors produce predominantly norepinephrine and normetanephrine (Larsen et al., 2003).

- *Neurofibromatosis type 1* (NF1) is an autosomal dominant disease characterized by neurofibromas, optic nerve gliomas, sphenoid dysplasia, café au lait spots, iris hamartomas, and axillary/inguinal freckling. This disorder is caused by a mutation in the NF1 gene located on chromosome 17, which causes a decreased production of neurofibromin (Walther et al., 1999).

- *Familial paraganglioma* is an autosomal dominant disorder characterized by paragangliomas localized in the head and neck. These tumors are usually benign. Symptoms depend on their local invasion and degree of vascularization. Around 10% have a malignant evolution. Prognosis depends on the extension of the disease at the time of diagnosis (Larsen et al., 2003).

- Finally, other neurocutaneous disorders associated with catecholamine-secreting tumors include ataxia-telangiectasia, tuberous sclerosis complex, and Sturge–Weber syndrome.

Clinical manifestations

Stressful stimuli such as anesthesia, hypoglycemia, or heart attacks increase the secretion of catecholamines, which have a very active role in the cardiovascular system and metabolic processes, increasing heart rate, blood pressure, myocardial contractility and cardiac conduction abnormalities. Clinical characteristics of pheochromocytomas are related to the catecholamines effects. The most common is arterial hypertension, which can be severe and can be accompanied by headaches, palpitations, and diaphoresis (Bravo and Gifford, 1984).

Tumors secreting norepinephrine usually produce severe sustained hypertension, whereas those that secrete primarily epinephrine produce episodic hypertensive crises. Other symptoms include increased sweating, tremors, weakness, and anxiety associated with palpitations. The triad of episodic headaches, diaphoresis, and palpitations has a specificity of over 60% for pheochromocytomas (Stein and Black, 1991).

Angina, nausea, constipation, hyperglycemia, diabetes, hypercalcemia, Raynaud phenomena, and livedo reticularis may be present in some patients. Hypertensive crisis may be precipitated by minor surgical procedures.

Neurologic manifestations of pheochromocytoma are usually caused by changes in blood pressure, and include episodic headaches and sometimes ischemic or hemorrhagic cerebrovascular events (Eclavea et al., 1997; Lehmann et al., 1999; Dagartzikas et al., 2002). Musculoskeletal pain, sometimes with radiculopathies, can be caused by bone metastasis (Lynn et al., 1987). Rarely, patients may have seizures caused by either severe hypertension or strokes (Leiba et al., 2003). Recurrent syncopal episodes may result from hypotension due to downregulation of catecholamine receptors caused by chronic exposure to the neurotransmitter and to volume depletion secondary to inhibition of the renin–angiotensin system (Young, 1993).

Differential diagnosis of pheocromocytoma is very extensive and includes hyperthyroidism, anxiety, panic attacks, migraines, and drug abuse. Pheocromocytomas may also produce somatostatin and ACTH, causing symptoms resembling those in Cushing syndrome (Larsen et al., 2003).

Diagnosis

Diagnosis of catecholamine-secreting tumors is based on measurement of catecholamines, particularly plasma and urine metanephrines (Leiba et al., 2003). Measurements of other catecholamines, including normetanephrine, is also is useful.

Other disorders can raise levels of catecholamines and metanephrines, and they should be considered in the interpretation of the tests. These include withdrawal from medications or drugs (e.g., clonidine, alcohol), subarachnoid hemorrhage, migraine headaches, preeclampsia, and the use of medications such as tricyclic antidepressants, levodopa, buspirone, prochlorperazine, and acetaminophen (Young, 1993).

The clonidine suppression test is highly sensitive to distinguish between pheochromocytoma and other causes of increased plasma catecholamines. Clonidine is a centrally acting α-adrenergic receptor agonist that normally suppresses the release of catecholamines from neurons, but does not affect the secretion from tumors. Catecholamine and metanephrine are measured before and after clonidine (0.3 mg) is administered orally (Sjoberg et al., 1992). In patients with essential hypertension, their concentrations decrease significantly, while in patients with pheochromocytoma the concentrations do not change (Sjoberg et al., 1992; Eisenhofer et al., 2001, 2004). Imaging techniques are used to localize the tumor and include CAT scan, MRI, and particularly the radioactive iodine with metaiodobenzylguanidine scan (Ilias and Pacak, 2004; Brink et al., 2005).

Treatment

Treatment of pheocromocytomas consists of complete surgical resection of the tumors. Because sustained hypertension during and after surgery is the most serious complication, a careful preoperative and pharmacological preparation is crucial. Presurgical preparation includes administration of an α-adrenergic blocker (e.g., phenoxybenzamine) for control of blood pressure and prevention of arrhythmias. A β-adrenergic antagonist also is used after α-adrenergic blockade is obtained. Metyrosine (α-methylparatyrosine) is also used in this setting because it is a catecholamine synthesis inhibitor with antihypertensive properties. This should be used with caution and only when other agents have been ineffective. Treatment also includes acute management of hypertensive crisis with short-acting antihypertensive drugs (Larsen et al., 2003).

ACKNOWLEDGEMENTS

The authors would like to thank Dr. Joseph Fisher for reviewing the manuscript, Kay Daughterty for editorial help, and Cindy Culver for help in typing the manuscript.

REFERENCES

Addison T (1855). On the Constitutional and Local Effects of Disease of the Supra-Renal Capsules. Highley, London.

Al Sabri AM, Smith N, Busuttil A (1997). Sudden death due to auto-immune Addison's disease in a 12-year-old girl. J Legal Med 110: 278–280.

Anglin RE, Rosebush PI, Mazurek MF (2006). The neuropsychiatric profile of Addison's disease: revising a forgotten phenomenon. J Neuropsychiatry Clin Neurosci 18: 450–459.

Arlt W, Allolio B (2003). Adrenal insufficiency. Lancet 361: 1881–1893.

Aubourg P (1996). X-linked adrenoleukodystrophy. In: HW Moser (Ed.), Neurodystrophies and Neurolipidoses. Handbook of Clinical Neurology, vol. 22 (66). Elsevier, Amsterdam, pp. 447–483.

Aubourg P (2007). X-linked adrenoleukodystrophy. Ann Endocrinol (Paris) 68: 403–411.

Aubourg P, Adamsbaum C, Lavallard-Rousseau MC et al. (1993). A two-year trial of oleic and erucic acids. ("Lorenzo's oil") as treatment for adrenomyeloneuropathy. N Engl J Med 329: 745–752.

Bakaeen FG, Walkes JC, Reardon MJ (2005). Heparin-induced thrombocytopenia associated with bilateral adrenal hemorrhage after coronary artery bypass surgery. Ann Thorac Surg 79: 1388–1390.

Barbieri F, Filla A, Grossi D et al. (1982). Clinical and computerized tomographic study of a case of Schilder's disease. Acta Neurol (Napoli) 4: 57–61.

Bautista J, Gil-Neciga E, Gil-Peralta A (1979). Hypokalemic periodic paralysis in primary hyperaldosteronism: subclinical myopathy with atrophy of the type 2A muscle fibers as the most pronounced alteration. Eur Neurol 18: 415–420.

Benvenga S, Rodolico C, Trimarchi F et al. (2001). Endocrine evaluation for muscle pain. J R Soc Med 94: 405–407.

Berenbaum SA, Snyder E (1995). Early hormonal influences on childhood sex-typed activity and playmate preferences: implications for the development of sexual orientation. Dev Psychol 31: 31–42.

Berneis K, Staub JJ, Gessler A et al. (2002). Combined stimulation of adrenocorticotropin and compound-S by single dose metyrapone test as an outpatient procedure to assess hypothalamic–pituitary–adrenal function. J Clin Endocrinol Metab 87: 5470–5475.

Bertorini TE, Perez AS, Tammaa M (2008). Disorders of the adrenal glands and neuroendocrine tumors. In: J Biller (Ed.), The Interface of Neurology and Internal Medicine. Lippincott Williams and Wilkins, Philadelphia, pp. 482–496.

Betterle C, Dal Pra C, Mantero F et al. (2002). Autoimmune adrenal insufficiency and autoimmune polyendocrine syndromes: autoantibodies, autoantigens, and their applicability in diagnosis and disease prediction. Endocr Rev 23: 327–364.

Bhuwan PG, Omkar NM, William ED et al. (1983). Evoked response studies in patients with adrenoleukodystrophy and heterozygous relatives. Arch Neurol 40: 356–359.

Bishop MF (1949). The history of the discovery of Addison's disease. Proc R Soc Med 43 (October 26).

Bolton CF (2005). Neuromuscular manifestations of critical illness. Muscle Nerve 32: 140–163.

Bravo EL, Gifford RW (1984). Current concepts Pheochromocytoma: diagnosis, localization and management. N Engl J Med 311: 1298–1303.

Brian P, O'Neill MD, Hugo W et al. (1984). Adrenoleukodystrophy: clinical and biochemical manifestations in carriers. Neurology 34: 798–801.

Brink I, Hoegerle S, Klisch J et al. (2005). Imaging of pheochromocytoma and paraganglioma. Fam Cancer 4: 61–68.

Brown JJ, Davies DL, Ferriss JB et al. (1972). Comparison of surgery and prolonged spironolactone therapy in patients with hypertension, aldosterone excess, and low plasma renin. BMJ 2: 729.

Brown-Séquard CE (1856). Recherches expérimentales sur la psysiologie et la pathologie des capsules surrénales. Arch Gen Med 5: 385–401.

Budka H, Sluga E, Heiss WD (1976). Spastic paraplegia associated with Addison's disease: adult variant of adrenoleukodystrophy. J Neurol 213: 237–250.

Carey R (1997). The changing clinical spectrum of adrenal insufficiency. Ann Intern Med 127: 1103–1105.

Carling T (2005). Multiple endocrine neoplasia syndrome: genetic basis for clinical management. Curr Opin Oncol 17: 7–12.

Choy EH, Corkill MM, Gibson T et al. (1991). Isolated ACTH deficiency presenting with bilateral frozen shoulder. Br J Rheumatol 30: 226–227.

Coco G, Dal Pra C, Presotto F et al. (2006). Estimated risk for developing autoimmune Addison's disease in patients with adrenal cortex autoantibodies. J Clin Endocrinol Metab 91: 1637–1645.

Cohen SI, Marks IM (1961). Prolonged organic psychosis with recovery in Addison's disease. J Neurol Neurosurg Psychiatry 24: 366–368.

Conn JW, Knopf RF, Nesbit RM (1964). Clinical characteristics of primary aldosteronism from an analysis of 145 cases. Am J Surg 107: 159–172.

Cushing H (1932). The basophil adenomas of the pituitary body and their clinical manifestations (pituitary basophilism). Bull John Hopkins Hosp 50: 137–195.

Dagartzikas MI, Sprague K, Carter G et al. (2002). Cerebrovascular event, dilated cardiomyopathy, and pheochromocytoma. Pediatr Emerg Care 18: 33–35.

Danon MJ, Carpenter S (1991). Myopathy with thick filament (myosin) loss following prolonged paralysis with vecuronium during steroid treatment. Muscle Nerve 14: 1131–1139.

Danon MJ, Edinger J (1999). Steroid induced quadriplegic myopathy with selective thick filament loss: elevated proteasoma content suggestive of increased proteolysis of myosin (abstract). Neurology 52 (Suppl. 2): S123.

David N (1995). Cushing's syndrome. N Engl J Med 332: 791–803.

Di Giovanni S, Molon A, Broccolini A et al. (2004). Constitutive activation of MAPK cascade in acute quadriplegic myopathy. Ann Neurol 55: 195–206.

Dickstein G, Shechner C, Nicholson WE et al. (1991). Adrenocorticotropin stimulation test: effects of basal cortisol level, time of day, and suggested new sensitive low dose test. J Clin Endocrinol Metab 72: 773–778.

Dittmann RW, Kappes MH, Kappes ME et al. (1990). Congenital adrenal hyperplasia II: gender-related behavior and attitudes in female salt-wasting and simple-virilizing patients. Psychoneuroendocrinology 15: 421–434.

Dökmetas HS, Kilicli F, Korkmaz S et al. (2006). Characteristic features of 20 patients with Sheehan's syndrome. Gynecol Endocrinol 22: 279–283.

Dorin RI, Qualls CR, Crapo LM (2003). Diagnosis of adrenal insufficiency. Ann Intern Med 139: 194–204.

Duncan JL 3rd, Fuhrman GM, Bolton JS et al. (2000). Laparoscopic adrenalectomy is superior to an open approach to treat primary hyperaldosteronism. Am Surg 66: 932–935.

Eclavea A, Gagliardi JA, Jezior J et al. (1997). Phaeochromocytoma with central nervous system manifestations. Australas Radiol 41: 373–376.

Eekhoff EM, van der Lubbe PA, Breedveld FC (1998). Flexion contractures associated with a malignant neoplasm: "A Paraneoplastic Syndrome?". Clin Rheumatol 17: 157–159.

Eisenhofer G, Hunynh TT, Hiroi M et al. (2001). Understanding catecholamine metabolism as a guide to the biochemical diagnosis of pheochromocytoma. Rev Endocr Metab Disord 2: 297–311.

Eisenhofer G, Kipin IJ, Goldstein DS (2004). Catecholamine metabolism: a contemporary view with implications for physiology and medicine. Pharmacol Rev 56: 331–349.

Emma F, Pizzini C, Tessa A et al. (2006). "Bartter-like" phenotype in Kearns–Sayre syndrome. Pediatr Nephrol 21: 355–360.

Ernst M, Maheu FS, Schroth E et al. (2007). Amygdala function in adolescents with congenital adrenal hyperplasia: a model for the study of early steroid abnormalities. Neuropsychologia 45: 2104–2113.

Eustachius B (1774). Tabulae Anatomicae. In: B Lancicius (Ed.), Amsterdam.

Falorni A, Laureti S, Nikoshkov A et al. (1997). 21-hydroxylase autoantibodies in adult patients with endocrine autoimmune diseases are highly specific for Addison's disease Belgian Diabetes Registry. Clin Exp Immunol 107: 341–346.

Falorni A, Laureti S, De Bellis A et al. (2004). Italian Addison network study: update of diagnostic criteria for the etiological classification of primary adrenal insufficiency. J Clin Endocrinol Metab 89: 1598–1604.

Ferguson G, Irvin C, Cherniack R (1990). Effect of corticosteroids on respiratory musclehistopathology. Am Rev Respir Dis 142: 1047–1052.

Fiad TM, Kirby JM, Cunningham SK et al. (1994). The overnight single-dose metyrapone test is a simple and reliable index of the hypothalamic–pituitary–adrenal axis. Clin Endocrinol (Oxf) 40: 603–609.

Findling JW, Doppman JL (1994). Biochemical and radiologic diagnosis of Cushing's syndrome. Endocrinol Metab Clin North Am 23: 511–537.

Findling JW, Raff H, Aron DC (2004). The low-dose dexamethasone suppression test: a reevaluation in patients with Cushing's syndrome. J Clin Endocrinol Metab 89: 1222–1226.

Finucane FM, Liew A, Thornton E et al. (2008). Clinical insights into the safety and utility of the insulin tolerance test (ITT) in the assessment of the hypothalamo–pituitary–adrenal axis. Clin Endocrinol (Oxf) 69: 603–607.

Frankel F (1984). Classics in oncology A case of bilateral completely latent adrenal tumor and concurrent nephritis with changes in the circulatory system and retinitis, 1886. CA Cancer J Clin 34: 93–106.

Fujihara K, Miyoshi T, Yamaguchi Y et al. (1990). Tetany as a sole manifestation in a patient with Bartter's syndrome and successful treatment with indomethacin. Rinsho Shinkeigaku 30: 519–532.

Gambelunghe G, Falorni A, Ghaderi M et al. (1999). Microsatellite polymorphism of the MHC class I chain-related (MIC-A and MIC-B) genes marks the risk for autoimmune Addison's disease. J Clin Endocrinol Metab 84: 3701–3707.

Gonzalbez J, Villabona C, Ramon J et al. (2000). Establishment of reference values for standard dose short Synacthen test (250 microgram), low dose short Synacthen test (1 microgram) and insulin tolerance test for assessment of the hypothalamo–pituitary–adrenal axis in normal subjects. Clin Endocrinol (Oxford) 53: 199–204.

Gould E, Cameron HA, Daniels DC et al. (1992). Adrenal hormones suppress cell division in the adult rat dentate gyrus. J Neurosci 12: 3642–3650.

Griffin JW, Goren E, Schaumburg H (1977). Adrenomyeloneuropathy: a probable variant of adrenoleukodystrophy I Clinical and endocrinologic aspects. Neurology 27: 1107–1113.

Griffing GT, Aurecchia SA, Sindler BH et al. (1982). The effect of amiloride on the renin–aldosterone system in primary hyperaldosteronism and Bartter's syndrome. J Clin Pharmacol 22: 505–512.

Grinspoon SK, Biller BM (1994). Clinical review 62: laboratory assessment of adrenal insufficiency. J Clin Endocrinol Metab 79: 923–931.

Guo W, Burris TP, McCabe ER (1995). Expression of DAX-1, the gene responsible for X-linked adrenal hypoplasia congenital and hypogonadotropic hypogonadism, in the hypothalamic–pituitary–adrenal/gonadal axis. Biochem Mol Med 56: 8–13.

Harris GW (1948). Neural control of the pituitary gland. Physiol Rev 28: 139–179.

Hayashi Y, Hiyoshi T, Takemura T et al. (1989). Focal lymphocytic infiltration in the adrenal cortex of the elderly: immunohistological analysis of infiltrating lymphocytes. Clin Exp Immunol 77: 101–105.

Henkin RI (1970). The effects of corticosteroids and ACTH on sensory systems. Prog Brain Res 32: 270–294.

Henkin RU, Gill JR, Warmolts JR et al. (1963). Steroid-dependent increase of nerve conduction velocity in adrenal insufficiency. J Clin Invest 42: 941.

Henkin RI, Gill JR, Bartter FC (1973). Studies on taste thresholds in normal man and in patients with adrenal cortical insufficiency: the role of adrenal cortical steroids and of serum sodium concentration. J Clin Invest 42: 727–735.

Horita Y, Inenaga T, Nakahama H et al. (2001). Cause of residual hypertension after adrenalectomy in patients with primary aldosteronism. Am J Kidney Dis 37 (5): 884–889.

Huebner A, Elias L, Clark A (1999). ACTH resistance syndromes. J Pediatr Endocrinol Metab 12 (Suppl. 1): 277–293.

Husebye E, Lovas K (2009). Pathogenesis of primary adrenal insufficiency. Best Pract Res Clin Endocrinol Metab 23: 147–157.

Igarashi M, Belchis D, Suzuki K (1976). Fatty acid abnormality in adrenoleukodystrophy. J Neurochem 26: 851–860.

Ilias I, Pacak K (2004). Current approaches and recommended algorithm for the diagnostic localization of pheochromocytoma. J Clin Endocrinol Metab 89: 479–491.

Jennings CE, Owen CJ, Wilson V et al. (2005). A haplotype of the CYP27B1 promoter is associated with autoimmune Addison's disease but not with Graves' disease in a UK population. J Mol Endocrinol 34: 859–863.

Kaga M, Furushima W, Inagaki M et al. (2009). Early neuropsychological signs of childhood adrenoleukodystrophy (ALD). Brain Dev 31: 558–561.

Kelestimur F (2003). Sheehan's syndrome. Pituitary 6: 181–188.

Köhler B, Lin L, Ferraz-de-Souza B et al. (2008). Five novel mutations in steroidogenic factor 1 (SF1, NR5A1) in 46, XY patients with severe underandrogenization but without adrenal insufficiency. Hum Mutat 29: 59–64.

Korenke GC, Hunneman DH, Kohler J et al. (1995). Glyceroltrioleate/glyceroltrierucate therapy in 16 patients with X-chromosomal adrenoleukodystrophy/adrenomyeloneuropathy: effect on clinical, biochemical and neurophysiological parameters. Eur J Pediatr 154: 64–70.

Kriegel MA, Lohmann T, Gabler C et al. (2004). Defective suppressor function of human CD4+CD25+ regulatory T cells in autoimmune polyglandular syndrome type II. J Exp Med 199: 1285–1291.

Lacomis D, Giuliani MJ, Van Cott A et al. (1996). Acute myopathy of intensive care: clinical, electrommyographic and pathological aspects. Ann Neurol 40: 645–654.

Larsen PR, Kronenberg HM, Melmed S (Eds.), (2003). The Adrenal Cortex, and Endocrine Hypertension. Williams Textbook of Endocrinology. Saunders, Philadelphia, pp. 491–585.

Laureti S, Aubourgh P, Calcinaro F et al. (1998). Etiological diagnosis of primary adrenal insufficiency using an origin flowchart of immune and biochemical markers. J Clin Endocrinol Metab 83: 3163–3168.

Lehmann H, Nair NPV, Kline NS (1979). Beta-endorphin and naloxone in psychiatric patients: clinical and biological effects. Am J Psychiatry 136: 762–766.

Lehmann FS, Weiss P, Ritz R et al. (1999). Reversible cerebral ischemia in patients with pheochromocytoma. J Endocrinol Invest 22: 212–214.

Leiba A, Bar-Dayan Y, Leker RR et al. (2003). Seizures as a presenting symptom of pheochromocytoma in a young solider. J Hum Hypertens 17: 73–75.

Lever EG, Stansfeld SA (1983). Addison's disease, psychosis, and the syndrome of inappropriate secretion of ADH. Br J Psychiatry 143: 406–410.

Li CH, Simpson ME, Evans HM (1943). Adrenocorticotrophic hormone. J Biol Chem 149: 413–424.

Lim PO, Young WF, MacDonald TM (2001). A review of the medical treatment of primary aldosteronism. J Hypertens 19: 353–361.

Lindstrom LH, Widerlov E, Gunne LM et al. (1978). CSF: clinical correlations to some psychotic states. Acta Psychiatr Scand 57: 153–164.

Lloyd TE, Chaudhry V (2011). Treatment and management of hereditary neuropathies. In: TE Bertorini (Ed.), Neuromuscular Disorders: Treatment and Management. Elsevier, Philadelphia, pp. 191–213.

Lloyd RV, Tischer AS, Kimura N et al. (2004). Adrenal tumors: introduction. In: RA DeLellis, RV Lloyd, PU Heitz et al. (Eds.), World Health Organization Classification of Tumours: Pathology and Genetics of Tumours of Endocrine Organs. International Agency for Research on Cancer Press, Lyons, France, pp. 136–138.

Loes DJ, Stillman AE, Hite S et al. (1994). Childhood cerebral form of adrenoleukodystrophy: short-term effect of bone marrow transplantation on brain MR observations. AJNR Am J Neuroradiol 15: 1767–1771.

Lopez ER, Zwermann O, Segni M et al. (2004). A promoter polymorphism of the CYP27B1 gene is associated with Addison's disease, Hashimoto's thyroiditis, Graves' disease and type 1 diabetes mellitus in Germans. Eur J Endocrinol 151: 193–197.

Loriaux LD (2008). Jerome W Conn (1907–1994) Historical note. Endocrinologist 18: 159–160.

Lovas K, Husebye ES, Holsten F et al. (2003). Sleep disturbances in patients with Addison's disease. Eur J Endocrinol 148: 449–456.

Lynn MD, Braunstein EM, Shaprio B (1987). Pheochromocytoma presenting as musculoskeletal pain from bone metastases. Skeletal Radiol 16: 552–555.

McFarland HR (1963). Addison's disease and related psychoses. Compr Psychiatry 4: 90–95.

McNeill TH, Masters JN, Finch CE (1991). Effect of chronic adrenalectomy on neuron loss and distribution of sulfated glycoprotein-2 in the dentate gyrus of prepubertal rats. Exp Neurol 111: 140–144.

Mamoli B, Graf M, Toifl K (1979). EEG, pattern-evoked potentials and nerve conduction velocity in a family with adrenoleukodystrophy. Electroencephalogr Clin Neurophysiol 47: 411–419.

Manger WM, Gifford RW (1996). Background and importance and diagnosis. In: WM Manger, RW Gifford (Eds.), Clinical and Experimental Pheochromocytoma. 2nd edn Blackwell Science, Cambridge, pp. 1–7, 205–332.

Marx SJ (2005). Molecular genetics of multiple endocrine neoplasia types 1 and 2. Nat Rev Cancer 5: 367–375.

Mauri M, Sinforiani E, Bono G et al. (1993). Memory impairment in Cushing's disease. Acta Neurol Scand 87: 52–55.

Mayenknecht J, Diederich S, Bahr V et al. (1998). Comparison of low and high dose corticotropin stimulation tests in patients with pituitary disease. J Clin Endocrinol Metab 83: 1558–1562.

Medvei VC (1991). The history of Cushing's disease: a controversial tale. J R Soc Med 84: 363–366.

Meyer-Bahlburg HE (2011). Brain development and cognitive, psychosocial, and psychiatric functioning in classical 21-hydroxylase deficiency. Endocr Dev 20: 88–95.

Michiels C (2004). Physiological and pathological responses to hypoxia. Am J Pathol 164: 1875–1882.

Milsom SR, Espiner EA, Nicholls MG et al. (1986). The blood pressure response to unilateral adrenalectomy in primary hyperaldosteronism. QJM 61: 1141–1151.

Minowada S, Fujimura T, Takahashi N et al. (2003). Computed tomography-guided percutaneous acetic acid injection therapy for functioning adrenocortical adenoma. J Clin Endocrinol Metab 88: 5814–5817.

Mizoguchi K, Ishige A, Takeda S et al. (2004). Endogenous glucocorticoids are essential for maintaining prefrontal cortical cognitive function. J Neurosci 24: 5492–5499.

Momose KJ, Killberg RN, Kilman B (1971). High incidence of cortical atrophy of the cerebral and cerebellar hemispheres in Cushing's disease. Radiology 99: 341–348.

Moritz ML, Ayus CJ (2003). The pathophysiology and treatment of hyponatraemic encephalopathy: an update. Nephrol Dial Transplant 18: 2486–2491.

Moser AB, Moser HW (1999). The prenatal diagnosis of X-linked adrenoleukodystrophy. Prenat Diagn 19: 46–48.

Moser HW, Moser A, Powers JM et al. (1982). The prenatal diagnosis of adrenoleukodystrophy Demonstration of increased hexacosanoic acid levels in cultured amniocytes and fetal adrenal gland. Pediatr Res 16: 172–175.

Moser HW, Moser AE, Trojak JE et al. (1983). Identification of female carriers of adrenoleukodystrophy. J Pediatr 103: 54–59.

Moser HW, Raymond GV, Dubey P (2005a). Adrenoleukodystrophy: new approaches to a neurodegenerative disease. JAMA 294: 3131–3134.

Moser HW, Raymond GV, Lu SE et al. (2005b). Follow-up of 89 asymptomatic patients with adrenoleukodystrophy treated with Lorenzo's oil. Arch Neurol 62: 1073–1080.

Mosser J, Douar AM, Sarde CO et al. (1993). Putative X-linked adrenoleukodystrophy gene shares unexpected homology with ABC transporters. Nature 361: 726–730.

Myhre AG, Undlien DE, Lovas K et al. (2002). Autoimmune adrenocortical failure in Norway autoantibodies and human leukocyte antigen class II associations related to clinical features. J Clin Endocrinol Metabol 23: 618–623.

Myhre AG, Aarsetoy H, Undlien DE et al. (2003). High frequency of celiac disease among patients with autoimmune adrenocortical failure. Scand J Gastroenterol 38: 511–515.

Nakamagoe K, Ohkoshi N, Ishii A et al. (1994). Syndrome of contracture facio-brachio-abdomino-crurale en flexion in a case of isolated ACTH deficiency – biopsy findings of muscle and nerve. Rinsho Shinkeigaku 34: 250–254.

Nass R, Heier L, Moshang T et al. (1997). Magnetic resonance imaging in the congenital adrenal hyperplasia population: increased frequency of white-matter abnormalities and temporal lobe atrophy. J Child Neurol 12: 181–186.

Nejentsev S, Howson JM (2007). Localization of type 1 diabetes susceptibility to the MHC class I genes HLA-B and HLA-A. Nature 450: 887–892.

Nerup J, Andersen V, Bendixen G (1969). Anti-adrenal, cellular hypersensitivity in Addison's disease. Clin Exp Immunol 4: 355–363.

Nerup J, Andersen V, Bendixen G (1970). Anti-adrenal cellular hypersensitivity in Addison's disease IV In vivo and in vitro investigations on the mitochondrial fraction. Clin Exp Immunol 6: 733–739.

Nieman LK (2013a). Clinical Manifestations of Cushing's Syndrome. In: UpToDate, BD Rose (Eds.), UpToDate. Copyright @ 2007 UptoDate, Inc, Waltham, MA.

Nieman LK (2013b). Establishing the Diagnosis of Cushing's Syndrome. In: UpTo Date, BD Rose (Eds.), UpToDate. Copyright @ 2007 UptoDate, Inc, Waltham, MA.

Nieman LK (2013c). Establishing the Cause of Cushing's Syndrome. In: UpTo Date, BD Rose (Eds.), UpToDate. Copyright @ 2007 UptoDate, Inc, Waltham, MA.

Nieman LK (2013d). Clinical Manifestations of Adrenal Insufficiency in adults. In: A Lacroix, KA Martin (Eds.), Copyright 2013, UptoDate, Inc, Waltham, MA.

Nishikawa T (2003). Flexion contractures possibly reflect the existence of hypocortisolism (editorial). Intern Med 42: 629–631.

Odagaki T, Noguchi Y, Fukui T (2003). Flexion contractures of the legs as the initial manifestation of adrenocortical insufficiency. Intern Med 42: 710–713.

Osler W (1896). On six cases of Addison's disease with the report of a case greatly benefited by the use of suprarenal extract. Internat Med Mag 5: 3–11.

Pani MA, Seissler J, Usadel KH et al. (2002). Vitamin D receptor genotype is associated with Addison's disease. Eur J Endocrinol 147: 635–640.

Peczkowska M, Januszewicz A (2005). Multiple endocrine neoplasia type 2. Fam Cancer 4: 25–36.

Piedrola G, Casado JL, Lopez E et al. (1996). Clinical features of adrenal insufficiency in patients with acquired immunodeficiency syndrome. Clin Endocrinol (Oxf) 45: 97–101.

Powers JM, Schaumburg HH (1973). The adrenal cortex in adreno-leukodystrophy. Arch Pathol 96: 305–310.

Powers JM, Schaumburg HH (1974). Adrenoleukodystrophy: similar ultrastructural changes in adrenal cortical and Schwann cells. Arch Neurol 30: 406–408.

Presotto F, Fornasini F, Betterle C et al. (2005). Acute adrenal failure as the heralding symptom of primary antiphospholipid syndrome: report of a case and review of the literature. Eur J Endocrinol 153: 507–514.

Rajathurai A, Chazan BI, Jeans JE (1983). Self-mutilation as a feature of Addison's disease. Br Med J 287: 1027.

Raux-Demay MC, Girard F (1985). The physiology of corticotropin-releasing factor (CRF). Reprod Nutr Dev 25: 931–943.

Reutens AT, Achermann JC, Ito M et al. (1999). Clinical and functional effects on mutations in the DAX-1 gene in patients with adrenal hypoplasia congenital. J Clin Endocrinol Metab 84: 504–511.

Reynolds RM, Stewart PM, Seckl JR et al. (2006). Assessing the HPA axis in patients with pituitary disease: a UK survey. Clin Endocrinol (Oxf) 64: 82–85.

Romney SJ, Chik LC (2001). Frozen shoulders: an endocrine disease? A case report of isolated ACTH deficiency. Endocrinologist 11: 429–431.

Salvatori R (2005). Adrenal insufficiency. JAMA 294: 2481–2488.

Sanaker PS, Husebye ES, Fondenes O et al. (2007). Clinical evolution of Kearns–Sayre syndrome with polyendocrinopathy and respiratory failure. Acta Neurol Scand Suppl 187: 64–67.

Sauter NP, Toni R, McLaughlin CD et al. (1990). Isolated adrenocorticotropin deficiency associated with autoantibody to a corticotroph antigen that is not adrenocorticotropin or other proopiomelanocortin-derived peptides. J Clin Endocrinol Metab 70: 1391–1397.

Sawczuk IS, Reitelman C, Libby C et al. (1986). CT findings in Addison's disease caused by tuberculosis. Urol Radiol 8: 44–45.

Schaumburg HH, Powers JM, Raine CS et al. (1975). Adrenoleukodystrophy: a clinical and pathological study of 17 cases. Arch Neurol 32: 577–591.

Shapiro E, Krivit W, Lockman L et al. (2000). Long-term effect of bone-marrow transplantation for childhood-onset cerebral X-linked adrenoleukodystrophy. Lancet 356: 713–718.

Sjarif DR, Ploos van Amstel JK, Duran M et al. (2000). Isolated and contiguous glycerol kinase gene disorders: a review. J Inherit Metab Dis 23: 529–547.

Sjoberg RJ, Simcic KJ, Kidd GS (1992). The clonidine suppression test for pheochromocytoma A review of its utility and pitfalls. Arch Intern Med 152: 1193–1197.

Skinningsrud B, Husebye ES, Gervin K et al. (2008). Mutation screening of PTPN22: association of the 1858T-allele with Addison's disease. Eur J Hum Genet 16: 977–982.

Sloviter RS, Sollas AL, Dean E et al. (1993). Adrenalectomy-induced granule cell degeneration in the rat hippocampal dentate gyrus: characterization of an in vivo model of controlled neuronal death. J Comp Neurol 330: 324–336.

Smith CM (1958). Paranoid behavior in Addison's disease: report of a case. Can Psychiatr Assoc J 3: 145–154.

Speiser PW, White PC (2003). Congenital adrenal hyperplasia. N Engl J Med 349: 776–788.

Spoto B, Furlo G, Gervasi A et al. (2004). Familial hyperaldosteronism. G Ital Nefrol 21: 139–143.

Spurek M, Taylor-Gjevre R, Van Uum S et al. (2004). Adrenomyeloneuropathy as a cause of primary adrenal insufficiency and spastic paraparesis. CMAJ 171: 1073–1077.

Starkman MN, Gebarski SS, Berent S et al. (1992). Hippocampal formation volume, memory dysfunction, and cortisol levels in patients with Cushing's syndrome. Biol Psychiatry 32: 756–765.

Stein PP, Black HR (1991). A simplified diagnostic approach to pheochromocytoma: a review of the literature and report of one institution's experience. Medicine 70: 46–66.

Steinpresis RE (1996). The behavioral and neurochemical effects of phencyclidine in humans and animals: some implications for modeling psychosis. Behav Brain Res 74: 45–55.

Stewart PM (2003). The adrenal cortex. In: PR Larsen, HM Kronenberg, S Melmed, KS Polonski (Eds.), Williams Textbook of Endocrinology. Saunders, Philadelphia, pp. 491–585.

Syriou V, Moisidis A, Tamouridis N et al. (2008). Isolated adrenocorticotropin deficiency and flexion contractures syndrome. Hormones 7: 320–324.

Talib A, Mahmood K, Jairmani KL et al. (2004). Hypokalemic quadriparesis with normotensive primary hyperaldosteronism. J Coll Physicians Surg Pak 14: 492–493.

Ten S, New M, Maclaren N (2001). Clinical review 130: Addison's disease 2001. J Clin Endocrinol Metabol 86: 2909–2922.

Thompson WF (1973). Psychiatric aspects of Addison's disease: report of a case. Med Ann Dist Columbia 42: 62–64.

Ubogu EE, Ruff RL, Kaminski HJ (1994). Endocrine myopathy. In: A Engel, C Franzizi-Armstrong (Eds.), Myopathy. McGraw-Hill, New York, pp. 1713–1738.

van Geel BM, Assies J, Haverkort E et al. (1999). Progression of abnormalities in adrenomyeloneuropathy and neurologically asymptomatic X-linked adrenoleukodystrophy despite treatment with "Lorenzo's oil". J Neurol Neurosurg Psychiatry 67: 290–299.

Varadaraj R, Cooper AJ (1986). Addison's disease presenting with psychiatric symptoms. Am J Psychiatry 143: 553–554.

Vendrame F, Segni M, Grassetti D et al. (2006). Impaired caspase-3 expression by peripheral T cells in chronic autoimmune thyroiditis and in autoimmune polyendocrine syndrome-2. J Clin Endocrinol Metabol 91: 5064–5068.

Walther MM, Herring JC, Enquist EE et al. (1999). von Recklinghausen's disease and pheochromocytoma: Literature review. J Urol 162: 1582–1586.

Weber KT, Singh KD, Hey JC (2002). Idiopathic intracranial hypertension with primary aldosteronism: report of 2 cases. Am J Med Sci 324: 45–50.

Winqvist O, Karlsson FA (1992). 21-Hydroxilase, a major autoantige in idiopathic Addison's disease. Lancet 339: 1559–1562.

Wolfgang O (1996). Adrenal insufficiency. N Engl J Med 335: 1206–1212.

Young WF Jr (1993). Pheocromocytoma 1926–1993. Trends Endocrinol Metab 4: 122–127.

Yu L (1999). DRB1*04 and DQ alleles: expression of 21-hydroxilase autoantibodies and risk of progression to Addison's disease. J Clin Endocrinol Metab 84: 328–335.

Zucker KJ, Bradley SJ, Oliver G et al. (1996). Psychosexual development of women with congenital adrenal hyperplasia. Horm Behav 30: 300–318.

Handbook of Clinical Neurology, Vol. 120 (3rd series)
Neurologic Aspects of Systemic Disease Part II
Jose Biller and Jose M. Ferro, Editors
© 2014 Elsevier B.V. All rights reserved

Chapter 51

Diabetic neuropathy

GERALD CHARNOGURSKY*, HONG LEE, AND NORMA LOPEZ
Division of Endocrinology and Metabolism, Loyola University Chicago, Stritch School of Medicine, Maywood, IL, USA

HISTORY AND EPIDEMIOLOGY

Diabetes mellitus (DM) is a disorder characterized by impaired carbohydrate, protein, and fat metabolism that is due to either the insufficient production of insulin in type 1 DM or to target tissue insulin resistance and impaired insulin response in type 2 DM. The American Diabetes Association estimates over 8.3% of the US population had diabetes in 2011 including both children and adults. The prevalence of diabetes varies depending on the type of diabetes and the age of the patients. The prevalence at any given time is likely underestimated given that type 2 DM and impaired glucose tolerance often remain undiagnosed for many years. Complications from diabetes include heart disease and stroke, blindness, kidney disease, neuropathy, and limb amputations. The American Diabetes Association estimated that the cost of treating the disease in 2007 was US$174 billion.

Peripheral diabetic neuropathy is defined as the presence of symptoms and or signs of peripheral nerve dysfunction in people with diabetes after other causes of the dysfunction have been excluded. Boulton and colleagues describe diabetic neuropathy as consisting of a minimum of two of the following abnormalities: symptoms, signs, nerve conduction abnormalities, quantitative sensory test results, or a quantitative autonomic test result. For clinical studies, they suggest a system requiring that one of the two abnormalities include quantitative test results or electrophysiology findings (Boulton et al., 2004, 2005).

Neuropathy resulting from diabetes is estimated to affect 60–70% of people with diabetes if mild to severe forms of nervous system damage are included. The prevalence varies among series depending on the definition used. Dyck and colleagues found that some form of neuropathy – peripheral or autonomic – was present in 66% of all diabetic patients in their series (Dyck et al., 1993) using a definition based on symptoms, signs, nerve conductions studies, sensory testing, and autonomic testing. Prevalence estimates vary due to differences

in age, duration of diabetes, the definition of neuropathy used, presence or absence of pain, and whether or not other forms of neuropathy are excluded. Prevalence of painful diabetic neuropathy is estimated to be 10–20% (Galer et al., 2000).

Prospective studies confirming the relationship between impaired glucose tolerance (IGT) and neuropathy are lacking but some studies suggest that IGT may lead to neuropathy. Prevalence of IGT varied from 34% to 56% in two studies of patients with idiopathic peripheral neuropathy, as high as three times the prevalence of age-matched controls with normal glucose tolerance (Sumner et al., 2003; Singleton and Smith, 2007). While some studies do suggest IGT is an important cause of polyneuropathy, other studies do not confirm this relationship, possibly due the disparity in patient populations, controls, and the assessment of glycemic exposure and diabetic complications (Dyck et al., 2007). The MONIKA/KORA Augsburg surveys S_2 and S_3 revealed polyneuropathy in 28% of diabetics, 13% of patients with impaired glucose tolerance, 11.3% of patient with impaired fasting glucose and 7.4% of subjects with normal glucose tolerance (Ziegler et al., 2008).

Diabetic autonomic neuropathy (DAN) prevalence also varies depending on the study, from as low as 8% in new type 1 diabetics (Ziegler et al., 1992) to as high as 80% and 90% in early type 2 diabetics and in insulin-dependent potential pancreas transplant recipients (Zhong et al., 1981; Kennedy et al., 1995). Differences in the definition of DAN, testing modalities, duration and type of diabetes, patient cohort and glycemic control are some of the confounders reported. Ziegler studied over 1000 diabetic patients from over 20 centers in Europe and found that 25% of type 1 and 34% of type 2 diabetics had abnormal findings in more than two out of six autonomic function tests (Ziegler et al., 1992).

Prevalence studies have found differences in neuropathic abnormalities according to ethnicity. Diabetic neuropathy in non-Hispanic whites compared to

*Correspondence to: Gerald Charnogursky, M.D., Division of Endocrinology and Metabolism, Loyola University Stritch School of Medicine, 2160 S. First Ave., Maywood, IL 60153, USA. Tel: +1-708-216-6252, Fax: +1-708-216-5936, E-mail: gcharno@lumc.edu

African Americans was 47% versus 37%, respectively, in one series ($p < 0.01$) (Cohen et al., 1998). The UKPDS trial showed an increase in prevalence in both male and female Caucasians compared to Asian and Afro-Caribbean, 13% versus 4% and 6%, respectively, for males and 6% versus 4% and 2%, respectively, for females ($p < 0.001$) (UKPDS, 1994). There was no difference in the prevalence among Hispanics and non-Hispanic whites in one study (Hamman et al., 1991).

CLASSIFICATION AND CLINICAL FINDINGS

Diabetic peripheral polyneuropathy is the most common neuropathy in diabetics, with a prevalence as high as 54% in type 1 DM and 45% in type 2 DM (Dyck et al., 1993). Mixed syndromes of diabetic neuropathy may account for the differences in classifications that have been developed.

Symmetric polyneuropathies can be divided into sensory or sensorimotor polyneuropathy, selective small fiber polyneuropathy, and autonomic neuropathy.

Sensory or sensorimotor polyneuropathy

Distal sensory neuropathy with an insidious onset is the most common neuropathy in diabetic patients. The earliest symptoms involve the toes and then ascend upward in a "stocking and glove" pattern of sensation loss, the distal portions of the longest nerves being the first affected. Patients describe numbness or tingling mainly of the toes and feet. Upper extremity involvement occurs less commonly, later, and is usually less severe. Pain may be one the dominant features. Bilateral foot pain may be described as sharp, stabbing, burning, or aching in character. Many patients describe a worsening of the pain at night. Weakness and gait ataxia due to sensory loss may be the predominant symptoms in some patients.

Neurologic examination demonstrates reduced or absent ankle jerks. There may be varying degrees of sensory loss and distal muscle weakness mainly of toe and foot dorsiflexion. Distal weakness is typically mild and a less common presentation. Impairment of vibration and joint position suggest large fiber neuropathy. Sensorimotor neuropathy has features of both axon loss and demyelization on electromyography (EMG). The earliest and most sensitive findings are a reduction in conduction velocity and a decrease in signal amplitude on the EMG. Complete disappearance of a sensory response may be seen as the neuropathy becomes more severe. Motor nerve studies may be abnormal showing some slowing of nerve conduction waves even in asymptomatic patients.

Selective small fiber polyneuropathy

Small fiber neuropathies are characterized by pain and diminished thermal and pain perception. The pain is described as burning, pricking, stabbing, jabbing, or a tight, band-like pressure. Patients often experience dysesthesias. The dysesthesias are more commonly and initially in the toes but may spread to the legs and upper extremities as well. Strength, vibration, proprioception, and tendon reflexes are preserved in small fiber polyneuropathy. Electromyography and nerve conduction studies are useful for following progression of small fiber syndromes but not diagnostically. Nerve conduction study abnormalities may appear if a large fiber component of the neuropathy develops and progresses. Testing of autonomic function and of thermal sensitivity is used to test small fiber function.

Autonomic neuropathy

Autonomic neuropathy is defined as subclinical or clinical depending on the absence or presence of overt symptoms. Diabetic autonomic neuropathy (DAN) can affect all parts of the autonomic nervous system. Signs and symptoms of DAN may manifest as cardiovascular, gastrointestinal, genitourinary, metabolic, sudomotor, or pupillary disturbances. The clinical manifestations of cardiovascular autonomic neuropathy include resting tachycardia, exercise intolerance, and orthostatic hypotension. Autonomic neuropathy affecting the gastrointestinal system may manifest as esophageal dysmotility, gastroparesis diabeticorum, constipation, diarrhea, or fecal incontinence. Neurogenic bladder, erectile dysfunction, retrograde ejaculation, and female sexual dysfunction are all some of the clinical manifestations of autonomic neuropathy affecting the genitourinary system. Metabolic derangements seen with autonomic neuropathy include hypoglycemia unawareness. Anhidrosis, heat intolerance, and gustatory sweating may be clinical manifestations of sudomotor dysfunction due to autonomic neuropathy (Vinik et al., 2003).

Cardiovascular autonomic neuropathy (CAN) can contribute to silent myocardial infarctions. Many studies have suggested that cardiovascular autonomic neuropathy may contribute to an increase in silent myocardial infarcts in diabetics compared to nondiabetics and increased mortality in these patients. A 27% mortality in diabetic patients with CAN compared with 8% in those without CAN ($p > 0.01$) was found in one study (Ewing et al., 1991). Another study found 40% mortality versus 4% in patients with and without CAN ($p < 0.01$) (Jermendy et al., 1991). Other investigators found mortality rates of 23–40% in patients with CAN compared to a rate of 3–12% in patients without

CAN (Rathmann et al., 1993; Navarro et al., 1996; Chen et al., 2001).

Investigations examining the association of CAN and mortality vary in the tests of autonomic function used, the definition of CAN, and the subjects studied, but overall they provide consistent evidence that there is an increase in mortality among diabetic individuals with CAN compared to diabetics without it One study found increased 10 year mortality in type 1 diabetics with CAN only in those with symptoms and not in asymptomatic individuals (Sampson et al., 1990).

Meta-analysis of 15 studies with follow-up from 1 to 16 years concluded that the pooled estimate of the relative risk of death based on 2900 subjects was 2.14 for subjects with CAN at baseline compared to those with a normal baseline assessment. On multivariate analysis CAN was the most important independent predictor of mortality, with a cumulative 5 year mortality increased over five fold in type 1 diabetics with cardiovascular autonomic neuropathy (Vinik et al., 2007). The causative relationship between CAN and mortality, however, remains speculative. Studies have given alternative possible explanations for the increased mortality in diabetics with CAN including increased occurrence of silent myocardial ischemia (Niakan et al., 1986), asymptomatic ischemia leading to lethal arrhythmias (Rathmann et al., 1993), impaired hypoglycemic awareness (O'Brien et al., 1991), and an increased occurrence of concomitant disorders and other diabetic complications (Orchard et al., 1996). Other studies have cited prolongation of the QT interval (Sampson et al., 1990) and interrelationships with other cardiovascular risk factors (Maser et al., 1990; Spallone et al., 1997).

Focal and multifocal neuropathies

Focal and multifocal neuropathies can be divided into cranial neuropathy, limb mononeuropathy (compression and entrapment neuropathies), trunk mononeuropathy, and asymmetric lower limb motor neuropathy (amyotrophy).

Cranial neuropathy

The most common cranial neuropathy in diabetics is a mononeuropathy involving the third cranial nerve presenting as sudden onset of double vision, drooping of one eyelid and/or pain in the head or behind the affected eye. Patients may exhibit dysconjugate gaze, with the affected eye deviating laterally, and impaired movement of the gaze medially and vertically. Pupil reaction may be normal or abnormal. Cranial neuropathies involving other nerves are less common. Bell's palsy appears to be more common in diabetics than in patients with normoglycemia (Gilden, 2004). A study of 126 patients with Bell's palsy revealed 39% had evidence of biochemical or overt diabetes (Pecket and Schattner, 1982). Patients with Bell's palsy may complain of weakness or paralysis of all the muscles on one side of the face. On examination, the facial crease and nasolabial fold and forehead furrow of the affected side disappear, the corner of the mouth droops, the eyelid may not close and the lower lid may sag. Impairment in taste is less common in diabetics compared to patients without diabetes which suggests that the lesion in diabetic facial nerve palsy is distal to the chorda tympani. The treatment of Bell's palsy in diabetics does not differ from the treatment in patients without diabetes except for caution if steroids are used given the risk of steroid-exacerbated hyperglycemia.

Limb mononeuropathy (compression and entrapment neuropathies)

There is an increased frequency of compression neuropathy such as carpal tunnel syndrome (CTS) in diabetic patients. Dyck et al. found that although only 9% of type 1 diabetics and 6% of type 2 diabetics were symptomatic, as many as 27% and 35% of type 1 and type 2 diabetics had electrophysiologic evidence of CTS (Dyck et al., 1993). Data analysis of a large registry in the UK of 2655 diabetic and prediabetic patients found that the incidence of CTS in patients with prediabetes was increased, with a relative risk of 1.63. CTS can precede the diagnosis of diabetes by up to 10 years (Gulliford et al., 2006).

A study to investigate frequency of symptomatic mononeuropathies in diabetic patients found that only focal limb neuropathies due to external compression appear to be more common. Of 642 consecutive patients with various acute symptomatic mononeuropathies, patients with radial, ulnar neuropathy and peroneal neuropathy had rates of diabetes significantly higher than those anticipated according to the frequency of diabetes in the general population (Stamboulis et al., 2005). In this study patients with CTS and Bell's palsy had rates of diabetes similar to the general population.

Trunk mononeuropathy

Diabetic truncal neuropathy usually occurs in older patients and presents as dysesthesia in one or more of the thoracic dermatomes or as radicular thoracic pain. Stewart described 17 episodes of diabetic truncal neuropathy among seven diabetic patients and found varying combinations of sensory deficits, including but not limited to dysesthesia of a complete dermatomal band, involvement of adjacent main spinal nerves, and most commonly deficits restricted to the distribution of the ventral and dorsal rami of the spinal nerves or branches of the rami (Stewart, 1989). A series of 15 new cases of diabetic thoracic radiculopathy describes patients presenting with severe abdominal pain or chest pain and often weight loss. This condition generally carried a good prognosis for recovery (Kikta et al., 1982).

Asymmetric lower limb motor neuropathy (amyotrophy)

Amyotrophy is an asymmetric lower limb motor neuropathy also known as diabetic lumbosacral plexus neuropathy and Bruns-Garland syndrome. Patients typically present with an asymmetric, painful muscle wasting and weakness affecting the lower limbs and loss of reflexes and objective weakness on examination. Patients may describe a sudden onset of sharp pain in the hip and thigh that can spread to the opposite side over weeks to months, generally in a stepwise and steady progression affecting both proximal and distal muscles (Barohn et al., 1991). Amyotrophy is more likely to affect middle to older aged patients. Electrodiagnostic studies are useful in ruling out other conditions that may account for the symptoms of amytrophy.

LABORATORY INVESTIGATIONS

Methodologies used in studies that define diabetic neuropathy vary considerably. Methods range from relying on symptoms to including neurologic exams and using more quantitative sensory testing.

Evaluation of sensory function includes thresholds for vibration, assessment of light touch, joint position, and pinprick. Feldman described a population-based study in which 66% of patients with diabetes exhibited a decline in vibratory sense of the feet over time which was associated with diabetic neuropathy morbidity including foot ulcerations, infections, and foot amputations (Feldman et al., 1994). Sequential examination of vibration, touch, joint position, and pinprick is a practical clinical approach for following individual patients. Kincaid and colleagues suggest that vibratory quantitative sensory testing and nerve conduction studies have a low to moderate correlation suggesting the tests do not replace one another but are complementary (Kincaid et al., 2007). Comparisons of the clanging tuning fork (CTF) test to the 10 g Semmes-Weinstein monofilament test found the tuning fork to be reproducible, accurate, and able to detect neuropathy even in the presence of a normal monofilament test (Oyer et al., 2007). These investigators recommended replacing the monofilament test with the CTF technique for detection of DPN.

Electrophysiologic tests are a sensitive, objective, and reproducible way of diagnosing and following diabetic neuropathy. A long-term follow-up of 114 patients with diabetic neuropathy reported significant correlations between neuropathy disability scores (NDS) and alterations in motor nerve conduction velocities (Negrin and Zara, 1995). Other studies have confirmed these findings (Onde et al., 2008). Electrophysiologic tests may be abnormal in asymptomatic patients, revealing early stages of neuropathy and subclinical involvement, and they help provide objective measures of diabetic neuropathy diagnosis and severity (Dyck et al., 1991, 1992).

Newer methods of screening for diabetic neuropathy have been reported. A new indicator test based on the measurement of sweat production after exposure to dermal foot perspiration had a sensitivity of 86% for detecting sensorimotor polyneuropathy and 80.9% for detecting autonomic neuropathy, with specificity of 67% and 50%, respectively (Liatis et al., 2007). Researchers have also investigated a new technique in assessing possible nerve fiber repair in type 1 diabetics after pancreas transplant using a noninvasive technique of corneal confocal microscopy and found that small fiber repair can be detected 6 months after transplant using this novel technique (Mehra et al., 2007). In a study using corneal confocal microscopy to evaluate 101 diabetic patients compared to 17 controls, investigators found corneal sensation, nerve fiber density and length, and nerve branch density all decreased with increased neuropathic severity and correlated with neuropathy disability scores (Tavakoli et al., 2010). The investigators conclude that corneal confocal microscopy may be a promising noninvasive tool in the detection of diabetic neuropathy.

RISK FACTORS

Epidemiologic studies have identified duration and severity of hyperglycemia as the major risk factors for the development of diabetic neuropathy in patients with both type 1 and type 2 diabetes (Genuth, 2006). The Diabetes Complications and Control Trial (DCCT) showed that intensive glycemic control reduced the prevalence of autonomic dysfunction by 53% and clinical neuropathy by 60-69% (DCCT Research Group, 1995). The European Diabetes (EURODIAB) Prospective Complications Study demonstrated that in addition to glycemic control and duration of diabetes, traditional markers of macrovascular disease appear to be important in the pathogenesis of diabetic peripheral neuropathy (DPN). A total of 1172 patients with type 1 diabetes mellitus and no baseline DPN were enrolled from 31 centers and followed for 7.3 years to study the risk factors for the development of DPN. The cumulative incidence of DPN was 23.5%. After adjusting for duration of diabetes and glycosylated hemoglobin, an association was observed between modifiable cardiovascular risk factors and incidence of DPN. DPN developed more frequently when patients had hypertension (odds ratio (OR), 1.92), elevated triglyceride levels (OR, 1.35), smoking (OR, 1.55), or obesity (OR, 1.4). Microvascular disease at baseline (e.g., albuminuria (OR, 1.48) and retinopathy (OR, 1.7)) was also associated with an increased incidence of DPN. Cardiovascular disease at baseline independently doubled the risk of neuropathy (OR, 2.74).

PATHOPHYSIOLOGY

Diabetic neuropathy occurs when there is an imbalance between nerve fiber damage and repair. The nerve damaging process preferentially affects autonomic and distal sensory fibers, leading to the progressive loss of sensation. Besides metabolic factors listed above, ischemic factors and inflammation also contribute to the development of diabetic neuropathies. Metabolic factors seem to prevail in length-dependent diabetic polyneuropathy, whereas inflammation superimposed on ischemic nerve lesions is found in severe forms of focal neuropathies. The thickening and hyalinization of the walls of small blood vessels due to the reduplication of the basal lamina around endothelial cells suggests a role for nerve ischemia in diabetic neuropathy. There is also a reduction in endoneurial oxygen tension in the sural nerves of diabetic patients with advanced polyneuropathy (Newrick, 1986).

Possible mechanisms for neuropathy development include oxidative stress, nonenzymatic glycation, the polyol pathway, the hexosamine pathway, protein kinase C pathway, poly (ADP-ribose) polymerase and the reduction of neurotrophic factors (Table 51.1). These various pathogenetic factors may act synergistically to cause DPN

Oxidative stress

Elevated glucoses can increase oxidative stress by glucose auto-oxidation and production of advanced glycosylation end products and activation of the polyol pathway. Oxidative stress can also lead to activation of cytokoines, vascular adhesion molecules, endothelium-1 and procoagulant tissue factor . Oxidative stress also reduces endothelial production of nitric oxide which leads to impairment of endothelial function and reduced capillary vasodilation. This ultimately contributes to nerve hypoxia.

Table 51.1

Pathogenetic mechanisms of neuropathy

Oxidative stress with nitric oxide depletion
Advanced glycosylated end products
Activation of the polyol pathway
Activation of the hexosamine pathway
Excessive protein kinase C activity
Activation of poly(ADP-ribose) polymerase
Diminished neurotrophic peptide factors

The AGE pathway

Advanced glycosylation end products (AGEs) from chronic hyperglycemia play an important role in diabetic neuropathy and microvascular complications (Thornalley, 2002; Sugimoto et al., 2008). Excess glucose combines with amino acids on circulating or tissue proteins to form AGEs. AGEs do not resolve when hyperglycemia is corrected. These AGE peptides cross-link strongly with collagen *in vitro*, damaging nerve fibers. AGEs also bind to and activate the cell surface receptor called RAGE(Receptor for Advanced Glycation Endproducts). RAGE proteins are proinflammatory and expressed on endothelial cells, fibroblasts, mesangial cells, and macrophages. Endothelial cells with RAGE internalize AGEs into subepithelium enhancing permeability and endothelium-dependent coagulant activity which can contribute to vascular injury and endoneural hypoxia (Singh et al., 2001).

The polyol pathway

Excess glucose is shunted into the polyol pathway and converted to sorbitol by aldose reductase and then to fructose by sorbitol dehydrogenase. Increased activity of this metabolic pathway depletes the nicotinamide adenine dinucleotide phosphate hydrogen (NADPH) needed to regenerate the antioxidant glutathione. Without adequate glutathione, nerves are less able to scavenge reactive oxygen species, thus promoting oxidative stress in the nerve. The excess fructose and sorbitol also decrease expression of the sodium/myoinositol cotransporter, leading to a reduction in cellular uptake of myoinositol. Decreased levels of intracellular myoinositol subsequently lower the levels of its metabolite phosphoinositide. Consequently, the phosphoinositide signaling pathway is impaired, interfering with activation of the transmembrane sodium pump and decreasing nerve sodium/potassium ATPase activity. This results in slowed nerve conduction and with chronic exposure neuronal membrane breakdown ensues.

The hexosamine pathway

The glycolytic intermediates of excess glucose are also shunted into the hexosamine pathway. Fructose-6-phosphate is converted to N-acetylglucosamine-6-phosphate by glutamine: fructose-6-phosphate amidotransferase (GFAT). N-Acetylglucosamine-6-phosphate is then converted to N-acetylglucosamine-1,6-phosphate and to uridine diphosphate-N-acetyl glucosamine (UD-PGlcNAc). UD-PGlcNAc modifies gene expression and protein production essential for normal cell function. Many of the proteins produced in this pathway are inflammatory intermediates that promote neuropathy and include plasminogen-activator inhibitor, which inhibits normal blood clotting and increases vascular complications (Brownlee, 2001).

Protein kinase C (PKC) pathway and poly (ADP-ribose) polymerase (PARP)

Protein kinase C (PKC) is involved in controlling the function of proteins through the phosphorylation of hydroxyl groups of serine and threonine amino acid residues on these proteins. PKC is responsible for the activation of essential proteins and lipids in cells that are needed for cell survival (Vincent et al., 2004). Nevertheless, excessive PKC can be harmful to the nervous system. Its contribution to diabetic neuropathy is likely through effects on vascular blood flow and microvascular disease rather than directly on neuronal cells. Glucose is converted to diacylglycerol which activates PKC. PKC then activates the mitogen-activated protein kinases (MAPK) which phosphorylate transcription of stress genes such as heat shock proteins and c-Jun kinases that can lead to cell apoptosis or vascular atherosclerosis (Tomlinson, 1999). The inhibition of PKC reduces oxidative stress and normalizes blood flow and nerve conduction deficits in diabetic rats (Ishii et al., 1998; Cameron and cotter, 2002). Poly (ADP-ribose) polymerase (PARP) is activated in response to hyperglycemia. Overactivation of PARP results in increased free radical formation, enhanced protein kinase C activity, and AGE formation (Pacher et al., 2005). Each promotes nerve damage through the metabolic pathways described above.

Neurotrophic factors and nerve repair

The neurotrophic factors comprise a group of endogenous proteins essential to the health and survival of certain populations of neurons. These neurotrophic peptides include nerve growth factor, brain-derived neurotrophic factor, neurotrophin-3, the insulin-like growth factors (IGF), and vascular endothelial growth factors. They are important for the maintenance of nerve structure and function as well as repair following injury. Impaired peripheral nerve repair in diabetes may be due to diabetes-induced loss of these peptides (Kennedy, 2000, 2005). Insulin also functions as a neurotrophic factor to peripheral neurons, and thus loss of insulin in diabetics may compromise nerve viability and repair. Intrathecal delivery of low-dose insulin has reversed the slowing of motor and sensory nerve conduction velocity. Insulin and IGF-1 have also been shown to reverse atrophy in myelinated sensory axons in the sural nerve (Brussee et al., 2004).

TREATMENT OF DIABETIC NEUROPATHIES

Disease state modifiers

The treatment of diabetic peripheral and autonomic neuropathies has largely been directed at control of symptoms rather than treatment of the underlying pathologic mechanisms with the exception of control of hyperglycemia. The Diabetes Control and Complications Trial (DCCT) outcomes regarding neuropathy have been discussed above. The Epidemiology of Diabetes Interventions and Complications(EDIC) followed a cohort of 1257 DCCT participants for 8 years after completion of the trial and revealed ongoing limitation of neuropathy, based upon patient questionnaire and structured foot exam, even though the glycemic control of the previously intensively treated group approached that of the prior DCCT conventional care group (Martin et al., 2006). Further study of these patients by both clinical examination and nerve conduction studies at 13–14 years post close of DCCT revealed the former intensive treatment group had a 25% prevalence of neuropathy compared to 35% in the former conventional group, supporting the concept of metabolic memory in neuropathy development (Albers et al., 2010). In combined pancreas and kidney transplant patients with type 1 diabetes, correction of glucose abnormalities by successful transplantation has led to corneal small fiber nerve repair documented by confocal microscopy (Mehra et al., 2007). Significant improvement was seen in corneal nerve fiber density and nerve fiber length at 6 months post transplant.

The United Kingdom Prospective Diabetes Study (UKPDS) evaluated newly diagnosed type 2 diabetes patients, comparing intensive treatment with insulin, sulfonylurea, or metformin versus standard care with diet. The intensive care group had a 25% risk reduction in microvascular end points (neuropathy , retinopathy, and nephropathy) after 10 years and a 60% relative risk reduction in neuropathy at year 15 (UKPDS Study Group, 1998). More recent glycemic control studies, though not having long-term extension arms, have failed to show differences in progression of neuropathy with tight glycemic control. The Veterans Affairs Diabetes Trial (VADT) failed to show any decrease in neuropathic outcomes, including autonomic neuropathy, peripheral neuropathy, and mononeuropathy, in patients receiving tight glycemic control versus standard care groups with the median observation period of 5.6 years (Duckworth et al., 2009). Similarly, the Action in Diabetes and Vascular Disease (ADVANCE) trial failed to show limitation of new or worsening neuropathy in the setting of tight glycemic control over a median of 5 years observation (Patel et al., 2008). In both of these recent diabetes intervention studies, other vascular factors were also well managed in both treatment and control groups. Patients in these studies generally had more established diabetic end injury and vascular risk factors in the setting of a greater duration of diabetes at study onset. Patients in the VADT had an average duration of diabetes 11.5 years while those in the ADVANCE trial had been diabetic for 8 years at study onset. This compares to the UKPDS and DCCT wherin patients were either newly diagnosed with DM2 (UKPDS) or young healthy patients with DM1 (DCCT).

Attempts to treat other proposed pathogenetic mechanisms including protein kinase C activation via hyperglycemia-induced elevation of diacylglycerol, accumulation of advanced glycation end products, aldose reductase activation through the polyol pathway and increased activity of the hexosamine pathway have shown limited success except for the use of α-lipoic acid (ALA) to treat oxidative stress. ALA, also known as thioctic acid, is an antioxidant scavenger of reactive oxygen species. These free radicals can cause endoneurial hypoxia and impair nerve conduction in experimental diabetic neuropathy models (Low et al., 1997a). The Alpha-Lipoic Acid in Diabetic Neuropathy (ALADIN) studies (Ziegler et al., 1995, 1999; Reljanovic et al., 1999) evaluated parenteral, oral and sequential parenteral followed by oral treatments with α-lipoic acid revealing reduced neuropathic symptoms in ALADIN (parenteral 100–1220 mg daily for 3 weeks) and improved NIS (Neuropathy Impairment Score) in ALADIN III (parenteral followed by oral α-lipoic acid 600 mg orally three times daily). It is noteworthy that there were discrepant results between the reduction in subjective clinical neuropathic symptoms and the objective NIS in ALADIN III, raising concerns by the authors regarding the use of clinical symptoms as primary end points. ALA appears safe when used in daily 600 mg intravenous doses for 3 weeks (Ziegler et al., 2004), but parenteral ALA is not available in the US. The Symptomatic Diabetic Neuropathy(SYDNEY) 2 trial showed improvement in both clinical symptoms and NIS after a 5 week course of daily oral α-lipoic acid in 600–1800 mg/day doses (Ziegler et al., 2006).Oral ALA was well tolerated, with nausea the most common side-effect. The nausea appeared dose-dependent and since there was no incremental benefit in neuropathic symptom relief with higher doses, the ALA 600 mg/day regimen appears to be the optimal dose. However, the SYDNEY and ALADIN trials were limited by short study durations. The Neurological Assessment of Thioctic Acid in Diabetic Neuropathy (NATHAN) 1 trial evaluated 460 diabetic patients with mild to moderate distal symmetric sensory motor polyneuropathy, randomized to receive oral ALA 600 mg once daily versus placebo for 4 years (Ziegler et al., 2011). The study showed no significant change in the primary end point composite score

(NIS, NIS-Lower Limbs (NIS-LL), and seven neurophysiologic tests) between treatment and control groups group. When evaluating individual tests, patients on ALA did better on NIS, NIS-LLE and muscular weakness subscores when compared to placebo patients. Nerve conduction and QST results did not worsen in a placebo group over the 4 years observation, pointing to the slow progression of peripheral neuropathy even in the control patients.

Modifiers of the polyol pathyway including aldose reductase inhibitors (ARIs) have been in development for decades and only epalrestat is now available in Japan and India. Ranirestat is currently in clinical trials with a recent study showing no significant improvement in clinical symptoms compared to placebo as both trial groups had improved symptom profiles. After 52 weeks of therapy, ranirestat showed improvement in summed motor nerve conduction velocities (NCV), but did not show significant changes in summed sensory NCV (Bril et al., 2009). Use of other ARIs has been limited either by toxicity (tolrestat) or lack of clinical efficacy.

Treatment with protein kinase C β-inhibitor ruboxistaurin showed no differences versus placebo in vibration detection threshold or neuropathy total symptom scores in a 52 week study, but a subgroup with less severe symptomatic diabetic peripheral neuropathy did show improvement in these study parameters (Vinik et al., 2005). Vascular endothelial growth factor (VEGF) has been found to be reduced in diabetic nerves (Quattrini et al., 2008). Injection of plasmid VEGF into standardized areas around peripheral nerves did improve symptoms but did not improve nerve conduction velocities (Ropper et al., 2009).

Medical foods such as folate and B vitamins have been used in the treatment of peripheral neuropathies. L-methylfolate and 5-methyl tetrahydrofolate have been associated with improvement in nitric oxide levels, free radical scavenging, and thusly improved endothelial dysfunction (van Etten et al., 2002; Verhaar et al., 2002). Evaluation for B_{12} deficiency is of particular importance in patients on metformin as this first-line agent for type 2 diabetes has been associated with low B_{12} levels, elevated methylmalonic acid and homocysteine levels, and higher scores on neuropathy screening tools than matched patients who had not received metformin (Wile and Toth, 2010). This study, however, did not look at intervention with B_{12} replacement. While controlled trials using the B vitamins have been limited by small numbers and short study durations with equivocal clinical results, a single noncontrolled and nonblinded study of 20 patients with type 2 diabetes and peripheral neuropathy who received the combination of L-methylfolate, methylcobalamin, and pyridoxal 5-phosphate daily for 52 weeks showed improvement in 1-point tactile and 2-point discriminatory testing (Walker et al., 2010).

In the treatment of painful peripheral diabetic neuropathies, it is important to rule out other causes of neuropathy as up to 15% of cases can have etiologies other than solely diabetes. The evaluation should include complete blood count, erythrocyte sedimentation rate, comprehensive metabolic panel, thyroid function tests, B_{12} and serum protein electrophoresis (England et al., 2009). In addition to simply ameliorating symptoms with medications, treatment of other underlying metabolic issues associated with diabetes and also prediabetes may be helpful in controlling neuropathy (Tesfaye et al., 2005). Interventions include cessation of cigarette smoking and controlling hypertension, weight, and lipids in addition to glycohemoglobin.

Pain-controlling agents

Medications for diabetic peripheral neuropathic pain include tricyclic antidepressants, selective serotonin norepinephrine reuptake inhibitors, antiseizure agents including calcium channel α 2-γ ligands and sodium channel blockers, lidocaine and capsaicin topicals, opioids, and tramadol. Pharmacotherapies for pain control currently approved in the US include duloxetene and pregabalin. These medications as monotherapies or in combinations generally lead to amelioration but not resolution of pain symptoms. Most agents require 4–6 week trials to assess efficacy. Formal clinical trials of medications for neuropathic pain frequently have difficulty showing statistical significance of clinical symptom scores, neurologic standardized examination scores, or electrodiagnostic parameters as placebo groups can show stabilization or improvement in the setting of better diabetes, lipid, and hypertension control.

Pain control algorithms generally begin with tricyclics including amitriptyline, imipramine, nortriptyline, and desipramine .The tricyclics can treat concurrent depression along with the neuropathic pain. These agents are economical but side-effects can limit effective dosing. Dry mouth, urinary retention, and orthostatic hypotension are common anticholinergic side-effects. Drowsiness caused by these agents can be helpful in improving sleep but may be bothersome if somnolence lingers into daytime. The selective dual serotonin and norepinephrine reuptake inhibitor antidepressants duloxetine and venlafaxine have shown efficacy in controlled trials in painful diabetic neuropathy. Duloxetine in 60–120 mg daily doses has been shown in *post hoc* analysis of three double-blind, placebo-controlled 12 week trials to reduce average 24 hour pain scores with efficacy apparent after 1 week of treatment (Kajdasz et al., 2007). Side-effects including nausea, somnolence, dizziness, and anorexia appear more commonly with the higher 120 mg/day dosing and can be limited by

beginning with duloxetine 30 mg/day and titrating upward. Venlafaxine extended release showed reduction in multiple pain score scales over a 6 week trial (Rowbotham et al., 2004). Most common side-effects of venlafaxine were nausea and somnolence.

Anticonvulsants which modulate calcium channel activity include gabapentin and pregabalin. These agents bind to the α 2-γ subunit of calcium channels and inhibit neurotransmitter release. Side-effects of somnolence and dizziness are seen in both. Gabapentin decreased scores for daily pain severity and sleep interference and improved quality of life scores in a double-blind, placebo-controlled study (Backonja et al., 1998). This agent is given three or more times daily with dosing and subsequent pain relief often limited by dizziness and somnolence. Gabapentin doses $\geq$ 1800 mg/day are generally needed for pain relief (Backonja and Glanzman, 2003). An extended release gabapentin has been shown to be effective compared to placebo in reducing average daily pain scores in once or twice daily regimens (Sandercock et al., 2009). Pooled data from seven randomized controlled trials of pregabalin (Freeman et al., 2008) revealed significant reductions in pain and sleep interference end points. The pregabalin 600 mg/day dosing showed efficacy when divided into twice daily doses while lower daily doses required three times daily dosing. In addition to dizziness and somnolence, peripheral edema was also a common side-effect. Symptom improvement was seen in 5 days or less with doses 300 mg/day or greater.

Among anticonvulsants which block the sodium channels, lacosamide in doses of 400–600 mg/day in an 18 week study has been shown to decrease average daily pain score more than placebo, but statistical significance was not achieved (Ziegler et al., 2010). The authors suspected improved pain scores in the placebo group contributed to the lack of significance in this primary end point.

Topical therapies including capsaicin and lidocaine 5% patches or gel have also been useful in decreasing pain. As these agents exert their effects locally and without significant systemic absorption, they are limited to treatment of focal painful areas. Local irritation is the most common adverse effect. Capsaicin acts by depleting tissue substance P and has shown modest efficacy over short-term use (Zhang and Wan, 1994), but requires four times daily local application. A new high concentration 8% capsaicin patch has shown efficacy in postherpetic neuralgia and HIV neuropathy with a single 60 minute application in a 12 week study (Backonja et al., 2008).

Tramadol and opioids are efficacious in controlling diabetic neuropathic pain. Tramadol is a weak opioid receptor agonist which also inhibits norepinephrine and serotonin reuptake. This agent is less potent than the opioids. Side-effects of both groups include sedation, constipation, and nausea. Due to the potential for dependency with these agents, their use should limited to those patients who have failed trials of the other medications discussed above.

Medications for neuropathic pain

See Table 51.2.

Treatment of autonomic neuropathy

The clinical manifestations of diabetic autonomic neuropathy (DAN) are listed in Table 51.1. Treatment of hyperglycemia and other metabolic factors including hypertension and hyperlipidemia can help limit DAN. The Steno-2 study followed 160 type 2 DM patients with microalbuminuria for over 13 years of treatment with renin–angiotensin system blockers, aspirin and lipid lowering agents in additional to glucose controlling agents (Gaede et al., 2008). Progression of DAN, measured by electrocardiogram RR intervals during paced breathing and orthostatic hypotension, was noted in 39 patients on intensive therapy and 52 in the conventional treatment group ($p = 0.004$).

Treatments for DAN can be directed at abnormalities in the cardiovascular, gastrointestinal, and genitourinary systems. The major treated cardiovascular complication is orthostatic hypotension. Nonpharmacologic interventions include gradual position changes, $10–20°$ head of bed elevation, isotonic exercise, graded compression stockings, and abdominal binders. Removal of pharmacotherapies known to cause orthostasis can also be helpful. Unfortunately, many of the agents used to treat the peripheral neuropathic pain including tricyclics, duloxetine and anticonvulsants can also cause orthostasis. The mineralocorticoid fludrocortisone at doses of 0.1–0.5 mg daily plus high salt diet or salt tablets can assist

in volume expansion , but peripheral edema, congestive heart failure, hypokalemia, and supine hypertension can limit dose escalation. Midodrine, an α_1 adrenoreceptor agonist, at doses up to 10 mg three times a day, has been effective in increasing standing blood pressure (Low et al., 1997b; Wright et al., 1998) but has adverse effects of supine hypertension and urinary retention. Midodrine and fludrocortisone are frequently used in combination, yet supine hypertension can limit dose escalation. Pyridostigmine, a cholinestesterase inhibitor, increases diastolic blood pressure without causing supine hypertension. The baroreceptor efferent limb synapses at the autonomic ganglion with acetylcholine as the neurotransmitter. Singer et al. postulated that since autonomic ganglion activity is low when supine, this agent should not cause supine hypertension Their randomized four way crossover study evaluated pyridostigmine 60 mg alone and with varied doses of midodrine. The fall in standing diastolic blood pressure and orthostatic symptoms were reduced with treatment with pyridostigmine alone and in combination with midodrine 5 mg (Singer et al., 2006).

Yohimbine, an α_2 adrenergic receptor antagonist, can increase residual sympathetic tone in patients with autonomic failure by increasing norepinephrine release from sympathetic nerves. Shibao et al. studied 31 patients with severe autonomic failure. They postulated that yohimbine and pyridostigmine, due to their differing mechanisms of actions, might have a synergistic effect in ameliorating orthostatic hypotension. Patients received pyridostigmine 60 mg, yohimbine 5.4 mg, or a combination of both agents in a single-blind, randomized, placebo-controlled crossover study. Yohimbine improved standing diastolic pressure measured 60 minutes after drug administration. Contrary to the Singer study noted above, pyridostigmine did not increase diastolic blood pressure significantly in these patients. No evidence of synergy was found in

Table 51.2

Medications for neuropathic pain

Class	Agents	Common side-effects
Tricyclic antidepressants	Nortriptyline, desimipramine, amitriptyline, imipramine	Anticholinergic effects, somnolence, orthostasis
Selective serotonin and norepinephrine reuptake inhibitors	Duloxetine Venlafaxine	Nausea, somnolence, anorexia, dizziness
Anticonvulsants	Gabapentin Pregabalin	Somnolence, dizziness, leg edema
Topical medications	5% lidocaine patch Capsaicin	Local irritation
Opioid agonists	Tramadol Morphine, oxycodone, codeine	Nausea, somnolence, constipation

patients receiving both pyridostigmine and yohimbine (Shibao et al., 2010). Authors postulated that patients in the Singer trial may have had less severe autonomic dysfunction function with greater reserve.

Nonsteroidal anti-inflammatory drugs can help orthostasis by inducing volume expansion and also by antagonizing vasodilating prostaglandins. Erythropoietin has been helpful in patients with both anemia and orthostatic hypotension (Hoeldtke and Streeten, 1993).

Gastrointestinal neuropathy can affect any part of the bowel from esophagus to anus. Esophageal reflux can be treated with histamine-2 blockers and proton pump inhibitors. Gastroparesis can be worsened by acute hyperglycemia and can contribute to glucose lability by causing delayed and unpredictable delivery of nutrients to the small bowel and also by impeding absorption of oral diabetes medications. Incretin-modulating agents including exenatide and liraglutide and the amylin analog pramlintide can slow gastric emptying and should be avoided in patients with gastroparesis. Effective gastric prokinetic agents are limited. Cisapride, a stimulator of 5-HT$_4$ receptors, is no longer readily available in the US due to risk of cardiac rhythm disturbances. Domperidone, a dopamine antagonist which binds to the D$_2$ and D$_3$ dopamine receptors, has both prokinetic and antiemetic properties, but is not available in the US. Intravenous erythromycin lactobionate can be used to stimulate gastric emptying (Janssens et al., 1990) while oral forms of this agent have been less effective (Maganti et al., 2003). This macrolide antibiotic should be used only sporadically due to potential for GI side-effects including nausea and colitis. When used with CYP3A4 inhibitors, the drug can also cause QT interval prolongation with cardiac rhythm disturbances. Metoclopramide, a dopamine D$_2$ receptor antagonist and 5-HT$_4$ receptor agonist, improves gastric emptying and is also antiemetic. This agent is available for both oral and intravenous use and has been associated with extrapyramidal side-effects and tardive dyskinesia. An oral rapidly dissolving form is also available which requires no water or swallowing. Jejunostomy tube placement may be needed for nutritional support in patients who are unresponsive to the above described interventions. Gastrostomy tubes are rarely required for decompression in patients with persistent vomiting or distension. Gastric electrical stimulation has very limited availability and can improve gastroparesis symptoms without increasing gastric emptying.

Genitourinary neuropathy can present as bladder and erectile dysfunction. Cystopathy can be treated with timed voiding, intermittent self-catheterization, and cholinergic agents. Erectile dysfunction in diabetic male patients can be multifactorial so evaluation for hypogonadism, elevated prolactin, thyroid disease, and confounding medications should be performed. If no readily treatable etiologies are found, phosphodiesterase 5 inhibitors can be initiated. Sildenafil, vardenafil and tadalafil limit breakdown of cyclic guanosine monophosphate in the penile corpora cavernosa and increase penile blood flow and thus erection. Side-effects can include headache, impaired color vision, lightheadedness, syncope, hearing and vision loss. Tadalafil has a greater than 24 hour duration of action. While each agent is approved for intermittent use around the time of sexual relations, tadalafil, in doses of 2.5–5 mg, is also approved for scheduled daily dosing. Intraurethral prostaglandin E$_1$ (alprostadil), intracavernosal injections of papaverine, phentolamine and alprostadil and penile suction devices have also shown efficacy in treating erectile dysfunction.

CONCLUSIONS

While the pathophysiology of diabetic neuropathies is now reasonably well understood, clinicians are still limited in therapies directed at correcting the underlying etiologies. Other than control of glycemia and other vascular risk factors and antioxidants such as α-lipoic acid, specific effective agents are not available. Treatments for diabetic autonomic neuropathies such as orthostatic hypotension are directed largely at treating the end result of the condition rather than the etiology. Medications directed at neuropathic pain control are able to partially ameliorate symptoms rather than give complete resolution. Treatments are needed both to correct the pathologic mechanisms and to control pain and autonomic consequences in a way that will be safe for long-term use in chronic diabetes mellitus.

REFERENCES

Albers J, Herman W, Pop-Busai R et al. (2010). Effect of prior intensive insulin treatment during the Diabetes Control and Complications Trial (DCCT) on peripheral neuropathy in type 1 diabetes during the Epidemiology of Diabetes Interventions and Complications (EDIC) study. Diabetes Care 33: 1090–1096.

Backonja M, Glanzman R (2003). Gabapentin dosing for neuropathic pain: evidence from randomized, placebo-controlled clinical trials. Clin Ther 25: 81–104.

Backonja M, Beydoun A, Edwards K et al. (1998). Gabapentin for the symptomatic treatment of painful neuropathy in patients with diabetes mellitus: a randomized controlled trial. JAMA 280: 1831–1836.

Backonja M, Wallace M, Blonsky E et al. (2008). NGX-4010, a high-concentration capsaicin patch, for the treatment of post herpetic neuralgia: a randomized, double-blind study. Lancet Neurol 7: 1102–1112.

Barohn R, Sahenk Z, Warmolts J et al. (1991). The Bruns–Garland syndrome (diabetic amyotrophy). Revisited 100 years later. Arch Neurol 48 (11): 1130–1135.

Boulton A, Malik R, Arezzo J et al. (2004). Diabetic somatic neuropathies. Diabetes Care 27: 1458–1486.

Boulton A, Vinik A, Arezzo J et al. (2005). Diabetic neuropathies: a statement by the American Diabetes Association. Diabetes Care 28: 956–962.

Bril V, Hirose T, Tomioka S et al. (2009). Ranirestat for the management of diabetic sensorimotor polyneuropathy. Diabetes Care 32: 1256–1260.

Brownlee M (2001). Biochemistry and molecular cell biology of diabetic complications. Nature 414: 813–820.

Brussee V, Cunningham F, Zochodne D (2004). Direct insulin signaling of neurons reverses diabetic neuropathy. Diabetes 53: 1824–1830.

Cameron N, Cotter M (2002). Effects of protein kinase C beta inhibition on neurovascular dysfunction in diabetic rats: interaction with oxidative stress and essential fatty acid metabolism. Diabetes Metab Res Rev 18: 315–323.

Chen H, Hwu C, Kuo B et al. (2001). Abnormal cardiovascular reflex tests are predictors of mortality in type 2 diabetes mellitus. Diabet Med 18: 268–273.

Cohen J, Jeffers B, Faldut D et al. (1998). Risks for sensorimotor peripheral neuropathy and autonomic neuropathy in non-insulin-dependent diabetes mellitus (NIDDM). Muscle Nerve 21: 72–80.

Diabetes Control and Complications Trial Research Group (1995). The effect of intensive diabetes therapy on the development and progression of neuropathy. Ann Intern Med 122: 561–568.

Duckworth W, Abraira C, Moritz T et al. (2009). Glucose control and vascular complications in veterans with type 2 diabetes. N Engl J Med 360: 129–139.

Dyck P, Kratz K, Lehman K et al. (1991). The Rochester Diabetic Neuropathy Study: design, criteria for types of neuropathy, selection bias, and reproducibility of neuropathic tests. Neurology 41: 799–807.

Dyck P, Karnes J, O'Brien P et al. (1992). The Rochester Diabetic Neuropathy Study: reassessment of tests and criteria for diagnosis and staged severity. Neurology 42: 1164–1170.

Dyck P, Kratz K, Karnes J et al. (1993). The prevalence by staged severity of various types of diabetic neuropathy, retinopathy, and nephropathy in a population-based cohort: the Rochester Diabetic Neuropathy Study. Neurology 43: 817–824.

Dyck P, Dyck P, Klein C et al. (2007). Does impaired glucose metabolism cause polyneuropathy? Review of previous studies and design of a prospective controlled population-based study. Muscle Nerve 36: 536–541.

England J, Gronseth G, Franklin G et al. (2009). Practice parameter: evaluation of distal symmetric polyneuropathy: role of laboratory and genetic testing (an evidence-based review): report of the American Academy of Neurology, American Association of Neuromuscular and Electrodiagnostic Medicine, and American Academy of Physical Medicine and Rehabilitation. Neurology 72: 185–192.

Ewing D, Boland O, Neilson J et al. (1991). Autonomic neuropathy, QT interval lengthening, and unexpected deaths in male diabetic patients. Diabetologia 34: 182–185.

Feldman E, Stevens M, Thomas P et al. (1994). A practical two-step quantitative clinical and electrophysiological assessment for the diagnosis and staging of diabetic neuropathy. Diabetes Care 17: 1281–1289.

Freeman R, Durso-DeCruz E, Emir B (2008). Efficacy, safety, and tolerability of pregabalin treatment for painful diabetic peripheral neuropathy. Diabetes Care 31: 1448–1454.

Gaede P, Lund-Andersen H, Parving H et al. (2008). Effect of a multifactoral intervention on mortality in type 2 diabetes. N Engl J Med 358: 580–591.

Galer B, Gianas A, Jensen M (2000). Painful diabetic polyneuropathy: epidemiology, pain description, and quality of life. Diabetes Res Clin Pract 47: 123–128.

Genuth S (2006). Insights from the diabetes control and complications trial/epidemiology of diabetes interventions and complications study on the use of intensive glycemic treatment to reduce the risk of complications of type 1 diabetes. Endocr Pract 12 (Suppl 1): 34–41.

Gilden DH (2004). Clinical practice. Bell's palsy. N Engl J Med 351: 1323–1331.

Gulliford M, Latinovic R, Charlton J et al. (2006). Increased incidence of carpal tunnel syndrome up to 10 years before diagnosis of diabetes. Diabetes Care 29: 1929–1930.

Hamman R, Franklin G, Mayer E et al. (1991). Microvascular complications of NIDDM in Hispanics and non-Hispanic whites. San Luis Valley Diabetes Study. Diabetes Care 14: 655–664.

Hoeldtke R, Streeten D (1993). Treatment of orthostatic hypotension with erythropoietin. N Engl J Med 329: 611–615.

Ishii H, Koya D, King G (1998). Proteins kinase C activation and its role in the development of vascular complications in diabetes mellitus. J Mol Med (Berl) 76: 21–31.

Janssens J, Peeters T, Vantrappen G et al. (1990). Improvement of gastric emptying in diabetic gastroparesis by erythromycin. N Engl J Med 32: 1028–1031.

Jermendy G, Toth L, Voros P et al. (1991). Cardiac autonomic neuropathy and QT interval length. A follow-up study in diabetic patients. Acta Cardiol 46: 189–200.

Kajdasz D, Iyengar S, Desaiah D et al. (2007). Duloxetine for the management of diabetic peripheral neuropathic pain: evidence-based findings from post hoc analysis of three multicenter, randomized, double-blind, placebo-controlled, parallel-group studies. Clin Ther 29: 2536–2546.

Kennedy J, Zochodne D (2000). The regenerative deficit of peripheral nerves in experimental diabetes: its extent, timing and possible mechanisms. Brain 123: 2118–2129.

Kennedy J, Zochodne DW (2005). Impaired peripheral nerve regeneration in diabetes mellitus. J Peripher Nerv Syst 10: 144–157.

Kennedy W, Navarro X, Sutherland D (1995). Neuropathy profile of diabetic patients in a pancreas transplantation program. Neurology 45: 773–780.

Kikta DG, Breuer AC, Wilbourn AJ (1982). Thoracic root pain in diabetes: the spectrum of clinical and electromyographic findings. Ann Neurol 11: 80–85.

Kincaid J, Price K, Jimenez M et al. (2007). Correlation of vibratory quantitative sensory testing and nerve conduction studies in patients with diabetes. Muscle Nerve 36: 821–827.

Liatis S, Marinou K, Tentolouris N et al. (2007). Usefulness of a new indicator test for the diagnosis of peripheral and autonomic neuropathy in patients with diabetes mellitus. Diabet Med 24: 1375–1380.

Low P, Nickander K, Tritcshler H (1997a). The role of oxidative stress and antioxidant treatment in experimental diabetic neuropathy. Diabetes 46: S38–S42.

Low P, Gilden J, Freeman R et al. (1997b). Efficacy of midodrine vs placebo in neurogenic orthostatic hypotension: a randomized, double-blind multicenter study. JAMA 277: 1046–1051.

Maganti K, Onyemere K, Jones M (2003). Oral erythromycin and symptomatic relief in gastroparesis: a systematic review. Am J Gastroenterol 98: 259–263.

Martin C, Albers J, Herman W et al. (2006). The DCCT/EDIC research group. Neuropathy among the diabetes control and complications trial cohort 8 years after trial completion. Diabetes Care 29: 340–344.

Maser R, Pfeifer M, Dorman J et al. (1990). Diabetic autonomic neuropathy and cardiovascular risk. Pittsburgh Epidemiology of Diabetes Complications Study III. Arch Intern Med 150: 1218–1222.

Mehra S, Tavakoli M, Kallinikos P et al. (2007). Corneal confocal microscopy detects early nerve regeneration after pancreas transplantation in patients with type 1 diabetes. Diabetes Care 30: 2608–2612.

Navarro X, Kennedy W, Aeppli D et al. (1996). Neuropathy and mortality in diabetes: influence of pancreas transplantation. Muscle Nerve 19: 1009–1016.

Negrin P, Zara G (1995). Conduction studies as prognostic parameters in the natural history of diabetic neuropathy: a long-term follow-up of 114 patients. Electromyogr Clin Neurophysiol 35: 341–350.

Newrick P, Wilson A, Jakubowski J et al. (1986). Sural nerve oxygen tension in diabetes. Br Med J (Clin Res Ed) 293: 1053–1054.

Niakan E, Harati Y, Rolak L et al. (1986). Silent myocardial infarction and diabetic cardiovascular autonomic neuropathy. Arch Intern Med 146: 2229–2230.

O'Brien IA, McFadden JP, Corrall RJ (1991). The influence of autonomic neuropathy on mortality in insulin-dependent diabetes. Q J Med 79: 495–502.

Onde M, Ozge A, Senol M et al. (2008). The sensitivity of clinical diagnostic methods in the diagnosis of diabetic neuropathy. J Int Med Res 36: 63–70.

Orchard T, Lloyd C, Maser R et al. (1996). Why does diabetic autonomic neuropathy predict IDDM mortality? An analysis from the Pittsburgh Epidemiology of Diabetes Complications Study. Diabetes Res Clin Pract 34 (Suppl): S165–S171.

Oyer D, Saxon D, Shah A (2007). Quantitative assessment of diabetic peripheral neuropathy with use of the clanging tuning fork test. Endocr Pract 13: 5–10.

Pacher P, Obrosova I, Mabley J et al. (2005). Role of nitrosative stress and peroxynitrite in the pathogenesis of diabetic complications. Emerging new therapeutical strategies. Curr Med Chem 12: 267–275.

Patel A, MacMahon S, Chalmers J et al. (2008). Intensive blood glucose control and vascular outcomes in patients with type 2 diabetes. N Engl J Med 358: 2560–2572.

Pecket P, Schattner A (1982). Concurrent Bell's palsy and diabetes mellitus: a diabetic mononeuropathy? J Neurol Neurosurg Psychiatry 45: 652–655.

Quattrini C, Jeziorska M, Boulton A et al. (2008). Reduced vascular endothelial growth factor expression and intraepidermal nerve fiber loss in human diabetic neuropathy. Diabetes Care 31: 140–145.

Rathmann W, Ziegler D, Jahnke M et al. (1993). Mortality in diabetic patients with cardiovascular autonomic neuropathy. Diabet Med 10: 820–824.

Reljanovic M, Reichel G, Rett K et al. (1999). Treatment of diabetic polyneuropathy with antioxidant thioctic acid (α-lipoic acid): a two-year multi-center randomized double-blind placebo-controlled trial (ALADIN II). Alpha Lipoic Acid in Diabetic Neuropathy. Free Radic Res 31: 171–179.

Ropper A, Gorson K, Gooch C et al. (2009). Vascular endothelial growth factor gene transfer for diabetic polyneuropathy: a randomized, double-blinded trial. Ann Neurol 65: 386–393.

Rowbotham M, Goli V, Kunz N et al. (2004). Venlafaxine extended release in the treatment of painful diabetic neuropathy: a double-blind, placebo- controlled study. Pain 110: 697–706.

Sampson M, Wilson S, Karagiannis P et al. (1990). Progression of diabetic autonomic neuropathy over a decade in insulin-dependent diabetics. Q J Med 75: 635–646.

Sandercock D, Cramer M, Wu J et al. (2009). Gabapentin extended release for the treatment of painful diabetic neuropathy. Diabetes Care 32: e20.

Shibao C, Okamoto L, Gamboa A et al. (2010). Comparative efficacy of yohimbine against pyridostigmine for the treatment of orthostatic hypotension in autonomic failure. Hypertension 56: 847.

Singer W, Sandroni P, Opfer-Gehrking T et al. (2006). Pyridostigmine treatment trial in heneurogenic orthostatic hypotension. Arch Neurol 63: 513.

Singh R, Barden A, Mori T et al. (2001). Advanced glycation end products: a review. Diabetologia 44: 129–146.

Singleton J, Smith A (2007). Neuropathy associated with prediabetes: what is new in 2007? Curr Diab Rep 7: 420–424.

Spallone V, Maiello M, Cicconetti E et al. (1997). Autonomic neuropathy and cardiovascular risk factors in insulin-dependent and non insulin-dependent diabetes. Diabetes Res Clin Pract 34: 169–179.

Stamboulis E, Vassilopoulos D, Kalfakis N (2005). Symptomatic focal mononeuropathies in diabetic patients: increased or not? J Neurol 252: 448–452.

Stewart JD (1989). Diabetic truncal neuropathy: topography of the sensory deficit. Ann Neurol 25: 233–238.

Sugimoto K, Yasujima M, Yagihashi S (2008). Role of advanced glycation end products in diabetic neuropathy. Curr Pharm Des 14: 953–961.

Sumner C, Sheth S, Griffin J et al. (2003). The spectrum of neuropathy in diabetes and impaired glucose tolerance. Neurology 60: 108–111.

Tavakoli M, Quattrini C, Abbot D (2010). Corneal confocal microscopy. A novel noninvasive test to diagnose and stratify the severity of human diabetic neuropathy. Diabetes Care 22: 1792–1797.

Tesfaye S, Chaturvedi N, Eaton S et al. (2005). Vascular risk factors and diabetic neuropathy. N Engl J Med 352: 341–350.

Thornalley P (2002). Glycation in diabetic neuropathy: characteristics, consequences, causes, and therapeutic options. Int Rev Neurobiol 50: 37–57.

Tomlinson D (1999). Mitogen-activated protein kinase C as glucose transducers for diabetic complications. Diabetologia 42: 1271–1281.

UK Prospective Diabetes Study Group (UKPDS) (1994). XI. Biochemical risk factors in type 2 diabetic patients at diagnosis compared with age-matched normal subjects. Diabet Med 11: 534–544.

UK Prospective Diabetes Study (UKPDS) Group (1998). Intensive blood-glucose control with sulphonylureas or insulin compared with conventional treatment and risk of complications in patients with type 2 diabetes (UKPDS 33). Lancet 352: 837–853.

Van Etten R, deKoning F, Verhaar M et al. (2002). NO-dependent vasodilation in patients with type II non-insulin-dependent diabetes mellitus is restored by acute administration of folate. Diabetologia 45: 1004–1010.

Verhaar M, Stroes E, Rabelink T (2002). Folates and cardiovascular disease. Arterioscler Thromb Vasc Biol 22: 6–11.

Vincent A, Russell J, Low P et al. (2004). Oxidative stress in the pathogenesis of diabetic neuropathy. Endocr Rev 25: 612–628.

Vinik AI, Ziegler D (2007). Diabetic cardiovascular autonomic neuropathy. Circulation 115: 387–397.

Vinik A, Maser R, Mitchell B et al. (2003). Diabetic autonomic neuropathy. Diabetes Care 26: 1553–1579.

Vinik A, Bril V, Kempler P et al. (2005). Treatment of symptomatic diabetic peripheral neuropathy with the protein kinase C β-inhibitor ruboxistaurin mesylate during a 1-year, randomized, placebo-controlled, double-blind clinical trial. Clin Ther 27: 1164–1180.

Walker M, Morris L, Cheng D (2010). Improvement of cutaneous sensitivity in diabetic peripheral neuropathy with combination L-methylfolate, methylcobalamin and pyridoxal 5-phosphate. Rev Neurol Dis 7: 132–139.

Wile D, Toth C (2010). Association of metformin, elevated homocysteine, and methylmalonic acid levels and clinically worsened diabetic peripheral neuropathy. Diabetes Care 33: 156–161.

Wright R, Kaufmann H, Perera R et al. (1998). A double-blind, dose-response study of midodrine in neurogenic orthostatic hypotension. Neurology 51: 120–124.

Zhang W, Wan Po A (1994). The effectiveness of topically applied capsaicin: a meta analysis. Eur J Clin Pharmacol 45: 517–522.

Zhong X, Zheng B, Hu G et al. (1981). Peripheral and autonomic nerve function tests in early diagnosis of diabetic neuropathy: correlation between motor nerve conduction velocity and fasting plasma glucose. Chin Med J (Engl) 94: 495–502.

Ziegler D, Gries F, Spuler M et al. (1992). The epidemiology of diabetic neuropathy. Diabetic Cardiovascular Autonomic Neuropathy Multicenter Study Group. J Diabetes Complications 6: 49–57.

Ziegler D, Hanefeld M, Ruhnau K et al. (1995). Treatment of symptomatic diabetic peripheral neuropathy with the antioxidant α-lipoic acid. A three-week multicentre randomized controlled trial (ALADIN study). Diabetologia 38: 1425–1433.

Ziegler D, Hanefeld M, Ruhnau K (1999). Treatment of symptomatic diabetic polyneuropathy with the antioxidant alpha-lipoic acid: a 7-month multicenter randomized controlled trial (ALADIN III study). Diabetes Care 22: 1296–1301.

Ziegler D, Nowak H, Kempler P (2004). Treatment of symptomatic diabetic polyneuropathy with the antioxidant alpha-lipoic acid: a meta analysis. Diabet Med 21: 114–121.

Ziegler D, Ametov A, Barinov A et al. (2006). Oral treatment with alpha lipoic acid improves symptomatic diabetic polyneuropathy-the SYDNEY 2 trial. Diabetes Care 29: 2365–2370.

Ziegler D, Rathmann W, Dickhaus T et al. (2008). Prevalence of polyneuropathy in pre-diabetes and diabetes is associated with abdominal obesity and macroangiopathy: the MONICA/KORA Augsburg surveys S2 and S3. Diabetes Care 31: 464–469.

Ziegler D, Hidvegi T, Gurieva I et al. (2010). Efficacy and safety of lacosamide in painful diabetic neuropathy. Diabetes Care 33: 838–841.

Ziegler D, Low P, Litchy W et al. (2011). Efficacy and safety of antioxidant treatment with alpha lipoic acid over 4 years in diabetic polyneuropathy. The NATHAN 1 trial. Diabetes Care 34: 2054–2060.

Handbook of Clinical Neurology, Vol. 120 (3rd series)
Neurologic Aspects of Systemic Disease Part II
Jose Biller and Jose M. Ferro, Editors

Chapter 52

Neurologic disorders associated with disease of the ovaries and testis

JORGE C. KATTAH[1]* AND WILLIAM C. KATTAH[2]

[1]*Department of Neurology, University of Illinois College of Medicine, Peoria, IL, USA*

[2]*Endocrinology Department, University of the Andes, Bogota, Colombia*

INTRODUCTION

Whereas cerebral metastases are a known, albeit uncommon, complication of endothelial ovarian cancer (Pectasides et al., 2006), germ cell tumors of the testis rarely metastasize to the brain. Tumors of the testis and ovaries may also be associated with paraneoplastic encephalitis with well-defined clinical phenotypes and serum and CSF markers. These paraneoplastic neurologic syndromes are frequently the initial symptom of these tumors and may represent a formidable diagnostic and treatment challenge The first reported paraneoplastic syndrome due to ovarian cancer was a progressive cerebellar degeneration associated with the anti-Yo tumor marker, often reported among women in the sixth decade and associated with epithelial carcinoma of the ovaries (Greenlee and Brashear, 1983). Subsequently, the anti-Ma-2 serum marker was identified in patients with testicular germ cell tumors and three clinical phenotypes were recognized: limbic encephalitis, hypothalamic hypersomnia (narcolepsy/cataplexy), and a slowly progressive upper brainstem ophthalmoplegia (Voltz et al., 1999; Dalmau et al., 2004; Tenner and Einhorn, 2009). More recently, an anti-N-methyl-D-aspartate (NMDA) receptor encephalitis associated with ovarian teratoma was described (Dalmau et al., 2007; Dalmau et al., 2008; Florance et al., 2009; Tuzun et al., 2009; Lancaster et al., 2010). Less common manifestations of the anti-NMDA antibody syndrome include status epilepticus, dyskniesias of the trunk and face, and jaw dystonia.

HISTORY

Neurologic complications of tumors of the ovaries and testis represent the most common interface between neurologists, gynecologic oncologists and urologic oncologists. From 1993 to 1996, 4% of all ovarian cancer patients evaluated at Memorial Sloan-Kettering Cancer Center, 83, had 121 neurologic consultations. Causes for consultation were iatrogenic complications ($n = 38$), metastasic disease ($n = 27$), cerebrovascular disease ($n = 14$), and paraneoplastic syndromes ($n = 4$). More than half of the patients had improvement following neurologic intervention (Abrey and Dalmau, 2000).

Non-seminomatous tumors are more likely to be associated with cerebral metastases (Bokemeyer et al., 1997), and a brain hemorrhage may be a complication of metastatic choriocarcinoma of the testis (Salvati and Cervoni, 1994; Fadul, 2008). Following radiotherapy of testicular tumors, lumbosacral plexus and lower spinal cord syndromes may develop with a variable latency. Neurologic complications of radiotherapy of the testis are probably more frequent than other postradiation complications such as *de novo* pelvic and other neoplasms or accelerated iliofemoral atherosclerosis.

Neurologic phenotypes of paraneoplastic syndromes associated with cancer of the ovaries and testis are summarized in Table 52.1. These syndromes may precede tumor diagnosis in more than half of the cases. The neurologic syndrome combined with a lymphocytic cerebrospinal fluid (CSF) reaction, increased IgG synthetic rate,

---

*Correspondence to: Jorge C. Kattah, M.D., Department of Neurology, University of Illinois College of Medicine at Peoria and the Illinois Neurological Institute at OSF Saint Francis Medical Center, 530 NE Glen Oak Avenue, Peoria, IL 61637, USA. E-mail: kattahj@uicomp.uic.edu

Table 52.1

Paraneoplastic syndromes associated with cancer of the ovary and the testis

Antibody	Syndrome	Target	CNS pathology	MRI findings	CSF	Common tumors	Treatment
Anti-Yo	Pure cerebellar degeneration	CDR2 protein in cytoplasm Purkinje cells	Loss of Purkinje cells Inflammation	1. Normal early 2. Cerebellar atrophy late	Lymphocytic Pleocytosis OCB* High protein	Ovarian cancer Breast cancer	Oncotherapy Immunoglobulin Steroids Cytoxan
Anti-Ma-2	1. Limbic encephalitis 2. Narcolepsy 3. Vertical gaze palsy 4. Ataxia Parkinsonism	Unknown cytoplasmic neuronal protein	Perivascular lymphocytic cuffing Variable gliosis Neuronal degeneration	Increased signal in hippocampus diencephalon upper brainstem	Lymphocytic Pleocytosis OCB* High protein	Germ cell tumor of testis Lung cancer	Orchidectomy Oncotherapy Immunotherapy
Anti-NMDA	Progressive encephalopathy Delirium psychosis Involuntary facial movement Hypoventilation Dysautonomia	NR1 + NR2 NMDA** receptor in hippocampus, forebrain, basal ganglia spinal cord	Loss of neurons in hippocampus Gliosis IgG deposits T cells infrequent	Loss of pyramidal cells in hippocampus Gliosis Cerebellum is spared	Lymphocytic Pleocytosis OCB* High Protein	Teratoma of the ovary in females over 18	Immunotherapy Oncotherapy Tumor resection

*OCB, oligoclonal bands.

**NMDA, N-methyl-D-aspartate receptor.

and oligoclonal bands may prompt the astute neurologist to order a clinical pelvic examination or testicular examination, serum and CSF ovarian and testis markers, and pertinent imaging studies, thus, neurologists may have a very important role to play in these patients, as often gynecologists, oncologists, and urologists may be skeptical about the potential significance of clinical and serum makers and the need for urgent diagnosis and intervention. In these instances, neurologists must convincingly argue the potential relationship between the observed phenotype and a primary gonadal tumor.

The annual incidence of epithelial ovarian carcinoma in the US has been estimated to be 12.9/100 000 among women aged 50–54 years. The annual incidence of newly detected testicular tumors in the US has been estimated at between 7500 and 8000. Over a lifetime, the risk of testicular carcinoma is approximately 1 in 250 (0.4%). Testicular tumors are the most common solid tumors in men between the ages of 15 and 34 years (Bosl and Motzer, 1997).

CLINICAL FINDINGS

Local pelvic neurologic symptoms of ovarian tumors.
Unilateral lumbar plexus syndromes could be seen as a late complication of ovarian carcinoma (Beatrous et al., 1990). Patients typically develop severe pelvic pain, unilateral painful weakness of the iliopsoas and quadriceps muscles, edema of the lower extremity, and foot drop. Isolated malignant infiltration of the psoas muscle may also occur with ovarian tumors. A late lumbosacral plexopathy secondary to irradiation, characterized by painless weakness and atrophy of the lower extremities, may be seen in patients with ovarian carcinoma; this is often seen several years after initial irradiation (Numaba et al., 1990).

Brain metastases of ovarian carcinoma are uncommon and usually associated with poor prognosis (Pectasides et al., 2006). The approximate incidence of cerebral metastases is ~1%,(0.4–6 %). Most patients with CNS metastases have stage III and IV disease. Isolated brain relapse may be seen in a third of the patients. Single metastases occur in one-third of cases. Multiple metastases occur in the rest. Most lesions are located in the cerebral hemispheres. The median interval between initial tumor diagnosis and brain metastases ranges from 15 to 70 months. Hemiparesis and altered mental status are the most common finding (Pectasides et al., 2006).

Early pelvic complications of tumors of the testis are distinctly uncommon; however, late complications from radiotherapy may occur with greater frequency, particularly if the average total radiation dose exceeds 40 Gy. Following a variable latency, the clinical picture involves progressive lower extremity flaccid weakness and atrophy with sparing of sphincters function

(Greenfield and Stark, 1948; Bowen et al., 1996; Knap et al., 2007).

Approximately 10% of all nonmetastatsic neurologic complications in patients with cancer are paraneoplastic (Tenner and Einhorn, 2009). In two-third of cases, the neurologic syndrome precedes the diagnosis of ovarian or testicular tumor (Table 52.1). A progressive cerebellar degeneration is typical in cases of the anti-Yo antibody syndrome (Figs 52.1 and 52.2). The majority of anti-Yo cases are characterized by a pure, progressive limb and truncal cerebellar ataxia (Hudson et al., 1993; Abrey and Dalmau, 2000; Keime-Guibert et al., 2000; Dorn et al., 2003). Common paraneoplastic neuroophthalmologic manifestations of gonadal tumors are listed in Table 52.2 and include ophthalmoplegia, opsoclonus, nystagmus, and fixation intrusions, etc. (Ko et al., 2008). Clinical manifestations of the anti-Ma-2 antibody syndrome associated with germ cell tumors of the testicles include three characteristic clinical phenotypes: (1) limbic encephalitis with short-term memory loss, altered mental status, and psychomotor seizures; (2) hypothalamic syndromes with excessive daytime sleepiness, cataplexy, hypnagogic hallucinations, hyperthermia, and endocrinopathies; (3) vertical gaze palsy. Less common presentations include brainstem encephalitic syndromes with encephalopathy, long tract signs, ophthalmoparesis, vestibular dysfunction, nystagmus, ataxia, and cranial neuropathies. Overlap syndromes with simultaneous limbic system, diencephalon, and brainstem structures are less common (Dalmau et al., 2004; Ko et al., 2008). The anti-NMDAR antibody syndrome is characterized by a viral prodrome, prominent psychiatric symptoms, encephalopathy, abnormal facial and jaw movements, autonomic instability, and central hypoventilation requiring frequent intubation (Dalmau et al., 2007, 2008; Florance et al., 2009; Tuzun et al., 2009; Lancaster et al., 2010).

NATURAL HISTORY

Pelvic complications of tumors of the ovaries or testis represent late complications of irradiation and are far more common with testicular tumors (Greenfield and Stark, 1948; Numaba et al., 1990; Bowen et al., 1996; Knap et al., 2007). Single metastatic ovarian carcinoma to the brain may transiently respond favorably to surgical resection, irradiation, and chemotherapy, with average survival rates varying from 16 to 27 months (Cormio et al., 2003; D'Andrea et al., 2004; Pectasides et al., 2006). In general, paraneoplastic syndromes without treatment cause death from either oncologic or neurologic causes within a few months from initial symptoms. Whereas the anti-Yo antibody has poor prognosis, favorable response of tumor treatment with human

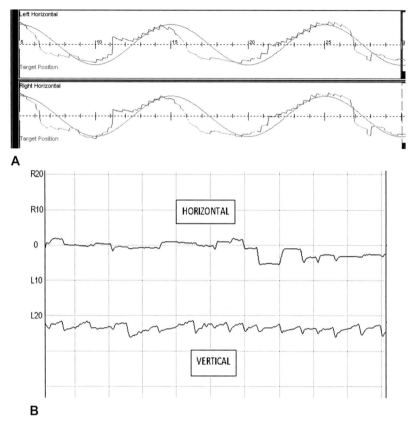

Fig. 52.1. (**A**) Observe saccadic horizontal (h) pursuit when the patient tracks a target toward her right and to a lesser extent to the left. Tracings were obtained in a 67-year-old woman with an acute vestibular syndrome, saccadic horizontal pursuit and downbeat nystagmus. The workup showed a positive anti-Yo antibody and she was found to have stage 3B ovarian carcinoma. (**B**) Observe a 10 second recording of central fixation in the same patient. Downbeat nystagmus in the primary position of gaze; frequency: 1.5 Hz, amplitude 3 degrees and velocity 3 degrees/sec is observed in the vertical V tracing.

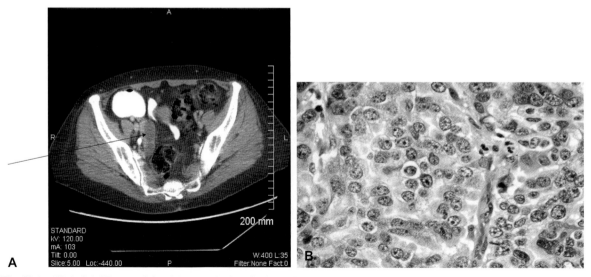

Fig. 52.2. (**A**) Axial CT scan of the abdomen obtained in the patient described in Figures 52.1 (A and B). It demonstrates a cystic mass involving the right ovary (arrow). Histopathologic examination established a diagnosis of carcinoma of the ovary. (**B**) Ovarian cancer in patient with anti-Yo syndrome described in Figure 52. 1A. H&E ×400. Observe large nuclei and multinucleated cells. Mitosis can be observed in several cells.

Table 52.2

Neuro-ophthalmologic paraneoplastic syndromes in tumors of the ovary and testis

Syndrome	Neurophthalmologic findings	Tumor
Anti-Yo antibody	Downbeat nystagmus Direction changing Horizontal nystagmus Saccade dysmetria Saccadic pursuit	Epithelial cancer of the ovary
Anti-Ma-2	Vertical gaze palsy* Complete gaze palsy Hearing loss/vertigo OTR/skew INO/sixth nerve palsy Up and downbeat nystagmus Opsoclonus/ocular flutter Positional central nystagmus**	Germinoma of the testis
Anti-NMDA antibody	Visual hallucinations Oculogyric crisis Opsoclonus	Teratoma of the ovary

*Vertical gaze abnormalities are frequent in the anti-Ma-2 antibody syndrome and the differential frequently includes Whipple's disease (Dalmau et al., 2004; Ko et al., 2008).

**Patient with a paraneoplastic cerebellar degeneration and testicular neoplasia presented with episodic vertigo and positional central nystagmus, he had a negative anti-Ma-2 antibody, was found to have a germinoma in undescended testis, and improved following bilateral orchidectomy and immunotherapy (Tafur et al., 2008).

immunoglobulin has been reported (Keime-Guibert et al., 2000; Dorn et al., 2003). The anti-NMDAR antibody syndrome responds well to tumor resection and immunosuppression (Ferioli et al., 2010; Kurlan et al., 2010). Likewise, the anti-Ma-2 antibody syndrome responds to orchidectomy, even in cases of testicular germinoma *in situ* (Dalmau et al., 2004).

LABORATORY INVESTIGATIONS

Ovarian cancer tumor markers are indicated when there is a clinical suspicion that a pelvic lesion is a primary tumor of the ovary. CA 125 may be elevated in 83% of women with ovarian cancer. When a teratoma of the ovary is suspected, α-fetoprotein, human choriogonadotropic hormone (h-CGD), and lactate dehydrogenase can be confirmatory. When suspecting germ cell tumors of the testicle, α-fetoprotein, h-CGD, and lactate dehydrogenase may also be helpful (Bosl and Motzer, 1997). Investigation for paraneoplastic syndromes includes a panel of antibodies ordered on the basis of the clinical phenotype. Anti-Yo (PCA-1) antibodies, anti-Ma-2 protein antibodies and anti-NMDA receptor antibodies are known serum/CSF markers associated with the tumors under consideration in this chapter. However, since the clinical findings may not be fully defined at the time of the initial workup, a more extensive panel of antibodies is often requested,

including anti-Tr and mGUR1 antibodies, anti-ANNNA-1, ANNA-2, ANNA-3, CV2/CRMP-5, antiphysin and voltage gated calcium channel (VGCC) antibodies. A more recently introduced anti-LGI1 antibody may be added, particularly in cases thought to have anti-voltage gated K-channel antibodies (Meizan et al., 2010). CSF examination includes determination of protein content, glucose, and cell count, including cytology, CSF IgG, IgG synthetic rate, oligoclonal bands, and tumor markers for paraneoplastc syndromes.

NEUROIMAGING INVESTIGATIONS

1. *Tumor diagnosis localized to the pelvis.* Ovarian tumors are first investigated with ultrasonography, computed tomography (CT) scan of the abdomen, or magnetic resonance imaging (MRI) with contrast. These investigations may provide an idea of the extent of tumor invasion (Fig. 52.2A) and are helpful in staging and surgery planning. Imaging and tumor markers are also helpful in differentiating benign versus malignant tumors. Testicular tumors are best differentiated from chronic orchitis and epididymitis with ultrasound. The typical germ cell tumor is intratesticular and has microcalcifications (one or more hypoechoic masses). More extensive testicular tumors are usually investigated with

pre- and postcontrast CT scan, MRI, and positron emission tomography (PET) scans which will be also useful for staging and treatment planning. In the event of lumbar or sacral plexus dysfunction these techniques may also show tumoral invasion of retroperitoneal structures. In cases of delayed postirradiation neurologic syndromes, there may be contrast enhancement of the cauda equina and lumbar and sacral roots (Bowen et al., 1996).

2. *Cerebral metastases of ovarian carcinoma.* MRI with contrast is the most sensitive test in patients with suspected metastatic ovarian carcinoma. Characteristic imaging findings include multiple lesions, localization at the gray–white matter junction, and small tumor focus with significant vasogenic edema.

3. *Neuroimaging findings of paraneoplastic syndromes.* The anti-Yo antibody syndrome is usually associated with a normal MRI in the initial phase; cerebellar atrophy develops in later stages. The anti-Ma-2 antibody syndrome may be associated with asymmetric areas of increased signal in the temporal lobes, particularly the hippocampi, hypothalamus, and upper brainstem. These lesions typically enhance following contrast administration. Simultaneous multifocal lesions of the diencephalon and brainstem may also be found. PET scan may show areas of hypometabolism (Dalmau et al., 2004). Patients with the anti-NMDAR antibody syndrome may have areas of increased signal abnormalities in different locations of the cerebrum on long T2 and fluid attenuated inversion recovery (FLAIR) sequences scans (Lancaster et al., 2010).

PATHOLOGY

Metastasic tumors of the ovaries to the brain. The histopathologic findings in metastatic tumor of the ovaries to the brain involve the characteristic findings of the primary tumor, associated with congestion and edema.

The histopathologic findings in the late, postirradiation lower motor neuron syndrome following testicular and rarely with ovarian tumors has been reported in detail. Gross examination of the cauda equina shows irregular thickening with focal areas of hemorrhage. Microscopically, clusters of dilated vascular channels with thickened hyalinized walls are found with sparing of anterior horn cells (Bowen et al., 1996). On the basis of these neuropathologic findings, the term "postirradiation lumbosacral radiculopathy" has been proposed (Bowen et al., 1996; Knap et al., 2007).

Paraneoplastic anti-Yo antibody syndrome. Neuropathologic examination of the cerebellum in patients with epithelial carcinomas of the ovaries show severe loss of Purkinje cells with proliferation of Bergmann glia

and infiltrates of inflammatory cells in the deep cerebellar nuclei. The actual mechanism of neuronal injury in this syndrome is not quite clear. The cytoplasmic Yo protein found in normal Purkinje and in ovarian carcinoma cells represent 34, 52, and 62 kDa cytoplasmic proteins known to interact with c-Myc. The disruption of the normal c-Myc cytoplasmic pathway leads to accelerated neuronal apoptosis. Anti-Yo antibodies may be seen in ovarian cancer, breast cancer, and at least one report of transitional cancer of the bladder. The anti-Yo antibody may also be present in patients with ovarian neoplasm without neurologic symptoms for prolonged follow-up periods.

Anti-Ma-2 antibody syndrome. The neuropathology of the anti Ma-2 antibody syndrome associated with germ cell tumors of the testis involves perivascular lymphocytic cuffing, lymphocytic interstitial infiltrates, variable gliosis and neuronal degeneration; The majority of lymphocytes are T cells with a smaller number of B cells, macrophages, plasma cells, and microglia (Dalmau et al., 2004). The predominant pathogenic mechanism, hypothesizes that the neurologic deficit is mediated by cytotoxic T cells attacking neurons. The initial event is triggered by apoptotic tumor cells which are captured by tissue dendritic cells, generating a specific T cell-mediated response. The dendritic cells in turn activate CD8+ and CD4-helper cells in lymph nodes, targeting cytoplasmic Ma proteins which are presumably involved in neuronal apoptosis prevention. (Tenner and Einhorn, 2009). The Ma-2 antibody has been found in other neoplasms, including lung, and in a recent report of hypothalamic neurosarcoidosis (Desestret et al., 2010).

Anti-N-methyl-D-aspartate receptor (anti-NMDAR) antibody encephalitis. Extensive neuronal loss, microgliosis, T lymphocytes, IgG deposits, and rare inflammation are the most distinctive characteristics. Preferential CNS involvement include the hippocampi, forebrain, basal ganglia, and spinal cord (Tuzun et al., 2009). The Purkinje cells are relatively spared, and cells expressing T cell markers of cytotoxicity are infrequent. The histopathology of the ovarian teratomas studied in this syndrome contain nervous tissue (mature and immature neurons) confirmed by their morphologic characteristics and neuronal markers (microtubule-associated protein-2). The absence of "encephalitis" on clinical grounds contrasts with the vigorous macrophage and T lymphocyte inflammatory reaction found on pathologic examination (Dalmau et al., 2008; Tuzun et al., 2009).

MANAGEMENT

Management of cerebral metastases of carcinoma of the ovaries depends on number and locations of these lesions. Solitary metastases in noneloquent brain areas are best treated with surgical resection followed by whole brain irradiation (Salvati and Cervoni, 1994; Cormio et al., 2003; Pectasides et al., 2006). Surgical resection followed by whole brain irradiation and platinum-based chemotherapy has been advocated (Cormio et al., 2003). However, the role of chemotherapy has not been studied in detail.

Platinum chemotherapy may be associated with transient neurologic deficits, including status epilepticus and cortical blindness and posterior reversible encephalopathy syndrome (Kattah et al., 1987). Moreover, platinum treatment is frequently associated with peripheral neuropathy and nephropathy.

The management of the paraneoplastic syndromes associated with tumors of the ovaries and testes involve optimal oncologic management with resection of the primary tumor and/or immunotherapy. In the anti-Ma-2 (Dalmau et al., 2004) and the anti-NMDAR syndromes (Dalmau et al., 2007, 2008), neurologic improvement is possible and frequent. The anti-Yo syndrome may be more difficult to treat (Keime-Guibert et al., 2000). However, chemotherapy and, more recently, rituximab have been shown to be helpful (Shams'ili et al., 2006; Esposito et al., 2008; Goret et al., 2008). Successful management of the anti-NMDA antibody syndrome can also be accomplished in pregnant women with ovarian teratomas with a good outcome for the mother and neonate (Kumar et al., 2010).

INFERTILITY, INFECUNDITY, ANDROGEN RECEPTOR INSENSITIVITY SYNDROME, AND PRIMARY OVARIAN FAILURE IN PATIENTS WITH NEUROLOGIC DISORDERS

Approximately 5–15% of couples in the reproductive age are unable to either become pregnant or maintain pregnancy to full term. Most cases (56%) relate to female infertility, about 25% to male infertility, and have a mixed cause in the remainder. Infertility deserves expert consultation after a period exceeding 1 year without successful pregnancy. Predictably, individuals in their thirties and forties have higher rates of infertility than the younger counterparts. A number of genetic X-linked neurologic disorders are associated with androgen receptor insensitivity (ARI), leading to testicular atrophy, oligospermia/azoospermia, gynecomastia and infertility in males and primary ovarian failure (POF) in carrier females. Other non-X chromosome genetic neurologic disorders, neuroendocrine syndromes, and commonly acquired neurologic syndromes, such as spinal cord injury and multiple sclerosis, among others, may affect male fertility.

Common, non-neurologic causes of infertility in males and females

Female "causes" for infertility include sequelae from sexually transmitted diseases, endometriosis, ovulatory dysfunction, poor nutrition, hormone imbalance, ovarian cysts, pelvic infection, tumors, or blockage of transport from the cervix through the fallopian tubes. Common "male" causes for infertility include testicular tumors, varicoceles, testicular atrophy, low sperm volume, low concentration or absence of sperm per milliliter of semen (oligospermia, azoospermia), or low sperm motility. Once preliminary tests have been conducted, when screening men and women for potential infertility causes the cervical mucus penetration assay test is performed. If less than 5–20% of uncovered hamster eggs are penetrated by spermatozoa, infertility is diagnosed (Healy et al., 1999; Montella et al., 2000; Bhasin, 2007).

From the aforementioned it is clear to neurologists that only a few neurologic disorders will be associated with AIS or POF. However, awareness of the possible association may be helpful in the patient's management and may lead to proper gynecologic, urologic, and genetic counseling. Table 52.3 is a list of the most common neurologic entities associated with POF and AIS. These are discussed briefly as they are associated with AIS in males and POF in females.

Fragile X syndrome

Introduction

The fragile X syndrome results from an expansion of CGG repeats in the *FMR1* gene which encodes the FMRP protein critical for intellectual development. Individuals with CGG repeats from 55 to 200 are considered premutation (carriers). More than 200 CGG repeats are associated with the fragile X syndrome (Hagerman and Hagerman, 2004; Wattendorf and Muenke, 2005).

History

The fragile X syndrome is the most common cause of inherited mental retardation with a variable phenotype depending on number of trinucleotide repeats in the X chromosome. Male adults with low CGG repeat expansion may have late onset ataxia and tremor (fragile X-associated tremor/ataxia syndrome, FXTAS). Women carriers may present with POF. A high number of CGG repeat expansion causes the full fragile X phenotype. It is possible that the father, and to a lesser extent the mother, of fragile X syndrome patients may develop late-onset FXTAS.

Table 52.3

Testicular atrophy, azoospermia, primary ovarian failure in common neurologic disorders

Disease and androgen receptor (AR) gene expansion*	Primary ovarian failure (POF)	Testis	Male phenotype	Infertility
Fragile X syndrome CGG repeats Kennedy's syndrome CAG repeats	+	Macroorchidism	Normal	Common in males POF in females**
Mild CAG repeats in AR < 28 repeats	Moderate androgen receptor insensitivity (ARI)	Gynecomastia Micropenis Testicular atrophy	Undervirilization Gynecomastia Female phenotype	Fertility possible Infertility
Severe >28 CAG repeats	Severe ARI			
Myotonic dystrophy CAG/CTG repeats	Possible	Phenotypically female. Testis in abdomen. Ambiguous genitalia Testicular atrophy Azoospermia in > than 18 CAG/CTG repeats	Gynecomastia	Infertility depends on CAG/CTG repeats
Machado Joseph's spinocerebellar ataxia	Unknown	Depends on CAG repeats Azoospermia > than 29 repeats	Normal	Infertility edepends on CAG repeats
3 CAG repeats Mitochondrial disorders	Possible	Normal	Normal	Infertility due to decreased spermatozoa mobility
Spinal cord injury + myelopathy	Not present	Normal	Normal	Sperm abnormal Spermatozoa normal

*Idiopathic azoospermia = 31 CAG repeats in the AR.
**POF in premutation females = 55–200 CAG repeats.

CLINICAL FINDINGS

Mental retardation, autism-like picture, and attention deficit hyperactivity disorder (ADHD), behavioral changes, a typical facies, scoliosis, and significant macrorchidism are common findings in the fragile X syndrome. Seizures in the late-onset form are common. Ataxia and tremor may be observed. Young patients with limited CGG repeats may be fertile and become infertile over time. Females may have POF (Sherman, 2000; Welt et al., 2004; Sullivan, 2005).

NATURAL HISTORY

Rate of progression of neurologic findings depends on the number of CGG repeats (usually greater than 200). The phenotype of a male with a smaller number of repeats is associated with a more benign clinical course which may manifest as late-onset essential type tremor and ataxia (FXTAS).

PATHOLOGY

Histopathologic studies show no gross structural abnormalities, despite the profound degree of mental retardation (Nelson, 1998). Microscopic examination shows eosinophilic intranuclear inclusions in neuron and astrocytes throughout the cortex, subcortical structures and brainstem (Chaussenot et al., 2008), abnormal dendrite spine morphology with preservation of neuronal density in the neocortex may be found (Hinton et al., 1991).

LABORATORY INVESTIGATIONS

The cause of the fragile X syndrome is a defect in the synthesis of the fragile X mental retardation protein (FMRP), a regulatory protein in neurons and dendrites required for normal neuronal maturation. The presence of expanded CGG repeats interferes with the synthesis and action of FMRP, which has a role in ctytoplasmic mRNA metabolism (Nelson, 1998).

1. DNA testing is recommended. The exact number of CGG repeats in the *FMR1* gene may be determined by Southern blot or polymerase chain reaction (PCR). The normal number of CGG repeats vary from 5 to 54. More than 55 CGG repeats are considered premutation. More than 200 CGG repeats define a full mutation. Mosaic patterns are common. Mothers of fragile X males have a premutation. Females with fragile X are less severely affected. Germane to this topic, premutation females may present with isolated POF. In fragile X-phenotype males and females CGG expansion may not be found, but point mutation in the *FMR1* gene may be identified.
2. MRI of the brain in the FXTAS shows cerebral and cerebellar atrophy, and nonspecific increased signal in the white matter, including the symmetric middle cerebellar peduncle sign (Berry-Kravis et al., 2007).

MANAGEMENT

Symptomatic treatment of the neurologic manifestations and genetic counseling are the main treatment options (Berry-Kravis et al., 2007).

Kennedy's Disease

INTRODUCTION

Also known as spinobulbar muscular atrophy (SBMA), this is an X-linked spinal bulbar neuronopathy associated with androgen receptor insensitivity (La Spada et al., 1991).

HISTORY

Muscle weakness and wasting are usually present between the ages of 15 and 60 years. Muscle weakness is mostly proximal. Fasciculations involving the facial muscles and bulbar musculature are common. Insensitivity to male hormones, gynecomastia, microrchidism, infertility and impotence may be present in the teenage years or develop in the forties or fifties. In some cases with milder forms, fertility may be normal. Diabetes mellitus may also be present (Kennedy et al., 1968).

NATURAL HISTORY

The natural history varies with the degree of CAG repeats in the androgen receptor located in chromosome Xq 11-12 which causes progressive loss of motoneurons (normal CAG repeats: 17–26). An unstable expansion of the CAG repeat in exon 1 of the androgen receptor (AR) gene is the pathogenic mechanism. Progressive spinal atrophy may lead to an inability to ambulate. Bulbar musculature compromise may cause slowly progressive swallowing difficulties and dysarthria. In milder forms, the patient may be able to walk even in the fourth to fifth decades (Kennedy et al., 1968; Sperfeld et al., 2002). During puberty, overt signs of undervirilization may be noted, but the more severe forms of ARI are not associated with this disease (Nistche and Hiort, 2000; Wisniewski et al., 2000).

PATHOLOGY

Muscle biopsy shows predominant neurogenic and, to a lesser extent, myopathic changes.

LABORATORY INVESTIGATIONS

Testosterone levels are decreased, estradiol may be increased, and luteinizing hormone (LH) may be increased. All of these hormonal levels correlate with the amount of CAG repeats in the AR. Men with greater than 28 repeats have increased risk of impaired spermatogenesis. However, if clinical signs of AR develop in the fourth or fifth decade then they may able to procreate; 72% report having children. PCR for CAG repeats in exon 1 of the AR gene will demonstrate a diagnostic expansion (greater than 26 CAG repeats).

MANAGEMENT

Other than symptomatic treatment and genetic counseling, there is little else to offer to these patients.

Myotonic dystrophy

INTRODUCTION

Myotonic dystrophy (MD). The most frequent cause of muscular dystrophy in adults (Harper, 2001) is an autosomal dominant inherited disorder characterized by muscle weakness and wasting (dystrophy) and sustained involuntary muscle contractions (myotonia). Systemic manifestations of MD may be seen chiefly with cardiac, endocrine, and multiorgan compromise.

HISTORY

Initial manifestations often occur in teenagers in the form of distal muscle weakness, atrophy, and myotonia. Both males and females are affected. Testicular atrophy, impotence, and loss of sex drive develops among MD males. Females often report loss of sex drive, premature menopause, and habitual abortions. Myotonia may be symptomatic. Cataracts may occasionally be the first manifestation; their features may be quite characteristic by slit lamp examination (Christmas tree, multicolored iridescent). Gynecomastia and lack of male sexual development, impotence, and infertility may be initial complaints (Fig. 52.3). Diabetes mellitus, glucose intolerance, respiratory failure, and cardiac arrhythmias/insufficiency may be late manifestations (Harper, 2001).

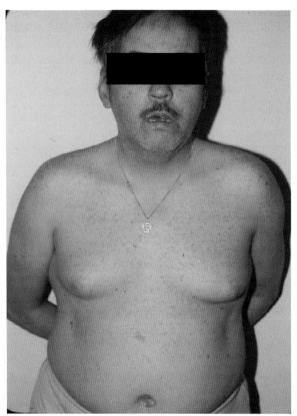

Fig. 52.3. Observe gynecomastia in a patient with myotonic dystrophy and a complaint of infertility. He had low serum testosterone levels, testicular atrophy, and erectile dysfunction.

NATURAL HISTORY

Clinical signs vary with the number of CTG trinucleotides in the myotonic dystrophy protein kinase (*DMPK*) gene (normal 5–30 repeats). The gene normally encodes the myotonic dystrophy protein kinase (myotininkinase), which is expressed primarily in muscle. Loss of DMPK results in altered muscle-specific chloride channel function. The gene is located in the short arm of chromosome 19 (19q). MD tends to be more severe with subsequent generations. The cause for infertility in males with MD is not clearly defined. Decreased sperm function has been found in the ejaculates of sterile MD patients (Hortas et al., 2000). However, infertility is not universal in MD males. Females may have higher risk of complications during pregnancy. A relationship between the number of CTG repeats and sterility has been reported (Hsiao, 2002). Increased CTG/CAG repeats in the androgen receptor have been identified in MD and Machado Joseph's disease (Pan et al., 2002).

LABORATORY INVESTIGATIONS

The clinical characteristics are usually diagnostic. However, a genetic diagnosis provides 100% sensitivity and specificity (Shelbourne et al., 1993). EMG and muscle biopsy can offer diagnostic information but genetic testing is the recommended choice if possible. Prenatal and preimplantation diagnosis is possible and genetic intervention may be successful (Sermon et al., 1997; Kakorou et al., 2007).

TREATMENT

Symptomatic treatment is the only therapeutic alternative. Management of systemic complications involves multiple specialists and from the aforementioned, genetic counseling is critical in this disorder.

Miscellaneous

There are several genetic and acquired disorders of the hypothalamus and pituitary gland that result in secondary gonadal atrophy and infertility in addition to neurologic abnormalities. The main congenital disorders include: (1) Praeder–Labhart–Willi syndrome: congenital deficiency of gonadal releasing hormone (GnRH) with hypogonadism, mental retardation, facial dysmorphism and obesity (Ledbetter et al., 1981); (2) Kallmann syndrome: decreased GnRh and anosmia ataxia, hearing loss (Kallmann et al., 1943); (3) Laurence–Moon–Bardet–Biedl syndrome with hypogonadism, retinitis pigmentosa, obesity, and polydactyly (McLouglin and Shanklin, 1967; Laurence and Moon, 1886; Qureshi et al., 2003).

Acquired causes of hypothalamic and pituitary gland dysfunction include pituitary tumors, craniopharyngioma, germinomas, granulomatous disorders, hystiocytosis and s/p therapeutic radiation (Kattah and Kattah, 2008).

Infertility may also be a complication of mitochondrial disorders with reduced sperm motility (Folgero et al., 1993). Patients with spinal cord injury besides erectile dysfunction may also have abnormal semen, most likely due to denervation of the seminal vesicles and prostate with diminished sperm motility (Kafetsoulis et al., 2006; Brackett et al., 2010). Although sperm may be obtained without major difficulty, in these patients a successful pregnancy rate is low (Yamamoto et al., 1997).

REFERENCES

Abrey LE, Dalmau JO (2000). Neurologic complications of ovarian carcinoma. Cancer 85: 127–133.

Beatrous TE, Choyke PL, Frank JA (1990). Diagnostic evaluation of cancer patients with pelvic pain: comparison of scintigraphy, CT and MR imaging. AJR Am J Roentgenol 155: 85–88.

Berry-Kravis E, Abrams L, Coffey SM et al. (2007). Fragile X-associated tremor/ataxia syndrome: clinical features, genetics, and testing guidelines. Mov Disord 22: 2018–2030.

Bhasin S (2007). Approach to infertility man. Clin Endocrinol Metab 92: 1995–2004.

Bokemeyer C, Nowak P, Haupt A (1997). Treatment of brain metastases in patties with testicular cancer. J Clin Oncol 15: 1449–1454.

Bosl GJ, Motzer RJ (1997). Testicular germ cell tumors. N Engl J Med 337: 242–254.

Bowen J, Gregory R, Squier M et al. (1996). The post-irradiation lower motor neuron syndrome neuropathy or radiculopathy. Brain 119: 1429–1439.

Brackett NL, Lynne CM, Ibrahim E et al. (2010). Treatment of infertility in men with spinal cord injury: semen abnormalities. Nat Rev Urol 7: 162–172.

Chaussenot A, Borg M, Bayreuther C et al. (2008). Late cerebellar ataxia associated with fragile X premutation. Rev Neurol 164: 957–963.

Cormio G, Maneo A, Colamaria A et al. (2003). Surgical resection of solitary brain metastasis from ovarian carcinoma: an analysis of 22 cases. Gynecol Oncol 89: 116–119.

D'Andrea GD, Roperto R, Dinia L et al. (2004). Solitary cerebral metastases from ovarian epithelial carcinoma: 11 cases. Neurosurg Rev 28: 120–123.

Dalmau J, Graus F, Villarejo A et al. (2004). Clinical analysis of anti-Ma2-associated encephalitis. Brain 127: 1831–1844.

Dalmau JO, Tuzun E, Wu HY et al. (2007). Paraneoplastic anti-N-methyl aspartate receptor encephalitis associated with ovarian teratoma. Ann Neurol 61: 25–36.

Dalmau JO, Gleichman AJ, Hughes EG et al. (2008). Anti-NMDA receptor encephalitis: case series and analysis of the effect of antibodies. Lancet Neurol 7: 1091–1098.

Desestret V, Didelot A, Meyronet D et al. (2010). Neurosarcoidosis with diencephalitis and anti-Ma2 antibodies. Neurology 74: 772–774.

Dorn C, Knobloch C, Kupka M et al. (2003). Paraneoplastic neurological syndrome: patient with anti-Yo antibody and breast cancer: a case report. Arch Gynecol Obstet 269: 62–65.

Esposito M, Penza P, Orefice G et al. (2008). Successful treatment of paraneoplastic cerebellar degeneration with rituximab. J Neurooncol 86: 363–364.

Fadul CE (2008). Testis and ovaries. In: J Biller (Ed.), The Interface of Neurology and Internal Medicine. Wolters Kluwer/Lippincott, Williams and Wilkins, Philadelphia, pp. 502–507.

Ferioli S, Dalmau J, Kobet CA et al. (2010). Anti-N-methyl-D aspartate receptor encephalitis. Arch Neurol 67: 250–251.

Florance NR, Davis RL, Lam C et al. (2009). Anti-N-methyl-D-aspartate receptor (NMDAR) encephalitis in children and adolescents. Ann Neurol 66: 11–18.

Folgero T, Bertheussen K, Lindal S (1993). Andrology: mitochondrial disease and reduced sperm motility. Hum Reprod 11: 1863–1993.

Goret F, Bosca I, Fratalia L et al. (2008). Long-lasting remission after rituximab treatment in a case of anti-HU associated neuronopathy and gastric pseudoobstruction. J Neurooncol 93: 421–423.

Greenfield MM, Stark FM (1948). Post-irradiation neuropathy. Am J Roentgenol 60: 617–622.

Greenlee JE, Brashear HR (1983). Antibodies to cerebellar Purkinje cells in patients with paraneoplastic cerebellar degeneration and ovarian carcinoma. Ann Neurol 14: 609–613.

Hagerman PJ, Hagerman RJ (2004). The fragile-X premutation: a maturing perspective. Am J Hum Genet 74: 805–816.

Harper PS (2001). Myotonic Dystrophy. 3rd edn WB Saunders, London.

Healy DL, Trounson AO, Anderson AN et al. (1999). Female infertility: causes and treatment. Lancet 343: 1539–1544.

Hinton VJ, Brown WT, Wisnieswski K et al. (1991). Analysis of neocortex in three males with the fragile x-syndrome. Am J Med Genet 41: 289–294.

Hortas ML, Castilla JA, Gil MT et al. (2000). Decreased sperm function of patients with myotonic dystrophy. Hum Reprod 15: 445–448.

Hsiao KM (2002). Reported relationship between increased CTG repeat lengths in myotonic dystrophy and azoospermia. Hum Reprod 17: 1578–1583.

Hudson CN, Curling M, Potsides P et al. (1993). Paraneoplastic syndromes in patients with ovarian neoplasia. J R Soc Med 86: 202–204.

Kafetsoulis A, Brackett NL, Ibrahim E et al. (2006). Current trends of infertility in men with spinal cord injury. Fertil Steril 86: 781–789.

Kakorou G, Dhnajal S, Daphni D et al. (2007). Preimplantation genetic diagnosis for myotonic dystrophy type 1: detection of crossover between the gene and the linked marker APOC2. Prenat Diagn 27: 111–116.

Kallmann FJ, Schonfeld WA, Barrera SE et al. (1943). The genetic aspects of primary eunuchoidism. Am J Ment Defic 48: 203–206.

Kattah JC, Kattah WC (2008). Pituitary and hypothalamus. In: J Biller (Ed.), The Interface of Neurology and Internal Medicine. Wolters Kluwer/Lippincott, Williams and Wilkins, Philadelphia, pp. 465–470.

Kattah JC, Potolicchio SJ, Kotz HL et al. (1987). Cortical blindness and occipital lobe seizures induced by cys-platinum. Neurophthalmology 7: 99–104.

Keime-Guibert F, Graus F, Fleury A et al. (2000). Treatment of paraneoplastic neurological syndromes with antineuronal antibodies (Anti-Hu, anti-Yo) with a combination of immunoglobulins, cyclophosphamide, and methylprednisolone. J Neurol Neurosurg Psychiatry 68: 479–482.

Kennedy WR, Alter M, Sung JH et al. (1968). Progressive proximal spinal and bulbar muscular atrophy of late onset: a sex-linked recessive trait. Neurology 18: 671–680.

Knap MM, Bentzen SM, Overgaard J (2007). Late neurological complications after irradiation of malignant tumors of the testis. Acta Oncol 46: 497–503.

Ko MW, Dalmau J, Galetta S (2008). Neuro-ophthalmologic maanifestations of paraneoplastic syndromes. J Neuroophthalmol 28: 58–68.

Kumar MA, Jain A, Dechant VE et al. (2010). Anti-N-methyl-D aspartate receptor encephalitis during pregnancy. Arch Neurol 67: 884–887.

Kurlan M, Lalive PH, Dalmau JO et al. (2010). Opsoclonus-myoclonus syndrome in anti-methyl-D-aspartate receptor encephalitis. Arch Neurol 67: 118–121.

La Spada AR, Wilson EM, Lubahn DB et al. (1991). Androgen receptor gene mutation in X-linked spinal and bulbar muscular atrophy. Nature 352: 77–79.

Lancaster E, Lai M, Peng X (2010). Antibodies to the GABA_B receptor in limbic enecephalitis with seizures: case series and characterization of the antigen. Lancet Neurol 9: 67–76.

Laurence JZ, Moon RC (1886). Four cases of retinitis pigmentosa occurring in the same family and accompanied by general imperfections of metabolism. Ophthalmol Rev 2: 32.

Ledbetter DH, Riccardi VM, Airhart SD et al. (1981). Deletion of chromosome 15 as a cause Praeder–Willi syndrome. N Engl J Med 304: 325–329.

McLouglin TG, Shanklin JR (1967). Pathology of Laurence–Moon–Bardet–Biedl syndrome. J Pathol 93: 65–79.

Meizan L, Maarteje GMH, Lancaster E et al. (2010). Investigation of LGI1 as the antigen in límbic encephalitis previously attributed to potassium channels: a case series. Lancet Neurol 9: 776–785.

Montella K, Keekly E, Laifer S et al. (2000). Evaluation and management of infertility in women: the internist role. Ann Intern Med 132: 974–981.

Nelson DL (1998). Molecular Basis of Mental Retardation: Fragile X-Syndrome. In: JB Martin (Ed.), Molecular Neurology. Scientific American, New York, pp. 19–35.

Nitsche EM, Hiort O (2000). The molecular basis of androgen insensitivity. Horm Res 54: 327–333.

Numaba K, Ito M, Uchiyama S (1990). A case of delayed radiation lumbosacral plexopathy. No To Shinkei 42: 629–633.

Pan H, Li Y, Li T (2002). Increased (CTG/CAG) lengths in myotonic dystrophy type 1 and Machado–Joseph disease genes in idiopathic azoospermia patients. Hum Reprod 17: 1578–1583.

Pectasides D, Pectasides M, Econoopoulos T (2006). Brain metastases from epithelial ovarian cancer: a review of the literature. Oncologist 11: 252–260.

Qureshi T, Nasti AR, Ashai M (2003). Laurence, Moon, Bardet, Biedl syndrome. JK Practitioner 10: 217–218.

Salvati M, Cervoni L (1994). Solitary metastasis from ovarian carcinoma: report of 4 cases. J Neurooncol 19: 75–77.

Sermon K, Lissens W, Jones S (1997). Clinical application of preimplanatation diagnosis for myotonic dystrophy. Prenat Diagn 17: 925–932.

Shams'ili S, Beukelaar J, Willem Gartama J et al. (2006). An uncontrolled trial of rituximab for antibody associated paraneoplastic neurologic syndromes. J Neurol 253: 16–20.

Shelbourne P, Davies J, Baxton J et al. (1993). Direct diagnosis of myotonic dystrophy with a disease-specific DNA marker. N Engl J Med 328: 471–475.

Sherman SL (2000). Primary ovarian failure in the fragile x-syndrome. Am J Med Genet 3: 189–194.

Sperfeld AD, Karitzky J, Brummer D et al. (2002). X-linked bulbospinal neuronopathy. Arch Neurol 59: 1921–1926.

Sullivan AK (2005). Association of FMR1 repeats size with ovarian dysfunction. Hum Reprod 20: 402–412.

Tafur AJ, Baumann Kreuzinger LM, Quevedo F et al. (2008). 28-year-old man with severe vertigo. Mayo Clin Proc 83: 1070–1073.

Tenner L, Einhorn L (2009). Ma-2 paraneoplastic encephalitis in the presence of bilateral testicular cancer. J Clin Oncol 27: e57–e58.

Tuzun E, Zhou L, Baehring JM (2009). Evidence for antibody-mediated pathogenesis in anti-NMDAR encephalitis associated with ovarian teratoma. Acta Neuropathol 118: 737–743.

Voltz R, Gultekin SH, Rosenfeld MR et al. (1999). A serologic marker of paraneoplastic limbic and brainstem encephalitis in patients with testicular cancer. N Engl J Med 340: 1788–1795.

Wattendorf DJ, Muenke M (2005). Diagnosis and management of fragile X-syndrome. Am Fam Physician 2005: 111–113.

Welt CK, Smith PC, Taylor AE (2004). Evidence of early ovarian aging in fragile-X premutation carriers. J Clin Endocrinol Metab 9: 4569–4574.

Wisniewski AB, Migeon CJ, Meyer-Bahlburg HF et al. (2000). Complete androgen insensitivity syndrome: long term medical, surgical and psychosexual outcome. J Clin Endocrinol Metab 85: 2664–2669.

Yamamoto N, Yamada K, Hirata N et al. (1997). Electroejaculation and assisted reproductive techniques in patients with spinal cord injury. Nippon Heikatsukin Gakkai Zasshi 88: 420–426.

Handbook of Clinical Neurology, Vol. 120 (3rd series)
Neurologic Aspects of Systemic Disease Part II
Jose Biller and Jose M. Ferro, Editors

Chapter 53

Neurologic complications of multiple endocrine syndromes

JORGE C. KATTAH[1]* AND WILLIAM C. KATTAH[2]

[1]*Department of Neurology, University of Illinois College of Medicine, Peoria, IL, USA*

[2]*Endocrinology Department, University of the Andes, Bogota, Colombia*

INTRODUCTION

The neurologic manifestations of different endocrine syndromes may be classified according to specific hormone production changes and target tissue receptor response. Central nervous system (CNS) and peripheral nervous system (PNS) abnormalities are common manifestations of endocrine disorders. This chapter reviews the CNS and PNS manifestations of multiple endocrine syndromes (MES). MES account for a group of uncommon, familial disorders with polyglandular abnormalities, occurring in two main clinical contexts. The first involves *autoimmune-mediated* destruction of glandular tissue with decreased or absent hormone production: polyendocrine autoimmune syndromes (APS) acknowledge clinical phenotypes, type I and II involving adrenal insufficiency and type III sparing the adrenal glands. A second relates to *familial oncogene* derangements associated with multiple endocrine neoplasia (MEN), types 1 and 2. CNS and PNS abnormalities may be seen with both autoimmune and neoplastic MES and represent the subject of this chapter. Although the pathogenesis of the neurologic abnormalities associated with MES frequently involves endocrine and metabolic-mediated CNS and PNS alterations, independent autoimmune neurologic syndromes due to antineuronal antibodies may also be observed in the autoimmune polyglandular syndrome.

AUTOIMMUNE POLYGLANDULAR SYNDROME TYPE I

(Table 53.1)

Introduction

The endocrine characteristics define autoimmune polyglandular syndrome (APS) I. The pathogenesis involves antibody production against glandular surface cellular receptors, intracellular enzymes, and secreted proteins. APS I has no known HLA association. It is inherited as a sporadic, autosomal recessive (AR) trait. The genetic locus resides in the short arm of chromosome 21. A monogenic change of the AIRE-1 (autoimmune regulator-1) gene causes decreased immune tolerance leading to multiple endocrine glandular dysfunctions. The *AIRE* gene controls the expression of a tissue-specific substance in the thymus that controls autoimmune tolerance. Different mutations, deletions and insertions of the *AIRE* gene are responsible for the development of APS I (Balazs and Feher, 2009). The disorder is considered very uncommon. Given its AR inheritance, it is clustered in communities with high rates of consanguinity (Neufeld et al., 1981; Heino et al., 1999).

History

Typical initial manifestations are observed among young children beginning from ages 3–5 years to early adolescence. The three cardinal manifestations include: mucocutaneous candidiasis; clinical manifestations consistent with hypoparathyroidism with tetany and encephalopathy in childhood or adolescence; Addison's disease occurring in the first two decades of life, with encephalopathy, arterial hypotension, hypoglycemia, shock, and other manifestations of Addison's disease. Additional multiple endocrinopathies may develop in

---

*Correspondence to: Jorge C. Kattah, M.D., Department of Neurology, University of Illinois College of Medicine at Peoria and the Illinois Neurological Institute at OSF Saint Francis Medical Center, 530 NE Glen Oak Avenue, Peoria, IL 61637, USA. E-mail: kattahj@uicomp.uic.edu

Table 53.1

Polyendocrine autoimmune syndromes

Type	Clinical manifestations	Genetics	Neurologic manifestations
1	Mucocutaneous candidasis Hypoparathyroidism Addison's disease	Autosomal recessive	Movement disorders Ataxia Tetany

2	Addison's disease
	Type 1 diabetes mellitus
	Autoimmune thyroid
	  disease
		Polygenic	Related to diabetes mellitus
			  and hypothyroidism

3	Normal adrenal function Autoimmune thyroiditis Type 1 diabetes mellitus	Autosomal dominant	Related to diabetes mellitus and hyopothyroidism

older patients with APS I. Addison's disease may be categorized by age of onset (Carey, 1997). The association with recurrent candidiasis and absence of overt neurologic and neuro-ophthalmologic abnormalities is the best way to separate this syndrome from the childhood-onset, sex-linked variant of adrenoleukodystrophy (Moser et al., 2004).

Clinical findings

APS I should be suspected in any patient with autoimmune Addison's disease; genetic testing may be used for confirmation. Evidence of recurrent mucocutaneous candidiasis is a frequent finding in these patients and is present in the first year of life. The defining cardinal manifestations occur within the first 20 years of life. Hypocalcemia results from parathyroid hypoplasia or DiGeorge syndrome. Carpopedal spasm, paresthesias, seizures, laryngospasm, cataracts, papilledema, and encephalopathy may be observed. The electrocardiogram may show prolonged QT interval. Addison's disease is usually the last endocrinopathy to occur in patients with APS I. Orthostatic intolerance, weakness, and fatigue are early signs. Additional features include hypogonadism, malabsorption, pernicious anemia, alopecia, and vitiligo. Late neurologic abnormalities include a single case report of a Miller Fisher syndrome with spontaneous recovery followed by progressive autoimmune spinocerebellar syndrome (Berger et al., 2008), a case of choreoathetosis and hemibalismus (Baumert et al., 1993), and a familial, limb girdle, muscular dystrophy in three sisters with APS I who had trabecular fibers in muscle biopsy, cataracts, epilepsy, and intracranial basal ganglia calcifications (Gazulla et al., 2005).

Natural history

Laboratory investigations

To confirm the autoimmune etiology of the endocrinopathies, an investigation for organ-specific antibodies is required. Autoantibodies against the parathyroid glands and/or the calcium sensor may be present. The 21-hydroxylase (OH) is the principal target antigen in cases of autoimmune Addison's disease, found in 85% of patients with APS I (Kahaly, 2009). Specific AIRE-1 genetic testing for symptomatic patients may confirm the clinical suspicion. Patients with APS I should be routinely monitored for the emergence of new endocrine and systemic autoimmune complications.

Neurologic abnormalities may be potential manifestations of this syndrome, particularly in patients with circulating antibodies which may precede clinically detectable abnormalities. Common antibodies directed to specific neurotransmitters found in these patients include: aromatic L-amino acid decarboxylase antibodies (AADC), tyrosine hydroxilase (TH), tryptophan hydroxylase (TPH), glutamic acid decarboxylase (GAD), and γ-aminobutyric acid (GABA). Antibodies against dopamine, serotonin, and noradrenaline may also be found (Fettisov et al., 2009). Although antibodies against enzymes involved in monoamine neurotransmitter synthesis are found in these patients, they do not always cause clinical manifestations.

Neuroimaging

No specific cerebral imaging abnormalities are found in patients with APS I. Cerebral calcinosis may be found in some cases, probably related to hypoparathyroidism (Gass, 1962; Baba et al., 2005).

Pathology

Lymphocytic infiltration of affected endocrine glands is associated with functional loss of epithelial cells and scarring. A dominance of T-helper cells and deficiency of suppressor T cells has been demonstrated in endocrine autoimmunity. No specific report of neuropathologic findings among APS I have been reported to our knowledge (Kahaly, 2009).

Management

The individual endocrine syndrome is managed as usual. Antifungal therapy is used as needed for recurrent candidiasis. Ketoconazole should be avoided, however, due to its potential effect on endocrine function. Calcium, vitamin D, and parathyroid hormone (PTH) are provided as needed. A major challenge is to anticipate the future development of additional endocrine failure. In general, antibodies against 21-hydroxylase (OH) represent an indication for treatment. Genetic counseling may be advisable.

AUTOIMMUNE POLYGLANDULAR SYNDROME TYPE II

Introduction

Also known as Schmidt's syndrome, APS type II is characterized by the association of Addison's disease, type 1 diabetes mellitus (DM), and autoimmune thyroid disease. Adrenal insufficiency is present in a high percentage of cases. APS II is more common in women and is far more frequent than APS I. The prevalence of APS II has been estimated at 1.4–2/100 000 and occurs most frequently in the third to fourth decades. Type 1 DM is one of the earliest manifestation of APS II. APS type II is inherited as an autosomal dominant (AD) trait with incomplete penetrance. HLA antigens and their IR genes are decisive in the pathogenesis of this disease (Balazs and Feher, 2010). HLA-DR3 and HLA-DR4 are more common in APS II. The pathogenesis of APS II is unknown. A familial defect of immunoregulation is likely (Dittmar and Kahaly, 2003).

History

Clinical manifestations depend on the specific hormone deficiency. Diagnosis is suspected when there is a combination of type 1 DM, adrenal insufficiency, and autoimmune thyroiditis or Graves' disease. Neurologic abnormalities may result from complications of DM, adrenal disease, or autoimmune thyroiditis. Graves' disease and ophthalmopathy may occur. A paraneoplastic syndrome with neuropathy and ataxia was reported in a patient with APS II and small cell carcinoma of the lung (Watanabe et al., 2008). An APS II patient with low serum vitamin B_{12} and antiparietal cell antibodies had fluctuating neurologic symptoms and a radiologic picture resembling multiple sclerosis (Hosseini et al., 1998).

In large published series from the University of Gutemberg, concerning 15 000 patients with different endocrine disorders, 360 were diagnosed with APS II and 151 of them were followed for ~13 years (Dittmar and Kahaly, 2003). Autoimmune thyroid disease was observed in 65% of cases. Autoimmune thyroiditis and Graves' disease occurred with the same frequency. Type 1 DM occurred in 60% of cases. Addison's disease was found in 18.5% and gonadal failure in 5.3% of cases. Nonendocrine manifestations included vitiligo, alopecia, and pernicious anemia. The interval between the different clinical APS II manifestations was variable, but usually no longer than 10 years. In the Gutemberg series, the presence of endocrine autoantibodies generally predicted eventual clinical manifestations of glandular failure.

Clinical findings

The systemic and neurologic findings in these patients are related to the underlying single or multiple endocrinopathies present (Heuss et al., 1995).

Besides APS-II, common causes of concurrent endocrine and neurologic disorders include the following: (1) multiple endocrine neoplasia; (2) autoimmune thyroid disease (Brain et al., 1966; Flanagan et al., 2010); (3) Graves' disease; (4) mitochondrial disorders; (5) DM, diabetes insipidus, optic atrophy, and sensorineural deafness in cases of Wolfram's syndrome; (6) polyglandular endocrine failure may also be seen in association with panhypopituitarism and hypothalamic disorders (Kattah and Kattah, 2008); (7) endocrinopathy associated with plasma cell dyscrasia and circulating cytokines (IL-1β), characterized clinically by organomegaly, adenopathy, monoclonal gammopathy syndrome and known by the acronym POEMS (Ghandi et al., 2007).

Natural history

Most of the clinical manifestations of APS II are treated with hormonal replacement. Patients must be monitored for additional endocrine and other systemic autoimmune disorders.

Laboratory investigations

An autoimmune etiology should be considered in any patient with type 1 DM, thyroid failure, Graves' disease, or adrenal failure. Antibodies against thyroid peroxidase (TPO), thyroglobulin (TG), and thyroid stimulating immunoglobulin may be ordered for patients with clinical signs of thyroid dysfunction. Anti-GAD and anti-insulin antibodies may be requested to diagnose type 1

DM. The 21-hydroxylase (OH), the 17-α-(OH) and the side chain cleavage enzyme antibodies should be requested to confirm autoimmune Addison's disease. Genetic testing is not available as this is a polygenic disorder. HLA typing could be requested in selected cases.

Neuroimaging and pathology

Neuroimaging or neuropathologic findings in APS II are not available to our knowledge. In general, the pathologic findings in the endocrine glands of these patients are similar in all APS syndromes and overlap with those found in single autoimmune endocrine syndromes. We report in this chapter typical clinical and brain MRI findings in a patient with APS II with acute limbic encephalitis (Fig. 53.1). Immunosuppression improved the clinical and imaging abnormalities.

Management

Management of APS II involves hormonal replacement. Therapy for syndromic endocrine failure is similar to isolated endocrine failure. Normalization of adrenal failure must precede thyroid replacement when managing simultaneous adrenal and thyroid dysfunction. Life-threatening

adrenal failure may develop as a result of increased hepatic corticosteroid metabolism due to the replaced thyroid hormone (Majeroni and Patel, 2007).

AUTOIMMUNE POLYGLANDULAR SYNDROME TYPE III

Introduction

The characteristic phenotype of this syndrome includes polyglandular failure with autoimmune thyroiditis, type 1 DM, and other autoimmune disorders with absence of adrenal insufficiency. Autoimmune thyroiditis or Graves' disease may occur, usually in the third decade of life. The precise pathogenesis of this disorder is unknown. APS III has been reported in monozygotic twins (Ugur et al., 2004). The HLA DRB-1 is found in this group of patients. The presumed pathogenesis involves a similar mechanism to APS II. The diagnosis of APS III followed treatment with interferon-α. (Sasso et al., 2003). This raises the possibility of viral-mediated mechanisms, molecular mimicry, or permanent autoimmunity. Adrenal failure would be distinctly uncommon in this syndrome in contrast to APS I and APS II. APS III is rare. No epidemiologic data are currently

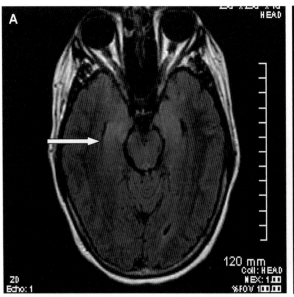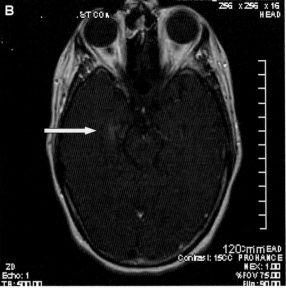

Fig. 53.1. Axial MRI obtained on a patient with a long-standing history of polyglandular dysfunction. She was initially diagnosed as having Hashimoto's thyroiditis in her twenties. This was followed a few years later by autoimmune adrenal failure. Positive antibodies against 21-hydroxylase were detected with a 27.3 U/mL serum titer (normal: <1 U/mL), and ovarian failure in her thirties. She has a + HLA DR3 and DR4. Clinical and HLA findings are diagnostic of polyendocrine autoimmune syndrome (APS) II. She presented at age 38 with acute delirium, a lymphocytic CSF reaction and an initial normal MRI (not shown). HSV PCR was negative. She improved on steroids; 6 weeks later a diagnosis of temporal lobe epilepsy was made. Three years later a syndrome of recent memory loss occurred and a second MRI showed bilateral increased signal in the hippocampi (**A**, arrow). Local disruption of the blood–brain barrier is observed in the right mesial temporal lobe (**B**). A diagnosis of recurrent autoimmune limbic encephalitis was made. The patient has done well for the last decade on 20 mg of methotrexate per week. To our knowledge this is the first description of an autoimmune encephalitis associated with APS II.

available. The disease is generally symptomatic among middle-aged patients and more frequent in women. An AD inheritance with incomplete penetrance is the cause of this disorder.

History

Generally symptoms of hyper- or hypothyroidism may be present and may be followed by type 1 DM.

Clinical findings

Clinical and neurologic findings are discussed in other chapters in this volume. Abnormalities associated with vitamin B_{12} deficiency and celiac disease may be observed. Single case reports of neurologic syndromes observed in APS III include: myasthenia gravis (Lubinsk et al., 2007), a multiple sclerosis mimic in two different reports (Donadio et al., 2001; Boz et al., 2003), and a patient with Tolosa–Hunt syndrome (Cesareo et al., 1995).

Natural history

Most of the clinical manifestations of APS III are treated with hormonal replacement. Patients must be monitored for additional endocrine and other systemic autoimmune disorders.

Laboratory investigations

Antithyroglobulin antibodies, antithyroid receptor antibodies, antithyroid microsomal antibodies (also known as antithyro peroxidase antibodies) can be ordered. In addition, if type 1 DM is present, anti-islet cell and anti-GAD antibodies may be requested. Antiparietal cell antibodies are useful to screen for the possibility of celiac disease if clinically warranted. HLA typing is not generally recommended.

Neuroimaging and pathology

In general, imaging findings may be similar to those found in single endocrine deficiencies. The same applies to the pathologic findings in the affected endocrine glands.

Management

Management goals are to provide appropriate hormonal replacement. In addition, it is imperative to be aware of new clinical findings due to emerging endocrine or systemic abnormalities and to treat them in timely fashion. Normal life expectancy is likely if the multiple syndrome complications are properly managed.

MULTIPLE ENDOCRINE NEOPLASIA

Table 53.2

Introduction

Disorders of oncogene regulation result in development of multiple benign and malignant tumors of endocrine glands with increased single or multiple hormonal production and skin tumors. In addition, melanomas and benign CNS tumors may be identified in multiple endocrine neoplasia (MEN). Neural crest-derived secretory cells known as "amine, precursor uptake and decarboxylase" (APUD) cells proliferate in MEN. The normal function of AUPD cells is the synthesis of polypeptide hormones, and includes the chromaffin cells in the adrenal medulla, the intestinal chromaffin cells, the pituitary

Table 53.2

Multiple endocrine neoplasia

Type	Clinical manifestations	Genetics	CNS manifestations and neoplasms
1	Parathyroid adenomas Skin lesions Pancreatic adenomas	Autosomal dominant MENIN mutation	Pituitary adenomas Hyperparathyroidism-related meningiomas
2A	Medullary carcinioma thyroid Bilateral pheochromocytomas Hyperthroidism Cutaneous lesions	RET proto-oncogene Autosomal dominant	Hypertensive crisis Hypercalcemia
2B	Medullary carcinoma thyroid Marfanoid features Abnormal facial features Megacolon	RET proto-oncogene	Peripheral neuropathy Pes cavus Hypertrophic corneal nerves (pathognomonic)

corticotrophs and melanotrophs, the pancreatic islet cells A and D, and the thyroid C cells (Pearse, 1974).

In MEN type 1 (Wermer's syndrome), parathyroid adenomas, pituitary adenomas (frequently prolactinomas), and pancreatic endocrine tumors develop. In MEN type 2A, medullary carcinoma of the thyroid, pheochromocytoma, and hyperparathyroidism are the most frequent neoplasms found. MEN type 2B has a readily recognizable phenotype including medullary carcinoma of the thyroid with gastrointestinal tumors and Marfan-like body build (Dyck et al., 1979). Familial medullary thyroid carcinoma may represent another type of MEN.

Each of the two major types of MEN affects an estimated 1 in 30 000 people. Type 2B is relatively uncommon and amounts to only 5% of type 2 MEN cases.

MEN type 1 is caused by a mutation in the *MEN1* gene which encodes a nuclear protein (MENIN). It acts as a regulator of cell growth. The gene is located in chromosome 11 band q13. Unlike other AD inherited diseases, both alleles of the gene must mutate for oncogenesis to occur. Thus, besides the inherited mutant allele, the noninherited *MEN1* allele must also spontaneously mutate. In the lifetime of an individual with MEN 1, a small number of cells have the two mutant alleles, with a greater frequency in the parathyroid, endocrine, pancreas, and pituitary gland.

Type 2 MEN is the result of mutation in the RET proto-oncogene involved in cell signaling. It promotes or inhibits cell division. A mutation of the *RET* gene causes increased signaling leading to uncontrolled cellular growth, particularly in the parathyroid gland, the adrenal medulla, and the C cells of the thyroid gland.

Most affected individuals inherit a mutated MEN gene. The remaining cases probably represent new mutations.

Multiple endocrine neoplasia: MEN type 1

HISTORY

Skin lesions, chronic hypercalcemia, neprolithiasis, and chronic renal failure may be the presenting findings. Recurrent gastric and duodenal ulcers may be found in the Zollinger–Ellison syndrome (ZES). Amenorrhea, galactorrhea, and sterility may be the first sign of a prolactinoma. A positive family history suggestive of MEN 1 may also be present.

CLINICAL FINDINGS

The majority of symptoms first appear in adolescent years. Skin lesions, angiofibromas, characterized by 1–4 mm brown papules with facial predilection, occur in a large percentage of patients. They are typically smaller than angiofibromas observed in patients with tuberous sclerosis complex. Lipomas and café au lait spots (usually < 3) may also occur (Darling et al., 1997; Asgharian et al., 2004a). Parathyroid adenomas are the most common tumor in MEN 1; usually all four parathyroid glands are affected. Typically, chronic and clinically silent hypercalcemia may be present for years. Osteopenia and kidney stones may be advanced at time of the initial diagnosis. In a series of 74 MEN 1 patients, 98% had parathyroid hyperplasia (Asgharian et al., 2004b). Tumors of the endocrine pancreas may give rise to insulinomas, glucagonomas, gastrinomas, and somastatin-secreting tumors. About one-third of patients with MEN 1 have gastrinomas (ZES), presenting with gastric and duodenal ulcers. Insulinomas may be associated with significant neurologic findings, including episodic seizures, tremor, irritability, weakness, diaphoresis, tachycardia, personality change, confusion, and coma. In contrast to the sporadic insulinomas, most cases of syndromic insulinomas have a known diagnosis of MEN 1.

Pituitary tumors also occur in MEN 1. Neurologic, endocrine, and neuro-ophthalmologic symptoms of pituitary tumors may be observed in MEN type 1. In a 19 year prospective series of 74 MEN 1 patients who underwent protocol-designed, annual, clinical, and neuroimaging evaluations at the US National Institutes of Health (NIH), roughly 40% of 74 patients had pituitary adenomas. An 8% incidence of supra- and infratentorial meningiomas was also found. The meningioma patients in this MEN 1 series also had ZES (Asgharian et al., 2004b).

NATURAL HISTORY

Management of the specific tumor/tumors of the multiple parathyroid adenomas involves surgical resection of the three largest glands and a partial resection of the fourth or resection of all of them with PTH and calcium replacement (Norton et al., 2008). Pituitary adenomas are frequent, and patients should be monitored. Whereas prolactinomas may respond to dopaminergic agonist therapy, other pituitary tumors may require transsphenoidal resection. Eventually, about half of the MEN type 1 cases developed a cancerous pancreatic or carcinoid tumor (thymus, lung, gastric). Metastatic cervical spine carcinoid was reported in a MEN 1 patient (Tanabe et al., 2008).

LABORATORY INVESTIGATIONS

Screening for parathyroid adenomas, the initial endocrine manifestation in MEN 1, often takes place between ages 5 and 50 years. Hyperparathyroidism occurring beyond age 50 is not likely to be associated with MEN 1. Investigation for ZES and pituitary adenomas may be initiated when one of the first endocrine symptoms appears, or when typical skin lesions are recognized or a positive family history of endocrine disorders is present. Genetic testing is possible and should be performed in affected individuals, as well as their relatives at risk. Identified MEN 1 mutations require frequent surveillance for evolving endocrine and other tumors.

NEUROIMAGING

Annual surveillance of MEN 1 patients will likely detect pituitary adenomas in 40% of cases and cranial meningiomas in 8% (Asgharian et al., 2004b). This study provides a solid basis for the early detection of intracranial lesions and timely intervention. The imaging characteristics of the intracranial MEN 1 lesions are not different from those observed with sporadic pituitary adenomas and meningiomas.

NEUROPATHOLOGY

The histopathology of MEN 1 intracranial tumors is not different from findings observed with sporadic intracranial pituitary tumors. In a resected MEN 1 meningioma, gene testing in tumor cells showed a unique genetic signature. Two major abnormalities were observed: (1) loss of heterozigosity at the 11q13 locus (MEN 1 mutation); (2) gene mutations in chromosome 1 (including p 73) frequently found in sporadic meningiomas. In contrast, there were none of the gene changes in chromosome 22 that are frequently found in neurofibromatosis type 2 (Asgharian et al., 2004b).

MANAGEMENT

Patients and family members must be kept under observation for possible endocrine tumor development. Parathyroid adenomas are usually surgically treated, with PTH and calcium replacement possibly needed after surgery. Pituitary adenomas may be medically treated (e.g., prolactinoma) or surgically resected. Other intracranial tumors may be observed and treated as needed. The management of pancreatic tumors may be more controversial. The ZES may be treated with proton pump inhibitors or surgically resected. Insulinomas must be surgically resected. Given the AD inheritance, all relatives of MEN 1 must be screened for the mutation. Genetic counseling is advisable.

Multiple endocrine neoplasia: MEN type 2A

HISTORY

The main endocrine abnormalities that define this syndrome include medullary carcinoma of the thyroid (MCT), pheochromocytoma, and hyperparathyroidism. Accordingly, symptoms of chronic hypercalcemia with nephrolithiasis and chronic renal failure may occur early in childhood or adolescence. Hypertensive crisis, frequently paroxysmal, generally secondary to bilateral pheochromocytomas, may be the first manifestation of MEN 2A. Paradoxically profound hypotensive crisis associated with tachycardia may be seen in association with pheochromocytomas secreting primarily epinephrine (Page et al., 1969; Aronoff et al., 1980). A thyroid mass may be the first sign of MCT (Sipple, 1961; Williams and Pollock, 1966). Cutaneous lesions (lichen amyloidosis) may be found frequently on the interscapular or extensor surfaces).

In MEN 2A, complications from pheochromocytoma may cause headaches, palpitations, diaphoresis, arterial hypertension, focal neurologic symptoms, altered mental status, and seizures. Sudden death is a potential complication. Focal transient or permanent neurologic signs have been reported in MEN 2A patients; these may relate to hypercalcemia or secretion of vasoactive substances (Bruyland et al., 1983).

In MEN 2A C cell thyroid hyperplasia is observed at an early age (3–5 years), and may be present at birth. A neck mass may be found between the ages of 15 and 20 years. By then, 50% of cases already have lymph node metastases. Rarely, metastatic MCT to the brain have been reported. In one instance, parenchymal brain metastases occurred 25 years after total thyroidectomy (Pitale et al., 1999).

NATURAL HISTORY

Prolonged survival is possible with appropriate management. Timely identification of MCT with early thyroidectomy is probably the most important variable to ensure a good outcome. Surgical resection of bilateral pheochromocytomas and parathyroid adenomas may also be required. In addition, these patients should be followed for the emergence of additional nonendocrine tumors.

LABORATORY INVESTIGATIONS

Pheochromocytomas in MEN 2A are bilateral, and unlike sporadic pheochromocytomas, they most frequently secrete epinephrine. Determination of 24 hour metanephrine urine levels, preferably after a hypertensive crisis, is the most specific screening laboratory test for a pheochromocytoma.

MCT can be screened with serum levels of calcitonin, which serves a tumor marker. Pentagastrin-stimulated calcitonin probably identifies all potential MCT cases.

NEUROIMAGING

Brain imaging is often normal in patients with MEN type 2A. Neurologic complications of pheochromocytoma may rarely include parenchymal or subarachnoid hemorrhage. Half of the pheochromocytomas involve one of the adrenal glands (usually nonsyndromic), 25% involve both adrenal glands (usually syndromic), and in 25% of cases, the tumor is extra-adrenal. Approximately 10% of pheochromocytomas are malignant. Besides MEN type 2A, bilateral pheochromocytomas may also occur in Von Hippel–Lindau syndrome and neurofibromatosis type 1.

MANAGEMENT

Early identification of patients with germline *RET* mutation before symptoms develop is desirable. Screening for hyperparathyroidism and pheochromocytoma and a prophylactic thyroidectomy, preferably at the C cell hyperplasia stage, are the main goals of treatment.

Management of pheochromocytomas, if present, takes priority. Surgical resection is the goal. Bilateral adrenalectomy should be considered. Careful management with both α- and β-blockers is required preoperatively to control blood pressure prior to surgical resection. Treatment at specialized centers is recommended. Total thyroidectomy should be performed at the C cell hyperplasia or microscopic MCT stage (Bruyland et al., 1983).

Multiple endocrine neoplasia: MEN type 2B

HISTORY

Patients with MEN type 2B primarily report gastrointestinal, neurologic, ocular, or cosmetic symptoms. Constipation or recurrent diarrhea results from intestinal ganglioneuromas. Neuropathic and myopathic manifestations may be present. Gait difficulty may result from pes cavus. Patients may experience failing vision and occasionally may request consultation for their abnormal facial features. Everted, fleshy lips and small white nodules, probably neuromas of the tongue and mucosal surface of the lips, may be present in adolescents, but may be rather inconspicuous in younger children. Patients with MEN 2B also have a high incidence of thyroid mass lesions. In a series of 11 MEN type 2B, MCT was present at initial evaluation in 10 patients (Dyck et al., 1979).

Neurologic and ophthalmologic abnormalities in these patients have been studied and classified (Schweitzer and Van Der Pol, 1977; Dyck et al., 1979). A typical marfanoid phenotype and coarse facial features are typical. Peripheral neuropathy with moderate weakness and denervation features in EMG may be found. Although pes cavus and hammer toes may be present, there is no frank foot drop. Constipation and other signs of dysautonomia, including megacolon, may be found (Dyck et al., 1979). Visual blurring is caused by hypertrophy of corneal nerves, a pathognomonic feature

of this disorder (Schweitzer and Van Der Pol, 1977). In addition, patients may have yellowish tumors of the lid margins or the canthus which may be pedunculated. Dry eyes and pupillary abnormalities may also be observed.

NATURAL HISTORY

Early death may result from MCT metastases. A diligent identification of C cell thyroid hyperplasia with the pentagastrin stimulation test is an indication for thyroidectomy. Not all patients with familial MCT have the MEN 2A or 2B mutations, and they should be monitored for other potential complications.

LABORATORY INVESTIGATIONS

Genetic identification of the *RET* gene mutation for type 2B MEN confirms the diagnosis. Similar to MEN type 2A, these patients also have pheochromocytomas and MCT. Therefore, similar investigations and follow-up are required. Testing should be considered in patients with pheochromocytomas, multiple mucosal neuromas, or hypertrophic corneal nerves.

NEUROIMAGING

CNS complications of MEN 2B could potentially show abnormalities on brain and spinal cord imaging. Manifestations from pheochromocytoma-related arterial hypertensive complications with intracerebral hemorrhages are possible. Metastasic MCT is also a possibility.

NEUROPATHOLOGY

Details from postmortem examination in one MEN 2B patient consisted of plaque-like brainstem lesions with proliferation of neural tissue. Invasion of the pia was observed. Similar extramedullary lesions were present in spinal cord and spinal roots. Schwannomas of peripheral nerves (Antoni type A and B cells) were also present. Focal changes were identified in the sciatic and vagus nerves and the cauda equina (Dyck et al., 1979). Sural nerve biopsies also showed decreased number of myelinated fibers per square millimeter.

MANAGEMENT

Management of patients with MEN 2B involves early thyroidectomy. Resection of pheochromocytomas and management of gastrointestinal and ocular complications are tailored for the specific patient needs.

REFERENCES

Aronoff ST, Passami E, Borowsky BA et al. (1980). Norepinephrine and epinephrine secretion from a clinically secreting chromocytoma. Am J Med 69: 321–324.

Asgharian B, Turner ML, Gibril F et al. (2004a). Cutaneous tumors in patients with multiple neoplasm type 1 (MEN 1) and gastrinomas, prospective study of frequency and development of criteria with high sensitivity and specificity MEN 1. J Clin Endocrinol Metab 89: 5328–5336.

Asgharian B, Chen YJ, Patronas NJ et al. (2004b). Meningiomas may be a component tumor of multiple endocrine neoplasia type 1. Clin Cancer Res 10: 869–880.

Baba Y, Broderick DF, Uitti RJ (2005). Heredofamilial brain calcinosis syndrome. Mayo Clin Proc 80: 641–651.

Balazs C, Feher J (2009). Associations of autoimmune endocrine diseases. Orv Hetil 150: 1589–1597.

Baumert T, Kleber G, Schwarz J et al. (1993). Reversible hyperkinesia in a patient with autoimmune polyglandular syndrome type 1. Clin Investig 71: 924–927.

Berger JR, Weaver A, Greenlee J (2008). Neurologic consequences of autoimmune polyglandular syndrome type 1. 70: 2248–2252.

Boz C, Velioglu S, Altunayoglu V (2003). Central nervous system involvement in autoimmune polyglandular syndrome. Clin Neurol Neurosurg 105: 102–104.

Brain L, Jellinek EH, Ball K (1966). Hashimoto's disease and encephalopathy. Lancet 2: 512–514.

Bruyland M, Verbruggen E, Maes R et al. (1983). An unusual cause of attacks of focal cerebral symptoms: multiple endocrine neoplasia type II A. Clin Neurol Neurosurg 85: 49–55.

Carey RM (1997). The changing clinical spectrum of adrenal insufficiency. Ann Intern Med 127: 1103–1105.

Cesareo R, Reda G, Verallo O (1995). Sindrome di Tolosa Hunt e syndrome polighlandolare autoimmune. Un caso raro clinico. Minerva Endocrinol 20: 149–152.

Darling TN, Waskarulis MC, Steimberg SM et al. (1997). Multiple facial angiofibromas and collagenomas in patients with multiple endocrine neoplasia type 1. Arch Dermatol. 133: 853–857.

Dittmar M, Kahaly G (2003). Polyglandular autoimmune syndromes, immunogenetics and long term follow-up. J Clin Endocrinol Metab 88: 2983–2992.

Donadio V, Cortelli P, Liquori R (2001). Multiple-sclerosis-like disease in polyglandular autoimmune syndrome. J Neurol 248: 61–62.

Dyck PJ, Carney JA, Sizemore GW et al. (1979). Multiple endocrine neoplasia, type 2b: phenotype recognition; neurologic features and their pathologic basis. Ann Neurol 6: 302–314.

Fettisov SO, Bensing S, Mulder J (2009). Autoantibodies in autoimmune polyglandular syndrome type 1 patients react with major brain neurotransmitter systems. J Comp Neurol 513: 1–20.

Flanagan EP, McKeon A, Lennon VA (2010). Autoimmune dementia. Clinical course and predictors of immunotherapy response. Mayo Clin Proc 85: 881–897.

Gass JD (1962). The syndrome of keratoconjunctivitis, superficial moniliasis, idiopathic hypoparathyroidism and Addison's disease. Am J Ophthalmol 54: 660–674.

Gazulla AJ, Benavente Aguilar I, Ricoy Campo JR (2005). Myopathy with trabecular fibers associated with familiar autoinmune polyglandular syndrome type I. Neurologia 20: 702–704.

Ghandi G, Basu R, Dispenzeri A et al. (2007). Endocrinopathy in POEMS syndrome The Mayo Clinic experience. Mayo Clin Proc 82: 836–842.

Heino M, Scott HS, Chen Q et al. (1999). Mutation analysis of North-American APS-1 patients. Hum Mutat 13: 69–74.

Heuss D, Engelhardt A, Gobel H (1995). Myopathological findings in interstitial myositis type II polyendocrine autoimmune syndrome. Neurol Res 17: 233–237.

Hosseini H, Tourbah A, Levy R (1998). Ataxia revealing Biermer's disease associated with autoimmune polyendocrinopathy. Rev Neurol 154: 706–707.

Kahaly GJ (2009). Polyglandular autoimmune syndromes. Eur J Endocrinol 161: 11–20.

Kattah JC, Kattah WC (2008). Pituitary and hypothalamus. In: J Biller (Ed.), The Interface of Neurology and Internal Medicine. Wolters Kluwer, Lippincott, Williams and Wilkins, Philadelphia, ch. 76, pp. 465–470.

Lubinsk M, Swiatowska-Stolduska R, Kazimierk E et al. (2007). Acquired von Willebrand's syndrome in a patient with severe primary hypothyroidism associated with myasthenia gravis in the course of autoimmune polyglandular syndrome type 3. Hemophilia 13: 675–676.

Majeroni BA, Patel P (2007). Autoimmune polyglandular syndrome type II. Am Fam Physician 75: 667–670.

Moser H, Dubey P, Fatemi A (2004). Progress in X-linked adrenoleukodystrophy. Curr Opin Neurol 17: 263–269.

Neufeld M, Maclaren NK, Blizzard M (1981). Two types of autoimmune Addison's associated with different polyglandular autoimmune (PGA) syndromes. Medicine 60: 355–362.

Norton JA, Venzon DJ, Berna MJ et al. (2008). Prospective study of surgery for primary hyperparathyroidism (HPT) in multiple endocrine neoplasia-type 1 (MEN), and Zollinger Ellison's syndrome (ZERS): long-term outcome of a more virulent form of HPT. Ann Surg 247: 501–510.

Pearse AGE (1974). The AUPD cell concept and its implications in pathology. In: SC Sommmers (Ed.), Pathology Annual. Appleton-Century-Croft, New York, pp. 27–41.

Pitale ES, Melian E, Thomas C (1999). Brain metastases from medullary thyroid carcinoma in a patient with multiple endocrine neoplasia type 2A. Thyroid 9: 1123–1125.

Sasso FC, Carbonara O, DiMicco P (2003). A case of autoimmune polyglandular syndrome developed after interferon alpha therapy. Br J Clin Pharmacol 56: 238–239.

Schweitzer NMJ, Van Der pol BAE (1977). Multiple mucosal neuroma (MMM) or multiple endocrine neoplasia (MEN) type 3 syndrome Ocular manifestations, a case report. Doc Ophthalmol 44: 151–159.

Sipple JH (1961). The association of pheochromocytoma with carcinoma of the thyroid gland. Am J Med 31: 163–166.

Tanabe M, Akatsuka K, Umeda S et al. (2008). Metastasis of carcinoid to the arch of the axis in multiple endocrine neoplasia patient, a case report. Spine J 8: 841–844.

Ugur AB, Arikan E, Guldiken S et al. (2004). Autoimmune polyglandular syndrome type III in monozygot
ic twins, a case report. Acta Clin Belg 59: 225–228.

Watanabe S, Tanaka J, Ohta T (2008). Paraneoplastic neurologic syndrome and polyglandular autoimmune syndrome type 2 in a case of small cell lung cancer. Thorax 63: 1118–1119.

Williams ED, Pollock DJ (1966). Multiple mucosal neuromata with endocrine tumours: a syndrome allied to von Recklinghausen's disease. J Pathol Bacteriol 91: 71–80.

Handbook of Clinical Neurology, Vol. 120 (3rd series)
Neurologic Aspects of Systemic Disease Part II
Jose Biller and Jose M. Ferro, Editors

Chapter 54

Commonly used endocrine drugs

MÁRIO MIGUEL ROSA[1]* AND TERESA DIAS[2]

[1]*Neurology Department, Hospital de Santa Maria, Lisbon, Portugal*

[2]*Endocrinology, Diabetes and Metabolism Unit, Hospital de Santa Maria, Lisbon, Portugal*

INTRODUCTION

Endocrine disorders are unique in the sense that treatment can be targeted directly to the malfunctioning path. Hormone therapy replacement in hypofunction diseases and specific antihormone treatment in hyperfunction disorders are the hallmark of endocrine treatment. It might then be expected that endocrine drugs would be among the safest in the therapeutic arsenal, at least the most commonly used. But although less risky than some groups, such as chemotherapy agents or anticoagulants, they are also related to significant neurologic adverse events (AEs). In this chapter we will provide an overview of the common neurologic AEs of endocrine drugs. Other chapters have dealt with some agents commonly used in endocrinology, such as corticosteroids or sexual hormones, and will not be discussed here.

As a rule, adverse events occur independently of the indication for which the drug is used. On the other hand, some drugs, in spite of being hormones or antihormones, are not just used to treat endocrine diseases. A good example is antiandrogen use for prostate cancer. Taking this into consideration, we will not discuss agents that have been referred to elsewhere. We will thus focus on agents related to hypothalamus, pituitary, thyroid, and parathyroid hormones, and finally, diabetes mellitus (DM).

Our chapter aims to summarize the most commonly used drugs in endocrinology. In order to facilitate thorough access and quick information, we provide references with the links to product information of the most relevant drugs discussed, particularly from the European Medicines Agency (EMA) and the US Food and Drug Administration (FDA). In the rare instances where product information is not available on these sites, national drug authorities that have product information in English are also referred to.

In accordance with World Health Organization (WHO) guidance, adverse reactions are listed under headings of frequency (number of patients expected to experience the reaction), using the following categories: very common ($\geq 10\%$); common ($\geq 1\%$ to $< 10\%$); uncommon ($\geq 0.1\%$ to $< 1\%$); rare ($\geq 0.01\%$ to $< 0.1\%$); very rare ($< 0.01\%$).

Unlike common drugs, endocrine drugs cause rather repetitive neurologic AEs such as headache, nausea, and vomiting. On occasion, new and serious AEs may be identified, leading to reassessment of the benefit to risk ratio. This is why postmarket reporting of new or serious adverse events is of paramount importance in iatrogenic neurology.

HYPOTHALAMIC AND PITUITARY HORMONES AND ANALOGS

Hormones are neurotransmitter equivalents, but have a much longer lasting and distant effect.

The most commonly used hypothalamic/pituitary hormones in endocrinology are listed in Table 54.1.

Hypothalamic hormones and analogs

Synthetic thyrotropin-releasing hormone (TRH), growth hormone-releasing hormone (GHRH), gonadotropin-releasing hormone (GnRH), and corticotropin-releasing hormone (CRH) are used as endocrine tests of hypothalamic-pituitary function (TRH and GHRH are rarely indicated today). GnRH analogs are used in

---

*Correspondence to: Mário Miguel Rosa, M.D., Neurology Consultant, Neurology Department, Hospital de Santa Maria, Avenida Professor Egas Moniz, 1649-035 Lisbon, Portugal. Tel: +35-196-648-9287, E-mail: mario.miguel.rosa@gmail.com

Table 54.1

Pituitary and hypothalamic hormones and analogs

Drug name	Indication	Neurologic adverse events*
Bromocriptine	Hyperprolactinemia	Very common: nausea, headache, dizziness Common: fatigue, light-headedness, vomiting, drowsiness
Cabergoline	Hyperprolactinemia	Very common: headache, dizziness
Conivaptan	Euvolemic and hypervolemic hyponatremia (hospitalized patients)	Very common: headache Common: nausea, vomiting, confusion, insomnia
Desmopressin (DDAVP)	Central cranial diabetes insipidus and temporary polyuria and polydipsia following head trauma or surgery in the pituitary Primary nocturnal enuresis	Common: headache, dizziness, asthenia Rare: convulsions due to dilution hyponatremia
Lanreotide	Acromegalia	Very common: nausea Common: headache
Mecasermin	Severe primary IGFD	Common: dizziness, muscle cramps, flank pain, hypoglycemic seizures, intracranial hypertension
Octreotide	Acromegaly; carcinoid syndrome; acute variceal bleeding	Very common: nausea Common: headaches, dizziness
Pasireotide	Cushing disease	Very common: nausea, headache, fatigue
Pegvisomant	Second-line treatment of acromegaly	Common: headache, asthenia
Quinagolide	Hyperprolactinemia	Very common: dizziness, fatigue, nausea, vomiting, headache Common: muscular weakness Rare: somnolence
Somatropin	GHD	Common: stiffness in the extremities, arthralgia, myalgia; paraesthesia, headache Uncommon: CTS Rare: benign intracranial hypertension
Tolvaptan	Hypervolemic and euvolemic hyponatremia (serum sodium < 125 mEq/L or less marked hyponatremia that is symptomatic and has resisted correction with fluid restriction), including patients with heart failure, cirrhosis, and SIADH (in Europe, SIADH is single indication)	Common: xerostomia, orthostatic hypotension Uncommon: dysgeusia

CTS, carpal tunnel syndrome; GHD, growth hormone deficiency; IGFD, insulin-like growth factor-1 deficiency; SIADH, syndrome of inappropriate antidiuretic hormone.

*Frequency (number of patients expected to experience the reaction) of adverse reactions is given, using the following categories: very common ($\geq 1/10$); common ($\geq 1/100$, $<1/10$); uncommon ($\geq 1/1000$, $<1/100$); rare ($\geq 1/10000$, $<1/1000$); very rare ($<1/10000$).

endocrinology to treat patients with sex hormone-dependent disorders such as precocious puberty. Central nervous system adverse reactions include dizziness, lethargy, insomnia, headache, depression, emotional lability, and memory disorders, but peripheral neuropathy and myalgia have also been reported (FDA leuprolide adults label, 2011; FDA leuprolide pediatrics label, 2012).

SOMATOSTATIN AND SOMATOSTATIN ANALOGS

Somatostatin inhibits growth hormone (GH) and thyroid-stimulating hormone (TSH) pituitary secretion and, under certain conditions, prolactin (PRL) and adrenocorticotropic hormone (ACTH) pituitary secretion as well. In many endocrine-secreting tumors (insulinomas, glucagonomas,

VIPomas, some gastrinomas, and carcinoid tumors), somatostatin blocks their hormone release. Somatostatin analogs include octreotide, lanreotide, vapreotide, and pasireotide.

Octreotide is a potent inhibitor of growth hormone, glucagon, and insulin. It is indicated for symptomatic treatment of acromegaly, carcinoid syndrome, and acute esophageal variceal bleeding.

Long-acting lanreotide is used in the management of acromegaly and symptoms caused by neuroendocrine tumors, most notably carcinoid syndrome. Vapreotide is used for esophageal variceal bleeding.

Octreotide is usually used in its long-acting formulation, allowing a single intramuscular injection per month. Neurologic AEs include nausea (16%), headache (6%), and dizziness (5%) (FDA octreotide label, 2012).

Lanreotide is available for the long-term treatment of acromegalic patients, administered by sc injection every 4 weeks. Neurologic symptoms include nausea (11%) and headache (7%) (FDA lanreotide label, 2011). Pasireotide is recently available for Cushing disease in adults for whom surgery is not an option or for whom surgery has failed. Neurologic AEs include nausea (52%), headache (28%) and fatigue (19%) (FDA pasireotide label, 2012).

DOPAMINE AND DOPAMINE AGONISTS

Dopamine is the primary prolactin-inhibitory hormone. Bromocriptine, cabergoline, pergolide, and quinagolide are dopamine agonist drugs, used in hyperprolactinemic disorders.

Dopamine agonists are first-line treatment for patients with hyperprolactinemia disorders, either idiopathic or due to pituitary adenomas. Bromocriptine and cabergoline are the most commonly used dopamine agonist drugs in endocrinology.

Bromocriptine has been marketed for over three decades and was the first effective medical therapy for hyperprolactinemia. It is an ergot derivative and is administered orally, in divided doses. Very common central nervous system adverse effects are: nausea (49%), headache (19%), and dizziness (17%); fatigue (7%), light-headedness (5%), vomiting (5%), drowsiness (3%), and orthostatic hypotension (2%) are common (FDA bromocriptine label, 2012). Most side-effects occur at the start of treatment, but they can usually be avoided by starting with a low dose at bedtime and then gradually increasing it over days to weeks, or by using alternative intravaginal administration (Kletzky and Vermesh, 1989).

Bromocriptine has also recently been marketed in the US for the treatment of type 2 diabetes mellitus (T2DM) (FDA bromocriptine label, 2011).

Cabergoline is a more potent and much longer-acting ergot dopamine agonist, and better tolerated than bromocriptine. Since its introduction about 15 years ago, it has surpassed bromocriptine and therefore become the first-line therapeutic choice for most patients. Very common central nervous system AEs include headache (26%) and dizziness (15% to 17%). To reduce AEs, treatment may be slowly started (FDA cabergoline label, 2011). At high doses, such as those used for the treatment of Parkinson disease (PD), cabergoline may be associated with an increased risk of valvular heart disease, along with other dopamine agonists.

Pergolide, a dopamine agonist ergot derivative was used primarily to treat PD, but also for the treatment of hyperprolactinemia. However, due to the cardiac valve AEs it has become a second-line approach for Parkinson disease, and has been discontinued in several countries, including US.

Quinagolide is available in Europe for the treatment of hyperprolactinemia. It is administered once a day. Very common neurologic AEs are dizziness, fatigue, nausea, vomiting, and headache; muscular weakness, anorexia, insomnia, and orthostatic hypotension are common; somnolence is rare (Swedish Medical Products Agency quinagolide product information, 2009).

CSF leakage with nasal discharge may occur during dopamine agonist treatment for very large lactotroph adenomas that extend inferiorly and invade the floor of the sella (Davis et al., 1990; Leong et al., 2000). Although uncommon, early recognition and evaluation is important due to the potential risk of meningitis.

Anterior pituitary lobe hormones and analogs

Synthetic forms of corticotropin (ACTH) and thyrotropin (TSH) will not be discussed since they are available for single administrations either for diagnosis or, in the case of thyrotropin, to potentiate radioactive iodine in the treatment of thyroid cancer. Human recombinant gonadotropins, luteinizing hormone (LH) or follicle stimulating hormone (FSH), are endocrine drugs whose use is reserved for reproductive medicine.

SOMATROPIN (GROWTH HORMONE) AND SOMATROPIN AGONISTS

Growth hormone (GH) therapy is indicated for short stature in children and adolescents due to GH deficiency (GHD), associated with Turner syndrome, associated with chronic renal insufficiency, born small who failed to show catch-up growth by 4 years of age or later, associated with Noonan syndrome, with idiopathic short stature, and in Prader–Willi syndrome. It is also indicated as replacement therapy in adults with pronounced growth hormone deficiency.

The GH replacement therapy was done initially with human cadaver pituitary-derived GH (hGH). Because of the association between its use and Creutzfeldt–Jakob disease (CJD), natural growth hormone was halted in 1985 and replaced by recombinant human growth hormone (rhGH). CJD has been reported to start at 4–30 years after therapy with cadaveric somatropin (Brown et al., 1992) so that new cases may still occur (Gibbons et al., 2000).

In adult patients, myalgia is very common, and is related to fluid retention. In pediatric patients this undesirable effect is common. Paresthesias and headache are common AE and the latter may be an early indicator of the rare complication benign intracranial hypertension. Carpal tunnel syndrome (CTS) is uncommon AE with somatropin (EMA somatropin product information, 2011, 2012; FDA somatropin label, 2012).

Mecasermin is a somatropin analog produced as recombinant DNA-derived human insulin-like growth factor-1(IGF-1). It is approved for the long-term treatment of growth failure in children and adolescents with severe primary insulin-like growth factor-1 deficiency (primary IGFD), but is also used in children with primary GHD who have developed neutralizing antibodies to GH (Collett-Solberg and Misra, 2008). It is administered twice daily subcutaneously. Hypoglycemia is the most frequently reported adverse drug reaction (40%), with hypoglycemic seizures accounting for 5% (Chernausek et al., 2007), but headache (18%) is also very common. Roncopathy, generally beginning in the first year of treatment, was reported in 22%. Hypoacusis occurs in 20%. Dizziness, muscle cramps, and flank pain are common, as well as intracranial hypertension, which occurs in 4% (FDA mecasermin label, 2012; EMA mecasermin product information, 2012).

SOMATROPIN (GROWTH HORMONE) ANTAGONISTS

Pegvisomant is a GH receptor antagonist used in the treatment of acromegaly for patients that have not responded to other treatments. Occasionally tumors that secrete growth hormone (GH) may expand and cause serious complications. Pegvisomant is usually administered as a daily subcutaneous injection. Headache (6%) and asthenia (6%) are common AEs (FDA pegvisomant label, 2012; EMA pegvisomant product information, 2012).

Posterior pituitary hormones

VASOPRESSIN AND ANALOGS

Arginine vasopressin is the human antidiuretic hormone. Vasopressin analogs such as the longer-acting desmopressin are thoroughly used by endocrinologists but also neurologists and neurosurgeons.

Desmopressin or DDAVP is indicated as antidiuretic replacement therapy in the management of central diabetes insipidus and for management of temporary polyuria and polydipsia following head trauma or surgery in the pituitary region, and in primary nocturnal enuresis. It is contraindicated in patients with moderate to severe renal impairment, or a history of hyponatremia. The dose must be individually adjusted to the patient, with special attention in the very young to the danger of an extreme variation in plasma osmolality, with resulting convulsions. There have also been rare reports of hyponatremic convulsions associated with concomitant use of oxybutynin or imipramine. Besides this, dizziness is the single neurologic adverse event

reported with high doses of desmopressin (FDA desmopressin label, 2003, 2007).

VASOPRESSIN ANTAGONISTS

Vasopressin antagonists are indicated for the treatment of clinically significant hypervolemic and euvolemic hyponatremia.

Tolvaptan is a selective vasopressin V_2-receptor antagonist used in hypervolemic and euvolemic hyponatremia, including patients with heart failure, cirrhosis, and syndrome of inappropriate antidiuretic hormone (SIADH). Oral treatment should be initiated in hospital due to need for dose titration with close monitoring of serum sodium and volume status.

Tolvaptan is mostly metabolized via CYP3A, and drugs that modify CYP3A activity heavily interact with tolvaptan.

Neurologic AEs include: very common xerostomia (13%) and common: dysgeusia, orthostatic hypotension, and asthenia (EMA tolvaptan product information, 2012; FDA tolvaptan label, 2012).

Conivaptan is a nonpeptide, V_{1A} and V_2-receptor antagonist of arginine vasopressin (AVP) indicated for the treatment of hospitalized patients.

Headache is a very common adverse event (10%); vomiting (7%), orthostatic hypotension (6%), nausea (5%), confusion (5%), and insomnia (4%) are common (FDA conivaptan label, 2012).

THYROID AND PARATHYROID AGENTS

Thyroid hormones

Thyroid hormones have a common indication for the treatment of hypothyroidism. There are two drugs currently available in the world: levothyroxine and liothyronine. Levothyroxine is the stereoisomer of thyroxine (T_4), the endogenous hormone. Liothyronine is a stereoisomer of the endogenous hormone triiodothyronine (T_3). T_4 is the drug of choice to treat hypothyroidism and to suppress the production of TSH in patients with thyroid carcinoma since it has a long half-life and is metabolized to T_3 in the peripheral tissues. Therapeutic use of T_3 is therefore generally only recommended when T_4 therapy needs to be interrupted for administration of ^{131}I in the treatment of thyroid cancer.

In some countries there are also natural preparations available, extracted from beef or hog thyroids, but their use is no longer recommended.

When administered in excessive amounts, adverse events mimic the effects of T_4 and T_3 endogenous overproduction (Table 54.2). In standard doses, however, they usually do not cause significant AEs.

Table 54.2

Thyroid hormones, antithyroid agents, parathyroid hormone and analog

Drug name	Indication	Neurologic adverse events*
Levothyroxine sodium	Hypothyroidism	Tremor, nervousness, irritability, headache, insomnia, behavior disturbance (increased appetite), leg cramps, nausea/vomiting
Liothyronine sodium	Hypothyroidism	Same as levothyroxine
Parathyroid hormone	Osteoporosis in population at increased/high risk of fractures	Very common: nausea Common: headache
Potassium perchlorate	Hyperthyroidism	Nausea/vomiting
Propylthiouracil	Hyperthyroidism	Nausea/vomiting, ageusia, arthralgias/myalgia, paresthesias, headaches
Teriparatide	Osteoporosis in women at high risk of fractures	Very common: feeling sick, pain in limb, headache, dizziness Common: nausea, depression, muscle cramps
Thiamazole	Hyperthyroidism	Nausea/vomiting, ageusia, dizziness, arthralgias/myalgia, paresthesias, headaches

*Frequency (number of patients expected to experience the reaction) of adverse reactions is given, using the following categories: very common ($\geq 1/10$); common ($\geq 1/100$, $<1/10$); uncommon ($\geq 1/1000$, $<1/100$); rare ($\geq 1/10000$, $<1/1000$); very rare ($<1/10000$).

In differentiated thyroid carcinoma remnants, a T_4 suppressive dose is used, which may induce subclinical hyperthyroidism.

The most important neurologic side-effects are: moderate to high frequency postural tremor (Deuschl et al., 1998; Elble et al., 1996); headaches (migraine), fatigue, nausea/vomiting, diaphoresis, nervousness/irritability, anxiety, insomnia, and leg cramps.

Thyroid hormone clearance may be increased with hepatic inducers like a few antiepileptic drugs (barbiturates, carbamazepine, primidone) and, most important, some β-blockers that may be used concomitantly. Special attention must be paid when starting treatment on an orally anticoagulated patient, for thyroid hormones increase the activity of oral anticoagulants (FDA levothyroxine label, 2009; FDA liothyronine label, 2012).

In critically ill patients, thyroid dysfunction may occur despite normal levels of thyroxine. Independently from the mechanism that causes euthyroid sick syndrome or nonthyroidal illness, special care should be taken when using agents that may interfere with thyroxine/liothyronine efficacy, such as dopaminergics and somatostatin (Mebis and Van den Berghe, 2009).

Antithyroid preparations

This group comprises preparations used in the treatment of thyrotoxicosis. It includes thionamides and perchlorates.

Most antithyroid agents have more than 60 years in the market. Therefore the type of adverse events is known, but data on frequency is not available.

THIONAMIDES

Propylthiouracil (PTU) and methimazole (MMI) are the two thionamides widely available.

Methylthiouracil is also a thionamide, closely related to PTU, not clinically used in most of the Western countries. The same applies to benzylthiouracil.

Carbimazole is a prodrug, as after absorption it is converted to the active form, MMI. It is still used in some countries, and has the same adverse event profile as MMI (eMC carbimazole discontinued product information, 2012).

PTU and MMI have similar efficacy in reducing overproduction of thyroid hormones, but PTU is reserved for: (1) life-threatening thyrotoxicosis or thyroid storm, because of PTU's ability to inhibit peripheral conversion of T_4 to T_3; (2) first trimester pregnancy, due to MMI toxicity: aplasia cutis, choanal and esophageal atresias (Clementi et al., 1999); (3) patients with adverse reactions to MMI. MMI is now the drug of choice for all other circumstances, due to less toxicity. In fact, although marketed for over 60 years, PTU is an example that significant adverse drug reactions may be easily overlooked, particularly when not frequent. In 2009 both FDA and EMA published alerts notifying healthcare professionals of the risk of serious liver injury, including liver failure and death, in patients taking PTU (Benyounes et al., 2006; FDA propylthiouracil Drug Safety Communication, 2009; FDA propylthiouracil Information for Healthcare Professionals, 2009; EMA propylthiouracil risk, 2009).

Both PTU and MMI neurologic side-effect are rare, but include nausea/vomiting, ageusia, arthralgias, or myalgia, paresthesia, and headaches. Agranulocytosis (0.5%) (Andersohn et al., 2007) and vasculitis – particularly with PTU – are rare but serious AEs (FDA methimazole label, 2001).

Perchlorates

Potassium perchlorate is an iodide transport inhibitor which can be used as an alternative to thionamides in cases of allergy. It has also been used to treat iodine-induced forms of thyrotoxicosis, such as type 1 hyperthyroidism due to amiodarone. It has been discontinued in most Western countries due to potential bone marrow toxicity. It also causes nausea/vomiting in up to 10% of cases (Crooks and Wayne, 1960; Morgans and Trotter, 1960; Fumarola et al., 2010).

Parathyroid hormones and analogs

Parathyroid hormone (PTH) is the primary regulator of calcium and phosphate metabolism in bone and kidney. PTH increases serum calcium, partially accomplishing this by increasing bone resorption. Thus, chronically elevated PTH will deplete bone stores. However, intermittent exposure to PTH will activate osteoblasts more than osteoclasts. This is the rationale for use of parathyroid hormone (84 amino acids) or more recently a fraction of total PTH (sequence 1 through 34) called teriparatide. Teriparatide is indicated for the treatment of osteoporosis in postmenopausal women and in men at high risk of fracture, and osteoporosis associated with sustained systemic glucocorticoid therapy in women and men at high risk for fracture. Parathyroid hormone is indicated for women at high risk of fractures with postmenopausal osteoporosis. Teriparatide and PTH are administered subcutaneously once daily. The very commonly reported AEs for parathyroid hormone are hypercalciuria (39%), hypercalcemia (25%), and nausea (13%); headache (9%) is common. The very common AEs reported for teriparatide are indeed neurologic: feeling sick, pain in limb, headache and dizziness; nausea, depression, and muscle cramps are common (FDA teriparatide label, 2009); EMA parathyroid hormone product information, 2012; EMA teriparatide product information, 2012).

Antiparathyroid agents, namely calcitonin, elcatonin, cinacalcet, and paricalcitol, are mostly used by either rheumatologists or nephrologists, and will not be referred to here.

DRUGS USED IN DIABETES

Drugs for diabetes are extensively used by several medical specialties, particularly general and internal medicine and endocrinology.

Although treatment of DM does not only mean glucose control, optimal glucose control in both type 1 and type 2 diabetic patients reduces the risk for complications such as retinopathy, nephropathy, and neuropathy. Glucose lowering agents such as insulin is also used in critically ill patients not previously diagnosed as diabetics, to reduce Intensive Care Unit major complications like polyneuropathy or myopathy (Hermans et al., 2008b; Van den Berghe et al., 2009).

Insulins and analogs

Insulin is used as substitution therapy for patients with an absolute or relative deficiency of the hormone. Insulin replacement is therefore lifesaving for type 1 diabetes (T1DM) and also needed for achieving a good glucose control in T2DM.

This group comprises both human and animal insulins. In most Western countries, animal-derived insulins were discontinued, in favor of the much safer human insulin and human insulin analogs, produced by DNA recombinant technologies. Animal-derived insulins are nevertheless still used to treat diabetes in many developing countries, being the only available alternative to a significant part of the world population.

Insulin preparations differ in respect of their time of onset and duration of action. Four types of insulins are available: (1) rapid-acting insulin analogs; (2) short-acting regular human insulin; (3) intermediate-acting human insulin; (4) long-acting insulin analogs. Current insulin characteristics and bioavailability are summarized in Table 54.3, and their schematic pharmacokinetic profile is shown in Fig. 54.1.

Premixed combination of human insulins (regular + neutral protamine Hagedorn (NPH)) and of insulin analogs (rapid-acting analog + same protaminated analog) are currently available in fixed proportions (FDA regular and NPH human insulin fixed combination label, 2010; EMA regular human insulin and fixed combinations regular and NPH product information, 2011, 2012).

Current regimens try to mimic physiological insulin secretion by injection of delayed action (basal) insulin for basal insulin supply, and rapid-acting insulins for food intake control, the so-called "basal-bolus" regimen.

Not all insulins are approved to be used in children below certain ages: insulin aspart may be used in children of 2 years old or above; insulin detemir, glargine, and glulisine is used in children of 6 years or above. All other insulins (lispro, NPH, and regular) do not have age constraints.

Until 1980, insulins contained a significant amount of impurities (300–10 000 parts per million), leading to immune reactions. New, more efficient and economical filters were developed and safer insulins, with virtually no contaminants and ≤ 10 parts per million of proinsulin

Table 54.3

Current insulin structure and bioavailability characteristics

Insulin type	Onset of action	Peak action	Duration
Aspart	10–30 min	0.5–1.5 h	3–4 h
Glulisine			
Lispro			
Regular	30–60 min	2–4 h	6–8 h
NPH	2–4 h	6–10 h	10–20 h
Detemir	1–2 h	No clear peak	6–24 h
Glargine	1–2 h	No clear peak	20–24 h

NPH, neutral protamine Hagedorn; onset of action, peak action and duration time spans based on SmPC/labels of different agents, doses, and indications (T1DM or T2DM).

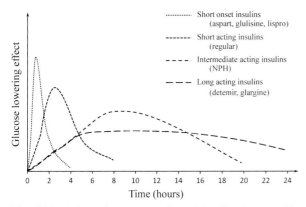

Fig. 54.1. Schematic representation of insulin pharmacokinetics.

emerged. All human insulins and analogs are purified. In spite of so many advances, AEs are common. We will discuss the most common neurologic AEs (Table 54.4).

Hypoglycemia is the most frequently occurring undesirable effect in insulin treatment. It may occur if the insulin dose is too high in relation to the insulin requirement. In clinical trials and after marketing authorization, the frequency of hypoglycemia varies with patient population and dose regimens. Therefore, no specific frequency can be presented. Severe hypoglycemia may lead to unconsciousness and/or convulsions and may result in temporary or permanent impairment of brain function or even death. Hypoglycemic encephalopathy has a distinctive imagiological pattern (Fujioka et al., 1997; Ma et al., 2009). Computed tomography (CT) scan shows symmetrical persistent low-density lesions, with enhancement in cerebral cortex, caudate, and lenticular nuclei decreasing after 2 weeks. Magnetic resonance imaging (MRI) reveals persistent symmetrical lesions hyperintense on T1 and hypointense on T2, in the caudate and lenticular nuclei, cerebral cortex, substantia nigra, and/or hippocampus from 8 days to 12 months after onset. White matter is very sensitive to hypoglycemia, and diffuse, extensive injury observed on the diffusion-weighted imaging (DWI) predicts a poor neurologic outcome. Regional minor hemorrhages on MRI typical of postischemic-anoxic encephalopathy are absent in hypoglycemic encephalopathy.

Hypoglycemia in the conscious patient may be associated with listlessness, confusion, palpitations, headache, sweating, visual refraction disorders, and vomiting. Peripheral neuropathies are rare. In fact, in T2DM, occurrence of peripheral neuropathy may indeed be a reason to start insulin therapy. A usually self-limited and reversible "acute painful neuropathy" (APN), also known as insulin neuritis (Caravati, 1933), has been described in patients in whom a rapid glycemic control is achieved. It is characterized by acute, severe pain, peripheral nerve degeneration, and autonomic dysfunction after intensive glycemic control (Gibbons and Freeman, 2010). All patients with APN have more severe autonomic dysfunction than patients with generalized diabetic peripheral neuropathy. APN is more frequent in the longer-acting formulations (EMA long-acting human insulin product information, 2012).

In intensive care, patients are much less able to signal adverse events, and carers must thus pay special attention to small signs of hypoglycemia and to the mastering of glucose monitoring. This is particularly important, since intensive glucose control is commonly practiced in ICUs. Strict glucose monitoring is important not only to prevent hypoglycemia, but also to improve overall prognosis. In fact there is evidence that critical illness polyneuropathy and myopathy may be prevented under intensive insulin therapy (Hermans et al., 2008a, b, 2009).

SHORT- AND RAPID-ACTING INSULINS

Regular or short-acting human insulin is a soluble insulin with a short-acting onset. To achieve quicker onset, modifications were made in the insulin molecule to prevent it from forming hexamers or polymers that slow absorption and delay action (Barnett and Owens, 1997;

Table 54.4

Drugs used in diabetes: insulins and analogs

Drug name	Indication	Neurologic adverse events*
Insulins as a whole	DM, where treatment with insulin is required (age restrictions apply for some insulins)	Very common: hypoglycemia – may induce several neurologic symptoms: listlessness, confusion, palpitations, headache, sweating, impaired consciousness, convulsions, encephalopathy, death Uncommon: visual refractory disorders, peripheral neuropathy, including acute painful neuropathy Special attention must be paid to the comatose or sedated patient, as in ICU

DM, diabetes mellitus; ICU, intensive care unit.

*Frequency (number of patients expected to experience the reaction) of adverse reactions is given, using the following categories: very common ($\geq 1/10$); common ($\geq 1/100$, $<1/10$); uncommon ($\geq 1/1000$, $<1/100$); rare ($\geq 1/10000$, $<1/1000$); very rare ($<1/10000$).

Zib and Raskin, 2006). This led to the development of rapid-action insulin analogs: aspart, glulisine, and lispro.

Rapid-onset insulins enable physicians to intensify mealtime insulin treatment, without increasing the risk of hypoglycemia or other adverse events (FDA aspart insulin label, 2009; FDA glulisine insulin label, 2009; EMA glulisine insulin product information, 2011; EMA lispro insulin product information, 2011; EMA aspart insulin product information, 2012; FDA lispro insulin label, 2012).

INTERMEDIATE AND LONG-ACTING INSULINS

Intermediate-acting insulins are insulins associated to neutral pH protamine (also called NPH insulin). This preparation has been used since 1946 (Fisher and Scott, 1933; Scott and Fisher, 1935). Protamine releases insulin slowly, with a smaller and more protracted peak but longer duration of action.

Headache and worsening diabetic neuropathy are uncommon neurologic events (FDA NPH insulin label, 2010; EMA long-acting human insulin product information, 2012; EMA NPH insulin product information, 2012).

Human insulins associated to excess zinc in an acetate buffer (insulin ultralente) are long acting insulins (Fisher and Scott, 1935; Scott and Fisher, 1938; EMA ultralente insulin product information, 2008). Due to their inconsistent insulin action and very long duration, their use has been replaced by the more recent long-acting insulin analogs detemir and glargine. These long-acting insulin analogs may have some clinical advantages over NPH, namely less nocturnal hypoglycemia, but are of higher cost (EMA detemir insulin product information, 2012; FDA detemir insulin label, 2012).

Insulin glargine has a higher affinity to the human IGF-1 receptor than other insulins. Theoretically, this could alter mitogenic activity (Zib and Raskin, 2006), increasing the risk of cancer and, most important, the risk of retinopathy. Clinical data, however, are still lacking (FDA glargine insulin label, 2009; EMA glargine insulin product information, 2010).

Noninsulin blood glucose-lowering drugs

Except for a few agents in restricted indications, noninsulin glucose-lowering drugs are indicated just for T2DM. Therapeutic regimens in patients with T2DM have long included noninsulin drugs. All available data demonstrate the need for polypharmacy in the majority of patients with T2DM, in order to achieve target glycemic control. Noncompliance is a major healthcare problem, with estimates ranging from 30% to 60%. In T2DM, compliance with sulfonylureas (SU) or metformin monotherapy is 36% higher than dual treatment with SU plus metformin with single agent pills (Dailey et al., 2001). Compliance can be promoted by the use of a single pill combining two different classes of antihyperglycemic agents (Halimi et al., 2001).

For decades, oral agents were confined to biguanides and sulfonylureas. In the past 20 years several new agents have emerged in the market (Table 54.5).

BIGUANIDES

Biguanides do not affect the output of insulin; unlike other hypoglycemic agents such as sulfonylureas and meglitinides. They do not cause hypoglycemia *per se*. Phenformin and buformin are being discontinued due to the risk of lactic acidosis, fatal in many cases.

Table 54.5

Drugs used in diabetes: noninsulin blood glucose-lowering drugs

Drug name	Indication	Neurologic adverse events*
Acarbose	T2DM	Common: hypoglycemia (when combined with sulfonylurea or insulin)
Exenatide	T2DM not adequately controlled in combination with metformin, and/or sulfonylureas	Very common: hypoglycemia, nausea, vomiting Common: headache, dizziness, asthenia, feeling jittery
Glibenclamide (glyburide)	T2DM	Common: hypoglycemia
Gliclazide	T2DM	Common: hypoglycemia Uncommon: nausea
Glimepiride	T2DM	Common: dizziness, headache, hypoglycemia
Liraglutide	T2DM not adequately controlled in dual therapy with metformin or sulfonylurea, or triple therapy with metformin and sulfonylurea or metformin and thiazolidinedione	Very common: hypoglycemia, headache, nausea, vomiting Common: dizziness, fatigue
Metformin	T2DM in adults	Very common: hypoglycemia (only when combined with other glucose-lowering agent, namely sulfonylureas) Common: dysgeusia (metallic taste)
Miglitol	T2DM	Common: hypoglycemia (when combined with sulfonylurea or insulin)
Nateglinide	T2DM inadequately controlled with metformin	Very common: hypoglycemia Common: nausea Uncommon: vomiting
Pioglitazone	T2DM (monotherapy only if metformin not indicated)	Very common: hypoglycemia Common: hypoesthesia, headache, dizziness
Pramlintide	T1DM or T2DM treated with mealtime insulin, not adequately controlled	Very common: nausea; headache, inflicted injury, vomiting, hypoglycemia (in combination with insulin) Common: fatigue, dizziness
Repaglinide	T2DM inadequately controlled in monotherapy and with dual oral therapy with metformin	Common: hypoglycemia
Saxagliptin	T2DM (as dual oral therapy if metformin, sulfonylurea or thiazolidinedione not indicated)	Very common: hypoglycemia Common: headache, dizziness, myalgia, fatigue, vomiting
Sitagliptin	T2DM (monotherapy only if metformin not indicated)	Very common: hypoglycemia Common: nausea, vomiting Uncommon: xerostomy
Vildagliptin	T2DM (as dual oral therapy if metformin, sulfonylurea or thiazolidinedione not indicated)	Common: hypoglycemia, tremor, headache, nausea, asthenia, dizziness Uncommon: fatigue

T2DM, type 2 diabetes mellitus; T1DM, type 1 diabetes mellitus.
*Frequency (number of patients expected to experience the reaction) of adverse reactions is given, using the following categories: very common ($\geq 1/10$); common ($\geq 1/100$, $<1/10$); uncommon ($\geq 1/1000$, $<1/100$); rare ($\geq 1/10\,000$, $<1/1000$); very rare ($<1/10\,000$).

Metformin is the gold standard oral medication agent in T2DM. Consensus statements from the American Diabetes Association and the European Association for the Study of Diabetes recommend that metformin should be initiated from the time of T2DM diagnosis, in the absence of contraindications (Nathan et al., 2009).

Metformin is also considered for the treatment of polycystic ovary syndrome (AACE, 2005).

The mechanism of action of metformin is not fully understood. However, it is thought that the main mode of action includes a reduction in hepatic glucose production through inhibition of gluconeogenesis and glycogenolysis. Other effects are that it delays intestinal glucose absorption and increases insulin sensitivity and glucose uptake into cells, particularly muscle. Metformin stimulates intracellular glycogen synthesis and increases the transport capacity of specific types of membrane glucose transporters (GLUT-1 and GLUT-4). Clinical studies have demonstrated a favorable effect on lipid metabolism independent of its glucose-lowering effect (Giugliano et al., 1993; Fanghänel et al., 1996), and there is still debate on whether it has a macrovascular sparing effect (UKPDS 33, 1998; UKPDS 34, 1998).

The most common side-effects are diarrhea and dyspepsia, occurring in up to 30% of patients; the most feared AE is lactic acidosis which is very rare (0.3/10 000). Dysgeusia, with patients reporting a metallic taste in the mouth, is also commonly found, and may explain decreased appetite. One rare but neurologically significant event (Liu et al., 2006) is that metformin decreases absorption of vitamin B_{12}, thus increasing the risk of subacute combined degeneration. The risk of megaloblastic anemia may be higher in patients with inadequate vitamin B_{12} or calcium intake or absorption. Some amino acids and folic acid may also have their absorption reduced (FDA metformin label, 2008).

SULFONAMIDES, UREA DERIVATIVES

All sulfonylureas contain a central *S*-phenylsulfonylurea structure, hence their name. Sulfonylureas bind to an ATP-dependent K^+ (KATP) channel on the cell membrane of pancreatic β cells. The rise in intracellular calcium leads to increased fusion of insulin granule with the cell membrane, and secretion of (pro)insulin. There is some evidence that sulfonylureas also sensitize β cells to glucose, limit glucose production in the liver, decrease lipolysis, and decrease clearance of insulin by the liver.

Sulfonylureas are divided into three groups: the first generation includes acetohexamide, chlorpropamide, tolazamide, and tolbutamide; the second generation comprises glibenclamide (glyburide), gliclazide, glipizide, gliquidone, and glyclopyramide (used in Japan); the third generation is represented by glimepiride (Hamaguchi et al., 2004).

First-generation sulfonylureas are less safe for they have long half-lives, are 90% protein bound in plasma, and have low albumin affinity, increasing the risk of drug interactions. Their use is limited worldwide.

Among the second generation, the most used are glibenclamide and gliclazide. Hypoglycemia is the most frequent and important AE. It may be severe and often prolonged. Shorter-acting sulfonylureas such as gliclazide and glipizide and the third generation glimepiride are less likely to cause hypoglycemia than the older ones (eMC gliclazide product information, 2012).

Most sulfonylureas are excreted by the kidney. Glibenclamide is excreted by both the liver and the kidney, and therefore mild to moderately renally impaired patients can be treated with a sulfonylurea (FDA glyburide (glibenclamide) label, 2009).

Glimepiride is a potent medium- to long-acting sulfonylurea (EMA glimepiride opinion following referral, 1998; eMC glimepiride product information, 2012; FDA glimepiride label, 2012). Glimepiride is also excreted by liver and kidney. The risk of hypoglycemia throughout the treatment is increased in the first weeks of treatment. Hypoglycemia (2%), dizziness, asthenia, and headache are common, transient visual disturbances and hypersensitivity reactions are rare.

Gliclazide and glimepiride offer protection against coronary artery disease while there is a controversy on whether glibenclamide and glipizide may increase cardiovascular risk (Harrower, 2000; Ueba et al., 2005).

All sulfonylureas are associated with cumulative weight gain as soon as treatment is started. Drug interactions are frequent: the hypoglycemic action of sulfonylureas may be potentiated by certain drugs including nonsteroidal anti-inflammatory agents, ACE inhibitors, disopyramide, fluoxetine, clarithromycin, and other drugs that are highly protein-bound, salicylates, sulfonamides, chloramphenicol, probenecid, monoamine oxidase inhibitors, and β-adrenergic blocking agents.

α-GLUCOSIDASE INHIBITORS

α-Glucosidase inhibitors include acarbose, miglitol, and voglibose. Their antihyperglycemic action results from competitive, reversible, membrane-bound intestinal α-glucoside hydrolase enzymes. Pancreatic α-amylase hydrolyzes complex starches to oligosaccharides in the lumen of the small intestine, while the membrane-bound intestinal α-glucosidases hydrolyze oligosaccharides, trisaccharides, and disaccharides to glucose and other monosaccharides in the brush border of the small intestine. In diabetic patients, this enzyme inhibition results in a delayed glucose absorption and a lowering of postprandial hyperglycemia. Because their mechanism of action is different, it has an additive effect on sulfonylureas, insulin, or metformin when used in combination. In addition, α-glucosidase inhibitors diminish the insulinotropic and weight-increasing effects of sulfonylureas.

Since acarbose prevents the degradation of complex carbohydrates into glucose, the carbohydrates will remain in the intestine. In the colon, bacteria will digest the complex carbohydrates, causing GI side-effects flatulence (78%) and diarrhea (14%). Acarbose is not absorbed, and its action is topical in the gut. Beside the action at the intestinal brush border, it also inhibits pancreatic α-amylase, having a double action on complex carbohydrates. In order to avoid intestinal related AEs, the drug is to be taken at the start of main meals (with the first bite of a meal three times daily) (FDA acarbose label, 2012); eMC acarbose product information, 2012).

Miglitol also has an antihyperglycemic action that results from a reversible inhibition of membrane-bound intestinal α-glucoside hydrolase enzymes. Unlike acarbose, this agent is absorbed, although saturable at high doses: a dose of 25 mg is completely absorbed, whereas a dose of 100 mg is only 50–70% absorbed. For all doses, peak concentrations are reached in 2–3 hours. There is no evidence that systemic absorption of miglitol contributes to its therapeutic effect, and its effect is also mainly topical (FDA miglitol label, 2012).

Voglibose is marketed in Japan. It may have fewer side-effects but has less fast glycemic and HbA1c control.

Theoretically α-glucosidase inhibitors should not induce hypoglycemia in the fasted or postprandial state as single agents. However, since most of the patients are also treated with other hypoglycemic drugs such as sulfonylureas or insulin, there is an increased risk of hypoglycemia when α-glucosidase inhibitors are added, and hypoglycemia becomes common.

It must be stressed that oral glucose (dextrose), whose absorption is not delayed by α-glucosidase inhibitors, should be used instead of sucrose (cane sugar) in the treatment of mild to moderate hypoglycemia in patients treated with α-glucosidase inhibitors. Sucrose, whose hydrolysis to glucose and fructose is inhibited by α-glucosidase inhibitors, is unsuitable for the rapid correction of hypoglycemia. Severe hypoglycemia may require the use of either intravenous glucose infusion or glucagon injection.

Thiazolidinediones

Thiazolidinediones act by binding to PPARs (peroxisome proliferator-activated receptors), a group of receptor molecules inside the cell nucleus, specifically PPAR-γ. The ligands for these receptors are free fatty acids (FFAs) and eicosanoids. When activated, the receptor migrates to the DNA, activating transcription of a number of specific genes. They work as insulin sensitizers, by binding to the PPAR receptors in fat cells and making the cells more responsive to insulin. There are several modes of action for thiazolidinediones by activating PPAR-γ: (1) insulin resistance is decreased; (2) adipocyte differentiation is modified; (3) vascular endothelial growth factor-induced angiogenesis is inhibited; (4) leptin levels are decreased (leading to an increased appetite); (5) levels of certain interleukins (e.g., IL-6) fall; (6) adiponectin levels rise.

There are three agents in this class: troglitazone, rosiglitazone and pioglitazone. Troglitazone was taken off market due to fatal hepatitis in some cases. Rosiglitazone was withdrawn due to increased cardiovascular risk (EMA recommends suspension of Avandia, Avandamet and Avaglim (2010).

Pioglitazone is contraindicated in patients with New York Heart Association (NYHA) class III and IV heart failure. It may cause edema or worsen heart failure. Postmarketing reports of new-onset or worsening diabetic macular edema, with decreased visual acuity, have also been reported. There was evidence of dose-related weight gain, which was greater when used in combination with insulin, but weight gain is a result of subcutaneous and not visceral fat accumulation. Pioglitazone treatment is associated with a dose-related reduction of hemoglobin levels. In patients with low hemoglobin levels before initiating therapy, there is an increased risk of anemia during treatment. Patients receiving pioglitazone in combination with a sulfonylurea or insulin therapy may be at risk for dose-related hypoglycemia.

Pioglitazone tablets are taken orally once daily with or without food.

The same concerns about cardiovascular risk apply to pioglitazone, but in this case risk seems lower as recent evidence suggests (Graham et al., 2010; FDA pioglitazone label, 2011; EMA metformin-pioglitazone product information, 2012; EMA pioglitazone product information, 2012; FDA metformin-pioglitazone label, 2012). There are new restrictions on the use of pioglitazone due to increased risk of bladder cancer (EMA recommends new contra-indications and warnings for pioglitazone to reduce small increased risk of bladder cancer, 2011).

Dipeptidyl peptidase 4 (DPP-4) inhibitors

Inhibitors of dipeptidyl peptidase 4 (DPP-4 inhibitors) are a class of oral hypoglycemics that block DPP-4. DPP-4 breaks down the incretins GLP-1 and GIP, gastrointestinal hormones that are released in response to a meal. By preventing GLP-1 and GIP inactivation, GLP-1 and GIP are able to potentiate the secretion of insulin and suppress the release of glucagon by the pancreas. This drives blood glucose levels toward normal. As the blood glucose level approaches normal, the amounts of insulin released and glucagon suppressed diminishes, thus tending to prevent an "overshoot" and subsequent low blood sugar (hypoglycemia) which is seen with some other oral hypoglycemic agents.

The DPP-4 enzyme is known to be involved in the suppression of certain malignancies, particularly in limiting the tissue invasion of these tumors. Inhibiting the DPP-4 enzymes may allow some cancers to progress. A study of DPP-4 inhibition in human non-small cell lung cancer (NSCLC) concluded that DPP-4 acts as a tumor suppressor, and its downregulation may contribute to the loss of growth control in NSCLC cells (Wesley et al., 2004). The risk of cancer suppression with DPP-4 downregulation applies to all marketed DPP-4 inhibitors.

The three available DPP-4 inhibitors are sitagliptin, vildagliptin, and saxagliptin. All the three are taken once daily and may be used in monotherapy, or in dual therapy either with metformin, a sulfonylurea, or pioglitazone. Hypoglycemia is common or very common in dual or triple therapy, but not in monotherapy. Their main difference is in the safety profile. Sitagliptin common AEs are nausea and vomiting. Headache is common in triple therapy (EMA metformin-sitagliptin product information, 2012; EMA sitagliptin product information, 2012; FDA metformin-sitagliptin label, 2012; FDA sitagliptin label, 2012).

Vildagliptin, unlike most other glucose lowering agents, commonly induces neurologic AEs: tremor, headache, dizziness, asthenia, and nausea. Fatigue is uncommon (EMA metformin-vildagliptin product information, 2012; EMA vildagliptin product information, 2012).

Saxagliptin has as common AEs headache and vomiting (FDA saxagliptin label, 2011; EMA saxagliptin product information, 2012).

Meglitinides

Meglitinides are secretagogues like sulfonylureas, although not structurally related. They induce insulin secretion from pancreas, with a different mechanism of action from sulfonylureas.

There are three available drugs: repaglinide, nateglinide, and mitiglinide. All of them are given before main meals.

Repaglinide can be administered alone or with metformin. Repaglinide is primarily excreted via the bile, and excretion is not affected by renal disorders. It should not be used with gemfibrozil. Hypoglycemia is a common AE, whereas nausea and vomiting are rare (EMA repaglinide product information, 2012; FDA repaglinide label, 2012).

Nateglinide is indicated as add-on therapy with metformin. It has a quicker onset and shorter duration of action than repaglinide. Its effect is quite specific in lowering postprandial glucose, and has little effect in lowering fasting plasma glucose. It can be used in moderate liver and renal impaired patients. Hypoglycemia is a very common AE (15%) and nausea is common (EMA nateglinide product information, 2011; FDA nateglinide label, 2012).

Mitiglinide was developed and is available in Japan.

Glucagon-like peptide-1 (GLP-1) receptor analog (incretin mimetics)

The rationale for the development of incretin mimetics was that, for patients with T2DM who are no longer achieving good glycemic control on oral agents, an effective and safe alternative to insulin could be beneficial. Endogenous incretins, such as glucagon-like peptide 1 (GLP-1), facilitate insulin secretion following their release from the gut into the circulation in response to food intake.

There are two incretin mimetics: exenatide and liraglutide. Incretin mimetics have multiple antihyperglycemic actions that mimic some of the effects of GLP-1. The main disadvantage of these agents is that they cannot be administered orally, and must be injected like insulin. There is also some concern regarding drug interactions, which involve a significant number of drugs.

Exenatide is approved as adjunctive therapy to improve glycemic control in patients with T2DM who are taking metformin, or a combination of metformin and a sulfonylurea, without adequate glycemic control. It has now been approved in some countries for use in monotherapy or with pioglitazone. Exenatide is administered twice daily, immediately before meals, and raises insulin levels quickly (within about 10 minutes). The effects on blood sugar last for 6–8 hours though insulin levels subside after 2 hours. Common AEs are: nausea, vomiting, hypoglycemia, feeling jittery, dizziness, and headache. Nausea usually decreases over time.

Liraglutide can be administered once a day. It can be used in monotherapy, or in combination with one or more oral antidiabetic drugs (metformin, sulfonylureas, or pioglitazone) when there is not adequate glycemic control. The most frequently reported adverse reactions during clinical trials were GI disorders. Headache is also common. Furthermore, hypoglycemia is common, and very common and more serious when liraglutide is used in combination with a sulfonylurea (FDA exenatide label, 2011; EMA exenatide product information, 2012; EMA liraglutide product information, 2012).

Amylin analog

Pramlintide is a synthetic analog of human amylin, a naturally occurring neuroendocrine hormone synthesized by pancreatic β cells that contributes to glucose control during the postprandial period. Amylin is cosecreted with insulin by pancreatic β cells in response to food intake. Amylin and insulin show similar fasting and postprandial patterns in healthy individuals. The gastric emptying rate is an important determinant of the postprandial rise in plasma glucose. Pramlintide slows the rate at which food leaves the stomach to the small intestine following a meal and thus reduces the initial postprandial increase in plasma glucose. This effect lasts for approximately 3 hours following pramlintide administration. It does not alter the net absorption of ingested carbohydrate or other nutrients. Pramlintide has been shown to decrease postprandial glucagon concentrations in insulin-using patients. Administered prior to a meal, it has been shown to reduce total caloric intake. This effect appears to be independent of the nausea that can accompany treatment. Pramlintide is indicated for patients with T1DM and insulin-treated T2DM. It is administered subcutaneously at meal time. T1DM patients occasionally exhibit severe hypoglycemia. When this occurs, it is seen within 3 hours following pramlintide injection. Nausea is very common. Inflicted injury (a new and troublesome AE), fatigue, and vomiting are also common AEs (FDA pramlintide label, 2007).

ALDOSE REDUCTASE INHIBITORS

Tolrestat is an aldose reductase inhibitor that was approved for the control of certain diabetic complications. It was discontinued in 1997 due to toxicity.

REFERENCES

AACE (2005). AACE Position statement on metabolic and cardiovascular consequences of polycystic ovary syndrome. American Association of Clinical Endocrinologists. Endocr Pract 11: 126–134.

Andersohn F, Konzen C, Garbe E (2007). Systematic review: agranulocytosis induced by nonchemotherapy drugs. Ann Intern Med 146: 657–665.

Barnett AH, Owens DR (1997). Insulin analogues. Lancet 349: 47–51.

Benyounes M, Sempoux C, Daumerie C et al. (2006). Propylthiouracyl-induced severe liver toxicity: an indication for alanine aminotransferase monitoring? World J Gastroenterol 12: 6232–6234.

Brown P, Preece MA, Will RG (1992). "Friendly fire" in medicine: hormones, homografts and Creutzfeldt–Jakob disease. Lancet 340: 24–27.

Caravati CM (1933). Insulin neuritis: a case report. Va Med Monthly 59: 745–746.

Chernausek SD, Backeljauw PF, Frane J et al. (2007). Long-term treatment with recombinant insulin-like growth factor (IGF-I) in children with severe IGF-I deficiency due to growth hormone insensitivity. J Clin Endocrinol Metab 92: 902–910.

Clementi M, Di Gianantonio E, Pelo E et al. (1999). Methimazole embryopathy: delineation of the phenotype. Am J Med Genet 83: 43–46.

Collett-Solberg PF, Misra M (2008). The role of recombinant human insulin-like growth factor-I in treating children with short stature. J Clin Endocrinol Metab 93: 10–18.

Crooks J, Wayne EJ (1960). A comparison of potassium perchlorate, methylthiouracil, and carbimazole in the treatment of thyrotoxicosis. Lancet 1: 401–404.

Dailey G, Kim MS, Lian JF (2001). Patient compliance and persistence with antihyperglycemic drug regimens: evaluation of a Medicaid patient population with type 2 diabetes mellitus. Clin Ther 23: 1311–1320.

Davis JR, Sheppard MC, Heath DA (1990). Giant invasive prolactinoma: a case report and review of nine further cases. Q J Med 74: 227–238.

Deuschl G, Bain P, Brin M (1998). Consensus statement of the Movement Disorder Society on Tremor. Mov Disord 13 (Suppl 3): 2–23.

Elble RJ, Brilliant M, Leffler K et al. (1996). Quantification of essential tremor in writing and drawing. Mov Disord 11: 70–78.

EMA aspart insulin product information (2012). European Medicines Agency (EMA), viewed 30OCT2012: http://www.ema.europa.eu/docs/en_GB/document_library/EPAR_-_Product_Information/human/000258/WC500030372.pdf

EMA detemir insulin product information (2012). EMA, viewed 30OCT2012: http://www.ema.europa.eu/docs/en_GB/document_library/EPAR_-_Product_Information/human/000528/WC500036662.pdf.

EMA exenatide product information (2012). EMA, viewed 30OCT2012: www.ema.europa.eu/docs/en_GB/document_library/EPAR_-_Product_Information/human/000698/WC500051845.pdf.

EMA glargine insulin product information (2010). EMA, viewed 30OCT2012: http://www.ema.europa.eu/docs/en_GB/document_library/EPAR_-_Product_Information/human/000284/WC500036082.pdf.

EMA glimepiride opinion following referral (1998). EMA, viewed 30OCT2012: http://www.emea.europa.eu/docs/en_GB/document_library/Referrals_document/Amaryl_29/WC500011177.pdf.

EMA glulisine insulin product information (2011). EMA, viewed 30OCT2012: http://www.ema.europa.eu/docs/en_GB/document_library/EPAR_-_Product_Information/human/000557/WC500025250.pdf.

EMA lispro insulin product information (2011). EMA, viewed 30OCT2012: http://www.ema.europa.eu/docs/en_GB/document_library/EPAR_-_Product_Information/human/000088/WC500050332.pdf.

EMA long-acting human insulin product information (2012). EMA, viewed 30OCT2012: http://www.ema.europa.eu/docs/en_GB/document_library/EPAR_-_Product_Information/human/000441/WC500033307.pdf.

EMA liraglutide product information (2012). EMA, viewed 30OCT2012: http: //www.ema.europa.eu/docs/en_GB/document_library/EPAR_-_Product_Information/human/001026/WC500050017.pdf.

EMA mecasermin product information (2012). EMA, viewed 30OCT2012: http://www.emea.europa.eu/docs/en_GB/document_library/EPAR_-_Product_Information/human/000704/WC500032225.pdf.

EMA metformin-pioglitazone product information (2012). EMA, viewed 30OCT2012: http://www.ema.europa.eu/docs/en_GB/document_library/EPAR_-_Product_Information/human/000655/WC500032620.pdf.

EMA metformin-sitagliptin product information (2012). EMA, viewed 30OCT2012: http://www.ema.europa.eu/docs/en_GB/document_library/EPAR_-_Product_Information/human/000861/WC500038805.pdf.

EMA metformin-vildagliptin product information (2012). EMA, viewed 30OCT2012: http://www.ema.europa.eu/

docs/en_GB/document_library/EPAR_-_Product_Information/human/000807/WC500030594.pdf.

EMA nateglinide product information (2011). EMA, viewed 30OCT2012: http://www.ema.europa.eu/docs/en_GB/document_library/EPAR_-_Product_Information/human/000335/WC500057862.pdf.

EMA NPH insulin product information (2012). EMA, viewed 30OCT2012: http://www.ema.europa.eu/docs/en_GB/document_library/EPAR_-_Product_Information/human/000442/WC500044920.pdf.

EMA parathyroid hormone product information (2012). EMA, viewed 30OCT2012: http://www.emea.europa.eu/docs/en_GB/document_library/EPAR_-_Product_Information/human/000659/WC500041343.pdf.

EMA pegvisomant product information (2012). EMA, viewed 30OCT2012: http://www.emea.europa.eu/docs/en_GB/document_library/EPAR_-_Product_Information/human/000409/WC500054629.pdf.

EMA pioglitazone product information (2012). EMA, viewed 30OCT2012: http://www.ema.europa.eu/docs/en_GB/document_library/EPAR_-_Product_Information/human/000285/WC500021386.pdf.

EMA propylthiouracil risk (2009). EMA - Pharmacovigilance Working Party, viewed 30OCT2012: http://www.emea.europa.eu/docs/en_GB/document_library/Report/2009/12/WC500016972.pdf.

EMA recommends new contra-indications and warnings for pioglitazone to reduce small increased risk of bladder cancer (2011). Viewed 30OCT2012: http://www.ema.europa.eu/docs/en_GB/document_library/Press_release/2011/07/WC500109176.pdf

EMA recommends suspension of Avandia, Avandamet and Avaglim (2010). Viewed 30OCT2012: http://www.ema.europa.eu/docs/en_GB/document_library/Press_release/2010/09/WC500096996.pdf.

EMA regular human insulin and fixed combinations regular and NPH product information (2012). EMA, viewed 30OCT2012: http://www.ema.europa.eu/docs/en_GB/document_library/EPAR_-_Product_Information/human/000761/WC500033441.pdf

EMA regular human insulin and fixed combinations regular and NPH product information (2011). EMA, viewed 30OCT2012: http://www.ema.europa.eu/docs/en_GB/document_library/EPAR_-_Product_Information/human/000201/WC500033784.pdf

EMA repaglinide product information (2012). EMA, viewed 30OCT2012: http://www.ema.europa.eu/docs/en_GB/document_library/EPAR_-_Product_Information/human/000362/WC500041220.pdf.

EMA saxagliptin product information (2012). EMA, viewed 30OCT2012: http://www.ema.europa.eu/docs/en_GB/document_library/EPAR_-_Product_Information/human/001039/WC500044316.pdf.

EMA sitagliptin product information (2012). EMA, viewed 30OCT2012: http://www.ema.europa.eu/docs/en_GB/document_library/EPAR_-_Product_Information/human/000722/WC500039054.pdf.

EMA somatropin product information (2012). EMA, viewed 30OCT2012: http://www.emea.europa.eu/docs/en_GB/document_library/EPAR_-_Product_Information/human/000607/WC500043695.pdf.

EMA somatropin product information (2011). EMA, viewed 30OCT2012: http://www.emea.europa.eu/docs/en_GB/document_library/EPAR_-_Product_Information/human/000315/WC500040084.pdf.

EMA teriparatide product information (2012). EMA, viewed 30OCT2012: http://www.emea.europa.eu/docs/en_GB/document_library/EPAR_-_Product_Information/human/000425/WC500027994.pdf.

EMA tolvaptan product information (2012). EMA, viewed 30OCT2012: http://www.emea.europa.eu/docs/en_GB/document_library/EPAR_-_Product_Information/human/000980/WC500048716.pdf.

EMA ultralente insulin product information (2008). EMA, viewed 30OCT2012: http://www.ema.europa.eu/docs/en_GB/document_library/EPAR_-_Product_Information/human/000439/WC500058877.pdf.

EMA vildagliptin product information (2012). EMA, viewed 30OCT2012: http://www.ema.europa.eu/docs/en_GB/document_library/EPAR_-_Product_Information/human/001048/WC500038241.pdf.

eMC acarbose product information (2012). The electronic Medicines Compendium (eMC) UK, viewed 30OCT2012: http://www.medicines.org.uk/guides/download/acarbose/Diabetes/acarbose%20100mg%20tablets.

eMC carbimazole discontinued product information (2012). eMC UK, viewed 30OCT2012: http://www.medicines.org.uk/emc/medicine/14594.

eMC gliclazide product information (2012). eMC UK, viewed 30OCT2012: http://www.medicines.org.uk/EMC/medicine/1942/SPC/Diamicron/.

eMC glimepiride product information (2012). eMC UK, viewed 30OCT2012: http://www.medicines.org.uk/EMC/medicine/27034/SPC/Amaryl+1mg+Tablets/.

Fanghänel G, Sánchez-Reyes L, Trujillo C et al. (1996). Metformin's effects on glucose and lipid metabolism in patients with secondary failure to sulfonylureas. Diabetes Care 19: 1185–1189.

FDA acarbose label (2012). Food and Drug Administration (FDA), viewed 30OCT2012: http://www.accessdata.fda.gov/drugsatfda_docs/label/2012/020482s025lbl.pdf.

FDA aspart insulin label (2009). FDA, viewed 30OCT2012: http://www.accessdata.fda.gov/drugsatfda_docs/label/2009/019938s064,019959s067,019991s068,020986s055-lbl.pdf.

FDA bromocriptine label (2011). FDA, viewed 30OCT2012: http://www.accessdata.fda.gov/drugsatfda_docs/label/2011/020866s002lbl.pdf.

FDA bromocriptine label (2012). FDA, viewed 30OCT2012: http://www.accessdata.fda.gov/drugsatfda_docs/label/2012/017962s065s068lbl.pdf.

FDA cabergoline label (2011). FDA, viewed 30OCT2012: http://www.accessdata.fda.gov/drugsatfda_docs/label/2011/020664s012lbl.pdf.

FDA conivaptan label (2012). FDA, viewed 30OCT2012: http://www.accessdata.fda.gov/drugsatfda_docs/label/2012/021697s003lbl.pdf.

FDA desmopressin label (2003). FDA, viewed 30OCT2012: http://www.accessdata.fda.gov/drugsatfda_docs/label/2003/21333slr001_Minirin_lbl.pdf.

FDA desmopressin label (2007). FDA, viewed 30OCT2012: http://www.accessdata.fda.gov/drugsatfda_docs/label/2007/017922s038,018938s027,019955s013lbl.pdf.

FDA detemir insulin label (2012). FDA, viewed 30OCT2012: http://www.accessdata.fda.gov/drugsatfda_docs/label/2012/021536s041lbl.pdf.

FDA exenatide label (2011). FDA, viewed 30OCT2012: http://www.accessdata.fda.gov/drugsatfda_docs/label/2011/021773s029s030lbl.pdf.

FDA glargine insulin label (2009). FDA, viewed 30OCT2012: http://www.accessdata.fda.gov/drugsatfda_docs/label/2009/021081s034lbl.pdf.

FDA glimepiride label (2012). FDA, viewed 30OCT2012: http://www.accessdata.fda.gov/drugsatfda_docs/label/2012/020496s022lbl.pdf.

FDA glulisine insulin label (2009). FDA, viewed 30OCT2012: http://www.accessdata.fda.gov/drugsatfda_docs/label/2009/021629s008lbl.pdf.

FDA glyburide also known as glibenclamide label (2009). FDA, viewed 30OCT2012: http://www.accessdata.fda.gov/drugsatfda_docs/label/2009/017532s030lbl.pdf.

FDA lanreotide label (2011). FDA, viewed 30OCT2012: http://www.accessdata.fda.gov/drugsatfda_docs/label/2011/022074s003lbl.pdf.

FDA leuprolide pediatrics label (2012). FDA, 30OCT2012: http://www.accessdata.fda.gov/drugsatfda_docs/label/2012/019943s031,020011s038,020708s031lbl.pdf.

FDA leuprolide adults label (2011). FDA, viewed 30OCT2012: http://www.accessdata.fda.gov/drugsatfda_docs/label/2011/019010s035lbl.pdf.

FDA levothyroxine label (2009). FDA, viewed 30OCT2012: http://www.accessdata.fda.gov/drugsatfda_docs/label/2009/021292s002lbl.pdf.

FDA liothyronine label (2012). FDA, viewed 30OCT2012: http://www.accessdata.fda.gov/drugsatfda_docs/label/2002/10379s47lbl.pdf.

FDA lispro insulin label (2012). FDA, viewed 30OCT2012: http://www.accessdata.fda.gov/drugsatfda_docs/label/2012/020563s123lbl.pdf.

FDA mecasermin label (2012). FDA, viewed 30OCT2012: http://www.accessdata.fda.gov/drugsatfda_docs/label/2012/021839s010lbl.pdf.

FDA metformin label (2008). FDA, viewed 30OCT2012: http://www.accessdata.fda.gov/drugsatfda_docs/label/2008/020357s031,021202s016lbl.pdf.

FDA metformin-pioglitazone label (2012). FDA, viewed 30OCT2012: http://www.accessdata.fda.gov/drugsatfda_docs/label/2012/021842s008s010lbl.pdf.

FDA metformin-sitagliptin label (2012). FDA, viewed 30OCT2012: http://www.accessdata.fda.gov/drugsatfda_docs/label/2012/022044s026lbl.pdf.

FDA methimazole label (2001). FDA, viewed 30OCT2012: http://www.accessdata.fda.gov/drugsatfda_docs/label/2001/007517s022lbl.pdf.

FDA miglitol label (2012). FDA, viewed 30OCT2012: http://www.accessdata.fda.gov/drugsatfda_docs/label/2012/020682s010lbl.pdf.

FDA nateglinide label (2012). FDA, viewed 30OCT2012: http://www.accessdata.fda.gov/drugsatfda_docs/label/2011/021204s014lbl.pdf.

FDA NPH insulin label (2010). FDA, viewed 30OCT2012: http://www.accessdata.fda.gov/drugsatfda_docs/label/2010/018781s114lbl.pdf.

FDA octreotide label (2012). FDA, viewed 30OCT2012: http://www.accessdata.fda.gov/drugsatfda_docs/label/2012/019667s061lbl.pdf.

FDA pasireotide label (2012). FDA viewed 15OCT2013: http://www.accessdata.fda.gov/drugsatfda_docs/label/2012/200677lbl.pdf.

FDA pegvisomant label (2012). FDA, viewed 30OCT2012: http://www.accessdata.fda.gov/drugsatfda_docs/label/2012/021106s031lbl.pdf.

FDA pioglitazone label (2011). FDA, viewed 30OCT2012: http://www.accessdata.fda.gov/drugsatfda_docs/label/2011/021073s043s044lbl.pdf.

FDA pramlintide label (2007). FDA, viewed 30OCT2012: http://www.accessdata.fda.gov/drugsatfda_docs/label/2007/021332s006lbl.pdf.

FDA propylthiouracil Drug Safety Communication (2009). FDA, viewed 30OCT2012: http://www.fda.gov/Drugs/DrugSafety/PostmarketDrugSafetyInformationforPatientsandProviders/ucm209023.htm.

FDA propylthiouracil Information for Healthcare Professionals (2009). FDA, viewed 30OCT2012: http://www.fda.gov/Drugs/DrugSafety/PostmarketDrugSafetyInformationforPatientsandProviders/DrugSafetyInformationforHeathcareProfessionals/ucm162701.htm

FDA regular and NPH human insulin fixed combination label (2010). FDA, viewed 30OCT2012: http://www.accessdata.fda.gov/drugsatfda_docs/label/2010/019717s0 94lbl.pdf.

FDA repaglinide label (2012). FDA, viewed 30OCT2012: http://www.accessdata.fda.gov/drugsatfda_docs/label/2012/020741s040lbl.pdf.

FDA saxagliptin label (2011). FDA, viewed 30OCT2012: http://www.accessdata.fda.gov/drugsatfda_docs/label/2011/022350s004lbl.pdf.

FDA sitagliptin label (2012). FDA, viewed 30OCT2012: http://www.accessdata.fda.gov/drugsatfda_docs/label/2012/021995s025lbl.pdf.

FDA somatropin label (2012). FDA, viewed 30OCT2012: http://www.accessdata.fda.gov/drugsatfda_docs/label/2012/020280s072lbl.pdf.

FDA teriparatide label (2009). FDA, viewed 30OCT2012: http://www.accessdata.fda.gov/drugsatfda_docs/label/2009/021318s012lbl.pdf.

FDA tolvaptan label (2012). FDA, viewed 30OCT2012: http://www.accessdata.fda.gov/drugsatfda_docs/label/2012/022275s005lbl.pdf.

Fisher AM, Scott DA (1933). An attempt at peptic synthesis of insulin. J Gen Physiol 16: 741–755.

Fisher AM, Scott DA (1935). Zinc content of bovine pancreas. Biochem J 29: 1055–1058.

Fujioka M, Okushi K, Hiramatsu K et al. (1997). Specific changes in human brain after hypoglycemic injury. Stroke 28: 584–587.

Fumarola A, Di Fiore A, Dainelli M et al. (2010). Medical treatment of hyperthyroidism: state of the art. Exp Clin Endocrinol Diabetes 118: 678–684.

Gibbons CH, Freeman R (2010). Treatment-induced diabetic neuropathy: a reversible painful autonomic neuropathy. Ann Neurol 67: 534–541.

Gibbons RV, Holman RC, Belay ED et al. (2000). Creutzfeldt–Jakob disease in the United States: 1979–1998. JAMA 284: 2322–2323.

Giugliano D, Rosa ND, Maro GD et al. (1993). Metformin improves glucose, lipid metabolism, and reduces blood pressure in hypertensive, obese women. Diabetes Care 16: 1387–1390.

Graham DJ, Ouellet-Hellstrom R, MaCurdy T et al. (2010). Risk of acute myocardial infarction, stroke, heart failure, and death in elderly Medicare patients treated with rosiglitazone or pioglitazone. JAMA 304: 411–418.

Halimi S, Charpentier G, Grimaldi A et al. (2001). Effect on compliance, acceptability of blood glucose self-monitoring and HbA(1c) of a self-monitoring system developed according to patient's wishes. The ACCORD study. Diabetes Metab 27: 681–687.

Hamaguchi T, Hirose T, Asakawa H et al. (2004). Efficacy of glimepiride in type 2 diabetic patients treated with glibenclamide. Diabetes Res Clin Pract 66 (Suppl 1): S129–S132.

Harrower AD (2000). Comparative tolerability of sulphonylureas in diabetes mellitus. Drug Saf 22: 313–320.

Hermans G, De Jonghe B, Bruyninckx F et al. (2008a). Clinical review: critical illness polyneuropathy and myopathy. Crit Care 12: 238.

Hermans G, Schetz M, Van den Berghe G (2008b). Tight glucose control in critically ill adults. JAMA 300: 2725–2726.

Hermans G, De Jonghe B, Bruyninckx F et al. (2009). Interventions for preventing critical illness polyneuropathy and critical illness myopathy. Cochrane Database Syst Rev 1, CD006832.

Kletzky OA, Vermesh M (1989). Effectiveness of vaginal bromocriptine in treating women with hyperprolactinemia. Fertil Steril 51: 269–272.

Leong KS, Foy PM, Swift AC et al. (2000). CSF rhinorrhoea following treatment with dopamine agonists for massive invasive prolactinomas. Clin Endocrinol (Oxf) 52: 43.

Liu KW, Dai LK, Jean W (2006). Metformin-related vitamin B12 deficiency. Age Ageing 35: 200–201.

Ma J, Kim Y, Yoo W et al. (2009). MR imaging of hypoglycemic encephalopathy: lesion distribution and prognosis prediction by diffusion-weighted imaging. Neuroradiology 51: 641–649.

Mebis L, Van den Berghe G (2009). The hypothalamus–pituitary–thyroid axis in critical illness. Neth J Med 67: 332–340.

Morgans ME, Trotter WR (1960). Potassium perchlorate in thyrotoxicosis. Br Med J 2: 517–518.

Nathan DM, Buse JB, Davidson MB et al. American Diabetes Association, European Association for Study of Diabetes (2009). Medical management of hyperglycemia in type 2 diabetes: a consensus algorithm for the initiation and adjustment of therapy: a consensus statement of the American Diabetes Association and the European Association for the Study of Diabetes. Diabetes Care 32: 1327–1334.

Scott DA, Fisher AM (1935). Crystalline insulin. Biochem J 29: 1048–1054.

Scott DA, Fisher AM (1938). The insulin and the zinc content of normal and diabetic pancreas. J Clin Invest 17: 725–728.

Swedish Medical Products Agency quinagolide product information (2009). Sweden Medical Products Agency viewed 15OCT2013: http://www.lakemedelsverket.se/SPC_PIL/Pdf/enhumspc/Norprolac%20tablet%20ENG%20SmPC.doc

Ueba H, Kuroki M, Hashimoto S et al. (2005). Glimepiride induces nitric oxide production in human coronary artery endothelial cells via a PI3-kinase-Akt dependent pathway. Atherosclerosis 183: 35–39.

UKPDS 33 (1998). Intensive blood-glucose control with sulphonylureas or insulin compared with conventional treatment and risk of complications in patients with type 2 diabetes (UKPDS 33). UK Prospective Diabetes Study (UKPDS) Group. Lancet 352: 837–853, erratum Lancet (1999) 354: 602.

UKPDS 34 (1998). Effect of intensive blood-glucose control with metformin on complications in overweight patients with type 2 diabetes (UKPDS 34). UK Prospective Diabetes Study (UKPDS) Group. Lancet 352: 854–865, erratum Lancet 352: 1558.

Van den Berghe G, Bouillon R, Mesotten D (2009). Glucose control in critically ill patients. N Engl J Med 361: 89.

Wesley UV, Tiwari S, Houghton AN (2004). Role for dipeptidyl peptidase IV in tumor suppression of human non small cell lung carcinoma cells. Int J Cancer 109: 855–866.

Zib I, Raskin P (2006). Novel insulin analogues and its mitogenic potential. Diabetes Obes Metab 8: 611–620.

Section 7

Neurologic aspects of metabolic diseases

Handbook of Clinical Neurology, Vol. 120 (3rd series)
Neurologic Aspects of Systemic Disease Part II
Jose Biller and Jose M. Ferro, Editors
© 2014 Elsevier B.V. All rights reserved

Chapter 55

Disorders of purines and pyrimidines

ROGER E. KELLEY[1]* AND HANS C. ANDERSSON[2]

[1]*Department of Neurology, Tulane University School of Medicine, New Orleans, LA, USA*

[2]*Hayward Genetics Center, Tulane University School of Medicine, New Orleans, LA, USA*

OVERVIEW

Purines and pyrimidines are vital constituents of nucleic acids as well as other substrates of lipid and carbohydrate metabolism. Purines are derived either from dietary ingestion of purine-containing compounds or by *de novo* synthesis. Pyrimidines result from the combination of carbamylphosphate and aspartate to form orotic acid along with the key nucleotide substrate uridine 5'-monophosphate (UMP).

Purine and pyrimidine nucleotides are synthesized by two different pathways: a *de novo* pathway which produces these phosphorylated ring structures from simple precursors which include CO_2, glutamine, and glycine, while salvage pathways reconstitute already produced purine and pyrimidine bases (Nyhan, 2005). For purine metabolism, inosine monophosphate (IMP), also known as inosinic acid, is the central product of both the *de novo* and salvage pathways and is intimately involved in the conversion of purine nucleotides to adenine and guanine nucleotides. These are essential precursors for the synthesis of DNA, RNA, energy transducers, metabolic signaling pathways, growth regulators, and essential coenzymes. There appear to be distinct patterns for purine metabolism depending upon the organ involved, with the central nervous system more heavily dependent on the salvage pathway.

The intracellular concentration of purine is dependent upon the balance between anabolic and catabolic processes (Bzowska et al., 2000). Although the *de novo* and salvage pathways of purine nucleotide syntheses are regulated by end product feedback, purine catabolism appears to be a function of the availability of substrates. Fluctuations in the synthesis or breakdown of purine nucleotides can significantly affect intracellular function. The end product of purine catabolism is uric acid

and metabolic disorders of purine pathways often result in either hyperuricemia or hypouricemia.

Pyrimidine *de novo* synthesis is initiated with a carbamylphosphate synthetase reaction. The central compound of such a reaction is UMP. Two catalytic enzymes, orotic acid phophoribosyltransferase (OPRT) and orotidine monophosphate decarboxylase (OPD), are involved in the synthesis of UMP. Their activities are combined in a single protein, the enzyme UMP synthase, which is coded for by a single gene (Nyhan, 2005). The OPRT component serves in both the *de novo* synthesis and salvage pathways for pyrimidine.

DISORDERS OF PURINE METABOLISM

These disorders are summarized in Table 55.1, with identification of the presumptive pathogenetic mechanism, based upon presently available information, and are discussed below.

Gout

The most commonly encountered disorder of purine metabolism is gout. This affects roughly 1–2% of the population and is characterized by hyperuricemia with urate crystal deposition resulting in nephrolithiasis and inflammatory arthritis (Schlesinger, 2010). The development of gout is multifactorial in pathogenesis although an autosomal dominant juvenile gouty nephropathy has been reported (Calabrese et al., 1990). This genetically mediated disorder is related to reduced urate renal clearance and not to impaired purine metabolic pathways. There have been identified mutations of the *UMOD* gene which encodes uromodulin, also known as Tamm–Horsfall glycoprotein (Turner et al., 2003). There is eventual development of end stage

---

*Correspondence to: Roger E. Kelley, M.D., Department of Neurology, Tulane University School of Medicine, 1430 Tulane Avenue, New Orleans, LA 70112, USA. Tel: +1-504-988-1133, Fax: +1-504-988-9197, E-mail: rkelley2@tulane.edu

Table 55.1

Disorders of purine metabolism

Disorder	Manifestations	Etiological factors
Gout	Inflammatory arthritis Hyperuricemia Nephrolithiasis	Familial Multifactorial Autosomal dominant juvenile form with nephropathy

Phosphoribosyl- pyrophosphate
    synthetase (PRPS)
    hyperactivity
	Hyperuricemia with gout
	Sensorineural hearing loss
	Mental retardation
	Hypotonia
		X-linked with PRPS point mutations

PRPS deficiency	Mental retardation
	Hypouricemia
	Charcot–Marie–Tooth = CMTX5 with
	    peripheral neuropathy, hearing loss
	    and optic atrophy
		X-linked with *PRPS1* gene

Arts syndrome	Early onset with hypotonia Mental retardation Motor development delay Ataxia Hearing loss Optic atrophy Susceptibility to recurrent infection	X-linked with missense mutation resulting in loss of PRPS1 actvity

Hypoxanthine-guanine
    phosphoribosyl transferase
    (HRPT) deficiency (Lesch–
    Nyhan disease)
	Hyperuricemia
	Mental retardation
	Behavioral disturbance with self-mutilation
	Extrapyramidal syndrome with dystonia
	    and opisthotonic posturing
	Long tract signs
		X-linked with single gene mutation on
		    chromosome Xq26-27

Milder forms of HRPT deficiency (Lesch–Nyhan variants)	Cognitive impairment Dystonia Long tract signs	X-linked
Adenyl succinate lyase (ADSL) deficiency	Developmental delay Communication deficits Hypotonia Impaired muscle energy metabolism	Autosomal recessive

5-Amino-4-imidazole-
    carboxamide ribotide
    transformylase/IMP
    cyclohydrolase (ATIC)
    deficiency
	Profound intellectual disability
	Epilepsy
	Congential blindness
	Facial dysmorphism
		Frameshift and K426R gene mutation

5′-Nucleotidase pervasive
    developmental disorder
    (NAPDD)
	Language delay
	Behavioral disturbance
	Epilepsy
	Ataxia
	Absent manual dexterity
	Recurrent infection
		Unknown

Purine nucleosidase
    phosphorylase deficiency
	Autoimmune disorder with
	    hemolytic anemia
	Severe combined immune
	    deficiency (SCID)
	Developmental delay
	Sensorineural hearing loss
	Spasticity
	Hypouricemia
		Autosomal recessive

Table 55.1

Continued

Disorder	Manifestations	Etiological factors
Adenosine deaminase deficiency	SCID Hearing loss Epilepsy Cognitive impairment Motor dysfunction Behavioral disturbance	Affected gene on chromosome 20q13.11
Deoxyguanosine kinase deficiency	Liver failure with hepatocerebral syndrome	Chromosome 2013 with mitochondrial DNA depletion
Xanthine oxidase deficiency- hereditary xanthinuria	Hypouricemia Renal calculus formation Myalgia/muscle cramps	C682G gene mutations
Molybdenum cofactor deficiency	Hypouricemia Severe neonatal seizures Facial dysmorphism Lack of neurodevelopment Ophthalmic abnormalities	Mutations of MOCS1 locus on chromosome 6
Myoadenylate deaminase deficiency	Muscle cramps/myalgias after exercise	Homozygous C to T transition at nucleoside 34
Glucose-6-phosphatase deficiency (von Gierke disease)	Hypoglycemia Organomegaly Growth retardation Hyperuricemia Lactic acidemia Secondary metabolic encephalopathy	Autosomal recessive GSD-la and GSD lb mutation localized to chromosome 17-bound G6Pase gene and chromosome 11-bound G6PT gene

renal disease associated with the formation of renal medullary cysts.

Other than impaired purine metabolic pathways and reduced renal clearance of uric acid, other explanations for the hyperuricemia seen in gout include size of the purine nucleotide pool, enhanced catabolism of purine analogs including nucleic acids, increased turnover of preformed purines, and comorbid conditions associated with increased uric acid levels, such as morbid obesity, hyperlipidemia, malignancy, sickle cell disease, glycogen storage disease, diet (meat, seafood, beer, spirits), as well as familial predisposition.

Gout is not typically directly associated with neurologic disease. However, there can be secondary effects. For example, UMOD-related kidney disease can lead to uremic encephalopathy if not properly treated with hemodialysis. Furthermore, the so-called risk triad for the promotion of atherosclerosis in patients with gout includes inflammation, oxidative stress, and hyperlipidemia (Krishnan et al., 2008). This can enhance the risk of cerebrovascular disease as a complication of this triad.

The treatment of gout includes prevention with a low purine diet and the agent allopurinol, which blocks the conversion of hypoxanthine to the less soluble xanthine via inhibition of xanthine oxidase. Acute attacks are typically treated with either colchicine or nonsteroidal anti-inflammatory agents.

Phosphoribosylpyrophosphate synthetase

In the salvage pathway, purine nucleotides are assembled from preformed nucleobases and 5-phosphoribosyl-1-pyrophosphate (PRPP). The synthesis of PRPP from Mg-ATP and ribose-5-phosphate is catalyzed by a family of the isoforms of the enzyme phosphoribosylpyrophosphate synthetase (PRPS) (Fox and Kelley, 1972). There is an X-linked disorder of purine metabolism related to increased activity of PRPS (Becker et al., 1988a) resulting in uric acid overproduction with gout. Neurologic manifestations can include sensorineural hearing loss as well as mental retardation and hypotonia (Becker et al., 1988b). Three isoforms of PRPS have been identified and mutant PRPS1s isoforms have been reported in six hemizygous unrelated males who had PRPS hyperactivity associated with impaired responsiveness to purine nucleotide inhibitor (Becker et al., 1995).

Five of the six were reported to have neurodevelopmental delay. The cells of affected individuals were characterized by accelerated PRPP and purine synthesis as biochemical hallmarks (Becker et al., 1987).

Conversely, there have been reports of PRPS deficiency. Wada et al. (1974) reported an infant with mental retardation, hypouricemia and a defect of erythrocytic PRPS. Charcot–Marie–Tooth inherited neuropathy (CMTX5), including peripheral neuropathy, hearing loss, and optic atrophy has been attributed to diminished PRPS1 activity (Kim et al., 2007). This X-linked disorder, attributed to mutations in the *PRPS1* gene, was detected by a roughly 50% reduction in enzymatic activity of PRPS in the patient's fibroblasts. There was no associated mental retardation with CMTX5, and the uric acid level was normal.

Arts syndrome is an X-linked disorder characterized by early-onset hypotonia, mental retardation, ataxia, motor development delay, hearing loss, optic atrophy, and susceptibility to recurrent infections. The latter manifestation typically leads to early death. The serum uric acid level is low while urinary purine profiles in this disorder are typified by undetectable hypoxanthine with normal xanthine and uric acid levels. From a genetic standpoint, this is associated with missense mutations in L152P and Q133P causing loss of PRPS1 activity, as has been reported by De Brouwer et al. (2007). These authors found that the greater severity of this disorder, compared to CMTX5, was attributed to quantitatively less PRPS activity, which was found to be absent in erythrocytes and of the order of 0–10% in fibroblasts compared to controls.

In summary, the phenotypic manifestations of *PRPS1* gene mutations can reflect either genotypic hyper- or hypoactivity of this enzyme and appear to be a function of the degree of the residual enzymatic activity.

Hypoxanthine-guanine phosphoribosyltransferase deficiency

Hypoxanthine-guanine phosphoribosyltransferase (HPRT) is the enzyme which catalyzes salvage of the purine bases guanine and hypoxanthine into their respective monophosphate nucleoside i.e., guanylic monophosphate (GMP) and inosine monophosphate (IMP). This is a PRPP-dependent reaction and HPRT is encoded by a single structural gene located on the X chromosome (Xq26-27). The entire HPRT gene has been sequenced and several different alterations in the coding region have been identified as contributing to HPRT deficiency (Camici et al., 2010). There is a spectrum of disorders related to HPRT deficiency and the three major clinical features are: (1) hyperuricemia, (2) neurologic

manifestations, and (3) behavioral disturbance. The disorder that has achieved the most attention is Lesch–Nyhan disease, originally described in 1964 (Lesch and Nyhan, 1964). The expression of this disorder is almost exclusively recessive, but the small number of females reported is presumably related to nonrandom (skewed) inactivation of the normal X chromosome (Nyhan, 2005).

The myriad manifestations of Lesch–Nyhan disease include motor development retardation, extrapyramidal manifestations with dystonia, chorea, and athetosis, long tract signs with hyperreflexia, and positive Babinski response. The neurologic picture can mimic athetoid type of cerebral palsy. However, the hallmarks of self-injurious behavior (Fig. 55.1) and opisthotonic arching of the back usually allow clinical diagnosis of the

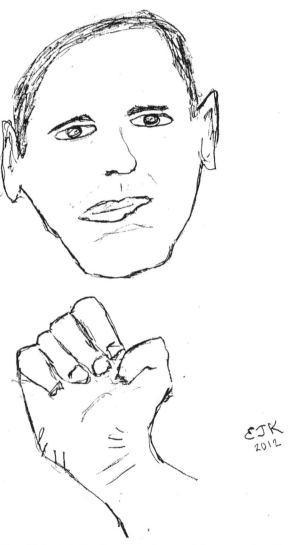

Fig. 55.1. Artist's drawing of potential areas of self-mutilation in Lesch–Nyhan syndrome, with involvement of lips and fingers.

disorder in older children. In addition to the self-injurious behavior, there is often cognitive impairment as well as aggressive and impulsive behavior. Physiologically, there is typically hyperuricemia and uricosuria, which may lead to gouty arthritis, tophus formation, hematuria, kidney stones, urinary tract infection, and renal failure. There is a spectrum of disease, reflective of the activity of HPRT, and, in this disorder, the erythrocyte activity is essentially undetectable.

The prevalence of Lesch–Nyhan disease is estimated to be approximately 1/380 000 live births, making it quite rare. Typically, affected patients have a normal prenatal and perinatal course followed by evolution of manifestations usually within 3–6 months. Most patients live no longer than 40 years and complications of hyperuricemia and complications of mobility restriction appear to be the main contributing factors to diminished longevity (Camici, 2010).

Pathophysiologically, Lesch–Nyhan disease involves other metabolic abnormalities reported in addition to the well recognized increased *de novo* purine synthesis. There have been a number of enzymes reported to display heightened activation and there may well be disturbed pyrimidine metabolism. Jinnah et al. (2006) have highlighted the impact on neurotransmitters in this disorder, including decreased striatal dopaminergic function along with increased levels of serotonin and 5-hydroxyindolacetate. Alteration of the dopaminergic pathways have been demonstrated *in vivo* with cerebral positron emission tomographic (PET) scanning (Wong et al., 1996). However, no clear pathophysiologic understanding exists currently to explain how the disturbed purine and pyrimidine metabolism leads to basal ganglionic damage.

Milder forms of HPRT have been recognized including cases with no neurologic disability (Kelley et al., 1969). Milder neurologic manifestations can include varying degrees of cognitive impairment, long tract signs, and dystonia. These have been referred to as "Lesch–Nyhan variants," reflecting this potential spectrum of manifestations (Jinnah et al., 2006) reflective of the level of HPRT enzyme activity (Page et al., 1981). A potential contributor to such variations presumably lies in the realm of the genetic expression of HPRT. Nguyen et al. (2012) reported on a normal HPRT DNA coding region for two subjects with Lesch–Nyhan syndrome but with significantly reduced HPRT messenger RNA expression.

Adenylsuccinate lyase deficiency

Adenylsuccinate lyase (ADSL) catalyzes two steps in the *de novo* synthesis of purine nucleotides (Crifò et al., 2005). Deficiency of ADSL is an autosomal recessive disorder associated with severe neurologic impairment including developmental delay, restricted communication suggesting autism, seizures, and hypotonia. ADSL deficiency impacts on glucose metabolism as demonstrated by reduced glucose uptake seen *in vivo* on cerebral PET scan (De Volder et al., 1988). In view of this finding, Salerno et al. (1999) reported a reduction in seizure frequency with administration of D-ribose and D-glucose in a patient with ADSL deficiency. The human ADSL gene has been located on chromosome 22q13.1-13.2; missense mutations and a promoter mutation have been described in numerous European populations with little genotype-phenotype correlation (Spiegel et al., 2006). In addition to the potential for severe CNS involvement, the role of ADSL in the Krebs cycle, in terms of the maintenance of the ATP/AMP ratio, has been cited as an explanation for ADSL deficiency being associated with impairment of muscle energy metabolism (Salerno et al., 1997).

In terms of the pathogenesis of ADSL deficiency and the effect on the CNS, Crifò et al. (2005) reported that compound heterozygosity for the P100A/D422Y mutations of the ADSL gene results in a defective enzyme which is inhibited by micromolar concentrations of trans-4-hydroxy-2-nonenal (HNE). HNE is a major product of membrane peroxidation that accumulates in the brain in neurodegenerative disorders. Based upon this association, it was theorized that inactivation of defective ASDL by HNE in the brain may account for the neurologic deficits observed.

This disorder is associated with a positive Bratton–Marshall reaction which is a test originally designed for detection of sulfonamide. However, both ADLS deficiency and ATIC deficiency (see below) can be associated with a positive Bratton–Marshall reaction which is unique among purine metabolism disorders.

5-Amino-4-imidazolecarboxamide ribotide transformylase/IMP cyclohydrolase deficiency

This single polypeptide acts as a bifunctional enzyme, AICAR transformylase/IMP cyclohydrolase (ATIC), in *de novo* purine synthesis. The human ATIC gene has been located to chromosome 2q35 (Camici, 2010). Marie et al. (2004) reported a female patient with profound mental retardation, epilepsy, congenital blindness, and dysmorphic features associated with severe deficiency of ATIC. Of note, there was a positive urinary Bratton–Marshall test for diazotizable amines (Laikind et al., 1986), which is indicative of accumulation of 5AICA-riboside which is a distinctive feature of ADSL deficiency. However, further analysis revealed a large accumulation of AICAR as well as its di- and triphosphate derivatives, which supports this enzyme deficiency as a primary component and which was also supported by sequencing of the ATIC gene.

This sequencing revealed a frameshift mutation in exon 2 of one allele, also found in the mother's DNA, resulting in mRNA instability. Furthermore, in the other allele, a K426R mutation identified in exon 13, which is part of the AICAR transformylase domain, was also present in the father. There are also increased levels of AICAR, and its triphosphate, in Lesch–Nyhan syndrome (Sidi and Mitchell, 1985), although to a lesser extent than in the patient reported by Marie et al. (2004).

5′-Nucleotidase

Nucleotidase associated pervasive developmental disorder (NAPDD) was first described by Page et al. (1997) and this is associated with a roughly 10-fold increase in purine and pyrimidine 5′-nucleotidase activity. There are myriad neurologic manifestations associated with this disorder including language delay or actual mutism, behavioral disturbance with impulsivity, hyperactivity, attention deficit, aggressiveness, social maladaption, as well as epilepsy, incoordination, ataxic gait, and problems with dexterity. There is a propensity to recurrent sinus and ear infection although laboratory studies tend to be normal outside of low immunoglobulins, low urinary urate level, and, on occasion, low T cell function. Of particular note, patients routinely have normal purine and pyrimidine nucleotide levels. In one patient (Trifilo and Page, 2000), there was increased 5′-nucleotidase activity in the fibroblasts which was associated with hyperexpression of the membrane-bound enzyme. However, a specific gene defect has not yet been identified. In terms of overlap with other disorders of purine metabolism, increased enzyme activity has been described in patients with Lesch–Nyhan syndrome (Pesi et al., 2000).

Purine nucleoside phosphorylase deficiency

Purine nucleoside phosphorylase (PNP) is an enzyme which catalyzes the first step in either purine base salvage or nucleoside catabolism. Specifically, PNP catalyzes the reversible cleavage of inosine to hypoxanthine and guanosine to guanine. PNP deficiency is associated with neurologic manifestations in roughly two-thirds of affected patients (Giblett et al., 1975; Markert, 1994), while one-third have autoimmune disorders with autoimmune hemolytic anemia as the most common. There is a severe combined immunodeficiency (SCID) reported in 4% of patients (Dalal et al., 2001) specifically involving cell-mediated immunity. Neurologic involvement can include mild to severe developmental delay with mental retardation, sensorineural deafness and motor findings including severe spasticity. This rare disorder is autosomal recessive and the gene has been localized to 14q13.1.

Unlike other immunodeficiency disorders associated with purine metabolism, PNP deficiency is associated with hypouricemia and reduction in urinary excretion of uric acid.

Adenine deaminase deficiency

Adenine deaminase (ADA) is expressed by a gene located on chromosome 20q13.11 (Markert, 1994). This enzyme catalyzes the hydrolytic deamination of adenosine to form inosine and deoxyadenosine to deoxyinosine. Deficiency of this enzyme results in accumulation of deoxyadenosine and deoxyadenosine triphosphate (dATP) with interference in normal DNA synthesis (Hirschhorn, 1993). There are severe lymphotoxic effects associated with ADA deficiency with susceptibility to SCID (Giblett et al., 1972). In the neurologic realm, motor and cognitive impairment is reported as well as hearing loss and seizures (Hirschhorn, 1980). As with other purine metabolism disorders, autistic-like behavior has been observed as well as attention deficit, learning disability and hyperactivity. The neurologic manifestations tend to develop beyond the neonatal period and increase in severity with age (Rogers et al., 2001). The phenotypic expression tends to be quite variable. Bone marrow transplantation is reported to help the immunologic manifestations, but not necessarily the neurologic deficits (Nofech-Mozes et al., 2007). Furthermore, efforts at enzyme replacement therapy as well as stem cell transplant have actually been reported to aggravate neurologic manifestations, rather than ameliorate them (Rogers et al., 2001) as was originally reported by Hirschhorn et al. (1980).

Deoxyguanosine kinase deficiency

Deoxyguanosine kinase (dGK) is an enzyme associated with phosphorylation of purine deoxynucleotides and their analogs (Eriksson et al., 2002). The human deoxyguanosine kinase gene (DGUOK) has been localized to chromosome 2p13 and the enzyme is mitochondrial in location (Johansson et al., 1996). Deficiency of this enzyme is rare and is associated with mitochondrial DNA (mtDNA) depletion syndromes with a reduction in mtDNA copy number (Mandel et al., 2001). dGK is an essential component of the mitochondrial deoxynucleoside triphosphate salvage pathway. The presentation is typically one of liver failure and neurologic manifestations in neonates along with a profound elevation of lactic acid in the serum. This resultant "hepatocerebral" syndrome is characterized, neurologically, by severe developmental retardation along with prominent multidirectional nystagmus (Labarthe et al., 2005). Eriksson and Wang (2008) have summarized molecular mechanisms of mitochondrial DNA depletion diseases associated with enzyme deficiency and report 22 point mutations to date in the *DGUOK* gene. The typical course is one of severe CNS and liver involvement, with death within the first year. However, compound heterozygosity, with missense mutations, can result in less severe organ involvement and longer survival (Salviati et al., 2002).

Xanthine oxidase deficiency (hereditary xanthinuria)

Deficiency of xanthine oxidase, also known as xanthine dehydrogenase, results in hypouricemia and susceptibility to renal calculus formation. There can also be deposition of xanthine crystals within the muscles of affected patients associated with myalgia and cramps (Chalmers et al., 1969). This disorder is usually detected by the assay of xanthine in the urine as well as by biopsy of the liver or intestine or by response to oral tetrahydrobiopterin (Blau et al., 1996). Two mutations for the xanthine oxidase gene, located at chromosome 2p22, have been reported in Japanese patients. These include a C682T mutation, which changed arginine 228 to a stop codon, and deletion of cytosine at position 2567 predicted to result in premature termination (Ichida et al., 1997).

Molybdenum cofactor deficiency

Deficiency of the xanthine oxidase cofactor, molybdenum, is caused by impaired processing to mature cofactor and leads to deficient activity of xanthine oxidase, sulfite oxidase, and aldehyde oxidase. Deficient xanthine oxidase is also associated with hypouricemia, the biochemical hallmark. However, of much greater clinical consequence are the severe neurologic manifestations thought to be due to sulfite oxidase deficiency which results in severe neonatal seizures, often with status epilepticus, and typically a very poor prognosis for both neurodevelopment and survival (Wadman et al., 1983). Less severe mutations are recognized and have been reported in association with facial dysmorphism, subluxed ocular lenses, and other ophthalmic abnormalities (Endres et al., 1988). The disorder can be detected by fibroblast assay of sulfite oxidase and can be made in the prenatal period (Johnson, 2003). The majority of deleterious mutations have been at the MOCS1 locus on chromosome 6. A number of mutations have been reported including a frameshift deletion (Nyhan, 2005).

Myoadenylate deaminase deficiency

Myoadenylate deaminase (AMP deaminase) catalyzes the conversion of adenosine monophosphate to inosine monophosphate and ammonia. Enzyme deficiency can result in muscle cramps and pain after exercise resembling McArdle's disorder of glycogenesis, but no specific neurologic abnormalities. Unlike McArdle's disease, the forearm ischemic test reveals a normal rise in serum lactic acid level, but not in ammonia level (Fishbein et al., 1978). To date, affected individuals have had a homozygous C to T transition at nucleotide 34 (Morisaki et al., 1992).

Glucose-6-phosphatase deficiency

Deficiency of glucose-6-phosphatase (G6Pase) results in a glycogen storage disease (GSD) type I, also known as von Gierke disease, and is associated with *de novo* overproduction of purine as well as gout in childhood or adolescence (Nyhan, 2005). G6Pase is an autosomal recessive disorder with an incidence of roughly 1 in 100 000 (Chou et al., 2002). There are two major gene mutation subtypes: (1) GSD-la, caused by a deficiency in glucose-6-phosphatase, and (2) GSD-lb caused by a deficiency in the glucose-6-phosphate transporter (G6PT). These two components maintain glucose homeostasis. Involvement of either subtype results in growth retardation, hypoglycemia, organomegaly, hyperuricemia, lactic acidemia, hyperlipidemia as well as was neutropenia. The neurologic sequelae are secondary to the associated metabolic disturbances. A number of mutations (primarily missense) have been identified (Janecke et al., 2001), and reliable carrier testing and prenatal diagnosis is now available with mutation analyses of the G6Pase gene (chromosome 17q21) and the G6PT gene (chromosome 11q23). There are experimental models of gene therapy for G6Pase deficiency (Chou and Mansfield, 2007), with some potential for this disorder.

DISORDERS OF PYRIMIDINE METABOLISM

Disorders of pyrimidine metabolism are summarized in Table 55.2, including the presumptive pathogenetic mechanism, based upon presently available information, and are discussed below.

Orotic aciduria

Orotic aciduria results in megaloblastic anemia and crytalluria (Huguley et al., 1959). The enzyme urindine-5-monophosphate (UMP) synthase contains, in a single protein, the activities of both phosphoribosyltransferase (OPRT) and ortoidine-5′-monophosphate (OMP) decarboxylase. These enzymes catalyze the last two steps of UMP synthesis (Smith et al., 1961).

A single gene codes for UMP synthase (Suchi et al., 1997). In terms of phenotypic expression, crystals of orotic acid can cause urethral and ureteral obstruction resulting in hematuria and renal impairment. Neurologically, one can see physical and mental development

Table 55.2

Disorders of pyrimidine metabolism

Disorder	Manifestations	Etiological factors
Orotic aciduria	Megaloblastic anemia Crystalluria Hematuria Renal impairment Susceptibility to severe infections Neurodevelopmental delay	Single gene point mutations
Pyrimidine nucleotide depletion and overactive cytosolic 5′-nucleotidase	Neurobehavioral disorder Seizures Neurodevelopmental delay Lack of fine motor skills Ataxia Alopecia Susceptibility to recurrent infection	Unknown
Dihydropyramidase deficiency	Epilepsy Mental retardation Microcephaly Can be asymptomatic	Gene mutations mapped to chromosome 8q22
Ureidoproprionase deficiency	Neurodevelopmental delay Epilepsy Dystonia	Three gene mutations identified to date affecting the β-ureidoproprionase gene (*UPB1*)

impairment with or without anemia. Early life megaloblastic anemia can result in susceptibility to severe infections with myriad consequences.

Deficiency of OPRT and OMP decarboxylase can be detected in red and white blood cells as well as cultured fibroblasts. Various point mutations have been identified in the gene on chromosome 3q13 (Suchi et al., 1997). Of particular importance is the recognition of this disorder in affected patients as uridine supplementation, at dose of 50–300 mg/kg/day, results in complete suppression of this metabolic disturbance (Sumi et al., 1997).

Pyrimidine nucleotide depletion and overactive cytosolic 5′-nucleotidase

This is another important disorder to recognize in light of its response to uridine supplementation as well (Nyhan, 2005). There is increased degradation of purine and pyrimidine nucleotides associated with increased enzymatic activity of 5′-nucleotidase as measured in cultured fibroblasts (Page et al., 1997). This can result in seizure, neurodevelopmental delay, lack of fine motor control, ataxia as well as alopecia and susceptibility to recurrent infections. What was initially reported to be autistic-like communication disturbance is now viewed as a more distinct neurobehavioral impairment including aggressive behavior, hyperactivity, language difficulty, and impaired reasoning.

Dihydropyrimidine dehydrogenase deficiency

The enzyme dihydropyrimidine dehydrogenase (DPD) catalyzes the first step in the breakdown of uracil and thymine. The products of this first step are dihydrouracil and dihydrothymine with 5-fluorouracil (5-FU) also a substrate. This latter feature can lead to excessive toxicity for 5-FU in cancer patients undergoing chemotherapy with this agent when there is coexistent DPD deficiency (Salgueiro et al., 2004). Enzyme assay can be accomplished on erythrocytes or cultured fibroblasts (Bakkeren et al., 1984). The screening for such DPD deficiency, to potentially avoid 5-FU toxicity, has resulted in recognition that many people with DPD deficiency are asymptomatic. However, there is the potential for epilepsy and neurodevelopment delay in infants and children with such an enzyme deficiency (Berger et al., 1984). Such patients are typically homozygous with the involved gene at chromosome 1p22. Screening for potential 5-FU toxicity can now be accomplished through an available test for a mutation at exon 14 which results in loss of a restriction site (Meinsma et al., 1995).

Dihydropyrimidinase deficiency (dihyropyrimidinuria)

Dihydropyrimidinase (DHP) is an enzyme responsible for the catalytic conversion of dihydrouracil and dihydrothymine to ureidoproprionic and ureidobutyric acids. Deficiency of this enzyme results in increased urinary excretion of dihydrouracil and dihydrothymine as well as uracil and thymine. DPH deficiency can lead to epilepsy, mental retardation, and microcephaly, although others are asymptomatic (Van Gennip et al., 1997). The responsible gene has been mapped to chromosome 8q22 with several potential mutations identified including both missense and frameshift types (Hamajima et al., 1998).

Ureidopropionase deficiency

β-Ureidopropionase deficiency can result in neurodevelopmental delay, epilepsy, and dystonia (van Kuilenburg et al., 2004; Nyhan, 2005). This enzyme catalyzes the conversion of ureidopropionic and ureidobutyric acids to β-alanine and β-aminoisobutyric acid. Enzyme deficiency has been detected by liver biopsy assay with various mutations identified (Van Gennip et al., 1997; van Kuilenburg et al., 2004). The affected gene is the β-ureidopropionase gene (*UPB1*). Mutations identified to date include two splice site mutations and one missense mutation. There is associated elevation of levels of *N*-carbamyl-β-alanine and N-carbamyl-β-aminoisobutyric acid in body fluids, including the cerebrospinal fluid, which can help in the detection of this disorder. In addition, detection of this disorder of pyrimidine catabolism has been reported with *in vitro* H-NMR spectroscopy (Assmann et al., 1998). In addition, proprionic acidemia can promote ureidopropionic aciduria through inhibition of ureidopropionase by propionic acid.

Less well-defined pyrimidine catabolic disorders

Other pyrimidine catabolic enzymatic pathway deficiencies have been reported, in isolated fashion, resulting in mental retardation, epilepsy, or both (Nyhan, 2005). This is reflective of the expanding scope of newer methods for identification for what were previously unexplained metabolic disorders.

SUMMARY

There is obviously an expanding array of knowledge in such inborn errors of metabolism as discussed here. The breadth of information being generated in terms of potential interactions of genotype and phenotype is truly staggering. However, several patterns appear to

Table 55.3

Potential indicators of purine or pyrimidine inborn errors of metabolism

1. Early age of onset
2. Hyper- or hypouricemia
3. Immunodeficiency
4. Unexplained neurodevelopmental delay
5. Seizure disorder which may be intractable
6. Sensorineural deafness
7. Autistic-like behavioral disturbance
8. Self-mutilating behavior such as in Lesch–Nyhan disease

be present in disorders of purine and pyrimidine metabolism which provide some level of comfort in terms of recognition (Table 55.3). Certainly there is variability in the degree of phenotypic expression as exemplified by Lesch–Nyhan disease versus Lesch–Nyhan variants. The enzymatic defect can manifest either underactivity, e.g., hypoxanthine phosphoribosyl transferase deficiency, versus overactivity, such as is seen with phosphoribosylpyrophosphate synthetase. Multiple interactive factors may play some role as illustrated by the spectrum of involvement in dihydropyrimidine dehydrogenase deficiency where a large proportion of those with the deficiency are asymptomatic. Some of the purine metabolic disorders are associated with hyperuricemia while others, including molybdenum cofactor deficiency, PRPP synthetase deficiency, purine nucleotide phosphorylase deficiency, and xanthine oxidase deficiency, are associated with hypouricemia.

Severe immunodeficiency can have a catastrophic outcome and be present in both purine metabolic disorders, such as adenosine deaminase deficiency and purine nucleoside phosphorylase deficiency, as well as disorders of pyrimidine metabolism such as orotic aciduria and pyrimidine nucleotide depletion syndrome. In terms of neurologic manifestations, when present, these tend to occur early on and are characterized by developmental delay, tendency toward seizures, sometimes to a severe, intractable degree, sensorineural deafness, along with neurobehavioral manifestations that can be suggestive of autism. Certain hallmarks are easily committed to memory such as the tendency toward self-mutilation in Lesch–Nyhan disease. One can also see ataxia, long tract signs, as well as dystonia and other extrapyramidal features in certain of these metabolic types. Facial dysmorphism can be seen in of some of these disorders, along with ophthalmologic abnormalities, and also microcephaly. Features such as liver and renal abnormalities, as well as myalgia and cramps, remind us of the potential for multiple organ involvement in disorders of purine and pyrimidine metabolism.

REFERENCES

Assmann B, Gohlich-Ratmann G, Brautigam L et al. (1998). Presumptive ureidopropionase deficiency as a new defect in pyrimidine catabolism found with in vitro H-NMR spectroscopy. J Inherit Metab Dis 21 (Suppl. 2): 1.

Bakkeren JAJM, De Abreau RA, Sengers RCA et al. (1984). Elevated urine, blood and cerebrospinal fluid levels of uracil and thymine in a child with dihydrothymine dehydrogenase deficiency. Clin Chim Acta 140: 247–254.

Becker MA, Losman MJ, Kim M (1987). Mechanism of accelerated purine nucleotide synthesis in human fibroblasts with superactive phosphoribosylpyrophosphate synthetase. J Biol Chem 262: 5596–5602.

Becker MA, Losman MJ, Wilson J et al. (1988a). Superactivity of phosphoribosylpyrophosphate synthetase due to altered regulation by nucleotide inhibitors and inorganic phosphate. Biochim Biophys Acta 882: 168–176.

Becker MA, Puig JG, Mateos FA et al. (1988b). Inherited superactivity of phosphoribosylpyrophosphate synthetase: association of uric acid overproduction and sensorial deafness. Am J Med 85: 383–390.

Becker MA, Smithy PR, Taylor W et al. (1995). The genetic and functional basis of purine nucleotide feedback-resistant phosphoribosylpyrophosphate synthetase superactivity. J Clin Invest 96: 2133–2141.

Berger R, Stoker-de Vries SA, Wadman SK et al. (1984). Dihydropyrimidine dehydrogenase deficiency leading to thymine-uraciluria. An inborn error of pyrimidine metabolism. Clin Chim Acta 141: 227–234.

Blau N, de Klerk KJ, Thony B et al. (1996). Tetrahydrobiopterin loading test in xanthine dehydrogenase and molybdenum cofactor deficiencies. Biochem Mol Med 58: 199–206.

Bzowska A, Kulikowska E, Shugar D (2000). Purine nucleoside phosphorylases: properties, functions, and clinical aspects. Pharmacol Ther 88: 349–425.

Calabrese G, Simmonds HA, Cameron JS et al. (1990). Precocious familial gout with reduced fractional urate clearance and normal purine enzymes. Q J Med 75: 441–450.

Camici M, Micheli V, Ipata PL et al. (2010). Pediatric neurological syndromes and inborn errors of purine metabolism. Neurochem Int 56: 367–378.

Chalmers RA, Watts RW, Bitensky J et al. (1969). Microscopic studies on crystals in skeletal muscle from two cases of xanthinuria. J Pathol 99: 45–49.

Chou JY, Mansfield BC (2007). Gene therapy for type I glycogen storage diseases. Curr Gene Ther 7: 79–88.

Chou JY, Matern D, Mansfield BC et al. (2002). Type I glycogen storage diseases: disorders of the glucose-6-phosphatase complex. Curr Mol Med 2: 121–143.

Crifò C, Siems W, Soro S et al. (2005). Inhibition of defective adenylsuccinate lyase by HNE: a neurological disease that may be affected by oxidative stress. Biofactors 24: 131–136.

Dalal I, Grunebaum E, Cohen A et al. (2001). Two novel mutations in a purine nucleoside phosphorylase (PNP)-deficient patient. Clin Genet 59: 430–437.

De Brouwer APM, Williams KL, Duley JA et al. (2007). Arts syndrome is caused by loss-of-function mutations in PRPS1. Am J Hum Genet 81: 507–518.

De Volder AG, Jaeken J, Van den Berghe G et al. (1988). Regional brain glucose utilization in adenylosuccinase-deficient patients measured by positron emission tomography. Pediatr Res 24: 238–242.

Endres W, Shin YS, Gunther R et al. (1988). Report on a new patient with combined deficiencies of sulphite oxidase and xanthine dehydrogenase due to molybdenum cofactor deficiency. Eur J Pediatr 148: 246–252.

Eriksson S, Wang L (2008). Molecular mechanism of mitochondrial DNA depletion diseases caused by deficiencies in enzymes in purine and pyrimidine metabolism. Nucleosides Nucleotides Nucleic Acids 27: 800–808.

Eriksson S, Munch-Petersen B, Johansson K et al. (2002). Structure and function of cellular deoxyribonucleoside kinases. Cell Mol Life Sci 59: 1327–1346.

Fishbein WN, Armbrustmacher VW, Griffin JL (1978). Myoadenylate deaminase deficiency: a new disease of muscle. Science 200: 545–551.

Fox IH, Kelley WN (1972). Human phosphoribosylpyrophosphate synthetase. Kinetic mechanism and end product inhibition. J Biol Chem 247: 2126–2131.

Giblett ER, Anderson JE, Cohen F et al. (1972). Adenosine deaminase deficiency in two patients with severely impaired cellular immunity. Lancet 2: 1067–1072.

Giblett ER, Amman AJ, Wara DW et al. (1975). Nucleoside phosphorylase deficiency in a child with severely defective T cell immunity and normal B cell immunity. Lancet 1: 1010–1013.

Hamajima N, Kouwaki M, Vreken P et al. (1998). Dihydropyrimidinase deficiency: structural organization, chromosomal localization, and mutation analysis of the human dihydropyrimidinase gene. Am J Hum Genet 63: 717–728.

Hirschhorn R (1993). Overview of biochemical abnormalities and molecular genetics of adenosine deaminase deficiency. Pediatr Res 33: 35–41.

Hirschhorn R, Papageorgiou PS, Kesarwala HH (1980). Amelioration of neurological abnormalities after enzyme replacement of adenosine deaminase deficieincy. N Engl J Med 303: 377–380.

Huguley C, Bain J, Rivers R et al. (1959). Refractory megaloblastic anaemia associated with excretion of orotic acid. Blood 14: 615–618.

Ichida K, Amaya Y, Kamatani N et al. (1997). Identification of two mutations in human xanthine dehydrogenase gene responsible for classical type I xanthinuria. J Clin Invest 99: 2391–2399.

Janecke AR, Mayatepek E, Utermann G (2001). Molecular genetics of type 1 glycogen storage disease. Mol Genet Metab 73: 117–125.

Jinnah HA, Visser JE, Harris JC et al. (2006). Delineation of the motor disorder of Lesch–Nyhan disease. Brain 129: 1201–1217.

Johansson M, Bajalic-Lagercrantz S, Lagercrantz J et al. (1996). Localization of the human deoxyguanosine kinase gene (*DGUOK*) to chromosome 2p13. Genomics 38: 450–451.

Johnson J (2003). Prenatal diagnosis of molybdenum cofactor deficiency and isolated sulphite oxidase deficiency. Prenat Diagn 23: 6–9.

Kelley WN, Greene ML, Rosenbloom FM et al. (1969). Hypoxanthine-guanine phosphoribosyltransferase deficiency in gout. Ann Intern Med 70: 155–206.

Kim H-J, Sohn K-M, Shy ME et al. (2007). Mutations in PRPS1, which encodes the phosphoribosyl pyrophosphate synthetase enzyme critical for nucleotide biosynthesis, cause hereditary peripheral neuropathy with hearing loss and optic atrophy (CMTX5). Am J Hum Genet 81: 552–558.

Krishnan E, Svendsen K, Neaton JD et al.MRFIT Research Group (2008). Long-term cardiovascular mortality among middle-aged men with gout. Arch Intern Med 168: 1104–1110.

Labarthe F, Dobbelaere D, Devisma L et al. (2005). Clinical, biochemical and morphological features of hepatocerebral syndrome with mitochondrial DNA depletion due to deoxyguanosine kinase deficiency. J Hepatol 43: 333–341.

Laikind PK, Seegmiller JE, Gruber HE (1986). Detection of 5′-phosphoribosyl-4-(N-succinylcarboxamide)-5-aminoimidazole in urine by use of the Bratton–Marshall reaction: identification of patients deficient in adenylosuccinate lyase activity. Analyt Biochem 156: 81–90.

Lesch M, Nyhan WL (1964). A familial disorder of uric acid metabolism and central nervous system function. Am J Med 36: 561–567.

Mandel H, Szargel R, Labay V et al. (2001). The deoxyguanosine kinase gene is mutated in individuals with depleted hepatocerebral mitochondrial DNA. Nat Genet 29: 337–341.

Marie S, Heron P, Bitoun P et al. (2004). AICA-ribosiduria: a novel, neurologically devastating inborn error of purine biosynthesis caused by mutation of *ATIC*. Am J Hum Genet 74: 1276–1281.

Markert ML (1994). Molecular basis of adenosine deaminase deficiency. Immunodeficiency 5: 141–145.

Meinsma R, Fernandez-Salguero P, Van Kuilenburg A et al. (1995). Human polymorphism in drug metabolism: mutation in the dihydropyrimidine dehydrogenase gene results in exon skipping and thymine uraciluria. DNA Cell Biol 14: 1–7.

Morisaki T, Gross M, Morisaki H et al. (1992). Molecular basis of AMP deaminase deficiency in skeletal muscle. Proc Natl Acad Sci 89: 6457–6461.

Nguyen KV, Naviaux RK, Paik KK et al. (2012). Lesch–Nyhan syndrome: mRNA expression of HPRT in patients with enzyme proven deficiency of HPRT and normal HPRT coding region of the DNA. Mol Genet Metab 106: 498–501.

Nofech-Mozes Y, Blaser SI, Kobayashi J et al. (2007). Neurologic abnormalities in patients with adenosine deaminase deficiency. Pediatr Neurol 37: 218–221.

Nyhan WL (2005). Disorders of purine and pyrimidine metabolism. Mol Genet Metab 86: 25–33.

Page T, Bakay B, Nissinen E et al. (1981). Hypoxanthine guanine phosphoribosyl transferase variants: correlation of clinical phenotype with enzyme activity. J Inherit Metab Dis 4: 203–207.

Page T, Yu A, Fontanesi J et al. (1997). Developmental disorder associated with increased cellular nucleotidase activity. Proc Natl Acad Sci U S A 94: 11601–11606.

Pesi R, Micheli V, Jacomelli G et al. (2000). Cystolic 5′-nucleotidase hyperactivity in erythrocytes of Lesch-Nyhan syndrome patients. Neuroreport 11: 1827–1831.

Rogers MH, Lwin R, Fairbanks L et al. (2001). Cognitive and behavioral abnormalities in adenosine deaminase deficient severe combined immunodeficiency. J Pediatr 139: 44–50.

Salerno C, Iotti R, Lodi R et al. (1997). Failure of muscle energy metabolism in a patient with adenylosuccinase deficiency An in vivo study by phosphorus NMR spectroscopy. Biochim Biophys Acta 1360: 271–276.

Salerno C, D'Eufemia P, Finocchiaro R et al. (1999). Effect of D-ribose on purine synthesis and neurological symptoms in a patient with adenylosuccinase deficiency. Biochim Biophys Acta 1453: 135–140.

Salgueiro N, Veiga I, Fragoso M et al. (2004). Mutations in exon 14 of dihydropyridimine dehydrogenase and 5′-fluorouracil toxicity in Portuguese colorectal cancer patients. Genet Med 6: 102–107.

Salviati L, Sacconi S, Mancuso M et al. (2002). Mitochondrial DNA depletion and dGK gene mutations. Ann Neurol 52: 311–317.

Schlesinger N (2010). Diagnosing and treating gout: a review to aid primary care physicians. Postgrad Med 122: 157–161.

Sidi Y, Mitchell BS (1985). Z-nucleotide accumulation in erythrocytes from Lesch–Nyhan patients. J Clin Invest 76: 2416–2419.

Smith LJ, Sullivan M, Huguley C (1961). Pyrimidine metabolism in man IV The enzymatic defect of orotic aciduria. J Clin Invest 40: 656–661.

Spiegel EK, Colman RF, Patterson D (2006). Adenylosuccinate lyase deficiency. Mol Genet Metab 89: 19–31.

Suchi M, Mizuno H, Kawai Y et al. (1997). Molecular cloning of the human UMP synthase gene and characterization of point mutations in two hereditary orotic aciduria families. Am J Hum Genet 60: 525–539.

Sumi S, Suchi K, Kidouchi H et al. (1997). Pyrimidine metabolism in hereditary orotic aciduria. J Inherit Metab Dis 20: 104–105.

Trifilo M, Page T (2000). NAPDD patients exhibit altered electrophoretic mobility of cytosolic 5′nucleotidase. Adv Exp Med Biol 486: 87–90.

Turner JJ, Stacey JM, Harding B et al. (2003). UROMODULIN mutations cause familial juvenile hyperuricemic nephropathy. J Clin Endocrinol Metab 88: 1398–1401.

Van Gennip A, Abeling N, Vreken P et al. (1997). Inborn errors of pyrimidine degradation: clinical, biochemical and molecular aspects. J Inherit Metab Dis 20: 203–208.

van Kuilenburg ABP, Meinsma R, Beke E et al. (2004). B-ureipropionase deficiency: an inborn error of pyrimidine degradation associated with neurological abnormalities. Hum Mol Genet 13: 2793–2801.

Wada Y, Nishimura Y, Tanabu M et al. (1974). Hypouricemic mentally retarded infant with a defect of 5-phosphoribosyl-1-pyrophosphate synthetase of erythrociytes. Tohoku J Exp Med 113: 149–157.

Wadman SK, Duran M, Beemer FA et al. (1983). Absence of hepatic molybdenum cofactor: an inborn error of metabolism leading to a combined deficiency of suphite oxidase and xanthine dehydrogenase. J Inherit Metab Dis 6 (Suppl 1): 78.

Wong DF, Harris JC, Naidu S et al. (1996). Dopamine transporters are markedly reduced in Lesch–Nyhan disease in vivo. Proc Natl Acad Sci U S A 93: 5539–5543.

Handbook of Clinical Neurology, Vol. 120 (3rd series)
Neurologic Aspects of Systemic Disease Part II
Jose Biller and Jose M. Ferro, Editors

Chapter 56

Porphyria and its neurologic manifestations

JENNIFER A. TRACY AND P. JAMES B. DYCK*
Mayo Clinic, Department of Neurology, Rochester, MN, USA

INTRODUCTION

Porphyrias are rare disorders of heme metabolism, each characterized by a defect in an enzyme required for the synthesis of heme. These disorders can produce disturbances of multiple organ systems, including the skin, liver, and central and peripheral nervous systems. The types of porphyria typically implicated in neurologic disease are acute intermittent porphyria, hereditary coproporphyria, and variegate porphyria, which are all autosomal dominant inherited conditions. These are generally characterized by neuropsychiatric symptoms with mood disorder and/or psychosis, peripheral neuropathy (generally motor-predominant), gastrointestinal disturbances, and (in the case of variegate porphyria and sometimes hereditary coproporphyria) photosensitivity and other cutaneous manifestations. The best management of these disorders is through the prevention of acute attacks (e.g., avoidance of cytochrome P450-inducing agents and periods of fasting), but intravenous hematin and glucose should be considered in the context of an acute attack.

BACKGROUND

Neurologic manifestations of porphyria have been recognized for over a century, with cases reported as far back as 1890 (Ranking and Pardington, 1890), and many detailed descriptions of individual cases have been reported since then. There has been postulation of major historical figures having this disorder, including the British King George III as well as other members of royal families (Macalpine and Hunter, 1966). Early descriptions of the disorder, prior to intensive biochemical analysis, have reported on the characteristic reddish-purple discoloration of urine after prolonged exposure to light and air (which represents porphyrins in the specimen). Subsequent research has helped elucidate the biochemical processes of porphyrin formation and the defects along the heme biosynthetic pathway.

The porphyrias are disorders of heme metabolism, caused by a defect in an enzyme responsible for the synthesis of the heme molecule, which in turn is necessary for the production of hemoglobin, myoglobin, and cytochromes. Heme is an oxygen carrier, and is essential for aerobic respiration and adenosine triphosphate (ATP) production via the electron transport chain. Cytochrome production is necessary for metabolism of multiple drugs within the body, most notably through the cytochrome P450 system, and also mediates the removal of some toxic substances. Adequate heme formation is extremely important for the health of the individual, both in terms of energy production and metabolism, and abnormalities can have a profound impact. Heme formation occurs primarily in the bone marrow and in the liver, but synthesis does take place in all cells. Heme production in the liver is closely linked to a negative feedback mechanism regulated by the presence of heme, which has important treatment implications for porphyria. The production of heme is necessary for life, but partial defects in heme synthesis can be compatible with life, resulting in significant disease in some patients.

The heme biosynthetic pathway (Fig. 56.1) starts in the mitochondria, with the production of δ-aminolevulinic acid from glycine and succinyl-CoA, which is catalyzed by the pyridoxine-dependent enzyme δ-aminolevulinic acid synthase (ALAS). This is the rate-limiting step in heme production and is the site of feedback inhibition, with inhibition of ALAS by heme, the end product of this pathway. The next step occurs in the cytoplasm and is the formation of porphobilinogen (catalyzed by δ-aminolevulinate dehydratase), followed by the formation of hydroxymethylbilane (catalyzed by porphobilinogen deaminase), followed by the formation

---

*Correspondence to: P. James B. Dyck, M.D., Mayo Clinic, Department of Neurology, 200 First Street SW, Rochester, MN 55905. USA. Tel: +1-507-284-3250, E-mail: dyck.pjames@mayo.edu

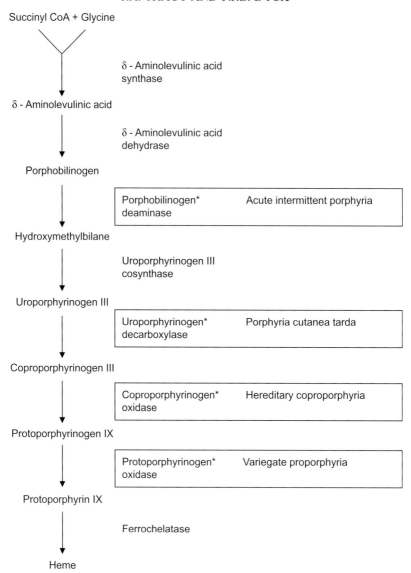

Fig. 56.1. The metabolic pathway of hepatic heme synthesis. Deficiencies of the outlined enzymes are responsible for the clinical types of porphyria. PBG deaminase (uroporphyrinogen I synthase), coproporphyrinogen oxidase, and protoporphyrinogen oxidase are usually deficient on a genetic basis and are associated with acute attacks of neurologic disease. Uroporphyrinogen decarboxylase deficiency may exist on a genetic basis or occur secondarily to toxic (usually alcohol-induced) liver disease. Porphyria cutanea tarda is not associated primarily with neurologic disease. The enzymes marked with an asterisk may be routinely assayed in erythrocytes in reference laboratories. (Reproduced from: Windebank and Bonkovsky, 2005.)

of uroporphyrinogen III (catalyzed by uroporphyrinogen III cosynthase), followed by the formation of coproporphyrinogen (catalyzed by uroporphyrinogen decarboxylase). The next step, which occurs in the mitochondria, is the production of proptoporphyrinogen IX (catalyzed by coproporphyrinogen oxidase), followed by the formation of protoporphyrin IX (catalyzed by protoporphyrinogen oxidase), and ultimately the production of heme (catalyzed by ferrochelatase, and utilizing iron). There are some differences in heme production between liver and bone marrow, with the liver

production being regulated by the presence of heme, which inhibits the activity of ALAS and decreases further production of heme. In contrast, in the bone marrow the formation of heme is driven by cellular response to erythropoietin (Puy et al., 2010).

There are eight specific types of porphyria, each resulting from a defect along the heme synthetic pathway; the only one of the heme biosynthetic enzymes for which deficiency is not associated with porphyria is ALA synthase. These defects lead to accumulation of toxic precursors within the body. Traditionally, these disorders are separated out into the erythropoietic and the hepatic porphyrias, depending on the major site of enzymatic expression. Porphyrias can cause pathology of multiple organ systems, including neurologic (central and/or peripheral), dermatologic, and gastrointestinal. The erythropoietic porphyrias mainly manifest with skin findings without associated neurologic disease and will not be extensively discussed in this chapter. There are four main types of hepatic porphyria, acute intermittent porphyria, hereditary coproporphyria, variegate porphyria, and porphyria cutanea tarda, all of which are implicated in neurologic disease except for porphyria cutanea tarda. The three hepatic porphyrias with potential neurologic manifestations are all autosomal dominant disorders and all present with acute attacks of illness. Another type of hepatic porphyria, caused by deficiency in δ-aminolevulinate dehydratase, can cause severe neurologic dysfunction but is extremely rare and will not feature in the following discussion.

CLINICAL PRESENTATION

Most porphyrias have an autosomal dominant inheritance pattern with incomplete penetrance. They affect approximately 0.5–10 per 100 000 people (Anderson et al., 2001). The prevalence within various populations can be difficult to accurately ascertain, given the frequency of asymptomatic cases, as will be described later. While there are multiple types of porphyria, not all cause neurologic dysfunction. Porphyria cutanea tarda, which is the most common type of porphyria, and erythropoietic protoporphyria typically have cutaneous manifestations and usually are not associated with clinical neurological disease. The types of porphyria which characteristically cause neurologic disease are acute intermittent porphyria, hereditary coproporphyria, and variegate porphyria (all of which fall under the classification of acute porphyrias). Patients with these types of porphyrias have an approximately 50% reduction in the affected enzyme for their respective disorders. These porphyrias are characterized by relatively quiescent phases interspersed with attacks of the disease, often precipitated by drug or toxin exposure or hormonal changes, and occur more commonly in women. When the heme biosynthetic pathway is activated, there is a massive toxic buildup of heme precursors, which are toxic to the nervous system.

Acute intermittent porphyria (AIP) results from a partial defect of porphobilinogen deaminase, which is the third enzyme in the heme biosynthetic pathway, caused by a mutation in the hydroxymethylbilane synthase gene. While this is an autosomal dominant disorder it is classically not fully penetrant, and it is estimated that less than 10% of people who carry this mutation become symptomatic throughout their life

(Sassa, 2006). Attacks of AIP typically produce severe and acute abdominal pain in association with neuropsychiatric symptoms. Patients will often also have a motor predominant neuropathy with proximal and distal components (such as is seen in acute inflammatory demyelinating polyneuropathy (AIDP) or chronic inflammatory demyelinating polyneuropathy (CIDP)), though prominently axonal. Autonomic involvement is also common. This is the most common type of acute hepatic porphyria, occurring most frequently in Scandinavia, Britain, and Ireland, though it can occur in any ethnic group (Albers and Fink, 2004). It is common in Sweden, with a prevalence of 1 in 10 000, though its rate of clinical penetrance can be variable. The W198X mutation is the most common within that population due to a founder effect, though many other mutations in the porphobilinogen deaminase gene have been described (Floderus et al., 2002). A large retrospective study of 356 AIP gene carriers from Sweden (Bylesjo et al., 2009) showed that just under half had clinical manifestations (42%), with attacks occurring more frequently and more severely in women. Some 89% of the patients in this study had the W198X mutation. They noted that half of the patients using medications were using agents that were considered unsafe in porphyria, most commonly medications for hypertension. Andersson et al. (2000) found a higher rate of clinical penetrance with the W198X and R173W mutations, as well as greater number and duration of attacks when compared with the R167W mutation.

Hereditary coproporphyria is also an autosomal dominant disorder, characterized by a defect in coproporphyrinogen oxidase, which can produce attacks of gastrointestinal and neuropsychiatric symptoms and signs and less commonly, skin changes. The presentation is very similar to AIP but is typically milder. Brodie et al. (1977) reviewed 111 cases of patients with hereditary coproporphyria and found that 23% had neurologic involvement, 23% had psychiatric symptoms, 29% had photosensitivity, and 80% had abdominal pain. He notes a relative increase in female gender compared to males in both acute attacks and latent cases. Similar to the other porphyrias described, drug use was felt to be a specific precipitant in 54% of the attacks. In a study by Kühnel et al. (2000) of hereditary coproporphyria attacks, the most frequent symptoms were abdominal pain (89%), neurologic (33%), and psychiatric (28%).

Variegate porphyria results from a defect in protoporphyrinogen oxidase and is also an autosomal dominant disease. Attacks are generally less severe and less frequent than in AIP. Variegate porphyria is much less common than AIP and the prevalence in Europe is approximately 0.5 per 100 000 (Elder et al., 1997). This form of porphyria is more common in the white South African population due to a founder effect, which appears to derive from a Dutch settler in South Africa (Dean, 1971). Hift and Meissner (2005) described 112 porphyric attacks in South Africa (25 with variegate porphyria and 87 with AIP) and found that the relative risk of an acute AIP attack compared to a variegate porphyria attack was 14.3, the median age of first attack was higher in patients with variegate porphyria than in AIP (30 versus 23.5 years old), the gender ratio was equal, and exposure to drugs was a common precipitant of variegate porphyria attacks (16 of the 25 attacks). Von und zu Fraunberg et al. (2002) evaluated the outcomes of 103 Finnish patients diagnosed with variegate porphyria and found that only 52% had clinical symptoms and 27% had acute attacks. They found that the specific mutation was important for prognosis, noting that patients with the I12T mutation, one of the three most common mutations causing variegate porphyria in Finland, had no photosensitivity and only 8% of this group had acute attacks.

Skin manifestations do not occur in acute intermittent porphyria but gastrointestinal and neuropsychiatric manifestations are prominent. Skin changes are much more common in variegate porphyria and can sometimes occur in hereditary coproporphyria. From a gastrointestinal and neuropsychiatric perspective, however, the attacks are very similar in these three types of porphyria. These attacks typically present with gastrointestinal distress with severe pain, though generally there are no objective signs of an "acute abdomen." Psychiatric and central nervous system manifestations can occur. Neuropsychiatric symptoms can vary markedly in severity from mild changes in affect, such as anxiety, but can also include psychosis and hallucinations. Seizure activity can also occur in a minority of patients, though management can be complicated by the limitations on safe medications in porphyria (Bylesjo et al., 1996).

Autonomic features, including tachycardia, constipation, and hypertension, are common. In general, peripheral neurologic manifestations occur later, within a few days or so of symptom onset. Peripheral neuropathy is typically motor predominant and asymmetric; it can involve proximal and distal muscles as well as cranial nerves. It can clinically resemble AIDP but with more abdominal pain and psychiatric symptoms. Sensory manifestations are often less evident or overlooked given the severity of the motor and autonomic changes, though various types of pain are commonly reported. The syndrome of inappropriate antidiuretic hormone secretion (SIADH) has been reported in patients with porphyric attacks (Chogle et al., 1980; Muraoka et al., 1995) and should be considered as possible contributing factor to changes in cognition and/or seizure activity.

The classic description of the reddish discoloration of urine may be helpful diagnostically during an attack; however, initially the urine will appear normal and it is only after prolonged observation with oxidation of porphyrin precursors that this color change can be observed; hence it can easily be missed in the hospital setting. In general, if an individual survives an attack there is good resolution of most symptoms with a more delayed, and sometimes incomplete, improvement of neuropathic weakness. Jeans et al. (1996) reviewed survival for patients hospitalized for AIP attacks from 1940 to 1988 and found the standardized mortality ratio for these patients to be 3.2, compared to age-matched hypothetical controls using census data, and noted that most deaths were due to an acute attack.

Several atypical manifestations have been described, including presentation with bilateral radial neuropathies (King et al., 2002) and subarachnoid hemorrhage due to transient hypertension from porphyria (van Heyningen and Simms, 2008). Andersson et al. (2002) described a patient with porphyria who had varying attacks over the years, including isolated weakness without gastrointestinal symptoms. Greenspan and Block (1981) reported on two patients with AIP whose diagnosis occurred in the context of respiratory insufficiency.

Psychiatric manifestations may be common in porphyria patients as a group. Tishler et al. (1985) screened 3867 psychiatry inpatients for intermittent acute porphyria and found eight patients who met criteria for this diagnosis, with a 0.21% positivity rate, noting that this is higher than expected for the general population. Millward et al. (2005) evaluated 90 patients with porphyria and felt that anxiety was a "relatively stable personality trait," with 46% of their group self-reporting some problem with anxiety and/or depression. Another long-term concern is the potential risk of carcinogenesis. Kauppinen and Mustajoki (1988) reviewed case histories of 82 deceased Finnish patients with acute hepatic porphyria and found that the cause of death in seven was hepatocellular carcinoma, noting that this risk was much higher than that of the general population. This finding of risk of hepatocellular carcinoma in acute hepatic porphyria was also reported by Andant et al. (2000), who recommended periodic screening in these patients.

RISK FACTORS FOR ATTACKS

Attacks in porphyria can be induced by a number of different factors. While it is clear that in many cases the precipitant of a specific attack cannot be identified, known factors in the induction of attacks include hormonal factors, nutritional factors, alcohol, and the use of drugs which induce the heme production pathway, thus leading to an overabundance of toxic heme precursors. The main risk factor for the development of attacks is the use of drugs which stimulate heme production, in particular those which require metabolism throughout the cytochrome P450 system leading to excess production of heme precursors and inducing an attack.

Because of the increased incidence of acute porphyric attacks in women, as well as the rarity of symptom onset prior to puberty, the role of sex hormones has been reviewed. The hormones estrogen, progesterone, and testosterone all cause increased ALA synthase activity (Windebank, 2003). One study found that 12 out of 50 women with AIP using oral contraceptives reported that oral contraceptives precipitated AIP attacks, and it precipitated the first attack in nine of those 12. In addition, of 22 women using hormone replacement therapy after menopause, no AIP attacks were induced (Andersson et al., 2003). Another group reviewed female patients with either AIP or variegate porphyria and recurrent menstrual-associated attacks who were treated with gonadotropin-releasing hormone (GnRH) agonists; they were also given low-dose estradiol and usually progesterone. Attacks were fewer and less severe in most of these women, though in some the estradiol and progesterone induced attacks (Innala et al., 2010). Treatment with a luteinizing hormone-releasing hormone agonist was found to reduce perimenstrual AIP attacks in women (Anderson et al., 1984).

Lip et al. (1991), through a questionnaire given to patients with AIP, found no difference in proportions of patients with latent or active disease who were smokers or nonsmokers, but did identify that of patients with active disease, smokers were more likely to have had more than one attack than nonsmokers. This was attributed to stimulation of the P450 system by elements of cigarette smoke and also to altered balance of steroid hormones in smokers. Alcohol use can induce a porphyric attack through inhibition of uroporphyrinogen decarboxylase and thus further accumulation of porphyrin precursors. In addition, decreased glucose to the liver can result in upregulation of ALA synthase activity, which can lead to an attack (Windebank, 2003). High carbohydrate diets cause reduction in porphobilinogen (PBG) excretion (Welland et al., 1964).

MECHANISMS OF NERVOUS SYSTEM DYSFUNCTION

The actual mechanisms of damage to nervous system tissue in porphyria are poorly understood and may be varied. The central and the peripheral nervous systems are both affected by porphyria. Because of the structural similarities of aminolevulinic acid (ALA) and γ-aminobutyric acid (GABA), it has been postulated that its accumulation may impair normal GABA function in the nervous system, leading to some of the central nervous system manifestations (Windebank, 2003). Other possible mechanisms described include direct toxicity of

the heme metabolites to nervous system tissue, direct effects of inadequate heme synthesis in the brain, secondary effects on brain heme synthesis from defective hepatic heme synthesis, and biochemical pathways leading to elevated synthesis of 5-hydroxytryptamine (Sassa, 2006). It has been suggested that the development of SIADH in some of these patients may be due to a direct toxic effect of the CNS by porphyrin precursors (Desaga et al., 1985).

King and Bragdon (1991) described a patient with porphyria, hallucinations, and seizures with brain lesions on MRI, which resolved along with her symptoms after treatment, and felt there was likely a vascular etiology. Aggarwal et al. (1994) described a patient with porphyric encephalopathy with MRI findings of diffuse predominantly gyriform cortical enhancement in both cerebral hemispheres; the findings resolved over time as the patient clinically improved. Kupferschmidt et al. (1995) described two patients with porphyria who developed cortical blindness, both with bilateral occipital lobe lesions which were felt to be consistent with vasospasm-induced ischemic lesions, though it has been suggested (Sze, 1996) that these may have represented findings of hypertensive encephalopathy. Central nervous system pathologic findings, similar to those of the peripheral nervous system, are not specific for porphyria and data are limited. In the 1950s, Gibson and Goldberg examined brains of patients with porphyrias and found evidence of axonal loss and perivascular demyelination in the cerebellum and white matter (Gibson and Goldberg, 1956).

The mechanism of the damage to the peripheral nervous system is not well understood, but axonal degeneration appears to predominate over segmental demyelination (Fig. 56.2). The enzyme defect causes a deficiency in the production of heme containing proteins for oxygen transport, electron transport, and the cytochrome P450 system. These abnormalities may disrupt axonal transport leading to axonal degeneration. The first autopsy case of porphyria was an acute polyneuritis following sulfophonal administration, in which Wallerian degeneration was described (Erbsloh, 1903).

In 1945, Denny-Brown and Sciarra (1945) reported segmental demyelination in porphyric nerve, suggesting that the primary source of pathology was in the myelin, but teased nerve fiber preparations were not done. Anzil and Dozic (1978) evaluated a sural nerve biopsy of a patient with porphyric neuropathy, by both light and electron microscopy, and found damage to both myelin and axons, and noted both myelin ovoids and mild evidence of segmental demyelination on teased fiber preparations. Felitsyn et al. (2008) exposed Schwann cells and sensory neurons in culture to δ-aminolevulinate and found that this was associated with lower levels of myelin-associated proteins and lipids.

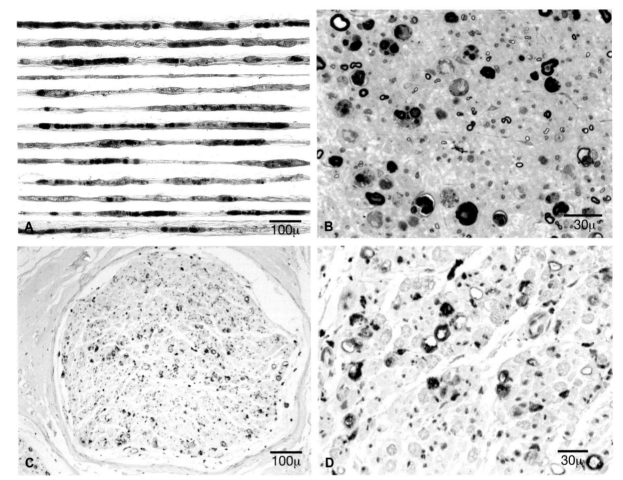

Fig. 56.2. Sural nerve biopsy showing fulminant axonal degeneration from a 33-year-old woman with 2 years of episodic abdominal pain, nausea, and vomiting, with acute onset of lower limb pain and weakness, vomiting, and anxiety. Urine porphobilinogen levels were elevated. (**A**) Teased nerve fiber preparations showing all myelinated fibers undergoing early axonal degeneration at the same stage (implying a common insult). (**B**) Semithin epoxy section stained with methylene blue showing most myelinated nerve fibers are degenerating. (**C**) Low and (**D**) high power of CD68 immunostain that reacts with macrophages. There are frequent macrophages at sites of axonal degeneration. These findings show the widespread acute axonal degeneration that can occur in an attack of acute porphyria.

Most pathologic and electrophysiologic studies suggest that the axon and not the myelin is the main target of porphyric neuropathy. Albers et al. (1978) reported on the electrophysiologic features of 11 patients with acute quadriparesis from AIP and found that eight had low amplitude compound action potentials with preserved conduction velocities, as well as fibrillations on electromyography consistent with a primarily axonal process. Cavanagh and Mellick (1965) performed detailed autopsy studies of nerve, muscle, spinal root, and cord of four patients with AIP and found no evidence of a primary demyelinating process but rather found evidence of an axonal process with motor fibers affected more significantly than sensory fibers. Thorner et al. (1981) described a patient with acute neuropathy from variegate porphyria for whom autopsy material was available,

showing evidence of a primary axonopathy with a dying-back phenomenon. Yamada et al. (1984) studied an autopsy case of a patient with acute porphyria and also found evidence consistent with a primary process of axonal degeneration with loss of axons and myelin in the peripheral nervous system and central chromatolysis of anterior horn cells in the spinal cord. Furthermore, they performed biochemical analyses on the sciatic nerve and reported increased ALA-S activity and decreased uroporphyrinogen I synthetase and ferrochelatase activities. These findings of primary axonal pathology are most in keeping with the classic electrophysiologic features described.

Lin et al. (2008) performed excitability measurements of peripheral motor axons in AIP subjects and found different responses to hyperpolarizing currents compared to controls. Their belief is that AIP neurotoxicity causes a decreased hyperpolarizing activated conductance in axons of patients without neuropathy and that membrane depolarization from decreased sodium/potassium pump activity results in porphyric neuropathy.

DIAGNOSIS

The diagnosis of porphyria can be challenging unless a high clinical suspicion is present. The presence of a family history of similar symptoms can be extremely helpful, but often this is not present. A history of discolored urine can also be helpful. In the context of an acute attack of porphyria, the diagnosis is often less complicated than when a patient presents after an attack has occurred but in an asymptomatic state.

The primary tool for diagnosis is measurement of porphyrin levels in urine, stool, and blood; these are most useful in the acutely symptomatic state as excretion of porphyrins is highest under that condition. In an acute attack of acute intermittent porphyria, there is elevated urinary excretion of aminolevulinic acid (ALA), porphobilinogen (PBG), uroporphyrin, and coproporphyrin; erythrocyte PBG deaminase may be normal or decreased. In the asymptomatic phase, in between attacks of acute intermittent porphyria, there can be decreased erythrocyte PBG deaminase or the value can be normal, urine excretion of the aforementioned compounds is generally normal or mildly elevated In hereditary coproporphyria, urine coproporphyrin, ALA, uroporphyrin and PBG levels are increased during an attack, and fecal coproporphyrin in particular can be quite increased during attacks; coproporphyrin is usually increased in urine and feces in between attacks as well. Variegate porphyria usually has increased levels of urine and fecal porphyrins during an attack, but generally urine porphyrin levels are normal in the latent phase of disease, aside from the possibility of increased coproporphyrin.

It should be remembered that there are other causes of increased porphyrin levels aside from porphyria, as these can be elevated in patients taking medications that induce the cytochrome P450 system, but these levels should normalize after discontinuation of the suspected offending drug (Windebank, 2003).

DNA testing is available for AIP, hereditary coproporphyria, and variegate porphyria and should be considered after initial screening tests are performed. There are many different mutations described in the respective genes for these disorders (Puy et al., 1997; Rosipal et al., 1999; Whatley et al., 1999), requiring careful screening. This testing is usually employed after suggestive findings on the testing previously described, or when an affected family member is identified and asymptomatic individuals want to be screened.

The differential for this disorder can be broad and includes acute inflammatory demyelinating polyradiculoneuropathy (AIDP, Guillain–Barré syndrome), which can appear similar to a porphyric attack. AIDP is characterized by an ascending, motor-predominant polyradiculoneuropathy, sometimes with associated sensory and autonomic symptoms and signs. This disorder can be associated with gastrointestinal symptoms, such as diarrhea. However, important differentiating characteristics include the lack of central nervous system manifestations, such as seizures or psychiatric symptoms in AIDP, as well as primary demyelinating features on nerve conduction studies, as opposed to the axonal pattern seen in porphyria. A variant of Guillain–Barré syndrome, acute motor axonal neuropathy (AMAN), can present with axonal features on EMG but again should not have central nervous system symptoms or findings. Porphyria should be at least considered in patients who have multiple episodes of acute to subacute weakness that have previously been labeled as Guillain–Barré syndrome.

There are many other motor-predominant neuropathies, including multifocal motor neuropathy, chronic inflammatory demyelinating polyradiculoneuropathy (CIDP) and POEMS (polyneuropathy, organomegaly, endocrinopathy, M-protein, skin changes) syndrome, but these should be ruled out due to their generally slower time course.

Other considerations for acute motor-predominant neuropathies should include infectious and inflammatory conditions such as Lyme disease, West Nile virus, enterovirus and herpesvirus-mediated polyradiculoneuropathies, and vasculitic neuropathies. Differentiation should be aided by attaining good exposure histories and appropriate serologies and CSF analyses. The association of an attack of weakness with either hormonal factors or medication use may be of help. Lead poisoning, which can produce both severe motor neuropathy as well as abdominal pain, should be considered in patients with risk for exposure, either occupationally or through hobbies, and certainly should be considered in children with a porphyria-like clinical presentation. In suspicious cases, blood lead levels should be obtained. As always in the case of acute weakness, one must always consider the possibility of acute presentations of neuromuscular junction disorders such as myasthenia gravis or of myopathies (such as toxic myopathies).

One must also be careful not to overinterpret less classic features seen in porphyria and attribute them to other disease processes. As previously noted, there are reports of patients with brain lesions in the context of an acute porphyric attack. Bylesjo et al. (2004) reported on the frequency of white matter T2 hyperintense lesions in patients with AIP. He found four of 16 AIP carriers (two with prior AIP attacks and two without) had such white matter lesions; however, he noted that all of these patients had CSF analysis which did not show oligoclonal bands, distinguishing these from multiple-sclerosis type patients. He also found that seven of these 16 patients had a hemoglobin A lc level over 6.0, suggesting chronically elevated blood sugars.

TREATMENT

The most important management strategy in patients with porphyria is prevention of acute attacks. Activation of the cytochrome P450 system uses up heme in the production of cytochromes, and the reduced heme supply reduces the inhibition on δ-aminolevulinic acid, thereby upregulating the heme production cycle, and in the case of porphyria, increases the production of toxic intermediates. Any medications that induce the cytochrome P450 system have the potential to induce an attack of porphyria. The use of alcohol can induce attacks as can many other pharmacologic agents, and any medication used in a patient with porphyria should be selected with care. While evaluation of the safety of any drug should be evaluated individually between a patient and his/her health care professional, there are useful guides available, including an online database provided through the American Porphyria Foundation's website (http://www.porphyriafoundation.com/drug-database). It is important to note that there may be a time lag for assessing the safety of newer medications for patients with porphyria, so caution must always be employed in treatment decisions. Prolonged fasting should be avoided. In addition, care needs to be taken in prescribing hormone therapy.

Once a porphyric attack is established, understanding of the biochemical pathways is helpful in determining treatment. From a biochemical perspective, heme serves as an inhibitor of ALAS in the liver and so artificially introducing heme can suppress the biosynthetic pathway of heme and thus reduce the amount of toxic metabolites produced in a patient with porphyria, which makes it an attractive option for the management of an acute porphyric attack.

For management of the underlying disorder, intravenous hematin should be given with a daily dose of 2–5 mg/kg given for 3–14 days. Mustajoki and Nordmann (1993) treated 51 acute porphyric attacks (in 22 patients with AIP and two with variegate porphyria) with heme arginate at either 250 mg or 3 mg/kg infusions for 4 days in almost all cases, with good clinical response in all patients, and with a mean duration of pain 2.5 days after the first infusion (which in nearly three-quarters of cases was given within 24 hours of admission). Potential side-effects of hematin administration include renal failure, phlebitis, and coagulopathy (Morris et al., 1981).

Nutritional supplementation is also crucial as the lack of sufficient glucose can increase the ALA synthase activity and thus increase porphyrin accumulation, worsening the attack. Intravenous glucose supplementation is advised with a recommendation of 3–500 g intravenously per 24 hours (Bonkovsky, 1990; Windebank, 2003).

While hematin is considered the standard of care, there are also limited reports of liver transplantation essentially rendering patients free of acute exacerbations (Seth et al., 2007). Soonawalla et al. (2004) described a 19-year-old patient with AIP and frequent exacerbations who underwent an orthotopic liver transplant, with no recurrent attacks over the 1.5 year period of follow-up. Stojeba et al. (2004) described a 46-year-old man with variegate porphyria and liver failure (with chronic alcohol abuse), who had a successful liver transplantation with no porphyria relapse over 3 months and normal uroprotoporphyrinogen and fecal protoporphyrin levels.

The importance of choosing medications that will not activate the heme biosynthetic pathway in patients with porphyria requires vigilance on the part of the treating physician. This adds a layer of complexity to the treatment of symptoms once a porphyric attack has occurred, as one must be careful not to cause pharmacologic worsening. Seizures in the context of a porphyric attack pose particular challenges. Bylesjo et al. (1996) carried out an epidemiologic study in which 10 of 268 AIP patients in Sweden reported having had seizures – six with tonic-clonic seizures and four with partial seizures with secondary generalization. Review of patient records indicated that six of these patients had a seizure in the context of an acute porphyric attack, with an estimate of a lifetime prevalence of 2.2% of patients with AIP-induced seizures.

Seizures are difficult to treat as phenytoin, phenobarbital, clonazepam, and valproic acid all have the potential to worsen a porphyric attack, though individual reports exist supporting the safety and efficacy of clonazepam. Bromides have been used with success in an attempt to avoid other enzyme-inducing antiepileptic drugs (Magnussen et al., 1975). Hahn et al. (1997) used a cell culture model of chicken embryo liver cells and induced a partial block in heme synthesis to simulate changes seen in porphyria, treated them with varying doses of vigabatrin, gabapentin, felbamate, lamotrigine, tiagabine, and phenobarbital, and found that vigabatrin and gabapentin did not lead to increased porphyrin accumulation while the other agents led to increased porphyrin production.

Taylor (1981) has reported on the use of intravenous magnesium for seizures in AIP. Zaatreh (2005) described a patient with AIP and status epilepticus, who was successfully treated acutely with a combination of intravenous magnesium and oral levetiracetam, and was maintained thereafter on oral gabapentin and levetiracetam without side-effects. Another case (Bhatia et al., 2008) of a 12-year-old boy with AIP and status epilepticus reported resolution with intravenous propofol (in addition to continuation of the gabapentin and levetiracetam he was on at the time of the episode of status epilepticus). Another patient with AIP was given propofol induction twice for anesthesia with no disease exacerbation (Mitterschiffthaler et al., 1988). Weir and Hodkinson (1988) described a patient with variegate porphyria for whom propofol induction was used, with a subsequent increase in urinary porphyrins, but no associated clinical symptoms. One case report (Asirvatham et al., 1998) adds a note of caution as they describe a patient treated with propofol for a cardiac procedure, who had prolonged impaired consciousness and elevated urinary porphyrins, suspected to be a case of previously asymptomatic coproporphyria.

Tatum and Zachariah (1995) described good seizure control using gabapentin in two patients with AIP, without induction of acute attacks. Krauss et al. (1995) reported on a patient with porphyria cutanea tarda with complex partial seizures, who became seizure free on gabapentin monotherapy (1800 mg/day) without recurrent manifestations of porphyria. Zadra et al. (1998) reported on a female patient with AIP who had both partial and generalized seizures, who had porphyric attacks with the use of phenytoin, carbamazepine, and valproic acid, but who remained seizure-free and attack-free on monotherapy with gabapentin. Another report (Paul and Meencke, 2004) of a patient with hereditary coproporphyria treated with levetiracetam reported no porphyric exacerbations.

There are also individual reports of patients with types of porphyria without neurologic manifestations who have coexisting seizure disorders, commenting on drug efficacy and safety in this context. Bilo et al. (2006) reported on a patient with idiopathic generalized epilepsy and porphyria cutanea tarda with full seizure control and no induction of porphyric attacks on levetiracetam monotherapy. There is also a report of a patient with porphyria cutanea tarda with partial seizures, who had good seizure control with oxcarbazepine without elevation of liver function tests, and it was suggested that with the lower hepatic enzyme induction of oxcarbazepine (as opposed to carbamazepine) may render this agent a safer alternative (Gaida-Hommernick et al., 2001).

CONCLUSIONS

Porphyrias are disorders of the heme biosynthetic pathway. A limited number of these can cause significant neurologic deficit (AIP, hereditary coproporphyria,

variegate porphyria) with autonomic symptoms, motor-predominant peripheral neuropathy, gastrointestinal distress, and sometimes cutaneous manifestations. An accurate diagnosis can be made through routine testing for overproduction of porphyrins during an acute attack, but this may be more difficult during a quiescent phase of disease. The most important factor for making the correct diagnosis is a high index of suspicion and awareness of the diversity of clinical manifestations. DNA testing is also available for the diagnosis. Treatment, based upon knowledge of the biochemical pathways of porphyria, can be very effective for management of acute attacks, including hematin as well as glucose supplementation and prohibition of drugs that may worsen an attack. For long-term management, careful modification of risk factors, in particular the avoidance of drugs that stimulate the heme biosynthetic pathway is crucial.

REFERENCES

Aggarwal A, Quint DJ, Lynch JP, 3rd (1994). MR imaging of porphyric encephalopathy. AJR Am J Roentgenol 162: 1218–1220.

Albers JW, Fink JK (2004). Porphyric neuropathy. Muscle Nerve 30: 410–422.

Albers JW, Robertson WC, Jr. Daube JR (1978). Electrodiagnostic findings in acute porphyric neuropathy. Muscle Nerve 1: 292–296.

Andant C, Puy H, Bogard C et al. (2000). Hepatocellular carcinoma in patients with acute hepatic porphyria: frequency of occurrence and related factors. J Hepatol 32: 933–939.

Anderson KE, Spitz IM, Sassa S et al. (1984). Prevention of cyclical attacks of acute intermittent porphyria with a long-acting agonist of luteinizing hormone-releasing hormone. N Engl J Med 311: 643–645.

Anderson KE, Sassa S, Bishop DF et al. (2001). Disorders of heme biosynthesis: X-linked sideroblastic anemia and the porphyrias. In: CR Scriver, A Beaudet, WS Sly et al. (Eds.), The Metabolic and Molecular Bases of Inherited Disease. 8th edn. McGraw-Hill, New York, pp. 2991–3062.

Andersson C, Floderus Y, Wikberg A et al. (2000). The W198X and R173W mutations in the porphobilinogen deaminase gene in acute intermittent porphyria have higher clinical penetrance than R167W. A population-based study. Scand J Clin Lab Invest 60: 643–648.

Andersson C, Nilsson A, Backstrom T (2002). Atypical attack of acute intermittent porphyria – paresis but no abdominal pain. J Intern Med 252: 265–270.

Andersson C, Innala E, Backstrom T (2003). Acute intermittent porphyria in women: clinical expression, use and experience of exogenous sex hormones. A population-based study in northern Sweden. J Intern Med 254: 176–183.

Anzil AP, Dozic S (1978). Peripheral nerve changes in porphyric neuropathy: findings in a sural nerve biopsy. Acta Neuropathol 42: 121–126.

Asirvatham SJ, Johnson TW, Oberoi MP et al. (1998). Prolonged loss of consciousness and elevated porphyrins following propofol administrations. Anesthesiology 89: 1029–1031.

Bhatia R, Vibha D, Srivastava MV et al. (2008). Use of propofol anesthesia and adjunctive treatment with levetiracetam and gabapentin in managing status epilepticus in a patient of acute intermittent porphyria. Epilepsia 49: 934–936.

Bilo L, Meo R, Fulvia de Leva M (2006). Levetiracetam in idiopathic generalised epilepsy and porphyria cutanea tarda. Clin Drug Investig 26: 357–359.

Bonkovsky H (1990). Porphyrin and heme metabolism and the porphyrias. In: D Zakim, T Boyer (Eds.), Hepatology: A Textbook of Liver Disease. 2nd edn. WB Saunders, Philadelphia, pp. 378–424.

Brodie MJ, Thompson GG, Moore MR et al. (1977). Hereditary coproporphyria. Demonstration of the abnormalities in haem biosynthesis in peripheral blood. Q J Med 46: 229–241.

Bylesjo I, Forsgren L, Lithner F et al. (1996). Epidemiology and clinical characteristics of seizures in patients with acute intermittent porphyria. Epilepsia 37: 230–235.

Bylesjo I, Brekke OL, Prytz J et al. (2004). Brain magnetic resonance imaging white-matter lesions and cerebrospinal fluid findings in patients with acute intermittent porphyria. Eur Neurol 51: 1–5.

Bylesjo I, Wikberg A, Andersson C (2009). Clinical aspects of acute intermittent porphyria in northern Sweden: a population-based study. Scand J Clin Lab Invest 69: 612–618.

Cavanagh JB, Mellick RS (1965). On the nature of the peripheral nerve lesions associated with acute intermittend porphyria. J Neurol Neurosurg Psychiatry 28: 320–327.

Chogle AR, Shetty RN, Joshi VR et al. (1980). Acute intermittent porphyria with the syndrome of inappropriate ADH secretion (SIADH) (a report of two cases). J Assoc Physicians India 28: 379–382.

Dean G (1971). The Porphyrias. A Study of Inheritance and Environment. Pittman Medical: London.

Denny-Brown D, Sciarra D (1945). Changes in the nervous system in acute porphyria. Brain 68: 1–16.

Desaga U, Leonhardt KF, Frahm H et al. (1985). Clinical and experimental investigations of vasopressin secretion in acute porphyrias. Exp Clin Endocrinol 86: 79–86.

Elder GH, Hift RJ, Meissner PN (1997). The acute porphyrias. Lancet 349: 1613–1617.

Erbsloh W (1903). [Pathology and pathological anatomy of toxic polyneuritis after application of sulfonal]. Dtsch Z Nervenheilkd 23: 197–204.

Felitsyn N, McLeod C, Shroads AL et al. (2008). The heme precursor delta-aminolevulinate blocks peripheral myelin formation. J Neurochem 106: 2068–2079.

Floderus Y, Shoolingin-Jordan PM, Harper P (2002). Acute intermittent porphyria in Sweden. Molecular, functional and clinical consequences of some new mutations found in the porphobilinogen deaminase gene. Clin Genet 62: 288–297.

Gaida-Hommernick B, Rieck K, Runge U (2001). Oxcarbazepine in focal epilepsy and hepatic porphyria: a case report. Epilepsia 42: 793–795.

Gibson JB, Goldberg A (1956). The neuropathology of acute porphyria. J Pathol Bacteriol 71: 495–509.

Greenspan GH, Block AJ (1981). Respiratory insufficiency associated with acute intermittent porphyria. South Med J 74 (954–956): 959.

Hahn M, Gildemeister OS, Krauss GL et al. (1997). Effects of new anticonvulsant medications on porphyrin synthesis in cultured liver cells: potential implications for patients with acute porphyria. Neurology 49: 97–106.

Hift RJ, Meissner PN (2005). An analysis of 112 acute porphyric attacks in Cape Town, South Africa: evidence that acute intermittent porphyria and variegate porphyria differ in susceptibility and severity. Medicine 84: 48–60.

Innala E, Backstrom T, Bixo M et al. (2010). Evaluation of gonadotropin-releasing hormone agonist treatment for prevention of menstrual-related attacks in acute porphyria. Acta Obstet Gynecol Scand 89: 95–100.

Jeans JB, Savik K, Gross CR et al. (1996). Mortality in patients with acute intermittent porphyria requiring hospitalization: a United States case series. Am J Med Genet 65: 269–273.

Kauppinen R, Mustajoki P (1988). Acute hepatic porphyria and hepatocellular carcinoma. Br J Cancer 57: 117–120.

King PH, Bragdon AC (1991). MRI reveals multiple reversible cerebral lesions in an attack of acute intermittent porphyria. Neurology 41: 1300–1302.

King PH, Petersen NE, Rakhra R et al. (2002). Porphyria presenting with bilateral radial motor neuropathy: evidence of a novel gene mutation. Neurology 58: 1118–1121.

Krauss GL, Simmons-O'Brien E, Campbell M (1995). Successful treatment of seizures and porphyria with gabapentin. Neurology 45: 594–595.

Kühnel A, Gross U, Doss MO (2000). Hereditary coproporphyria in Germany: clinical-biochemical studies in 53 patients. Clin Biochem 33: 465–473.

Kupferschmidt H, Bont A, Schnorf H et al. (1995). Transient cortical blindness and biooccipital brain lesions in two patients with acute intermittent porphyria. Ann Intern Med 123: 598–600.

Lin CS, Krishnan AV, Lee MJ et al. (2008). Nerve function and dysfunction in acute intermittent porphyria. Brain 131: 2510–2519.

Lip GY, McColl KE, Goldberg A et al. (1991). Smoking and recurrent attacks of acute intermittent porphyria. BMJ 302: 507.

Macalpine I, Hunter R (1966). The "insanity" of King George 3d: a classic case of porphyria. Br Med J 1: 65–71.

Magnussen CR, Doherty JM, Hess RA et al. (1975). Grand mal seizures and acute intermittent porphyria. The problem of differential diagnosis and treatment. Neurology 25: 121–125.

Millward LM, Kelly P, King A et al. (2005). Anxiety and depression in the acute porphyrias. J Inherit Metab Dis 28: 1099–1107.

Mitterschiffthaler G, Theiner A, Hetzel H et al. (1988). Safe use of propofol in a patient with acute intermittent porphyria. Br J Anaesth 60: 109–111.

Morris DL, Dudley MD, Pearson RD (1981). Coagulopathy associated with hematin treatment for acute intermittent porphyria. Ann Intern Med 95: 700–701.

Muraoka A, Suehiro I, Fujii M et al. (1995). Delta-aminolevulinic acid dehydratase deficiency porphyria (ADP) with syndrome of inappropriate secretion of antidiuretic hormone (SIADH) in a 69-year-old woman. Kobe J Med Sci 41: 23–31.

Mustajoki P, Nordmann Y (1993). Early administration of heme arginate for acute porphyric attacks. Arch Intern Med 153: 2004–2008.

Paul F, Meencke HJ (2004). Levetiracetam in focal epilepsy and hepatic porphyria: a case report. Epilepsia 45: 559–560.

Puy H, Deybach JC, Lamoril J et al. (1997). Molecular epidemiology and diagnosis of PBG deaminase gene defects in acute intermittent porphyria. Am J Hum Genet 60: 1373–1383.

Puy H, Gouya L, Deybach JC (2010). Porphyrias. Lancet 375: 924–937.

Ranking J, Pardington G (1890). Two cases of haematoporphyria in the urine. Lancet 607–609.

Rosipal R, Lamoril J, Puy H et al. (1999). Systematic analysis of coproporphyrinogen oxidase gene defects in hereditary coproporphyria and mutation update. Hum Mutat 13: 44–53.

Sassa S (2006). The hematologic aspects of porphyria. In: M Lichtman, E Beutler, K Kaushansky et al. (Eds.), Williams Hematology. 7th edn. McGraw-Hill, Chicago, pp. 703–720.

Seth AK, Badminton MN, Mirza D et al. (2007). Liver transplantation for porphyria: who, when, and how? Liver Transpl 13: 1219–1227.

Soonawalla ZF, Orug T, Badminton MN et al. (2004). Liver transplantation as a cure for acute intermittent porphyria. Lancet 363: 705–706.

Stojeba N, Meyer C, Jeanpierre C et al. (2004). Recovery from a variegate porphyria by a liver transplantation. Liver Transpl 10: 935–938.

Sze G (1996). Cortical brain lesions in acute intermittent porphyria. Ann Intern Med 125: 422–423.

Tatum WO IVth, Zachariah SB (1995). Gabapentin treatment of seizures in acute intermittent porphyria. Neurology 45: 1216–1217.

Taylor RL (1981). Magnesium sulfate for AIP seizures. Neurology 31: 1371–1372.

Thorner PS, Bilbao JM, Sima AA et al. (1981). Porphyric neuropathy: an ultrastructural and quantitative case study. Can J Neurol Sci 8: 281–287.

Tishler PV, Woodward B, O'Connor J et al. (1985). High prevalence of intermittent acute porphyria in a psychiatric patient population. Am J Psychiatry 142: 1430–1436.

van Heyningen C, Simms DM (2008). Acute intermittent porphyria presenting with a subarachnoid haemorrhage. Ann Clin Biochem 45: 610–611.

von und zu Fraunberg M, Timonen K, Mustajoki P et al. (2002). Clinical and biochemical characteristics and genotype-phenotype correlation in Finnish variegate porphyria patients. Eur J Hum Genet 10: 649–657.

Weir PM, Hodkinson BP (1988). Is propofol a safe agent in porphyria? Anaesthesia 43: 1022–1023.

Welland FH, Hellman ES, Gaddis EM et al. (1964). Factors affecting the excretion of porphyrin precursors by patients with acute intermittent porphyria. I. The effect of diet. Metabolism 13: 232–250.

Whatley SD, Puy H, Morgan RR et al. (1999). Variegate porphyria in Western Europe: identification of PPOX gene mutations in 104 families, extent of allelic heterogeneity, and absence of correlation between phenotype and type of mutation. Am J Hum Genet 65: 984–994.

Windebank AJ (2003). Porphyria. In: JH Noseworthy (Ed.), Neurological Therapeutics: Principles and Practice. Martin Dunitz Taylor and Francis Group, New York, pp. 2181–2187.

Windebank AJ, Bonkovsky HL (2005). Porphyric neuropathy. In: PJ Dyck, PK Thomas (Eds.), Peripheral Neuropathy. 4th edn. Elsevier, Philadelphia, pp. 1883–1892. www.porphyriafoundation.com/drug-database.

Yamada M, Kondo M, Tanaka M et al. (1984). An autopsy case of acute porphyria with a decrease of both uroporphyrinogen I synthetase and ferrochelatase activities. Acta Neuropathol 64: 6–11.

Zaatreh MM (2005). Levetiracetam in porphyric status epilepticus: a case report. Clin Neuropharmacol 28: 243–244.

Zadra M, Grandi R, Erli LC et al. (1998). Treatment of seizures in acute intermittent porphyria: safety and efficacy of gabapentin. Seizure 7: 415–416.

Handbook of Clinical Neurology, Vol. 120 (3rd series)
Neurologic Aspects of Systemic Disease Part II
Jose Biller and Jose M. Ferro, Editors

Chapter 57

Disorders of heavy metals

FRANCE WOIMANT* AND JEAN-MARC TROCELLO
French National Wilson's Disease Centre (CNR Wilson), Lariboisière Hospital, Paris, France

INTRODUCTION

Heavy metals and trace elements play an important role in relation to the physiology and pathology of the nervous system. Metals are present in air, water, and diet. Input sources in humans are mainly respiratory and digestive and rarely dermal. Some metals have no biologic function but are toxic where there is excessive exposure (e.g., cadmium, lead, aluminum, mercury, manganese). The main features of these metal toxicities are summarized in Table 57.1. Other metals, such as iron and copper, are involved in biologic processes as cofactors of numerous enzymes. Disorders of metabolism of these metals will lead to various neurologic diseases.

COPPER DISORDERS

Copper is an essential trace element, necessary for the activity of many key enzymes including superoxide dismutase, lysyloxidase, dopamine β-hydroxylase, cytochrome oxidase, and ceruloplasmin.

Copper disorders can be divided into two groups:

- ATP7A- or ATP7B-related inherited copper transport disorders
- acquired diseases associated with copper deficiency or copper excess.

Copper metabolism

The main regulators of cellular copper metabolism are the copper-transporting P-type ATPases: ATP7A and ATP7B. Their transport activity is crucial for central nervous system (CNS) development, liver function, connective tissue formation, and many other physiologic processes (Barnes et al., 2005). The physiologic importance of Cu-ATPases is illustrated by the deleterious consequences of mutations or deletions in the gene encoding these proteins,

essentially Menkes disease for ATP7A and Wilson disease for ATP7B. Both Cu-ATPases have two main roles in cells, namely to provide copper to essential cuproenzymes and to mediate the excretion of excess intracellular copper (Lutsenko et al., 2007). They are expressed in most tissues. Their roles are probably not the same in all organs. In intestine where the two Cu-ATPases are expressed, ATP7B does not compensate for the deficiency of ATP7A function (Menkes disease). In contrast, in the cerebellum of ATP7B−/− mice, ATP7A appears to substitute for missing ATP7B (Barnes et al., 2005).

The daily intake of copper is about 3 mg. Copper is absorbed by the intestinal cells and stored with metallothioneins in a nontoxic form (Fig. 57.1). It is exported from the enterocytes into the blood by Cu-ATPase ATP7A and transported via the portal vein to the liver, which is the main organ responsible for copper homeostasis. In hepatocytes and other cells, copper is absorbed by copper transporter 1 (CTR1) (Vulpe et al., 1993). In the cytoplasm, it is bound to metallothionein or to copper-specific chaperone proteins (CCS, ATOX 1, and COX17). Thus, cells are protected from the toxic effects of free copper. CCS and COX17 guide copper to mitochondria and ATOX1 to the trans-Golgi network (TGN). Under basal conditions, ATP7A and ATP7B are essentially localized within the TGN. Under increased copper concentrations, ATP7A is translocated to the vesicles or to the plasma membranes, allowing excretion of excess intracellular copper; in hepatocytes, ATP7B is relocalized toward canalicular membrane allowing excretion of copper into the bile and subsequently to feces (de Bie et al., 2007). In liver, ATP7B mediates also the incorporation of copper into the copper-dependant ferroxydase ceruloplasmin (CP), which is subsequently secreted into the blood. CP is the major copper-containing protein; however, it does not seem to play an essential role in copper metabolism (Valentine and Gralla, 1997).

---

*Correspondence to: Dr France Woimant, Neurology Department, CNR Wilson, Lariboisière Hospital, 2 rue Ambroise Paré. 75010 Paris, France. Tel: +33-1-49-95-65-27, Fax: +33-1-49-95-65-34, E-mail: france.woimant@lrb.aphp.fr

Table 57.1

Main features of excessive exposure to heavy metals

Metal	Mode of intoxication	General features	Neurological features	Diagnosis
Cadmium (Sethi and Khandelwal, 2006)	Inhalation of fumes	Nephropathy Decreased bone density	Neuropsychiatric manifestations, polyneuropathy	Urinary cadmium level
Lead (Brodkin et al., 2007)	Occupational exposure, (manufacturing of batteries, pigments, solder . . .) Diet	Abdominal pain, anorexia, nausea and constipation, nephropathy, anemia with basophilic stippling	Headache, concentration and memory difficulties, sleep disturbances, peripheral neuropathy	Blood lead level
Mercury (Brodkin et al., 2007)	Dental amalgam Fish consumption	Gingivitis, stomatitis, hypersalivation, metallic taste, nephropathy	Irritability, concentration and memory difficulties, sleep disturbances, sensory peripheral neuropathy	Blood and urine mercury levels
Aluminum (Letzel et al., 2000; Yong et al., 2006)	Occupational exposure Dialysis Intravenous boiled methadone	Bone pain, ostemalacia, pathological fractures, microcytic anemia	Seizures, myoclonus, personality changes, tremor, ataxia	Serum aluminium level
Manganese (Jog and Lang, 1995; Stepens et al., 2008)	Intravenous methcathinone Inhalation of fumes Acquired hepatocerebral degeneration (CAHD)	Weakness	Personality changes, irritability, sleep disturbances, Parkinsonism, chorea, dystonia, ataxia, tremor, myoclonus	Serum manganese level Hypersignal on T1-weighted brain MRI in globus palidus

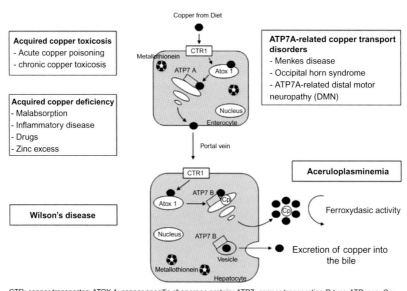

CTR: copper transporter; ATOX 1: copper specific chaperone protein; ATP7: copper-transporting P-type ATPases; Cp: ceruloplasmin (Apoceruloplasmin, without copper, holoceruloplasmin with copper)

Fig. 57.1. Copper metabolism and disorders.

ATP7A- or ATP7B-related inherited copper transport disorders

ATP7A-RELATED COPPER TRANSPORT DISORDERS

Menkes disease (MD), occipital horn syndrome (OHS), and ATP7A-related distal motor neuropathy are caused by mutations in the *ATP7A* gene, which is located on the long arm of the X chromosome (Xq13.1-q2). Over 200 mutations have been identified, among which are small deletions/insertions, nonsense mutations, missense mutations, and splice site mutations. In one-third of cases, MD is caused by *de novo* mutations. Splice site mutations appear to be over-represented in patients with OHS (de Bie et al., 2007). ATP7A-related distal motor neuropathy involves unique missense mutations (Kennerson et al., 2010).

Menkes disease (MD), also known as kinky hair disease, was first described by Menkes in 1962 (Menkes et al., 1962). Some 10 years later, Danks et al. (1972) found serum copper and ceruloplasmin levels to be reduced and suggested that the primary defect in Menkes disease involved copper metabolism. In 1993, three teams isolated the gene that encodes Cu-ATPase, the *ATP7A* gene (Chelly et al., 1993; Mercer et al., 1993; Vulpe et al., 1993).

Defective ATP7A function results in:

- dysfunction of several copper-dependant enzymes, due to inability to load these enzymes with copper
- reduction of elimination of copper from cells, and almost all the tissues except for liver and brain will accumulate copper to abnormal levels. As intestinal copper absorption is impaired, the copper level does not reach a toxic state (Tümer and Møller, 2010). In the liver, low levels of copper are explained by the fact that ATP7A is not the main liver copper transporter.

The incidence of MD is estimated to range between 1:40 000 and 1:350 000. (Møller et al., 2009). Clinical features include progressive neurologic deterioration and marked connective tissue dysfunction. As in linked-X disease, MD typically occurs in males. Usually, patients are born at term. Developmental regression appears within the first 2 months of life as axial hypotonia, seizures, and psychomotor retardation. The appearance of the hair is often remarkable, being sparse, hypopigmented, and kinky (pili torti). Ligamentous hyperlaxity, skin hyperelasticity, and bladder and ureter diverticula are often associated. Skeletal findings are metaphyseal spurs and long bone fractures. Autonomic dysfunction, including temperature instability and hypoglycemia, may be present in the neonatal period. Because of abnormal development of the vessel walls (fragmentation of the internal elastic lamina and thickening of the intima), arterial tortuosities and aneurysms are frequent, leading to cerebral infarcts and intracranial and intestinal bleeds (Horn et al., 1992). There is important variability in the severity of clinical expression of MD. Mild MD forms with later onset, moderate symptoms, and longer survival are observed in 5–10% of the patients.

Diagnosis of MD can be established by detecting low levels of copper (and ceruloplasmin) in the serum, and high levels in cutaneous fibroblasts (Table 57.2). However, in the neonatal period serum copper and ceruloplasmin should be interpreted with caution, as their levels are low in healthy newborns. In this period, plasma catecholamine analysis (ratio of dihydroxyphenylalanine to dihydroxyphenylglycol) indicative of dopamine β-hydroxylase deficiency allows a rapid diagnosis (Tümer and Møller, 2010). The diagnosis can be confirmed by identification of the gene mutation, but because of the large size of the gene and the high number of mutations, genetic analysis may take time. Genetic analysis also allows screening of carrier females and antenatal diagnosis through chorionic villus sampling.

Parenteral administration of histidine-copper improves the neurologic outcome and increases lifespan. The prognosis remains inevitably poor. The age at which treatment is started, the severity of the disease, and the presence of at least partially functional ATP7A seem to be among the main determinants for the prognosis. Death usually occurs by 3 years of age, but some patients survive to 10 years or even more (Tümer and Møller, 2010).

Occipital horn syndrome (or X-linked cutis laxa, or Ehlers–Danlos syndrome type 9) is a less severe allelic

Table 57.2

Cupric tests in copper disorders

	Menkes disease	Occipital horn disease	ATP7A related neuropathy	Wilson's disease	Copper deficiency	Aceruloplasminemia
Serum Cu	↘	NI / ↘	NI	↘	↘	↘
Urinary Cu	↘	NI / ↘	NI	↗	↘	NI
Serum Cp	↘	NI / ↘	NI	↘	↘	↘↘

Cu: copper; Cp: ceruloplasmin

variant of the MD syndrome (Kaler, 1998). Its incidence is unknown. Individuals typically live to at least mid-adulthood. Its principal clinical features are related to connective tissue, with bladder diverticula, inguinal hernias, skin laxity and hyperelasticity. Neurologic abnormalities are far less severe or even absent. Characteristic is the formation of occipital exostoses resulting from calcification of the trapezius and sternocleidomastoid muscles at their attachments to the occipital bone (Peltonen et al., 1983). The symptoms result from alterations in the function of copper-dependant enzymes, in particular that of lysyloxidase. Serum copper and ceruloplasmin levels are normal or low (Table 57.2).

A newly discovered allelic variant associated with ATP7A is *ATP7A-related distal motor neuropathy (DMN)*. It is an adult-onset distal motor neuropathy resembling Charcot–Marie–Tooth disease, and characterized by atrophy and weakness of distal muscles in hands and feet. There is no sign of systemic copper deficiency. Serum copper and ceruloplasmin levels are normal (Table 57.2) (Kaler, 2010).

ATP7B-RELATED COPPER TRANSPORT DISORDERS

Wilson disease (WD) is caused by mutations in the *ATP7B* gene, located on chromosome 13 (q14.3.-q21.1). Although missense mutations are most frequent, deletions, insertions, nonsense, and splice site mutations have been reported. More than 400 mutations and 100 polymorphisms have been documented. In the US and northern Europe, two mutations, His1069Gln and Gly1267Arg, represent 38% of identified mutations (Thomas et al., 1995). The worldwide prevalence of WD is estimated in the order of 30 per 1 million, with a carrier frequency of approximately 1 in 90. WD is more frequent in countries in which consanguineous marriages are common (Figus et al., 1995).

In 1912, in a doctoral thesis published in *Brain*, S.A. Kinner Wilson gave a very detailed description of both the clinical and pathologic characteristics of "Progressive lenticular degeneration: a familial nervous disease associated with cirrhosis of the liver" (Wilson, 1912; Walshe, 2006). The therapeutic area of WD began with Cumings in 1948; he suggested an etiologic role for copper and proposed chelating therapy with British anti-Lewisite (BAL or dimercaptopropanol) (Cumings, 1948). In 1956, Walshe proposed the use of D-penicillamine (Walshe, 1956), and in 1961, Schouwink the use of zinc salts as decoppering agents (Hoogenraad, 2001). In 1985, Frydman reported that the WD gene was located on chromosome 13 (Frydman et al., 1985). The identification of the gene, *ATP7B*, was realized by three separate teams during year 1993 (Bull et al., 1993; Tanzi et al., 1993; Yamaguchi et al., 1993).

Physiopathology

Defective ATP7B function leads a reduction of conversion of apoceruloplasmin into ceruloplasmin and of copper release into the bile, resulting in important copper accumulation in the liver, very low levels of copper-bound ceruloplasmin in the serum, and low biliary copper. When the hepatic copper storage capacity into metallothioneins is exceeded, unbound copper spills out of the liver and is deposited in other organs and tissues (Trocello et al., 2010a).

Clinical features

WD begins with a presymptomatic period during which there is accumulation of copper in the liver that will cause hepatitis and, without treatment, will progress to liver cirrhosis and development of extrahepatic symptoms. In our series of 385 patients, the initial manifestations are hepatic dysfunction in 44% of cases, and neurologic or neuropsychiatric symptoms in 39%. Other patients present with Kayser–Fleischer rings, hematologic or renal syndromes. The mean age of first hepatic symptoms is 17 years and for initial neurologic symptoms 23 years. It is rare that the first symptoms appear before 5 years, but WD has been diagnosed as early as 2 years (Beyersdorff and Findeisen, 2006), and as late as 72 years in a patient with Kayser–Fleischer rings (Czonkowska et al., 2008).

WD can be asymptomatic with abnormal serum aminotransferases or hemolytic anemia found incidentally. Isolated splenomegaly or thrombopenia due to clinical unapparent cirrhosis with portal hypertension or detection of Kayser–Fleischer rings can also reveal the disease. Nonspecific symptoms are often the first manifestations: nausea, anorexia, fatigue, abdominal pain, amenorrhea, or repeated miscarriages. Disease may also present as acute transient hepatitis that can mimic autoimmune hepatitis, as chronic liver disease and cirrhosis either compensated or decompensated, or as fulminant hepatic failure with an associated Coombs-negative hemolytic anemia and acute renal failure (Ala et al., 2007).

First neurologic symptoms of WD include changes in behavior, deterioration in school or professional work, in handwriting, dysarthria, drooling, tremor, or dystonia. The main neurologic manifestations can be roughly distinguished in three movement disorder syndromes (Trocello and Woimant, 2008):

- dystonic syndrome characterized by choreoathetosis and dystonic postures (Lorincz, 2010). It starts with focal signs or functional dystonia and may progress to generalized dystonia. It often affects facial muscles, resulting in a fixed sardonic smile. Dystonic dysarthria affects laryngeal or pneumophonatory muscles. Choreic movements are often associated.

- parkinsonian syndrome with rigidity and akinesia. Hypomimia is present, as well as dysarthria with hypophonia, tachylalia. Gait is unsteady with small steps, reduced postural reflexes, festination, and freezing. Rest tremor is rarely isolated.
- postural and action tremor with high amplitude and low frequency. Its proximal component can be well observed when a patient's arms are outstretched, showing the "wing-beating tremor." It is sometimes associated with cerebellar syndrome.

Behavioral abnormalities are common at diagnosis, particularly in case of neurologic presentation. Symptoms are apathy, irritability, aggressive behavior, obsession, and disinhibition. A recent study reported psychiatric disorders in 24% of patients: bipolar affection (18%), major depression (4%), and dysthymia (2%) (Shanmugiah et al., 2008). The frontier between subcortical disorders and psychiatric disease is imprecise. Many patients suffer from a dysexecutive syndrome linked to subcorticofrontal lesions. Corneal Kayser–Fleischer (KF) rings are detected by slit-lamp examination (Fig. 57.2). They are, in our experience, invariably present in patients with neurologic symptoms. They are detected in 42–62% of the hepatic forms (Roberts and Schilsky, 2008). They are very suggestive of WD, even if they are also seen in other chronic hepatopathies (Suvarna, 2008). Other ophthalmic findings are sunflower cataracts that do not impair vision and oculomotor abnormalities; vertical eye movements, in particular vertical pursuits, are often impaired (Ingster-Moati et al., 2007). Other extrahepatic features include renal manifestations (as lithiasis), osteoarticular disorders, myocardial abnormalities, endocrine disturbances (Hoogenraad, 2001).

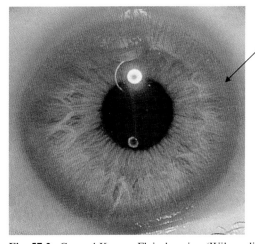

Fig. 57.2. Corneal Kayser–Fleischer ring (Wilson disease).

Wilson disease diagnosis

There is no single test for the diagnosis of WD; its assessment should include history, clinical, biologic, radiologic and sometimes histologic data. WD is characterized by low serum ceruloplasmin and total copper concentrations and increased urinary copper excretion (Table 57.2). Normal serum ceruloplasmin concentration does not exclude the diagnosis, since about 10% of WD patients and up to 50% of patients with severe liver disease have normal serum ceruloplasmin (Steindl et al., 1997). The level of serum ceruloplasmin is low in healthy newborns, and in Menkes disease, aceruloplasminemia, nephritic syndrome, copper deficiencies, and severe chronic liver disease of any cause (Pfeiffer, 2007). Some 20% of subjects heterozygous for the Wilson disease gene have reduced levels. In contrast, serum ceruloplasmin concentrations are elevated by inflammation states, by estrogen supplementation, and during pregnancy. Therefore, the interpretation of serum ceruloplasmin is often difficult (Chappuis et al., 2005). Serum copper level measures bound and free serum copper. Copper bound to ceruloplasmin normally represents about 90% of total serum copper. In WD, the total serum copper is usually decreased in proportion to the decreased ceruloplasmin. In cases of acute hepatitis or hemolysis, however, the total serum copper concentration can be increased due to important release of copper from liver or red blood cells. It has been proposed that the level of free copper should be calculated using the following formula: nonbound ceruloplasmin copper (μmol/L) = total serum copper (μmol/L) − 0.047 × serum holoceruloplasmin (mg/L). The result is dependent on the adequacy of the methods for measuring both serum copper and ceruloplasmin (Twomey et al., 2008) and so this method is not of great value in WD diagnosis or in monitoring therapy. Relative exchangeable copper (REC) (exchangeable copper/total serum copper) is probably the most useful screening method (El Balkhi et al., 2011). The majority of patients with WD have a level of urinary copper above 100 μg by 24 hours. Increased urinary copper levels are not specific for WD; they can be found in disorders with severe proteinuria and in heterozygotes for the Wilson disease gene. A provocative test for urinary copper excretion using D-penicillamine can be a useful diagnostic adjunctive test (Foruny et al., 2008). In suspected WD, if the clinical and biochemical parameters are not supportive, a hepatic biopsy with a measurement of its copper content can be carried out. The hepatic copper value in untreated WD patients is above 250 μg by gram of dry weight. Interpretation can be difficult because increased liver copper concentrations can be seen in long-term cholestasis, and hepatic copper concentrations can be falsely low in patients with extensive fibrosis (Ferenci et al., 2005).

ATP7B mutation analysis makes an important contribution to the diagnosis. Unfortunately, the sequencing of the complete coding sequence and of the intron-exon junction of the gene allows confirmation of the diagnosis of WD in only 80% of the cases (Trocello et al., 2009).

In our experience, brain magnetic resonance imaging (MRI) is always abnormal in patients with neurologic symptoms. It reveals widespread atrophy and on T2-weighted, FLAIR, and diffusion sequences shows bilateral, symmetric high-signal intensity mainly in the globus pallidus, putamen, thalamus, mesencephalon, pons, and dentate nucleus (Fig. 57.3) (Sener, 2003). A characteristic feature is the "face of the giant panda" sign on FLAIR and T2-weighted images of the midbrain. White matter changes are observed in about 25–40% of patients, often asymmetric with frontal predilection; when these lesions are extensive, they are associated with worse prognosis (Mikol et al., 2005). Abnormalities in the posterior part of the corpus callosum are frequent, observed in 23% of cases (Trocello et al., 2010b). Cortical lesions are infrequent. In patients with hepatic symptoms, a decrease of the apparent diffusion coefficient in the putamen can be detected before the occurrence of neurologic manifestations (Favrole et al., 2006). Patients with hepatic insufficiency may have high-signal intensity lesions in the basal ganglia on T1-weighted images (van Wassenaer-van Hall et al., 1996).

Wilson disease treatment

Wilson disease was fatal before the use of the first chelating agents. Low copper diet is recommended; chocolate, liver, nuts, and shellfish containing high concentrations of copper should be avoided, as should alcohol because of its liver toxicity. The drug treatment is particularly effective if it is administered at an early stage of the disease and followed for life. It is based on the use of copper chelators to promote copper excretion from the body (D-penicillamine and

triethylenetetramine or Trientine) and zinc salts (Wilzin®) to reduce copper absorption. The improvement is not immediate and may appear only after 3–6 months of therapy. Furthermore, at the institution of treatment there is a risk of a worsening of the hepatic and/or neurologic disease (Woimant et al., 2006). This deterioration is observed with all treatments, more frequently under D-penicillamine (13.8%) than under triethylenetetramine (8%) or zinc salts (4.3%) (Merle et al., 2007). A gradual institution of treatment might prevent this. Initial neurologic worsening could be due to the mobilization of hepatic copper into the circulation and its redistribution in the brain. It can also be observed in very acute forms as treatment might act too slowly. In rare cases, this deterioration is not reversible, the disease continuing to evolve under treatment. Tetratiomolybdate could have a lower risk of neurologic deterioration since it acts by forming a tripartite complex with copper and protein, either in the intestinal lumen where it prevents copper absorption or in the circulation where it makes the copper unavailable for cellular uptake (Brewer et al., 2006). This drug remains an experimental agent and is unavailable for general use.

The usual daily dose of D-penicillamine is 750–1500 mg/day. Regular monitoring of full blood count and urinary protein is recommended because of possible side-effects which occur in 30% of patients. Most of them are reversible when the drug is withdrawn. Early sensitivity reactions, with fever, rash, lymphadenopathy, proteinuria, or bone marrow depression with neutropenia, and thrombocytopenia, may occur during the first weeks. Later adverse effects include lupus-like syndrome, Goodpasture's syndrome, and myasthenia gravis. Long-term use of D-penicillamine induces changes in elastic tissues and in collagen and might cause skin lesions including elastosis perforans serpiginosa. The usual daily dose of triethylenetetramine is 750–1500 mg/day. Side-effects are rare but include lupus-like reactions and reversible sideroblastic anaemia (Pfeiffer,

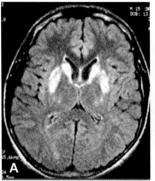 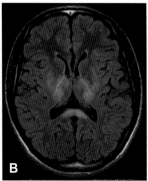 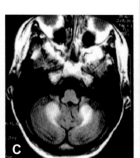 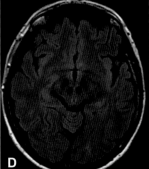

Fig. 57.3. Wilson disease, FLAIR MRI. Hypersignals in lenticular and caudate nuclei (**A**), thalami and corpus callosum (**B**), dentate nuclei (**C**), and mesencephal aspect of the "face of the giant panda" sign (**D**).

2007). The dose of zinc for adults is 150 mg/day of elemental zinc. Zinc is generally well tolerated although dyspepsia may occur; elevation in serum amylase and lipase, without clinical and radiologic evidence of pancreatitis, has been reported.

These treatments are monitored by measuring 24 hour urinary copper excretion: high during D-penicillamine and Trientine therapy, and less than 2 micromoles per day during zinc therapy.

The best therapeutic approach remains controversial because no controlled trials have compared these treatments. A recent systematic review showed no obvious differences in clinical efficacy of D-penicillamine and zinc as initial therapy in WD. The two drugs controlled the disease effectively in a majority of patients, with the best results being in presymptomatic patients (Wiggelinkhuizen et al., 2009). Therefore, the choice of drug varies from center to center, based on the opinion of the physicians and on drug availability and costs. When the disease is stabilized after several years of treatment, the initial treatment with chelator may be continued on a lower dosage or shifted to treatment with zinc salts because they are better tolerated. During pregnancy, the treatment by chelating agents or zinc salts must be maintained; however, dosages of drugs should be reduced and adapted to copper urinary excretion.

The most difficult question is how to manage patients who deteriorate despite medical therapy. Liver transplantation is the treatment for acute fulminant liver failure and for decompensated cirrhosis unresponsive to medical treatment. In cases of neurologic deterioration, the decision on whether to continue with the chosen treatment or change to adding another agent is difficult. Indication of liver transplantation is still a matter of controversy in cases of neurologic worsening without liver failure. In the study by Medici and colleagues, 70% of these patients improved after transplantation (Medici et al., 2005).

The follow-up of WD patients is essential to make sure of observance, efficiency, and tolerance of the treatment. A clinical or biologic deterioration may provoke poor compliance with treatment. In the longer term, patients may develop hepatocellular carcinoma (Walshe et al., 2003).

Family screening is essential in this autosomal recessive disease; indeed, early diagnosis of WD is essential as treatment is more effective if initiated early. The probability of finding a homozygote in siblings is 25%. The interpretation of cupric analysis can be difficult in WD heterozygotes and therefore molecular genetic analyses are very important. For families in which both mutations have been detected in the index patient, these mutations are researched in siblings. In the absence of indications on the mutations, haplotype analysis of markers around the *ATP7B* gene on chromosome 13 is used (Chappuis et al., 2005).

Acquired diseases associated with copper deficiency or copper excess

ACQUIRED COPPER DEFICIENCY

Copper deficiency is exceptional in developed countries because copper is present in numerous foods. However, nutritional copper deficiency is well documented in premature newborns and in patients maintained on parenteral nutrition for long periods of time without copper supplementation. Copper malabsorption is observed in other conditions such as upper gastrointestinal surgery or inflammatory bowel disease. An unusual cause of acquired copper deficiency is excess zinc intake, for example chronic use of denture cream containing zinc (Nations et al., 2008; Trocello et al., 2011).

Manifestations of acquired copper deficiency are almost always neurologic and hematologic (Madsen and Gitlin, 2007). Patients present with a spastic gait and prominent sensory ataxia related to a myelopathy, similar to subacute combined degeneration observed in vitamin B_{12} deficiency. Associated peripheral neuropathy is common. Spinal MRI typically shows a longitudinal high T2 signal lesion in the dorsal cervical and thoracic cord. Cytopenias are found in 78% of cases, particularly anemia. Low serum copper and ceruloplasmin levels confirmed the diagnosis and, in contrast to WD, urinary copper levels were typically low (Table 57.2). Copper supplementation resolves the anemia and neutropenia promptly and completely. But, improvement of neurologic deficits is slight and often subjective (Jaiser and Winston, 2010).

ACQUIRED COPPER TOXICOSIS

The first case of fatal copper intoxication was reported by Percival in 1785. Acute copper poisoning may occur accidentally or intentionally with suicidal objective, although the lethal dose is about 1000 times normal dietary intakes (Bremner, 1998). It manifests by a metallic taste, vomiting, diarrhea, gastrointestinal bleeding, hemolysis, oliguria, hematuria, seizures, coma, and death.

The low incidence of chronic copper toxicosis reflects the efficiency of the copper homeostatic control mechanisms. Nevertheless, copper poisoning can develop under certain conditions. Liver copper accumulation has been observed in Indian childhood cirrhosis, non-Indian disease termed idiopathic copper toxicosis, and Tyrolean childhood cirrhosis. D-penicillamine, if given early, reduces mortality. The excess copper found in these childhood types of cirrhosis was believed to be due to increased dietary intake of copper associated with an autosomal recessive inherited defect in copper metabolism; this genetic disorder is as yet uncharacterized (Haywood et al., 2001).

IRON DISORDERS

Iron is essential in multiple functions in CNS, including DNA synthesis, gene expression, myelinization, neurotransmission, and mitochondrial functions. Either brain accumulation or depletion of intracellular iron may impair normal function and promote cell death (Benarroch, 2009).

Iron brain disorders can be divided into:

- genetic neurodegeneration with brain iron accumulation
- genetic systemic iron accumulation with neurologic features (hemochromatosis)
- acquired neurodegenerative disorders such as Alzheimer disease and Parkinson disease
- acquired diseases associated with iron excess (superficial siderosis) or iron deficiency (restless leg syndrome).

Iron metabolism

(Fig. 57.4)

Dietary iron (Fe^{3+}) is first reduced to Fe^{2+} by duodenal cytochrome B (DcytB), a ferrireductase present on the apical membranes of enterocytes. Fe^{2+} then enters the enterocytes by divalent metal transporter-1 (DMT1) expressed on the apical membrane. Once inside, Fe^{2+} can be stored as ferritin or can leave the enterocyte through ferroportin (Fpn, Iregl, MTP1), expressed on the basolateral membrane. Prior to the transport of iron outside the cell, intracellular iron must be converted to Fe^{3+} via either hephaestin or ceruloplasmin, both of which have ferroxidase activity (Mills et al., 2010).

Intracellular iron is regulated by the IRE (iron regulatory element)–IRP (iron regulatory proteins) system. So, in case of elevation of intracellular iron, and particularly of the LIP (labile iron pool), the synthesis of ferritin is increased (allowing the storage of the overload iron) and the expression of the receptor for transferrin (RTf1) reduced (limiting the entrance of iron to the cell). Hepcidin produced by hepatocytes is an important regulator of cellular iron export by controlling the amount of ferroportin that is the primary determinant of gastrointestinal absorption and iron release from reticuloendothelial stores. Ceruloplasmin is a major copper-containing protein in the serum (Lutsenko et al., 2007). This α-2-glycoprotein is synthesized in the hepatic microsomes, as apoceruloplasmin. Loaded with six copper atoms per molecule, it is excreted into the circulation as holoceruloplasmin. Its essential function is a ferroxidase activity which is necessary to release iron from storage.

The cellular and intercellular iron transport mechanisms in the CNS are still poorly understood. Blood–brain barrier limits iron entry to the brain from the blood, so disturbances of systemic iron homeostasis exhibit minimal effects on CNS iron content or metabolism (Moos and Morgan, 2004). Molecular mechanisms of iron transport seem similar to those described in the peripheral tissues; ferritine, DMT 1, ferroportine, hephaestine, and ceruloplasmin are all expressed in the CNS. Brain endothelial cells express the transferrin receptor 1 in their luminal membrane; this receptor binds iron-loaded transferrin and internalizes this complex in endosomes. Then ceruloplasmin, which acts as a ferroxidase, oxidizes ferrous iron to ferric iron, which binds to the transferrin in brain interstitial fluid (Benarroch, 2009).

Disorders

INHERITED NEURODEGENERATION WITH BRAIN IRON ACCUMULATION

Inherited neurodegeneration with brain iron accumulation (NBIA) includes neurologic progressive disorders with basal ganglia iron accumulation and axonal dystrophy (spheroid bodies).

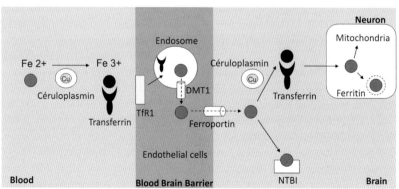

TfR1r: Transferrin receptor 1; DMT1: Divalent metal transporter 1; NTBI: Non transferrin bound iron; Fe2+: ferrous iron; FE3+: ferric iron.

Fig. 57.4. Brain iron metabolism.

NBIA type 1: pantothenate kinase-associated neurodegeneration

In 1922, Hallervorden and Spatz described the Hallervorden–Spatz disease (HSD) (Hallervorden and Spatz, 1922). Since the discovery of the *PANK2* gene, the eponym HSD is no longer used. Classic pantothenate kinase-associated neurodegeneration (PKAN) begins with gait abnormalities, usually before 6 years of age. Dystonia, often asymmetric, is the major feature. Others symptoms include dysarthria, extrapyramidal syndrome, cognitive deterioration, or psychiatric disorder. About two-thirds of patients have clinical or electroretinographic evidence of retinopathy (Gregory et al., 2009). Death occurs about 30 years of age, related to decubitus complications. Approximately 25% of affected individuals have an atypical presentation with later onset (teenage) and slower progression. Presenting features include speech difficulties and extrapyramidal syndrome; psychiatric disorders are more prominent than in the classic form of the disease, including depression, emotional lability and impulsivity (Gregory et al., 2010). PKAN gene mutations have also been described in the HARP syndrome (hypo-β-lipoproteinemia, acanthocyosis, retinitis pigmentosa and pallidal degeneration) (Ching et al., 2002). Iron tests are normal. Classic and atypical PKAN patients show the same brain MRI findings. In globus pallidus, the "eye of the tiger" sign consists of bilateral areas of hyperintensity (corresponding to necrosis tissue) surrounded by a ring of hyposignal (high iron) on T2*-weighted sequences (Fig. 57.5) (Angelini et al., 1992; Grabli et al., 2011). Hypointensity of the substantia nigra and dentate nucleus are also described.

PKAN is a recessive autosomal disease caused by a mutation of the gene (20p13-p12.3) encoding pantothenate kinase 2 (*PANK2*), an essential mitochondrial enzyme involved in coenzyme A biosynthesis (Zhou et al., 2001). Pantothenate kinase deficiency is thought to cause accumulation of N-pantothenoyl-cysteine and pantetheine, which may cause cell toxicity directly or via free radical damage as chelators of iron (Yoon et al., 2000). *PANK2* mutations (essentially missense) are present in all patients with the classic form of the disease and in one-third of those with atypical disease and late onset (Hayflick et al., 2003).

NBIA type 2: classic infantile neuroaxonal dystrophy and atypical neuroaxonal dystrophy

Infantile neuroaxonal dystrophy (INAD), sometimes called Seitelberger disease, was considered for a long time as an early form of Hallervorden–Spatz disease. The classic form begins generally in early childhood, before the age of 2 years, mostly with a regression of

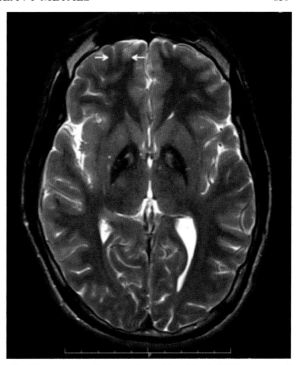

Fig. 57.5. PKAN disease. T2-weighted brain MRI. Aspect of the "eye of the tiger" sign (Grabli© 2010, Elsevier Masson SAS).

psychomotor acquisitions, delayed walking, or gait disturbance. Other presenting signs are cerebellar syndrome with ataxia, pyramidal signs, and bulbar dysfunction. Disease progression is rapid with axial hypotonia and severe spastic tetraparesis. Strabismus, nystagmus, and optic atrophy are common. Death occurs generally during the first decade, but some patients can survive up to the age of 20 years (Aicardi and Castelein, 1979; Kurian et al., 2008). In the atypical form of INAD (ANAD), the onset is often later and the evolution slower. Ataxia remains the main symptom (Kurian et al., 2008).

Denervation atrophy is seen on the electromyogram (Johnson et al., 2004). T2-weighted MRI demonstrates cerebellar cortical atrophy, white matter abnormalities, and corpus callosum changes. T2*-weighted MRI can show hypointense globus pallidus and substantia nigra (indicating iron accumulation). These abnormalities are more severe with increasing age (Kurian et al., 2008). Biological investigations do not indicate the presence of a metabolic disorder.

Before the finding of the *PLA2G6* gene, the diagnosis of INAD was established by tissue biopsy (sural nerve, skin, muscles, rectal). Indeed, unlike the neurodegeneration associated with pantothenate-kinase deficit, typical dystrophic axons are not limited to the CNS.

INAD is inherited in an autosomal recessive manner related to mutations in the *PLA2G6* gene (22q13.1) encoding a calcium-independent phospholipase A2 group VI that is thought to play a key role in cell membrane homeostasis. The sequencing of the gene allows detecting approximately 85% of the mutations. The less severe atypical NAD phenotype is caused by compound heterozygosity for missense mutations (Gregory et al., 2008).

Idiopathic neurodegeneration with brain iron accumulation

In recent years, progress has been made in the discovery of gene mutations and phenotypes. However, a large population of idiopathic cases caused by undiscovered genes remains to be investigated.

Neuroferritinopathy

Neuroferritinopathy was described for the first time in 2001 in a family from the north of England; it results from mutations in the ferritin light polypeptide gene (FTL) encoding the light chain of ferritin (Curtis et al., 2001). Clinical onset is around 40–50 years of age, with chorea, dystonia, and extrapyramidal syndrome. A cerebellar syndrome is sometimes associated (Ory-Magne et al., 2009). The evolution of the disease is slowly progressive; the majority of patients develop a characteristic orofacial dystonia leading to dysarthrophonia,and the gait is generally lost more than 20 years after the first symptoms.

Serum ferritin concentrations are low (<20 µg/L) in the majority of males and postmenopausal females but within normal limits for premenopausal females. Serum iron concentrations are usually normal (Chinnery et al., 2007). All affected individuals have evidence of excess brain iron accumulation. In presymptomatic patients, T2* MRI demonstrates hyposignals of substantia nigra and red nuclei related to iron deposits. In symptomatic patients, T2* hyposignals are described in caudate, globus pallidus, putamen, thalami, and dentate nuclei. Cortical cerebellar atrophy is sometimes present. At a later stage, cystic cavitation in the caudate and putamen appears on T2-weighted sequences as a hypersignal surrounded with a hypointense ring and on T1-weighted sequences as a hyposignal (Chinnery et al., 2007). This image is very close to "the eye of tiger" described in PKAN.

Neuroferritinopathy is an autosomal dominant disease. *FTL*, located on chromosome 19, is the only gene currently known to be associated with neuroferritinopathy. *FTL* mutations are known to alter the structure of E-helices, thereby leading to the release of free iron and excessive oxidative stress (Harrison and Arosio, 1996).

Iron depletion therapy by iron chelation in symptomatic patients has not been shown to be beneficial.

Aceruloplasminemia

Miyajima et al. described in 1987 the first case of aceruloplasminemia (Miyajima et al., 1987). Since then, about 40 families have been reported. This disease is clinically characterized by the triad of retinal degeneration, diabetes mellitus, and neurologic symptoms, including dystonia, chorea, blepharospasm, tremor, cerebellar ataxia, and cognitive deterioration (Miyajima, 2003). Anemia is often present, prior to onset of diabetes mellitus. The age at diagnosis ranged from 16 to 71 years with a mean of 51. Prognosis depends on heart disease due to cardiac iron overload, control of diabetes, and severity of neurologic impairment. Treatment is based on iron chelators (deferiprone or deferasirox). Heterozygous patients have a partial CP deficiency; some develop a less severe disease with cerebellar ataxia, tremor, or choreaathetosis (McNeill et al., 2008a).

Diagnosis is based on the absence of serum ceruloplasmin and low serum copper concentration, low serum iron concentration, high serum ferritin concentration, as well as hepatic iron overload (Table 57.2). MRI findings are abnormal T2* hyposignals reflecting iron accumulation in the brain (striatum, thalamus, dentate nucleus) and liver (McNeill et al., 2008b).

Genetic testing can confirm the diagnosis. Aceruloplasminemia is a rare autosomal recessive disorder caused by mutations in the *CP* gene (3q23-q24). The absence of ceruloplasmin and its ferroxidase activity leads to pathologic iron overload in the brain and other organs (McNeill et al., 2008a).

GENETIC SYSTEMIC IRON ACCUMULATION WITH NEUROLOGIC FEATURES

Hereditary hemochromatosis (HH) is an autosomal recessive condition in which excessive intestinal iron absorption leads to iron deposition in systemic tissues. The most common form, especially in populations of Northern European origin, is caused by mutations in *HFE*. Presenting features are chronic asthenia, arthropathies, impotence, hyperpigmentation, liver abnormalities (hepatomegaly, slight hypertransaminasemia), diabetes, cardiomyopathy, and hyperferritinemia. Neurologic manifestations are rarely described in HH. Tremor, myoclonus, cerebellar ataxia, cervical dystonia, or parkinsonism have occasionally reported. Brain MRI suggests excessive iron in the basal ganglia of these patients. However, the CNS damage in hemochromatosis remains a subject for discussion and Russo suggests that such patients should be thoroughly investigated for another cause of neurologic disorders (Russo et al., 2004).

Restless legs syndrome (RLS) in patients with hemochromatosis occurred predominantly in patients with serum ferritin levels below 50 ng/mL. The emergence of RLS symptoms was most likely when ferritin fell below 25 ng/mL and indicates that iron removal has been excessive in such patients. Nevertheless, RLS can occur in patients with iron overload, as prior to diagnosis and treatment of HH (Shaughnessy et al., 2005). Polyneuropathy has also been reported (Hermann et al., 2002).

ACQUIRED NEURODEGENERATIVE DISORDERS SUCH AS ALZHEIMER DISEASE AND PARKINSON DISEASE

Iron accumulates in the brain as a function of age, primarily in the form of ferritin, particularly in the microglia and astrocytes, but also in oligodendrocytes. Imbalance in iron homeostasis leading to either excessive accumulation of free cytosolic iron or decreased iron availability for critical enzymes is suggested as a precursor to the neurodegenerative processes. Increased iron concentrations are reported in the cortex and cerebellum from cases of preclinical Alzheimer disease (AD) and mild cognitive impairment (Smith et al., 2010). Iron may have a direct impact on plaque formation through its effects on amyloid precursor protein. Parkinson disease (PD) is characterized by iron accumulation in dopaminergic neurons of the substantia nigra (Benarroch, 2009). This iron accumulation is probably not causal but secondary to the disease process.

ACQUIRED DISEASES ASSOCIATED WITH IRON EXCESS OR IRON DEFICIENCY

Superficial siderosis (SS) of the CNS is caused by repeated slow hemorrhage into the subarachnoid space with resultant hemosiderin deposition in the subpial layers of the brain and spinal cord. It is characterized by deafness and cerebellar ataxia. Less frequently, it is also associated with bladder disturbance, anosmia, ocular palsies, anisocoria, dementia, or myelopathy. Gradient-echo T2-weighted MRI shows a rim of hypointensity (due to hemosiderin deposition) around the cerebellum, brainstem, and spinal cord; it may also involve the cortical sulci, sylvian fissure, and interhemispheric fissure. Cerebrospinal fluid analysis may show xanthochromia and an increased number of red blood cells (Kumar, 2007). The causes of SS include history of trauma, aneurysms, or other vascular malformations, CNS tumors, and cerebral amyloid angiopathy (Vernooij et al., 2009). In most cases, however, despite extensive investigations, the cause of bleeding remains undetermined. Therapy is treatment for of the cause of the bleeding when this is possible. In the absence of a curable cause, medical treatments are proposed (copper or iron chelators) but their effectivenes remains low.

RESTLESS LEGS SYNDROME

All studies of CNS iron have consistently shown iron insufficiency in restless legs syndrome (RLS) (Allen et al., 2001). Autopsy analysis revealed that the immunostaining for iron management proteins was altered in the substantia nigra of RLS brains and the profile of proteins responsible for iron management in the neuromelanin cells indicated iron deficiency (Connor et al., 2003). Iron supplementation improves the symptoms (Allen et al., 2001).

REFERENCES

Aicardi J, Castelein P (1979). Infantile neuroaxonal dystrophy. Brain 102: 727–748.

Ala A, Walker AP, Ashkan K et al. (2007). Wilson's disease. Lancet 369: 397–408.

Allen RP, Earley CJ (2001). Restless legs syndrome. A review of clinical and pathophysiologic features. J Clin Neurophysiol 18: 128–147.

Angelini L, Nardocci N, Rumi V et al. (1992). Hallervorden-Spatz disease : clinical and MRI study of 11 cases diagnosed in life. J Neurol 239: 417–425.

Barnes N, Tsivkovskii R, Tsivkovskaia N et al. (2005). The copper-transporting ATPases, Menkes and Wilson disease proteins, have distinct roles in adult and developing cerebellum. J Biol Chem 280: 9640–9645.

Benarroch EE (2009). Brain iron homeostasis and neurodegenerative disease. Neurology 72: 1436–1440.

Beyersdorff A, Findeisen A (2006). Morbus Wilson: case report of a two-year-old child as first manifestation. Scand J Gastroenterol 41: 496–497.

Bremner I (1998). Manifestations of copper excess. Am J Clin Nutr 67: 1069S–1073S.

Brewer GJ, Askari F, Lorincz MT et al. (2006). Treatment of Wilson disease with ammonium tetrathiomolybdate: IV. Comparison of tetrathiomolybdate and trientine in a double-blind study of treatment of the neurologic presentation of Wilson disease. Arch Neurol 63: 521–527.

Brodkin E, Copes R, Mattman A et al. (2007). Lead and mercury exposures: interpretation and action. CMAJ 176: 59–63.

Bull PC, Thomas GR, Rommens JM et al. (1993). The Wilson disease gene is a putative copper transporting P-type ATPase similar to the Menkes gene. Nat Genet 5: 327–337.

Chappuis P, Bost M, Misrahi M et al. (2005). Wilson disease: clinical and biological aspects. Ann Biol Clin (Paris) 63: 457–466.

Chelly J, Tümer Z, Tønnesen T et al. (1993). Isolation of a candidate gene for Menkes disease that encodes a potential heavy metal binding protein. Nat Genet 3: 14–19.

Ching KH, Westaway SK, Gitschier J et al. (2002). HARP syndrome is allelic with pantothenate kinase-associated neurodegeneration. Neurology 58: 1673–1674.

Chinnery PF, Crompton DE, Birchall D et al. (2007). Clinical features and natural history of neuroferritinopathy caused by the FTL1 460InsA mutation. Brain 130: 110–119.

Connor JR, Boyer PJ, Menzies SL et al. (2003). Neuropathological examination suggests impaired brain iron acquisition in restless legs syndrome. Neurology 61: 304–309.

Cumings JN (1948). The copper and iron content of brain and liver in the normal and in hepato-lenticular degeneration. Brain 71: 410–415.

Curtis AR, Fey C, Morris CM et al. (2001). Mutation in the gene encoding ferritin light polypeptide causes dominant adult-onset basal ganglia disease. Nat Genet 28: 350–354.

Członkowska A, Rodo M, Gromadzka G (2008). Late onset Wilson's disease: therapeutic implications. Mov Disord 23: 896–898.

Danks DM, Campbell PE, Stevens BJ et al. (1972). Menkes's kinky hair syndrome. An inherited defect in copper absorption with widespread effects. Pediatrics 50: 188–201.

de Bie P, Muller P, Wijmenga C et al. (2007). Molecular pathogenesis of Wilson and Menkes disease: correlation of mutations with molecular defects and disease phenotypes. J Med Genet 44: 673–688.

El Balkhi S, Trocello JM, Poupon J et al. (2011). Relative exchangeable copper: a new highly sensitive and highly specific biomarker for Wilson's disease diagnosis. Clin Chim Acta 412: 2254–2260.

Favrole P, Chabriat H, Guichard JP et al. (2006). Clinical correlates of cerebral water diffusion in Wilson disease. Neurology 66: 384–389.

Ferenci P, Steindl-Munda P, Vogel W et al. (2005). Diagnostic value of quantitative hepatic copper determination in patients with Wilson's disease. Clin Gastroenterol Hepatol 3: 811–818.

Figus A, Angius A, Loudianos G et al. (1995). Molecular pathology and haplotype analysis of Wilson disease in Mediterranean populations. Am J Hum Genet 57: 1318–1324.

Foruny JR, Boixeda D, López-Sanroman A et al. (2008). Usefulness of penicillamine-stimulated urinary copper excretion in the diagnosis of adult Wilson's disease. Scand J Gastroenterol 43: 597–603.

Frydman M, Bonne-Tamir B, Farrer L et al. (1985). Assignment of the gene for Wilson disease to chromosome 13: linkage to the esterase D locus. Proc Natl Acad Sci U S A 82: 1819–1821.

Grabli D, Auré K, Roze E (2011). Movement disorders and neurometabolic diseases. Rev Neurol (Paris) 167: 123–134.

Gregory A, Hayflick SJ (1993–2002 [updated 2010]). Pantothenate kinase-associated neurodegeneration. In: RA Pagon, TC Bird, CR Dolan et al. (Eds.), GeneReviews, [Internet]. University of Washington, Seattle.

Gregory A, Westaway SK, Holm IE et al. (2008). Neurodegeneration associated with genetic defects in phospholipase A(2). Neurology 71: 1402–1409.

Gregory A, Polster BJ, Hayflick SJ (2009). Clinical and genetic delineation of neurodegeneration with brain iron accumulation. J Med Genet 46: 73–80.

Hallervorden J, Spatz H (1922). Eigenartige Erkrankung im extrapyramidalen System mit besonderer Beteilgung des Globus pallidus und der Substantia nigra: ein Beitrag zu den Beziehungen zwischen diesen beiden Zentren. Z Ges Neurol Psychiat 79: 254–302.

Harrison PM, Arosio P (1996). The ferritins: molecular properties, iron storage function and cellular regulation. Biochim Biophys Acta 1275: 161–203.

Hayflick SJ, Westaway SK, Levinson B et al. (2003). Genetic, clinical, and radiographic delineation of Hallervorden–Spatz syndrome. N Engl J Med 348: 33–40.

Haywood S, Muller T, Muller W et al. (2001). Copper-associated liver disease in North Ronaldsay sheep: a possible animal model for non Wilsonian hepatic copper toxicosis of infancy and childhood. J Pathol 195: 264–269.

Hermann W, Guenther P, Clark D et al. (2002). Polyneuropathy in idiopathic haemochromatosis. J Neurol 249: 1316–1317.

Hoogenraad T (2001). Wilson's Disease. Internal Medical Pubishers, Amsterdam.

Horn N, Tønnesen T, Tümer Z (1992). Menkes disease: an X-linked neurological disorder of the copper metabolism. Brain Pathol 2: 351–362.

Ingster-Moati I, Bui Quoc E, Pless M et al. (2007). Ocular motility and Wilson's disease: a study on 34 patients. J Neurol Neurosurg Psychiatry 78: 1199–1201.

Jaiser SR, Winston GP (2010). Copper deficiency myelopathy. J Neurol 257: 869–881.

Jog MS, Lang AE (1995). Chronic acquired hepatocerebral degeneration: case reports and new insights. Mov Disord 10: 714–722.

Johnson MA, Kuo YM, Westaway SK et al. (2004). Mitochondrial localization of human PANK2 and hypotheses of secondary iron accumulation in pantothenate kinase-associated neurodegeneration. Ann N Y Acad Sci 1012: 282–298.

Kaler SG (1993–2003 [updated 2010]]). ATP7A-related copper transport disorders. In: RA Pagon, TC Bird, CR Dolan et al. (Eds.), GeneReviews. [Internet]. University of Washington, Seattle, .

Kaler SG (1998). Metabolic and molecular bases of Menkes disease and occipital horn syndrome. Pediatr Dev Pathol 1: 85–98.

Kennerson ML, Nicholson GA, Kaler SG et al. (2010). Missense mutations in the copper transporter gene ATP7A cause X-linked distal hereditary motor neuropathy. Am J Hum Genet 86: 343–352.

Kumar N (2007). Superficial siderosis: associations and therapeutic implications. Arch Neurol 64: 491–496.

Kurian MA, Morgan NV, MacPherson L et al. (2008). Phenotypic spectrum of neurodegeneration associated with mutations in the PLA2G6 gene (PLAN). Neurology 70: 1623–1629.

Letzel S, Lang CJ, Schaller KH et al. (2000). Longitudinal study of neurotoxicity with occupational exposure to aluminum dust. Neurology 54: 997–1000.

Lorincz MT (2010). Neurologic Wilson's disease. Ann N Y Acad Sci 1184: 173–187.

Lutsenko S, Barnes NL, Bartee MY et al. (2007). Function and regulation of human copper-transporting ATPases. Physiol Rev 87: 1011–1046.

Madsen E, Gitlin JD (2007). Copper deficiency. Curr Opin Gastroenterol 23: 187–192.

McNeill A, Pandolfo M, Kuhn J et al. (2008a). The neurological presentation of ceruloplasmin gene mutations. Eur Neurol 60: 200–205.

McNeill A, Birchall D, Hayflick SJ et al. (2008b). T2* and FSE MRI distinguishes four subtypes of neurodegeneration with brain iron accumulation. Neurology 70: 1614–1619.

Medici V, Mirante VG, Fassati LR et al. (2005). Monotematica AISF 2000 OLT study group. Liver transplantation for Wilson's disease: the burden of neurological and psychiatric disorders. Liver Transpl 11: 1056–1063.

Menkes JH, Alter M, Steigleder GK et al. (1962). A sex-linked recessive disorder with retardation of growth, peculiar hair, and focal cerebral and cerebellar degeneration. Pediatrics 29: 764–779.

Mercer JF, Livingston J, Hall B et al. (1993). Isolation of a partial candidate gene of Menkes disease by positional cloning. Nat Genet 3: 20–25.

Merle U, Schaefer M, Ferenci P et al. (2007). Clinical presentation, diagnosis and long-term outcome of Wilson's disease: a cohort study. Gut 56: 115–120.

Mikol J, Vital C, Wassef M et al. (2005). Extensive cortico-subcortical lesions in Wilson's disease: clinico-pathological study of two cases. Acta Neuropathol 110: 451–458.

Mills E, Dong XP, Wang F et al. (2010). Mechanisms of brain iron transport: insight into neurodegeneration and CNS disorders. Future Med Chem 2: 51.

Miyajima H (2003). Aceruloplasminemia, an iron metabolic disorder. Neuropathology 23: 345–350.

Miyajima H, Nishimura Y, Mizoguchi K et al. (1987). Familial apoceruloplasmin deficiency associated with blepharospasm and retinal degeneration. Neurology 37: 761–767.

Møller LB, Mogensen M, Horn N (2009). Molecular diagnosis of Menkes disease: genotype-phenotype correlation. Biochimie 91: 1273–1277.

Moos T, Morgan EH (2004). The metabolism of neuronal iron and its pathogenic role in neurological disease: review. Ann N Y Acad Sci 1012: 14–26.

Nations SP, Boyer PJ, Love LA et al. (2008). Denture cream: an unusual source of excess zinc, leading to hypocupremia and neurologic disease. Neurology 71: 639–643.

Ory-Magne F, Brefel-Courbon C, Payoux P et al. (2009). Clinical phenotype and neuroimaging findings in a French family with hereditary ferritinopathy (FTL498-499InsTC). Mov Disord 24: 1676–1683.

Peltonen L, Kuivaniemi H, Palotie A et al. (1983). Alterations in copper and collagen metabolism in the Menkes syndrome and a new subtype of the Ehlers–Danlos syndrome. Biochemistry 22: 6156–6163.

Pfeiffer RF (2007). Wilson's disease. Semin Neurol 27: 123–132.

Roberts EA, Schilsky ML (2008). American association for study of liver diseases (AASLD). Diagnosis and treatment of Wilson disease: an update. Hepatology 47: 2089–2111.

Russo N, Edwards M, Andrews T et al. (2004). Hereditary haemochromatosis is unlikely to cause movement disorders – a critical review. J Neurol 251: 849–852.

Sener RN (2003). Diffusion MR imaging changes associated with Wilson disease. AJNR Am J Neuroradiol 24: 965–967.

Sethi PK, Khandelwal D (2006). Cadmium exposure: health hazards of silver cottage industry in developing countries. J Med Toxicol 2: 14–15.

Shanmugiah A, Sinha S, Taly AB et al. (2008). Psychiatric manifestations in Wilson's disease: a cross-sectional analysis. J Neuropsychiatry Clin Neurosci 20: 81–85.

Shaughnessy P, Lee J, O'Keeffe ST (2005). Restless legs syndrome in patients with hereditary hemochromatosis. Neurology 64: 2158.

Smith MA, Zhu X, Tabaton M et al. (2010). Increased iron and free radical generation in preclinical Alzheimer disease and mild cognitive impairment. J Alzheimers Dis 19: 363–372.

Steindl P, Ferenci P, Dienes HP et al. (1997). Wilson's disease in patients presenting with liver disease: a diagnostic challenge. Gastroenterology 113: 212–218.

Stepens A, Logina I, Liguts V et al. (2008). Parkinsonian syndrome in methcathinone users and the role of manganese. N Engl J Med 358: 1009–1017.

Suvarna JC (2008). Kayser–Fleischer ring. J Postgrad Med 54: 238–240.

Tanzi RE, Petrukhin K, Chernov I et al. (1993). The Wilson disease gene is a copper transporting ATPase with homology to the Menkes disease gene. Nat Genet 5: 344–350.

Thomas GR, Roberts EA, Walshe JM et al. (1995). Haplotypes and mutations in Wilson disease. Am J Hum Genet 56: 1315–1319.

Trocello JM, Woimant F (2008). Case study 3. In: A Schapira, A Hartmann, Y Agid (Eds.), Parkinsonian disorders in clinical practice. Wiley-Blackwell, Oxford, pp. 74–78.

Trocello JM, Chappuis P, Chaine P et al. (2009). Wilson disease. Presse Med 38: 1089–1098.

Trocello JM, Chappuis P, El Balkhi S et al. (2010a). Abnormal copper metabolism in adult. Rev Med Interne 31: 750–756.

Trocello JM, Guichard JP, Leyendecker A et al. (2010b). Corpus callosum abnormalities in Wilson's disease. J Neurol Neurosurg Psychiatry 82: 1119–1121.

Trocello JM, Hinfray S, Sanda N et al. (2011). An unrecognized cause of myclopathy associated with copper deficiency: the use of denture cream. Rev Neurol (Paris) 167: 537–540.

Tümer Z, Møller LB (2010). Menkes disease. Eur J Hum Genet 18: 511–518.

Twomey PJ, Viljoen A, Reynolds TM et al. (2008). Non-ceruloplasmin-bound copper in routine clinical practice in different laboratories. J Trace Elem Med Biol 22: 50–53.

Valentine JS, Gralla EB (1997). Delivering copper inside yeast and human cells. Science 278: 817–818.

van Wassenaer-van Hall HN, van den Heuvel AG, Algra A et al. (1996). Wilson disease: findings at MR imaging and CT of the brain with clinical correlation. Radiology 198: 531–536.

Vernooij MW, Ikram MA, Hofman A et al. (2009). Superficial siderosis in the general population. Neurology 73: 202–205.

Vulpe C, Levinson B, Whitney S et al. (1993). Isolation of a candidate gene for Menkes disease and evidence that it encodes a copper-transporting ATPase. Nat Genet 3: 7–13.

Walshe JM (1956). Penicillamine, a new oral therapy for Wilson's disease. Am J Med 21: 487–495.

Walshe JM (2006). History of Wilson's disease: 1912 to 2000. Mov Disord 21: 142–147.

Walshe JM, Waldenström E, Sams V et al. (2003). Abdominal malignancies in patients with Wilson's disease. QJM 96: 657–662.

Wiggelinkhuizen M, Tilanus ME, Bollen CW et al. (2009). Systematic review: clinical efficacy of chelator agents and zinc in the initial treatment of Wilson disease. Aliment Pharmacol Ther 29: 947–958.

Wilson SAK (1912). Progressive lenticular degeneration: a familial nervous disease associated with cirrhosis of the liver. Brain 34: 295–507.

Woimant F, Chaine P, Favrole P et al. (2006). Wilson disease. Rev Neurol (Paris) 162: 773–781.

Yamaguchi Y, Heiny ME, Gitlin JD (1993). Isolation and characterization oh a human liver cDNA as a candidate gene for Wilson disease. Biochem Biophys Res Commun 197: 271–277.

Yong RL, Holmes DT, Sreenivasan GM (2006). Aluminum toxicity due to intravenous injection of boiled methadone. N Engl J Med 354: 1210–1211.

Yoon SJ, Koh YH, Floyd RA et al. (2000). Copper, zinc superoxide dismutase enhances DNA damage and mutagenicity induced by cysteine/iron. Mutat Res 448: 97–104.

Zhou B, Westaway SK, Levinson B et al. (2001). A novel pantothenate kinase gene (PANK2) is defective in Hallervorden–Spatz syndrome. Nat Genet 28: 345–349.

Handbook of Clinical Neurology, Vol. 120 (3rd series)
Neurologic Aspects of Systemic Disease Part II
Jose Biller and Jose M. Ferro, Editors
© 2014 Elsevier B.V. All rights reserved

Chapter 58

Disorders of bone and bone mineral metabolism

MONICA KOMOROSKI[1], NASRIN AZAD[2], AND PAULINE CAMACHO[1]*

[1]*Loyola University Osteoporosis and Metabolic Bone Disease Center, Loyola University Medical Center, Maywood, IL, USA*

[2]*Edward Hines Jr. VA Hospital, Hines, IL, USA*

CALCIUM AND PARATHYROID HORMONE DISORDERS

Introduction

Calcium is the third most abundant ion in the body and plays an important role regarding normal cell function, neural transmission, membrane stability, bone structure, blood coagulation, and intracellular signaling (Liamis et al., 2009). Parathyroid hormone (PTH) is an important hormone involved in the regulation of calcium and phosphorus homeostasis. PTH is synthesized by the parathyroid glands and is then processed and stored in secretory granules as a mature 84 residue hormone. Once released, the circulating 84 amino acid protein has a short half-life of 2–4 minutes. It is through the effects of PTH that the serum calcium concentration is maintained within normal limits (Al Zahrani and Levine, 1997).

Most of total-body calcium (99%) is in the form of hydroxyapatite in the skeleton, and the rest is in extracellular fluids and soft tissues. It is the extracellular concentration of ionized calcium that is the most important determinant of PTH secretion. The rate of PTH secretion is controlled by the interaction of extracellular calcium with specific calcium-sensing receptors present on the plasma membrane of the parathyroid cell. Hypocalcemia stimulates PTH synthesis and secretion. Hyperphosphatemia and severe hypomagnesemia also stimulate PTH secretion. PTH acts via direct and indirect mechanisms to increase serum calcium. Within minutes, PTH directly increases renal calcium reabsorption and decreases renal phosphorus reabsorption in the distal tubule. PTH also directly stimulates osteoclasts, leading to bone resorption. This process releases calcium and phosphorus from the bone into the circulation. PTH also increases 1α-hydroxylase activity in the kidney which converts calcidiol to calcitriol, which in turn increases intestinal absorption of calcium and phosphorus. This process takes about 1–2 days. Overall, PTH acts to raise serum calcium concentrations and to lower serum phosphorous concentrations (Al Zahrani and Levine, 1997).

Vitamin D is also important in the regulation of calcium. It is synthesized in the skin or can be obtained through dietary sources; it is carried in the bloodstream to the liver, where it is converted into calcidiol. Calcidiol can then be metabolized by the kidney, via 1α-hydroxylase, to the biologically active form of vitamin D, calcitriol, which then acts throughout the body and essentially functions as a hormone. The most important function is exerted on the small intestine, where calcitriol regulates the intestinal reabsorption of calcium and, to a lesser degree, phosphorus. Calcitriol inhibits PTH secretion. In summary, the integrated actions of PTH and vitamin D on target tissues gives precise control of serum concentrations of calcium and phosphorous (Al Zahrani and Levine, 1997).

HYPERCALCEMIA

Many disorders are associated with hypercalcemia. However, there are a limited number of mechanisms contributing to the hypercalcemia which include the following: increased bone resorption, increased gastrointestinal absorption of calcium, or decreased renal excretion of calcium.

Classification

The most common causes of hypercalcemia are malignancy and primary hyperparathyroidism (Riggs, 2002). Hypercalcemic disorders can be divided into two major groups, PTH-mediated and non-PTH-mediated.

*Correspondence to: Pauline M. Camacho, MD, FACE, Associate Professor of Medicine, Program Director, Endocrinology Fellowship Program, Director, Loyola University Osteoporosis and Metabolic Bone Disease Center, Loyola University Medical Center, 2160 S. First Avenue, Maywood, IL 60153, USA. Tel: +1-708-216-0160, Fax: +1-708-216-5936, E-mail: pcamach@lumc.edu

PTH- mediated hypercalcemic disorders can be distinguished by an elevated or inappropriately normal PTH lèvel in the setting of hypercalcemia. These include primary hyperparathyroidism (secondary to parathyroid adenoma or hyperplasia), lithium-associated hypercalcemia, and familial hypercalcemic hypocalciuria. Non-PTH-mediated hypercalcemic disorders are characterized by a suppressed PTH in the setting of hypercalcemia. These include hypercalcemia of malignancy (secondary to bony metastases, PTHrP or other humoral factors), vitamin D intoxication (from ingestion of supraphysiologic doses of vitamin D or increased synthesis of calcitriol from macrophages in granulomatous disease), milk-alkali syndrome, conditions associated with high bone turnover (including hyperthyroidism, immobilization, vitamin A intoxication), conditions associated with renal failure (tertiary hyperparathyroidism, aluminum intoxication, excessive calcium and vitamin D intake), and medications (thiazides and theophylline).

Clinical features

Mild hypercalcemia may be asymptomatic or may be associated with vague, nonspecific symptoms such as fatigue, difficulty concentrating, personality changes, irritability, anxiety, and depression. Alterations in mental status, including progressive lethargy, confusion, and ultimately coma, are common in severe hypercalcemia, defined as serum calcium levels greater than 14 mg/dL or in acute hypercalcemia . Headache, elevated cerebrospinal fluid protein, and seizures may also occur in patients with hypercalcemia (Riggs, 2002).

The kidney is the only route of calcium elimination. Hypercalcemia impairs glomerular filtration rate. As a result, the urinary concentrating ability is impaired which leads to dehydration. This further compromises renal calcium clearance.

Treatment

The treatment of hypercalcemia includes medical and surgical strategies, and the severity and chronicity influence management. In all situations, drugs contributing to hypercalcemia should be discontinued. The goal of treatment in symptomatic hypercalcemia is to increase renal excretion of calcium in attempts to decrease serum calcium level. Intravenous fluids, preferably normal saline, should be administered at a rapid rate (200–300 cc/hour) to reverse intravascular volume contraction and to promote renal excretion of calcium. Loop diuretics can also be employed to reduce the risk of volume overload and to inhibit calcium resorption in the loop of Henle (Ariyan and Sosa, 2004). Calcitonin, administered subcutaneously, acts quickly (within 24–48 hours) to lower serum calcium and can be used in the acute setting. Intravenous bisphosphonates may also be used to lower serum calcium but they may take up to 1 week to exert maximal effect.

Some of the other treatments for hypercalcemia are dependent upon the etiology of the hypercalcemia. Parathyroidectomy is the recommended treatment for primary hyperparathyroidism. Glucocorticoids are effective in managing hypercalcemia secondary to sarcoidosis, where hypercalcemia stems from vitamin D toxicity. These agents inhibit the effects of vitamin D, reduce intestinal calcium absorption, and increase renal calcium excretion. Surgery, radiation, and/or chemotherapy are effective treatments in hypercalcemia related to malignancy.

PRIMARY HYPERPARATHYROIDISM

Introduction

Primary hyperparathyroidism (PHPT) is characterized by excessive secretion of parathyroid hormone (PTH) and consequent hypercalcemia. Before routine measurement of serum calcium concentration was available, PHPT was thought to be an uncommon metabolic disorder that was typically associated with pronounced metabolic bone disease and renal stones. PHPT is now a common metabolic disorder most often diagnosed after the incidental discovery of hypercalcemia in an asymptomatic patient. There has been a marked reduction in the classic signs and symptoms of primary hyperparathyroidism. Although PHPT can occur at any age, it is most common in the fifth and sixth decades. The disorder is also two to three times more common in women than in men, and this difference increases with age.

Etiology

More than 80% of cases of primary hyperparathyroidism are secondary to a single parathyroid adenoma. Multiple adenomas are uncommon. Diffuse hyperplasia of all parathyroid glands account for 15–20% of cases. Half of these are part of a familial syndrome (multiple endocrine neoplasia I or IIb). Parathyroid cysts are uncommon and parathyroid carcinoma is very rare (0.5% of primary hyperparathyroidism) (Bilezikian et al., 2005).

Diagnosis

Hypercalcemia is the biochemical hallmark of primary hyperparathyroidism and is an essential diagnostic criterion. Hypercalcemia may be mild or even intermittent in some patients, and PTH is either elevated or is inappropriately normal (Al Zahrani and Levine, 1997). The serum phosphate concentration is usually in the low or low normal range; there may be a mild hyperchloremic acidosis as well (Al Zahrani and Levine, 1997).

Clinical features

Primary hyperparathyroidism (PHP) has been associated with skeletal, renal, gastrointestinal, cardiovascular, neuromuscular, and neuropsychiatric manifestations. Most of the following manifestations are seen in moderate and severe hyperparathyroidism. However, some skeletal, cardiovascular, and neuropsychiatric features have been described in mild hyperparathyroidism, which is the most common form seen today. The symptoms and signs of PHP are, in part, related to the degree of hypercalcemia.

Skeletal manifestations

Osteitis fibrosa cystica is the classic bone disease of primary hyperparathyroidism but now occurs in < 10% of patients. Features include subperiosteal resorption (at the radial aspects of the middle phalanges or the distal phalanges), distal tapering of the clavicles, and a "salt and pepper" appearance of the skull. Bone cysts and brown tumors are locally destructive lesions that occur in more advanced stages of hyperparathyroid bone disease (Al Zahrani and Levine, 1997). Histologically, there is an increase in the number of osteoclasts, marrow fibrosis, and cystic lesions that may contain fibrous tissue. This condition is associated with bone pain and pathologic fractures.

Osteoporosis, fractures, pseudogout (Geelhoed and Kelly, 1989), bone and joint pains are the other skeletal manifestations of primary hyperparathyroidism. These features have been described in mild PHPT. Unlike other disorders causing osteoporosis, hyperparathyroidism often results in cortical bone loss (Khan and Bilezikian, 2000). The most common site of skeletal involvement is the distal third of the radius, a site of cortical bone. The lumbar spine is made up mostly of cancellous bone and therefore is only minimally reduced. The hip region is a mixture of cortical and cancellous bone and bone density is intermediate between the radius and spine. Trabecular/cancellous bone mass and strength are relatively maintained in mild hyperparathyroidism. Therefore, one would expect the spine to be relatively resistant to fractures. The above densitometric profile though is not always seen in PHPT. In some patients, cancellous bone density of the lumbar spine can be substantially reduced (Khan and Bilezikian, 2000). Back pain and vertebral crush fractures can be a presenting feature of PHPT (Dauphine et al., 1975).

Renal manifestations

Nephrolithiasis is the classic renal disease, which occurred in about 40% of cases but now occurs in about 15–20% of cases (Al Zahrani and Levine, 1997).

Hypercalciuria has been implicated in the pathogenesis of nephrolithiasis. Nephrocalcinosis is the diffuse deposition of calcium and phosphate throughout the kidneys, which can also occur in patients with PHP. Nephrocalcinosis may be associated with stones but it is rare; progressive renal insufficiency, however, is not uncommon. Chronic hypercalcemia can compromise the renal concentrating ability, contributing to polyuria and as a result polydipsia.

Cardiovascular manifestations

Studies have revealed the effects of hyperparathyroidism on the heart. The development of coronary artery disease has been associated with elevated calcium and PTH levels. Hypertension (HTN) is frequently seen in association with PHPT, even among those with mild disease. Left ventricular hypertrophy, independent of HTN, is also seen in association with PHPT in most but not all studies across a wide range of calcium levels (10.5–12 mg/dL). PTH seems to increase intracellular levels of calcium that subsequently activates protein kinase C, thereby initiating hypertrophic processes such as protein synthesis. Hyperparathyroidism has been associated with diastolic filling impairment but not with systolic dysfunction (Andersson et al., 2004). Myocardial and valvular calcifications have clearly been demonstrated in PHPT patients with marked hypercalcemia but not in mild or moderate hypercalcemia. In patients with severe hypercalcemia (12.1 mg/dL or above), serum calcium levels correlated positively with T wave duration and negatively with QT interval. Studies from Scandinavia have documented an increased mortality from cardiovascular disease in severe and moderately severe PHPT. Several studies of patients with mild PHPT have not found an increased cardiovascular mortality (Silverberg et al., 2009).

Gastrointestinal manifestations

Dyspepsia, nausea, and constipation all occur, probably as a consequence of hypercalcemia. There is probably no increase in peptic ulcer disease except in patients with multiple endocrine neoplasia (Silverberg, 2002; Bilezikian et al., 2005).

Neuromuscular and neuropsychiatric manifestations

Hypercalcemia reduces neuromuscular excitability and may cause muscle weakness. Easy fatigability and muscle weakness are more common in hyperparathyroidism than in other hypercalcemic disorders (Riggs, 2002). Von Recklinghausen and Vical were the first to describe neuromuscular involvement in primary hyperparathyroidism. Primary hyperparathyroidism should be in the differential diagnosis of those presenting with symptoms consistent with motor neuron disease (Delmont et al., 2001; Carvalho et al., 2005). The clinical features of hyperparathyroid myopathy include proximal muscle weakness and wasting with preserved or even brisk reflexes and mild nonspecific myopathic features on electromyogram and muscle biopsy. Aside from hypercalcemia, vitamin D deficiency, chronic phosphate deficiency, or neuropathy may contribute to myopathy (Riggs, 2002). Carpal tunnel syndrome has occasionally been associated with hyperparathyroidism (Palma, 1983).

Calcium is critical to neurotransmitter function and elevations in serum calcium have been postulated to have either a direct or indirect effect on cerebral function. PTH is also elevated in the cerebrospinal fluid of patients with hyperparathyroidism compared with controls, although it is uncertain if this contributes to the neuropsychiatric manifestations. Neuropsychiatric manifestations of primary hyperparathyroidism range from subtle personality changes to stupor and coma. Memory problems, dementia, confusion, delirium, and obtundation have been reported. In addition, psychotic behavior, catatonia, and mania have been described. A Creutzfeldt–Jakob-like syndrome, manifesting with subacute dementia and a gait disorder, has also been described in primary hyperparathyroidism (Chadenat et al., 2009).

Hyperparathyroidism has also rarely been associated with severe CNS dysfunction, including ataxia, internuclear ophthalmoplegia, corticospinal tract dysfunction, dysarthria, and dysphagia.

Classic neuromuscular and neuropsychiatric disease are rare in mild PHPT, although weakness and easy fatigability remain common complaints. Other common complaints include depression, cognitive impairment, loss of initiative, anxiety, irritability, sleep disturbances, and somatization (Walker and Silverberg, 2007; Silverberg et al., 2009). These nonspecific symptoms may or may not improve with surgery (Silverberg, 2002)

Data regarding the presence, extent, and reversibility of psychological and cognitive features of primary hyperparathyroidism (PHPT) are conflicting. Multiple trials have also shown variable results in terms of functional/physical functioning. One study sought to clarify the nature of cognitive and affective impairments in PHPT and changes postparathyroidectomy. Of 111 patients with PHPT who underwent neuropsychological evaluation prior to parathyroidectomy, 68 returned for an early postsurgical evaluation. In a subset of patients, assessment revealed a significant pattern of cognitive slowing, reductions in psychomotor speed, memory impairment, and depression prior to parathyroidectomy. Postsurgical evaluations revealed a trend for improvements on timed tests and depression but a decline in memory. Older patients and the patients with more

dramatic changes in biochemical status following surgery responded less well to surgical intervention. One prospective study looked at patients with PHPT and evaluated them pre- and postoperatively with validated psychometric and neurocognitive testing to determine whether learning, memory, or concentration improved after parathyroidectomy. Analysis revealed that a spatial learning deficit and delayed processing occurred in patients with primary hyperparathyroidism and these improved after parathyroidectomy. In addition, individuals with a greater change in PTH were more likely to improve in their learning efficiency postparathyroidectomy and there were no differences in depressive symptoms or verbal memory in the pre- versus postoperative groups (Roman et al., 2005).

One study looked at 18 asymptomatic older (>50 years) patients with biochemically confirmed PHPT who did not meet US National Institutes of Health (NIH) consensus conference criteria for undergoing a parathyroidectomy. They were randomly assigned to either a surgical group (parathyroidectomy) or a control group (observation). All patients were functionally similar at baseline; all underwent functional testing which included a 6 minute walk test at baseline/presurgery and at 6 weeks and 6 months after surgery or baseline. Six minute walk distance increased in the surgery group by 184 feet, a distance that is both significant ($p < 0.05$) and clinically meaningful. The improvement in 6 minute walk distance observed in the surgery group suggests that parathyroidectomy can improve functional capacity, and hence the performance of activities of daily living in asymptomatic, older PHPT patients (Morris et al., 2010).

Another study looked at the impact of parathyroidectomy (PTX) on brain function and sleep in 18 "asymptomatic" PHPT patients. These patients were randomly assigned to parathyroidectomy versus observation. Functional magnetic resonance imaging (MRI) of the brain, sleep assessment, and validated neuropsychological battery were performed at baseline, 6 weeks, and 6 months. This study revealed that decreased serum PTH levels correlated with improved sleep and that parathyroidectomy decreased sleepiness (which correlated with better performance on executive function) in patients with asymptomatic PHPT (Perrier et al., 2009). Another nonrandomized study also revealed increased sleep disturbance and neurocognitive impairment in patients with PHPT, with improvement after parathyroidectomy (Mittendorf et al., 2007).

A large, controlled, multinational study randomized 191 patients with asymptomatic mild hyperparathyroidism to either parathyroidectomy or medical observation to study the effects on morbidity, quality of life (QOL) and psychiatric symptoms. The SF-36 and comprehensive psychopathologic rating scale (CPRS) are validated and reliable methods that were used to assess symptoms. CPRS can be used to screen for the presence and severity of psychotic, mood, and neurotic disorders. At baseline, the patients had significantly lower QOL and more psychological symptoms, compared with age- and sex-matched healthy subjects. However, in this study, surgery did not provide consistent improvement over medical observation in terms of psychological domains of functioning or psychiatric symptoms (Bollerslev et al., 2007). A prospective study also revealed significantly decreased quality of life (assessed by a mental and physical functioning score) in the group with primary hyperparathyroidism versus controls. Preoperative neuropsychological symptoms were related to the serum calcium levels. In this study, however, postoperative health-related QOL improved significantly in addition to symptoms of depression and anxiety (Weber et al., 2007). Another prospective randomized study looked at 50 patients with mild asymptomatic hyperparathyroidism and tried to determine if there was any benefit in terms of BMD and also QOL. These 50 patients were randomly assigned to parathyroidectomy or no parathyroidectomy and were evaluated at 6 months and at 1 year. This study revealed a significant improvement in BMD at the hip and spine and QOL (based on four QOL measures: bodily pain, vitality, general health, and mental health) in patients with mild asymptomatic PHPT who underwent a parathyroidectomy (Ambrogini et al., 2007).

One case-control study revealed that at baseline, women with PHPT had significantly higher symptom scores for depression and anxiety than controls and worse performance on tests of verbal memory and nonverbal abstraction. Depressive symptoms, nonverbal abstraction, and some aspects of verbal memory improved after parathyroidectomy (Walker et al., 2009).

Management

Parathyroidectomy is the definitive therapy for primary hyperparathyroidism. The procedure is curative-in > 90% of individuals in the hands of an experienced parathyroid surgeon (Bilezikian, 2000). However, the decision to operate on all patients with primary hyperparathyroidism is controversial, especially in the setting of asymptomatic hyperparathyroidism. This is because a number of prospective, nonrandomized studies have suggested that bone mineral density, renal function, serum calcium, and PTH levels remain stable in the majority of asymptomatic patients during periods of observation as long as 10 years. Bisphosphonates, hormone replacement therapy, and calcimimetics are alternative options for those who have mild disease,

those who have persistent disease, those who are poor surgical candidates, and those who decline surgery.

The Third International Workshop on Primary Hyperparathyroidism held in 2008 recommended surgery for the following situations: a calcium level more than 1 mg/dL above the upper limit of normal; creatinine clearance less than 60 mL/minute; age less than 50 years; T score less than −2.5 at the spine, hip, and/or radius or history of fragility fracture. For less severe bone disease, antiresorptive therapy is an alternative to surgical intervention. A meta-analysis looking at the optimal management of the skeletal consequences of mild primary hyperparathyroidism (PHPT) revealed that surgical treatment and antiresorptive therapies increase BMD in mild PHPT to a similar degree, and each represents a reasonable option in a patient with mild PHPT and low BMD. Untreated subjects had significant bone loss; the rates of loss ranged from 0.6% to 1.0% per year. Analysis of studies reporting data beyond 2 years of follow-up demonstrated stable increases in BMD after surgery and stable BMD or slow loss (0.1–0.3%/year) in untreated PHPT (Sankaran et al., 2010).

Urinary calcium excretion > 400 mg/day is no longer an indication for surgery as it was in the 1990 and 2002 consensus panel guidelines. This is because urinary calcium excretion has low precision and varies with age, sex, race, and dietary calcium intake and vitamin D status as well as glomerular filtration rate. Moreover, urinary calcium is only one of multiple risk factors affecting the development of kidney stones. The other risk factors include urinary volume, oxalate levels, uric acid, pH, and citrate. In addition, a high urinary calcium is not associated with the development of stones in patients who have not yet formed stones (Silverberg et al., 2009).

Some have argued that cardiovascular effects in mild PHPT should be included in the criteria for surgery referral. However, studies looking at cardiovascular manifestations in mild disease have been inconsistent. Also, studies looking at surgery and resolution of cardiovascular manifestations in mild PHPT have been inconsistent. HTN does not resolve after parathyroidectomy. Left ventricular hypertrophy (LVH) has been found to regress after parathyroidectomy in some but not all studies. Also, several studies of patients with mild PHPT have not found an increased cardiovascular mortality (Silverberg et al., 2009).

Neuropsychiatric symptoms were not added as an indication for parathyroidectomy because of inconsistent data on their precise nature, association with underlying disease, and reversibility. In addition, these symptoms are difficult to quantify. The current NIH guidelines for curative, surgical intervention of PHPT exclude the 80% of patients with asymptomatic hyperparathyroid disease who have subjective neurobehavioral and physical symptoms affecting quality of life.

Some have argued that neuromuscular and neuropsychiatric effects should be included in the criteria for surgery referral. However, studies looking at surgery and resolution of neuromuscular and neuropsychiatric manifestations have been inconsistent (Coker et al., 2005; Silverberg et al., 2009). Moreover, most studies looking at the reversibility of cognitive effects with surgery in mild hyperparathyroidism are suboptimal, limited by observational design, small sample sizes, inclusion of subjects with symptomatic hyperparathyroidism, lack of appropriate control groups, lack of objective testing, or short follow-up time. Others are suboptimal as a result of the nonspecific effects of surgery, selection bias, or confounding factors.

Two major studies doing an extensive literature review have suggested improvement in quality of life after parathyroidectomy; psychiatric and cognitive benefits are more variable. Coker et al. (2005) did an electronic search reviewing prospective studies in which cognitive functioning was measured with formal neuropsychological (NP) testing and health-related quality of life (HRQL) was measured with valid and reliable instruments before and following parathyroidectomy for PHPT. Six small studies of cognitive functioning report inconsistent findings. Seven well-designed studies of HRQL report improvement across multiple domains following surgery. The authors concluded that formal NP testing and evaluation of HRQL are useful tools that may assist physicians in choosing whom to refer for parathyroidectomy. Roman and Sosa (2007) also performed a rigorous review of the most recent advances and studies that measured health-related quality of life, neurocognitive and psychiatric changes, as well as neurophysiologic imaging in patients with primary hyperparathyroidism undergoing parathyroidectomy. In studies conducted pre- and postparathyroidectomy, six studies have described improvements in health-related quality of life. Five studies included evaluations with validated psychiatric and cognitive tests in prospective case-control trials, but showed varied improvements in depression, memory, and concentration after parathyroidectomy.

HYPOCALCEMIA

Classification

Hypocalcemia can result from a failure to secrete PTH, altered responsiveness to PTH, a deficiency of vitamin D, or a resistance to vitamin D. Hypocalcemia may also occur secondary to abnormal magnesium metabolism or in clinical situations in which multiple factors (pancreatitis, sepsis, and critical illness) play contributing roles. Severe acute hypocalcemia most frequently occurs after thyroid or parathyroid surgery (Cooper and Gittoes, 2008).

Clinical features

Most patients who have mild hypocalcemia are asymptomatic, but large or abrupt changes in ionized calcium may lead to symptoms (Moe, 2008). Most of the signs and symptoms of hypocalcemia occur secondary to increased neuromuscular excitability (Riggs, 2002). The increased neuromuscular reactivity manifest as hyperactive deep tendon reflexes, Chvostek's and Trousseau's signs (Moe, 2008). Chvostek's sign refers to twitching or spasm of the facial muscles elicited by tapping on the facial nerve in front of the earlobe. Trousseau's sign refers to the spasm of the outstretched hand that occurs after 3 minutes of inflating a blood pressure cuff 20 mmHg above the systolic blood pressure. Trousseau's sign is more specific than Chvostek's (Moe, 2008). Positive Trousseau's sign can be seen in 4% and Chvostek's sign in up to 25% of normal individuals.

Clinically, the hallmark of severe hypocalcemia is tetany, a state of spontaneous tonic muscular contraction. Tetany originates in the peripheral nerve axon and is caused by spontaneous, irregular, repetitive nerve action potentials. The classic presentation is carpopedal spasm which is preceded by perioral and acral numbness. Opisthotonos may occur if spasms involve the trunk. Bronchospasm and laryngeal stridor may ultimately occur.

Hypocalcemia may predispose to central nervous system effects, including irritability, anxiety, agitation, confusion, delirium, delusions, hallucinations, psychosis, depression, focal or generalized seizures, pseudotumor cerebri, papilledema, confusion, and organic brain syndrome. Longstanding hypocalcemia, even without neuromuscular symptoms, is associated with neuropsychiatric symptoms and occasionally raised intracranial pressure (Cooper and Gittoes, 2008). Chronic hypocalcemia in children may lead to mental retardation.

The other signs and symptoms attributable to hypocalcemia occur secondary to deposition of calcium into soft tissues such as the pancreas (contributing to pancreatitis), the eyes (contributing to cataract formation), the basal ganglion (contributing to movement disorders such as chorea and parkinsonism).

Treatment

Intravenous calcium gluconate is recommended in those presenting with acute hypocalcemia and neuromuscular irritability. In milder hypocalcemia, the treatment depends upon the underlying etiology. Vitamin D supplementation, in the form of cholecalciferol or ergocalciferol, is needed in vitamin D deficiency. Vitamin D supplementation, in the form of calcitriol, is needed in hypoparathyroidism since there is no conversion from inactive to active vitamin D without PTH (Cooper and Gittoes, 2008).

HYPOPARATHYROIDISM AND PSEUDOHYPOPARATHYROIDISM

Hypoparathyroidism may be surgical, idiopathic, familial, autoimmune, infiltrative, or idiopathic. The hallmarks are hypocalcemia, hyperphosphatemia, and an inappropriately low or normal PTH, with a few exceptions. When PTH is normal, it is usually within the lower part of the reference range (Cooper and Gittoes, 2008). Hypoparathyroidism causes hypocalcemia because PTH secretion is inadequate; calcium cannot be mobilized from the bone or reabsorbed from the distal nephron; in addition, there is no activation of renal 1α-hydroxylase activity and as a result, there is insufficient 1,25-dihydroxyvitamin D, which leads to decreased intestinal absorption of calcium (Shoback, 2008).

The most common cause of hypoparathyroidism is surgery on the neck, with removal or destruction of the parathyroid glands. Tetany occurs 1–2 days postoperatively. Postoperatively, there may be impaired blood supply to the parathyroid gland, often referred to as stunning, which results in inadequate PTH secretion. However, PTH secretion may resolve when the gland recovers its blood supply. Because of this phenomenon, half of the patients with hypoparathyroidism after surgery will not need permanent treatment.

Parathyroidectomy for primary hyperparathyroidism in those with severe hyperparathyroid bone disease may result in hypocalcemia. This phenomenon of "hungry bone syndrome" is because calcium and phosphate are avidly taken up by the bone and the parathyroids cannot compensate. This condition can be distinguished from the above based on elevated PTH and low phosphorus.

Aside from surgery, destruction of the parathyroid glands may also occur secondary to an autoimmune or infiltrative process. Type I polyglandular autoimmune syndrome includes hypoparathyroidism, adrenal insufficiency, and mucocutaneous candidasis. In this syndrome, hypoparathyroidism results from the formation of antibodies against the parathyroid glands and typically occurs about 5–9 years of age. This syndrome is also associated with adrenal insufficiency and mucocutaneous candidiasis. Hypoparathyroidism can also be caused by accumulation of iron (in hemochromatosis or transfusion-dependent thalassemia) or copper (in Wilson disease) in the parathyroid glands or metastatic infiltration of the parathyroid glands by tumor. Iodine 131 therapy for thyroid disease is a rare cause of hypoparathyroidism.

Both hypomagnesemia and acute severe hypermagnesemia may be responsible for the development of functional hypoparathyroidism. They can impair release of PTH and lead to hypocalcemia; in addition, hypomagnesemia and hypermagnesemia can blunt the peripheral actions of PTH. Cisplatin, aminoglycosides, and amphotericin are the most common causes of drug-induced hypomagnesemia; loop diuretics can also contribute to hypomagnesemia. Long-term use of magnesium-containing drugs such as antacids and laxatives, in the setting of renal failure, are common causes of hypermagnesemia (Liamis et al., 2009).

Hypoparathyroidism may also be secondary to genetic disorders of PTH biosynthesis and parathyroid gland development. Etiologies include *PTH* gene mutations, mutations or deletions in transcription factors and other regulators of the development of the parathyroid glands, and mitochondrial gene mutations. Features such as growth failure, congenital anomalies, hearing loss, or retardation point to a genetic disease (Shoback, 2008).

Pseudohypoparathyroidism is the term used to describe a group of rare disorders characterized by hypocalcemia and hyperphosphatemia but elevated PTH, indicating unresponsiveness or resistance to PTH at the tissue level (Moe, 2008). The most common form of pseudohypoparathyroidism is type Ia, Albright's hereditary osteodystrophy. This disease is characterized by short stature, round facies, obesity, mental retardation, brachydactyly, frontal bossing, and ectopic ossifications (Shoback, 2008).

Clinical manifestations

The neurologic manifestations of hypoparathyroidism resulting from primary, secondary, or pseudohypoparathyroidism (parathyroid hormone-resistant syndromes) largely reflect hypocalcemia (refer to section on hypocalcemia). The duration, severity, and rate of development of hypocalcemia determine the clinical presentation. Hypoparathyroidism may present as reversible peripheral neuropathy (Goswami et al., 2002). Chronic hypoparathyroidism may present with extensive intracranial calcifications of the basal ganglia (Kowdley et al., 1999; Jabr et al., 2004; Mejdoubi and Zegermann, 2006); involvement of the basal ganglia may present as tetany and seizures in addition to parkinsonism and dementia (Verulashvili et al., 2006).

Hypocalcemia secondary to hypoparathyroidism is a rare cause of reversible congestive heart failure; it must be considered in the differential diagnosis in someone presenting with heart failure that is not responding to traditional treatment; cardiac function improves after restoration of normocalcemia (Altunbas et al., 2003; Kazmi and Wall, 2007).

Treatment

Hypermagnesemia and severe magnesium depletion should be ruled out first as these could cause reversible impairment of PTH secretion. Slightly low serum calcium levels with a detectable but inappropriately low PTH may indicate hypomagnesemia (Shoback, 2008). Severe magnesium depletion should be treated; dialysis may be indicated in hypermagnesemia. In all other situations of hypoparathyroidism, the only mechanism to increase serum calcium in hypoparathyroidism is via intestinal absorption. This is achieved by the administration of vitamin D (preferably the active form, calcitriol, because of its potency and its rapid onset of action) and oral calcium (Moe, 2008; Shoback, 2008). When parathyroid hormone is absent or nonfunctional, hypercalciuria may occur. Therefore, thiazide diuretics may be indicated to increase the renal tubular reabsorption of calcium, reducing hypercalciuria (Marx, 2000). Intravenous calcium therapy is only indicated in severe symptomatic hypocalcemia (i.e., seizures, laryngospasm, bronchospasm, significant electrocardiographic changes, cardiac failure, and altered mental status). If hyperphosphatemia is a problem, dietary restriction of phosphorus or phosphate binders are acceptable options (Shoback, 2008).

MAGNESIUM AND PHOSPHORUS DISORDERS

Magnesium

Some 66% of the total body stores of magnesium are in bone, 33% in the intracellular compartment, and 1% in the extracellular compartment. Magnesium homeostasis (in addition to calcium and phosphorus) is controlled by serum concentrations of the ion and regulating hormones (i.e., PTH) that act on three target organs: bone, intestine, and kidney. Severe hypomagnesemia stimulates PTH secretion which in turn increases bone resorption by multiple mechanisms. However, hypomagnesemia may also impair synthesis or secretion of PTH or contribute to end organ resistance to the action of PTH and contribute to worsening hypomagnesemia. Magnesium supplementation in this situation leads to a rapid rise in plasma PTH (Weisinger and Bellorin-Font, 1998).

Dietary intake of magnesium is a critical determinant of magnesium levels (Dacey, 2001) as intestinal magnesium absorption is a passive process. Renal magnesium absorption involves both passive and active processes. Most absorption occurs in the proximal tubule and the thick ascending limb of the loop of Henle with only 5% occurring in the distal tubule.

CLASSIFICATION OF HYPOMAGNESEMIA

Hypomagnesemia is very common. One study found that 7–12% of inpatients and 20% of ICU patients had hypomagnesemia. Hypomagnesemia is commonly associated with other electrolyte abnormalities including hypokalemia (in up to 40–60%), hypocalcemia (Weisinger and Bellorin-Font, 1998), hyponatremia (Topf and Murray, 2003), and hypophosphatemia.

The differential diagnosis of hypomagnesemia involves four main categories: (1) reduced intake secondary to starvation, alcohol abuse, or prolonged postoperative state; (2) acute intracellular shift of magnesium secondary to metabolic acidosis, insulin administration for DKA, hungry bone syndrome after parathyroidectomy, catecholamine excess states including alcohol withdrawal, and acute pancreatitis; pancreatitis can lead to hypomagnesemia because of sequestration of magnesium-rich fluid within the pancreas combined with losses through nasogastric suctioning and diarrhea; (3) reduced absorption which includes a specific gastrointestinal magnesium malabsorption syndrome (secondary to a rare inborn error of metabolism) or generalized malabsorption syndrome (secondary to extensive bowel resection), diffuse bowel disease and/or chronic diarrhea; (4) extrarenal factors that increase magnesuria which include drugs (diuretics, aminoglycosides, antibiotics, digoxin, cisplatin, amphotericin B, foscarnet, and ciclosporin), hormones (hyperaldosteronism, hyperthyroidism, and hypoparathyroidism, syndrome of inappropriate antidiuretic hormone secretion (SIADH)), hypercalcemia, hypophosphatemia, and alcohol ingestion. Any acute renal injury, particularly renal tubular injury, may promote wasting of magnesium (Dacey, 2001). There are also two congenital conditions associated with a primary renal tubular magnesium wasting. Both are characterized by hypokalemia, metabolic alkalosis, and normotension. Bartter's syndrome is also characterized by hypercalciuria, nephrocalcinosis, and a tubular acidification defect; Gitelman's syndrome is associated with hypocalciuria and a defect in the gene encoding for the thiazide-sensitive Na+/Cl− cotransporter (Weisinger and Bellorin-Font, 1998).

Hypomagnesemia may also be secondary to correction of chronic systemic acidosis, postobstructive nephropathy, renal transplantation, and the diuretic phase of acute tubular necrosis. Magnesium wasting in these clinical situations is due to tubular dysfunction in the recovering kidney. Diabetes mellitus is the most common cause of hypomagnesemia (Mouw et al., 2005), secondary to glycosuria and osmotic diuresis.

CLINICAL MANIFESTATIONS OF HYPOMAGNESEMIA

Magnesium has a profound effect on neural excitability; the most characteristic signs and symptoms of magnesium deficiency are produced by neural and neuromuscular hyperexcitability. The neurologic manifestations of hypomagnesemia are similar to those of hypocalcemia and include hyperirritability with agitation, apathy, depression, delirium, confusion, convulsions, generalized muscle weakness, tremors of extremities and of the tongue, Chvostek's sign, paresthesias, and tetany. A tetany syndrome has been described, which encompasses a constellation of clinical findings including muscle spasms, cramps, hyperarousal, hyperventilation, and asthenia in addition to Chvostek's and Trousseau's. Other features of this syndrome may include migraine attacks, transient ischemic attacks, sensorineural hearing loss, and convulsions (Galland, 1991). Other manifestations of hypomagnesemia include vertigo, nystagmus, myoclonus, and hyperreflexia. These signs and symptoms typically occur when serum magnesium is less than 0.8 mEq/L. Cortical blindness has also been associated with hypomagnesemia (Al-Tweigeri et al., 1999). Occasionally, focal neurologic signs may be seen in patients with hypomagnesemia.

Magnesium is vital to carbohydrate metabolism. Magnesium influences glucose and insulin homeostasis, and hypomagnesemia is associated with the metabolic syndrome (Volpe, 2008). Hypomagnesemia could potentially increase the risk of atherosclerosis, since experimental magnesium deficiency has resulted in hypertriglyceridemia and hypercholesterolemia.

Hypomagnesemia has cardiovascular effects. Hypomagnesemia enhances arterial sensitivity to vasoconstrictor agents, attenuates responses to vasodilators, promotes vasoconstriction and increases peripheral resistance, leading to hypertension (Sontia and Touyz, 2007). Hypomagnesemia is associated with a prolonged PR interval, prolonged QRS interval, T wave inversion, and the appearance of U waves (Topf and Murray, 2003). Hypomagnesemia has been implicated in severe ventricular arrhythmias, especially in the settings of acute ischemic heart disease, congestive heart failure, torsades de pointes, after cardiopulmonary bypass, in the acutely ill patient in the intensive care unit, and as a risk factor for developing coronary heart disease (Agus and Agus, 2001). Chronic hypomagnesemia has also been associated with a cardioskeletal mitochondrial myopathy.

Persistent magnesium deficiency has been implicated as a risk factor for osteoporosis and osteomalacia, especially in patients with chronic alcoholism, diabetes mellitus, and malabsorption syndromes (Rude and Olerich, 1996).

TREATMENT

The choice of route of magnesium repletion depends on the severity of the clinical findings. When convulsions occur in patients with hypomagnesemia, intravenous magnesium sulfate is required. However, an acute infusion of magnesium could decrease magnesium reabsorption in the loop of Henle, with most of the infused magnesium excreted in the urine. For this reason, oral replacement is usually preferred, especially in the symptom-free patients (Weisinger and Bellorin-Font, 1998).

Hypermagnesemia

Magnesium is regulated by the kidneys. The kidney responds rapidly to elevated serum magnesium levels. Therefore, hypermagnesemia is uncommon and is primarily seen in the setting of renal failure with excessive magnesium intake. Excessive magnesium intake can occur by the oral, intravenous route or by means of enema.

Massive oral ingestion can exceed renal excretory capacity, especially if there is underlying renal failure. Magnesium is found in over-the-counter antacids, in many laxatives, in enemas, and in herbal supplements. Severe hypermagnesemia has been described with accidental poisoning with Epsom salts, in laxative abusers, and in those receiving magnesium as catharsis for drug overdose. In addition, those with active gastrointestinal disease (including peptic ulcer disease, gastritis, colitis) can have enhanced magnesium absorption with subsequent hypermagnesemia. Substantial quantities of magnesium can also be absorbed from the large bowel following a magnesium enema. Intravenous magnesium is commonly used to decrease neuromuscular excitability in pregnant women with severe pre-eclampsia or eclampsia.

Mild hypermagnesemia (defined as magnesium < 3 mEq/L) can occur in a variety of other clinic settings including some cases of primary hyperparathyroidism, familial hypocalciuric hypercalcemia, diabetic ketoacidosis, hypercatabolic states (such as in tumor lysis syndrome), lithium ingestion, milk-alkali syndrome, and adrenal insufficiency.

CLINICAL MANIFESTATIONS

In contrast to hypomagnesemia, the neurologic manifestations of hypermagnesemia are characterized by nervous system depression (Riggs, 2002). Clinical manifestations of hypermagnesemia typically correlate with the degree of hypermagnesemia. Nausea, flushing, headache, lethargy, drowsiness, and diminished deep tendon reflexes may be seen with a plasma magnesium concentration of 4–6 mEq/L. Somnolence and absent deep tendon reflexes may be seen with a plasma concentration of 6–10 mEq/L. Hypermagnesemia at this level may also inhibit PTH secretion and lead to hypocalcemia. Muscular paralysis, which is the result of neuromuscular transmission blockade, is the predominant neurologic manifestation in severe hypermagnesemia. When the respiratory muscles are involved, subsequent hypoxia, hypercarbia, coma, and ultimately death ensues.

Intracellular magnesium profoundly blocks several cardiac potassium channels which accounts for the cardiac manifestations. Hypotension, bradycardia, electrocardiographic features such as an increase in the PR interval, QRS duration and QT interval may be seen with a plasma concentration of 6–10 mEq/L. Further prolongation of the QT interval can lead to complete heart block and cardiac arrest.

TREATMENT

The treatment in hypermagnesemia-induced arrhythmias is calcium; hemodialysis is indicated in symptomatic hypermagnesemia (characterized by refractory hypotension, mental obtundation, and respiratory arrest) (Hirose et al., 2002).

Congenital and acquired phosphorus disorders

Approximately 85% of the total adult body store of phosphorus is contained in bone in the form of hydroxyapatite. Of the remainder, 14% is intracellular and only 1% is extracellular.

Inorganic phosphorus is critical for numerous normal physiologic functions including skeletal development, mineral metabolism, energy transfer through mitochondrial metabolism, cell membrane phospholipid content and function, cell signaling, and even platelet aggregation. Between 60% and 70% of dietary phosphorus is absorbed by the gastrointestinal tract, in all segments. Phosphorus absorption depends on passive transport (related to the concentration in the intestinal lumen) and on active transport (stimulated by calcitriol). In the kidney, approximately 70–80% of the filtered load of phosphorus is reabsorbed in the proximal tubule, which serves as the primary regulated site of the kidney. The remaining approximately 20–30% is reabsorbed in the distal tubule.

Vitamin D, 1,25 OH and PTH are key hormone players in phosphorus regulation. When serum phosphorus levels decrease, the kidneys secrete 1α-hydroxylase, increasing the conversion of inactive to active vitamin D (calcitriol), which in turn increases intestinal phosphorus absorption and decreases urinary phosphorus excretion. When serum phosphorus levels increase, PTH is increased which increases urinary excretion of phosphorus.

Hypophosphatemia

CLASSIFICATION

Hypophosphatemia is often graded as mild (phosphorus < 3.5 mg/dL), moderate (phosphorus < 2.5 mg/dL) or severe (phosphorus < 1 mg/dL). Hypophosphatemia may occur secondary to internal redistribution of phosphorus from the extracellular fluid into the cell. Glycolysis leads to redistribution of phosphorus into the cell by formation of phosphorylated glucose compounds, with resultant hypophosphatemia. Glycolysis is stimulated in the following conditions: respiratory alkalosis secondary to hyperventilation, recovery from malnutrition, recovery from diabetic ketoacidosis, and insulin administration. Internal redistribution of phosphorus also occurs in parathyroidectomy for primary hyperparathyroidism. Phosphorus moves into the bone, contributing to hypophosphatemia (Weisinger and Bellorin-Font, 1998). Hypophosphatemia may also occur secondary to increased urinary excretion of phosphorus. This can occur in the following clinical conditions: primary hyperparathyroidism; secondary hyperparathyroidism in as a result of decreased vitamin D synthesis, or vitamin D resistance; familial disorders of vitamin D metabolism including vitamin D-dependent rickets and X-linked hypophosphatemic rickets; kidney transplant; malabsorption; renal tubular defects such as in Fanconi's syndrome; alcohol abuse, and metabolic or respiratory acidosis (Weisinger and Bellorin-Font, 1998). Finally, hypophosphatemia can occur secondary to decreased intestinal absorption. This can occur in the following clinical conditions: severe dietary phosphorus restriction, antacid abuse, and chronic diarrhea. Vitamin D deficiency secondary to malabsorption of vitamin D that occurs with diarrhea may exacerbate hypophosphatemia by enhancing phosphaturia (Weisinger and Bellorin-Font, 1998).

Pseudohypoparathyroidism encompasses a group of rare disorders characterized by hypocalcemia and hypophosphatemia but elevated PTH, indicating unresponsiveness to PTH at the tissue level.

CLINICAL MANIFESTATIONS

Hypophosphatemia contributes to altered bone and mineral metabolism and disorders of the skeletal muscle, cardiac, respiratory, hematologic, and central nervous systems. Many of these manifestations are related to decreased intracellular adenosine triphosphate. Common skeletal/smooth muscle manifestations include myopathy, dysphagia, and ileus; respiratory failure occurs with respiratory muscle involvement; depressed cardiac contractility occurs with cardiac muscle involvement. Rhabdomyolysis may occur in severe hypophosphatemia, especially in alcoholics. Hematologic manifestations include hemolysis, thrombocytopenia, impaired phagocytosis, and granulocyte chemotaxis. Neurologic manifestations, secondary to tissue ischemia, include irritability, confusion/encephalopathy, and even coma.

TREATMENT

Oral phosphorus is recommended in the treatment of hypophosphatemia. Intravenous phosphorus carries a high risk of severe hypocalcemia; however, intravenous phosphorus is indicated in severe symptomatic hypophosphatemia (Weisinger and Bellorin-Font, 1998).

Hyperphosphatemia

CLASSIFICATION

Hyperphosphatemia can occur from increased intestinal absorption, cellular release or rapid intracellular to extracellular shifts, or decreased renal excretion (Moe, 2008). Increased intestinal absorption is caused by large intake of phosphorus-containing laxatives or enemas, or by vitamin D overdose. Increased cellular release can occur in acute tumor lysis syndrome (most commonly after the initiation of cytotoxic therapy in patients with hematologic malignancies such as lymphoma, leukemia, and multiple myeloma (Liamis et al., 2009)), bowel infarction, rhabdomyolysis, hemolysis, hyperthermia, profound catabolic stress; these disorders can lead to renal injury further exacerbating hyperphosphatemia. Rapid cellular shifts can occur in acid–base disorders such as lactic acidosis, diabetic ketoacidosis, and respiratory acidosis (Weisinger and Bellorin-Font, 1998). Hypoparathyroidism, acromegaly, and thyrotoxicosis can also cause hyperphosphatemia by reducing urinary phosphorus excretion (Weisinger and Bellorin-Font, 1998). The kidneys respond rapidly to elevated phosphorus levels after dietary ingestion by excreting urinary phosphorus. Therefore, sustained hyperphosphatemia occurs predominantly in the setting of renal disease.

CLINICAL MANIFESTATIONS

Acute hyperphosphatemia generally does not cause symptoms. It is the resultant hypocalcemia (which occurs when excess phosphorus complexes with calcium and deposits in the soft tissues) that contributes to symptoms. The calcium phosphate depositions also contribute to symptoms by impairing the proper function of the heart, kidneys, vasculature, and other soft tissues. Signs and symptoms include decreased mental status, seizures, dysrhythmia, weakness, cramps, hyperreflexia, tetany, anorexia, nausea, vomiting, decreased visual acuity, conjunctivitis, renal failure, and papular eruptions (Shiber and Mattu, 2002).

TREATMENT

Hyperphosphatemia is best managed by treating the underlying disorder (i.e., administering intravenous fluids for rhabdomyolysis). No treatment is usually needed in the setting of normal renal function as hyperphosphatemia is self-resolving. Limiting dietary phosphate intake (by reducing protein intake) and blocking intestinal phosphate absorption with phosphate binders is indicated in mild persistent asymptomatic hyperphosphatemia in the setting of mild to moderate renal failure. Common oral phosphate binders include calcium carbonate, calcium acetate, and sevelamer (Moe, 2008). Hemodialysis may be required for severe hyperphosphatemia with symptomatic hypocalcemia (Shiber and Mattu, 2002).

OSTEOPOROSIS

Introduction

Osteoporosis is a skeletal disease in which reduced bone strength results in an increase in bone fragility and thus increases susceptibility to fractures. Bone strength takes into account not only bone mineral density (the amount of bone tissue) but also bone quality (the structure and material composition of bone) (Becker, 2008). Osteoporosis is defined by the World Health Organization in postmenopausal women as a bone mineral density 2.5 standard deviations below peak bone mass (the standard is the average bone density of a 20-year-old healthy female) as measured by dual energy X-ray absorptiometry (DXA). Bone quality includes other properties of bone including macroarchitecture (shape and geometry), microarchitecture (trabecular and cortical), matrix and mineral composition, as well as the degree of mineralization, microdamage accumulation, and the rate of bone turnover. These are not visualized on the DXA scan but do affect the structural and material properties of bone. These components must also be included in the algorithms of fracture detection. Fractures of the hip, vertebral body, and distal forearm are the typical osteoporotic fractures although there is an increased risk of almost any type of fracture. Worldwide, elderly people represent the fastest growing age group, and the yearly number of fractures is likely to rise substantially with continued aging of the population.

Etiology

Low peak bone mass, excessive bone resorption, or inadequate bone formation are the major processes that lead to osteoporosis. Estrogen deficiency, calcium deficiency, vitamin D deficiency, and hyperparathyroidism are the major underlying etiologies (Becker, 2008). Other etiologies include hypercalciuria, hyperthyroidism, testosterone deficiency, hypercortisolism, and multiple myeloma.

Clinical manifestations

Osteoporosis is generally a silent disease until a fragility fracture occurs. There is a high frequency of spinal fractures secondary to osteoporosis. Most spinal fractures usually show no serious spinal canal compromise or spinal instability. Most spinal fractures resulting from osteoporosis usually do not manifest with immediate neurologic deficits but they may lead to a gradual collapse of the vertebrae, ultimately resulting in progressive kyphosis, prolonged back pain and/or paraparesis (Ito et al., 2002). In particular, fractures of the middle vertebral column can lead to retropulsion of vertebral body fragments with significant canal compromise and neurologic injury; surgical intervention may be indicated. It is important to assess a patient with an osteoporotic fracture for neurologic deterioration (Nguyen et al., 2003).

The majority of osteoporotic, spinal cord compressive, vertebral fractures occurs at the thoracolumbar junction level (Blondel et al., 2009). Most of the neurologic symptoms may develop late and manifest as radiculopathy (Tezer et al., 2006); a decompression procedure may be indicated in certain cases.

Burst fractures may occur after a fall in osteoporosis. A burst fracture is a type of traumatic spinal injury in which a vertebra breaks from a high-energy axial load, with pieces of vertebra shattering into surrounding tissues and sometimes the spinal canal. Immediate hospitalization is required, as such injuries may result in varying degrees of spinal cord injury with possible paralysis. A retrospective study was performed on the operative results following osteoporotic burst fractures with neurologic compromise; 70% of the fractures occurred at the thoracolumbar junction. All the patients were treated operatively with decompression and arthrodesis with a mean time to follow-up of 16 months. Neurologic recovery occurred in six of the 10 patients; however, significant disability secondary to pain was common (Nguyen et al., 2003). Despite surgical intervention and neurologic recovery, pain remains a persistent problem.

Multiple thoracic fractures can result in restrictive lung disease, progressive back pain, and disabling kyphosis. Other sequelae include constipation, abdominal pain and distention, reduced appetite, premature satiety, and weight loss (Becker, 2008).

Osteoporotic fractures of the sacrum have also been reported; the most common symptoms include sphincter dysfunction and lower limb paresthesias (Finiels et al., 2002).

In summary, osteoporotic fractures may contribute to neurologic deficits, pain, and physical limitations. In addition, osteoporotic fractures can contribute to changes in lifestyle and appearance which can have damaging psychological effects, including depression, loss of self-esteem, anxiety, fear, anger, and strained relationships with family and friends (Becker, 2008).

Treatment

The major target of treatment is the inhibition of bone resorption by osteoclasts. The main class of antiresorptives currently in use are bisphosphonates; they decrease the numbers of vertebral and nonvertebral fractures. Estrogen, calcium, selective estrogen receptor modulators (SERMs) and calcitonin are other antiresorptives (Reid, 2008). A newer antiresorptive, denosumab, is a human monoclonal antibody that inhibits osteoclastic-mediated bone resorption by binding to osteoblast-produced RANKL. By reducing RANKL binding to the osteoclast receptor RANK, bone resorption and turnover decrease. It has been shown to increase bone mineral density (BMD) and decrease fracture risk in postmenopausal women with osteoporosis (Lewiecki, 2009). It has been approved for the treatment of postmenopausal women who have a high risk for osteoporotic fractures, including those with a history of fracture or multiple risk factors for fracture, or those who have failed or are intolerant to other osteoporosis therapy. Another target of treatment is bone formation. Recombinant teriparatide is the only agent in this category. Current limitations include limited length of treatment (2 years) and a high cost of therapy. Therefore, teriparatide is best reserved for the treatment of patients with osteoporosis at high risk of fracture, or for patients with osteoporosis who have unsatisfactory responses to or intolerance of other osteoporosis therapies (Blick et al., 2008).

PAGET'S DISEASE

Introduction

Paget's disease is a metabolic bone disease characterized by increased and disorganized bone turnover which results in excessive and dense but structurally deficient and weak bones. Paget's disease rarely occurs before 30 years of age. Paget's disease may involve one (monostotic) or multiple bones (polyostotic). The monostotic form, found in 15% of patients, commonly affects the tibia, ilium, femur, and skull. The polyostotic form commonly affects the pelvis, spine, and skull. The hands, feet, ribs, and fibula are rarely involved (Hullar and Lustig, 2003). Highest prevalence occurs in the US, Germany, France, Austria, England, Australia, and New Zealand (Hullar and Lustig, 2003). Genetic and environmental factors have been implicated in the disease (Ralston, 2008).

Clinical manifestations

Symptomatic Paget's is only seen in 15–20% of affected individuals (Hullar and Lustig, 2003). Pain is the most common symptom. Pain may be secondary to direct pagetic involvement or osteoarthropathy. Pain in the extremities may be caused by expansion of bone with involvement of the periosteum, whereas in the lumbar spine, pain may result from vertebral expansion or collapse as a result of microfractures. In contrast to pain from degenerative joint disease, pagetic pain is typically increased at night, when the limbs are warm, and upon weight bearing. The structural changes from disrupted bone architecture can interact with the mechanical requirements of the affected bone and/or the function of adjacent organs and lead to various other complications, both structural and functional.

Orthopedic complications are common; oncologic complications are rare. Involvement of the skull may result in skull enlargement and pain. Enlargement of the skull can lead to leontiasis ossea, making it difficult for the patient to hold the head erect. Involvement of the spine may result in skeletal pain and altered posture, predominantly kyphosis. Involvement of the weight bearing long bones such as the tibia or fibula may lead to skeletal deformation, i.e., bowing of the lower extremities. This deformation may result in abnormal mechanical stress on the bone and may lead to fissure and compression fractures. In addition, the deformation may result in a gait disturbance which may accelerate degenerative joint disease in the hip and/or the knee. However, Paget's disease itself may involve subchondral areas resulting in damage to cartilage and leading to osteoarthritis. In addition to osteoarthritis /degenerative joint disease, acute gouty arthritis and other inflammatory arthritides have been associated with Paget's disease, including rheumatoid arthritis, psoriatic arthritis, and ankylosing spondylitis (Ankrom and Shapiro, 1998). Neoplastic degeneration of pagetic bone, or osteosarcoma, may also occur but it is rare (<1% of patients). Osteosarcomas tend to occur in patients with long-standing, polyostotic disease and tend to affect patients in their seventh decade. The spine is usually not involved; the pelvis, femur, humerus, and skull are the more common sites of involvement (Hansen et al., 2006). Other tumors have been reported when Paget's involves the temporal bone, including neuroma, fibroma, and spindle cell sarcoma (Shonka and Kesser, 2006). Involvement of the temporomandibular joint can cause dental problems, including loosening and loss of teeth or spreading of teeth and malocclusion (Ankrom and Shapiro, 1998).

Neurologic complications can occur secondary to pagetic impingement of neural structures. When the temporal bone is involved, patients may report tinnitus and balance problems (Hullar and Lustig, 2003). When the skull base is involved, platybasia may occur. Platybasia is the malformation of the skull base, which may result in the forward displacement of the upper cervical vertebrae and bony impingement on the brainstem. Neurologic presentation varies secondary to the degree of compression and also the structures affected. The most common symptoms are neck pain, often associated with a headache and also signs and symptoms of spinal cord compression. Compression of the C2 root and the greater occipital nerve leads to neck pain, oftentimes spreading to the arms and accompanied by an occipital headache. Spinal cord compression involves the upper cervical cord and may affect the motor tracts resulting in spastic paresis in the arms, legs or both; joint position and vibration sense (posterior column function) are commonly affected; pain and temperature sense (spinothalamic tract) are rarely affected. Brain compression may also occur in platybasia and may cause brainstem, cranial nerve, and cerebellar deficits (Poncelet, 1999; Beer et al., 2006). Brainstem and cranial nerve deficits include sleep apnea, internuclear ophthalmoplegia, downbeat nystagmus, hoarseness, dysarthria, and dysphagia. Cerebellar deficits lead to impaired coordination. Vertebrobasilar ischemia can be triggered by changing head position; symptoms include intermittent syncope, vertigo, confusion or altered consciousness, weakness and visual disturbance (Beer et al., 2006). Syringomyelia (Raubenheimer et al., 2002) and hydrocephalus (Meca et al., 1997; Raubenheimer et al., 2002) have also been reported. Cranial nerve deficits secondary to narrowing of the neural foramina have been described but are uncommon. Optic foramen involvement may result in optic atrophy and papilledema. Ophthalmoplegia, anosmia, trigeminal neuralgia, and facial and bulbar palsy have also been described (Bone, 2006). The spine is the second most commonly affected site with Paget's disease. Pagetic involvement of the cervical and thoracic spine is more commonly associated with neural symptoms than pagetic involvement of the lumbar spine. Some patients with spinal involvement exhibit symptoms of clinical stenosis. Clinical spinal stenosis can be categorized as lateral or central. Lateral spinal stenosis may manifest as constant or intermittent leg pain (worsened by walking) with radicular distribution and associated with paresthesias. The pain may be associated with motor weakness, reflex and sensory changes. Central stenosis may manifest as leg weakness, cramps, and pain (worsened by walking). Central stenosis with myelopathy is associated with upper motor neuron manifestations (Hadjipavlou et al., 2001). Patients may have both lateral and central stenosis. Pagetic involvement of the cervical and thoracic spine tends to present with clinical spinal stenosis along with myelopathy. Compressive myelopathy can occur secondary to pagetic bone overgrowth, intraspinal soft tissue overgrowth, ossification of epidural fat, spontaneous bleeding, sarcomatous degeneration, and vertebral fracture or subluxation (Hadjipavlou et al., 2001). A cervical lesion with or without an odontoid fracture is rare but may result in atlantoaxial instability with resultant progressive spinal cervical cord compression (Tessitore et al., 2008). Involvement of the vertebra may also result in a vascular "steal" syndrome whereby the hypervascular pagetic bone may divert blood away from the spinal cord leading to ischemia. This may result in quadriparesis or paraparesis, which is reversible with treatment (Bone, 2006). Progressive paraparesis with bladder and bowel involvement may also occur (Ankrom and Shapiro, 1998).

Hearing loss is common when Paget's involves the temporal bone, but it is not well understood. The deficit is often mixed, with a predominantly low-frequency conductive loss and a high frequency sensorineural component. Ossicular fixation is not universally found in cases of conductive hearing loss. The disease may affect the middle and outer ear through increased ossicular mass or fusion, round or oval window distortion or obliteration, or concentric growth of the tympanic bone resulting in tympanic annulus constriction and relaxation of the tympanic membrane (Hullar and Lustig, 2003). There seems to be a lack of evidence supporting auditory nerve dysfunction with more support toward a cochlear site of lesion. The cochlear capsule may contribute to the acoustic and/or electrical properties of the cochlea so that involvement of the cochlea with Paget's may lead to high frequency pure tone hearing loss (Monsell et al., 1999; Bone, 2006).

Cardiovascular complications have also been described. Paget's disease can lead to high-output cardiac failure when there is extensive skeletal involvement (Bone, 2006). Paget's disease can also contribute to arterial wall calcification and has been implicated in coronary artery disease and peripheral vascular disease (Ankrom and Shapiro, 1998).

Diagnosis

Diagnosis may be confirmed by X-rays and by an elevated serum alkaline phosphatase.

An elevated alkaline phosphatase occurs in as many as 85% of individuals with untreated active Paget's disease (Josse et al., 2007). Alkaline phosphatase can be normal in patients with monostotic disease or in those with metabolically inactive disease (Ralston, 2008). Urinary hydroxyproline may also be elevated in active disease. Radiographic features include cortical thickening, sclerotic changes, and osteolytic areas (V-shaped lesions or flame-shaped lesions occur proximal to the distal epiphysis of a long bone with gradual progression to the opposite end and osteoporosis circumscripta in the skull) (Delmas

and Meunier, 1997). Vertebral lesions may be mistaken for malignant lesions. With disease evolution, the ingrowth of fibrovascular tissue and a high rate of bone remodeling may lead to enlarged dense vertebral bodies (Ankrom and Shapiro, 1998). X-rays are helpful but radionuclide bone scanning is the most reliable means of identifying pagetic lesions and should be performed at the time of diagnosis (Delmas and Meunier, 1997).

Treatment

Treatment with a bisphosphonate (intravenous zoledronic acid, pamidronate or oral risedronate and alendronate) is indicated in patients with Paget's disease who have symptoms referable to active disease and are likely to respond to treatment, such as bone pain, joint pain, and neurologic complications (Siris et al., 2006). Randomized placebo-controlled clinical trials have shown that bisphosphonate therapy reduces bone turnover, improves bone pain, promotes healing of osteolytic lesions, and restores normal bone histology in Paget's disease (Ralston, 2008). Intravenous zoledronic acid has been shown to have superior effects when compared to the oral bisphosphonates. Surgery is indicated as a primary treatment when neural compression is secondary to pathologic fractures, dislocations, spontaneous epidural hematoma, syringomyelia, platybasia, or sarcomatous transformation (Hadjipavlou et al., 2001). Bisphosphonates may be used preoperatively to reduce intraoperative blood loss from highly vascular pagetic bone and also in the management of rare instances of immobilization hypercalcemia. Treatment is also indicated in those who have no symptoms but with active disease in areas of the skeleton with the potential to produce complications of clinical importance (Delmas and Meunier, 1997; Siris et al., 2006). The sites associated with an increased risk of complications are the base of the skull (because of the risk of hearing loss), the spine (because of the risk of spinal cord compression), the long bones of the lower limbs (because of the risk of fracture), and the hip or knee (because of the risk of secondary osteoarthritis). The sites associated with little or no risk of complications include the iliac crest, sacrum, scapula, upper limbs, and ribs (Delmas and Meunier, 1997). Other drugs that may be used in the treatment of Paget's disease include calcitonin, and very infrequently, plicamycin (mithramycin), and gallium nitrate (Delmas and Meunier, 1997; Hadjipavlou et al., 2001).

HYPOPHOSPHATASIA

Introduction

Hypophosphatasia is a rare inherited disorder of bone metabolism. It is characterized by defective bone mineralization due to the impaired activity of tissue-nonspecific isoenzyme of alkaline phosphatase and elevated concentrations of its substrates, including pyrophosphates (Beck et al., 2009).

Clinical manifestatations

Clinical presentation is highly variable, ranging from stillbirth without mineralized bone to pathologic fractures in late adulthood. There are currently six recognized clinical forms: perinatal (lethal), perinatal benign, infantile, childhood, adult, and odontohypophosphatasia. The lethal perinatal form presents with impaired mineralization *in utero*. The infantile form presents with respiratory complications, premature craniosynostosis, widespread demineralization, and rachitic changes in the metaphyses. Failure to thrive and hypotonia have also been reported in infantile hypophosphatasia (Chou et al., 2005). The childhood form presents with skeletal deformities, short stature, and a waddling gait. The adult form presents with stress fractures, thigh pain, chondrocalcinosis, and marked osteoarthropathy. Odontohypophosphatasia presents with dental abnormalities such as premature loss of dentition or severe dental caries but no skeletal abnormalities (Mornet, 2007). The constellation of chronic multifocal periarticular pain and soft tissue swelling has been reported in some children. Diagnosis after biopsies of affected bone and imaging revealed chronic nonbacterial osteomyelitis (Whyte et al., 2009). Seizures have been reported in lethal perinatal hypophoshatasia (Litmanovitz et al., 2002; Nunes et al., 2002; Smilari et al., 2005) and infantile hypophosphatasia (Yamamoto et al., 2004).

Affected children typically present with rickets, growth delay, and dental problems. Affected adults typically present with fractures and bone pain (Moulin et al., 2009); adults often present with slowly healing metatarsal stress fractures and proximal femur pseudofractures (Whyte et al., 2007).

Diagnosis

The biochemical diagnosis is based on measurement of low levels of serum alkaline phophatase and increased serum or urine concentrations of phosphoethalnolamine, pyridoxal 5′-phosphate and inorganic pyrophosphate. The diagnosis is also based on DNA sequencing/molecular analysis of the liver/bone/alkaline phosphatase (*ALPL*) gene; the diagnosis is supported by radiographic imaging. DNA sequencing can detect approximately 95% of mutations found in severe (perinatal and infantile) hypophosphatasia. Genetic counseling of the disease is complicated by the variable inheritance pattern (autosomal dominant or autosomal recessive), the existence of the uncommon prenatal benign form, and by incomplete penetrance of the trait (Mornet, 2007).

Treatment

There is no curative treatment at this time; enzyme replacement therapy is not yet available. Symptomatic support with nonsteroidal anti-inflammatories (NSAIDs) has been shown to be helpful (Girschick et al., 2006). Teriparatide treatment has been shown to improve biochemical markers of bone remodeling and increase skeletal mineralization (Whyte et al., 2007; Camacho et al., 2008).

VITAMIN D AND CENTRAL NERVOUS SYSTEM FROM FETAL LIFE TO AGING, AND FROM GOOD HEALTH TO ILLNESS

It has long been accepted that vitamin D plays a crucial role in calcium homeostasis and the classic target organs for vitamin D are bone, kidney, intestine, and parathyroid gland. However, during the past few decades a variety of additional roles have been recognized for vitamin D; among these is the effect of vitamin D on neurogenesis, secretion and metabolism of neuropeptides, on neuromuscular function, and its role as a neuroprotective against various neurotoxins and inflammatory processes. Moreover, the importance of vitamin D in the neuronal system is also important for its effect on calcium homeostasis. Vitamin D is produced in the neuronal system and its function on the nervous system is demonstrated by the presence of vitamin D receptors on various neuronal cells. Furthermore, many studies have associated a lack of vitamin D with a variety of neuronal disorders.

The major endogenous source of vitamin D is that produced in the skin by a UVB- mediated, photolytic, nonenzymatic reaction that converts 7-dehydrocholesterol to previtamin D_3. Previtamin D_3 undergoes a subsequent nonenzymatic reaction (thermal isomerization conversion) to vitamin D_3. Then vitamin D_3 from skin is transported to the liver and in hepatic parenchyma it is converted, by cytochrome P450, to 25 HO-vitamin D_3 ($25HD_3$). The active form of vitamin D, calcitriol (1,25 dihydroxyvitamin $D = 1,25(OH)_2D_3$) is the product of 1-dehydroxylase in the kidney (Heaney, 2007).

Production and presence of vitamin D and its receptor in the central nervous system

Human and rodent brain express 1α-hydroxylase (Miller and Portale, 2000), the enzyme responsible for hydroxylation of $25HO-D_3$ to active $1,25(OH)_2D_3$ which in turn is catbolized by 25-hydroxyvitamin D_3 to 24-hydroxylase to a more active form of vitamin D. Furthermore, brain also expresses the nuclear vitamin D receptor (VDR) that is responsible for genomic effect of vitamin D in the brain. This member of the steroid nuclear family is widely distributed in the central nervous system, such as rodent cortex, cerebellum, mesopontine area, diencephalon, spinal cord, amygdala, hypothalamus, and hippocampus, with strong nuclear staining in CA1, CA3, and CA4 areas. VDR and 1α-hydroxylase are codistributed throughout the human adult and the rodent adult (Musiol et al., 1992; Walbert et al., 2001) and fetal brain, as early as ED12 (Burkert et al., 2003). The brain distribution of VDR is similar in human and rodents. In addition, VDR has been detected in microglia, astrocytes, oligodendrocytes (the cells that produce myelin) and Schwann cells in both the central and the peripheral nervous systems (Prufer et al., 1999; Baas et al., 2000; Langub et al., 2001). Calcitriol (1,25(OH)$_2$D$_3$) is strongly concentrated in those regions of brain involved in memory and cognition in both humans and animals (Musiol et al., 1992).

Vitamin D and neurogenesis

A growing body of evidence demonstrates that vitamin D has an important role in the early development of the central nervous system and in neurogenesis during adulthood (Baas et al., 2000). Adult stem cells are located in various areas of the brain such as the subgranular zone of the hippocampus and the dentate gyrus where cells are differentiated into neural and glial cells. Stem cells are also found in the olfactory bulb but it is believed that they are originally located in the subventricular region of the forebrain then later migrate to the olfactory bulb (Taupin and Gage, 2002; Watts et al., 2005). Interestingly, VDR is also expressed in the area of the brain rich with stem cells and it is shown that it plays an essential role in cell growth and neuronal cell differentiation. Calcitriol, in brain, enhances gene expression and production of neurotrophins (Woo and Lu, 2006) and other neuronal growth factors such as NGF, NT-3, NT-4/5, GDNF, and TGF-α2. They are considered as target genes for vitamin D in the central nervous system (CNS). Neurotrophins (NGF, NT-3, NT-4/5, and GDNF) support the survival and differentiation of neurons and enhance their function. NGF is mainly present in the hippocampus and neocortex and influences neuronal plasticity and neurotransmission (Siegel et al., 1999). NT-3 enhances neuronal transmission in the hippocampus (Kang and Schuman, 1995) and NT-4/5 (Rose et al., 2003) and is involved in calcium signaling. GDNF is a member of transforming growth factor α (TGF-α) and increases survival and differentiation of dompaminergic neurons in developing striatum of rat fetus (Siegel et al., 1999). Fetuses and newborn rodents with vitamin D deficiency are found to have reduced levels of NGF and GDNF and they have larger brain ventricles and longer cortex. Furthermore, calibindin-D28K, parvalbumin, and calretinin, three major calcium-binding proteins, are uniquely distributed in the brain and exhibit a temporal pattern during brain development, and all three molecules are modulated by vitamin D. These binding proteins function as calcium buffers, protect the neurons, and are involved in brain function, for example, motor neuron activity, learning, and memory. They also modulate secretion of various neurotransmitters (DeViragh et al., 1989; Baimbridge et al., 1992).

Absence of vitamin D disrupts the normal sequence of apoptotic/mitotic activities during brain development by acting at the transcriptional level. Mitotic rate is definitely increased in maternally vitamin D-depleted animals and apoptosis becomes impaired in the offspring of mothers with vitamin D deficiency (Ko et al., 2004). Furthermore, rats with vitamin D deficiency demonstrate anatomic brain abnormalities similar to aging animals (Stio et al., 1993). These rats also have reduced expression of neurotrophins in addition to decreased phosphorus and increased citric acid concentration. These vitamin D-deficient rats express increased acetylcholinesterase, glucose-6-phosphate dehydrogenase, and acylphosphatase activities in cortical synaptosomes, coupled with increased NAD+-dependent isocitrate dehydrogenase in cortical mitochondria (Stio et al., 1993). None of these changes were found in animals on a normal vitamin D diet (Stio et al., 1993). Administration of calcitriol into the rat's brain causes increased density of neuronal cells in the hippocampus (Schaller et al., 2005; Christophersen et al., 2007) and providing a diet rich in vitamin D to these animals improves axonal outgrowth and neuronal function during the recovery phase after a peripheral nerve injury (Schwaller et al., 2002). Moreover, vitamin D treatment is shown to significantly increase dopamine levels in the brainstem and homovanillic acid in striatum and hypothalamus (Tekes et al., 2009). It is also shown that vitamin D protect neurons against neurotoxicity of glutamate exposure (Taniura et al., 2006).

Collectively, this evidence suggests that vitamin D may enhance neurogenesis in CNS by neuronal cell differentiation and maturation during the developmental period, in adulthood, and after nerve injury, probably by various neurotrophins. Vitamin D also improves and/or facilitates neuronal function and protects neurons from neurotoxins.

Vitamin D and disorders of the nervous system

There are some convincing data regarding the association of vitamin D deficiency and various neurologic disorders such as aging, dementia, depression, and multiple sclerosis.

VITAMIN D, NEUROCOGNITION, AND PREMATURE AGING

The association between vitamin D and cognition and aging in humans has been reported in several clinical and population studies. A positive association between vitamin D level and memory and cognitive performance, particularly with measures of executive function, was seen in an elderly population in a cross-sectional study (Buell et al., 2009). Another cross-sectional study, investigating elderly individuals receiving home care, demonstrates a correlation between vitamin D deficiency or insufficiency and all-cause dementia, Alzheimer's, and stroke (Buell et al., 2010). In addition, lower vitamin D is associated with significantly more cerebrovascular pathology found on MRI (Buell et al., 2010). Moreover, in animal studies, VDRKO mice (Tokyo knockout mice that are commonly used for aging studies) with significantly lower growth factors such as NF-κ B, Fgf-23, p53, and IGFR, exhibit more motor disability (Keisala et al., 2009). These VDRKO mice are also reported to have thalamic calcification, progressive hearing loss, and vestibular problems during aging (Zou et al., 2008).

Féron et al. extended their previous study (Eyles et al., 2003) and compared brain from vitamin D-deficient offspring at 10 weeks of age with those of controls. They observed that vitamin D_3 deficiency during early life increases the size of lateral ventricular and reduces nerve growth factor protein content couples with reduction in expression of number of genes involved in neuronal structure, i.e., neurofilament or MAP-2 or neurotransmission, i.e., GABA-A(a4) in various parts of rats' brains (Féron et al., 2005). The authors concluded that transient vitamin D deficiency in early life not only disrupts brain development but leads to persistent brain structural and functional changes similar to those seen in aged animals. It is known that FgF-23 produced in bone increases vitamin D_3 production and in conjunction with Klotho acts on kidney to decrease renal phosphorus reabsorption. But FgF-23 and Klotho are also recognized as antiaging factors for neuronal tissue (Kuro-o, 2008). Antiaging activity of Klotho is observed in mice and its level is significantly diminished in VDRKO mice (Kuro-o, 2008).

VITAMIN D AND PARKINSON DISEASE

Demonstration of very high immunohistochemical staining for both VDRs and enzymes involved in vitamin D synthesis in the hypothalamus and the large neurons of the substantia nigra suggest the presence of autocrine/paracrine properties for vitamin D in these areas of the CNS which are rich in dopamine and a crucial site for movement and hormonal production (Eyles et al., 2005). The role of vitamin D in regulating body movement not only by improving muscular function but by working on the central nervous system is further supported by a previous study showing the regulatory role of 1,25 vitamin D in metabolism of acetylcholine and dopamine (Garcion et al., 2002). Vitamin D is shown to increase dopamine synthesis in CNS (Baksi and Hughes, 1982). Collectively, therefore, this information makes a strong argument for the presence of an interrelation between vitamin D deficiency and Parkinson disease (PD).

VITAMIN D AND DEPRESSION

Several epidemiologic studies and many animal studies have demonstrated an association between vitamin D and depression in the past. VDR and 1α-hydroxylase, the enzyme capable of metabolizing 25(OH)D to 1,25 $(OH)_2$ D, are both present in various parts of the human brain such as the prefrontal cortex, hippocampus, cingulate, thalamus, hypothalamus, and substantia nigra (Eyles et al., 2003, 2005). Many of these areas of the brain are implicated in the pathophysiology of depression and it further suggests the importance of vitamin D in neuronal function and mood changes. The observation that vitamin D protects the neurons exposed to methamphetamine which results in preventing the decline of serotonin and dopamine in striatum and accumbens in rats (Cass et al., 2006) may further support the role of vitamin D in protecting brain from depression . Moreover, it has been shown that vitamin D increases expression of genes encoding tyrosine hydroxylase, the precursor of norepinephrine, in the adrenal glands (Garcion et al., 2002). In addition, some studies show the possible presence of cross-talk between vitamin D and glucocorticoids in the hippocampus where both hormones have receptors (Obradovic et al., 2006). All these findings further support the role of vitamin D in metabolism of stress-related neurotransmitters in strategic locations of the CNS that are important in regulation of mood and depression.

Data from the longitudinal Aging Study Amsterdam have shown the presence of a significant negative correlation between mean serum 25(OH)D and depression assessed by the Center for Epidemiologic Studies Depression (CES-D) scale. The correlation remains significant even after adjusting for various factors such as age, gender, body weight, smoking, etc. (Hoogendijk et al., 2008). Others, however, have not observed any relation between vitamin D and depression using almost the same measures (Pan et al., 2009). Using observational studies to assess the correlation between vitamin D and depression is tainted by various factors such as the effect of depression on nutrition and outdoor activities, the very two factors required for attaining normal vitamin D levels in the body. However, a large prospective randomized study shows administration of almost 40 000 units/week of vitamin D was able to significantly improve depression scores/measures. This improvement in cognitive-affective disorders is more significant in females, in older people, and in individuals with larger BMIs (Jorde et al., 2008).

These are some preliminary animal and observational human studies suggesting the possibility of the influence of vitamin D in depression but clearly more information is required for the final verdict.

VITAMIN D AND MULTIPLE SCLEROSIS

Combinations of genetic and environmental factors have been identified as underlying problems for multiple sclerosis (MS). Among environmental factors, several studies have demonstrated a possible link between vitamin D and MS. A number of epidemiologic studies suggest an association between MS and exposure to sun, latitude, and serum level of vitamin D. A low prevalence of MS has been observed in Ecuador (Abad et al., 2008), located very close to the equator with plenty of sunshine and higher blood vitamin D concentration. Interestingly, the prevalence of MS increases in residents of countries further away from equator (Pierrot-Deseilligny, 2009). Moreover, it has been shown that the serum vitamin D level is lower in patients with MS and increasing serum concentration of vitamin D to 100 nmol in young people decreases the future risk for MS by 10-fold (Munger et al., 2006).

The immunomodulatory and anti-inflammatory roles for vitamin D are well accepted. In a healthy person, regulatory T cells (Treg) regulate the quantity and quality of the immune response and consequently may improve autoimmune disease. Of interest, the capacity of Treg cells in patients with MS is significantly compromised but interestingly vitamin D replacement is shown to improve Treg function and cause Th1/Th2 balance toward Th2 (Smolders et al., 2009). This clinical observation suggests vitamin D is a promotor of T cell regulation in patients with MS.

VITAMIN D AND EPILEPSY

The relation between seizure disorder and vitamin D is complicated. Severe vitamin D deficiency results in hypocalcemia that may cause seizures. In addition, antiepileptic medications such as phenytoin, phenobarbital, carbamazepine, or oxcarbazepine induce the hepatic cytochrome P450 system (Mintzer et al., 2006; Menon and Harinaryan, 2010) and accelerate vitamin D metabolism, which in turn causes vitamin D deficiency and hypocalcemia which worsen seizure disorders. Hypocalcemia is extensively reviewed in the other section of this review and I will talk about vitamin D deficiency during fetal life. Briefly, hypocalcemia secondary to vitamin D deficiency during fetal life and/or infancy causes seizures in newborns as young as 1 week (Holick et al., 2009). Vitamin D deficiency is very common when infants are born to mothers with vitamin D deficiency and are being fed breast milk only (Camadoo et al., 2007).

Based on these studies and many other epidemiologic, clinical, and observational studies we learn that vitamin D is present, produced and plays and important role in neurogenesis from the early developmental period to old age. Lack of vitamin D is probably a partial culprit in many CNS disorders. But most available studies either do not have the power to effectively show the relation between vitamin D level and CNS disorders or they are tainted with some problem with the design or methodology. Hopefully, in the future we will have better answers to our numerous questions on the role vitamin D in general and on the CNS in particular.

REFERENCES

Abad EP, Perez M, Alarcon T et al. (2008). Epidemiological evidence of multiple sclerosis in Ecuador. Mult Scler 14 (Suppl 1): S55–S56.

Agus MS, Agus ZS (2001). Cardiovascular actions of magnesium. Crit Care Clin 17: 175–186.

Al Zahrani A, Levine MA (1997). Primary hyperparathyroidism. Lancet 349: 1233–1238.

Altunbas H, Balci MK, Yazicioglu G et al. (2003). Hypocalcemic cardiomyopathy due to untreated hypoparathyroidism. Horm Res 59: 201–204.

Al-Tweigeri T, Magliocco AM, DeCoteau JF (1999). Cortical blindness as a manifestation of hypomagnesemia secondary to cisplatin therapy: case report and review of literature. Gynecol Oncol 72: 120–122.

Ambrogini E, Cetani F, Cianferotti L et al. (2007). Surgery or surveillance for mild asymptomatic primary hyperparathyroidism: a prospective randomized clinical trial. J Clin Endocrinol Metab 92: 3114–3121.

Andersson P, Rydberg E, Willenheimer R (2004). Primary hyperparathyroidism and heart disease – a review. Eur Heart J 25: 1776–1787.

Ankrom MA, Shapiro JR (1998). Paget's disease of bone (osteitis deformans). J Am Geriatr Soc 46: 1025–1033.

Ariyan CE, Sosa JA (2004). Assessment and management of patients with abnormal calcium. Crit Care Med 32 (Suppl): S146–S154.

Baas D, Prufer K, Ittel ME et al. (2000). Rat oligodendrocytes express the vitamin D(3). receptor and respond to 125-dihydroxyvitaminD(3). Glia 31: 59–68.

Baimbridge KG, Celio MR, Rogers JH (1992). Calcium-binding proteins in the nervous system. Trends Neurosci 15: 303–308.

Baksi SN, Hughes MJ (1982). Chronic vitamin D deficiency in the weanling rat alters catecholamine metabolism in the cortex. Brain Res 242: 387–390.

Beck C, Morbach H, Stenzel M et al. (2009). Hypophosphatasia. Klin Padiatr 221: 219–226.

Becker C (2008). Pathophysiology and clinical manifestations of osteoporosis. Clin Cornerstone 9: 42–47.

Beer MH, Porter RS, Jones TV (2006). The Merck Manual of Diagnosis and Therapy.

Bilezikian JP (2000). Primary hyperparathyroidism. When to observe and when to operate. Endocrinol Metab Clin North Am 29: 465–478.

Bilezikian JP, Brandi ML, Rubin M et al. (2005). Primary hyperparathyroidism: new concepts in clinical densitometric and biochemical features. J Intern Med 257: 6–17.

Blick SK, Dhillon S, Keam SJ (2008). Teriparatide: a review of its use in osteoporosis. Drugs 68: 2709–2737.

Blondel B, Fuentes S, Metellus P et al. (2009). Severe thoracolumbar osteoporotic burst fractures: treatment combining open kyphoplasty and short-segment fixation. Orthopaedics and Traumatology Surgery and Research 95: 359–364.

Bollerslev J, Jansson S, Mollerup CL et al. (2007). Medical observation compared with parathyroidectomy for asymptomatic primary hyperparathyroidism: a prospective randomized trial. J Clin Endocrinol Metabol 92: 1687–1692.

Bone HG (2006). Nonmalignant complications of Paget's disease. J Bone Miner Res 21 (Suppl 2): P64–P68.

Buell JS, Scott TM, Dawson-Hughes B et al. (2009). Vitamin D is associated with cognitive function in elders receiving home health services. J Gerontol A Biol Sci Med Sci 64: 888–895.

Buell JS, Dawson-Hughes B, Scott TM et al. (2010). 25-Hydroxyvitamin D dementia and cerebrovascular pathology in elders receiving home services. Neurology 74: 18–26.

Burkert R, McGrath J, Eyles D (2003). Vitamin D receptor expression in the embryonic rat brain. Neurosci Res Comm 33: 63–71.

Camacho PM, Painter S, Kadanoff R (2008). Treatment of adult hypophosphatasia with teriparatide. Endocr Pract 14: 204–208.

Camadoo L, Tibbott R, Isaza F (2007). Maternal vitamin D deficiency associated with neonatal hypocalcemic convulsions. Nutr J 6: 23.

Carvalho AA, Vieira A, Simplicio H et al. (2005). Primary hyperparathyroidism simulating motor neuron disease: case report. Arq Neuropsiquiatr 63: 160–162.

Cass WA, Smith MP, Peters LE (2006). Calcitriol protects against the dopamine- and serotonin-depleting effects of neurotoxic doses of methamphetamine. Ann N Y Acad Sci 1074: 261–271.

Chadenat ML, Dalloz MA, D'Anglejean J et al. (2009). Primary hyperparathyroidism as a differential diagnosis of Creutzfeldt–Jakob disease. Rev Neurol (Paris) 165: 185–188.

Chou YY, Ou HY, Wu TJ et al. (2005). Hypophosphatasia in Taiwan: report of two cases. Kaohsiung J Med Sci 21: 134–137.

Christophersen NS, Gronborg M, Petersen TN et al. (2007). Midbrain expression of delta-like 1 homologue is regulated by GDNF and is associated with dopaminergic differentiation. Exp Neurol 204: 791–801.

Coker LH, Rorie K, Cantley L et al. (2005). Primary hyperparathyroidism cognition and health-related quality of life. Ann Surg 242: 642–650.

Cooper MS, Gittoes NJ (2008). Diagnosis and management of hypocalcaemia. BMJ 336: 1298–1302.

Dacey MJ (2001). Hypomagnesemic disorders. Crit Care Clin 17: 155–173.

Dauphine RT, Riggs BL, Scholz DA (1975). Back pain and vertebral crush fractures: an unemphasized mode of presentation for primary hyperparathyroidism. Ann Intern Med 83: 365–367.

Delmas PD, Meunier PJ (1997). The management of Paget's disease of bone. N Engl J Med 336: 558–566.

Delmont E, Roth S, Heudier P et al. (2001). Primary hyperparathyroidism a differential diagnosis of motor neuron diseases. Rev Med Interne 22: 1253–1255.

DeViragh PA, Haglid KG, Celio MR (1989). Parvalbumin increases in the caudate putamen of rats with vitamin D hypervitaminosis. Proc Natl Acad Sci U S A 86: 3887–3890.

Eyles D, Brown J, Mackay-Sim A et al. (2003). Vitamin D3 and brain development. Neuroscience 118: 641–653.

Eyles DW, Smith S, Kinobe R et al. (2005). Distribution of the vitamin D receptor and 1alpha-hydroxylase in human brain. J Chem Neuroanat 29: 21–30.

Féron F, Burne TH, Brown J et al. (2005). Developmental vitamin D3 deficiency alters the adult rat brain. Brain Res Bull 65: 141–148.

Finiels PJ, Finiels H, Strubel D et al. (2002). Spontaneous osteoporotic fractures of the sacrum causing neurological damage. Report of three cases. J Neurosurg 97 (Suppl): 380–385.

Galland L (1991). Magnesium stress and neuropsychiatric disorders. Magnes Trace Elem 10: 287–301.

Garcion E, Wion-Barbot N, Montero-Mcnei CN et al. (2002). New clues about vitamin D functions in the nervous system. Trends Endocrinol Metab 13: 100–105.

Geelhoed GW, Kelly TR (1989). Pseudogout as a clue and complication of in primary hyperparathyroidism. Surgery 106: 1036–1041.

Girschick HJ, Schneider P, Haubitz I et al. (2006). Effective NSAID treatment indicates that hyperprostaglandinism is affecting the clinical severity of childhood hypophosphatasia. Orphanet J Rare Dis 1: 24.

Goswami R, Bhatia M, Goyal R et al. (2002). Reversible peripheral neuropathy in idiopathic hypoparathyroidism. Acta Neurol Scand 105: 128–131.

Hadjipavlou AG, Gaitanis LN, Katonis PG et al. (2001). Paget's disease of the spine and its management. Eur Spine J 10: 370–384.

Hansen MF, Seton M, Merchant A (2006). Osteosarcoma in Paget's disease of bone. J Bone Miner Res 21 (Suppl 2): P58–P63.

Heaney R (2007). Vitamin D endocrine physiology. J Bone Miner Res 22 (Suppl 2): V25–V27.

Hirose M, Kobayashi M, Sudo S (2002). Hemodialysis for toxic hypermagnesemia caused by intravenous magnesium in a woman with eclampsia and renal insufficiency. A case report. J Reprod Med 47: 1050–1052.

Holick MF, Lim R, Dighe AS (2009). Case records of the Massachusetts General Hospital. Case 3-2009. A 9-month-old boy with seizures. N Engl J Med 360: 398–407.

Hoogendijk WJ, Lips P, Dik MG et al. (2008). Depression is associated with decreased 25-hydroxyvitamin D and increased parathyroid hormone levels in older adults. Arch Gen Psychiatry 65: 508–512.

Hullar TE, Lustig LR (2003). Paget's disease and fibrous dysplasia. Otolaryngol Clin North Am 36: 707–732.

Ito Y, Hasegawa Y, Toda K et al. (2002). Pathogenesis and diagnosis of delayed vertebral collapse resulting from osteoporotic spinal fracture. Spine J 2: 101–106.

Jabr FI, Matari HM, Prempeh AL (2004). Extensive intracranial bilateral symmetrical calcification secondary to hypoparathyroidism. Arch Neurol 61: 281.

Jorde R, Sneve M, Figenschau Y et al. (2008). Effects of vitamin D supplementation on symptoms of depression in overweight and obese subjects: randomized double blind trial. J Intern Med 264: 599–609.

Josse RG, Hanley DA, Kendler D et al. (2007). Diagnosis and treatment of Paget's disease of bone. Clin Invest Med 30: E210–E223.

Kang H, Schuman EM (1995). Long-lasting neurotrophin-induced enhancement of synaptic transmission in the adult hippocampus. Science 267: 1658–1662.

Kazmi AS, Wall BM (2007). Reversible congestive heart failure related to profound hypocalcemia secondary to hypoparathyroidism. Am J Med Sci 333: 226–229.

Keisala T, Minasyan A, Lou YR et al. (2009). Premature aging in vitamin D receptor mutant mice. J Steroid Biochem Mol Biol 115: 91–97.

Khan A, Bilezikian J (2000). Primary hyperparathyroidism: pathophysiology and impact on bone. CMAJ 163: 184–187.

Ko P, Burkert R, McGrath J et al. (2004). Maternal vitamin D3 deprivation and the regulation of apoptosis and cell cycle during rat brain development. Dev Brain Res 153: 61–68.

Kowdley KV, Coull BM, Orwoll ES (1999). Cognitive impairment and intracranial calcification in chronic hypoparathyroidism. Am J Med Sci 317: 273–277.

Kuro-o M (2008). Endocrine FGFs and Klothos: emerging concepts. Trends Endocrinol Metab 19: 239–245.

Langub MC, Herman JP, Malluche HH et al. (2001). Evidence of functional vitamin D receptors in rathippocampus. Neuroscience 104: 49–56.

Lewiecki EM (2009). Denosumab update. Curr opin Rheumatol 21: 369–373.

Liamis G, Milionis HJ, Elisaf M (2009). A review of drug-induced hypocalcemia. J Bone Miner Metab 27: 635–642.

Litmanovitz I, Reish O, Dolfin T et al. (2002). Glu274Lys/Gly309Arg mutation of the tissue-nonspecific alkaline phosphatase gene in neonatal hypophosphatasia associated with convulsions. J Inherit Metab Dis 25: 35–40.

Marx SJ (2000). Medical progress: hyperparathyroid and hypoparathyroid disorders. N Engl J Med 343: 1863–1875.

Meca JE, Molto-Jorda JM, Morales-Ortiz A et al. (1997). Neurological manifestations of Paget's disease: presentation of one case and review of the literature. Rev Neurol 25: 1076–1078.

Mejdoubi M, Zegermann T (2006). Neurological picture. Extensive brain calcification in idiopathic hypoparathyroidism. J Neurol Neurosurg Psychiatry 77: 1328.

Menon B, Harinaryan CV (2010). The effect of anti epileptic drug therapy on serum 25-hydroxyvitamin D and parameters of calcium and bone metabolism – a longitudinal study. Seizure 19: 153–158.

Miller WL, Portale AA (2000). Vitamin D 1 alphahydroxylase. Trends Endocrinol Metab 11: 315–319.

Mintzer S, Boppana P, Toguri J et al. (2006). Vitamin D levels and bone turnover in epilepsy patients taking carbamazepine or oxcarbazepine. Epilepsia 47: 510–515.

Mittendorf EA, Wefel JS, Meyers CA et al. (2007). Improvement of sleep disturbance and neurocognitive function after parathyroidectomy in patients with primary hyperparathyroidism. Endocr Pract 13: 338–344.

Moe SM (2008). Disorders involving calcium, phosphorus, and magnesium. Prim Care 35: 215–237.

Monsell EM, Cody DD, Bone HG et al. (1999). Hearing loss as a complication of Paget's disease of bone. J Bone Miner Res 14 (Suppl 2): 92–95.

Mornet E (2007). Hypophosphatasia. Orphanet J Rare Dis 2: 40.

Morris GS, Grubbs EG, Hearon CM et al. (2010). Parathyroidectomy improves functional capacity in asymptomatic older patients with primary hyperparathyroidism: a randomized control trial. Ann Surg 251: 832–837.

Moulin P, Vaysse F, Bieth E et al. (2009). Hypophosphatasia may lead to bone fragility: don't miss it. Eur J Pediatr 168: 783–788.

Mouw DR, Latessa RA, Hickner J (2005). Clinical inquiries. What are the causes of hypomagnesemia? J Fam Pract 54: 174–176.

Munger KL, Levin LI, Hollis BW et al. (2006). Serum 25-hydroxyvitamin D levels and risk of multiple sclerosis. JAMA 296: 2832–2838.

Musiol IM, Stumpf WE, Bidmon HJ et al. (1992). Vitamin D nuclear binding to neurons of the septal substriatal and amygdaloid area in the Siberian hamster (Phodopus sungorus) brain. Neuroscience 48: 841–848.

Nguyen HV, Ludwig S, Gelb D (2003). Osteoporotic vertebral burst fractures with neurologic compromise. J Spinal Disord Tech 16: 10–19.

Nunes ML, Mugnol F, Bica I et al. (2002). Pyridoxine-dependent seizures associated with hypophosphatasia in a newborn. J Child Neurol 17: 222–224.

Obradovic D, Gronemeyer H, Lutz B et al. (2006). Cross-talk of vitamin D and glucocorticoids in hippocampal cells. J Neurochem 96: 500–509.

Palma G (1983). Carpal tunnel syndrome and hyperparathyroidism. Ann Neurol 14: 592.

Pan A, Lu L, Franco OH et al. (2009). Association between depressive symptoms and 25-hydroxyvitamin D in middle-aged and elderly Chinese. J Affect Disord 118: 240–243.

Perrier ND, Balachandran D, Wefel JS et al. (2009). Prospective randomized controlled trial of parathyroidectomy versus observation in patients with asymptomatic primary hyperparathyroidism. Surgery 146: 1116–1122.

Pierrot-Deseilligny C (2009). Clinical implications of a possible role of vitamin D in multiple sclerosis. J Neurol 256: 1468–1479.

Poncelet A (1999). The neurologic complications of Paget's disease. J Bone Miner Res 14: 88–91.

Prufer K, Veenstra TD, Jirikowski GF et al. (1999). Distribution of 125-dihydroxyvitamin D3 receptor immunoreactivity in the rat brain and spinal cord. J Chem Neuroanat 16: 135–145.

Ralston SH (2008). Pathogenesis of Paget's disease of bone. Bone 43: 819–825.

Raubenheimer PJ, Taylor AG, Soule SG (2002). Paget's disease complicated by hydrocephalus and syringomyelia. Br J Neurosurg 16: 513–516.

Reid IR (2008). Anti-resorptive therapies for osteoporosis. Semin Cell Dev Biol 19: 473–478.

Riggs JE (2002). Neurologic manifestations of electrolyte disturbances. Neurol Clin 20: 227–239.

Roman S, Sosa JA (2007). Psychiatric and cognitive aspects of primary hyperparathyroidism. Curr Opin Oncol 19: 1–5.

Roman SA, Sosa JA, Mayes L et al. (2005). Parathyroidectomy improves neurocognitive deficits in patients with primary hyperparathyroidism. Surgery 138: 1121–1128; discussion 1128–1129.

Rose CR, Blum R, Pichler B et al. (2003). Truncated TrkB-T1 mediates neurotrophin- evoked calcium signalling in glia cells. Nature 426: 74–78.

Rude RK, Olerich M (1996). Magnesium deficiency: possible role in osteoporosis associated with gluten-sensitive enteropathy. Osteoporos Int 6: 453–461.

Sankaran S, Gamble G, Bolland M et al. (2010). Skeletal effects of interventions in mild primary hyperparathyroidism: a meta-analysis. J Clin Endocrinol Metabol 95: 1653–1662.

Schaller B, Andres RH, Huber AW et al. (2005). Effect of GDNF on differentiation of cultured ventral mesencephalic dopaminergic and non-dopaminergic calretinin-expressing neurons. Brain Res 1036: 163–172.

Schwaller B, Meyer M, Schiffmann S (2002). "New" functions for "old" proteins: the role of the calcium-binding proteins calbindin D-28k calretinin and parvalbumin in cerebellar physiology Studies with knockout mice. Cerebellum 1: 241–258.

Shiber JR, Mattu A (2002). Serum phosphate abnormalities in the emergency department. J Emerg Med 23: 395–400.

Shoback D (2008). Clinical practice. Hypoparathyroidism. N Engl J Med 359: 391–403.

Shonka DC Jr, Kesser BW (2006). Paget's disease of the temporal bone. Otol Neurotol 27: 1199–1200.

Siegel GJ, Agranoff BW, Albers RW et al. (1999). Basic Neurochemistry: Molecular Cellular and Medical Aspects. 6th edn. Lippincott Williams and Wilkins, Philadelphia.

Silverberg SJ (2002). Non-classical target organs in primary hyperparathyroidism. J Bone Miner Res 17 (Suppl 2): N117–N125.

Silverberg SJ, Lewiecki EM, Mosekilde L et al. (2009). Presentation of asymptomatic primary hyperparathyroidism: proceedings of the third international workshop. J Clin Endocrinol Metabol 94: 351–365.

Siris ES, Lyles KW, Singer FR et al. (2006). Medical management of Paget's disease of bone: indications for treatment and review of current therapies. J Bone Miner Res 21 (Suppl 2): P94–P98.

Smilari P, Romeo DM, Palazzo P et al. (2005). Neonatal hypophosphatasia and seizures. A case report. Minerva Pediatr 57: 319–323.

Smolders J, Thewissen M, Peelen E et al. (2009). Vitamin D status is positively correlated with regulatory T cell function in patients with multiple sclerosis. PLoS One 4: e6635.

Sontia B, Touyz RM (2007). Role of magnesium in hypertension. Arch Biochem Biophys 458: 33–39.

Stio M, Lunghi B, Iantomasi T et al. (1993). Effect of vitamin D deficiency and 125-dihydroxyvitamin D3 on metabolism and D-glucose transport in rat cerebral cortex. J Neurosci Res 35: 559–566.

Taniura H, Ito M, Sanada N et al. (2006). Chronic vitamin D3 treatment protects against neurotoxicity by glutamate in association with upregulation of vitamin D receptor mRNA expression in cultured rat cortical neurons. J Neurosci Res 83: 1179–1189.

Taupin P, Gage FH (2002). Adult neurogenesis and neural stem cells of the central nervous system in mammals. J Neurosci Res 69: 745–749.

Tekes K, Gyenge M, Folyovich A et al. (2009). Influence of neonatal vitamin A and vitamin D on the concentration of biogenic amines and their metabolites in the rat brain. Horm Metab Res 41: 277–280.

Tessitore E, Luzi M, Lobrinus JA et al. (2008). Cervical Paget disease of bone with spinal cord compression due to atlanto-axial instability: a case report and review of the literature. Spine 33: E85–E89.

Tezer M, Ozturk C, Erturer E et al. (2006). Bilateral L5 radiculopathy due to osteoporotic L1 vertebral fracture: a case report. J Spinal Cord Med 29: 430–435.

Topf JM, Murray PT (2003). Hypomagnesemia and hypermagnesemia. Rev Endocr Metab Disord 4: 195–206.

Verulashvili IV, Glonti LS, Miminoshvili DK et al. (2006). Basal ganglia calcification: clinical manifestations and diagnostic evaluation. Georgian Med News 140: 39–43.

Volpe SL (2008). Magnesium, the metabolic syndrome, insulin resistance, and type 2 diabetes mellitus. Crit Rev Food Sci Nutr 48: 293–300.

Walbert T, Jirikowski GF, Prufer K (2001). Distribution of 125-dihydroxyvitamin D3 receptor immunoreactivity in the limbic system of the rat. Horm Metab Res 33: 525–531.

Walker MD, Silverberg SJ (2007). Parathyroidectomy in asymptomatic primary hyperparathyroidism: improves bones but not psychic moans. J Clin Endocrinol Metabol 92: 1613–1615.

Walker MD, McMahon DJ, Inabnet WB et al. (2009). Neuropsychological features in primary hyperparathyroidism: a prospective study. J Clin Endocrinol Metabol 94: 1951–1958.

Watts C, McConkey H, Anderson L et al. (2005). Anatomical perspectives on adult neural stem cells. J Anat 207: 197–208.

Weber T, Keller M, Hense I et al. (2007). Effect of parathyroidectomy on quality of life and neuropsychological symptoms in primary hyperparathyroidism. World J Surg 31: 1202–1209.

Weisinger JR, Bellorin-Font E (1998). Magnesium and phosphorus. Lancet 352: 391–396.

Whyte MP, Mumm S, Deal C (2007). Adult hypophosphatasia treated with teriparatide. J Clin Endocrinol Metabol 92: 1203–1208.

Whyte MP, Wenkert D, McAlister WH et al. (2009). Chronic recurrent multifocal osteomyelitis mimicked in childhood hypophosphatasia. J Bone Miner Res 24: 1493–1505.

Woo NH, Lu B (2006). Regulation of cortical interneurons by neurotrophins: from development to cognitive disorders. Neuroscientist 12: 43–56.

Yamamoto H, Sasamoto Y, Miyamoto Y et al. (2004). A successful treatment with pyridoxal phosphate for West syndrome in hypophosphatasia. Pediatr Neurol 30: 216–218.

Zou J, Minasyan A, Keisala T et al. (2008). Progressive hearing loss in mice with a mutated vitamin D receptor gene. Audiol Neurootol 13: 219–230.

FURTHER READING

Agus ZS (1999). Hypomagnesemia. J Am Soc Nephrol 10: 1616–1622.

Alonso G, Varsavsky M, Munoz-Torres M (2009). Hypophosphatasia: new therapeutic approaches. Med Clin 132: 108–111.

Bilezikian JP, Silverberg SJ (2004). Clinical practice. Asymptomatic primary hyperparathyroidism. N Engl J Med 350: 1746–1751.

Brown EM (2002). The pathophysiology of primary hyperparathyroidism. J Bone Miner Res 17 (Suppl 2): N24–N29.

Chabas JO, Alluin O, Rao G et al. (2008). Vitamin D2 potentiates axon regeneration. J Neurotrauma 25: 1247–1256.

Chiang CY, Andrewes DG, Anderson D et al. (2005). A controlled prospective study of neuropsychological outcomes post parathyroidectomy in primary hyperparathyroid patients. Clin Endocrinol (Oxf) 62: 99–104.

Cianferotti L, Cox M, Skorija K et al. (2007). Vitamin D receptor is essential for normal keratinocyte stem cell function. Proc Natl Acad Sci U S A 104: 9428–9433.

Diercks DB, Shumaik GM, Harrigan RA et al. (2004). Electrocardiographic manifestations: electrolyte abnormalities. J Emerg Med 27: 153–160.

Eastell R, Arnold A, Brandi ML et al. (2009). Diagnosis of asymptomatic primary hyperparathyroidism: proceedings of the third international workshop. J Clin Endocrinol Metabol 94: 340–350.

Eigelberger MS, Cheah WK, Ituarte PH et al. (2004). The NIH criteria for parathyroidectomy in asymptomatic primary hyperparathyroidism: are they too limited? Ann Surg 239: 528–535.

Fawcett WJ, Haxby EJ, Male DA (1999). Magnesium: physiology and pharmacology. Br J Anaesth 83: 302–320.

Fraser WD (2009). Hyperparathyroidism. Lancet 374: 145–158.

Garg RK, Garg N, Tandon N et al. (1999). Idiopathic hypoparathyroidism presenting as epilepsy in a 40 years female. Neurol India 47: 244–245.

Gittoes NJ, Cooper MS (2010). Primary hyperparathyroidism – is mild disease worth treating? Clin Med 10: 45–49.

Gums JG (2004). Magnesium in cardiovascular and other disorders. Am J Health Syst Pharm 61: 1569–1576.

Hansen MF, Nellissery MJ, Bhatia P (1999). Common mechanisms of osteosarcoma and Paget's disease. J Bone Miner Res 14 (Suppl 2): 39–44.

Humes HDDuPont HL, Gardner LB et al. (Eds.), (2000). Kelley's Textbook of Internal Medicine. 4th edn. Lippincott Williams and Wilkins, Philadelphia.

Kaplan FS (1999). Surgical management of Paget's disease. J Bone Miner Res 14 (Suppl 2): 34–38.

Khan A, Grey A, Shoback D (2009). Medical management of asymptomatic primary hyperparathyroidism: proceedings of the third international workshop. J Clin Endocrinol Metabol 94: 373–381.

Khosla S, Riggs BL (2005). Pathophysiology of age-related bone loss and osteoporosis. Endocrinol Metab Clin North Am 34: 1015–1030.

Kifor O, Moore FD Jr, Delaney M et al. (2003). A syndrome of hypocalciuric hypercalcemia caused by autoantibodies directed at the calcium-sensing receptor. J Clin Endocrinol Metabol 88: 60–72.

Kochbati S, Daoud L, Zouaoui W et al. (2009). Spinal cord compression due to benign osteoporotic vertebral fracture. Tunis Med 87: 152–154.

Kramer JH, Spurney C, Iantorno M et al. (2009). Neurogenic inflammation and cardiac dysfunction due to hypomagnesemia. Am J Med Sci 338: 22–27.

Lal G, Clark OH (2003). Primary hyperparathyroidism: controversies in surgical management. Trends Endocrinol Metab 14: 417–422.

Mankin HJ, Hornicek FJ (2005). Paget's sarcoma: a historical and outcome review. Clin Orthop Relat Res 438: 97–102.

Maricic M (2006). The use of zoledronic acid for Paget's disease of bone. Curr Osteoporos Rep 4: 40–44.

Miller PD (2009). Denosumab: anti-RANKL antibody. Curr Osteoporos Rep 7: 18–22.

Mornet E (2008). Hypophosphatasia. Best Pract Res Clin Rheumatol 22: 113–127.

Nagano N (2006). Pharmacological and clinical properties of calcimimetics: calcium receptor activators that afford an innovative approach to controlling hyperparathyroidism. Pharmacol Ther 109: 339–365.

Noor M, Shoback D (2000). Paget's disease of bone: diagnosis and treatment update. Curr Rheumatol Rep 2: 67–73.

Noronha JL, Matuschak GM (2002). Magnesium in critical illness: metabolism assessment and treatment. Intensive Care Med 28: 667–679.

Prager G, Kalaschek A, Kaczirek K et al. (2002). Parathyroidectomy improves concentration and retentiveness in patients with primary hyperparathyroidism. Surgery 132: 930–935.

Ramage IJ, Howatson AJ, Beattie TJ (1996). Hypophosphatasia. J Clin Pathol 49: 682–684.

Rastogi R, Beauchamp NJ, Ladenson PW (2003). Calcification of the basal ganglia in chronic hypoparathyroidism. J Clin Endocrinol Metabol 88: 1476–1477.

Rodgers SE, Lew JI, Solorzano CC (2008). Primary hyperparathyroidism. Curr Opin Oncol 20: 52–58.

Rubin MR, Bilezikian JP, McMahon DJ et al. (2008). The natural history of primary hyperparathyroidism with or without parathyroid surgery after 15 years. J Clin Endocrinol Metabol 93: 3462–3470.

Saifuddin A, Hassan A (2003). Paget's disease of the spine: unusual features and complications. Clin Radiol 58: 102–111.

Sambrook P, Cooper C (2006). Osteoporosis. Lancet 367: 2010–2018.

Shalitin S, Davidovits M, Lazar L et al. (2008). Clinical heterogeneity of pseudohypoparathyroidism: from hyper- to hypocalcemia. Horm Res 70: 137–144.

Shankar S, Hosking DJ (2006). Biochemical assessment of Paget's disease of bone. J Bone Miner Res 21 (Suppl 2): P22–P27.

Silverberg SJ (2000). Natural history of primary hyperparathyroidism. Endocrinol Metab Clin North Am 29: 451–464.

Smith SE, Murphey MD, Motamedi K et al. (2002). From the archives of the AFIP. Radiologic spectrum of Paget disease of bone and its complications with pathologic correlation. Radiographics 22: 1191–1216.

Udelsman R, Pasieka JL, Sturgeon C et al. (2009). Surgery for asymptomatic primary hyperparathyroidism: proceedings of the third international workshop. J Clin Endocrinol Metabol 94: 366–372.

Verani RR (1992). Obesity-associated focal segmental glomerulosclerosis: pathological features of the lesion and relationship with cardiomegaly and hyperlipidemia. Am J Kidney Dis 20: 629–634.

Whitaker CH, Malchoff CD, Felice KJ (2000). Treatable lower motor neuron disease due to vitamin D deficiency and secondary hyperparathyroidism. Amyotroph Lateral Scler Other Motor Neuron Disord 1: 283–286.

Whyte MP (2006). Clinical practice. Paget's disease of bone. N Engl J Med 355: 593–600.

Section 8

Neurologic aspects of nutritional disorders

Handbook of Clinical Neurology, Vol. 120 (3rd series)
Neurologic Aspects of Systemic Disease Part II
Jose Biller and Jose M. Ferro, Editors

Chapter 59

Hydrosoluble vitamins

JASVINDER CHAWLA[1,2]* AND DAVID KVARNBERG[2]

[1]*Department of Neurology, Hines VA Hospital, Hines, IL, USA*

[2]*Department of Neurology, Loyola University Medical Center, Maywood, IL, USA*

HISTORY

Most of the work on vitamins goes back to the early twentieth century. Vitamin supplementation fell into dispute after the studies reported in the middle of the century. Very little clinical research has been done since then and major medical journals have consistently rejected what clinical research has been reported. The use of thiamin and its disulfide derivatives, in particular, is much neglected in Western medicine. Beriberi was described in the 17th century when Brontius in the Dutch East Indies reported cases of sensorimotor polyneuropathy. Thiamin was one of the earliest vitamins to be discovered and synthesized. It was originally spelled thiamine, and although this spelling is still often used, the alternative spelling of thiamin was adopted when it was found that it was not an amine. Thiamin deficiency is the major cause of beriberi, a disease that had affected humans for centuries. The name *Kakke* was the term used for the disease in Japan and this word can be found in documents as early as 808 (Inouye and Katsura, 1965). In 1890, Eijkman found that polished rice, given to pigeons, caused polyneuritis and the histopathology was similar to that seen in humans in beriberi. Funk and Cooper isolated an "antiberiberi factor" from rice polishing in 1910 and this was crystallized in 1926 and called Vitamin (Jansen and Donath, 1926). The first national statistics on mortality came from Japanese literature in 1920's and showed a death rate of 30 per 100,000. This dropped to 0.5 in 1959 after its nutritional association was discovered (Inouye and Kastura, 1965).

Pellagra was seemingly unknown prior to the introduction of maize into Europe from the New World. In the US, pellagra became epidemic among economically challenged inhabitants of some southern states in the early 20th century due to nutritionally inadequate diets as well as manufacturing methods that removed vitamins from processed grain. Vitamin fortification of foodstuffs during World War II ultimately eradicated endemic pellagra in the US. In the 1940s and 1950s, with advanced biochemical knowledge, pellagra was reformulated as a deficiency state resulting from inadequate niacin and its amino acid precursor tryptophan. Nicotinic acid is the oldest drug known to modify serum lipids and is the most effective drug currently available for the elevation of high-density lipoprotein (HDL).

Casimir Funk, in 1920, introduced the term vitamin C to indicate the nutritional factor necessary to prevent the pathologic state known as scurvy; however, the nature of the molecule was still unknown. When considering the history of vitamin C, and the names given to this molecule in early days, the Latin proverb *nomen est omen* suddenly comes to mind.

The impact of overt deficiency-associated disease was significant enough that the key discoveries in prevention and management received numerous Nobel prizes. Nowadays, almost half of Americans take vitamins and dietary supplements. As many as 80% of them consider vitamins and supplements safe, thus increasing the potential for vitamin toxicity. Animal data have added considerably to our clinical knowledge, but it still remains limited due to the difficulty in translating it successfully to naturally occurring disease in humans (Griffin and Hoffman, 2009; Kopelman et al., 2009). Table 59.1 gives an overview of the hydrosoluble vitamins and Table 59.2 summarizes hydrosoluble vitamin investigations.

---

*Correspondence to: Jasvinder Chawla, M.D., M.B.A., Chief of Neurology, Hines VA Hospital, Department of Neurology, Building 228, Room 5000, 5000 South 5th Avenue, Hines, IL 60141, USA. Tel: +1-708-202-2847, Fax: +-708-202-7936, E-mail: Jasvinder.chawla2@va.gov

Table 59.1

Hydrosoluble vitamins: an overview

Vitamin	Major functions	Recommended daily intake	Food sources	Deficiency	Toxicity	Stability in foods
Thiamin (vitamin B$_1$)	Important in function of nervous system. Helps release energy from foods; promotes normal appetite	Infants: 0.2–0.3 mg Children: 0.5–0.6 mg Adolescents: 0.9–1.2 mg Men: 1.2 mg Women: 1.1 mg Pregnant/lactating women: 1.4 mg	Pork/pork products, beef, liver, yeast/baked products, enriched and whole grain cereals, nuts, and seeds	Beriberi: anorexia, weight loss, weakness, peripheral neuropathy Wernicke–Korsakoff syndrome: gait ataxia, ophthalmoplegia, encephalopathy, dementia, memory loss	None reported	Losses depend on cooking method, length, alkalinity of cooking medium; destroyed by sulfite used to treat dried fruits such as apricots; dissolves in cooking water
Riboflavin (vitamin B$_2$)	Helps with vision, release energy from foods; healthy skin	Infants: 0.3–0.4 mg Children: 0.5–0.6 mg Adolescents: 0.9–1.3 mg Men: 1.3 mg Women: 1.1 mg Pregnant women: 1.4 mg Lactating women: 1.6 mg	Milk, eggs, mushrooms, whole grains, enriched grains, green leafy vegetables, yeast, liver, and oily fish	Ariboflavinosis: glossitis, cheilosis, dermatitis, growth retardation, conjunctivitis, neuropathy	None reported	Sensitive to light; unstable in alkaline solutions
Niacin (vitamin B$_3$)	Promotes healthy nerves, skin. Energy production from foods; aids digestion, promotes normal appetite	Infants: 2–4 mg Children: 6–8 mg Adolescents: 12–16 mg Men: 16 mg Women: 14 mg Pregnant women: 18 mg Lactating women: 17 mg	Meat, poultry, fish, yeast, enriched and whole grain breads and cereals, peanuts, mushrooms, milk, and eggs (tryptophan)	Pellagra: diarrhea, dematitis, dementia, and death	Flushing of skin, itching, nausea and vomiting, and liver damage occurs at intake over 35 mg/day from supplements	Not known
Pantothenic acid (vitamin B$_5$)	Aids in formation of hormones; involved in energy production	Infants: 1.7–1.8 mg Children: 2–3 mg Adolescents: 4–5 mg Men and women: 5 mg Pregnant women: 6 mg Lactating women: 7 mg	Widely distributed in foods	Rare	None reported	About half of pantothenic acid is lost in the milling of grains and heavily refined foods

Vitamin	Function	Recommended amounts	Sources	Deficiency	Toxicity	Stability
Pyridoxine (vitamin B_6)	Aids in protein metabolism, absorption; aids in red blood cell formation; helps body use fats	Infants: 0.1–0.3 mg Children: 0.5–0.6 mg Adolescents: 1.0 –1.3 mg Men and women (19–50 years): 1.3 mg Men over 50 years: 1.4 mg Women over 50 years: 1.3 mg Pregnant women: 1.9 mg Lactating women: 1.2 mg	Meat, fish, poultry, spinach, potatoes, bananas, avocados, sunflower seeds	Dermatitis, anemia, seizure, depression, encephalopathy, decline in immune function	None from foods, excess intake above 100 mg/day from supplements causes painful neuropathy and skin lesions	Considerable losses during cooking
Biotin (vitamin B_8)	Helps release energy from carbohydrates; aids in fat synthesis	Infants: 5–6 μg Children: 8–12 μg Adolescents: 20–25 μg Men and women: 30 μg Pregnant women: 30 μg Lactating women: 35 μg	Whole grains, eggs, nuts and seeds, widely distributed in small amounts	Infants: dermatitis, seizures, alopecia, neurological disorders, growth retardation	Not known	Not known
Ascorbic acid (vitamin C)	Formation of collagen; wound healing; maintaining blood vessels, bones, teeth; absorption of iron, calcium, folacin; production of neurohormones, immune factors; antioxidant	Infants: 40–50 mg Children: 15–25 mg Adolescents: 45–75 mg Men: 90 mg Women: 75 mg Pregnant women: 80–85 mg Lactating women: 115–120 mg Smokers: +35 mg	Citrus fruits, strawberries, broccoli, green vegetables	Scurvy: fatigue, poor wound healing, pinpoint hemorrhages around hair follicles on back of arms and legs, bleeding gums and joints	Megadoses over 2 g/day causes nausea, abdominal cramps, diarrhea and kidney stones	Most unstable under heat, drying, storage; very soluble in water, leaches out of some vegetables during cooking; alkalinity (baking soda) destroys vitamin C

Table 59.2

Hydrosoluble vitamins: investigations

Vitamin	Laboratory investigations	Neuroimaging	Genetics	Pathology
Thiamin (vitamin B$_1$)	No specific test Blood thiamin, pyruvate, α-ketoglutarate, lactate and glyoxylate levels Urinary excretion of thiamin and its metabolites Erythrocyte transketolase levels: normal values range from 0% to 15%; a value of 15–25% indicates thiamin deficiency > 25% indicates severe deficiency	T2 hyperintensities of bilateral thalami, mamillary bodies, tectal plate and periaqueductal area	No significant genetic association	Neuronal loss, gliosis, vascular damage in areas surrounding the 3rd and 4th ventricles, and aqueduct, mamillary bodies, thalamus and superior cerebellar vermis
Riboflavin (vitamin B$_2$)	Blood glutathione reductase activity Urinary riboflavin excretion	No specific findings	MADD is improved with riboflavin supplementation	Peripheral nerve demyelination in chickens
Niacin (vitamin B$_3$)	Serum niacin, tryptophan, NAD, NADP Urinary levels of N-methylnicotinamide and pyridone	No specific findings	Hartnup disease	Chromatylic changes in neurons of motor cortex Degeneration of spinal cord Patchy demyelination in peripheral nerves Nonspecific dermatitic changes (i.e., perivascular lymphohistologic infiltrate, mild edema, fibrosis)
Pantothenic acid (vitamin B$_5$)	No specific test is available	No specific neuroimaging findings	No specific genetic associations	No specific pathological findings
Pyridoxine (vitamin B$_6$)	Blood levels of pyridoxine Urinary excretion of 4-pyridoxic acid Erythrocyte aspartate aminotransferase (EAST) and EAST activation for long-term pyridoxine status	No specific neuroimaging findings	Pyridoxine-dependent seizures in newborns	Axonal degeneration of sensory nerve fibers with pyridoxine toxicity

Biotin (vitamin B8)	Serum biotinidase activity screening in newborns Excretion of 3-hydroxyisovaleric acid and biotin in urine Activity of propionyl-CoA carboxylase in lymphocytes	MRI findings of myelopathy MRI brain with leukoencephalopathy, low cerebral volume, ventriculomegaly, caudate and parieto-occipital cortical abnormalities MR spectroscopy with decreased NAA peaks, elevated lactate levels, and reversal of choline to creatine ratio	Biotinidase deficiency in newborns	Poorly delineated necrotic lesions with gliosis in the pons, hypothalamus, hippocampus, and medulla
Ascorbic acid (vitamin C)	WBC ascorbic acid levels. Plasma levels are not very helpful because they reflect recent dietary intake rather than tissue levels	Changes in bones seen on X-ray: cortical thinning, trabecular atrophy, corner sign of Park	No specific genetic associations	Rapidly growing tissues dependent on collagen synthesis are affected most. Hemorrhaging can occur in any organ. Bone contains subperiosteal hemorrhage and microscopic fractures

NAD, Nicotinamine adenine dinucleotide; NADP, Nicotinamine adenine dinucleotide phosphate; MADD, multiple acyl-CoA dehydrogenation deficiency; WBC, White blood cell; MRI, magnetic resonance imaging; NAA, N-acetyl-L-aspartate.

THIAMIN (VITAMIN B₁)

Biochemical function

Thiamin consists of a pyrimidine ring (2,5-dimethyl 1-6-aminopyrimidine) and a thiazolium ring (4-methyl-5-hydroxy ethyl thiazole) joined by a methylene bridge. Thiamin (or vitamin B_1) has an important role as a cofactor in several biochemical pathways, particularly the respiratory chain in oxidative metabolism. The best-characterized form is thiamin pyrophosphate, which is a coenzyme in carbohydrate and amino acid metabolism. In 1938, Minz first suggested a relationship between thiamin and nervous excitation when he observed that thiamin was released into the bathing medium when pneumogastric nerve from an ox was stimulated (Minz, 1938). In 1979, Cooper and Pincus reviewed the evidence that there was a possibility that thiamin has a function in the nervous system distinct from its activity as a cofactor to enzymes (Cooper and Pincus, 1979). Another important thiamin-dependent enzyme that is particularly vulnerable to thiamin deficiency is α-ketoglutarate dehydrogenase (KGDH) which also plays a key role in the regulation of glucose metabolism. The mitochondrial uncoupling that occurs as a result of thiamin deficiency results in oxidative stress, and this makes oxidative-dependent organs such as the nervous system and heart particularly vulnerable to damage (Hazell and Butterworth, 2009). Thiamin is also required in the biosynthesis of the neurotransmitters acetylcholine and γ-aminobutyric acid (GABA) and in myelin production. The increase in severity of the seizures and the prolongation beyond the normal period of audiogenic seizure initiation supported the role of thiamin in its stimulation of the cholinergic central nervous system activity. Two publications have indicated that thiamin supplementation has a mild clinical effect in Alzheimer's disease where the abnormality of cholinergic system is part of the pathophysiology (Blass et al., 1988; Meador et al., 1993). Thiamin deficiency in rats caused encephalopathy and DNA synthesis decreased significantly in cortex, subcortical structures, brainstem, and cerebellum. This was reversible by administration of thiamin (Henderson and Schenker, 1975).

Natural sources

Since the body does not produce thiamin, humans must consume it through food sources, with products such as enriched whole grains, lean meats, seafood, legumes, and spinach being the most important. Some preparation methods, such as heating, canning, or pasteurization, can denature the molecule and destroy its efficaciousness. Thiamin is absorbed in the proximal small intestine with a carrier-mediated mechanism, and excreted by the kidney. It is also produced by the normal microflora of the large intestine with efficient uptake in that region. It is mostly concentrated in the skeletal muscles. Other organs where thiamin is found are the brain, heart, liver, and kidneys. It has a biologic half-life of 10–20 days, and because of a limited storage capacity of up to 30 mg in the tissues, continuous dietary supplementation is required. Thiamin deficiency most commonly results from malnutrition or impaired absorption associated with chronic diseases, such as alcoholism, gastrointestinal diseases, AIDS, and diabetes.

Clinical findings

Symptoms suggestive of dysfunction of the central and peripheral nervous system generally precede by months the gross signs of neurologic dysfunction. Of neurologic interest, two distinct disorders related to thiamin deficiency are nutritional polyneuropathy and the Wernicke–Korsakoff syndrome. Other disorders due to some extent to lack of thiamin are also discussed.

NUTRITIONAL POLYNEUROPATHY

Nutritional polyneuropathy, or dry beriberi, is the most common of all nervous system nutritional disorders. Thiamin deficiency plays a dominant role in the pathogenesis of polyneuropathy among both the alcoholic and nonalcoholic population. It is uncertain whether dry beriberi relates to an isolated thiamin deficiency state or rather to a deficiency of multiple B vitamins, including pyridoxine (B_6) and pantothenic acid (B_5). Epidemics of beriberi have been known to occur in association with increased affluence simply because it was expensive to take the rice to the mill. Beriberi has no age, gender, or racial predilection (Rao et al., 2008; Fattal-Valevski et al., 2009; Masumoto et al., 2009).

Nutritional polyneuropathy most often presents as a symmetric, mixed sensorimotor polyneuropathy. Onset and progression of symptoms are usually slow. The distal portions of the limbs are characteristically involved. Symptoms include numbness or tingling distally in the limbs, frequently accompanied by dull pains and cramps in both feet and calves. Patients often complain of severe burning sensation in the feet. Examination demonstrates a variable degree of distal muscle weakness and atrophy, including bilateral foot drop. In the early stages, the muscles may be tender to palpation. The muscle stretch reflexes are reduced or absent. Sensory examination shows impaired proprioception (Howard et al., 2010). Electrophysiologic studies demonstrate findings of an axonal polyneuropathy; features of superimposed compressive mononeuropathies may be present.

Autonomic dysfunction is occasionally encountered, including hyperhidrosis of hands and feet, arterial hypotension, hoarseness, dysphagia, and pupillary abnormalities (Stamboulis et al., 2006). This was noted to be asymmetric in some cases, with symptoms including violent temper tantrums, migraine-like headaches, asymmetry in the pupils, change in color of one half of the body (similar to harlequin discoloration), lack of sweat on one side of the body, and lack of sleep spindles on one side of the brain (Lonsdale, 1987, 1990).

Infantile beriberi has been found among infants fed only with breast milk from mothers deficient in thiamin. An epidemic of infantile thiamin deficiency was reported among Israeli infants fed with a formula deficient in thiamin (Rao et al., 2008; Masumoto et al., 2009). Manifestations of infantile beriberi include high output congestive heart failure and absent muscle stretch reflexes (Rao et al., 2008). In cases of wet beriberi, clinical improvement is observed within 12 hours of treatment, with normalization of heart function and size occurring within 1 or 2 days. True beriberi heart disease is infrequent. Sudden death may occur from acute cardiovascular collapse, so-called shoshin beriberi (Loma-Osorio et al., 2008).

WERNICKE–KORSAKOFF SYNDROME

Wernicke's encephalopathy (WE) was first described in 1881 by Carl Wernicke as "superior acute hemorrhagic poliencephalitis" in two men with alcoholism and in a woman affected by pyloric stenosis (Wernicke, 1881), whereas the association of WE with thiamin deficiency was first suspected in the 1940s (Campbell and Russell, 1941). WE is an acute or subacutely evolving disorder. The disorder has no racial predilection, however, more common in men with a male to female ratio of 1.7 : 1. Average age at onset is approximately 50 years. A carbohydrate load is the immediate precipitating factor in some patients. Generally, there is a background of chronic and severe undernutrition, with some additional stressors including trauma or infection. In the Western world, thiamin deficiency is characteristically associated with chronic alcoholism (Attard et al., 2006). Other high-risk conditions for thiamin deficiency include hyperemesis gravidarum, malabsorption syndromes, celiac and tropical sprue, gastric resection, intestinal bypass, starvation states (anorexia nervosa, radical diets), long-term parenteral hyperalimentation, hemodialysis, leukemia, children with malignancy, hyperthyroidism, lactation, and certain dietary restrictions (e.g., flour not enriched with thiamin). A characteristic triad of clinical features including a global confusional state, ocular abnormalities, and ataxia is seen in only 30% of the cases, which explains at least in part why WE is often clinically underdiagnosed (Foster et al., 2005; Indraccolo et al., 2003; Ueda et al., 2006; Phayphet et al., 2007; Aasheim

et al., 2009; Sebastian et al., 2010). In view of the poor diagnostic performance of the classic triad, new classification criteria have been proposed. These criteria require two of four items including dietary deficiences, oculomotor abnormalities, cerebellar dysfunction, and altered mental state or mild memory impairment (Caine et al., 1997).

Mental status changes are the most frequently observed manifestations. Some patients appear apathetic and listless, with short attention span, reduced speech spontaneity, confusion, and drowsiness. The most common neuro-ophthalmologic manifestation is nystagmus (Donnino et al., 2007). Other neuro-ophthalmologic manifestations include bilateral sixth cranial nerve palsies and conjugate gaze palsies. Pupillary involvement is rare. Gait ataxia may also be a presenting symptom (Decker and Isaacman, 2000). The ataxia is multifactorial and likely the result of polyneuropathy, cerebellar damage, and vestibular paresis. In less severe cases, patients ambulate cautiously with a broad-based gait. Truncal ataxia may be noted with patient sitting or standing (Kim et al., 2009). Patients may also exhibit autonomic changes such as orthostatic hypotension, cardiac dysfunction and hypothermia (Loma-Osorio et al., 2008).

Korsakoff psychosis (amnestic confabulatory state; psychosis polyneuritica) is primarily characterized by a pervasive impairment regarding the acquisition of new information out of proportion to other cognitive functions in an otherwise alert and responsive patient. Patients also have some degree of retrograde amnesia. This amnesic disorder, like Wernicke disease, can be seen with a variety of disorders and most often associated with malnutrition and alcoholism. In the alcoholic, nutritionally deficient patient, the Korsakoff amnesic state is usually associated with Wernicke disease. Korsakoff psychosis is the psychic manifestation of Wernicke disease. Most patients with Wernicke disease or WE have a symptom complex including opthalmoparesis, nystagmus, variable gait ataxia, and an acute confusional state. If a long-term defect in the learning memory is added, the symptom complex is appropriately designated as the Wernicke–Korsakoff syndrome (Kopelman et al., 2009).

CORTICAL CEREBELLAR DEGENERATION

Thiamin deficit (and other nutritional deficiencies) is probably a determinant factor in cerebellar degeneration associated with alcohol consumption, as thiamin-deficient membranes are particularly susceptible to osmotic stress. Cortical cerebellar degeneration appears closely linked to Wernicke's encephalopathy. Examination demonstrates gait and truncal instability. A wide-based gait ataxia with ataxia of individual leg movements is characteristic. After stabilization, patients may show modest improvement as their nutrition improves, especially if supplemental vitamins are taken. However, a significant cerebellar deficit invariably remains and persists for years thereafter (Mancall and McEntee, 1965; Greenwood et al., 1984; Mulholland et al., 2005).

An epidemic of thiamin deficiency, and other B vitamins, on a background of excessive alcohol consumption and severe food shortages, occurred in Cuba in the early 1990s (Roman et al., 1985, 1994). The most common inciting factor precipitating Wernicke encephalopathy in the setting of thiamin deficiency is infection (Donnino et al., 2007).

Each year a large percentage of the population with morbid obesity has bariatric surgery. Patients undergoing bariatric surgery are at risk for various nutritional deficiencies including vitamins B_1, B_{12}, C, folate, A, D, and K, along with the trace minerals iron, selenium, zinc, and copper. Over-the-counter multivitamin and mineral supplements do not provide adequate amounts of certain nutrients and patients will require additional lifelong doses of prophylactic supplementation to maintain optimal micronutrient status. This issue becomes even more important in considering adequate prenatal supplementation for pregnant women who have undergone bariatric surgery. All bariatric surgery patients are best served by receiving regular monitoring of serum nutrient levels as mentioned above by starting at 3 months following surgery and periodically thereafter (Shankar et al., 2010; Bordalo et al., 2011). Thiamin deficiency tends to occur in the first weeks or months after surgery. Copper deficiency tends to be a late complication, developing several years to many years following surgery. For those patients who have had a bariatric procedure and then develop a neuropathy, evaluating levels of thiamin, copper, vitamin B_{12}, methylmalonic acid, and homocystine is indicated (Rudnicki, 2010). The 2007 Annual Report of the American Association of Poison Control Centers' National Poison Data System document the total number of exposures for each class of vitamins, the number of patients with major adverse outcomes, and the number of fatalities from that ingestion (Bronstein et al., 2008).

THIAMIN TOXICITY

Vitamin B_1 toxicity effects may be minimal and nonspecific, and may be characterized by tachycardia, hypotension, cardiac dysrhythmias, headaches, vasodilation, weakness, seizures, and even anaphylaxis (Mularski et al., 2006).

Laboratory investigations

The diagnosis of WE is mainly clinical. No specific laboratory test is available. Normal electrolyte levels may only give false reassurance and may delay therapy. Measurement of thiamin levels can be considered in cases of diagnostic uncertainty (Donnino et al., 2007).

If laboratory confirmation is needed, blood thiamin, pyruvate, α-ketoglutarate, lactate, and glyoxylate may be measured. Also, measurement of urinary excretion of thiamin and its metabolites may be useful (Lu and Frank, 2008). Erythrocyte transketolase levels reliably detect thiamin deficiency and the extent of deficiency is expressed in percentage stimulation compared with baseline levels. Normal values range from 0% to 15%; a value of 15–25% indicates thiamin deficiency, and greater than 25% indicates severe deficiency. A thiamin loading test is the best indicator of thiamin deficiency. An increase of more than 15% in enzyme activity is a definitive marker of deficiency. However, this test is expensive and time-consuming. Measurement of serum thyroid-stimulating hormone troponin I may be required in some cases (Tran, 2006). Magnesium depletion aggravates the clinical effects of thiamin deficiency. Magnesium and calcium deficiency affects the distribution of thiamin in rat brain (Dyckner et al., 1985). Magnesium deficiency has been reported in sudden infant death syndrome and the strong association with thiamin metabolism warrants checking its levels (Caddell, 1972).

Vitamin B_1 toxicity requires no specific laboratory tests. In suspected cases of thiamin toxicity, electrolytes should be checked in patients with severe vomiting or diarrhea (Popovich et al., 2009).

Neuroimaging

MRI demonstrates abnormal hyperintensities of the mammillary bodies and periaqueductal gray matter with associated abnormal enhancement on T1-weighted images (Antunez et al., 1998; Kaineg and Hudgins, 2005). However, a normal MRI does not exclude the diagnosis of Wernicke's encephalopathy (Antunez et al., 1998; Zuccoli and Pipitone, 2009) (Fig. 59.1A-E).

Genetics

No significant genetic association exists with thiamin-related disorders. However, in 1969, Cooper and colleagues (Cooper et al., 1969) published their finding of thiamin pyrophosphate (TPP) deficiency in Leigh's disease, also known as subacute necrotizing encephalopathy. The pathophysiology of this disease is similar but not identical to that of Wernicke's disease (Leigh et al., 1981; Nixon, 1984; Mukherjee et al., 1986; Alexander-Kaufman and Harper, 2009).

Pathology

Lesions typically involve the mammillary bodies, third ventricular walls, medial dorsal nucleus of the thalamus, periaqueductal gray matter, floor of the fourth ventricle, and superior cerebellar vermis.

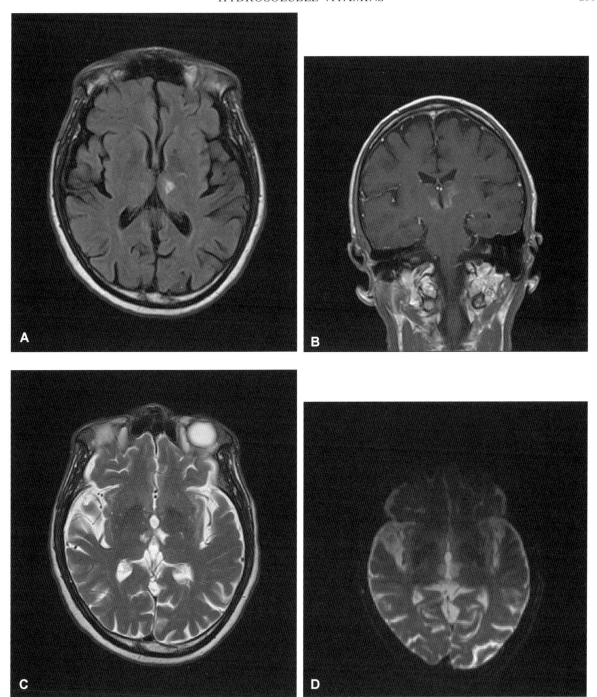

Fig. 59.1. MRI Wernicke's encephalopathy. (**A**) Axial T1 image with contrast enhancement of medial thalami. (**B**) Coronal T1 postcontrast image with enhancement of medial thalamus and periaqueductal gray matter. (**C**) T2-weighted image with increased signal in bilateral medial thalamus and periaqueductal gray region. (**D**) Axial diffusion-weighted image with hyperintensity of medial thalami and periaqueductal white matter adjacent to third ventricle.

Continued

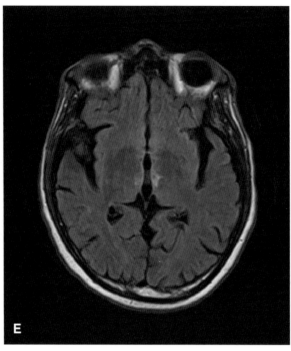

Fig. 59.1—cont'd (**E**) Axial fluid-attenuated inversion recovery (FLAIR) image showing increased signal in the medial thalami.

Inflammatory changes are present. In some instances, fresh petechial hemorrhages are found. The neuropathologic changes in Korsakoff's syndrome are essentially identical in distribution and histologic character to those of Wernicke's encephalopathy. In a large series of pathologically documented cases of Korsakoff's syndrome, compared to thalamic lesions, lesions of the mammillary bodies were not consistently observed.

Pathologic changes in alcoholic cortical cerebellar degeneration involve the anterior and superior portions of the cerebellar vermis and hemispheres. Occasional lesions are found elsewhere in the cerebellar cortex. Secondary changes may be found in the cerebellar white matter, deep cerebellar nuclei, and related brainstem nuclei, such as the olivary complex.

Management

SOURCES, DAILY REQUIREMENTS, AND TOXIC DOSAGES

WE is a medical emergency (Donnino et al., 2007). Poorly nourished patients should receive large doses of parenteral thiamin, particularly if intravenous glucose administration is necessary, even in the absence of symptoms and signs of WE (Fattal-Valevski et al., 2009). Restoration of a well-balanced diet with supplemental vitamins of the B group, especially thiamin, is the keystone of therapy.

If patients respond to vitamin replacement, it is safe to assume that thiamin deficiency was responsible for the condition. The parenteral use of thiamin is advisable in the early stages of treatment. Although the minimum adult daily requirement is approximately 1 mg, injections of 50–100 mg daily are often used early in therapy, with 50–100 mg subsequently taken orally several times daily. A maintenance dose of 2.5–5 mg per day orally is subsequently administered unless a malabsorption syndrome is suspected. Cardiovascular support may be necessary in cases of wet beriberi. Electrolyte abnormalities including hypomagnesemia should be corrected (Donnino et al., 2007). An open trial with thiamin tetrahydrofurfuryl disulfide (TTFD) was performed on 44 patients with polyneuropathy. Thirty-four patients showed improvement of motor function and some restoration of sensory function without any side-effects (Djoenaidi and Notermans, 1990).

If vigorous therapy with thiamin is instituted during the acute phase of the disease, one would anticipate a greater chance of either avoiding or appreciably lessening the ultimate memory defect. Unfortunately, this has not been well documented. Within hours of parenteral administration of 25–50 mg thiamin, the ophthalmoplegia improves, and ocular palsies generally disappear entirely within several days. The truncal ataxia also improves, but again rather slowly and often incompletely. In contrast, improvement in mental status is less predictable. Patients with a quiet confusional state or delirium tend to improve over a period of weeks. However, all too often, memory impairment appears in the course of recovery and may persist thereafter

(Victor et al., 1960; Thomson and Marshall, 2006). The possibility of thiamin deficiency secondary to diuretic therapy has received only scant attention. In patients with advanced congestive heart failure, particularly those receiving long-term furosemide therapy, thiamin deficiency is one determinant of their poor clinical status (Seligman et al., 1991).

In view of the widespread nature of marginal malnutrition in the US, where there is a heavy emphasis on sweet foods containing the simple carbohydrates, particularly sucrose and fructose, findings of this nature are often relevant. Limited data are available on the relation between thiamin requirements and the intake of simple carbohydrate in human physiology, but a study was reported that investigated the influence of stepwise increases of carbohydrate intake on the status of thiamin in healthy volunteers under isocaloric conditions (Elmadfa et al., 2001).

Thiamin, even at high concentrations, is not toxic in a person with normal renal function. No cases of thiamin toxicity have been reported from the use of thiamin at the dosages indicated, even in patients in critical condition (Lheureux et al., 2005).

RIBOFLAVIN (VITAMIN B₂)

Biochemical function

Riboflavin (7,8-dimethyl-10-ribitylisoalloxazine; vitamin B_2), like thiamin, is a water-soluble vitamin with an essential role as a cofactor in redox metabolic reactions involving energy production from carbohydrates, fats, ketone bodies, and proteins. The flavin coenzymes are also used in amino acid and fat metabolism. Effects of riboflavin deficiency on growth are classically related to flavin-dependent redox reactions in the pathways of intermediary metabolism but other mechanisms may also be involved. The oxidative folding of secretary proteins in the endoplasmic reticulum requires flavin dependent oxidases (Tu et al., 2000). The importance of riboflavin derivatives to mitochondrial function was demonstrated in the 1970s and 1980s in studies conducted in riboflavin-deficient animals. Additionally, riboflavin is necessary for the production of glutathione, which is a free radical scavenger.

Natural sources

Riboflavin is an essential nutrient that is unable to be produced by the body. However, it is produced by the normal microflora of the large intestine, with efficient uptake by the colonocytes. It is obtained from the diet as "free" riboflavin and in the forms of flavin mononucleotide (FMN) and flavin adenine dinucleotide (FAD). The main dietary sources are dairy, eggs, whole grains, green leafy vegetables, legumes, organ meats,

mushrooms, and almonds. Although it is heat stable, riboflavin is very light sensitive and easily destroyed with exposure to light. Like thiamin, it is absorbed via a carrier-mediated mechanism in the proximal small intestine and excreted in the urine, and it is not stored in the body in ample amounts, making a constant dietary supply a necessity. Primary riboflavin deficiency results when dietary sources are insufficient. Secondary deficiency can be a consequence of chronic diarrhea, intestinal malabsorption syndromes, liver disorders, hemodialysis, peritoneal dialysis, long-term use of barbiturates, and chronic alcoholism. Commonly, riboflavin deficiency is seen with deficiency of other vitamins, and it is rarely seen in isolation.

Genetics

One inherited form of flavoprotein dysfunction is multiple acyl-CoA dehydrogenation deficiency (MADD). MADD is an autosomal recessive disorder of fatty acid, amino acid, and choline metabolism that can result from defects in two flavoproteins, electron transfer flavoprotein (ETF) or ETF-ubiquinone oxidoreductase (ETF-QO). Some patients respond to pharmacologic doses of riboflavin. It is unknown whether these patients have defects in the flavoproteins themselves or defects in the formation of the cofactor, flavin adenine dinucleotide (FAD), from riboflavin. The deficiency also existed among those with congenital and acquired cardiac diseases (Steier et al., 1976).

Clinical findings

The most common symptoms or riboflavin deficiency are dermatologic, such as cracked red lips, inflamed oral mucosal tissue, and dry scaly skin. The main neurologic manifestation of riboflavin deficiency is a sensory or sensorimotor peripheral neuropathy that is similar to that seen in thiamin deficiency. However, since isolated riboflavin deficiency is rare, and it commonly occurs with other water-soluble B vitamins such as thiamin, the neuropathy that results may be a combination effect to a pan-deficiency of the B vitamins. There is an association of riboflavin deficiency in infants and children with poor growth, but this is likely to be a manifestation of numerous chronic nutrient deficiencies including riboflavin (Bates et al., 1982). Additionally, diabetic children may also be at risk for riboflavin deficiency. The percentage of diabetic children with riboflavin deficiency is fourfold greater than in nondiabetics (Cole et al., 1976).

The presentation of MADD, an inherited deficiency in electron transfer flavoprotein or ubiquinone oxidoreductase that can lead to dehydrogenase deficiency, is typically with nonspecific systemic symptoms of metabolic dysfunction in infancy. Generalized weakness, hypotonia, vomiting, hypoglycemia, and metabolic acidosis are common. The neurologic manifestation occurs with later onset as a lipid storage myopathy. A deficiency state usually occurring in the neonatal period can be easily treated by riboflavin and coenzyme Q10, and therefore should be included in the differential diagnosis of adult-onset painful myopathy (Kaminsky et al., 2011).

Although a riboflavin deficiency state has not been associated with migraines, riboflavin supplementation has been shown to play a role in the treatment of migraines. A randomized controlled trial of high dose riboflavin (400 mg) versus placebo in patients with migraine showed a significant beneficial effect in improvement of headache frequency and headache days (Schoenen et al., 1998). Additionally, acute stroke is another area in neurology where riboflavin treatment may play a role. Experimental evidence shows that riboflavin supplementation reduces oxidative damage and cerebral edema following acute stroke (Gariballa and Ullegaddi, 2007).

Toxicity

Riboflavin toxicity effects may be minimal and nonspecific. Riboflavin turns the urine yellow-orange and is essentially nontoxic (Mularski et al., 2006).

Laboratory investigations

Estimation of erythrocyte glutathione reductase activity accurately reflects riboflavin nutritional status in at-risk individuals (Petteys and Frank, 2011). Diagnosis can also be confirmed by a therapeutic trial or by measuring urinary excretion of riboflavin. Vitamins B_2 toxicity requires no specific laboratory tests (Popovich et al., 2009).

Neuroimaging

There are no characteristic imaging findings in patients with riboflavin deficiency.

Genetics

Maternal riboflavin deficiency enhanced the effects of the genetic trait and increased the frequency of cleft palate in the offspring. An interaction has been reported between the occurrence of cleft palate in genetically susceptible chickens and maternal riboflavin deficiency. (Juriloff and Roberts, 1975).

Pathology

A segmental demyelinating or tomaculous polyneuropathy has also been reported in chickens with riboflavin deficiency, suggesting a detrimental effect on Schwann cells (Cai et al., 2007).

Management

Sources, daily requirements, and toxic dosages

Riboflavin 5–10 mg/day orally is given until recovery. In addition to the stiffening of keratoconic and ectatic cornea, riboflavin-UVA treatment is effective in reducing corneal edema and has the potential to heal corneal ulcers (Ehlers et al., 2009). Management of riboflavin toxicity is mainly supportive.

NIACIN OR NICOTINIC ACID (VITAMIN B₃)

Biochemical function

Niacin (or vitamin B_3) is a water-soluble B vitamin that has multiple necessary biologic effects, particularly energy metabolism. Niacin is defined collectively as nicotinamide and nicotinic acid, both of which fulfill the vitamin functions of niacin carried out by the bioactive forms NAD(P). Niacin is converted to NAD, NADH, which serve necessary roles in oxidative respiration as electron carriers. NADP and NADPH are also niacin-dependant biomolecules which are important in synthesis of nucleic acids, fatty acids, and cholesterol. Therefore, it plays an important role in DNA repair and production of steroid hormones. Niacin could also have a major impact on decreasing the risk for cardiovascular disease as well as treatment of cancer.

Natural sources and history

Dietary sources of niacin include meat, fish, nuts, and green vegetables. Like the other B vitamins previously discussed, niacin is absorbed in the proximal small intestine via carrier-mediated process, is excreted by the kidneys, and is poorly stored in the body. However, alcohol, coffee, and excess carbohydrates interfere with its absorption. Niacin can also be produced within the liver from the essential amino acid tryptophan, but this process requires thiamin, pyridoxine, and riboflavin. Niacin is stable to common food processing techniques.

Niacin deficiency, when severe, causes a clinical syndrome known as pellagra. Niacin deficiency results from inadequate intake of either niacin or tryptophan, as seen in states of malnutrition or chronic alcoholism. Additionally, people who live in areas where corn or maize is a staple food are also vulnerable to niacin deficiency because corn is the only grain that is low in digestible niacin and tryptophan. The high incidence of pellagra in India among people who eat millet with a high leucine content has led to the hypothesis that amino acid imbalance may contribute to deficiency. Deficiencies of protein and many B vitamins commonly accompany primary niacin deficiency. Secondary deficiency may be due to diarrhea, cirrhosis, or alcoholism. Pellagra may also occur in carcinoid syndrome (tryptophan is diverted to form 5-hydroxytryptophan and serotonin) and in Hartnup disease (absorption of tryptophan by the intestine and kidneys is defective). Prolonged treatment with isoniazid, which interferes with the absorption of niacin, is also another important cause of niacin deficiency.

Clinical findings

A deficiency of nicotinic acid or tryptophan amino acid precursor is the cause of pellagra. Pellagra is uncommon in developed countries. Clinical manifestations include pigmented skin rash (dermatitis described as thick, scaly, and darkly pigmented rash; appearance of painful skin flushing with exposure to sun, heat or trauma to the skin), gastroenteritis (diarrhea), and widespread neurologic deficits, including cognitive decline (dementia). Diagnosis is mainly clinical and skin rashes are one of the diagnostic clues for a vitamin B_3 deficiency.

Evidence of central nervous system involvement includes irritability, insomnia, depression, mania, confusion, intellectual decline, and memory impairment. Typical central features of pellagra may also be observed among patients receiving isoniazid, along with the classic dermatologic and intestinal manifestations of the naturally occurring disease (Ishii and Nishihara, 1985). Optic neuropathy, extrapyramidal and cerebellar manifestations may develop. A mild polyneuropathy characterized by distal limb weakness and hypoactive muscle stretch reflexes is often present. Impaired proprioception and vibratory sense may reflect underlying neuropathy or associated myelopathy. Additional findings include glossitis, cheilosis, and seborrheic dermatitis (Pitche, 2005).

Jolliffe et al., in 1940, described nicotinic acid deficiency encephalopathy as acute cerebral edema in alcoholic patients. Symptoms consisted of clouding of consciousness progressing to coma, extrapyramidal rigidity, tremors and primitive reflexes including uncontrollable grasping and sucking. Most of their patients exhibited overt manifestation of Wernicke disease, pellagra, scurvy and polyneuropathy. The status of this syndrome in relation to pellagra is uncertain (Jolliffe et al., 1940).

Acute toxic injection of niacin causes prostaglandin-mediated reaction and include flushing, pruritus, wheezing, vasodilation, headache, increased intracranial blood flow, diarrhea, vomiting, and rarely acanthosis nigricans (Mularski et al., 2006). Serious hepatic toxicity from

niacin administration has been reported with the use of slow-release formulations. Niacin has been shown to induce insulin resistance in short-term trials, but the glycemic response in subjects with and without diabetes is usually minor. Rare, less well-defined side-effects of niacin include blurred vision due to cystoid macular edema, nausea and vomiting, and the exacerbation of peptic ulcers.

Laboratory investigations

Diagnosis of niacin deficiency is clinical and may be straightforward when skin lesions, diarrhea, delirium, and dementia occur simultaneously. Presentation may not be specific and on occasion differentiating the CNS changes from those in thiamin deficiency is difficult. A history of a diet lacking niacin and tryptophan may help establish the diagnosis. A favorable response to treatment with niacin can usually confirm it. If available, laboratory testing can help confirm the diagnosis, particularly when the diagnosis is otherwise unclear. Serum niacin, tryptophan, NAD, and NADP levels can be decreased. Urinary excretion of N-methylnicotinamide is decreased; <0.8 mg/day (<5.8 µmol/day) suggests a niacin deficiency. Laboratory abnormalities with niacin toxicity that are usually small and clinically unimportant include increased prothrombin time, increased uric acid, and decreases in platelet count and serum phosphorus (Guyton and Bays, 2007). Vitamin B_3 monitoring requires liver function tests, uric acid may be increased, leading to gouty arthritis, and in some cases elevated glucose levels can be seen.

Neuroimaging

There are no characteristic imaging findings in patients with niacin-associated disorders.

Genetics

Hartnup disease is an autosomal recessive disorder caused by the defective transport of neutral amino acids in the small intestine and kidneys. The causative gene, *SLC6A19,* is located on a locus on the short arm of chromosome 5 (band 5p15.33) which encodes a transporter. Patients with Hartnup disease present with pellagra-like skin eruptions, cerebellar ataxia, and aminoaciduria. Other skin conditions resembling this rash are seborrheic eczema, nutritional pellagra (where the staple diet is maize), congenital poikilodermas with photosensitivity, systemic lupus erythematosus, and carcinoid syndrome. An abnormality in tryptophan transport leads to niacin deficiency, which is responsible for the pellagra-like eruptions and photosensitivity. Amino acids (tryptophan) retained within the intestinal lumen are converted by bacteria to indolic compounds toxic to the nervous system. After absorption, indole is converted to 3-hydroxyindole (i.e., indoxyl, indican) in the liver where it is conjugated with potassium sulfate or glucuronic acid, then excreted by kidneys as indicanuria (Baron et al., 1956; Castiello and Lynch, 1972; Kraut and Sachs, 2005). In patients with Hartnup disease, the skin, psychiatric symptoms, and diarrhea respond well to niacin 50 mg twice a day. Some patients with autosomal recessive homocystinuria from cystathionine synthetase deficiency may be treated effectively with high doses of vitamin B_6.

Pathology

Pathologic changes are found in the cerebrum, spinal cord, peripheral nerves, and nerve roots. Chromatolytic changes in neurons are encountered, involving most prominently the large Betz cells of the motor cortex. Degenerative changes are found symmetrically in the posterior and lateral columns of the spinal cord. The peripheral nerves show a patchy loss of myelin and axons.

Management

SOURCES, DAILY REQUIREMENTS, AND TOXIC DOSAGES

Although the clinical manifestations of pellagra are due to niacin deficiency, the neurologic changes are remarkably resistant to treatment with niacin alone, even when 25 mg is administered intravenously twice daily. Because multiple deficiencies are common, a balanced diet, including other B vitamins (particularly riboflavin and pyridoxine), is needed.

The Framingham Heart Study has revealed that elevated low-density lipoprotein (LDL) and insufficient high-density lipoprotein (HDL) are independent risk factors for coronary artery disease. Nicotinic acid is the oldest drug known to modify the serum lipids and it is the most effective drug available for elevation of HDL. It also helps reduce cardiovascular risk by reducing serum LDL and triglyceride (TG). Besides over-the-counter sources, Niaspan is another source currently available in the market for nicotinic acid. The statin drugs on the other hand are effective in reducing LDL but they do not significantly raise HDL. At intermediate doses (1000 mg/day), triglyceride levels decrease 15–20%, and HDL cholesterol levels increase 15 –30%. Reductions in LDL cholesterol are modest (<10%). Higher doses of niacin (3000 mg/day) reduce LDL cholesterol 15–20% but may cause jaundice, abdominal discomfort, blurred vision, worsening of hyperglycemia, and precipitation of pre-existing gout. People with a liver disorder probably should not take high-dose niacin. Suspected cases of niacin toxicity require supportive management. Standard protocols indicate that nicotininc acid, combined with diet and exercise, should be the first agent used in an attempt to lower LDL, lower TG and raise HDL. Unfortunately, almost half of the patients discontinue oral nicotinic acid therapy in view of the side-effects of flushing, which drive patients to seek other options. While providing similar efficacy with oral and transdermal delivery, new research is looking into the transdermal delivery to avoid niacin concentration below the threshold for vasodilatation (LaRosa and LaRosa, 2000).

Nicotinamide is predominantly utilized to treat deficiency, because nicotinamide, unlike nicotinic acid (the most common form of niacin), does not cause flushing, itching, burning, or tingling sensations. Nicotinamide is given in doses ranging from 40 to 250 mg/day orally in 3–4 divided doses. Flushing is minimized if niacin is taken after meals or if aspirin is taken 30–45 minutes before niacin. The chance of severe flushing can be reduced by starting immediate-release niacin at a low dose (e.g., 50 mg three times a day) and increasing it very slowly.

PANTOTHENIC ACID (VITAMIN B_5)

Biochemical function

Pantothenic acid, a component of coenzyme A, is an essential nutrient that is required in the synthesis of acetylcholine and melatonin. Coenzyme A is also used as a means of transporting carbon atoms within the cell by catalyzing the production of acetyl-CoA. Therefore, it is important in the conversion of pyruvate to acetyl-CoA and α-ketoglutarate to succinyl-CoA which is necessary for the propagation of the tricarboxylic acid cycle in energy production. It is also needed for the synthesis of fatty acids.

Natural sources

Pantothenic acid is a necessary nutrient that must be obtained from dietary sources. Its name is derived from the Greek pantothen which means "from everywhere." Hence, small quantities of pantothenic acid are present in nearly every food source. The best food sources are avocado, yogurt, mushrooms, eggs, meat, whole grains, legumes, and cruciferous vegetables (such as broccoli or cauliflower). Pantothenic acid is relatively unstable in food. Cooking and commercial processing may result in significant losses of usable vitamin. It is absorbed in the small intestine through a sodium-dependent active transport system within the intestinal cells. No clear indices of pantothenic acid nutrition exist at present (Bender, 1999a).

Clinical findings

Since pantothenic acid is needed for a wide range of biochemical processes, deficiencies in pantothenic acid could potentially have wide-ranging systemic effects. However, naturally occurring pantothenic acid deficiency in humans is actually very rare and has been observed only in cases of severe malnutrition. Most information comes from case reports of severe malnutrition or from experimental animal research. The symptoms of deficiency are similar to other B vitamin deficiencies, which are primarily are due to impaired energy production. Nonspecific systemic symptoms commonly seen are fatigue, irritability, apathy, malaise, nausea, and abdominal cramps. Neurologically, acetylcholine synthesis can also be impaired, which may result in paresthesias or muscle cramps. In the severely malnourished World War II prisoners of the Philippines, Burma, and Japan, painful burning sensations in the feet were improved with administration of pantothenic acid (Bibile et al., 1957). Dogs with pantothenic acid deficiency can develop convulsions. As pantothenic deficiency progresses, more severe acetylcholine insufficiency develops, which can lead to prolonged tetanus (Fry et al., 1976; Bender, 1999a). Chickens develop nerve root damage associated with degeneration of myelin sheaths. Homopantothenate, a pantothenic acid antagonist with cholinergic effects, was used in Japan to enhance cognitive function, especially in Alzheimer's disease. A rare side-effect was the development of hepatic encephalopathy, which was reversible with pantothenic acid supplementation.

No significant pantothenic acid toxicity has been described with large doses of pantothenic acid. Massive doses (i.e., greater than 10 g/day) may cause mild intestinal distress or mild diarrhea.

Laboratory investigations

No confirmatory testing is existent. There are no characteristic imaging findings, known genetic association, or significant pathologic findings in patients with pantothenic acid-associated disorders.

Management

Sources, daily requirements, and toxic dosages

Pantothenic acid is widely distributed in foods and is an essential component of coenzyme A. No set adequate intake level has been determined thus far. Adults probably require about 5 mg/day. Suspected cases of toxicity may require supportive management, but as stated these are typically mild.

PYRIDOXINE OR PYRIDOXAL (VITAMIN B_6)

Biochemical function

Vitamin B_6 is a collective term for the family of 2-methyl-3-hydroxy-5-hydroxymethylpyridine compounds. There are six major derivatives; pyridoxine, pyridoxal, and pyridoxamine, and their phosphorylated derivatives, pyridoxine-5-phosphatase, pyridoxal-5-phosphatase, and pyridoxamine-5-phosphatase. Pyridoxine is a water-soluble vitamin that acts primarily as a necessary cofactor for over 100 enzymes that are mostly involved in amino acid metabolism, including transamination, deamination, and decarboxylation, in addition to being necessary in glycolysis and gluconeogenesis. It is also needed in the decarboxylation of some amino acids into neurotransmitters. Examples of these are the conversion of histidine to histamine, tryptophan to serotonin, glutamate to γ-aminobutyric acid (GABA), and dihydroxyphenylalanine to dopamine. Pyridoxine is also needed for the synthesis of sphingolipids, hemoglobin, and gene expression. Vitamin B_6 deficiency reduces the conversion from tryptophan to niacin and therefore and can induce niacin deficiency (Shibata et al., 1995). Because vitamin B_6 is one of the major determinants of total plasma homocysteine concentrations, a well-known predictor for atherosclerotic disease, the role of vitamin B_6 in coronary artery disease has been mostly addressed through its coenzymatic function for the degradation of homocysteine via transsulfuration pathway in one carbon metabolism (Selhub et al., 1993; Dalery et al., 1995; Stanger et al., 2003). Vitamin B_6 restores blood coagulation abnormalities in homocystinuric subjects and attenuates the formation of thrombin-antithrombin III complexes and prothrombin fragment in subjects treated for mild hyperhomocystinemia (Palareti et al., 1986). The impaired activity of lysyl oxidase, another vitamin B_6-dependent enzyme which is involved in the cross-linking of collagen and elastin, may favor arterial wall degeneration even in conditions of moderate vitamin B_6 deficiency (Murray and Levene, 1977). In addition, vitamin B_6 has been shown to have antioxidant effect by inhibiting superoxide radical generation, reducing lipid peroxidation, and by preventing damage to mitochondrial membrane integrity in a cell culture model (Stephens et al., 2006). By reducing the function of cystathione-β-synthase, vitamin B_6 deficiency causes accumulation of S-adenosylhomocysteine as well as export of homocysteine from the cell, leading to hyperhomocystinemia. This biochemical change induced by vitamin B_6 deficiency is quite similar to what is brought about by a well-known genetic disorder which is related to reduced cystathione-β-synthase activity and provokes premature atherosclerosis and thrombosis (McCully and Ragsdale, 1970).

Natural sources

Pyridoxine is found in a wide variety of food sources, the best ones being meats and fish, chickpeas, whole grains, nuts, potatoes, and bananas. It is also produced by normal microflora of the large intestine which contains mechanisms for efficient absorption. Vitamin B_6 in human breast milk is present mainly as pyridoxal and pyridoxal phosphate. In animal-derived foods, it is also present largely as pyridoxal phosphate and pyridoxamine phosphate, while in plant-derived foods vitamin B_6 is present mainly as pyridoxine, pyridoxine phosphate, and pyridoxine glucoside (Clayton, 2006). Processing of foods through cooking, freezing, or long-term storage can destabilize pyridoxine and significantly reduce its bioavailability. Pyridoxine is readily absorbed in the proximal small intestine, and excreted in the urine. Isolated deficiencies in pyridoxine are relatively uncommon, and deficiencies are usually in combination with the other B vitamins. Therefore, pyridoxine deficiency occurs most commonly with malnourishment, malabsorption states (e.g., celiac disease, Crohn's disease, and ulcerative colitis), and chronic alcoholism. Conditions of chronic illness, such as chronic renal insufficiency, hemodialysis patients, HIV, liver disease, sickle cell disease (Kelly et al., 2004), rheumatoid arthritis, hyperoxaluria types I and II, and tissue injury (Mydlik and Derzsiova, 2010) are also risk factors for pyridoxine deficiency. Certain medications, particularly isoniazid and hydrocortisone, interfere with the absorption of pyridoxine. Antiepileptics such as valproic acid, carbamazapine, and phenytoin, are known to increase the catabolic rate of pyridoxine. Other medications such as cyclosporin hydralazine, D-penicillamine, and pyrazinamide have also been implicated. Acute excessive alcohol ingestion and poisoning with gyromitra mushroom can also lead to a pyridoxine deficiency state. Inherited conditions, such as pyridoxine-dependent neonatal seizures (Khayat et al., 2008; Striano et al., 2009), as well as hereditary sideroblastic anemia, are also proposed etiologies (Morris et al., 2010). Chinese women appear to have an increased risk of developing pyridoxine deficiency. However, it remains unclear whether the increased risk is limited to women in China only or Chinese women around the world (Ronnenberg et al., 2000). Although pyridoxine deficiency can develop in people of any age, the elderly are at increased risk (Woolf and Manore, 2008).

Clinical findings

Pyridoxine deficiency may present with cardiovascular, dermatologic, gastrointestinal, hematologic, or neurologic symptoms. Mild deficiency in B_6 vitamin is a state that may be associated with an increased risk of cardiovascular disease. Cardiovascular abnormalities include early myocardial infarction, early stroke, and recurrent venous thromboembolism (Kelly et al., 2004). B_6 impairment is reported to be associated with higher risk for coronary artery disease (CAD) in patients with coronary atherosclerosis established by angiographic documentation (Robinson et al., 1995). The most convincing data regarding vitamin B_6 supplementation and cardiovascular disease prevention are from the heart outcomes prevention evaluation study (Lonn et al., 2006). Disturbance of cholesterol metabolism is a major risk factor for CAD and it has been suggested that low plasma concentrations of the active vitamin B_6 form, pyridoxal phosphate (PLP), may increase the risk of CAD by affecting the cholesterol metabolism. Selhub et al. described a relationship between lower vitamin B_6 levels and extracranial carotid artery stenosis, which diminished when adjusted for homocysteine levels (Selhub et al., 1995). Pyridoxine treatment has been observed to reduce plasma total cholesterol and low density lipoprotein cholesterol in atherosclerotic patients (Brattstrom et al., 1990). In a 12 week, open-label, randomized, placebo-controlled trial, vitamin B_6 supplementation in male patients with hypertriglyceridemia reduced plasma total cholesterol and HDL-C concentrations (Hlais et al., 2010).

Hematologic problems include anemia. Dermatologic symptoms include erythematous itching, burning, blisters, vesicles, hyperpigmentation, and thickening of skin, similar to those observed with vitamin B_2 or vitamin B_3 deficiencies. Gastrointestinal symptoms include nausea, diarrhea, abdominal discomfort, and pain (Nelson et al., 2002).

Central nervous system symptoms include depression, anxiety, irritability, confusion, and generalized seizures. Peripheral nervous system manifestations include a mixed distal symmetric painful polyneuropathy. Patients with tuberculosis treated with isoniazid, an agent that inhibits pyridoxine phosphorylation, may develop peripheral neuropathy if not given supplemental pyridoxine. In neonates and young infants, neurologic signs include hypotonia, irritability, restlessness, focal, bilateral motor, or myoclonic seizures, and infantile spasms. In addition, patients may have confusion, dementia, disorientation, and rigidity.

Epidemiologic and laboratory animal studies have suggested that the availability of vitamin B_6 modulates cancer risk. The most convincing data were obtained from a series of animal studies conducted in a chemical carcinogen model of colon cancer in mice, evaluating the effect of dietary vitamin B_6 on colonic carcinogenesis (Komatsu et al., 2001). Shimada et al. (2005) found high dietary pyridoxine (35 mg/kg) reduced tumor incidence compared to low dietary pyridoxine (7 mg/kg diet). The exact mechanism remains unclear but it has been reported that high dietary vitamin B_6 attenuates, and low dietary vitamin B_6 increases the risk of cancer.

Vitamin B_6 is usually safe at doses up to 200 mg per day in adults. When taken at higher doses over a long period of time, vitamin B_6 can produce a range of nonspecific systemic symptoms, including nausea, vomiting, diarrhea, tachypnea, and rash. Megadoses (greater than 2 g/day) of pyridoxine may cause a sensory neuronopathy with severe generalized sensory loss throughout the body (Parry and Bredesen, 1985; Dalton and Dalton, 1987; Castagnet et al., 2010). However, there have been a few case reports of patients developing sensory neuropathies at doses of less than 500 mg daily over a period of months (Bender, 1999b). Because placebo-controlled studies have generally failed to show therapeutic benefits of high doses of pyridoxine, there is little reason to exceed the UL of 100 mg/day. Muscle weakness has been described in a few patients.

Laboratory investigations

Pyridoxine deficiency is diagnosed by measuring pyridoxine blood levels. Levels of 4-pyridoxic acid can be measured in the urine and are normally 128–680 nmol per nmol of creatinine. Urine levels of 4-pyridoxic acid are lower in women and are also reduced in persons with riboflavin deficiency (Attard et al., 2008). The erythrocyte aspartate aminotransferase (EAST) and the EAST activation (EAST-AC) coefficient are valuable indicators of functional long-term pyridoxine status due to the 120 day lifespan of erythrocytes. A low EAST-AC value confirms a subacute to chronic deficiency state. The tryptophan loading test is most useful for monitoring an individual's response to pyridoxine supplementation. A tryptophan load of 50–100 mg/kg is administered, and the urinary excretion of tryptophan metabolites is measured. Hematologic indexes may indicate the presence of a hypochromic-microcytic anemia with normal iron levels. Patients with inherited sideroblastic anemias have marked red blood cell dimorphism, anisocytosis, and poikilocytosis. Concentration of plasma pyridoxal-5-phosphate (PLP) below the lowest 20th percentile for control subjects (<23.3 nmol/L) was associated with an increased risk for atherosclerosis and the relationship between vitamin B_6 and atherosclerosis was independent of traditional risk factors including plasma homocysteine levels (Robinson et al., 1998). The Framingham Heart Study cohort were analyzed precisely to explore a possible relationship between vitamin B_6 and a major marker of acute phase. This study highlighted an inverse correlation between plasma PLP and values of C-reactive protein (Friso et al., 2004).

EEG findings in pyridoxine-dependent seizures are characterized by repetitive runs of high-voltage, generalized, bilateral, synchronous 1–4 Hz spikes and sharp wave bursts. Normalization of EEG findings or seizure cessation by injecting 100 mg of intravenous pyridoxine identifies pyridoxine-dependent and pyridoxine-responsive seizures. EMG studies can demonstrate absent or severely reduced sensory nerve action potentials, with mild slowing of sensory nerve conduction velocities. Compound motor action potential and motor nerve conduction velocity are normal. Sural nerve biopsy shows axonal degeneration of both large- and small-diameter myelinated fibers (Schmitt et al., 2010).

Electrolytes should be checked in patients with severe vomiting or diarrhea. Vitamin B_6 toxicity does not require laboratory or other tests. Lumbar puncture (LP) may be considered to rule out other causes if the patient has a peripheral neuropathy (Popovich et al., 2009).

Neuroimaging

There are no characteristic imaging findings in a patient with pyridoxine-associated disorders.

Genetics

Pyridoxine-dependent seizures occur almost exclusively in children younger than 3 months of age, usually in the newborn period. Seizures presumably result from depletion of GABA and high glutamate levels. Inherited pyridoxine-dependent seizure is a rare autosomal recessive condition. Patients with pyridoxine-dependent seizures may exhibit developmental delay, particularly in language, irritability, tremulousness, and poor psychomotor development. The administration of pyridoxine arrests seizures and may also foster normal development. Vigilance is required injecting pyridoxine into an infant or neonate as it can cause a precipitous decrease in blood pressure (Khayat et al., 2008; Striano et al., 2009; Schmitt et al., 2010).

Pathology

The relationship between pyridoxine overdose levels and histologic damage has been well characterized (Windebank et al., 1985). Pyridoxine given in large doses is thought to selectively destroy the large-diameter peripheral sensory nerve fibers, leaving motor fibers intact. Diverse models have been used on a variety of animals, such as rats, dogs (Chung et al., 2008), guinea pigs (Xu et al., 1989) and cats (Stapley et al., 2002). In addition, new models of acute auditory neuropathy have been studied after massive administrations of pyridoxine (Hong et al., 2009).

Management

SOURCES, DAILY REQUIREMENTS, AND TOXIC DOSAGES

Neuropathy caused by isoniazid may be prevented by the concomitant administration of pyridoxine. Although the minimum daily requirement of pyridoxine is only approximately 2 mg in adults, 50 mg/day or more may be required for successful therapy in the deficiency states. Pyridoxine supplementation has been tried on people with sickle cell anemia; however, no changes were noted in these patients' hematologic indexes or disease activity. Oral pyridoxine supplementation with 120 mg/day for 5 weeks reduced serum folate concentration as well as total plasma homocysteine concentration in healthy subjects (Mansoor et al., 1999). Pyridoxine may have beneficial therapeutic effects in cardiovascular disease states and has previously been shown to increase endothelial NO biosynthesis (Wu et al., 2009). Current interest in vitamin B_6 focuses on its role in decreasing circulating homocysteine, a risk factor for vascular disease, or on its role in the risk of cancers. However, the B_6-related atherogenesis is still poorly understood. Seizures in infants who are pyridoxine-dependent must be treated using pharmacologic doses of pyridoxine (vitamin B_6), and lifelong therapy is required. Dosing in adults and pediatric populations is variable and based on underlying indications.

Pyridoxine has the highest adverse outcome per toxic exposure for any vitamin, although no deaths have been reported. There is currently no specific antidote for the treatment of pyridoxine intoxication; management is supportive (Lheureux et al., 2005).

ASCORBIC ACID (VITAMIN C)

Biochemical function

Ascorbic means "against scurvy," and scurvy is known to be mainly due to the inactivation of some important dioxygenases involved in the synthesis of a few key molecules, including several collagen forms (De Tullio, 2004). Ascorbic acid, also known as vitamin C, is a water-soluble vitamin that is most importantly needed as an enzymatic cofactor in the synthesis of collagen. Therefore, it is needed for the production and repair of skin, tendons, ligaments, and blood vessels. The basis of the neurologic disorders observed in scurvy is probably related to low activity of other ascorbic acid dependent enzymes. Indoleamine 2,3-dioxygenase, the first and rate-limiting enzyme in human tryptophan metabolism, has also been implicated in the pathogenesis of many diseases. This enzyme is necessary to form kynurenine, and its pathway regulates the metabolism of tryptophan to neuroactive compounds, and also seems to be a key factor in the communication between the nervous and immune systems (Widner et al., 2000; Stone and Darlington, 2002). Intracellular ascorbate serves several functions in the CNS, including antioxidant protection, peptide amidation, myelin formation, synaptic potentiation, and protection against glutamate toxicity. Whereas the whole brain ascorbate concentrations are 1–2 mM,

intracellular neuronal concentrations have been calculated to be much higher (Rice, 2000). Most of the ascorbate in brain is seen in the neurons. More recent investigations have localized high ascorbate concentrations to neuron-rich areas of the hippocampus and neocortex in normal human brain, where the ascorbate content is as much as twofold higher than in other brain regions (Mefford et al., 1981). Neuronal ascorbate content as maintained by this protein also has relevance for human disease. Ascorbate supplements decrease the infarct size in ischemia-reperfusion injury models of stroke, and ascorbate may protect neurons from oxidant damage associated with neurodegenerative disorders such as Alzheimer's, Parkinson's and Huntington's diseases.

Vitamin C experiences degradation directly related to heat exposure. Therefore, cooking and storage in a warm environment can reduce the vitamin C concentration of foods. Additionally, vitamin C can be leached out of foods when cooked in water, which is then poured away. Since the body can only store a certain amount of vitamin C, the body stores become depleted if the vitamin is not regularly consumed. Clinical symptoms of deficiency can develop in a couple of months with a completely vitamin C deficient diet.

Vitamin C deficiency causes a clinical syndrome known as scurvy. Inactivation of peptidyl-prolyl-4-hydroxylase (P4H) by ascorbic acid deficiency is the first identified cause of scurvy (Stone and Meister, 1962). It is rarely found in the US. However, the elderly, alcoholics, and those who subsist on diets devoid of fresh fruits and vegetables are most vulnerable. Infants and children on restrictive diets for medical, economic, or social reasons are at risk for scurvy. In one of the studies done in Thailand it was noted that prolonged consumption of heated milk (ultra-high temperature milk) and inadequate intake of vegetables and fruits were the risk factors for the development of scurvy (Ratanachu-Ek et al., 2003).

Clinical findings

The symptoms of scurvy result from the breakdown of tissues dependent on collagen. The signs of the disease are caused by alteration of the extracellular matrix in the blood vessels, bones, skin, gums, and tendons, which result in skin lesions, hemorrhages, and fragile bone (Fain, 2005). Symptoms of scurvy include lassitude, vision problems, and neurologic disorders. Neurologic symptoms associated with vitamin C deficiency are unusual. Although the disease has been associated with paraparesis in humans, death appears to be due to more to complications of systemic collagen dysfunction and not to a distinct neurologic syndrome (Hirschmann and Raugi, 1999). Most cases of infantile scurvy occur among infants aged 6–24 months. Scurvy is otherwise uncommon in the neonatal period. Initial symptoms are nonspecific and include loss of appetite, poor weight gain, diarrhea, tachypnea, and fever (Popovich et al., 2009). Examination often reveals an infant who is apprehensive, anxious, and progressively irritable. Severe thigh tenderness causing excruciating pain may result in a pseudoparalysis state. Infants often assume the frog leg posture for comfort. Subperiosteal hemorrhages are typical of infantile scurvy. The lower ends of the femur and tibia are the most frequently involved. Petechial hemorrhages of the skin and mucous membranes, including gums, can occur. Hematuria, hematochezia, and melena are rarely noted. Proptosis may result from orbital hemorrhage. Low-grade fever, anemia, and poor wound healing may be present (Ragunatha et al., 2008). Sudden death due to cardiac failure has been reported in infants and adults with scurvy. Predominant morbidity results from hemorrhage into various tissues. Recent laboratory data suggest that the neonatal brain is particularly susceptible to vitamin C deficiency and that this condition may adversely affect early brain development (Tveden-Nyborg and Lykkesfeldt, 2009). Ascorbic acid was also successfully used to induce myelination of the peripheral nerves in a mouse model of Charcot–Marie–Tooth disease; however, the underlying biochemical mechanism is not clear (Passage et al., 2004).

Toxicity associated with vitamin C is characterized by renal colic due to nephrolithiasis, diarrhea, and nausea, rebound scurvy in infants born to women taking high doses, hemolysis if glucose-6-phosphate dehydrogenase (G-6-PD) deficiency is present, possible dental decalcification, and increased estrogen levels. Findings may also include occult rectal bleeding.

Laboratory investigations

Laboratory tests are usually not helpful in diagnosis of scurvy. An infant presenting with the typical clinical and radiologic picture of scurvy, along with a supportive history of dietary deficiency of vitamin C, is often sufficient to diagnose infantile scurvy. A fasting serum ascorbic acid level greater than 0.6 mg/dL rules out scurvy. Serum ascorbic acid levels of 0.2 mg/dL or greater are considered nutritionally acceptable. Levels of 0.10–0.19 mg/dL are considered low. Levels less than 0.10 mg/dL are considered deficient. White blood cell (WBC) ascorbic acid concentration is a more accurate measure of a vitamin C nutritional state. A zero level indicates latent scurvy. Levels > 15 mg/dL reflect a state of nutritional adequacy. Levels of 8–15 mg/dL are considered low while levels of 0–7 mg/dL reflect a state of deficiency (Popovich et al., 2009).

Vitamin C toxicity requires urine analysis to rule out uricosuria. False-negative test results for glucosuria are possible. Renal function tests should be performed. Prothrombin time should be measured if the patient is taking warfarin; vitamin C may interfere with coumadin. Serum iron levels should also be measured since vitamin C also enhances the absorption of iron (Popovich et al., 2009).

Neuroimaging

Characteristic radiologic changes in scurvy occur at the growth cartilage-shaft junction of bones with rapid growth. The knee joints, wrists, and sternal ends of the ribs are typical sites of involvement. In the early phase of scurvy, the cortex becomes thin and the trabecular structure of the medulla atrophies and develops a ground-glass appearance. The zone of provisional calcification becomes dense and widened, and this zone is referred to as the white line of Frankel. The zone of rarefaction typically involves the lateral aspects of the white line, resulting in triangular defects called the corner sign of Park. With healing, they become calcified and are readily observed (Choi et al., 2007). A helical CT scan or an intravenous urogram (IVU) should be obtained for suspected nephrolithiasis in patients with vitamin C toxicity.

Genetics

No significant genetic association has been described either with vitamin C deficiency or with toxicity. However, both ascorbic acid deficiency and low expression of prolyl hydroxylase due to inherited defects or gene manipulation lead to the same results (Myllyharju and Kivirikko, 2001).

Pathology

The typical pathologic manifestations of vitamin C deficiency are noted in collagen-containing tissues and in organs and tissues such as skin, cartilage, dentine, osteoid, and capillary blood vessels. Pathologic changes are a function of the rate of growth of the affected tissues; hence, the bone changes are often observed only in infants during periods of rapid bone growth. The bony changes occur at the junction between the end of the diaphysis and growth cartilage (Popovich et al., 2009).

Management

SOURCES, DAILY REQUIREMENTS, AND TOXIC DOSAGES

Humans lack the ability to synthesize and make vitamin C and therefore depend on exogenous dietary sources to meet their vitamin C needs. Consumption of fruits and vegetables or diets fortified with vitamin C is essential to avoid ascorbic acid deficiency. Although scurvy is uncommon, it still occurs and can affect adults and children who have chronic dietary vitamin C deficiency. The dietary requirements for vitamin C sufficient to prevent deficiency vary with the age of the individual. Vitamin C administered by mouth or via the parenteral route is effective in curing infantile scurvy. All symptoms can be reversed with ascorbic acid administration.

Ascorbate supplements decrease the size of the infarct in animal studies. For example, in monkeys given 1 g/day of ascorbate parenterally for 6 days before middle cerebral artery occlusion, brain ascorbate was increased by 50%. Infarct size was decreased by 50% in the ascorbate-treated group compared to the control group (Ranjan et al., 1993). Orange juice is an effective dietary remedy for curing infantile scurvy and was the standard treatment before the discovery of vitamin C. Upon instituting dietary or pharmacologic treatment, the clinical recovery is impressive. The appetite of the infant is recovered within 24–48 hours. The symptoms of irritability, fever, tenderness upon palpation, and hemorrhage generally resolve within 7 days. The Food and Nutrition Board of the National Academy of Sciences (2012), National Research Council's minimum recommended daily dietary allowances of vitamin C for infants is 30–40 mg, for children and adults 45–60 mg, for pregnant women 70 mg, and for lactating mothers 90–95 mg (Popovich et al., 2009). Supplements are usually 100–2000 mg per capsule. Chronic toxic dose is more than 2 g/day.

Suspected toxicity with vitamin C requires supportive management.

CONCLUSIONS (INCLUDING FUTURE DIRECTIONS)

Worldwide nutritional disorders of the nervous system associated with vitamin deficiency states are common and diverse. In the US, many foods (but not alcoholic beverages) are supplemented with multiple vitamins and minerals. Fortifying alcoholic beverages with thiamin might lower healthcare costs. Depending on the cause of the vitamin deficiency, a referral to an alcohol dependency clinic may be needed. There is still much to learn about the interrelationships between vitamins and minerals in the overall management of oxidative metabolism. Follow-up care until delivery of current pregnancy, intensive care of advanced cardiomyopathy, definitive care for hyperthyroidism, or further workup of intestinal derangement may be warranted. Because of vitamin fortification of processed foods and the relative affluence of our present culture, we are not ready to consider that ambiguous symptoms, particularly those that are generally termed functional, are of dietary origin. Education should be provided to adults on serious adverse effects resulting from unintentional overdose on a megavitamin regimen.

REFERENCES

Aasheim ET, Bjorkman S, Sovik TT et al. (2009). Vitamin status after bariatric surgery: a randomized study of gastric bypass and duodenal switch. Am J Clin Nutr 90: 15–22.

Alexander-Kaufman K, Harper C (2009). Transketolase: observations in alcohol-related brain damage research. Int J Biochem Cell Biol 41: 717–720.

Antunez E, Estruch R, Cardenal C et al. (1998). Usefulness of CT and MR imaging in the diagnosis of acute Wernicke's encephalopathy. AJR Am J Roentgenol 171: 1131–1137.

Attard O, Dietemann JL, Diemunsch P et al. (2006). Wernicke encephalopathy: a complication of parenteral nutrition diagnosed by magnetic resonance imaging. Anesthesiology 105: 847–848.

Attard PJ, Eliseo AJ, DeNicola NG et al. (2008). Pyridoxine-related metabolite concentrations in normal and Down syndrome amniotic fluid. Fetal Diagn Ther 23: 254–257.

Baron DN, Dent CE, Harris H et al. (1956). Hereditary pellagra-like skin rash with temporary cerebellar ataxia, constant renal amino-aciduria and other bizarre biochemical features. Lancet 271: 421–428.

Bates CJ, Prentice A, Paul AA et al. (1982). Riboflavin status in infants born in rural Gambia and the effect of weaning food supplement. Trans R Soc Trop Med Hyg 76: 253–258.

Bender DA (1999a). Optimum nutrition: thiamin, biotin and pantothenate. Proc Nutr Soc 58: 427–433.

Bender DA (1999b). Non-nutritional uses of vitamin B6. Br J Nutr 81: 7–20.

Bibile SW, Lionel DW, Dunuwille R et al. (1957). Pantothenol and the burning feet syndrome. Br J Nutr 11: 434–439.

Blass JP, Gleason P, Brush D et al. (1988). Thiamin and Alzheimer's disease. Arch Neurol 45: 833–835.

Bordalo LA, Teixeira TF, Bressan J et al. (2011). Bariatric surgery: how and why to supplement. Rev Assoc Med Bras 57: 113–120.

Brattstrom L, Stavenow L, Galvard H et al. (1990). Pyridoxine reduces cholesterol and low-density lipoprotein and increases antithrombin III activity in 80-year-old men with low plasma pyridoxal 5-phosphate. Scand J Clin Lab Invest 50: 873–877.

Bronstein AC, Spyker DA, Cantilena LR Jr et al.American Association of Poison Control Centers (2008). 2007 Annual Report of the American Association of Poison Control Centers' National Poison Data System (NPDS): 25th Annual Report. Clin Toxicol (Phila) 46: 927–1057.

Caddell JL (1972). Magnesium deprivation in sudden unexpected infant death. Lancet ii: 258–262.

Cai Z, Blumbergs PC, Finnie JW et al. (2007). Novel fibroblastic onion bulbs in a demyelinating avian peripheral neuropathy produced by riboflavin deficiency. Acta Neuropathol 114: 187–194.

Caine D, Halliday GM, Kril JJ et al. (1997). Operational criteria for the classification of chronic alcoholics: identification of Wernicke's encephalopathy. J Neurol Neurosurg Psychiatry 62: 51–60.

Campbell ACP, Russell WR (1941). Wernicke's encephalopathy: the clinical features and their probable relationship to vitamin B deficiency. Q J Med 10: 41–64.

Castagnet S, Blasco H, Vourc'h P et al. (2010). [Chronic demyelinating polyneuropathy and B6 hypervitaminosis]. [Article in French], Rev Med Interne 31: e1–e33.

Castiello RJ, Lynch PJ (1972). Pellagra and the carcinoid syndrome. Arch Dermatol 105: 574–577.

Choi SW, Park SW, Kwon YS et al. (2007). MR imaging in a child with scurvy: a case report. Korean J Radiol 8: 443–447.

Chung JY, Choi JH, Hwang CY et al. (2008). Pyridoxine induced neuropathy by subcutaneous administration in dogs. J Vet Sci 9: 127–131.

Clayton PT (2006). B6-responsive disorders: a model of vitamin dependency. J Inherit Metab Dis 29: 317–326.

Cole HS, Lopez R, Cooperman JM (1976). Riboflavin deficiency in children with diabetes mellitus. Acta Diabetol Lat 13: 25–29.

Cooper JR, Pincus JH (1979). The role of thiamin in nervous tissue. Neurochem Res 4: 223–239.

Cooper JR, Itokawa Y, Pincus JH (1969). Thiamin triphosphate deficiency in subacute necrotizing encephalopathy. Science 164: 72–73.

Dalery K, Lussier-Cacan S, Selhub J et al. (1995). Homocysteine and coronary artery disease in French Canadian subjects: relation with vitamins B12, B6, pyridoxal phosphate, and folate. Am J Cardiol 75: 1107–1111.

Dalton K, Dalton MJ (1987). Characteristics of pyridoxine overdose neuropathy syndrome. Acta Neurol Scand 76: 8–11.

De Tullio MC (2004). How does ascorbic acid prevent scurvy? A survey of the nonantioxidant functions of vitamin C. In: H Asard, J May, N Smirnoff (Eds.), Vitamin C, its functions and biochemistry in animals and plants. Bios Scientific Publishers, Oxford, UK, pp. 159–172.

Decker MJ, Isaacman DJ (2000). A common cause of altered mental status occurring at an uncommon age. Pediatr Emerg Care 16: 94–96.

Djoenaidi W, Notermans SL (1990). Thiamin tetrahydrofurfuryl disulfide in nutritional polyneuropathy. Eur Arch Psychiatry Neurol Sci 239: 218–220.

Donnino MW, Vega J, Miller J et al. (2007). Myths and misconceptions of Wernicke's encephalopathy: what every emergency physician should know. Ann Emerg Med 50: 715–721.

Dyckner T, Elk B, Nyhlin H et al. (1985). Aggravation of thiamin deficiency by magnesium depletion. A case report. Acta Scan 218: 129–131.

Ehlers N, Hjortdal J, Nielsen K et al. (2009). Riboflavin-UVA treatment in the management of edema and nonhealing ulcers of the cornea. J Refract Surg 25: S803–S806.

Elmadfa I, Majchrzak D, Rust P et al. (2001). The thiamin status of adult humans depend on carbohydrate intake. Int J Vitam Nutr Res 71: 217–221.

Fain O (2005). Musculoskeletal manifestations of scurvy. Joint Bone Spine 72: 124–128.

Fattal-Valevski A, Azouri-Fattal I, Greenstein YJ et al. (2009). Delayed language development due to infantile thiamin deficiency. Dev Med Child Neurol 51: 629–634.

Foster D, Falah M, Kadom N et al. (2005). Wernicke encephalopathy after bariatric surgery: losing more than just weight. Neurology 65: 1987.

Friso S, Girelli D, Martinelli N et al. (2004). Low plasma vitamin B-6 concentrations and modulation of coronary artery disease risk. Am J Clin Nutr 79: 992–998.

Fry PC, Fox HM, Tao HG (1976). Metabolic response to a pantothenic acid deficient diet in humans. J Nutr Sci Vitaminol (Tokyo) 22: 339–346.

Gariballa S, Ullegaddi R (2007). Riboflavin status in acute ischaemic stroke. Eur J Clin Nutr 61: 1237–1240.

Greenwood J, Jeyasingham M et al. (1984). Heterogeneity of human erythrocyte transketolase: a preliminary report. Alcohol Alcohol 19: 123–129.

Griffin RM, Hoffman H (2009). Live well vitamins and supplements center. WebMD. Available at http://gnc.webmd.com/vitamin-facts.

Guyton JR, Bays HE (2007). Safety considerations with niacin therapy. Am J Cardiol 99 (6A): 22C–31C.

Hazell A, Butterworth R (2009). Update of cell damage mechanisms in thiamin deficiency: focus on oxidative stress, excitotoxicity and inflammation. Alcohol Alcohol 44: 141–147.

Henderson GI, Schenker S (1975). Reversible impairment of cerebral DNA synthesis in thiamin deficiency. J Lab Clin Med 86: 77–90.

Hirschmann JV, Raugi GJ (1999). Adult scurvy. J Am Acad Dermatol 41: 895–906.

Hlais S, Reslan DR, Sarieddine HK et al. (2010). Effect of lysine, vitamin B(6), and carnitine supplementation on the lipid profile of male patients with hypertriglyceridemia: a 12-week, open-label, randomized, placebo-controlled trial. Clin Ther 34: 1674–1682.

Hong BN, Yi TH, Kim SY et al. (2009). High-dosage pyridoxine-induced auditory neuropathy and protection with coffee in mice. Biol Pharm Bull 32: 597–603.

Howard AJ, Kulkarni O, Lekwuwa G et al. (2010). Rapidly progressive polyneuropathy due to dry beriberi in a man: a case report. J Med Case Reports 4: 409.

Indraccolo U, Gentile G, Pomili G et al. (2003). Thiamin deficiency and beriberi features in a patient with hyperemesis gravidarum. Nutrition 21: 967–968.

Inouye K, Katsura E (1965). Etiology and pathology of beriberi. In: Thiamin and Beriberi, Igaku Shoin, Tokyo, pp. 1–28.

Ishii N, Nishihara Y (1985). Pellagra encephalopathy among tuberculous patients: its relation to isoniazid therapy. J Neurol Neurosurg Psychiatry 48: 628–634.

Jansen BCT, Donath WF (1926). On the isolation of the antiberiberi vitamin. Proc I Acad Wei Amsterdam 29: 1390.

Jolliffe N, Bowman KM, Rosenblum LA et al. (1940). Nicotinic acid deficiency encephalopathy. JAMA 114: 307.

Juriloff DM, Roberts CW (1975). Genetics of cleft palate in chickens and the relationship between the occurence of the trait and maternal riboflavin deficiency. Poult Sci 54: 334–346.

Kaineg B, Hudgins PA (2005). Images in clinical medicine. Wernicke's encephalopathy. N Engl J Med 352: e18.

Kaminsky P, Acquaviva-Bourdain C, Jonas J et al. (2011). Subacute myopathy in a mature patient due to multiple acyl-coenzyme A dehydrogenase deficiency. Muscle Nerve 43: 444–446.

Kelly PJ, Kistler JP, Shih VE et al. (2004). Inflammation, homocysteine, and vitamin B6 status after ischemic stroke. Stroke 35: 12–15.

Khayat M, Korman SH, Frankel P et al. (2008). PNPO deficiency: an under diagnosed inborn error of pyridoxine metabolism. Mol Genet Metab 94: 431–434.

Kim E, Ku J, Namkoong K et al. (2009). Mammillothalamic functional connectivity and memory function in Wernicke's encephalopathy. Brain 132: 369–376.

Komatsu SI, Watanabe H, Oka T et al. (2001). Vitamin B-6 supplemented diets compared with a low vitamin B-6 diet suppress azoxymethane-induce colon tumorigenesis in mice by reducing cell proliferation. J Nutr 131: 2204–2207.

Kopelman MD, Thomson AD, Guerrini I et al. (2009). The Korsakoff syndrome: clinical aspects, psychology and treatment. Alcohol Alcohol 44: 148–154.

Kraut JA, Sachs G (2005). Hartnup disorder: unraveling the mystery. Trends Pharmacol Sci 26: 53–55.

LaRosa JH, LaRosa JC (2000). Enhancing drug compliance in lipid-lowering treatment. Arch Fam Med 9: 1169–1175.

Leigh D, McBurney A, McIlwain H (1981). Wernicke–Korsakoff syndrome in monozygotic twins: a biochemical peculiarity. Br J Psychiatry 139: 156.

Lheureux P, Penaloza A, Gris M (2005). Pyridoxine in clinical toxicology: a review. Eur J Emerg Med 12: 78–85.

Loma-Osorio P, Peñafiel P, Doltra A et al. (2008). Shoshin beriberi mimicking a high-risk non-ST-segment elevation acute coronary syndrome with cardiogenic shock: when the arteries are not guilty. J Emerg Med 41: e73–e77.

Lonn E, Yusuf S, Arnold MJ et al. (2006). Homocysteine lowering with folic acid and B vitamins in vascular disease. N Engl J Med 354: 1567–1577.

Lonsdale D (1987). Biochemical studies in functional dysautonomia. In: A nutritionist's guide to the clinical use of vitamin B1, Life Sciences Press, Tacoma, WA, pp. 78–115.

Lonsdale D (1990). Asymmetric functional dysautonomia. J Nutr Med 1: 59–61.

Lu J, Frank EL (2008). Rapid HPLC measurement of thiamin and its phosphate esters in whole blood. Clin Chem 54: 901–906.

Mancall EL, McEntee WJ (1965). Alteration of the cerebellar cortex in nutritional encephalopathy. Neurology 15: 303.

Mansoor MA, Kristensen O, Hervig T et al. (1999). Plasma total homocysteine response to oral doses of folic acid and pyridoxine hydrochloride (vitamine B6) in healthy individuals. Oral doses of vitamin B6 reduce concentrations of serum folate. Scand J Clin Lab Invest 59: 139–146.

Masumoto K, Esumi G, Teshiba R et al. (2009). Need for thiamin in peripheral parenteral nutrition after abdominal surgery in children. JPEN J Parenter Enteral Nutr 33: 417–422.

McCully KS, Ragsdale BD (1970). Production of arteriosclerosis by homocysteinemia. Am J Pathol 61: 1–11.

Meador KJ, Nichols ME, Franke P et al. (1993). Evidence for a central cholinergic effect of high dose vitamin. Ann Neurol 34: 724–726.

Mefford IN, Oke AF, Adams RN (1981). Regional distribution of ascorbate in human brain. Brain Res 212: 223–226.

Minz B (1938). Sur la libération de la vitamin par le tronc isole de nerf pheumogastrique soumis à l'excitation éléctrique. CR Soc Biol (Paris) 127: 1251–1253.

Morris MS, Sakakeeny L, Jacques PF et al. (2010). Vitamin B-6 intake is inversely related to, and the requirement is affected by, inflammation status. J Nutr 140: 103–110.

Mukherjee AB, Ghazanfari A, Svoronos S et al. (1986). Transketolase abnormality in tolazamide-induced Wernicke's encephalopathy. Neurology 36: 1508.

Mularski RA, Grazer RE, Santoni L et al. (2006). Treatment advice on the internet leads to a life-threatening adverse reaction: hypotension associated with niacin overdose. Clin Toxicol (Phila) 44: 81–84.

Mulholland PJ, Self RL, Stepanyan TD et al. (2005). Thiamin deficiency in the pathogenesis of chronic ethanol-associated cerebellar damage in vitro. Neuroscience 135: 1129–1139.

Murray JC, Levene CI (1977). Evidence for the role of vitamin B6 as a cofactor of lysyl oxidase. Biochem J 167: 463–467.

Mydlik M, Derzsiova K (2010). Vitamin B6 and oxalic acid in clinical nephrology. J Ren Nutr 20 (5 Suppl): S95–S102.

Myllyharju J, Kivirikko KI (2001). Collagens and collagen-related diseases. Ann Med 33: 7–21.

National Academy of Sciences (2012). Dietary Guidance: Dietary Reference Intake Reports. USDA National Agricultural Library. Available at http://fnic.nal.usda.gov/nal_display/index.php?info_center=4andtax_level=3andtax_subject=256andtopic_id=1342andlevel3_id=5141.

Nelson MC, Zemel BS, Kawchak DA et al. (2002). Vitamin B6 status of children with sickle cell disease. J Pediatr Hematol Oncol 24: 463–469.

Nixon PF (1984). Is there a genetic component to the pathogenesis of the Wernicke–Korsakoff syndrome? Alcohol Alcohol 19: 219.

Palareti G, Salardi S, Pizzi S et al. (1986). Blood coagulation changes in homocystinuria: effects of pyridoxine and other specific therapy. J Pediatr 109: 1001–1006.

Parry GJ, Bredesen DE (1985). Sensory neuropathy with low-dose pyridoxine. Neurology 35: 1466–1468.

Passage E, Norreel JC, Noack-Fraissignes P et al. (2004). Ascorbic acid treatment corrects the phenotype of a mouse model of Charcot–Marie–Tooth disease. Nat Med 10: 396–401.

Petteys BJ, Frank EL (2011). Rapid determination of vitamin B (riboflavin) in plasma by HPLC. Clin Chim Acta 412: 38–43.

Phayphet M, Rafat C, Andreux F et al. (2007). Hyperemesis gravidarum: a rare cause of Wernicke encephalopathy. Presse Med 36: 1759–1761.

Pitche PT (2005). Pellagra. Sante 15: 205–208.

Popovich D, McAlhany A, Adewumi AO et al. (2009). Scurvy: forgotten but definitely not gone. J Pediatr Health Care 23: 405–415.

Ragunatha S, Inamadar AC, Palit A et al. (2008). Diffuse non-scarring alopecia of scalp: an indicator of early infantile scurvy? Pediatr Dermatol 25: 644–646.

Ranjan A, Theodore D, Haran R et al. (1993). Ascorbic acid and focal cerebral ischaemia in a primate model. Acta Neurochir (Wien) 123: 87–91.

Rao SN, Mani S, Madap K et al. (2008). High prevalence of infantile encephalitic beriberi with overlapping features of Leigh's disease. J Trop Pediatr 54: 328–332.

Ratanachu-Ek S, Sukswai P, Jeerathanyasakun Y (2003). Scurvy in pediatric patients: a review of 28 cases. J Med Assoc Thai 86 (Suppl 3): S734–S740.

Rice ME (2000). Ascorbate regulation and its neuroprotective role in the brain. Trends Neurosci 23: 209–216.

Robinson K, Mayer EL, Miller DP et al. (1995). Hyperhomocysteinemia and low pyridoxal phosphate. Common and independent reversible risk factors for coronary artery disease. Circulation 92: 2825–2830.

Robinson K, Arheart K, Refsum H et al. (1998). Low circulating folate and vitamin B6 concentrations. Risk factors for stroke, peripheral vascular disease, and coronary artery disease. Circulation 97: 437–443.

Roman GC, Spencer PS, Schoenberg BS (1985). Tropical myeloneuropathies: the hidden endemic. Neurology 35: 1158.

Ronnenberg AG, Goldman MB, Aitken IW et al. (2000). Anemia and deficiencies of folate and vitamin B-6 are common and vary with season in Chinese women of childbearing age. J Nutr 130: 2703–2710.

Rudnicki SA (2010). Prevention and treatment of peripheral neuropathy after bariatric surgery. Curr Treat Options Neurol 12: 29–36.

Schmitt B, Baumgartner M, Mills PB et al. (2010). Seizures and paroxysmal events: symptoms pointing to the diagnosis of pyridoxine-dependent epilepsy and pyridoxine phosphate oxidase deficiency. Dev Med Child Neurol 52: e133–e142.

Schoenen J, Jacguy J, Lenaerts M (1998). Effectiveness of high-dose riboflavin in migraine prophylaxis. A randomized controlled trial. Neurology 50: 466–470.

Sebastian JL, JM V, Tang LW et al. (2010). Thiamin deficiency in a gastric bypass patient leading to acute neurologic compromise after plastic surgery. Surg Obes Relat Dis 6: 105–106.

Selhub J, Jacques PF, Wilson PW et al. (1993). Vitamin status and intake as primary determinants of homocysteinemia in an elderly population. JAMA 270: 2693–2698.

Selhub J, Jacques PF, Bostom AG et al. (1995). Association between plasma homocysteine concentrations and extracranial carotid-artery stenosis. N Engl J Med 332: 857–863.

Seligman H, Halkin H, Rauchfleisch S et al. (1991). Thiamin deficiency in patients with congestive heart failure receiving long-term furosemide therapy: a pilot study. Am J Med 91: 151–155.

Shankar P, Boylan M, Sriram K (2010). Micronutrient deficiencies after bariatric surgery. Nutrition 26: 1031–1037.

Shibata K, Mushiage M, Kondo T et al. (1995). Effects of vitamin B6 deficiency on the conversion ratio of tryptophan to niacin. Biosci Biotechnol Biochem 59: 2060–2063.

Shimada D, Fukuda A, Kawaguchi H et al. (2005). Effect of high dose of pyridoxine on mammary tumorigenesis. Nutr Cancer 53: 202–207.

Stamboulis E, Katsaros N, Koutsis G et al. (2006). Clinical and subclinical autonomic dysfunction in chronic inflammatory demyelinating polyradiculoneuropathy. Muscle Nerve 33: 78–84.

Stanger O, Herrmann W, Pietrzik K et al. (2003). DACH-LIGA homocystein e. V. DACH-LIGA homocystein (German, Austrian and Swiss homocysteine society): concensus paper on the rational clinical use of homocysteine, folic acid and B-vitamins in cardiovascular and thrombotic diseases: guidelines and recommendations. Clin Chem Lab Med 41: 1392–1403.

Stapley PJ, Ting LH, Hulliger M et al. (2002). Automatic postural responses are delayed by pyridoxine-induced somatosensory loss. J Neurosci 22: 5803–5807.

Steier M, Lopez R, Cooperman JM (1976). Riboflavin deficiency in infants and children with heart disease. Am Heart J 92: 139–143.

Stephens JW, Gable DR, Hurel SJ et al. (2006). Increased plasma markers of oxidative stress are associated with coronary heart disease in males with diabetes mellitus and with 10-year risk in a prospective sample of males. Clin Chem 52: 446–452.

Stone TW, Darlington LG (2002). Endogenous hynureines as targets for drug discovery and development. Nat Rev Drug Discov 1: 609–620.

Stone N, Meister A (1962). Function of ascorbic acid in the conversation of praline to collagen hydroxyproline. Nature 194: 555–557.

Striano P, Battaglia S, Giordano L et al. (2009). Two novel ALDH7A1 (antiquitin) splicing mutations associated with pyridoxine-dependent seizures. Epilepsia 50: 933–936.

Thomson AD, Marshall EJ (2006). The treatment of patients at risk of developing Wernicke's encephalopathy in the community. Alcohol Alcohol 41: 159–167.

Tran HA (2006). Increased troponin I in "wet" beriberi. J Clin Pathol 59: 555.

Tu BP, Ho-Schlyer SC, Travers KL et al. (2000). Biochemical basis of oxidative protein folding in the endoplasmic reticulum. Science 290: 1571–1574.

Tveden-Nyborg P, Lykkesfeldt J (2009). Does vitamin C deficiency result in impaired brain development in infants? Redox Rep 14: 2–6.

Ueda K, Takada D, Mii A et al. (2006). Severe thiamin deficiency resulted in Wernicke's encephalopathy in a chronic dialysis patient. Clin Exp Nephrol 10: 290–293.

Victor M, Mancall EL, Dreyfus PM (1960). Deficiency amblyopia in the alcoholic patient: a clinicopathological study. Arch Ophthalmol 64: 1.

Wernicke C (1881). Die akute hämorrhagische polioencephalitis superior. Fischer Verlag, Kassel. Lehrbuch der Gehirnkrankheiten für Ärzte und Studierende II: 229–242.

Widner B, Ledochowski M, Fuchs D (2000). Interferon-gamma-induced tryptophan degradation: neuropsychiatric and immunological consequences. Curr Drug Metab 1: 193–204.

Windebank AJ, Low PA, Blexrud MD et al. (1985). Pyridoxine neuropathy in rats: specific degeneration of sensory axons. Neurology 35: 1617–1622.

Woolf K, Manore MM (2008). Elevated plasma homocysteine and low vitamin B-6 status in nonsupplementing older women with rheumatoid arthritis. J Am Diet Assoc 108: 443–453.

Wu Y, Liu Y, Han Y et al. (2009). Pyridoxine increases nitric oxide biosynthesis in human platelets. Int J Vitam Nutr Res 79: 95–103.

Xu Y, Sladky JT, Brown MJ (1989). Dose-dependent expression of neuronopathy after experimental pyridoxine intoxication. Neurology 39: 1077–1083.

Zuccoli G, Pipitone N (2009). Neuroimaging findings in acute Wernicke's encephalopathy: review of the literature. AJR Am J Roentgenol 192: 501–508.

Handbook of Clinical Neurology, Vol. 120 (3rd series)
Neurologic Aspects of Systemic Disease Part II
Jose Biller and Jose M. Ferro, Editors
© 2014 Elsevier B.V. All rights reserved

Chapter 60

Neurologic aspects of cobalamin (B$_{12}$) deficiency

NEERAJ KUMAR*

Department of Neurology, Mayo Clinic, Rochester, MN, USA

INTRODUCTION

Optimal functioning of the central and peripheral nervous system is dependent on a constant supply of appropriate nutrients. Neurologic signs occur late in malnutrition. Deficiency diseases such as kwashiorkor and marasmus are endemic in underdeveloped countries. Individuals at risk in developed countries include the poor and homeless, the elderly, patients on prolonged or inadequate parenteral nutrition, individuals with food fads or eating disorders such as anorexia nervosa and bulimia, those suffering from malnutrition secondary to chronic alcoholism, and patients with pernicious anemia (PA) or other disorders that result in malabsorption such as sprue, celiac disease, and inflammatory bowel disease. Of particular concern in the developed world is the epidemic of obesity. The rising rates of bariatric surgery have been accompanied by neurologic complications related to nutrient deficiencies. The preventable and potentially treatable nature of these disorders makes this an important subject. Prognosis depends on prompt recognition and institution of appropriate therapy.

Particularly important for optimal functioning of the nervous system are the B group vitamins (vitamin B$_{12}$, thiamin, niacin, pyridoxine, and folic acid), vitamin E, and copper. Not infrequently multiple nutritional deficiencies coexist. This review deals with neurologic aspects of vitamin B$_{12}$ deficiency and attempts to highlight recent developments. A prior edition of *Handbook of Clinical Neurology* contains a more comprehensive account of historical and clinical aspects of the neurology of cobalamin (Cbl) deficiency (Cole, 1998). This chapter is biased toward more recent references. The interested reader is directed to some recent review articles and book chapters for detailed bibliographies (Tefferi and Pruthi, 1994; Green and Kinsella, 1995; Cole, 1998; Carmel, 2000, 2008; Ward, 2002; Carmel et al., 2003a; Alpers, 2005; Kumar, 2007; Dali-Youcef and Andrès, 2009; Quadros, 2009; Kumar, 2010).

Formulation of liver extract to treat pernicious anemia led to Minot, Murphy, and Whipple being awarded the Nobel Prize for Physiology/ Medicine in 1934 (Chanarin, 2000). Subsequent elucidation of the crystalline structure of vitamin B$_{12}$ led to Dorothy Hodgkins being awarded the Nobel Prize for Chemistry in 1964 (Chanarin, 2000).

COBALAMIN

TERMINOLOGY

Vitamin B$_{12}$ refers to a specific group of cobalt-containing corrinoids with biological activity in humans. Cobalt is responsible for the red color of this water-soluble vitamin. This group of corrinoids is also referred to as cobalamins. The main cobalamins in humans and animals are adenosylCbl, methylCbl, and hydroxoCbl. Food Cbl is hydroxoCbl. AdenosylCbl and methylCbl are the active coenzyme forms. In all tissues adenosylCbl is the predominant intracellular form and is located in the mitochondria. MethylCbl has a cytosolic localization. MethylCbl is a minor component of intracellular Cbl but is the major form of Cbl in plasma and is the form that is disproportionately reduced in Cbl deficiency. CyanoCbl is a stable synthetic pharmaceutical that also has to be converted to adenosylCbl or methylCbl to become metabolically active. Even though vitamin B$_{12}$ refers specifically to cyanoCbl, the terms Cbl, B$_{12}$, and vitamin B$_{12}$ are generally used interchangeably.

REQUIREMENT FOR AND SOURCES OF COBALAMIN

The recommended dietary allowance of Cbl for adults is 2.4 μg/day and the median intake from food in the US is

*Correspondence to: Neeraj Kumar, M.D., Department of Neurology, Mayo Clinic, 200 First St SW, Rochester, MN 55905, USA.
E-mail: kumar.neeraj@mayo.edu

3.5 µg/day for women and 5 µg/day for men. No adverse effects have been associated with excess Cbl intake. Cbl is synthesized solely by microorganisms. Ruminants obtain Cbl from the foregut. Foods of animal origin such as meat, eggs, and milk are the major dietary sources. The richest sources of Cbl include shellfish, organ meats such as liver, some game meat, and certain fish. In some countries Cbl-fortified cereals are particularly efficient sources.

FUNCTIONS AND KINETICS

In the stomach, Cbl bound to food is dissociated from proteins in the presence of acid and pepsin (Fig. 60.1). The released Cbl binds to haptocorrins (HC, encoded by the *TCN1* gene). The HC have been referred to in the literature as R proteins or R-binder or transCbl I

and III. The HC are secreted by many cell types including glandular cells (salivary glands, gastric mucosa, and others). In the small intestine, pancreatic proteases partially degrade the Cbl-HC complex at neutral pH and release Cbl which then binds with intrinsic factor (IF, encoded by the *GIF* gene). IF is a Cbl-binding glycoprotein secreted by parietal cells in the fundus of the stomach. The Cbl-IF complex binds to a specific receptor in the ileal mucosa called cubilin (CUB, encoded by the *CUBN* gene) and is then internalized (Christensen and Birn, 2002). The internalization of cubulin with Cbl-IF is facilitated by amnionless (AMN, encoded by the *AMN* gene), an endocytic receptor protein that directs sublocalization and endocytosis of CUB with its Cbl-IF complex (Fyfe et al., 2004). The megalin receptor (MAG, encoded by the *LRP-2* gene) may play a role in the stability of the cubilin/AMN complex. Like MAG, the receptor-associated protein (RAP) can interact with

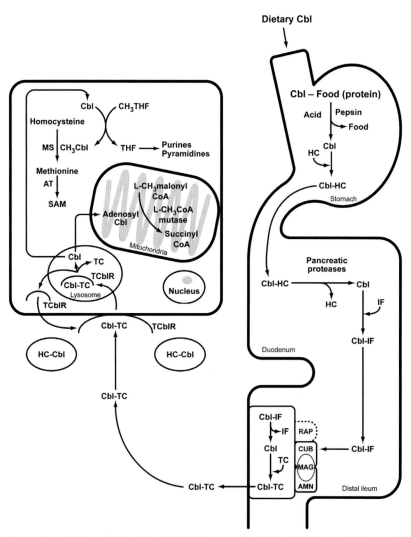

Fig. 60.1. Cbl absorption and metabolism. Cbl, cobalamin; HC, haptocorrin; IF, intrinsic factor; CUB, cubilin; AMN, amnionless; MAG, megalin; RAP, receptor-associated protein; TC, transcobalamin; TCblR, transcobalamin receptor; CH3, methyl; THF, tetrahydrofolate; MS, methionine synthetase; AT, adenosyl transferase; SAM, *S*-adenosylmethionine; CoA, coenzyme A.

CUB, but the precise role of these proteins in CUB-mediated Cbl-IF absorption has not been determined. The Cbl-IF complex enters the ileal cell where IF is destroyed. In addition to the IF-mediated absorption of ingested Cbl, there is a nonspecific absorption of free or crystalline Cbl that occurs by passive diffusion at all mucosal sites. This is a relatively inefficient process by which 1–2% of the ingested amount is absorbed.

TransCbl (TC, encoded by the *TCN2* gene) is a nonglycosylated plasma protein that carries 10–30% of the total Cbl. TC has been referred to in the literature as transCbl II. TC-bound Cbl (holotransCbl, holoTC) represents the active form of Cbl (Refsum et al., 2006). TC binds to and transports the newly absorbed Cbl in the distal ileum to cells throughout the body where it is internalized by receptor-mediated cellular uptake (Quadros et al., 2009). The gene encoding the transCbl receptor (TCblR), *CD320*, was identified from the human genome databank (Quadros et al., 2009). Following internalization, the Cbl-TC complex is degraded by the lysosome and the receptor is recycled to the plasma membrane. Intracellular lysosomal degradation releases Cbl (hydroxoCbl) for conversion to methylCbl in the cytosol or adenosylCbl in the mitochondria (Tefferi and Pruthi, 1994). TC reflects rapidly turning over B$_{12}$, while B$_{12}$ attached to HC in circulating plasma reflect tissue levels of B$_{12}$.

MethylCbl is a cofactor for a cytosolic enzyme, methionine synthase, in a methyl-transfer reaction which converts homocysteine (Hcy) to methionine. Methionine is adenosylated to *S*-adenosylmethionine (SAM), a methyl group donor required for neuronal methylation reactions involving proteins, nucleic acids, neurotransmitters, myelin, and phospholipids. Decreased SAM production possibly leads to reduced myelin basic protein methylation and white matter vacuolization in Cbl deficiency. The biologically active folates are in the tetrahydrofolate (THF) form. MethylTHF is the predominant folate and is required for the Cbl-dependent remethylation of Hcy to methionine. During the process of methionine formation methylTHF donates the methyl group and is converted into THF, a precursor for purine and pyrimidine synthesis. Methionine also facilitates the formation of formylTHF which is involved in purine synthesis. Impaired DNA synthesis could interfere with oligodendrocyte growth and myelin production. Methylation of deoxyuridylate to thymidylate is mediated by methyleneTHF. Impairment of this reaction results in accumulation of uracil which replaces the decreased thymine in nucleoprotein synthesis and initiates the process that leads to megaloblastic anemia. AdenosylCbl is a cofactor for mitochondrial L-methylmalonyl coenzyme A (CoA) mutase which catalyzes the conversion of L-methylmalonyl CoA to succinyl CoA in an isomerization reaction. Accumulation of methylmalonate and propionate may provide abnormal substrates for fatty acid synthesis.

Between 0.5 and 5.0 μg of Cbl enters the bile each day. This binds to IF. Most of the Cbl secreted in the bile is reabsorbed along with Cbl derived from sloughed intestinal cells. Reabsorption of biliary Cbl is intact in vegetarians. Hence, Cbl deficiency develops more rapidly with malabsorption than in vegetarians. The estimated daily losses of Cbl (mainly in the urine and feces) are minute (1–3 μg) compared with body stores (2–3 mg). The body does not have the ability to degrade Cbl. Hence, even in the presence of severe malabsorption, 2–5 years may pass before Cbl deficiency develops (Green and Kinsella, 1995).

CAUSES OF COBALAMIN DEFICIENCY

An acidic environment in the stomach is required for Cbl to be released from food protein. The incidence of atrophic gastritis increases with age. Atrophic gastritis is accompanied by hypochlorhydria. Cbl deficiency is particularly common in the elderly and is most likely due to the high incidence of atrophic gastritis and associated achlorhydria-induced food-Cbl malabsorption (Pennypacker et al., 1992; Carmel, 1995, 1997, 2000; Andrès et al., 2005). Other causes of Cbl deficiency (e.g. *Helicobacter pylori* infection, antacid therapy) may coexist (Andrès et al., 2005). Food-bound Cbl malabsorption does not affect free Cbl, including recycled biliary Cbl (Carmel, 1995). Food-Cbl malabsorption is insidious in onset and rarely associated with overt clinically significant deficiency. Though controversial, there has been recent concern that low Cbl levels in the elderly might cause nervous system damage, but studies specifically in the elderly have not consistently demonstrated improvements in neurologic function following therapy. This concern has led to the development of the controversial concept of subclinical or subtle Cbl deficiency (Carmel, 2000; Carmel et al., 2003b). The low Cbl levels commonly seen in elderly patients can be accompanied by elevated methylmalonic acid (MMA) and Hcy.

Many patients with clinically expressed Cbl deficiency have IF-related malabsorption such as that seen in pernicious anemia (Pruthi and Tefferi, 1994; Toh et al., 1997). Pernicious anemia is associated with IF antibodies. The literature suggests that it is more common in African Americans and in people with a northern European background. Onset is often after age 60, but may be earlier in African American and Hispanic women.

Cbl deficiency is commonly seen following gastric surgery (gastrectomy and bariatric surgery) (Juhasz-Pocsine et al., 2007). This may result from inadequate intake, impaired hydrolysis of vitamin B$_{12}$ from dietary protein, IF loss, or due to abnormal IF and vitamin B_{12} interaction.

Acid reduction therapy such as with H_2 blockers and prolonged use of drugs such as metformin can also cause Cbl deficiency (Marcuard et al., 1994; Ting et al., 2006). Cbl deficiency has also been reported in association with oral therapy with the multitargeted tyrosine kinase inhibitor sunitinib (Gillessen et al., 2007). Cbl malabsorption has been rarely reported with some other drugs but this is generally not clinically significant.

Other causes of Cbl deficiency include conditions associated with malabsorption such as ileal disease or resection, intestinal tuberculosis or lymphoma, celiac disease, Whipple's disease, inflammatory bowel disease, radiation enteritis, graft-versus-host disease, pancreatic disease, and tropical sprue (Carmel, 2000). Bacterial overgrowth can occur in jejunal diverticulosis, enteroanastomosis, strictures, fistulas, and operative procedures and result in Cbl malabsorption. The high acidity associated with the Zollinger–Ellison syndrome causes inactivation of pancreatic trypsin and prevents Cbl release from HC. *H. pylori* infection of the stomach may be associated with mucosal atrophy, hypochlorhydria, and impaired splitting of bound Cbl from food proteins. Competition for Cbl secondary to parasitic infestation by the fish tapeworm *Diphyllobothrium latum* may cause Cbl deficiency. This is not uncommon in the Baltic states, Finland, and Russia.

Certain hereditary enzymatic defects and mutations in genes encoding endocytic receptors involved in ileal absorption and cellular Cbl uptake can also manifest as disorders of Cbl metabolism (Alpers, 2005; Dali-Youcef and Andrès, 2009). Mutations in the gene encoding for the gastric IF (*GIF*) can cause hereditary Cbl deficiency (Tanner et al., 2005). Inborn errors of intrinsic factor are rare and range from a total lack of intrinsic factor to a nonfunctional protein. Mutations in *CUBN* and *AMN* genes have been associated with selective Cbl malabsorption and proteinuria (Imerslund–Gräsbeck syndrome) (Aminoff et al., 1999; Tanner et al., 2003; Fyfe et al., 2004). Low serum Cbl levels can be seen with HC deficiency but this is not clinically significant (Carmel, 2003). Mutation in *TCN2* leading to TC deficiency is clinically significant (Qian et al., 2002; Namour et al., 2003). Congenital abnormalities of TC include complete absence of TC, immunoreactive TC that does not bind to Cbl or does not bind to the receptor. Additional genetic defects of Cbl metabolism involve intracellular processing and utilization of Cbl and include lysosomal release of free Cbl and enzymes involved in synthesis and utilization of Cbl cofactors. Disorders involving the synthesis of Cbl cofactors are identified as cblA to cblG based on the order in which they were discovered (Coelho et al., 2008; Quadros,

2009). These disorders are rare and generally present in childhood with multisystem clinical abnormalities, including developmental, hematologic, and neurologic findings with methylmalonic aciduria or homocystinuria.

Increased prevalence of B_{12} deficiency has been recognized in HIV-infected patients with neurologic symptoms but the precise clinical significance of this is unclear (Kieburtz et al., 1991; Robertson et al., 1993). In AIDS-associated myelopathy the Cbl and folate-dependent transmethylation pathway is depressed and cerebrospinal fluid and serum levels of SAM are reduced (Di Rocco et al., 2002). Despite low B_{12} levels in many AIDS patients, Hcy and MMA levels are normal and Cbl supplementation fails to improve clinical manifestations.

Nitrous oxide (N_2O, "laughing gas") is a commonly used inhalational anesthetic that has been abused because of its euphoriant properties. N_2O irreversibly oxidizes the cobalt core of Cbl and renders methylCbl inactive. Clinical manifestations of Cbl deficiency appear relatively rapidly with N_2O toxicity because the metabolism is blocked at the cellular level. They may, however, be delayed up to 8 weeks (Marie et al., 2000). Postoperative neurologic dysfunction can be seen with N_2O exposure during routine anesthesia if subclinical Cbl deficiency is present (Kinsella and Green, 1995). N_2O toxicity due to inhalant abuse has been reported among dentists, other medical personnel, and university students (Ng and Frith, 2002).

Vitamin B_{12} deficiency is only rarely the consequence of diminished dietary intake. Strict vegetarians may rarely develop mild Cbl deficiency after years. The low vitamin B_{12} level noted in vegetarians is often without clinical consequences. Clinical manifestations are more likely when poor intake begins in childhood wherein limited stores and growth requirements act as additional confounders.

Not infrequently the cause of Cbl deficiency is unknown (Carmel, 2000; Andrès et al., 2005).

CLINICAL MANIFESTATIONS OF COBALAMIN DEFICIENCY

Neurologic manifestations may be the earliest and often the only manifestation of Cbl deficiency (Lindenbaum et al., 1988; Healton et al., 1991; Carmel et al., 2003a). The severity of the hematologic and neurologic manifestations may be inversely related in a particular patient. Relapses are generally associated with the same neurologic phenotype. The commonly recognized neurologic manifestations include a myelopathy with or without an associated neuropathy, optic neuropathy (impaired vision, optic atrophy, centrocecal scotomas), and paresthesias without abnormal signs.

The best characterized neurologic manifestation of Cbl deficiency is a myelopathy that has commonly been referred to as "subacute combined degeneration." The neurologic features typically include a spastic paraparesis, extensor plantar response, and impaired perception of position and vibration. Accompanying peripheral nerve or rarely optic nerve involvement may be present. Asymmetry should prompt search for other causes. Copper deficiency can cause a myeloneuropathy identical to the subacute combined degeneration seen with Cbl deficiency (Kumar et al., 2004).

Neuropsychiatric manifestations of Cbl deficiency include decreased memory, personality change, psychosis, emotional lability, and rarely delirium or coma (Kosik et al., 1980; Lindenbaum et al., 1988; Healton et al., 1991). A concomitant encephalopathy may obscure a coexisting myelopathy (Kosik et al., 1980). Cbl-responsive neuropsychiatric manifestations may be seen in patients without hematologic manifestations and in some patients with a low-normal Cbl level (Lindenbaum et al., 1988). In an individual patient with dementia and Cbl deficiency, the response of the cognitive complaints to Cbl administration is variable and may relate to duration of deficiency (Andrès and Kaltenbach, 2003; Andrès et al., 2005).

Epidemiologic data on Cbl deficiency and cognitive impairment is complex and often contradictory (Clarke, 2008; Vogel et al., 2009). The studies done (cross-sectional surveys, longitudinal studies, intervention studies) are heterogeneous in terms of design and populations studied. Variables include the basis on which Cbl deficiency and cognitive impairment are defined. Additional variables in intervention studies, mostly uncontrolled, include the dose, duration, and route of Cbl supplementation. Many, but not all, studies have shown a relationship between cognitive decline or cognitive deficits and Cbl deficiency. This relationship has been studied not only with vitamin B_{12} levels but also with Hcy or MMA levels, holoTC levels, and vitamin B_{12} intake. Some studies have also looked into rate of brain volume loss and white matter hyperintensities (Vogiatzoglou et al., 2008; de Lau et al., 2009). Despite these observations, the bulk of evidence suggests that vitamin B_{12} supplementation does not result in improved cognition or slowed cognitive decline despite normalization of Hcy or B_{12} levels (Vogel et al., 2009; Ford et al., 2010).

Unusual, and therefore poorly characterized, reported neurologic manifestations possibly related to Cbl deficiency include cerebellar ataxia, leukoencephalopathy, orthostatic tremors, myoclonus, ophthalmoplegia, catatonia, vocal cord paralysis, a syringomyelialike distribution of motor and sensory deficits, and autonomic dysfunction (Eisenhofer et al., 1982; Kandler and Davies-Jones, 1988; Benito-Leon and Porta-Etessam, 2000; Berry et al., 2003; Celik et al., 2003; Morita

et al., 2003; Ahn et al., 2004; Puri et al., 2004; Puri et al., 2006; Akdal et al., 2007). The pediatric literature makes note of involuntary movements and severe neurologic findings including hypotonia and developmental regression with delayed myelination and cerebral atrophy (Avci et al., 2003). Symptoms like fatigue, irritability, and lethargy are nonspecific but not uncommonly reported in the older literature.

Clinical, electrophysiologic, and pathologic involvement of the peripheral nervous system has been described with Cbl deficiency (McCombe and McLeod, 1984; Saperstein et al., 2003). In most cases the clinical features of a Cbl deficiency polyneuropathy are similar to those of a cryptogenic sensorimotor polyneuropathy. Clues to possible B_{12} deficiency in a patient with polyneuropathy included a relatively sudden onset of symptoms, findings suggestive of an associated myelopathy, onset of symptoms in the hands, concomitant involvement of upper and lower limbs, macrocytic red blood cells, and the presence of a risk factor for Cbl deficiency.

Serum Cbl can be normal in some patients with Cbl deficiency and serum MMA and total Hcy levels are useful in diagnosing patients with Cbl deficiency (Allen et al., 1990; Lindenbaum et al., 1990; Stabler et al., 1990; Savage et al., 1994; Green and Kinsella, 1995; Stabler, 1995). The sensitivity of the available metabolic tests for Cbl deficiency has facilitated the development of the concept of subclinical Cbl deficiency (Carmel, 2000; Carmel et al., 2003b). This refers to biochemical evidence of Cbl deficiency in the absence of hematologic or neurologic manifestations. These biochemical findings should respond to Cbl therapy if Cbl deficiency is their true cause (Stabler et al., 1990). If it is unclear whether an elevated MMA or Hcy is due to Cbl deficiency, the response to empirical parenteral B_{12} replacement can be assessed. The frequency of subclinical Cbl deficiency is estimated to be at least 10 times that of clinical Cbl deficiency and its incidence increases with age (Lindenbaum et al., 1994; Metz et al., 1996; Carmel et al., 2003b). The cause of subclinical Cbl deficiency includes food-bound Cbl malabsorption but is frequently unknown; the course is often stationary (Elwood et al., 1971; Waters et al., 1971). Some of these individuals may have subtle neurologic and neurophysiologic abnormalities of uncertain significance that may respond to Cbl therapy (Karnaze and Carmel, 1990; Carmel et al., 1995). The presence of a low Cbl in the association with neurologic manifestations does not imply cause and effect or indicate the presence of metabolic Cbl deficiency. The incidence of cryptogenic polyneuropathy, cognitive impairment, and Cbl deficiency increases with age and the latter may be a chance occurrence rather than causative (Lindenbaum et al., 1994). Further, though Cbl levels are frequently low in the elderly, up to a third are falsely low by clinical and metabolic criteria, and many of the remainder are clinically innocent (Lindenbaum et al., 1994; Carmel, 1997, 2008; Carmel et al., 1999). The clinical impact of subclinical Cbl deficiency and its appropriate management are uncertain.

INVESTIGATIONS

Serum Cbl determination has been the mainstay for evaluating Cbl status (Green and Kinsella, 1995; Snow, 1999; Carmel, 2008). The older microbiological and radioisotopic assays have been replaced by immunologically based chemiluminescence assays. Though a widely used screening test, serum Cbl measurement has technical and interpretive problems and lacks sensitivity and specificity for the diagnosis of Cbl deficiency (Lindenbaum et al., 1990; Moelby et al., 1990; Stabler et al., 1990; Lindenbaum et al., 1994; Matchar et al., 1994; Savage et al., 1994; Green and Kinsella, 1995; Stabler, 1995; Snow, 1999; Carmel, 2000; Carmel et al., 2003a; Solomon, 2005). A proportion of Cbl deficient patients may have Cbl levels that are on the lower side of the normal range (Lindenbaum et al., 1990). A proportion of patients with low Cbl levels are not Cbl deficient (Stabler et al., 1990; Matchar et al., 1994). Levels of serum MMA and plasma total Hcy are useful as ancillary diagnostic tests (Allen et al., 1990; Lindenbaum et al., 1990; Moelby et al., 1990; Stabler et al., 1990; Savage et al., 1994; Green and Kinsella, 1995; Stabler, 1995). They too have significant limitations (Chanarin and Metz, 1997). The specificity of MMA is superior to that of Hcy. Though Hcy is a very sensitive indicator of Cbl deficiency, its major limitation is its poor specificity. Table 60.1 indicates causes other than Cbl deficiency that can result in abnormal levels of Cbl, MMA, and Hcy (Snow, 1999; Carmel, 2000; Ward, 2002; Carmel, 2003; Carmel et al., 2003a). Low serum Cbl levels can be seen with HC deficiency but this is not clinically significant (Carmel, 2003). The highest levels of serum B_{12} reflect concomitant systemic disease in some individuals. Some authors suggest that low Cbl and increased MMA or Hcy levels may not be sensitive markers of Cbl-responsive

Table 60.1

Common causes, other than Cbl deficiency, for abnormal Cbl, MMA, and Hcy levels

Cbl	MMA	Hcy
Decrease (falsely low)	*Increase*	*Increase*
Pregnancy (third trimester)	Renal insufficiency	Renal insufficiency
Haptocorrin deficiency (also seen in sickle cell disease)	Volume contraction (possible)	Volume contraction
Folate deficiency	Bacterial contamination of gut (possible)	Folate deficiency
Other diseases: HIV infection and myeloma (abnormalities in Cbl binding proteins)	MMCoA mutase deficiency	Vitamin B_6 deficiency
Drugs: anticonvulsants, oral contraceptives, radionuclide isotope studies	Other MMA-related enzyme defects	Other diseases: hypothyroidism, renal transplant, leukemia, psoriasis, alcohol abuse
Idiopathic	Infancy, pregnancy	Inappropriate sample collection and processing
Increase (falsely normal)	*Decrease*	Drugs: isoniazid, colestipol, niacin, L-dopa, diuretics
Renal failure	Antibiotic-related reductions in bowel flora	Enzyme defects: cystathionine β-synthase deficiency, MTHFR deficiency
Intestinal bacterial overgrowth (measurement of biochemically inert B_{12} analogs)		Increased age, males, caffeine consumption, increased muscle mass
Increase haptocorrin concentration (seen in liver disease and myeloproliferative disorders such as polycythemia vera, chronic myelogenous leukemia, chronic myelofibrosis)		*Decrease*
		Drugs: estrogens, tamoxifen, statins

Cbl, cobalamin; MMA, methylmalonic acid; Hcy, homocysteine; HIV, human immunodeficiency virus; MTHFR, methylene tetrahydrofolate reductase.

disorders and MMA and Hcy may be normal in some patients with neurologic or hematologic abnormalities responsive to Cbl (Solomon, 2005). Further, short-term fluctuations of Cbl, MMA, and Hcy may obscure Cbl deficiency and lead to erroneous conclusions regarding response to therapy (Solomon, 2005). Measuring MMA and Hcy is also useful in patients with N$_2$O toxicity and some inherited disorders of Cbl metabolism. In these conditions vitamin B$_{12}$-dependent pathways are impaired despite normal vitamin B$_{12}$ levels.

Vitamin B$_{12}$ bound to TC (the Cbl-TC complex, also called holoTC) is the fraction of total vitamin B$_{12}$ available for tissue uptake. HoloTC concentration or TC saturation (holoTC:total TC) have been proposed by some as potentially useful alternative indicators of vitamin B$_{12}$ status (Pennypacker et al., 1992; Herbert, 1994; Hvas and Nexo, 2005; Morkbak et al., 2005; Miller et al., 2006; Refsum et al., 2006; Clarke et al., 2007; Brady et al., 2008). Its levels appear to fall before those of B$_{12}$ as measured by standard methods. A major limitation had been availability of sensitive and reproducible methods of detecting holoTC levels. Some recently published determination methods hold promise (Morkbak et al., 2005; Brady et al., 2008). The test is not available for clinical use and the clinical utility of the measurement awaits further studies (Carmel, 2002). Increase in urinary MMA after an oral dose of one of its precursors, usually valine, can indicate Cbl deficiency but this test is cumbersome and has limited sensitivity (Chanarin et al., 1973).

A rise in the mean corpuscular volume may precede development of anemia. The presence of neutrophil hypersegmentation may be a sensitive marker for Cbl deficiency and may be seen in the absence of anemia or macrocytosis. Megaloblastic bone marrow changes may be seen. The deoxyuridine suppression test measures the synthesis of thymidine and its incorporation into DNA by bone marrow cells. The incubation of nucleated hematopoietic cells with excessive deoxyuridine reduces the uptake of subsequently added titrated thymidine into DNA. This suppression is subnormal in patients with B$_{12}$ or folate deficiency. It is not available for clinical use.

In order to determine the cause of Cbl deficiency tests directed at determining the cause of malabsorption are undertaken. Concerns regarding cost, accuracy, and radiation exposure have led to a significant decrease in the availability of the Schilling test (Carmel, 2007). Further, the Schilling test is based on absorption of crystalline Cbl (with and without intrinsic factor) and does not detect food-Cbl malabsorption. Tests of food-cobalamin absorption using cobalamin bound to animal protein (eggs, salmon, trout, chicken serum) have been devised (Carmel, 2000; Andrès et al., 2003, 2005). The disparity between the abnormal results of these tests and the normal results with the Schilling test defines the disorder of food-cobalamin malabsorption. An elevated serum gastrin and decreased pepsinogen I is seen in 80–90% of patients with pernicious anemia but the specificity of these tests is limited (Carmel, 1988). Elevated gastrin levels are a marker for hypochlorhydria or achlorhydria which are invariably seen with pernicious anemia. Elevated serum gastrin levels may be seen in up to 30% of the elderly (Hurwitz et al., 1997). Elevated serum gastrin levels are approximately 70% specific and sensitive for PA (Miller et al., 1989). Anti-intrinsic factor antibodies are specific (over 95%) but lack sensitivity and are found in approximately 50–70% of patients with pernicious anemia (Carmel, 1992). Studies suggest that antiparietal cell antibodies may not be seen as commonly as was earlier believed and therefore have limited utility (Carmel, 1992). Further, false-positive results for the gastric parietal cell antibody are common. They may be seen in 10% of people over age 70 and are also present in other autoimmune endocrinopathies. A common approach is to combine the specific but insensitive intrinsic factor antibody test with the sensitive but nonspecific serum gastrin or pepsinogen level in patients with Cbl deficiency (Carmel, 2008).

Electrophysiologic abnormalities include nerve conduction studies suggestive of a sensorimotor axonopathy, and abnormalities on somatosensory evoked potentials, visual evoked potentials, and motor evoked potentials (McCombe and McLeod, 1984; Hemmer et al., 1998; Saperstein et al., 2003). Somatosensory evoked potential abnormalities may commonly be seen in patients with a Cbl-deficiency neuropathy and indicate a subclinical myelopathy. Quantitative sensory testing abnormalities are commonly seen but are not specific.

Magnetic resonance imaging (MRI) abnormalities in Cbl deficiency include a signal change in the posterior and lateral columns and less commonly subcortical white matter (Murata et al., 1994; Hemmer et al., 1998; Vry et al., 2005) (Fig. 60.2). Similar spinal cord MRI findings are seen with nitrous oxide toxicity (Ng and Frith, 2002). Contrast enhancement involving the dorsal or lateral columns may be present (Locatelli et al., 1999). The dorsal column may show a decreased signal on T1-weighted images (Locatelli et al., 1999). Other reported findings include cord atrophy and anterior column involvement (Bassi et al., 1999; Karantanas et al., 2000). Treatment may be accompanied by reversal of cord swelling, contrast enhancement, and signal change (Hemmer et al., 1998; Locatelli et al., 1999; Karantanas et al., 2000). Also reported are increased T2 signal involving the cerebellum (Katsaros et al., 1998; Morita et al., 2003). Rarely striking diffuse

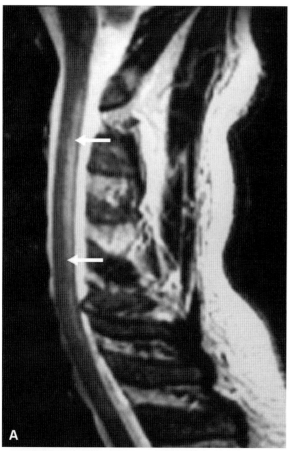

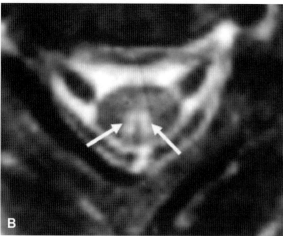

Fig. 60.2. Magnetic resonance imaging (MRI) in cobalamin deficiency. T2-weighted sagittal (**A**) and axial (**B**) MRI of the cervical spinal cord from a patient with myelopathy due to cobalamin deficiency showing increased signal involving the dorsal column. (Adapted from Hemmer et al., 1998, with permission.)

white matter abnormalities (supratentorial and very rarely infratentorial) suggestive of a leukoencephalopathy may be seen (Stojsavljevic et al., 1997; Su et al., 2000; Morita et al., 2003). Brain T2 hyperintensities seen in Cbl deficiency may show significant improvement with

vitamin B$_{12}$ replacement (Stojsavljevic et al., 1997; Su et al., 2000; Morita et al., 2003).

PATHOLOGY

The most severely involved regions in Cbl deficiency-related myelopathy are the cervical and upper thoracic posterior columns. Changes are also seen in the lateral columns. Involvement of the anterior columns is rare. The earliest change is in the dorsal columns and involves splitting and swelling of the myelin sheath which histologically manifests as vacuolization. There is myelin loss followed by axonal degeneration and gliosis. Nerve biopsies show evidence of axonal degeneration (Kosik et al., 1980; McCombe and McLeod, 1984).

MANAGEMENT

The goals of treatment are to reverse the signs and symptoms of deficiency, replete body stores, ascertain the cause of deficiency, and monitor response to therapy. With normal Cbl absorption, oral administration of 3–5 µg of vitamin B$_{12}$ may suffice. In patients with food-bound Cbl malabsorption due to achlorhydria 50–100 µg vitamin B$_{12}$ given orally is often adequate (Verhaeverbeke et al., 1997). More recent studies have shown blunted metabolic responses in elderly persons with subclinical deficiency until oral doses reached 500 µg or more (Eussen et al., 2005). Patients with Cbl deficiency due to achlorhydria-induced food-bound Cbl malabsorption show normal absorption of crystalline B$_{12}$ but are unable to digest and absorb Cbl in food due to achlorhydria.

The more common situation is one of impaired absorption where parenteral therapy is required. A short course of daily or weekly therapy is often followed by monthly maintenance therapy. A common regimen is 1000 µg intramuscular injections for 5–7 days followed by monthly 500–1000 µg intramuscular injections (Green and Kinsella, 1995).

If the oral dose is large enough, even patients with an absorption defect, including pernicious anemia, may respond to oral vitamin B$_{12}$ (Kuzminski et al., 1998; Bolaman et al., 2003; Butler et al., 2006; Andrès et al., 2010). The daily requirement for vitamin B$_{12}$ is 1–2 µg, and approximately 1% of orally administered vitamin B$_{12}$ can be absorbed by patients with pernicious anemia. Consequently an oral vitamin B$_{12}$ dose of 1000–2000 µg/day could suffice. This has been confirmed in clinical trials (Kuzminski et al., 1998; Bolaman et al., 2003; Butler et al., 2006). The role of oral therapy in patients with severe neurologic disease has not been well studied (Andrès et al., 2010).

Patients with pernicious anemia have a higher risk of gastric cancer and carcinoids and therefore should get an endoscopy (Kokkola et al., 1998). Patients with pernicious anemia also have a higher frequency of thyroid disease, diabetes, and iron deficiency and should be screened for these conditions (Carmel and Spencer, 1982; Carmel et al., 1987). A clinical relapse in pernicious anemia after interrupting vitamin B$_{12}$ therapy takes approximately 5 years before it is recognized.

Patients with Cbl deficiency are prone to develop neurologic deterioration following N$_2$O anesthesia. It is preventable by prophylactic vitamin B$_{12}$ given weeks before surgery in individuals with a borderline B$_{12}$ level who are expected to receive N$_2$O anesthesia. Intramuscular B$_{12}$ should be given to patients with acute N$_2$O poisoning. Methionine supplementation has also been proposed as a first-line therapy (Stacy et al., 1992). With chronic exposure, immediate cessation of exposure should be ensured.

In AIDS-associated myelopathy possible benefit of administration of the S-adenosyl methionine precursor, L-methionine, was suggested by a pilot study but not confirmed in a subsequent double-blind study (Di Rocco et al., 2004).

Response to treatment may relate to extent of involvement and delay in starting treatment (Healton et al., 1991). Remission correlates inversely with the time lapsed between symptom onset and therapy initiation. Response of the neurologic manifestations is variable, may be incomplete, often starts in the first week, and is complete in 6 months (Healton et al., 1991; Carmel, 2008). Approximately 2% of patients show a "coasting" phenomenon wherein sensory symptoms show an initial worsening (Healton et al., 1991). The neuropathy may be slow to respond or may not respond at all (McCombe and McLeod, 1984; Saperstein et al., 2003). This is not unexpected given the underlying axonal degeneration. Response of the hematologic derangements is prompt and complete. Reticulocyte count begins to rise within 3 days and peaks around 7 days. Red blood cell count begins to rise by 7 days and is followed by a decline in mean corpuscular volume, with normalization by 8 weeks. MMA and Hcy levels normalize by 10–14 days. If it is unclear whether an elevated MMA or Hcy indicated Cbl deficiency, empirical vitamin B$_{12}$ replacement therapy can be given and metabolite levels repeated after a few weeks. If an elevated MMA or Hcy is due to Cbl deficiency, these values will normalize after 1–2 weeks of replacement therapy (Stabler, 1995). Cbl and holoTC levels rise after injection regardless of the benefit. Hence MMA and Hcy are more reliable ways for monitoring response to therapy. In patients with severe Cbl deficiency, replacement therapy may be accompanied by hypokalemia due to proliferation of bone marrow cells

that utilize potassium. The clinical significance of this hypokalemia is unproven (Carmel, 2008).

HydroxoCbl is commonly used in parts of Europe. It is more allergenic but has superior retention and may permit injections every 2–3 months (Skouby, 1987). Compared with hydroxoCbl, cyanoCbl binds to serum proteins less well and is excreted more rapidly. Intranasal administration of hydroxoCbl has been associated with fast absorption and normalization of Cbl levels (Slot et al., 1997). Advantages of delivering Cbl by the nasal or sublingual route are unproven. Oral preparations of intrinsic factor are available but not reliable. Antibodies to intrinsic factor may nullify its effectiveness in the intestinal lumen.

For unclear reasons, neurologically affected patients with Cbl deficiency may have high folate levels (Carmel et al., 2003b; Quinlivan, 2008). Further, serum B$_{12}$ levels may be lowered in patients with established folate deficiency. Anemia due to Cbl deficiency often responds to folate therapy, but the response is incomplete and transient. Anecdotal evidence suggests that inappropriate folate therapy in patients with Cbl deficiency-related anemia may delay recognition of the Cbl deficiency and cause neurologic deterioration (Kosik et al., 1980). This is controversial, and it is unclear if routine folate supplementation may compromise the early diagnosis of the hematologic manifestations or worsen the neurologic consequences (Dickinson, 1995). Folate exposure has increased after food fortification but studies suggest that this has not resulted in masking of Cbl deficiency (Mills et al., 2003).

REFERENCES

Ahn TB, Cho JW, Jeon BS (2004). Unusual neurological presentations of vitamin B(12) deficiency. Eur J Neurol 11: 339–341.

Akdal GG, Yener G, Ada E et al. (2007). Eye movement disorders in vitamin B12 deficiency: two new cases and a review of the literature. Eur J Neurol 14: 1170–1172.

Allen RH, Stabler SP, Savage DG et al. (1990). Diagnosis of cobalamin deficiency I: usefulness of serum methylmalonic acid and total homocysteine concentrations. Am J Hematol 34: 90–98.

Alpers DH (2005). What is new in vitamin B(12)? Curr Opin Gastroenterol 21: 183–186.

Aminoff M, Carter JE, Chadwick RB et al. (1999). Mutations in CUBN encoding the intrinsic factor-vitamin B12 receptor cubilin cause hereditary megaloblastic anaemia 1. Nat Genet 21: 309–313.

Andrès E, Kaltenbach G (2003). Prevalence of vitamin B12 deficiency among demented patients and cognitive recovery with cobalamin replacement. J Nutr Health Aging 7: 309–310.

Andrès E, Noel E, Kaltenbach G et al. (2003). Vitamin B12 deficiency with normal Schilling test or non-dissociation of vitamin B12 and its carrier proteins in elderly patients A study of 60 patients. Rev Med Interne 24: 218–223.

Andrès E, Affenberger S, Vinzio S et al. (2005). Food-cobalamin malabsorption in elderly patients: clinical manifestations and treatment. Am J Med 118: 1154–1159.

Andrès E, Fothergill H, Mecili M (2010). Efficacy of oral cobalamin (vitamin B12) therapy. Expert Opin Pharmacother 11: 249–256.

Avci Z, Turul T, Aysun S et al. (2003). Involuntary movements and magnetic resonance imaging findings in infantile cobalamine (vitamin B12) deficiency. Pediatrics 112: 684–686.

Bassi SS, Bulundwe KK, Greeff GP et al. (1999). MRI of the spinal cord in myelopathy complicating vitamin B12 deficiency: two additional cases and a review of the literature. Neuroradiology 41: 271–274.

Benito-Leon J, Porta-Etessam J (2000). Shaky-leg syndrome and vitamin B12 deficiency. N Engl J Med 342: 981.

Berry N, Sagar R, Tripathi BM (2003). Catatonia and other psychiatric symptoms with vitamin B12 deficiency. Acta Psychiatr Scand 108: 156–159.

Bolaman Z, Kadikoylu G, Yukselen V et al. (2003). Oral versus intramuscular cobalamin treatment in megaloblastic anemia: a single-center prospective randomized open-label study. Clin Ther 25: 3124–3134.

Brady J, Wilson L, McGregor L et al. (2008). Active B12: a rapid automated assay for holotranscobalamin on the Abbott AxSYM analyzer. Clin Chem 54: 567–573.

Butler CC, Vidal-Alaball J, Cannings-John R et al. (2006). Oral vitamin B12 versus intramuscular vitamin B12 for vitamin B12 deficiency: a systematic review of randomized controlled trials. Fam Pract 23: 279–285.

Carmel R (1988). Pepsinogens and other serum markers in pernicious anemia. Am J Clin Pathol 90: 442–445.

Carmel R (1992). Reassessment of the relative prevalences of antibodies to gastric parietal cell and to intrinsic factor in patients with pernicious anaemia: influence of patient age and race. Clin Exp Immunol 89: 74–77.

Carmel R (1995). Malabsorption of food cobalamin. Baillieres Clin Haematol 8: 639–655.

Carmel R (1997). Cobalamin the stomach and aging. Am J Clin Nutr 66: 750–759.

Carmel R (2000). Current concepts in cobalamin deficiency. Annu Rev Med 51: 357–375.

Carmel R (2002). Measuring and interpreting holotranscobalamin (holo-transcobalamin II). Clin Chem 48: 407–409.

Carmel R (2003). Mild transcobalamin I (haptocorrin) deficiency and low serum cobalamin concentrations. Clin Chem 49: 1367–1374.

Carmel R (2007). The disappearance of cobalamin absorption testing: a critical diagnostic loss. J Nutr 137: 2481–2484.

Carmel R (2008). How I treat cobalamin (vitamin B12) deficiency. Blood 112: 2214–2221.

Carmel R, Spencer CA (1982). Clinical and subclinical thyroid disorders associated with pernicious anemia Observations on abnormal thyroid-stimulating hormone levels and on a possible association of blood group O with hyperthyroidism. Arch Intern Med 142: 1465–1469.

Carmel R, Weiner JM, Johnson CS (1987). Iron deficiency occurs frequently in patients with pernicious anemia. JAMA 257: 1081–1083.

Carmel R, Gott PS, Waters CH et al. (1995). The frequently low cobalamin levels in dementia usually signify treatable metabolic neurologic and electrophysiologic abnormalities. Eur J Haematol 54: 245–253.

Carmel R, Green R, Jacobsen DW et al. (1999). Serum cobalamin homocysteine and methylmalonic acid concentrations in a multiethnic elderly population: ethnic and sex differences in cobalamin and metabolite abnormalities. Am J Clin Nutr 70: 904–910.

Carmel R, Green R, Rosenblatt DS et al. (2003a). Update on cobalamin folate and homocysteine. Hematology Am Soc Hematol Educ Program 2003: 62–81.

Carmel R, Melnyk S, James SJ (2003b). Cobalamin deficiency with and without neurologic abnormalities: differences in homocysteine and methionine metabolism. Blood 101: 3302–3308.

Celik M, Barkut IK, Oncel C et al. (2003). Involuntary movements associated with vitamin B12 deficiency. Parkinsonism Relat Disord 10: 55–57.

Chanarin I (2000). Historical review: a history of pernicious anaemia. Br J Haematol 111: 407–415.

Chanarin I, Metz J (1997). Diagnosis of cobalamin deficiency: the old and the new. Br J Haematol 97: 695–700.

Chanarin I, England JM, Mollin C et al. (1973). Methylmalonic acid excretion studies. Br J Haematol 25: 45–53.

Christensen EI, Birn H (2002). Megalin and cubilin: multifunctional endocytic receptors. Nat Rev Mol Cell Biol 3: 256–266.

Clarke R (2008). B-vitamins and prevention of dementia. Proc Nutr Soc 67: 75–81.

Clarke R, Sherliker P, Hin H et al. (2007). Detection of vitamin B12 deficiency in older people by measuring vitamin B12 or the active fraction of vitamin B12 holotranscobalamin. Clin Chem 53: 963–970.

Coelho D, Suormala T, Stucki M et al. (2008). Gene identification for the cblD defect of vitamin B12 metabolism. N Engl J Med 358: 1454–1464.

Cole M (1998). Neurological manifestations of vitamin B12 deficiency. In: C Goetz, M Aminoff (Eds.), Handbook of Clinical Neurology: Systemic Diseases, Part II. Elsevier Science BV, Amsterdam.

Dali-Youcef N, Andrès E (2009). An update on cobalamin deficiency in adults. QJM 102: 17–28.

de Lau LML, Smith AD, Refsum H et al. (2009). Plasma vitamin B12 status and cerebral white-matter lesions. J Neurol Neurosurg Psychiatry 80: 149–157.

Di Rocco A, Bottiglieri T, Werner P et al. (2002). Abnormal cobalamin-dependent transmethylation in AIDS-associated myelopathy. Neurology 58: 730–735.

Di Rocco A, Werner P, Bottiglieri T et al. (2004). Treatment of AIDS-associated myelopathy with L-methionine: a placebo-controlled study. Neurology 63: 1270–1275.

Dickinson CJ (1995). Does folic acid harm people with vitamin B12 deficiency? QJM 88: 357–364.

Eisenhofer G, Lambie DG, Johnson RH et al. (1982). Deficient catecholamine release as the basis of orthostatic hypotension in pernicious anaemia. J Neurol Neurosurg Psychiatry 45: 1053–1055.

Elwood PC, Shinton NK, Wilson CI et al. (1971). Haemoglobin vitamin B12 and folate levels in the elderly. Br J Haematol 21: 557–563.

Eussen SJ, de Groot LC, Clarke R et al. (2005). Oral cyanocobalamin supplementation in older people with vitamin B12 deficiency: a dose-finding trial. Arch Intern Med 165: 1167–1172.

Ford AH, Flicker L, Alfonso H et al. (2010). Vitamins B(12) B(6) and folic acid for cognition in older men. Neurology 75: 1540–1547.

Fyfe JC, Madsen M, Højrup P et al. (2004). The functional cobalamin (vitamin B12)-intrinsic factor receptor is a novel complex of cubilin and amnionless. Blood 103: 1573–1579.

Gillessen S, Graf L, Korte W et al. (2007). Macrocytosis and cobalamin deficiency in patients treated with sunitinib. N Engl J Med 356: 2330–2331.

Green R, Kinsella LJ (1995). Current concepts in the diagnosis of cobalamin deficiency. Neurology 45: 1435–1440.

Healton EB, Savage DG, Brust JC et al. (1991). Neurologic aspects of cobalamin deficiency. Medicine (Baltimore) 70: 229–245.

Hemmer B, Glocker FX, Schumacher M et al. (1998). Subacute combined degeneration: clinical electrophysiological and magnetic resonance imaging findings. J Neurol Neurosurg Psychiatry 65: 822–827.

Herbert V (1994). Staging vitamin B-12 (cobalamin) status in vegetarians. Am J Clin Nutr 59 (5 Suppl.): 1213S–1222S.

Hurwitz A, Brady DA, Schaal SE et al. (1997). Gastric acidity in older adults. JAMA 278: 659–662.

Hvas AM, Nexo E (2005). Holotranscobalamin – a first choice assay for diagnosing early vitamin B deficiency? J Intern Med 257: 289–298.

Juhasz-Pocsine K, Rudnicki SA, Archer RL et al. (2007). Neurologic complications of gastric bypass surgery for morbid obesity. Neurology 68: 1843–1850.

Kandler RH, Davies-Jones GA (1988). Internuclear ophthalmoplegia in pernicious anaemia. BMJ 297: 1583.

Karantanas AH, Markonis A, Bisbiyiannis G (2000). Subacute combined degeneration of the spinal cord with involvement of the anterior columns: a new MRI finding. Neuroradiology 42: 115–117.

Karnaze DS, Carmel R (1990). Neurologic and evoked potential abnormalities in subtle cobalamin deficiency states including deficiency without anemia and with normal absorption of free cobalamin. Arch Neurol 47: 1008–1012.

Katsaros VK, Glocker FX, Hemmer B et al. (1998). MRI of spinal cord and brain lesions in subacute combined degeneration. Neuroradiology 40: 716–719.

Kieburtz KD, Giang DW, Schiffer RB et al. (1991). Abnormal vitamin B12 metabolism in human immunodeficiency virus infection Association with neurological dysfunction. Arch Neurol 48: 312–314.

Kinsella LJ, Green R (1995). "Anesthesia paresthetica": nitrous oxide-induced cobalamin deficiency. Neurology 45: 1608–1610.

Kokkola A, Sjoblom SM, Haapiainen R et al. (1998). The risk of gastric carcinoma and carcinoid tumours in patients with pernicious anaemia A prospective follow-up study. Scand J Gastroenterol 33: 88–92.

Kosik KS, Mullins TF, Bradley WG et al. (1980). Coma and axonal degeneration in vitamin B12 deficiency. Arch Neurol 37: 590–592.

Kumar N (2007). Nutritional neuropathies. Neurol Clin 25: 209–255.

Kumar N (2010). Neurologic presentations of nutritional deficiencies. Neurol Clin 28: 107–170.

Kumar N, Gross JB Jr, Ahlskog JE (2004). Copper deficiency myelopathy produces a clinical picture like subacute combined degeneration. Neurology 63: 33–39.

Kuzminski AM, Del Giacco EJ, Allen RH et al. (1998). Effective treatment of cobalamin deficiency with oral cobalamin. Blood 92: 1191–1198.

Lindenbaum J, Healton EB, Savage DG et al. (1988). Neuropsychiatric disorders caused by cobalamin deficiency in the absence of anemia or macrocytosis. N Engl J Med 318: 1720–1728.

Lindenbaum J, Savage DG, Stabler SP et al. (1990). Diagnosis of cobalamin deficiency: II Relative sensitivities of serum cobalamin methylmalonic acid and total homocysteine concentrations. Am J Hematol 34: 99–107.

Lindenbaum J, Rosenberg IH, Wilson PW et al. (1994). Prevalence of cobalamin deficiency in the Framingham elderly population. Am J Clin Nutr 60: 2–11.

Locatelli ER, Laureno R, Ballard P et al. (1999). MRI in vitamin B12 deficiency myelopathy. Can J Neurol Sci 26: 60–63.

Marcuard SP, Albernaz L, Khazanie PG (1994). Omeprazole therapy causes malabsorption of cyanocobalamin (vitamin B12). Ann Intern Med 120: 211–215.

Marie RM, Le Biez E, Busson P et al. (2000). Nitrous oxide anesthesia-associated myelopathy. Arch Neurol 57: 380–382.

Matchar DB, McCrory DC, Millington DS et al. (1994). Performance of the serum cobalamin assay for diagnosis of cobalamin deficiency. Am J Med Sci 308: 276–283.

McCombe PA, McLeod JG (1984). The peripheral neuropathy of vitamin B12 deficiency. J Neurol Sci 66: 117–126.

Metz J, Bell AH, Flicker L et al. (1996). The significance of subnormal serum vitamin B12 concentration in older people: a case control study. J Am Geriatr Soc 44: 1355–1361.

Miller A, Slingerland DW, Cardarelli J et al. (1989). Further studies on the use of serum gastrin levels in assessing the significance of low serum B12 levels. Am J Hematol 31: 194–198.

Miller JW, Garrod MG, Rockwood AL et al. (2006). Measurement of total vitamin B12 and holotranscobalamin singly and in combination in screening for metabolic vitamin B12 deficiency. Clin Chem 52: 278–285.

Mills JL, Von Kohorn I, Conley MR et al. (2003). Low vitamin B-12 concentrations in patients without anemia: the effect of folic acid fortification of grain. Am J Clin Nutr 77: 1474–1477.

Moelby L, Rasmussen K, Jensen MK et al. (1990). The relationship between clinically confirmed cobalamin deficiency and serum methylmalonic acid. J Intern Med 228: 373–378.

Morita S, Miwa H, Kihira T et al. (2003). Cerebellar ataxia and leukoencephalopathy associated with cobalamin deficiency. J Neurol Sci 216: 183–184.

Morkbak AL, Heimdal RM, Emmens K et al. (2005). Evaluation of the technical performance of novel holotranscobalamin (holoTC) assays in a multicenter European demonstration project. Clin Chem Lab Med 43: 1058–1064.

Murata S, Naritomi H, Sawada T (1994). MRI in subacute combined degeneration. Neuroradiology 36: 408–409.

Namour F, Helfer AC, Quadros EV et al. (2003). Transcobalamin deficiency due to activation of an intra exonic cryptic splice site. Br J Haematol 123: 915–920.

Ng J, Frith R (2002). Nanging. Lancet 360: 384.

Pennypacker LC, Allen RH, Kelly JP et al. (1992). High prevalence of cobalamin deficiency in elderly outpatients. J Am Geriatr Soc 40: 1197–1204.

Pruthi RK, Tefferi A (1994). Pernicious anemia revisited. Mayo Clin Proc 69: 144–150.

Puri V, Chaudhry N, Gulati P (2004). Syringomyelia-like manifestation of subacute combined degeneration. J Clin Neurosci 11: 672–675.

Puri V, Chaudhry N, Satyawani M (2006). Down beat nystagmus in vitamin B 12 deficiency syndrome. Electromyogr Clin Neurophysiol 46: 101–104.

Qian L, Quadros EV, Regec A et al. (2002). Congenital transcobalamin II deficiency due to errors in RNA editing. Blood Cells Mol Dis 28: 134–142, discussion 143–145.

Quadros EV (2009). Advances in the understanding of cobalamin assimilation and metabolism. Br J Haematol 148: 195–204.

Quadros EV, Nakayama Y, Sequeira JM (2009). The protein and the gene encoding the receptor for the cellular uptake of transcobalamin-bound cobalamin. Blood 113: 186–192.

Quinlivan EP (2008). In vitamin B12 deficiency higher serum folate is associated with increased homocysteine and methylmalonic acid concentrations. Proc Natl Acad Sci U S A 105: E7.

Refsum H, Johnston C, Guttormsen AB et al. (2006). Holotranscobalamin and total transcobalamin in human plasma: determination determinants and reference values in healthy adults. Clin Chem 52: 129–137.

Robertson KR, Stern RA, Hall CD et al. (1993). Vitamin B12 deficiency and nervous system disease in HIV infection. Arch Neurol 50: 807–811.

Saperstein DS, Wolfe GI, Gronseth GS et al. (2003). Challenges in the identification of cobalamin-deficiency polyneuropathy. Arch Neurol 60: 1296–1301.

Savage DG, Lindenbaum J, Stabler SP et al. (1994). Sensitivity of serum methylmalonic acid and total homocysteine determinations for diagnosing cobalamin and folate deficiencies. Am J Med 96: 239–246.

Skouby AP (1987). Hydroxocobalamin for initial and long-term therapy for vitamin B12 deficiency. Acta Med Scand 221: 399–402.

Slot WB, Merkus FW, Van Deventer SJ et al. (1997). Normalization of plasma vitamin B12 concentration by intranasal hydroxocobalamin in vitamin B12-deficient patients. Gastroenterology 113: 430–433.

Snow CF (1999). Laboratory diagnosis of vitamin B12 and folate deficiency: a guide for the primary care physician. Arch Intern Med 159: 1289–1298.

Solomon LR (2005). Cobalamin-responsive disorders in the ambulatory care setting: unreliability of cobalamin methylmalonic acid and homocysteine testing. Blood 105: 978–985.

Stabler SP (1995). Screening the older population for cobalamin (vitamin B12) deficiency. J Am Geriatr Soc 43: 1290–1297.

Stabler SP, Allen RH, Savage DG et al. (1990). Clinical spectrum and diagnosis of cobalamin deficiency. Blood 76: 871–881.

Stacy CB, Di Rocco A, Gould RJ (1992). Methionine in the treatment of nitrous-oxide-induced neuropathy and myeloneuropathy. J Neurol 239: 401–403.

Stojsavljevic N, Levic Z, Drulovic J et al. (1997). A 44-month clinical-brain MRI follow-up in a patient with B12 deficiency. Neurology 49: 878–881.

Su S, Libman RB, Diamond A et al. (2000). Infratentorial and supratentorial leukoencephalopathy associated with vitamin B12 deficiency. J Stroke Cerebrovasc Dis 9: 136–138.

Tanner SM, Aminoff M, Wright FA et al. (2003). Amnionless essential for mouse gastrulation is mutated in recessive hereditary megaloblastic anemia. Nat Genet 33: 426–429.

Tanner SM, Li Z, Perko JD et al. (2005). Hereditary juvenile cobalamin deficiency caused by mutations in the intrinsic factor gene. Proc Natl Acad Sci U S A 102: 4130–4133.

Tefferi A, Pruthi RK (1994). The biochemical basis of cobalamin deficiency. Mayo Clin Proc 69: 181–186.

Ting RZ, Szeto CC, Chan MH et al. (2006). Risk factors of vitamin B(12) deficiency in patients receiving metformin. Arch Intern Med 166: 1975–1979.

Toh BH, van Driel IR, Gleeson PAQ (1997). Pernicious anemia. N Engl J Med 337: 1441–1448.

Verhaeverbeke I, Mets T, Mulkens K et al. (1997). Normalization of low vitamin B12 serum levels in older people by oral treatment. J Am Geriatr Soc 45: 124–125.

Vogel T, Dali-Youcef N, Kaltenbach G et al. (2009). Homocysteine vitamin B12 folate and cognitive functions: a systematic and critical review of the literature. Int J Clin Pract 63: 1061–1067.

Vogiatzoglou A, Refsum H, Johnston C et al. (2008). Vitamin B12 status and rate of brain volume loss in community-dwelling elderly. Neurology 71: 826–832.

Vry MS, Haerter K, Kastrup O et al. (2005). Vitamine-B12-deficiency causing isolated and partially reversible leukoencephalopathy. J Neurol 252: 980–982.

Ward PC (2002). Modern approaches to the investigation of vitamin B12 deficiency. Clin Lab Med 22: 435–445.

Waters WE, Withey JL, Kilpatrick GS et al. (1971). Serum vitamin B 12 concentrations in the general population: a ten-year follow-up. Br J Haematol 20: 521–526.

Handbook of Clinical Neurology, Vol. 120 (3rd series)
Neurologic Aspects of Systemic Disease Part II
Jose Biller and Jose M. Ferro, Editors

Chapter 61

The neurology of folic acid deficiency

E.H. REYNOLDS*

Department of Clinical Neurosciences, King's College, London, UK

HISTORICAL BACKGROUND

Any modern understanding of the relationship of folic acid to nervous system disorders requires some consideration of the historical evolution of our concepts of the neurology of both folic acid and vitamin B_{12} deficiency. This is necessary because of (1) the intimate relationship between folic acid and vitamin B_{12} metabolism; (2) the morphologically indistinguishable megaloblastic anemias that can be caused by either deficiency state; (3) the overlapping neuropsychiatric syndromes and neuropathology associated with either deficiency or related inborn errors of metabolism.

In the late 19th century, the earliest accounts of the neurologic associations of megaloblastic anemia were by Leichtenstern (1884) ("Progressive pernicious anemia in tabetic patients") and Lichtheim (1887), who described typical lesions in the posterior and lateral columns of the spinal cord, for which Russell et al. (1900) coined the term "subacute combined degeneration of the cord" (SCD) when they reported the first full account of the disorder.

In the first third of the 20th century, before treatment became available in the form of liver extract, the neuropsychiatry and neuropathology of megaloblastic anemia was thoroughly documented by many authors (Woltmann, 1919; Ahrens, 1932; Kinnier Wilson, 1940). They recognized: (1) that the nervous system complications could be very varied and included peripheral nerve and psychiatric disorders as well as the classic cord syndrome (SCD); (2) there was often considerable dissociation between the hematologic and neuropsychiatric manifestations, either of which could precede the other. In the absence of treatment, however, patients with megaloblastic anemia would eventually almost all develop some nervous system involvement before death. At this time before the discovery of folic acid or vitamin B_{12} the separation of megaloblastic anemias had not begun and most were regarded as "pernicious anemia," which rested on the demonstration of achlorhydria. Kinnier Wilson (1940) noted that in neurologic series acid was found in the stomach in up to 25%.

Unfortunately folic acid was synthesized first in 1945, 3 years ahead of the isolation of vitamin B_{12}, and was immediately utilized in the treatment of "pernicious anemia" as the possibly deficient dietary factor (Chanarin, 1969). These trials were encouraged by some initially promising improvement in the megaloblastic anemia. However, over the subsequent 5 years and beyond there followed several disturbing reports of aggravation or precipitation of the neurologic complications of "pernicious anemia" by the vitamin (Hall and Watkins, 1947; Schwartz et al., 1950). In fact, folic acid was also often associated with later deterioration in the anemia after the initial improvement (Schwartz et al., 1950); and in some reports there was some temporary improvement in neurologic symptoms before the more florid deterioration (Hall and Watkins, 1947; Reynolds, 1976).

These developments in the period 1945–1950 had a profound effect on subsequent concepts. The introduction of vitamin B_{12} treatment, with its beneficial effects on both the blood and the nervous system, coincided with the height of concern about folic acid. In the third quarter of the 20th century it was therefore erroneously assumed: (1) that the neuropsychiatry of megaloblastic anemia, so carefully documented in the preceding half century, was that of vitamin B_{12} deficiency only; (2) that folic acid was only harmful to the nervous system and there was no neuropsychiatry of folic acid deficiency (see Reynolds, 1976, 1979a).

In the last third of the 20th century these deeply held misconceptions were slowly eroded with the application

---

*Correspondence to: Dr. E.H. Reynolds, Department of Clinical Neurosciences, King's College, Denmark Hill Campus, Weston Education Centre, 1 Cutcombe Road, London SE5 6PJ, UK. Tel: +44-1737-360867, Fax: +44-1737-363415, E-mail: reynolds@buckles.u-net.com

of folate and vitamin B_{12} assays and other techniques to neuropsychiatric patients with and without megaloblastic anemia (Chanarin, 1969; Reynolds, 1976; Botez and Reynolds, 1979), reinforced later by the introduction of homocysteine assays in the 1990s (Carmel and Jacobsen, 2001). Such is the interest now in the role of folates, vitamin B_{12}, and homocysteine in brain metabolism and function at all ages, especially in relation to nervous system development, repair, mood, aging, cognitive function, and dementia (Massaro and Rogers, 2002; Reynolds, 2002a, 2006; Bottiglieri and Reynolds; 2010; Morris and Jacques, 2010), that some have questioned whether folic acid ever had any harmful effects on the nervous system (Dickinson, 1995), another misconception because the vitamin, as with almost all treatments, is associated with benefits and some risks (Reynolds, 2002b).

FOLATE METABOLISM

Reviews of the structure, binding, absorption, transport, metabolism, and function of folates, including polymorphisms of folate-related enzymes and the interaction of folate and vitamin B_{12} metabolism, are the subject of textbooks (Chanarin, 1969; Bailey, 1995, 2010).

Folic acid, also known as pteroyglutamic acid, consists of a pteridine ring linked to p-aminobenzoic acid, in turn linked to glutamic acid. Biologically active folates are reduced by the addition of two or four hydrogen atoms and are referred to as dihydro- or tetrahydrofolates. Some intracellular folate derivatives have additional glutamic acid residues attached to the terminal glutamic acid to produce so-called folylpolyglutamates.

Central to our understanding of folate metabolism is the folate cycle (Fig. 61.1) in which tetrahydrofolate (THF)

accepts a single carbon unit from serine which is progressively reduced through formyl (CHO), methenyl (CH^+), and methylene (CH_2) derivatives, ultimately to 5-CH_3 tetrahydrofolate (5-MTHF). The latter gives up its methyl group to homocysteine to form methionine in an important enzymatic reaction mediated by methionine synthase and catalyzed by vitamin B_{12}, the key area of interaction between folate and vitamin B_{12} metabolism (Fig. 61.1). The released THF begins the cycle of methyl group synthesis all over again. The methyl groups are passed on from methionine to S-adenosylmethionine (SAM), which is the major donor of methyl groups in innumerable genomic and nongenomic methylation reactions in all tissues, including the nervous system, involving nucleoproteins, proteins, lipids, monoamines, etc. SAM also exerts feedback control on methionine synthase activity (Fig. 61.1).

The interconversion of the various carbon-linked folate derivatives in the folate cycle also provides carbon units for other important metabolic pathways. In particular, 5,10-methylene-THF is essential for the synthesis of purines and pyrimidines and therefore ultimately for nucleotide, DNA, and RNA synthesis and, therefore, genetic function. Epigenetic function is in turn also linked to methylation reactions involving SAM.

The circulating form of folate monoglutamates in body fluids including serum and cerebrospinal fluid (CSF) is 5-methyltetrahydrofolate (5-MTHF). Remarkably, folate levels are two to three times higher in CSF than in serum and a high degree of correlation between the two exists in controls and in neurologic and psychiatric patients (Reynolds et al., 1972). An active transport process for 5-MTHF across the blood–brain barrier via the choroid plexus has been confirmed (Spector and Lorenzo, 1975). The correlation between serum

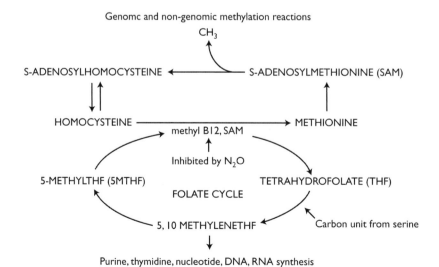

Fig. 61.1. Relationships between the folate cycle, vitamin B_{12}, methylation and nucleotide synthesis. SAM, S-adenosylmethionine; THF, tetrahydrofolate; N_2O, nitrous oxide.

and CSF folate is lost during clinical treatment with folic acid because the blood–brain barrier mechanism limits the entry of 5-MTHF, perhaps in part because of the convulsant properties of folate derivatives which have been demonstrated experimentally (Hommes et al., 1973; Reynolds, 1976).

Because mammalian cells are unable to synthesize folates *de novo* specialized carrier-mediated transport systems for the absorption and delivery of folate derivatives from food have been developed. The three main types of transport system are: the proton-coupled folate transporter (PCFT), the reduced folate carrier (RFC), and a small family of folate receptors (FRs), the latter encoded by three distinct genes i.e., $FR\alpha$, $FR\beta$ and FR_γ. Both $FR\alpha$ and RFC are involved in the transport process across the blood–brain barrier and into neuronal cells (Ramaekers et al., 2005; Wollack et al., 2008).

There has been increasing interest in the last decade in the role of genetic folate polymorphisms in human health, including vascular disease, cancer, and nervous system disorders, especially birth defects (Lucock, 2004; van der Linden et al., 2005; Christensen and Rozen, 2010). Particular attention has focused on MTHFR, especially the $677C \rightarrow T$ variant, and methionine synthase, but no folate enzyme is exempt. Large-scale epidemiologic studies are required to clarify the health impact of these polymorphisms which may assume greater significance only if they are severe or if there are additional nutritional deficiencies and/or other genetic predispositions.

The metabolic basis of megaloblastic anemia has been thoroughly studied and is similar in both folic acid and vitamin B_{12} deficiency (Stabler, 2010). The two basic mechanisms involve: (1) DNA synthesis, especially the impaired incorporation of thymidine and misincorporation of uracil into DNA; (2) methylation, especially impairment of SAM-dependent methylation of DNA (Fig. 61.1). The key metabolic reaction is the vitamin B_{12}-dependent methylation of homocysteine by methionine synthase to produce methionine. In folate deficiency there appears to be a failure in the supply of methyl groups. In vitamin B_{12} deficiency there appears to be a block in the utilization of methyl groups. As will be discussed in this review, these mechanisms involving DNA synthesis and genomic and nongenomic methylation appear also to be at the heart of the neurologic manifestations of these deficiency states.

THE NEUROLOGY OF FOLATE-DEFICIENT MEGALOBLASTIC ANEMIA

Our understanding of the neurology of folic acid or vitamin B_{12} deficiency is greatly influenced by the many clinical and pathologic descriptions in the first half of the 20th century of patients with neuropsychiatric associations of megaloblastic anemia, who usually progressed to death from either the anemia or the neurologic complications in the era before treatment became available, first with liver therapy and later folic acid or vitamin B_{12}. The best review of that older literature is by Kinnier Wilson (1940), who described the overlapping syndromes of SCD, peripheral neuropathy, autonomic dysfunction, optic atrophy, mood and behavior changes, psychosis, memory impairment, and cognitive decline.

Although for a period between the late 1940s and the 1960s it was widely assumed, for the reasons described in the historical introduction, that the older literature must have been synonymous with vitamin B_{12} deficiency, this misconception was gradually dispelled from the 1960s onwards as examples of the neurologic complications of megaloblastic anemia due to folic acid deficiency were increasingly recognized. Thus, Grant et al. (1965) described seven cases of spinal cord and peripheral nerve disease; Strachan and Henderson (1967) reported two patients with dementia; and Reynolds et al. (1968) described eight patients with a range of neuropsychiatric associations of anticonvulsant megaloblastic anemia.

In 1972, Pincus et al. described a patient with dementia and SCD. By 1979 Pincus reviewed 25 cases in the literature of SCD associated with folate deficiency. In a general medical hospital population Reynolds et al. (1973) compared the neurologic status of 24 patients with severe folate deficiency and 21 control patients with normal folate levels. A significant increase in organic brain syndrome and pyramidal tract damage was found in the vitamin-deficient group, which was independent of the degree of anemia. In 1976, Manzoor and Runcie reported 10 cases of folate-responsive SCD and neuropathy, some of whom had cognitive and other mental changes. A year later, Botez et al. (1977) summarized 16 cases of a range of peripheral nerve, spinal cord, and mental disorders responsive to folate therapy, most, but not all of whom had megaloblastic anemia. SCD is invariably accompanied by clinical and/or electrical evidence of peripheral neuropathy, but folate deficiency may also cause isolated peripheral neuropathy (Botez et al., 1979a; Shorvon and Reynolds, 1979).

In retrospect it was by now clear that the early 20th century literature must have included patients with megaloblastic anemia due to folate as well as vitamin B_{12} deficiency, as could also be suspected from the number of those earlier patients who had acid in their stomach and were therefore not suffering from "pernicious anemia." It therefore became important to compare the neurologic complications of the two deficiency states which could now be readily separated with vitamin assay techniques. Patients may present to hematologists and physicians with megaloblastic anemia or to neurologists and

Table 61.1

Neuropsychiatric findings in patients with megaloblastic anemia presenting to physicians (Shorvon et al., 1980)

	Vitamin B_{12} deficiency (%)	Folic acid deficiency (%)
Normal	32	35
Organic mental change	26	27
Affective disorder	20	56
Subacute combined degeneration	16	0
Peripheral neuropathy	40	18
Optic atrophy	2	0

Etiology			
	Number of cases		Number of cases
Pernicious anemia	32	Coeliac disease	16
Dietary	8	Dietary	8
Gastrointestinal	7	Malabsorption	8
Unexplained	3	Unexplained	2
	n = 50		n = 34

psychiatrists with predominantly nervous system symptoms. In a prospective study of patients with megaloblastic anemia Shorvon et al. (1980) compared 50 patients with vitamin B_{12} deficiency and 34 with folate deficiency. The neuropsychiatric findings and the causes of anemia are summarized in Table 61.1. The incidence of nervous system involvement was similar, occurring in about two-thirds of each series. About a quarter of each group had cognitive decline. However, peripheral neuropathy was twice as common in vitamin B_{12} deficiency than in folate deficiency. By contrast, depression was more than twice as common in folate deficiency than in vitamin B_{12} deficiency. SCD was uncommon in vitamin B_{12} deficiency but it was not seen at all in 34 patients with folate deficiency, although, as described above, it can be a rare complication of the latter deficiency.

This study confirmed yet again that there is a poor correlation between anemia and nervous system manifestations. As many as a third of each group with a severe deficiency state had no neuropsychiatric complications. There was a considerable overlap between the neuropsychiatric syndromes in the other two-thirds, with a greater emphasis on the spinal cord and peripheral nerves in vitamin B_{12} deficiency and more affective disorder in the folate-deficient group. Some of these differences may perhaps reflect the older age of the vitamin B_{12}-deficient patients, two-thirds of whom had pernicious anemia, whereas three-quarters of the folate-deficient

group had coeliac disease or other malabsorption syndromes, perhaps resulting in additional deficiency states contributing to the neurologic complications. Nevertheless it is clear that either deficiency state can produce very similar neuropsychiatric syndromes, as is also true of the hematologic manifestations.

NEUROPSYCHIATRIC DISORDERS WITHOUT ANEMIA OR MACROCYTOSIS

About a quarter of patients with folate-responsive neuropsychiatric disorders do not have anemia or macrocytosis when first seen (Bottiglieri et al., 1995), as is the case for vitamin B_{12} deficiency in about one-fifth of patients (Lindenbaum et al., 1988). There are other neuropsychiatric patients with low serum or red cell folate levels in whom the deficiency may be secondary to the neuropsychiatric disorder for dietary or other reasons but in whom the deficiency may be harmful in the longer term if uncorrected (Reynolds, 1976, 2002b).

Up to one-third of psychiatric, and especially psychogeriatric, hospital admissions have low serum or red cell folate, mostly without anemia or macrocytosis (Reynolds, 1976; Crellin et al., 1993; Bottiglieri et al., 1995). The cause of folate deficiency in these patients has been variously attributed to poor diet, chronic illness, drugs (e.g., barbiturates, alcohol), malabsorption, increased demand, or unknown (Carney and Sheffield, 1970; Bottiglieri et al., 1995). The corresponding incidence of low serum vitamin B_{12} levels is up to 5% in younger patients but between 10% and 20% in elderly patients (Clarke et al., 2004). Folate deficiency has been consistently associated with evidence of depression (Reynolds et al., 1970; Crellin et al., 1993; Reynolds, 2002a; Ramos et al., 2004; Lewis et al., 2006) and cognitive decline (Sneath et al., 1973; Crellin et al., 1993; Reynolds, 2002a; Ramos et al., 2005), whereas low vitamin B_{12} levels are associated mostly with cognitive impairment (Carney and Sheffield, 1970; Starr et al., 2005).

Neuropsychological studies have suggested general and specific impairments of intellectual function, including attention, episodic and visual spatial memory, and abstract reasoning, which were attributed to folate deficiency (Botez et al., 1979b; Goodwin et al., 1983; Wahlin et al., 2001). In the Kungsholmen (Stockholm) Community Aging and Dementia Project, the pattern of cognitive dysfunction resulting from folate deficiency was said to resemble that in normal aging, i.e., impairment in tasks that involve little structure, are unfamiliar and attention demanding, and involve complex processing of information (Hassing et al., 1999; Wahlin et al., 2001).

There has been continuing debate about the significance of folate deficiency without anemia or macrocytosis in the presence of psychiatric illness, including dementia. For those who have continued to doubt the existence of neuropsychiatric symptoms due to folate deficiency it has been all too easy to assume that the deficiency is secondary to the mental illness for dietary reasons, especially as apathy, withdrawal, and anorexia are common symptoms in depression and dementia. However, nutritional studies have not confirmed this oversimplistic interpretation (Bottiglieri et al., 1995) and it has long been apparent that even when folate deficiency is secondary to mental illness it is an aggravating factor that may lead eventually to a vicious circle of decline (Reynolds, 1976, 2006). Furthermore, impaired motivation and social withdrawal due to deficiency are some of the most folate-responsive symptoms (Reynolds, 1968, 2002b; Manzoor and Runcie, 1976; Botez et al., 1977). In the last two decades evidence of a direct causal link between folate metabolism and some depressions and dementias has been reinforced by studies of homocysteine metabolism.

FOLATE, HOMOCYSTEINE, DEPRESSION, DEMENTIA, AND AGING

Hyperhomocysteinemia has long been suspected as a possible risk factor for vascular disease (Clarke et al., 2002; McIlroy et al., 2002). However, the lowering of homocysteine concentrations by treatment with folic acid, vitamin B_{12}, or vitamin B_6 has not been convincingly shown to be effective in the secondary prevention of cardiovascular or cerebrovascular disease, but a possible role for the vitamins in primary prevention is still being evaluated (Kalin and Rimm, 2010). Following the earlier clinical reports, reviewed above, of an association between folate deficiency, depression, and dementia, most, but not all, community-based studies reviewed by Morris (2003) and Morris and Jacques (2010) have suggested that hyperhomocysteinemia and low folate levels are independent risk factors for depression and especially dementia, including both Alzheimer's disease and vascular dementia.

The large prospective Framingham community study indicated that a high plasma homocysteine concentration doubled the risk of developing either Alzheimer's disease or other dementias (Seshadri et al., 2002). Similarly, a Swedish community study suggested that low levels of serum folate or vitamin B_{12} doubled the risk of Alzheimer's disease (Wang et al., 2001). In a retrospective study of the survivors of the Scottish Mental Surveys of 1932 which included childhood IQ, plasma homocysteine concentration accounted for 7–8% of the variance in cognitive performance (Duthie et al., 2002). A prospective Italian population-based study confirmed that high plasma homocysteine and low serum folate values were independent predictors of dementia and Alzheimer's disease, whereas the association with vitamin B_{12} was not significant (Ravaglia et al., 2005). In the American Veteran Affairs Normative Aging Study high homocysteine and low folate levels predicted cognitive decline in aging men (Tucker et al., 2005). In a community study of 518 elderly patients without dementia in South Korea 45 (8.7%) developed dementia, three-quarters with Alzheimer's disease, over a prospective follow-up period of 2.4 years. Incident dementia was predicted by baseline low folate, but not by vitamin B_{12} or homocysteine levels. However, the onset of dementia was also more strongly associated with an exaggerated decline in folate and rise in homocysteine, although weakened by adjustment for weight loss (Kim et al., 2008). According to Morris and Jacques (2010), the few inconsistent epidemiologic studies appear explicable by selection factors, misclassification and confounding.

There is substantial overlap between Alzheimer's disease and vascular dementia, and the separation of these two diseases from each other and from other dementias is not easy in life even with the most sophisticated techniques (Neuropathology Group of the Medical Research Council's Cognitive Function and Ageing Study, 2001). Therefore neuropathologic studies are of particular importance. In a case controlled study of 164 patients with Alzheimer's disease, 76 of whom were confirmed neuropathologically, Alzheimer's disease was significantly associated with high plasma homocysteine and low serum folate and vitamin B_{12} (Clarke et al., 1998). Higher plasma homocysteine was associated with a more rapid atrophy of the medial temporal lobes over 3 years. In 12 patients high homocysteine was also significantly associated with confirmed vascular dementia. In people without dementia plasma homocysteine was inversely related to magnetic resonance imaging (MRI) measures of hippocampal and cortical volume (den Heijer et al., 2003). However, poor cognitive ability associated with high homocysteine concentrations was independent of structural brain changes on MRI (Prins et al., 2002). In a prospective study of 30 nuns from the same environmental and nutritional background who died at age 78–101 years, half had neuropathologic confirmation of Alzheimer's disease. Of 18 nutritional factors examined only serum folate was correlated with atrophy of the neocortex, especially in the 15 nuns with Alzheimer's disease but also in those with minimal atherosclerosis and no infarcts (Snowdon et al., 2000).

One reason for the apparently high incidence of folate deficiency and hyperhomocysteinemia in elderly people is that folate levels in serum and CSF fall and plasma homocysteine rises with age (Bottiglieri et al., 2000a; Seshadri et al., 2002; Serot et al., 2005), perhaps contributing to the aging process (Wahlin et al., 2001; Reynolds, 2002a, 2006). Interestingly the pattern of cognitive dysfunction associated with folate deficiency was noted to be similar to that in normal aging (Hassing et al., 1999; Wahlin et al., 2001), while the domains of cognitive function which improved in normal subjects with folate supplementation for 3 years were those that tend to decline with age (Durga et al., 2007a).

Raised plasma homocysteine levels have been observed in up to 30% of patients with severe depression (Fava et al., 1997; Bottiglieri et al., 2000b; Morris and Jacques, 2010). Bottiglieri et al. (2000b) have described a biological subgroup of depressed patients with high plasma homocysteine concentrations, folate deficiency, and impaired monoamine neurotransmitter metabolism. In an Australian study low folate and high homocysteine, but not vitamin B_{12}, were correlated with depressive symptoms in community-dwelling middle-aged individuals. The effects of folate and homocysteine were overlapping but distinct (Sachdev et al., 2005). In a large Norwegian community study hyperhomocysteinemia and the folate polymorphism MTHFR 677C→T were associated with depression, but not anxiety, in middle-aged, but not elderly, patients (Bjelland et al., 2003). The relationship of MTHFR 677C→T polymorphisms and depression was supported by Lewis et al. (2006), but this has also been noted with cognitive impairment (Durga et al., 2006).

FOLIC ACID AND EPILEPSY

Folate deficiency induced by some of the older antiepileptic drugs, e.g., phenytoin or barbiturates, was commonly associated with mental changes, especially depression, apathy, psychomotor retardation, and cognitive decline (Reynolds, 1968, 1976). Although folate deficiency in epileptic patients appears less common since the newer antiepileptic drugs, e.g., carbamazepine and valproate, have become available, more recent studies have revealed hyperhomocysteinemia in up to 40% of adults and 15% of children with epilepsy (Schwaninger et al., 1999; Huemer et al., 2005). High homocysteine levels are significantly related to antiepileptic medication and to low folate levels and are normalized by treatment with folic acid, 1 mg daily for 3 months (Huemer et al., 2005). Antiepileptic medication is associated with an increased risk of major congenital malformations, including neural tube defects (NTD), but it is unclear to what extent these birth defects are mediated by folate mechanisms or prevented by prophylactic periconceptual folic acid (Morrow et al., 2009) (see section below on neural tube defects).

Treatment of 26 patients with epilepsy and drug-induced folate deficiency with 15 mg of folic acid daily *for 1–3 years* resulted in improved drive, initiative, alertness, concentration, mood and sociability in most and an increase in seizure frequency in some (Reynolds, 1968). Controlled trials of folate therapy for *up to 3 months* produced inconsistent results, but there is abundant experimental evidence that folate derivatives have excitatory properties, especially when the efficient blood–brain barrier mechanism for the vitamin is circumvented (Reynolds et al., 1972; Reynolds, 1976; Hommes et al., 1979). In laboratory animals intravenous sodium folate will only induce seizures in very large doses; but if the blood–brain barrier is damaged locally by trauma or a heat lesion the dose required for an epileptogenic effect is much lower; and if the blood–brain barrier is circumvented by intraventricular or intracortical administration all folate derivatives are highly convulsant (Hommes et al., 1973, 1979). Furthermore the vitamin enhances the kindling model of epilepsy and can even be used to kindle seizures directly (Miller et al., 1979). It is uncertain how folates induce their excitatory effects but they may do so by blocking or reversing GABA-mediated inhibition (Davis and Watkins, 1973). Excitatory phenomena produced by folates resemble those induced by disinhibitory compounds such as bicuculline, penicillin, or picrotoxin (Hommes et al., 1979).

The risk of aggravating seizures in patients with epilepsy is small because the blood–brain barrier limits entry of folic acid, but the risk increases with larger doses over longer times (Reynolds, 1976,

2002b). The vitamin can also lower blood phenytoin levels which may be an additional possible aggravating mechanism (Rivey et al., 1984).

TREATMENT ISSUES

Reports from the 1960s and 1970s of folate-responsive neurologic disorders, usually but not always associated with megaloblastic anemia, have been described above. Considering that a third of patients with folate (or vitamin B$_{12}$) deficiency severe enough to produce anemia have no immediate nervous system involvement (Shorvon et al., 1980), the significance of folate deficiency in the presence of neuropsychiatric disorders without anemia or macrocytosis is not always clear, especially in the elderly (Bottiglieri et al., 1995; Reynolds, 2002a). However, if this deficiency, whether primary or secondary, is not already affecting the nervous system, it is highly likely to do so in the longer term if left untreated (Reynolds, 2002b, 2006).

The neurologic response to folate treatment is usually slow over many weeks and months, at least in part because of the efficient blood–brain barrier mechanism for this vitamin which limits entry, perhaps because of its excitatory properties (Hommes et al., 1973; Reynolds, 1976, 2002b). Treatment is recommended for at least

6 months, but some improvement should be detected within 2–3 months. The response and the degree of residual disability will be related to the duration and severity of nervous system manifestations before treatment.

Depression

In patients with depression the presence of folate deficiency is associated with a poorer response to standard antidepressant therapy (Reynolds et al., 1970; Papakostas et al., 2005). Six controlled trials for periods varying from 8 weeks to 1 year have confirmed an effect of folates on mood and social recovery either directly or mostly in addition to psychotropic treatment in psychiatric patients mainly with depression (Botez et al., 1979b; Coppen et al., 1986; Godfrey et al., 1990; Passeri et al., 1993; Coppen and Bailey, 2000; Papakostas et al., 2012). The details of the trials and outcomes are summarized in Table 61.2. The trials have utilized folic acid or more recently methylfolate, both with positive outcomes. Which formulation is best is uncertain but methylfolate is the transport form across the blood–brain barrier and has theoretical advantages.

Recently, Papakostas et al. (2012) reported that 7.5 mg of L-methylfolate for 30 days was ineffective but 15 mg for 60 days significantly improved mood

Table 61.2

Controlled clinical trials of folate in depressive disorders

Authors	Patients	Number	Trial design	Outcome
Botez et al., 1979	Depression Folate deficiency	24	Folic acid 15 mg daily versus placebo; 4 months	Improved mood, Wechsler IQ memory scale and Kohs block design
Coppen et al., 1986	Manic depression On lithium	102	Folic acid 200 µg daily versus placebo; 1 year	Lower affective morbidity index associated with higher end of trial serum folate levels
Godfrey et al., 1990	Major depression Schizophrenia Red cell folate < 200 µg/L On standard psychotropic medication	41	Methylfolate 15 mg daily versus placebo; 6 months	Enhanced clinical social recovery in depression and schizophrenia increasing over time
Passseri et al., 1993	Elderly depression with moderate dementia	96	Methylfolate 50 mg daily versus trazodone 100 mg daily; 8 weeks	Similar outcome in mood (Hamilton scale) in both groups
Coppen and Bailey 2000	Depression on fluoxetine	127	Folic acid 500 µg daily versus placebo; 10 weeks	Enhanced mood outcome, especially in women
Papakostas et al., 2012	Major depression SSRI-resistant	148	L-methylfolate 7.5 mg daily versus placebo; 30 days	No significant differences
		75	L-methylfolate 15 mg daily versus placebo; 60 days	Improved response rate and reduction in depression scores

and outcome in patients with major depression who were SSRI-resistant. Earlier Godfrey et al. (1990) had reported increasing clinical and social recovery over 6 months in major depressive and schizophrenic patients with definite or borderline folate deficiency, in whom 15 mg of methylfolate was added to standard psychotropic medication. The folate status of the patients in the trial by Papakostas et al. (2012) was not reported, but there is preliminary evidence of an antidepressant effect of methylfolate monotherapy in the absence of folate deficiency (Passeri et al., 1993; Bottiglieri et al., 1995), but with a greater rise in red cell folate in responders than nonresponders (Bottiglieri et al., 1995; Reynolds, 2006). An important clue is the mood-elevating properties of nitrous oxide, i.e., laughing gas. This euphoriant effect of nitrous oxide is very probably related to the instantaneous inactivation of methionine synthase leading to an acute rise in methylfolate in the brain (Reynolds, 2006). (See section on metabolic mechanisms, below).

Cognitive function

A few controlled trials, reviewed recently by Morris and Jacques (2010), of the effect of the vitamin on cognitive function in elderly patients, with or without impaired cognitive function, have been more inconsistent. The latter authors confirm the importance of separating studies of patients who are folate-deficient from those in whom the vitamin was given (usually together with vitamin B_{12} and vitamin B_6) to lower homocysteine levels, the latter mostly in the absence of cognitive impairment but with a view to preventing future deterioration. For example, in folate-deficient subjects with mild to moderate cognitive impairment Fioravanti et al. (1997) reported that folic acid 15 mg daily for 60 days significantly improved attention and memory recall in comparison to placebo. In the largest and longest study to date, Durga et al. (2007a), who also reviewed earlier trials, reported that in normal subjects aged 50–70 years with raised plasma homocysteine levels, supplementation with 800 µg folic acid daily for 3 years significantly improved memory, information processing speed and sensorimotor speed compared with placebo. They also noted that the improvements were in domains of cognitive function that tend to decline with age. Although 98% of subjects had normal folate levels at basline the cognitive benefits were generally 2–5 times greater in those with relatively lower red cell folate concentrations (Durga et al., 2007b).

Some of the inconsistencies in clinical trials are partly related to unsolved questions about dose and duration of therapy, whichever formulation is utilized. In experimental studies of repair in the adult nervous system

Iskandar et al. (2010) reported that regeneration of afferent spinal neurons was biphasic and dose-dependent, and correlated closely over its dose range with global and gene-specific DNA methylation. It is also relevant that the adverse neurologic effects of folic acid in the presence of vitamin B_{12} deficiency are related both to the dose and the duration of folate therapy (Schwartz et al., 1950; Savage and Lindenbaum, 1995). In clinical studies small doses of the vitamin over the longer term may be preferable to larger doses in the short or long term, not least because of the risks to the nervous system, especially in vitamin B_{12} deficiency and epilepsy (Reynolds, 2002b). A positive response is more likely in the presence of confirmed folate deficiency.

Studies of homocysteine lowering treatment with combined vitamin B_{12}, vitamin B_6, and folic acid are beyond the scope of this review, but it is of interest that treatment with this combination of vitamins for 2 years in the VITACOG trial has been reported to slow the rate of cognitive decline and brain atrophy in elderly subjects with mild cognitive impairment (de Jager et al., 2012).

NEURAL TUBE DEFECTS AND THEIR PREVENTION

Birth defects probably arise from a complex interplay of genetic, epigenetic, environmental, and lifestyle factors. The prevalence of neural tube defects (NTD) varies from 0.8 per 1000 births in areas of the US to 13.8 per 1000 in areas of China. Worldwide approximately 300 000 children are born each year with NTD (Hobbs et al., 2010).

Since the early reports of Hibbard (1964) and Smithells et al. (1981), abundant evidence has confirmed that impaired maternal folate intake and status, including the administration of folate antagonists, significantly increases the risk of NTD (MRC Vitamin Study Group, 1991; Hernandez-Diaz et al., 2000; Massaro and Rogers, 2002; Hobbs et al., 2010). This evidence has led to numerous case control and cohort studies as well as two nonrandomized and four randomized trials showing that periconceptual preventive administration of varying doses of folic acid significantly reduced the risk of NTD, but approximately one-third of NTD are not preventable by folic acid (MRC Vitamin Study Group, 1991; Hobbs et al., 2010). For the last two decades many countries have had a public policy of recommending 400 µg of folic acid prior to any pregnancy, especially in those deemed to be at special risk for genetic or nutritional reasons.

As many women either do not receive or do not accept this prophylactic advice several countries have, in the last 15 years, introduced mandatory fortification of grain, flour, or cereals. In the US, Canada, Chile, Costa Rica, and South Africa, many community studies, reviewed by Berry et al. (2010), have reported a reduction of the prevalence of NTD of between approximately 20% and 50%, on average about one-third. However, fortification has sometimes resulted in higher intake of folic acid than predicted (Choumenkovitch et al., 2002) and some countries, notably the UK and New Zealand, have refrained from fortification because of concerns about masking or aggravating vitamin B$_{12}$ deficiency in the elderly and uncertainty over cancer risks. A report from Chile questions a possible increase in the incidence of SCD (Nogales-Gaete et al., 2004).

The mechanisms by which impaired maternal folate status increase risk and prophylactic folic acid reduces risk, even in mothers with apparently normal folate status, are largely unknown (Massaro and Rogers, 2002; Wallis et al., 2010). The focus is again on genetic and epigenetic mechanisms involving nucleotide synthesis and/or DNA methylation. There is much interest in various genetic polymorphisms of folate enzymes, especially the MTHFR 677C→T variant, but also others (Blom et al., 2006; Van der Linden et al., 2006), the presence of which in the population increases the risk of NTD (Christensen and Rozen, 2010). Vitamin B$_{12}$ and homocysteine have also been implicated (Ray and Blom, 2003; Wallis et al., 2010). Autoantibodies to the folate receptor-α have been detected in up to three-quarters of mothers who had given birth to a child with a NTD (Rothenberg et al., 2004). It is clear that folate is critical to normal fetal development and the search is ongoing for the factors that might impair uptake or metabolism of folate by fetal cells (Wallis et al., 2010).

DISORDERS OF FOLATE METABOLISM IN INFANCY AND CHILDHOOD

An increasing number of rare inherited or acquired disorders of the absorption, transport, or metabolism of folate and vitamin B$_{12}$ have been recognized over several decades. This is a highly specialized subject requiring sophisticated metabolic and genetic services attached to centers of pediatric neurology or child health and is beyond the scope of this chapter. Good reviews are those of Rosenblatt and Fenton (2001), Surtees (2001), and Whitehead (2006).

The commonest inborn error of folate metabolism is methylenetetrahydrofolate reductase (MTHFR) deficiency due to several mutations of varying severity of the *MTHFR* gene. Others include hereditary folate malabsorption and glutamate formiminotransferase-cyclodeaminase deficiency, both autosomal recessive disorders. The most recent disorder is cerebral folate deficiency (Ramaekers and Blau, 2004), associated with normal blood levels of folate and homocysteine, due to a defect in the transport activity of folate receptor-α

Table 61.3

Clinical neurologic features in remethylation defects related to age of presentation (Ogier de Baulny et al., 1998)

1. **Neonatal and early infancy (<3 months):**
   Poor feeding
   Lethargy
   Hypotonia/hypertonia
   Seizures
   Coma
2. **Late infancy and early childhood (>3 months to <10 years):**
   Slow development
   Lethargy
   Mental deterioration
   Encephalopathy
   Seizures
   Spastic paresis (subacute combined degeneration)
   Extrapyramidal signs
   Neuropathy
3. **Late childhood and early adulthood (>10 years):**
   Previous mild retardation
   Mental deterioration
   Behavior disturbance
   Encephalopathy
   Myelopathy (subacute combined degeneration)
   Neuropathy

(FRα), in turn associated with circulating antibodies to the receptor (Rothenberg et al., 2004). Mutations in the *FOLR1* gene that expresses FRα have been identified in a few families (Cario et al., 2009; Steinfeld et al., 2009).

This subject is impossible to separate from that of inborn errors or vitamin B$_{12}$ metabolism, of which there are even more examples. Such is the clinical and metabolic overlap that some authors integrate most of the inborn errors of either vitamin under the heading of "defects in remethylation" (Ogier de Baulny et al., 1998). The similar clinical features of these genetically dissimilar disorders of either folate or vitamin B$_{12}$ metabolism are best categorized according to the age of presentation and are well summarized in Table 61.3 (Ogier de Baulny et al., 1998).

CLINICAL DISSOCIATION

For over a century it has been well documented that there is a poor correlation between the hematologic and neuropsychiatric manifestations of folic acid and vitamin B$_{12}$ deficiency, i.e., both before and after the two vitamin deficiencies were separated in the late 1940s (Kinnier Wilson, 1940; Schwartz et al., 1950; Chanarin, 1969; Reynolds, 1976; Shorvon et al.; 1980; Lindenbaum et al., 1988). There is no doubt that some patients may present to hematologists without any evidence of neuropsychiatric disorder (e.g., Shorvon et al., 1980) but that other patients present to neurologists or psychiatrists with no anemia or even macrocytosis (e.g., Lindenbaum et al., 1988). Many other patients present with varying degrees of involvement of both blood and nervous systems. This clinical dissociation has led to repeated suggestions that the nervous system complications must have a different mechanism to the megaloblastic anemia (Chanarin, 1969; Lindenbaum et al.; 1988; Healton et al., 1991). To some extent the dissociation is illusory and is influenced by the timing of the diagnosis, especially the relatively early modern diagnosis of hematologic involvement by screening techniques. In the first third of the 20th century, before any treatment was available, patients would eventually progress at different rates to nearly 100% association between anemia and neuropsychiatric disorder (Woltmann, 1919; Ahrens, 1932; Kinnier Wilson, 1940). Furthermore this clinical dissociation between two separate complications of a single metabolic disorder is not unique to folic acid or vitamin B_{12} deficiency, but seems common to all general metabolic disorders that also affect the nervous system (Reynolds, 1976). For example, Wilson's disease may present either to a neurologist or hepatologist with predominantly cerebral or hepatic involvement; likewise, hypothyroidism may present either to an endocrinologist, a neurologist or a psychiatrist. There are several possible reasons for these divergences including the highly specialized structure, environment and function of the nervous system in comparison to other organs, especially the blood, but they need not and usually do not imply any fundamental difference in the metabolic basis of the neural manifestations (Reynolds, 1976, 2006).

Misunderstandings arose in the late 1940s and early 1950s when it was noted that the administration of large doses of folic acid to patients with undoubted vitamin B_{12} deficiency was often associated with suboptimal improvement in the anemia, apparently associated with precipitation or aggravation of neurologic complications. This gave rise to the theory that the improvement in the anemia by the administration of folic acid masked and delayed the diagnosis of vitamin B_{12} deficiency, allowing the neurologic disorder to progress (Chanarin, 1969). However, this misinterpretation did not accurately reflect what was actually reported in the middle of the 20th century. Careful review of that literature shows that after giving folic acid to treat "pernicious anemia" there was sometimes brief temporary symptomatic neurologic improvement before the more florid and sometimes explosive deterioration (Hall and Watkins, 1947; Schwartz et al., 1950). Furthermore after the obvious but suboptimal hematologic improvement there was commonly a later insidious hematologic relapse (Hall and Watkins, 1947; Schwartz et al., 1950). Eventually similar numbers of patients have neurologic and hematologic

relapse, although often again dissociated (Schwartz et al., 1950). In other words, both the nervous system and the blood may show improvement and relapse but to different degrees and at different rates, which may in turn reflect profound differences in structure, function, and cellular turnover in the two tissues. Occasional reports of neurologic deterioration due to untreated vitamin B_{12} deficiency during folate treatment continue to occur (Dhar et al., 2003).

There is some evidence that in patients with vitamin B_{12} deficiency there is an inverse correlation between the degree of anemia and the degree of neurologic disability (Healton et al., 1991). Furthermore, patients with neurologic complications of vitamin B_{12} deficiency have significantly higher serum folate concentrations than those without nervous system disorders (Waters and Mollin, 1961; Reynolds, 1979b). In a large scale community-based study of elderly subjects in the US, Morris et al. (2007) reported a greater cognitive decline in patients with high serum folate levels associated with low serum vitamin B_{12} levels compared with those with more modest folate levels in association with vitamin B_{12} deficiency. This was not confirmed in a subsequent UK study where there is no folate fortification policy (Clarke et al., 2008). However, in a more recent prefortification prospective epidemiologic study in Framingham in the US, low or "low normal" plasma vitamin B_{12} levels in conjunction with high plasma folate or supplemental folate predicted especially rapid cognitive decline (Morris et al., 2012). The American studies were supported by evidence of increasing homocysteine and methylmalonic acid levels in patients with vitamin B_{12} deficiency and increasing folate levels (Selhub et al., 2007). All studies confirm an intimate relationship between folate and vitamin B_{12} in both blood and nervous system, but at the moment there is little reason to doubt that the nature of this relationship is fundamentally any different in blood and nervous system.

METABOLIC MECHANISMS

The key to the metabolic understanding of both the neurology and hematology of both folate and vitamin B_{12} deficiency is the synthesis of methionine from homocysteine by methionine synthase in which both 5-methyltetrahydrofolate and methyl vitamin B_{12} act as cofactors (Fig. 61.1). Failures in the availability, absorption and delivery of folate through the folate cycle and therefore the supply of methyl groups, or in the availability of vitamin B_{12}, would have similar and overlapping consequences on both blood and nervous system.

The megaloblastic anemia in either deficiency state is due to impairment of DNA synthesis, integrity and transcription, associated with failures in the synthesis of purines and especially thymidine (Chanarin, 1969; Stabler, 2010). In folate deficiency there is a failure of delivery of methyl folate; in vitamin B_{12} deficiency, especially pernicious anemia, there is a block in the utilization of methyl folate, commonly leading to a rise in plasma folate, the so-called methyl-folate trap. Either mechanism leads to a morphologically indistinguishable megaloblastic anemia.

There is evidence that similar mechanisms apply to the neurologic disorders in these two deficiency states (Reynolds, 1976, 2006). However, the nervous system is also much more complex and hierarchical than the hemopoietic system and includes metabolic pathways that have little or no role in the blood, e.g., in relation to myelin or mood. Nor should we assume that all neuropsychiatric complications have exactly the same metabolic basis, as the failure of methylation can involve numerous metabolic pathways that require a supply of methyl groups through the methyl donor S-adenosyl methionine, including the methylation of DNA which plays a vital part in gene expression and other epigenetic mechanisms (Rampersaud et al., 2000; Friso and Choi, 2002; Bottiglieri and Reynolds, 2010).

An important model is that of nitrous oxide, which in man can produce megaloblastic changes in bone marrow within hours of anesthesia and the full range of neuropsychiatric complications within weeks or months of abuse (Layzer, 1978; Nunn, 1987), and which has been studied in several species including monkeys, pigs, rats, and fruit bats (Scott et al., 1994). By oxidizing the cobalt atom of vitamin B_{12}, nitrous oxide mimics vitamin B_{12} deficiency, rapidly inactivating methionine synthase (Fig. 61.1). Methionine protects against nitrous oxide-induced subacute combined degeneration implying that methylation processes are important in this disorder (Scott et al., 1994). The methylation hypothesis is also supported by results of studies of demyelination in inborn disorders of remethylation (Surtees, 1998). I have suggested that the euphoriant laughing gas effect of nitrous oxide in man is due to the rapid raising of methyl folate concentrations in the nervous system, consequent upon the almost instantaneous inactivation of vitamin B_{12} (Reynolds et al., 1984; Reynolds, 2006).

Table 61.4 summarizes postulated mechanisms not only for the neuropsychiatric complications of folate and vitamin B_{12} deficiency but also for the possible protective effect of folate in some disorders not primarily due to deficiency. As already discussed, folic acid can reduce the incidence of neural tube defects in the early embryonic period even in the absence of folate deficiency (Massaro and Rogers, 2002; Hobbs et al., 2010). Iskandar et al. (2004, 2010) reported that folic acid significantly improved the regrowth of sensory axons in a spinal cord regeneration model and improved neurologic recovery from spinal cord contusion injury in rats. Furthermore such repair occurs at least in part through DNA methylation, implicating an epigenetic mechanism in CNS recovery (Kronenberg and Endres, 2010). Folates seem to be of fundamental importance in brain growth, differentiation, development, repair, mood, cognition

Table 61.4

Proposed metabolic mechanisms of folate/vitamin B_{12} neurologic disorders

	Clinical implications of folate/vitamin B_{12} deficiency or inborn errors	Postulated metabolic mechanisms
Embryo Fetus Infant Child	Disorders of CNS growth and fetal development	Impaired DNA synthesis, transcription; impaired genomic methylation and epigenetic mechanisms
Adult	SCD/neuropathy	As above and impaired nongenomic methylation, e.g., myelin proteins, phospholipids
	Depression/psychiatric disorders	Impaired genomic and nongenomic methylation, e.g., monoamines, biopterins. Impaired excitation
Elderly	Brain aging Cognitive decline Dementia	All the above mechanisms including DNA synthesis, genomic and nongenomic methylation, e.g., proteins, phospholipids, choline Failure of repair mechanisms
Other	Alzheimer's disease	All the above mechanisms, oxidative stress, and increased β-amyloid formation
	Cerebrovascular disease and stroke	Homocysteine-related vascular mechanisms

CNS, central nervous system; SCD, subacute combined degeneration of the cord.

and aging (Reynolds, 2002a, 2006; Massaro and Rogers, 2002; Mattson and Shea, 2003; Lucock, 2004; Bottiglieri and Reynolds, 2010). Many of these functions and their breakdown in folate and vitamin B_{12} deficiency are probably primarily mediated through nucleotide synthesis, DNA integrity and transcription, and epigenetic mechanisms including gene expression, involving DNA methylation. As in megaloblastosis these mechanisms are probably involved in most, if not all the neurologic complications of deficiencies or inborn errors of folic acid or vitamin B_{12}, a kind of "megaloblastosis" of the nervous system (Reynolds, 2006). However, in addition there is widespread failure of nongenomic methylation involving potentially numerous S-adenosyl methionine-mediated methylation reactions in many neural pathways (Bottiglieri et al., 1990, 1994; Bottiglieri and Reynolds, 2010). Possible examples are myelin basic protein and membrane phospholipids, which may perhaps contribute to demyelination (Surtees et al., 1991; Scott et al., 1994; Bottiglieri and Reynolds, 2010). Methylation and turnover of monoamines and biopterins have been implicated in depression and perhaps other psychiatric symptoms in the context of folate deficiency (Reynolds et al., 1970; Bottiglieri et al., 1992; Bottiglieri and Reynolds, 2010). There is clinical evidence that the turnover of monoamines is increased by both folic acid and S-adenosylmethionine (Bottiglieri et al., 1990, 2000b; Bottiglieri and Reynolds, 2010).

There is also widespread interest in the role of homocysteine in vascular disease and dementia including Alzheimer's disease (Morris, 2003; Irizarry et al., 2005; Ravaglia et al., 2005; Bottiglieri and Reynolds, 2010). It is therefore of interest in relation to aging, cognitive decline, and various forms of dementia that serum and CSF folate concentrations fall and serum homocysteine concentrations rise with age (Reynolds, 2006; Bottiglieri and Reynolds, 2010). It has also been suggested that homocysteine-related impairment of glutathione metabolism and oxidative stress (McCaddon et al., 2003) or impaired DNA methylation and associated epigenetic mechanisms may increase amyloid-β-peptide production and toxicity in Alzheimer's disease (Kruman et al., 2002; Fuso et al., 2005, 2008; Irizarry et al., 2005; Bottiglieri and Reynolds, 2010).

Vulnerability to all the above mechanisms will be increased in relation to both the severity and duration of either folic acid or vitamin B_{12} deficiency (Reynolds, 1976, 2002a; Shorvon et al., 1980; Bottiglieri et al., 1995), in the presence of predisposing genetic factors, including polymorphisms of folate and vitamin B_{12}-dependent enzymes, especially if the latter are additionally compromised by dietary factors, i.e., nutrigenomics (Friso and Choi, 2002; Lucock, 2004; Durga et al., 2006;

Bottiglieri and Reynolds, 2010), or in the presence of associated metabolic disorders, such as malabsorption, or pharmacologic stress, e.g., folate antagonists (Shorvon et al., 1980; Reynolds, 2006).

CONCLUSIONS

In the last 50 years there has been a remarkable transformation in our understanding of the role of folates in nervous system disorders. The misconceptions of the late 1940s and 1950s that there was no neurology of folic acid deficiency and that folic acid administration was only harmful to the nervous system, have gradually been replaced by a recognition that the neuropsychiatric manifestations of folic acid deficiency, with or without megaloblastic anemia or macrocytosis, overlap considerably with those associated with vitamin B_{12} deficiency, as is also the case for the megaloblastic anemias of either vitamin deficiency.

In the early stages there is often dissociation between the neuropsychiatric and hematologic expression of the vitamin deficiency, as occurs in other general metabolic disorders that affect the nervous system. The occurrence of nervous system complications is influenced by the duration as well as the severity of the deficiency, by predisposing genetic factors, including polymorphisms of folate-dependent enzymes, and by any associated metabolic disorders. The administration of folic acid in the presence of vitamin B_{12} deficiency may be harmful to the nervous system and ultimately to the blood. The vitamin should be used with caution in epilepsy. Overall the benefits greatly exceed the risks but the latter should not be dismissed as of no importance. Both benefits and risks are influenced by the dose and duration of treatment.

In the nervous system, as in the blood, failure or blocking of the supply of methyl groups will result in impaired purine, thymidine, nucleotide and DNA synthesis and in disruption of DNA transcription, gene expression, and other epigenetic mechanisms affecting fetal and tissue growth, differentiation, and repair. In addition, impaired methylation of proteins, lipids, and monoamines may contribute to the varied neuropsychiatric disorders, including depression and cognitive decline. There is now great interest in the role of folate and its related metabolic pathways in nervous system function and disease at all ages and the potential use of the vitamin in the prophylaxis of some disorders of nervous system development, mood, and cognition, including the aging process.

SUMMARY

The metabolism of folic acid and the metabolism of vitamin B_{12} are intimately linked such that deficiency of either vitamin leads to an identical megaloblastic anemia. The neurologic manifestations of folate deficiency overlap with those of vitamin B_{12} deficiency and include cognitive impairment, dementia, depression and, less commonly, peripheral neuropathy and subacute combined degeneration of the spinal cord. In both deficiency states there is often dissociation between the neuropsychiatric and the hematologic complications. There is a similar overlap and dissociation between neurologic and hematologic manifestations of inborn errors of folate and vitamin B_{12} metabolism.

Low folate and raised homocysteine levels are risk factors for dementia, including Alzheimer's disease, and depression. Even when folate deficiency is secondary to psychiatric illness due to apathy or poor diet it may eventually aggravate the underlying disorder in a vicious circle effect. Clinical responses to treatment with folates are usually slow, over weeks and months, probably due to the efficient blood–brain barrier mechanism for the vitamin, perhaps in turn related to the experimentally demonstrated excitatory properties of folate derivatives. The inappropriate administration of folic acid in the presence of vitamin B_{12} deficiency may lead to both neurologic and, later, hematologic relapse.

Impaired maternal folate intake and status increases the risk of neural tube defects. Periconceptual prophylactic administration of the vitamin reduces, but does not eliminate the risk of neural tube defects even in the absence of folate deficiency. Folates and vitamin B_{12} have fundamental roles in central nervous system function at all ages, especially in purine, thymidine, nucleotide, and DNA synthesis, genomic and nongenomic methylation and, therefore, in tissue growth, differentiation, and repair. There is interest in the potential role of both vitamins in the prevention of disorders of central nervous system development, mood, dementia, including Alzheimer's disease, and aging.

REFERENCES

Ahrens RS (1932). Neurologic aspects of primary anaemia. Arch Neurol Psychiatry 28: 92–109.

Bailey LB (Ed.), (1995). Folate in Health and Disease. Marcel Dekker, New York.

Bailey LB (Ed.), (2010). Folate in Health and Disease, 2nd edn CRC Press, Boca Raton.

Berry RJ, Mulinare J, Hamner HC (2010). Folic acid fortification: neural tube defect risk reduction – a global perspective. In: LB Bailey (Ed.), Folate in Health and Disease. CRC Press, Boca Raton, pp. 179–204.

Bjelland I, Tell GS, Vollset SE et al. (2003). Folate, vitamin B12, homocysteine, and the MTHFR 677C→T polymorphism in anxiety and depression: the Hordaland homocysteine study. Arch Gen Psychiatry 60: 618–625.

Blom HJ, Shaw GM, den Heijer T et al. (2006). Neural tube defects and folate: case far from closed. Nat Rev Neurosci 7: 724–731.

Botez MI, Reynolds EH (Eds.), (1979). Folic Acid in Neurology, Psychiatry and Internal Medicine. Raven Press, New York.

Botez MI, Fontaine F, Botez T et al. (1977). Folate-responsive neurological and mental disorders: report of 16 cases. Eur Neurol 16: 230–246.

Botez MI, Peyronnard JM, Charron L (1979a). Polyneuropathies responsive to folic acid therapy. In: MI Botez, EH Reynolds (Eds.), Folic Acid in Neurology, Psychiatry and Internal Medicine. Raven Press, New York, pp. 401–412.

Botez MI, Botez T, Léveillé J et al. (1979b). Neuropsychological correlates of folic acid deficiency: facts and hypotheses. In: MI Botez, EH Reynolds (Eds.), Folic Acid in Neurology, Psychiatry and Internal Medicine. Raven Press, New York, pp. 435–461.

Bottiglieri T, Reynolds E (2010). Folate in neurological disease: basic mechanisms. In: LB Bailey (Ed.), Folate in Health and Disease. CRC Press, Boca Raton, pp. 355–380.

Bottiglieri T, Godfrey P, Flynn T et al. (1990). Cerebrospinal fluid S-adenosylmethionine in depression and dementia: effects of treatment with parenteral and oral S-adenosylmethionine. J Neurol Neurosurg Psychiatry 53: 1096–1098.

Bottiglieri T, Hyland K, Laundy M et al. (1992). Folate deficiency, biopterin and monoamine metabolism on depression. Psychol Med 22: 871–876.

Bottiglieri T, Hyland K, Reynolds EH (1994). The clinical potential of ademethionine (S-adenosylmethionine) in neurological disorders. Drugs 48: 1137–1152.

Bottiglieri T, Crellin R, Reynolds EH (1995). Folate and neuropsychiatry. In: LB Bailey (Ed.), Folate in Health and Disease. Marcel Dekker, New York, pp. 435–462.

Bottiglieri T, Reynolds EH, Laundy M (2000a). Folate in CSF and Age. J Neurol Neurosurg Psychiatry 69: 562.

Bottiglieri T, Laundy M, Crellin R et al. (2000b). Homocysteine, folate, methylation and monoamine metabolism in depression. J Neurol Neurosurg Psychiatry 69: 228–232.

Cario H, Bode H, Debaton KM et al. (2009). Congenital null mutations of the FOLR1 gene: a progressive neurologic disease and its treatment. Neurology 73: 2127–2129.

Carmel R, Jacobsen DW (Eds.), (2001). Homocysteine in Health and Disease. Cambridge University Press, Cambridge.

Carney MWP, Sheffield BF (1970). Associations of subnormal folate and vitaminB12 values and effects of replacement therapy. J Nerv Ment Dis 150: 404–411.

Chanarin I (1969). The Megaloblastic Anaemias. Blackwell, Oxford.

Choumenkovitch SF, Selhub J, Wilson PWF et al. (2002). Folic acid intake from fortification in United States exceeds predictions. J Nutr 132: 2792–2798.

Christensen KE, Rozen R (2010). Genetic variation: effect on folate metabolism and health. In: LB Bailey (Ed.), Folate in Health and Disease. CRC Press, Boca Raton, pp. 75–110.

Clarke R, Smith AD, Jobst KA et al. (1998). Folate, vitamin B12, and serum total homocysteine levels in confirmed Alzheimer disease. Arch Neurol 55: 1449–1455.

Clarke R, Collins R, Lewington S (2002). Homocysteine and risk of heart disease and stroke: a meta-analysis. JAMA 288: 2015–2022.

Clarke R, Grimley Evans J, Schneede J et al. (2004). Vitamin B12 and folate deficiency in later life. Age Ageing 33: 34–41.

Clarke R, Sherliker P, Hin H et al. (2008). Folate and vitamin B12 status in relation to cognitive impairment and anaemia in the setting of voluntary fortification in the UK. Br J Nutr 100: 1054–1059.

Coppen A, Bailey J (2000). Enhancement of the antidepressant action of fluoxetine by folic acid: a randomised, placebo controlled trial. J Affect Disord 60: 121–130.

Coppen A, Chaudhry S, Swade C (1986). Folic acid enhances lithium prophylaxis. J Affect Disord 10: 9–13.

Crellin R, Bottiglieri T, Reynolds EH (1993). Folates and psychiatric disorders. Drugs 45: 623–636.

Davis J, Watkins JC (1973). Facilitatory and direct excitatory effects of folate and folinate on single neurons of cat cerebral cortex. Biochem Pharmacol 22: 1667–1668.

de Jager CA, Oulhaj A, Jacoby R et al. (2012). Cognitive and clinical outcomes of homocysteine-lowering B-vitamin treatment in mild cognitive impairment: a randomised controlled trial. Int J Geriatr Psychiatry 27: 592–600.

den Heijer T, Vermeer SE, Clarke R et al. (2003). Homocysteine and brain atrophy on MRI of non-demented elderly. Brain 126: 170–175.

Dhar M, Bellevue R, Carmel R (2003). Pernicious anaemia with neuropsychiatric dysfunction in a patient with sickle cell anaemia treated with folate supplementation. N Engl J Med 348: 2204–2207.

Dickinson CJ (1995). Does folic acid harm people with vitamin B12 deficiency? Q J Med 88: 357–364.

Durga J, van Boxtel MPJ, Schouten EG et al. (2006). Folate and the methylenetetrahydrofolate reductase 677C→T mutation correlate with cognitive performance. Neurobiol Aging 27: 334–343.

Durga J, van Boxtel MPJ, Schouten EG et al. (2007a). Effect of 3-year folic acid supplementation on cognitive function in older adults in the FACIT trial: a randomised, double blind, controlled trial. Lancet 369: 208–216.

Durga J, van Boxtel MP, Verhoef P et al. (2007b). Folate and ageing. Lancet 369: 1601–1602.

Duthie SJ, Whalley LJ, Collins AR et al. (2002). Homocysteine, B vitamin status, and cognitive function in the elderly. Am J Clin Nutr 75: 908–913.

Fava M, Borus JS, Alpert JE et al. (1997). Folate, vitamin B12, and homocysteine in major depressive disorder. Am J Psychiatry 154: 426–428.

Fioravanti M, Ferrario E, Massaia M et al. (1997). Low folate levels in the cognitive decline of elderly patients and the efficacy of folate as a treatment for improving memory deficits. Arch Gerontol Geriatr 26: 1–13.

Friso S, Choi S-W (2002). Gene nutrient interactions and DNA methylation. J Nutr 132: 2382S–2387S.

Fuso A, Seminara L, Cavallaro RA et al. (2005). S-adenosylmethionine/homocysteine cycle alterations modify DNA methylation status with consequent deregulation of PS1 and BACE and beta-amyloid production. Mol Cell Neurosci 28: 195–204.

Fuso A, Nicolia V, Cavallaro RA et al. (2008). B-vitamin deprivation induces hyperhomocysteinemia and brain S-adenosylhomocysteinemia, depletes brain S-adenosylmethionine, and enhances PS1 and BACE expression and amyloid-beta deposition in mice. Mol Cell Neurosci 37: 731–746.

Godfrey PSA, Toone BK, Carney MWP et al. (1990). Enhancement of recovery from psychiatric illness by methyl folate. Lancet 336: 392–395.

Goodwin JS, Goodwin JM, Garry PJ (1983). Association between nutritional status and cognitive functioning in a healthy elderly population. JAMA 249: 2917–2921.

Grant HC, Hoffbrand AV, Wells DG (1965). Folate deficiency and neurological disease. Lancet 2: 763–767.

Hall BE, Watkins CH (1947). Experience with pteroylglutamic (synthetic folic) acid in the treatment of pernicious anaemia. J Lab Clin Med 32: 622–634.

Hassing L, Wahlin A, Winblad B et al. (1999). Further evidence on the effects of vitamin B12 and folate levels on episodic memory functioning; a population-based study of healthy very old adults. Biol Psychiatry 45: 1472–1480.

Healton EB, Savage DG, Brust JCM et al. (1991). Neurologic aspects of cobalamin deficiency. Medicine 70: 229–245.

Hernandez-Diaz S, Werler MM, Walker AM et al. (2000). Folic acid antagonists during pregnancy and the risk of birth defects. N Engl J Med 343: 1608–1614.

Hibbard BM (1964). The role of folic acid in pregnancy, with particular reference to anaemia, abruption and abortion. J Obstet Gynaecol Br Commonw 71: 529–542.

Hobbs CA, Shaw GM, Werler M et al. (2010). Folate status and birth defect risk: epidemiological perspective. In: LB Bailey (Ed.), Folate in Health and Disease. CRC Press, Boca Raton, pp. 133–153.

Hommes OR, Obbens EAMT, Wijfels CCB (1973). Epileptogenic activity of sodium-folate and the blood brain barrier in the rat. J Neurol Sci 19: 63–71.

Hommes OR, Hollinger JL, Jansen MJT et al. (1979). Convulsant properties of folate compounds; some considerations and speculations. In: MI Botez, EH Reynolds (Eds.), Folic Acid in Neurology, Psychiatry and Internal Medicine. Raven Press, New York, pp. 285–316.

Huemer M, Ausserer B, Graninger G et al. (2005). Hyperhomocysteinemia in children treated with antiepileptic drugs is normalised by folic acid supplementation. Epilepsia 46: 1677–1683.

Irizarry MC, Gurol ME, Raju S et al. (2005). Association of homocysteine with plasma amyloid β protein in aging and neurodegenerative disease. Neurology 65: 1402–1408.

Iskandar BJ, Nelson A, Resnick D et al. (2004). Folic acid supplementation enhances repair in the adult central nervous system. Ann Neurol 56: 221–227.

Iskandar BJ, Rizk E, Meier B et al. (2010). Folate regulation of axonal regeneration in the rodent central nervous system through DNA methylation. J Clin Invest 120: 1603–1616.

Kalin SR, Rimm EB (2010). Folate and vascular disease: epidemiological perspective. In: LB Bailey (Ed.), Folate in Health and Disease. CRC Press, Boca Raton, pp. 263–290.

Kim JM, Stewart R, Kim SW et al. (2008). Changes in folate, vitamin B12 and homocysteine associated with incident dementia. J Neurol Neurosurg Psychiatry 79: 864–868.

Kinnier Wilson SA (1940). Neurology. Arnold, London, pp. 1339–1358.

Kronenberg G, Endres M (2010). Neuronal injury: folate to the rescue? J Clin Invest 120: 1383–1386.

Kruman II, Kumaravel TS, Lohani A et al. (2002). Folic acid deficiency and homocysteine impair DNA repair in hippocampal neurons and sensitize them to amyloid toxicity in experimental models of Alzheimer's disease. J Neurosci 22: 1752–1762.

Layzer RB (1978). Myeloneurophathy after prolonged exposure to nitrous oxide. Lancet 2: 1227–1230.

Leichtenstern O (1884). Progressive perniciöse anämie bei tabeskranken. Dtsch Med Wochenschr 10: 849–850.

Lewis SJ, Lawlor DA, Davey Smith G et al. (2006). The thermolabile variant of MTHFR is associated with depression in the British Women's Heart and Health Study and a metaanalysis. Mol Psychiatry 11: 352–360.

Lichtheim L (1887). Zur kenntniss der perniciösen anämie. Munch Med Wochenschr 34: 301–306.

Lindenbaum J, Healton EB, Savage DG et al. (1988). Neuropsychiatric disorders caused by cobalamin deficiency in the absence of anaemia or macrocytosis. N Engl J Med 318: 1720–1728.

Lucock M (2004). Is folic acid the ultimate functional food component for disease prevention? BMJ 328: 211–214.

Manzoor M, Runcie J (1976). Folate-responsive neuropathy: a report of ten cases. BMJ 1: 1176–1178.

Massaro EJ, Rogers JM (Eds.), (2002). Folate and Human Development. Humana Press, Totowa, New Jersey.

Mattson MP, Shea TB (2003). Folate and homocysteine metabolism in neural plasticity and neurodegenerative disorders. Trends Neurosci 26: 137–146.

McCaddon A, Hudson P, Hill D et al. (2003). Alzheimer's disease and total plasma aminothiols. Biol Psychiatry 53: 254–260.

McIlroy SP, Dynan KB, Lawson JT et al. (2002). Moderately elevated plasma homocysteine, methylenetetrahydrofolate reductase genotype, and risk for stroke, vascular dementia, and Alzheimer disease in Northern Ireland. Stroke 3: 2351–2356.

Miller AA, Goff D, Webster RA (1979). Predisposition of laboratory animals to epileptogenic activity of folic acid. In: MI Botez, EH Reynolds (Eds.), Folic Acid in Neurology, Psychiatry and Internal Medicine. Raven Press, New York, pp. 331–334.

Morris MS (2003). Homocysteine and Alzheimer's disease. Lancet Neurol 2: 425–428.

Morris MS, Jacques PF (2010). Folate and neurological function: epidemiological perspective. In: LB Bailey (Ed.), Folate in Health and Disease. CRC Press, Boca Raton, pp. 325–353.

Morris MS, Jacques PF, Rosenberg IH et al. (2007). Folate and vitamin B-12 status in relation to anaemia, macrocytosis, and cognitive impairment in older Americans in the age of folic acid fortification. Am J Clin Nutr 85: 193–200.

Morris MS, Selhub J, Jacques PF (2012). Vitamin B-12 and folate status in relation to decline in scores on the minimental state examination in the Framingham heart study. J Am Geriatr Soc 60: 1457–1464.

Morrow JI, Hunt SJ, Russell AJ et al. (2009). Folic acid use and major congenital malformations in offspring of women with epilepsy: a prospective study from the UK Epilepsy and Pregnancy Register. J Neurol Neurosurg Psychiatry 80: 506–511.

MRC Vitamin Study Group (1991). Prevention of neural tube defects: results of the Medical Research Council Vitamin Study. Lancet 338: 131–137.

Neuropathology Group of the Medical Research Council Cognitive Function and Ageing Study (MRC CFAS) (2001). Pathological correlates of late-onset dementia in a multicentre, community-based population in England and Wales. Lancet 357: 169–175.

Nogales-Gaete J, Jiménez PP, Garcia PF et al. (2004). Mielopatia por déficit de vitamina B12: caracterizatin clinica de 11 cases. Rev Med Chil 132: 1377–1382, 2004.

Nunn JF (1987). Clinical aspects of the interaction between nitrous oxide and vitamin B12. Br J Anaesth 59: 3–13, 1987.

Ogier de Baulny H, Gérard M, Saudubray JM et al. (1998). Remethylation defects: guidelines for clinical diagnosis and treatment. Eur J Pediatr 157: S77–S83.

Papakostas GI, Petersen T, Lebowitz BD et al. (2005). The relationship between serum folate, vitamin B12, and homocysteine levels in major depressive disorder and the timing of improvement with fluoxetine. Int J Neuropsychopharmacol 8: 1–6.

Papakostas GI, Shelton RC, Zajecka JM et al. (2012). L-methylfolate as adjunctive therapy for SSRI-resistant major depression. Am J Psychiatry 169: 1267–1274.

Passeri M, Cuciniotta D, Abate G et al. (1993). Oral 5'-methyltetrahydrofolic acid in senile organic mental disorders with depression: results of a double-blind multicenter study. Ageing Clin Exp Res 5: 63–71.

Pincus JH (1979). Folic acid deficiency: a cause of subacute combined degeneration. In: MI Botez, EH Reynolds (Eds.), Folic Acid in Neurology, Psychiatry and Internal Medicine. Raven Press, New York, pp. 427–433.

Pincus JH, Reynolds EH, Glaser GH (1972). Subacute combined system degeneration with folate deficiency. JAMA 221: 496–497.

Prins ND, den Heijer T, Hofman A et al. (2002). Homocysteine and cognitive function in the elderly: the Rotterdam scan study. Neurology 59: 1375–1380.

Ramaekers VT, Blau N (2004). Cerebral folate deficiency. Dev Med Child Neurol 46: 843–851.

Ramaekers VT, Rothenberg P, Sequeira JM et al. (2005). Autoantibodies to folate receptors in the cerebral folate deficiency syndrome. N Engl J Med 352: 1985–1991.

Ramos MI, Allen LH, Haan MN et al. (2004). Plasma folate concentrations are associated with depressive symptoms in elderly Latina women despite folic acid fortification. Am J Clin Nutr 80: 1024–1028.

Ramos MI, Allen LH, Mungas DM et al. (2005). Low folate status is associated with impaired cognitive function and dementia in the Sacramento area Latino study on aging. Am J Clin Nutr 82: 1346–1352.

Rampersaud GC, Kauwell GPA, Hutson AD et al. (2000). Genomic DNA methylation decreases in response to moderate folate depletion in elderly women. Am J Clin Nutr 72: 998–1003.

Ravaglia G, Forti P, Maioli F et al. (2005). Homocystine and folate as risk factors for dementia and Alzheimer disease. Am J Clin Nutr 82: 636–643.

Ray JG, Blom HJ (2003). Vitamin B12 insufficiency and the risk of foetal neural tube defects. QJ Med 96: 289–295.

Reynolds EH (1968). Mental effects of anticonvulsants, and folic acid metabolism. Brain 91: 197–214.

Reynolds EH (1976). Neurological aspects of folate and vitamin B12 metabolism. In: AV Hoffbrand (Ed.), Clinics in Haematology. Vol. 5. Saunders, London, pp. 661–696.

Reynolds EH (1979a). Folic acid, vitamin B12 and the nervous system: historical aspects. In: MI Botez, EH Reynolds (Eds.), Folic Acid in Neurology, Psychiatry, and Internal Medicine. Raven Press, New York, pp. 1–5.

Reynolds EH (1979b). Interrelationships between the neurology of folate and vitamin B12 deficiency. In: MI Botez, EH Reynolds (Eds.), Folic Acid in Neurology, Psychiatry and Internal Medicine. Raven Press, New York, pp. 501–515.

Reynolds EH (2002a). Folic acid, ageing, depression, and dementia. BMJ 324: 1512–1515.

Reynolds EH (2002b). Benefits and risks of folic acid to the nervous system. J Neurol Neurosurg Psychiatry 72: 767–771.

Reynolds E (2006). Vitamin B12, folic acid, and the nervous system. Lancet Neurol 5: 949–960.

Reynolds EH, Chanarin I, Matthews DM (1968). Neuropsychiatric aspects of anti-convulsant megaloblastic anaemia. Lancet 1: 394–397.

Reynolds EH, Preece JM, Bailey J et al. (1970). Folate deficiency in depressive illness. Br J Psychiatry 117: 287–292.

Reynolds EH, Gallagher BB, Mattson RH et al. (1972). Relationship between serum and cerebrospinal fluid folate. Nature 240: 155–157.

Reynolds EH, Rothfeld P, Pincus JH (1973). Neurological disease associated with folate deficiency. BMJ 2: 398–400.

Reynolds EH, Carney MWP, Toone BK (1984). Methylation and mood. Lancet 2: 196–198.

Rivey MP, Schottelius DD, Berg MJ (1984). Phenytoin-folic acid: a review. Drug Intell Clin Pharm 18: 292–301.

Rosenblatt DS, Fenton WA (2001). Inherited disorders of folate and cobalamin transport and metabolism. In: CS Scriver, AL Beaudet, WS Sly et al. (Eds.), The Metabolic Basis of Inherited Disease. 8th edn McGraw-Hill, New York, pp. 3897–3933.

Rothenberg SP, da Costa MP, Sequeria JM et al. (2004). Auto-antibodies against folate receptors in women with a pregnancy complicated by a neural-tube defect. N Engl J Med 350: 134–142.

Russell JSR, Batten FE, Collier J (1900). Subacute combined degeneration of the spinal cord. Brain 23: 39–110.

Sachdev PS, Parslow RA, Lux O et al. (2005). Relationship of homocysteine, folic acid and vitamin B12 with depression in a middle aged community sample. Psychol Med 35: 529–538.

Savage DG, Lindenbaum J (1995). Neurological complications of acquired cobalamin deficiency: clinical aspects. Bailliere's Clinical Haematology, vol. 8. Bailliere Tindall, pp. 657–678.

Schwaninger M, Ringleb P, Winter R et al. (1999). Elevated plasma concentrations of homocysteine in antiepileptic drug treatment. Epilepsia 40: 345–350.

Schwartz SO, Kaplan SR, Armstrong BE (1950). The long-term evaluation of folic acid in the treatment of pernicious anaemia. J Lab Clin Med 35: 894–898.

Scott JM, Molloy AM, Kennedy DG et al. (1994). Effects of the disruption of transmethylation in the central nervous system: an animal model. Acta Neurol Scand 154: 27S–31S.

Selhub J, Morris MS, Jacques PF (2007). In vitamin B12 deficiency, higher serum folate is associated with increased total homocysteine and methylmalonic acid concentrations. Proc Natl Acad Sci U S A 104: 19995–20000.

Serot JM, Barbe F, Arning E et al. (2005). Homocysteine and methylmolonic acid concentrations in cerebrospinal fluid: relation with age and Alzheimer's disease. J Neurol Neurosurg Psychiatry 76: 1585–1587.

Seshadri S, Beiser A, Selhub J et al. (2002). Plasma homocysteine as a risk factor for dementia and Alzheimer's disease. N Engl J Med 346: 476–483.

Shorvon SD, Reynolds EH (1979). Folate deficiency and peripheral neuropathy. In: MI Botez, EH Reynolds (Eds.), Folic Acid in Neurology, Psychiatry and Internal Medicine. Raven Press, New York, pp. 413–421.

Shorvon SD, Carney MWP, Chanarin I et al. (1980). The neuropsychiatry of megaloblastic anaemia. BMJ 281: 1036–1038.

Smithells RW, Sheppard S, Schorah CJ et al. (1981). Apparent prevention of neural tube defects by periconceptional vitamin supplementation. Arch Dis Child 56: 911–918.

Sneath P, Chanarin I, Hodkinson HM et al. (1973). Folate status in a geriatric population and its relation to dementia. Age Ageing 2: 177–182.

Snowdon DA, Tully CL, Smith CD et al. (2000). Serum folate and the severity of atrophy of the neocortex in Alzheimer disease: findings from the nun study. Am J Clin Nutr 71: 993–998.

Spector R, Lorenzo AV (1975). Folate transport in the central nervous system. Am J Physiol 229: 777–782.

Stabler SP (2010). Clinical folate deficiency. In: LB Bailey (Ed.), Folate in Health and Disease. CRC Press, Boca Raton, pp. 409–428.

Starr JM, Pattie A, Whiteman MC et al. (2005). Vitamin B12, serum folate, and cognitive change between 11 and 79 years. J Neurol Neurosurg Psychiatry 76: 291–292.

Steinfeld R, Grapp M, Kraetzner R et al. (2009). Folate receptor alpha defect causes cerebral folate transport deficiency: a treatable neurogenerative disorder associated with disturbed myelin metabolism. Am J Hum Genet 85: 354–363.

Strachan RW, Henderson JG (1967). Dementia and folate deficiency. Q J Med 36: 189–204.

Surtees R (1998). Demyelination and inborn errors of the single carbon transfer pathway. Eur J Pediatr 157: 118S–121S.

Surtees R (2001). Cobalamin and folate responsive disorders. In: P Baxter (Ed.), Vitamin Responsive Conditions in Paediatric Neurology. International Review of Child Neurology Series. MacKeith Press, London, pp. 96–108.

Surtees R, Leonard J, Austin S (1991). Association of demyelination with deficiency of cerebrospinal-fluid S-adenosylmethionine in inborn errors of methyl-transfer pathway. Lancet 338: 1550–1554.

Tucker KL, Qiao N, Scott T et al. (2005). High homocysteine and low B vitamins predict cognitive decline in aging men: the Veterans Affairs Normative Aging Study. Am J Clin Nutr 82: 627–635.

van der Linden IJ, Afman LA, Heil SG et al. (2005). Genetic variation in genes of folate metabolism and neural tube defect risk. Proc Nutr Soc 65: 1–12.

van der Linden IJ, den Heijer M, Afman LA et al. (2006). The methionine synthase reductase 66A→G polymorphism is a maternal risk factor for spina bifida. J Mol Med 84: 1047–1054.

Wahlin TBR, Wahlin A, Winblad B et al. (2001). The influence of serum vitamin B12 and folate status on cognitive functioning in very old age. Biol Psychol 56: 247–265.

Wallis D, Ballard JL, Shaw GM et al. (2010). Folate-related birth defects: embryonic consequences of abnormal folate transport and metabolism. In: LB Bailey (Ed.), Folate in Health and Disease. CRC Press, Boca Raton, pp. 155–178.

Wang H-X, Wahlin A, Basun H et al. (2001). Vitamin B12 and folate in relation to the development of Alzheimer's disease. Neurology 56: 1188–1194.

Waters AH, Mollin DL (1961). Studies on the folic acid activity of human serum. J Clin Pathol 14: 335–344.

Whitehead VM (2006). Acquired and inherited disorders of cobalamin and folate in children. Br J Haematol 134: 125–136.

Wollack JB, Makori B, Ahlawat S et al. (2008). Characterisation of folate uptake by choroid plexus epithelial cells in a rat primary culture model. J Neurochem 104: 1494–1503.

Woltmann HW (1919). The nervous symptoms in pernicious anaemia: an analysis of 150 cases. Am J Med Sci 157: 400–409.

Section 9

Neurologic aspects of environmental disorders

Handbook of Clinical Neurology, Vol. 120 (3rd series)
Neurologic Aspects of Systemic Disease Part II
Jose Biller and Jose M. Ferro, Editors

Chapter 62

Disorders of body temperature

CAMILO R. GOMEZ*

Neurological Institute of Alabama, Birmingham, AL, USA

INTRODUCTION

The human body, as a product of its metabolism, generates heat capable of raising body temperature by approximately 1°C per hour. However, since this would not be compatible with life, the body also promotes the transfer of excess body heat into the environment by means of a thermoregulatory system. The latter is sufficiently effective as to allow, under normal circumstances, only minimal daily temperature variations (i.e., approximately 0.6°C). The present chapter is a discussion of disorders resulting form abnormally high or low body temperature, leading to neurologic dysfunction and often posing a threat to life. Beforehand though, we must discuss some basic physiologic concepts regarding body temperature homeostasis.

MECHANISMS OF HEAT EXCHANGE

Approximately 90% of the excess body heat is dissipated into the environment via the skin while the remaining 10% is lost in exhaled gas. There are several ways in which body heat is exchanged:

- *Radiation*. This accounts for approximately 60% of the human body's heat loss, and it consists of the emanation of electromagnetic infrared heat rays.
- *Evaporation*. Normally accounting for about 20% of total heat loss, it results when: (1) water or sweat evaporates from the surface of the body, and (2) as insensible fluid losses through the lungs.
- *Conduction*. This represents only 15% of the heat loss from the human body. It consists of the transfer of heat, via kinetic energy, to an object of lower temperature than the body.
- *Convection*. This is the least active mechanism, accounting for only 5% of the heat loss. It relates

to the effect of air currents on the surface and blood flow underneath the skin in promoting differential temperatures that promote conductive heat loss.

BASIC PATHOGENESIS OF HYPERTHERMIA

In response to thermal stress (e.g., hot weather, exercise), maintenance of normal body temperature is primarily maintained by enhanced blood flow to the skin (i.e., convection) and loss of sweat (i.e., evaporation). The latter constitutes an extremely effective and powerful process, accounting for approximately 70% of the loss of body heat during periods of thermal stress. In fact, the evaporation of one liter of sweat results in the loss of 580 kilocalories (kcal) of heat, or about one-quarter of the daily heat production of the average adult.

Hyperthermia results from abnormal temperature regulation, leading to extremely elevated body temperature (i.e., hyperpyrexia), often above 40°C. Conversely, fever results from a normal thermoregulatory mechanism operating at a higher set point. The former leads to specific clinical syndromes which share, as a common denominator, the inability of the thermoregulatory mechanism to maintain a constant body temperature in response to: (1) thermal stress, or (2) the effect of certain drugs.

BASIC PATHOGENESIS OF HYPOTHERMIA

The reduction of body temperature to levels below 35°C, by definition hypothermia, results from: (1) environmental exposure, (2) metabolic disorders, or (3) as a result of therapeutic intervention. The response of the human

---

*Correspondence to: Camilo R. Gomez, M.D., M.B.A., Neurological Institute of Alabama, 509 Brookwood Blvd, Birmingham, AL 35209, USA. Tel: +1-205-874-8888, Fax: +1-205-874-8880, E-mail: crgomez@theani.org

body to significant decrease in temperature is not as efficient or effective as that to temperature elevations. Such response includes: (1) cutaneous vasoconstriction, and (2) shivering. Unfortunately, these adaptive mechanisms are only effective in cases of mild hypothermia and require behavioral responses (e.g., wearing warm clothing) to the cold environment in order to successfully protect the subject (Soteras Martinez et al., 2011).

HEAT-RELATED ILLNESS

Clinical features

The various different syndromes resulting from abnormal thermoregulation in response to environmental or exercise stress are listed in Table 62.1. Heat rash, also known as "prickly heat," is the mildest of these and results from very profuse sweating in response to very hot and humid weather, leading to blockage of sweat ducts. Most commonly found in children, the condition manifests itself as a pruritic cluster of small pimples or blisters, typically in the neck, chest, elbow creases and groin. Heat cramps affect individuals who exercise strenuously and, as a result, sweat significantly. This leads to marked losses of fluid and salt, with electrolytic changes that manifest themselves as muscle spasms or cramps. Neither of these two conditions is characteristically associated with neurologic involvement. We have included them in our discussion because, at least in the case of heat cramps, they may be considered part of a continuum. Failure to heed these early milder syndromes may result in worsening of the ill effects of heat exposure.

Heat exhaustion is the most common heat-related condition and results from volume depletion. These patients develop a clinical syndrome characterized by muscle cramps, nausea, malaise, and tachycardia. The degree of neurologic dysfunction, if any, is typically very mild.

Heat stroke, unlike the other three, is a life-threatening condition characterized by very high elevations of body temperature ($\geq 41°C$) accompanied by severe neurologic dysfunction, volume depletion, hemodynamic compromise, rhabdomyolysis, multiorgan failure, and disseminated intravascular coagulation (DIC). The failure of splanchnic organs is manifested by acute renal and hepatic dysfunction. Inability to produce sweat is a common feature of this condition, but it is not invariably present.

There two different types of heat stroke: classic and exertional. Classic heat stroke results from exposure to very high environmental temperature within confined spaces. This is most common in the elderly and those taking psychiatric medications, or using alcohol or drugs. Exertional heat stroke results from strenuous physical activity in a very hot environment. It is typically seen in athletes and military personnel and is usually more severe, with a higher incidence of multiorgan failure.

Laboratory studies

Patients with heat cramps may show evidence of volume contraction such as increased hematocrit, serum urea nitrogen (BUN) or BUN/creatinine (Cr) ratio. However, more likely than not, their laboratory studies will be normal. Such evidence of volume depletion is much more frequently found in patients with heat exhaustion, along with abnormalities of serum sodium. Patients who experience a net loss of free water will show hypernatremia, while those whose salt and water losses are replaced with water alone are more likely to show hyponatremia.

Patients with heat stroke, however, display numerous laboratory abnormalities. In addition to evidence of volume depletion, as noted earlier, the most salient laboratory findings include elevation of serum creatinine and liver transaminases, indicative of renal and hepatic dysfunction respectively. Skeletal muscle is particularly vulnerable to thermal stress, and injury of the myocytes results in release of creatine kinase (CK) into the bloodstream. Very high levels of CK, greater than 15 000 Units/L or so, are important because of the propensity of myoglobin to precipitate in the renal tubules and produce direct damage of the tubular epithelium, with consequent renal failure. The presence of myoglobin in

Table 62.1

Different types of heat-related illnesses and their defining features

Feature	Heat rash	Heat cramps	Heat exhaustion	Heat stroke
Body temperature	$<39°C$	$<39°C$	$39°C$	$\geq 41°C$
CNS dysfunction	No	No	Mild	Severe
Sweat production	++++	+++	++	±
Dehydration	Yes	Yes	Yes	Yes
Multiorgan dysfunction	No	No	No	Yes

urine can be easily determined by means of comparing a urine dipstick blood test in urine with the presence of blood cells: A positive dipstick with no red blood cells in urine is highly suggestive of myoglobinuria.

Management

The management of heat cramps and heat exhaustion includes cessation of strenuous activity, volume repletion, and simple cooling measures (e.g., cold shower). In addition, all strenuous activity should be avoided for at least a number of hours.

Heat stroke, however, must be always considered a medical emergency and its treatment requires aggressive cooling and volume repletion in order to prevent organ failure. External cooling methods are the most practical, including icepacks placed in the groins and axillae, cooling blankets to cover the entire body, and evaporative cooling by using fans to promote evaporation of skin surface water. The latter has the advantage that it can be used in field, and it is probably the most effective of the external cooling methods, achieving body temperature reductions of up to 0.3°C per minute. In the past, in communities where environmental heat waves were common, emergency departments often had bathtubs with ice water available during the summer months. More recently, technology has improved to the point of having external cooling devices available not only in the emergency departments but also for use by paramedics. We will discuss this new technology separately, since it can be used to treat different conditions and not only heat stroke.

Internal cooling methods include ice saline lavage of the stomach, bladder, or rectum. These methods reduce body temperature faster but they are more cumbersome and less practical. In the past, we have had bags of normal saline frozen in our intensive care unit. We have infused such fluid after placing the solid frozen bag in the microwave for a few minutes and found it to be effective in reducing body temperature. As noted earlier, modern technology exists to provide intravascular cooling and this will be discussed separately. Finally, the treatment of heat stroke requires constant monitoring of all organ functions, opportunistically treating any derangements that require attention (e.g., seizures, renal failure).

DRUG-INDUCED HYPERTHERMIA

Clinical features

There are three specific syndromes characterized by increased internal heat production as a result of the effects of certain drugs:

- *Malignant hyperthermia.* This is an inherited condition transmitted with an autosomal dominant pattern, affecting approximately 1 in 50 000 adults (about 1 in 15 000 anesthesia cases). There are at least six different forms of genetic susceptibility to malignant hyperthermia caused by mutations in different genes. Mutations in the ryanodine receptor (*RYR1*) gene result in a form of the condition known as MHS1, which accounts for the majority of cases. Another form of the condition, known as MHS5, results from mutations in the *CACN1S* gene. The proteins produced by the *RYR1* and *CACNS1* genes are involved in the release of calcium from the sarcoplasmic reticulum of skeletal muscle. Mutations result in the RYR1 channels opening more easily and closing more slowly in response to halogenated inhalational anesthetic agents (e.g., isoflurane) or depolarizing neuromuscular blocking agents (e.g., succinylcholine), with consequent excessive release of calcium (Adnet and Krivosic-Horber, 2000; Balog et al., 2000; Evans et al., 2002; Finsterer, 2002; Haslego, 2002). The overabundance of calcium in the cytoplasm leads to uncoupling of oxidative phosphorylation and marked increased in metabolic rate. Clinically, this results in muscle rigidity (i.e., rhabdomyolysis), increased body temperature, depressed consciousness (i.e., obtundation, coma) and autonomic instability (i.e., arrhythmias, shock) (Jurkat-Rott et al., 2000).

- *Neuroleptic malignant syndrome.* This is a condition similar to malignant hyperthermia, produced by drugs that influence dopamine-mediated neurotransmission within the brain. As its name denotes, it is most commonly associated with neuroleptic agents (i.e., antipsychotics), notorious for reducing dopaminergic conduction, but it can occur in response to discontinuation of drugs that facilitate dopamine release (Table 62.2) (Adnet et al., 2000; al-Waneen, 2000; Aydin et al., 2000; Bobolakis, 2000; Cassidy and O'Kearne 2000; Doan and Callaghan, 2000; Gupta and Racaniello, 2000; Iwuagwu et al., 2000; Jarventausta and Leinonen, 2000; Nimmagadda et al., 2000; Nyfort-Hansen and Alderman, 2000; Sechi et al., 2000; Stanfield and Privette, 2000; Stanley and Hunter, 2000; Goldney, 2001; Hall et al., 2001; Harradine et al., 2001; Ito et al., 2001; So, 2001; Aboraya et al., 2002; Caroff et al., 2002). Although a familial tendency has been noted, no specific pattern of inheritance has been defined. It is important to note that this syndrome represents an idiosyncratic drug reaction and, as such, its occurrence bears no relationship to the length of use of the medications noted. However, most cases occur within a few days of the onset of drug therapy and certainly almost all of them within 2 weeks. Its presence is characterized by increased

Table 62.2

Different drugs previously associated with neuroleptic malignant syndrome

Ongoing drug intake	
Antipsychotic agents	Haloperidol, phenothiazines, clozapine, olanzapine, risperidone
Antiemetic agents	Metoclopramide, droperidol, prochlorperazine
Stimulants	Amphetamines, cocaine
Other	Lithium, tricyclics

Discontinued drug intake	
Dopaminergic agents	Amantadine, bromocriptine, levodopa, ropirinole, pramipexole

Table 62.3

Different drugs known to be associated with serotonin syndrome

Class of drug	Specific drugs
Dietary supplements and herbal products	L-tryptophan, St John's wort, ginseng
Antibiotics	Ritonavir, linezolid
Stimulant drugs (legal or illegal)	Amphetamines, MDMA, cocaine, LSD
Antidepressants	SSRIs, TCAs, MAOIs, buspirone
Narcotics	Meperidine, fentanyl, tramadol
Cough suppressants	Dextromethorphan
Antiemetics	Ondansetron, metoclopramide
Antiepileptic agents	Valproic acid
Migraine abortive agents	Sumatriptan
Other	Lithium

MDMA, 3,4-lethylenedioxymethamphetamine; LSD, lysergic acid diethylamide; SSRI, selective serotonin reuptake inhibitor; TCA, tricyclic antidepressant; MAOI, monoamine oxidase inhibitor.

Table 62.4

Specific drug–drug interactions capable of producing the serotonin syndrome

Specific drug–drug interactions
Phenelzine and meperidine
Tranylcypromine and imipramine
Phenelzine and SSRIs
Paroxetine and buspirone
Linezolid and citalopram
Moclobemide and SSRIs
Tramadol, venlafaxine and mirtazapine

SSRI, selective serotonin reuptake inhibitor.

body temperature (>40°C, muscle rigidity, altered mentation (either agitation or obtundation) and autonomic instability (arrhythmias, shock).

- *Serotonin syndrome.* This condition results from overstimulation of serotonin receptors in the brain. It is characterized by the abrupt onset of altered mentation (e.g., confusion, delirium, coma), autonomic hyperactivity (e.g., tachycardia, hypertension, hyperthermia, diaphoresis), and neuromuscular abnormalities (e.g., hyperkinesis, muscle rigidity, hyperreflexia). Drugs associated with excessive serotoninergic activity, and therefore this clinical syndrome, are listed in Table 62.3 (Bhanji, 2000; Hamilton and Malone, 2000; Perry, 2000; Trakas and Shear, 2000; Voirol et al., 2000; Kaneda et al., 2001a, b; Lavery et al., 2001; McCue and Joseph, 2001; Wigen and Goetz, 2002; Kontaxakis et al., 2003; Ubogu and Katirji, 2003; Bryant and Kolodchak, 2004; Thomas et al., 2004; Paruchuri et al., 2006; Vizcaychipi et al., 2007; Canan et al., 2008; Evans, 2008; Hadikusumo and Ng, 2009; Quinn and Stern, 2009; Sansone and Sansone, 2009; Gombar and Bhatia, 2010; Kirschner and Donovan, 2010; Thorpe et al., 2010; Gelener et al., 2011; Miller and Lovell, 2011). In addition, however, there are a number of drug interactions that have also been associated with the production of this syndrome (Table 62.4) (Spirko and Wiley, 1999; Hamilton and Malone, 2000; Hinds et al., 2000; Manos, 2000; Margolese and Chouinard, 2000; Smith and Wenegrat, 2000; Vandemergel et al., 2000; Dams et al., 2001; Demers and Malone,

2001; DeSilva et al., 2001; Gillman, 2001; Isbister et al., 2001; Kaneda et al., 2001a, b; McCue and Joseph, 2001; Dimellis, 2002; Dougherty et al., 2002; Bernard et al., 2003; Hachem et al., 2003; Isbister, 2003; Mittino et al., 2004; Munhoz, 2004; Altman and Manos, 2007; Steinberg and Morin, 2007; Ishii et al., 2008; Margetic and Aukst-Margetic, 2008). These not only include drugs that augment serotoninergic transmission by directly affecting the synthesis (↑), breakdown (↓), release (↑), or reuptake (↓) of serotonin, but also their combination with drugs that inhibit cytochrome isoforms CYP2D6 and CYP3A4 (Kaneda et al., 2002). The clinical manifestations vary from mild to life-threatening, beginning with muscular hyperactivity and altered mentation, progressing to muscular hypertonicity, hyperthermia, autonomic instability, and frank shock. These patients also present rhabdomyolysis, renal failure, and metabolic acidosis. The onset is typically abrupt (as opposed to the neuroleptic malignant syndrome), and even one single dose of an offending agent may be sufficient to cause it.

Laboratory studies

In patients with malignant hyperthermia, an early elevation of the partial pressure of carbon dioxide (PCO_2), resulting from the excessive metabolic rate, is often first noted by end-tidal CO_2 monitoring in the operating room. This is followed, just as with heat stroke, by an increase in serum CK and urine myoglobin, which carries the impending risk of acute renal failure. Due to its genetic nature, relatives of patients who have suffered an episode of malignant hyperthermia must be considered for susceptibility tests, either the caffeine halothane contracture test (CHCT) (Ruffert et al., 2000; Snoeck et al., 2000) or *RYR1* gene sequencing (Chamley et al., 2000; Gencik et al., 2000; McCarthy et al., 2000; Steinfath et al., 2002; Loke et al., 2003; Urwyler et al., 2003).

Patients with neuroleptic malignant syndrome present with pronounced leukocytosis (even as high as $40\,000/\mu L$ and often with leftward shift) and significant increase in serum CK. It is in fact the latter that should alert the clinician to the presence of this condition, differentiating it from sepsis. The serotonin syndrome is also associated with similar changes in serum CK, urine myoglobin and serum creatinine. However, these patients are also prone to showing metabolic acidosis.

Management

The first step in managing patients with malignant hyperthermia is the discontinuation of the offending anesthetic agent. This should be quickly followed by the administration of dantrolene, an agent that blocks the release of calcium by the sarcoplasmic reticulum and can reduce the mortality from approximately 70% to about 10% (Gronert, 2000; Kobayashi et al., 2010). We favor a regimen of 2 mg/kg intravenously (IV) with repeated similar doses every 15 minutes if necessary, until muscle rigidity disappears or a total of 10 mg/kg has been administered. This must be followed by 3 days treatment with 1 mg/kg IV every 6 hours, closely monitoring liver enzymes, because of the risk of the drug producing hepatocellular injury. Along these lines, the presence of liver dysfunction must be considered a relative contraindication to the use of dantrolene.

The management of neuroleptic malignant syndrome also requires removal of the offending drug, or reintroduction of discontinued dopaminergic agents that can be slowly discontinued at a later date. These patients often also require fluid resuscitation and measures to reduce multiorgan injury. The use of dantrolene is also recommended and, although the best dosing regimen is not quite defined, we favor an approach similar to that used for malignant hyperthermia. The only exception is that of patients with evidence of liver dysfunction, in whom instead of dantrolene, treatment with bromocriptine 2.5–10 mg every 8 hours may be a reasonable alternative. In any case, treatment should be continued for up to 2 weeks, depending upon the clearance of the offending drug.

The treatment of patients affected by the serotonin syndrome involves, as with the other conditions, discontinuation of the offending drug or drugs. In addition, supportive treatment is geared at controlling agitation, decreasing body temperature, and providing hemodynamic support. The degree of aggressiveness of the treatment depends upon the severity of the illness. Agitation can be controlled with parenteral benzodiazepines, and hypotension may require vasopressors once euvolemia is assured. Typically, controlling muscular hyperactivity, body temperature, and hypotension will result in correction of the metabolic acidosis and prevention of multiorgan failure. Additionally, it is important to consider the use of serotonin antagonists in the treatment of these patients, particularly cyproheptadine. This medication, at an initial dose of 12 mg (orally or by nasogastric tube) followed by 2 mg every 2 hours as necessary, results in blockade of 85–95% of serotonin receptors. Whenever parenteral administration is preferred, the use of 50–100 mg of chlorpromazine intramuscularly may be considered.

Finally, in any of these conditions, treatment of the elevated body temperature should be carried out using a strategy similar to that described above for heat stroke. In severe cases, if the muscular hyperactivity causing the hyperthermia does not readily respond to benzodiazepines, intubations and nondepolarizing neuromuscular blocking agents may be used.

FEVER IN NEUROLOGIC PRACTICE

Clinical features

For the purposes of our discussion, our operational definition of fever is that of an abnormal body temperature above 38.3°C, deserving special attention and a search for a cause. This definition, although not perfect, is practical and in line with that adopted by the Society of Critical Care Medicine (SCCM).

Fever results from the release of inflammatory cytokines that act on the hypothalamus to elevate body temperature. Unlike hyperthermia, resulting from abnormal body temperature regulation, in the context of fever the thermoregulatory system is intact although it is working at a higher set point. It is, therefore, an adaptive response of the organism that allows it to respond to infections and other insults, by enhancing the immune response. Unfortunately, fever is pervasively common in neurointensive care units, having been found in up to 63% of patients with ischemic stroke, and up to 93% of those with intracerebral hemorrhage.

The presence of fever in neurologic patients poses a major dilemma in clinical practice. On one hand, the febrile response is considered a potentially beneficial answer to inflammation, improving the body's ability to fight certain detrimental stimuli by enhancing the immune response (i.e., increasing production of antibodies and cytokines, activating T lymphocytes, facilitating neutrophil chemotaxis, enhancing phagocytosis, inhibiting bacterial and viral replication). Conversely, there is also evidence that increased body temperature has a detrimental effect in patients with neurologic injuries, either traumatic or ischemic. The former argument suggests that active treatment of fever may not be necessary, while the latter underscores our current practice and recommendations. *Maintaining normothermia should be a major priority in the treatment of critically ill neurologic patients!*

In part, the problem of dealing with fever is the fact that it simply represents a physical finding with many potential causes, only some of which are infectious. Thus, the presence of fever should not automatically lead to the conclusion that an underlying infection is its cause. Rather, it should trigger a deliberate and organized examination of all potential causes present in any patient (Table 62.5), especially because if the cause can be found and corrected, not only will the body temperature be lowered but the apparent conflict related to its treatment will disappear.

The subject is further complicated because not only neurologic injury can be cause of increased body temperature (i.e., neurogenic fever) but there is sufficient evidence to conclude that fever is associated with worsening of neurologic outcomes. Neurogenic fever appears to be the result of direct injury to the hypothalamus, and is characterized by increased temperature, resistance to antipyretic agents, and decreased perspiration. Published data suggest that fever has multiple ill effects upon the injured brain, including increased blood volume and intracranial pressure, promoting neuronal loss, increasing metabolic rate (about 13% per every 1°C), and causing vasospasm. All these changes have been associated with prolonged stay in the intensive care and worse long-term outcomes.

Table 62.5

Causes of fever in hospitalized patients

Noninfectious causes

Postoperative fever
Hemodialysis
Bronchoscopy
Blood transfusion
Venous thromboembolism
Acalculous cholecystitis
Drug-related
Adrenal crisis
Ischemia and infarction

Nosocomial infections

Pneumonia
Urinary tract infection
Catheter-related infections
Wound infections
Sinusitis
Intra-abdominal infections

Laboratory findings

Patients with fever of uncertain cause must have, at a minimum, complete blood count with differential. The presence of leukocytosis, particularly if accompanied by a leftward shift, is suggestive of the presence of a nosocomial infection. Elevation of eosinophils, on the other hand, is more likely to be present as a result of an allergic or a drug reaction. Chest radiographs may show infiltrates that point to the presence of a pneumonic infectious process, but if obtained very early may not show any abnormalities. In cases where there is a urinary tract infection, examination of the urine may show the presence of leukocytes or even bacteria that may be further identified via gram staining and culture. Blood cultures should be obtained whenever an infection is suspected, even though the results are typically delayed for days. Their importance hinges on the ability to identify an infective organism and its antimicrobial susceptibility. In intubated patients, the sputum can also show the presence of leukocytes and bacteria. The latter can be further identified by gram stain and culture. Infections of the paranasal sinuses can be diagnosed by conventional radiographs but computed tomography is a much more sensitive technique, especially if the patient can be moved out of the nursing unit. Finally, abdominal ultrasound can easily allow the diagnosis of abdominal ultrasound, but abdominal computed tomography is necessary for more complex processes, including intra-abdominal infections.

Management

As noted earlier, in the context of neurologic injury (traumatic or ischemic), achieving normothermia should be one of the most important priorities of overall care. Traditionally, this has been easier said than done, as the use of antipyretic medications and external cooling methods (i.e., cooling blankets) has a very high failure rate. Newer technology, to be discussed later in this chapter, is much more effective and can facilitate treatment. The antipyretic agents available for treatment include aspirin, acetaminophen (paracetamol), and non-steroidal anti-inflammatory agents (e.g., ibuprofen). We favor rotating them every 4–6 hours, at doses of 650 mg orally or rectally. Cooling blankets can be used, either singly or by placing the patient between two cooling blankets. As noted, though, these techniques are labor-intensive and somewhat ineffective. Thus, we recommend aggressive management of the cause of fever PLUS early utilization of the newer techniques described below.

ACCIDENTAL HYPOTHERMIA

Clinical features

Excessively low body temperature ($<35°C$) can result from: (1) prolonged submersion in cold water; (2) exposure to cold wind; (3) impairment of physiologic responses to cold (e.g., effect of alcohol on shivering); (4) inability to seek protection against cold weather. Hypothermia can be classified based upon the magnitude of the reduction of body temperature (Table 62.6). It is important to note that standard thermometers only record temperatures down to approximately 34°C and, therefore, specialized thermometers designed to measure core body temperature (i.e., bladder, rectum) must be used in the management of these patients. In addition to the clinical manifestations listed in Table 62.6, patients with severe hypothermia also experience two distinct behavioral abnormalities: (1) paradoxical undressing, and (2) terminal burrowing. The former occurs as a result of the confusional state in approximately 25% of patients. The removal of clothing further increases heat loss and worsens the situation. Its cause is uncertain but cold-induced malfunction of the hypothalamus has been postulated as a possibility. Terminal burrowing, also known as "hide-and-die" syndrome, leads the subject to crawl into small and confined spaces.

Laboratory studies

The most prominent abnormalities found in hypothermic patients include a coagulopathy characterized by prolongation of the partial thromboplastin time (PTT) and

Table 62.6

Various levels of accidental hypothermia and their features

Classification	Temperature	Manifestations
Mild	32–35°C	Shivering, hypertension, tachycardia, tachypnea, vasoconstriction, cold diuresis, hyperglycemia, confusion
Moderate	28–32°C	Sluggishness, incoordination, worsening confusion, paleness
Severe	20–28°C	Bradycardia, hypotension, edematous skin, amnesia, irrational behavior, severe incoordination, organ failure, dilated pupils
Profound	$<20°C$	Apnea, asystole

the international normalized ratio (INR). Arterial blood gases typically show acidosis, either respiratory or metabolic, and serum electrolytes are characterized by hyperkalemia, presumably secondary to release of potassium by skeletal muscle as the result of shivering. Elevation of serum creatinine, indicating renal dysfunction, may be caused by cold diuresis.

One of the most characteristic and curious findings in these patients (about 80%) involves prominent J waves (known as Osborn waves) in the QRS-ST junction of the electrocardiogram (Fig. 62.1). These waves are not exclusive of hypothermia, having been described in association with subarachnoid hemorrhage, hypercalcemia, and myocardial ischemia. Additionally, all types of arrhythmias can be seen in these patients, including heart block, junctional bradycardia, premature contractions, and ventricular fibrillation.

Management

Rewarming of the patient with hypothermia is the principal step in treatment and how it is carried out largely depends on how critical the clinical situation is. In mild cases, passive external rewarming by means of moving the patient to a warm environment and covering him or her with warm dry clothes is usually sufficient. Active rewarming techniques can be external (e.g., Bair

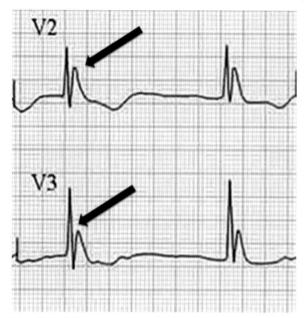

Fig. 62.1. Osborn waves (arrows) noted in the electrocardiogram of patients with hypothermia.

Hugger™) or internal. The latter can be accomplished by increasing the temperature of inhaled gases in intubated patients, by peritoneal lavage, or even by extracorporeal blood rewarming. At present, the use of newer technology, as described below, should always be considered early.

Finally, we must point out the active rewarming from moderate and severe hypothermia is often accompanied by shock. This results from a variety of factors, including volume depletion (following cold diuresis), myocardial depression, and vasodilation. These patients may require vasopressors, but the first step of treatment should be volume infusion with isotonic crystalloids administered through warming pump devices.

THERAPEUTIC BODY TEMPERATURE MANIPULATION: CURRENT TECHNOLOGY

Advances in technology, combined with an increasing interest in manipulating body temperature for therapeutic purposes, have resulted in the introduction of devices that facilitate the management of conditions associated with abnormal body temperature. As noted earlier, traditional methods of cooling or warming the body, both external and internal, have been repeatedly proved to be ineffective and impractical. In this section we will discuss the most important technology currently available for temperature control, and we will follow with a few comments about therapeutic hypothermia.

External methods

There are two systems that allow relatively rapid cooling of the body via external means, one based on the application of gel pads to areas of the patient's skin and circulating temperature-controlled water through them (Arctic Sun®, Medivance, Inc., Louisville, CO, USA). The other consists of a suit that allows immersing the patient into bath of circulating temperature-controlled water (ThermoSuit®, Life Recovery Systems, LLC, Kinnelon, NJ, USA). In both cases, the cooled water is circulated via an external pump that allows precise monitoring of the patient's core temperature and specific selection of the target therapeutic temperature. The differences between these two, and potential advantages of one versus the other, are not significant. From our point of view, the Arctic Sun® system has versatility to the point that can be applied and started quickly and in nearly any environment. On the other hand, the ThermoSuit® seems ideal for receiving patients in the emergency department, making it ideal for treating heat stroke in communities affected by severe heat waves.

Internal methods

The two systems available for internal temperature control consist of specialized intravascular catheters connected to an external pump that circulates temperature-controlled saline through catheter compartments, thereby changing the temperature of the blood circulating around the catheter. The one that has been available the longest is the Thermogard XP® (Zoll, Inc., Chelmsford, MA, USA) and will be the one we use as an example, although a second system (Reprieve®, Radiant Medical, Inc., Redwood City, CA, USA) shares many of its characteristics. The advantage of intravascular temperature control is that the system can be used to precisely achieve a target temperature and maintain it regardless of whether it involves cooling or warming of the body. The obvious disadvantage is that it is an invasive system, requiring intravascular access to the central venous system. The latter, however, is facilitated by the availability of different types of specialized catheters.

Therapeutic hypothermia

Although an exhaustive discussion of therapeutic hypothermia is beyond the scope of the present chapter, a discussion of body temperature changes in neurologic disorders would be incomplete without at least referring to this ever more popular form of treatment. The potential benefits of hypothermia as a neuroprotective strategy in patients with brain injury has been a subject of research for over two decades. The theoretical considerations of how hypothermia can lead to brain protection are

Table 62.7

Proposed neuroprotective mechanisms of hypothermia

Proposed neuroprotective mechanisms of hypothermia
Reduction of glutamate release
Reduction of calcium influx after glutamate
Reduction of inflammatory response to ischemia
Limit edema formation
Reduction of metabolic rate
Suppression of reactive oxygen species

numerous (Table 62.7) and have led to its study within the context of traumatic brain injury, ischemic stroke, increased intracranial pressure, and global brain ischemia resulting from cardiac arrest. At present, therapeutic hypothermia is being used in one or more of these clinical scenarios, the most frequent being following cardiac arrest (Eisenburger et al., 2001; Whitelaw and Thoresen, 2001; Darby, 2002; Gadkary et al., 2002; Marion, 2002; Feigin et al., 2003; Holzer and Sterz, 2003; Kochanek and Safar, 2003; McIntyre et al., 2003; Olsen et al., 2003; Bernard, 2004a, b, 2006; Moran and Solomon, 2004; Edwards and Azzopardi, 2006; Lyden et al., 2006).

CONCLUSIONS

Disorders of body temperature, either excessive elevation or severe reduction, are capable of producing significant neurologic disability and may carry a very high mortality. In general, these conditions are rather uncommon and effectively treatable if recognized early. In our opinion, the only exception is the serotonin syndrome, which we suspect to be very prevalent in milder forms due to the widespread use of the medications that can produce it. Any patient with increased body temperature should be considered at risk for neurologic dysfunction, and normothermia must be considered a high therapeutic priority for any neurologic patient. Finally, in specific circumstances (e.g., following cardiac arrest), controlled reduction of body temperature to approximately 33°C may be used in order to maximize the chances of a good neurologic outcome.

REFERENCES

Aboraya A, Schumacher J, Abdalla E et al. (2002). Neuroleptic malignant syndrome associated with risperidone and olanzapine in first-episode schizophrenia. W V Med J 98: 63–65.

Adnet P, Krivosic-Horber R (2000). Malignant hyperthermia and new halogen agents. Ann Fr Anesth Reanim 19: f115–f117.

Adnet P, Lestavel P, Krivosic-Horber R (2000). Neuroleptic malignant syndrome. Br J Anaesth 85: 129–135.

Altman EM, Manos GH (2007). Serotonin syndrome associated with citalopram and meperidine. Psychosomatics 48: 361–363.

al-Waneen R (2000). Neuroleptic malignant syndrome associated with quetiapine. Can J Psychiatry 45: 764–765.

Aydin N, Anac E, Caykoylu A et al. (2000). Neuroleptic malignant syndrome due to citalopram overdose. Can J Psychiatry 45: 941–942.

Balog EM, Enzmann NR, Gallant EM (2000). Malignant hyperthermia: fatigue characteristics of skeletal muscle. Muscle Nerve 23: 223–230.

Bernard S (2004a). New indications for the use of therapeutic hypothermia. Crit Care 8: E1.

Bernard SA (2004b). Therapeutic hypothermia after cardiac arrest. Med J Aust 181: 468–469.

Bernard S (2006). Therapeutic hypothermia after cardiac arrest. Neurol Clin 24: 61–71.

Bernard L, Stern R, Lew D et al. (2003). Serotonin syndrome after concomitant treatment with linezolid and citalopram. Clin Infect Dis 36: 1197.

Bhanji NH (2000). Serotonin syndrome following low-dose sertraline. Can J Psychiatry 45: 936–937.

Bobolakis I (2000). Neuroleptic malignant syndrome after antipsychotic drug administration during benzodiazepine withdrawal. J Clin Psychopharmacol 20: 281–283.

Bryant SM, Kolodchak J (2004). Serotonin syndrome resulting from an herbal detox cocktail. Am J Emerg Med 22: 625–626.

Canan F, Korkmaz U, Kocer E et al. (2008). Serotonin syndrome with paroxetine overdose: a case report. Prim Care Companion J Clin Psychiatry 10: 165–167.

Caroff SN, Rosenberg H, Mann SC et al. (2002). Neuroleptic malignant syndrome in the critical care unit. Crit Care Med 30: 2609, author reply 2609–2610.

Cassidy EM, O'Kearne V (2000). Neuroleptic malignant syndrome after venlafaxine. Lancet 355: 2164–2165.

Chamley D, Pollock NA, Stowell KM et al. (2000). Malignant hyperthermia in infancy and identification of novel RYR1 mutation. Br J Anaesth 84: 500–504.

Dams R, Benijts TH, Lambert WE et al. (2001). A fatal case of serotonin syndrome after combined moclobemide-citalopram intoxication. J Anal Toxicol 25: 147–151.

Darby JM (2002). Therapeutic hypothermia after cardiac arrest. N Engl J Med 347: 63–65, author reply 63–65.

Demers JC, Malone M (2001). Serotonin syndrome induced by fluvoxamine and mirtazapine. Ann Pharmacother 35: 1217–1220.

DeSilva KE, Le Flore DB, Marston BJ et al. (2001). Serotonin syndrome in HIV-infected individuals receiving antiretroviral therapy and fluoxetine. AIDS 15: 1281–1285.

Dimellis D (2002). Serotonin syndrome produced by a combination of venlafaxine and mirtazapine. World J Biol Psychiatry 3: 167.

Doan RJ, Callaghan WD (2000). Clozapine treatment and neuroleptic malignant syndrome. Can J Psychiatry 45: 394–395.

Dougherty JA, Young H, Shafi T (2002). Serotonin syndrome induced by amitriptyline meperidine and venlafaxine. Ann Pharmacother 36: 1647–1648.

Edwards AD, Azzopardi DV (2006). Therapeutic hypothermia following perinatal asphyxia. Arch Dis Child Fetal Neonatal Ed 91: F127–F131.

Eisenburger P, Sterz F, Holzer M et al. (2001). Therapeutic hypothermia after cardiac arrest. Curr Opin Crit Care 7: 184–188.

Evans RW (2008). Triptans and serotonin syndrome. Cephalalgia 28: 573–574, author reply 574–575.

Evans TJ, Parent CM, McGunigal MP (2002). Atypical presentation of malignant hyperthermia. Anesthesiology 97: 507–508.

Feigin V, Anderson N, Gunn A et al. (2003). The emerging role of therapeutic hypothermia in acute stroke. Lancet Neurol 2: 529.

Finsterer J (2002). Current concepts in malignant hyperthermia. J Clin Neuromuscul Dis 4: 64–74.

Gadkary CS, Alderson P, Signorini DF (2002). Therapeutic hypothermia for head injury. Cochrane Database Syst Rev: CD001048.

Gelener P, Gorgulu U, Kutlu G et al. (2011). Serotonin syndrome due to duloxetine. Clin Neuropharmacol 34: 127–128.

Gencik M, Gencik A, Mortier W et al. (2000). Novel mutation in the RYR1 gene (R2454C) in a patient with malignant hyperthermia. Hum Mutat 15: 122.

Gillman PK (2001). Comments on serotonin syndrome during treatment with paroxetine and risperidone. J Clin Psychopharmacol 21: 344–345.

Goldney RD (2001). Neuroleptic malignant syndrome: an underdiagnosed condition. Med J Aust 175: 501.

Gombar S, Bhatia N (2010). Serotonin syndrome in the perioperative period: role of tramadol. Anesth Analg 111: 1077.

Gronert GA (2000). Dantrolene in malignant hyperthermia (MH)-susceptible patients with exaggerated exercise stress. Anesthesiology 93: 905.

Gupta S, Racaniello AA (2000). Neuroleptic malignant syndrome associated with amoxapine and lithium in an older adult. Ann Clin Psychiatry 12: 107–109.

Hachem RY, Hicks K, Huen A et al. (2003). Myelosuppression and serotonin syndrome associated with concurrent use of linezolid and selective serotonin reuptake inhibitors in bone marrow transplant recipients. Clin Infect Dis 37: e8–e11.

Hadikusumo B, Ng B (2009). Serotonin syndrome induced by duloxetine. Aust N Z J Psychiatry 43: 581–582.

Hall KL, Taylor WH, Ware MR (2001). Neuroleptic malignant syndrome due to olanzapine. Psychopharmacol Bull 35: 49–54.

Hamilton S, Malone K (2000). Serotonin syndrome during treatment with paroxetine and risperidone. J Clin Psychopharmacol 20: 103–105.

Harradine PG, Williams SE, Doherty SR (2001). Neuroleptic malignant syndrome: an underdiagnosed condition. Med J Aust 174: 593–594.

Haslego SS (2002). Malignant hyperthermia: how to spot it early. RN 65: 31–35, quiz 36.

Hinds NP, Hillier CE, Wiles CM (2000). Possible serotonin syndrome arising from an interaction between nortriptyline and selegiline in a lady with parkinsonism. J Neurol 247: 811.

Holzer M, Sterz F (2003). Therapeutic hypothermia after cardiopulmonary resuscitation. Expert Rev Cardiovasc Ther 1: 317–325.

Isbister GK (2003). Comment: combination risperidone and SSRI-induced serotonin syndrome. Ann Pharmacother 37: 1531–1532, author reply 1532–1533.

Isbister GK, Dawson AH, Whyte IM (2001). Comment: serotonin syndrome induced by fluvoxamine and mirtazapine. Ann Pharmacother 35: 1674–1675.

Ishii M, Tatsuzawa Y, Yoshino A et al. (2008). Serotonin syndrome induced by augmentation of SSRI with methylphenidate. Psychiatry Clin Neurosci 62: 246.

Ito T, Shibata K, Watanabe A et al. (2001). Neuroleptic malignant syndrome following withdrawal of amantadine in a patient with influenza A encephalopathy. Eur J Pediatr 160: 401.

Iwuagwu CU, Riley D, Bonoma RA (2000). Neuroleptic malignant-like syndrome in an elderly patient caused by abrupt withdrawal of tolcapone a-catechol-o-methyl transferase inhibitor. Am J Med 108: 517–518.

Jarventausta K, Leinonen E (2000). Neuroleptic malignant syndrome during olanzapine and levomepromazine treatment. Acta Psychiatr Scand 102: 231–233.

Jurkat-Rott K, McCarthy T, Lehmann-Horn F (2000). Genetics and pathogenesis of malignant hyperthermia. Muscle Nerve 23: 4–17.

Kaneda Y, Ishimoto Y, Ohmori T (2001a). Mild serotonin syndrome on fluvoxamine. Int J Neurosci 109: 165–172.

Kaneda Y, Ohmori T, Okabe H (2001b). Possible mild serotonin syndrome related to co-prescription of tandospirone and trazodone. Gen Hosp Psychiatry 23: 98–101.

Kaneda Y, Kawamura I, Fujii A et al. (2002). Serotonin syndrome – "potential" role of the CYP2D6 genetic polymorphism in Asians. Int J Neuropsychopharmacol 5: 105–106.

Kirschner R, Donovan JW (2010). Serotonin syndrome precipitated by fentanyl during procedural sedation. J Emerg Med 38: 477–480.

Kobayashi S, Yano M, Uchinoumi H et al. (2010). Dantrolene a therapeutic agent for malignant hyperthermia inhibits catecholaminergic polymorphic ventricular tachycardia in a RyR2(R2474S/+) knock-in mouse model. Circ J 74: 2579–2584.

Kochanek PM, Safar PJ (2003). Therapeutic hypothermia for severe traumatic brain injury. JAMA 289: 3007–3009.

Kontaxakis VP, Havaki-Kontaxaki BJ, Christodoulou NG et al. (2003). Olanzapine-associated neuroleptic malignant syndrome: is there an overlap with the serotonin syndrome? Ann Gen Hosp Psychiatry 2: 10.

Lavery S, Ravi H, McDaniel WW et al. (2001). Linezolid and serotonin syndrome. Psychosomatics 42: 432–434.

Loke JC, Kraev N, Sharma P et al. (2003). Detection of a novel ryanodine receptor subtype 1 mutation (R328W) in a malignant hyperthermia family by sequencing of a leukocyte transcript. Anesthesiology 99: 297–302.

Lyden PD, Krieger D, Yenari M et al. (2006). Therapeutic hypothermia for acute stroke. Int J Stroke 1: 9–19.

Manos GH (2000). Possible serotonin syndrome associated with buspirone added to fluoxetine. Ann Pharmacother 34: 871–874.

Margetic B, Aukst-Margetic B (2008). Serotonin syndrome caused by olanzapine and clomipramine. Minerva Anestesiol 74: 445, author reply 446–447.

Margolese HC, Chouinard G (2000). Serotonin syndrome from addition of low-dose trazodone to nefazodone. Am J Psychiatry 157: 1022.

Marion DW (2002). Cytokines and therapeutic hypothermia. Crit Care Med 30: 1666–1667.

McCarthy TV, Quane KA, Lynch PJ (2000). Ryanodine receptor mutations in malignant hyperthermia and central core disease. Hum Mutat 15: 410–417.

McCue RE, Joseph M (2001). Venlafaxine- and trazodone-induced serotonin syndrome. Am J Psychiatry 158: 2088–2089.

McIntyre LA, Fergusson DA, Hebert PC et al. (2003). Prolonged therapeutic hypothermia after traumatic brain injury in adults: a systematic review. JAMA 289: 2992–2999.

Miller DG, Lovell EO (2011). Antibiotic-induced serotonin syndrome. J Emerg Med 40: 25–27.

Mittino D, Mula M, Monaco F (2004). Serotonin syndrome associated with tramadol-sertraline coadministration. Clin Neuropharmacol 27: 150–151.

Moran JL, Solomon PJ (2004). Application of therapeutic hypothermia in the intensive care unit. Intensive Care Med 30: 2288, author reply 2287.

Munhoz RP (2004). Serotonin syndrome induced by a combination of bupropion and SSRIs. Clin Neuropharmacol 27: 219–222.

Nimmagadda SR, Ryan DH, Atkin SL (2000). Neuroleptic malignant syndrome after venlafaxine. Lancet 355: 289–290.

Nyfort-Hansen K, Alderman CP (2000). Possible neuroleptic malignant syndrome associated with olanzapine. Ann Pharmacother 34: 667.

Olsen TS, Weber UJ, Kammersgaard LP (2003). Therapeutic hypothermia for acute stroke. Lancet Neurol 2: 410–416.

Paruchuri P, Godkar D, Anandacoomarswamy D et al. (2006). Rare case of serotonin syndrome with therapeutic doses of paroxetine. Am J Ther 13: 550–552.

Perry NK (2000). Venlafaxine-induced serotonin syndrome with relapse following amitriptyline. Postgrad Med J 76: 254–256.

Quinn DK, Stern TA (2009). Linezolid and serotonin syndrome. Prim Care Companion J Clin Psychiatry 11: 353–356.

Ruffert H, Olthoff D, Deutrich C et al. (2000). In vitro contracture test and gene typing in diagnosing malignant hyperthermia Each as an appropriate complement to the other method. Anaesthesist 49: 113–120.

Sansone RA, Sansone LA (2009). Tramadol: seizures, serotonin syndrome, and coadministered antidepressants. Psychiatry (Edgmont) 6: 17–21.

Sechi G, Agnetti V, Masuri R et al. (2000). Risperidone neuroleptic malignant syndrome and probable dementia with Lewy bodies. Prog Neuropsychopharmacol Biol Psychiatry 24: 1043–1051.

Smith DL, Wenegrat BG (2000). A case report of serotonin syndrome associated with combined nefazodone and fluoxetine. J Clin Psychiatry 61: 146.

Snoeck MM, Gielen MJ, Tangerman A et al. (2000). Contractures in skeletal muscle of malignant hyperthermia susceptible patients after in vitro exposure to sevoflurane. Acta Anaesthesiol Scand 44: 334–337.

So PC (2001). Neuroleptic malignant syndrome induced by droperidol. Hong Kong Med J 7: 101–103.

Soteras Martinez I, Subirats Bayego E, Reisten O (2011). Accidental hypothermia. Med Clin (Barc) 137: 171–177.

Spirko BA, Wiley JF 2nd (1999). Serotonin syndrome: a new pediatric intoxication. Pediatr Emerg Care 15: 440–443.

Stanfield SC, Privette T (2000). Neuroleptic malignant syndrome associated with olanzapine therapy: a case report. J Emerg Med 19: 355–357.

Stanley AK, Hunter J (2000). Possible neuroleptic malignant syndrome with quetiapine. Br J Psychiatry 176: 497.

Steinberg M, Morin AK (2007). Mild serotonin syndrome associated with concurrent linezolid and fluoxetine. Am J Health Syst Pharm 64: 59–62.

Steinfath M, Seranski P, Singh S et al. (2002). Evidence for a spontaneous C1840-T mutation in the RYR1 gene after DNA fingerprinting in a malignant hyperthermia susceptible family. Naunyn Schmiedebergs Arch Pharmacol 366: 372–375.

Thomas CR, Rosenberg M, Blythe V et al. (2004). Serotonin syndrome and linezolid. J Am Acad Child Adolesc Psychiatry 43: 790.

Thorpe EL, Pizon AF, Lynch MJ et al. (2010). Bupropion induced serotonin syndrome: a case report. J Med Toxicol 6: 168–171.

Trakas K, Shear NH (2000). Serotonin syndrome risk with antiobesity drug. Can J Clin Pharmacol 7: 216.

Ubogu EE, Katirji B (2003). Mirtazapine-induced serotonin syndrome. Clin Neuropharmacol 26: 54–57.

Urwyler A, Halsall PJ, Mueller C et al. (2003). Ryanodine receptor gene (RYR1) mutations for diagnosing susceptibility to malignant hyperthermia. Acta Anaesthesiol Scand 47: 492, author reply 493.

Vandemergel X, Beukinga I, Neve P (2000). Serotonin syndrome secondary to the use of sertraline and metoclopramide. Rev Med Brux 21: 161–163.

Vizcaychipi MP, Walker S, Palazzo M (2007). Serotonin syndrome triggered by tramadol. Br J Anaesth 99: 919.

Voirol P, Hodel PF, Zullino D et al. (2000). Serotonin syndrome after small doses of citalopram or sertraline. J Clin Psychopharmacol 20: 713–714.

Whitelaw A, Thoresen M (2001). Clinical experience with therapeutic hypothermia in asphyxiated infants. Dev Med Child Neurol Suppl 86: 30–31.

Wigen CL, Goetz MB (2002). Serotonin syndrome and linezolid. Clin Infect Dis 34: 1651–1652.

Handbook of Clinical Neurology, Vol. 120 (3rd series)
Neurologic Aspects of Systemic Disease Part II
Jose Biller and Jose M. Ferro, Editors
© 2014 Elsevier B.V. All rights reserved

Chapter 63

Neurology and diving

E. WAYNE MASSEY[1]* AND RICHARD E. MOON[2]

[1]*Department of Neurology, Duke University Medical Center, Durham, NC, USA*

[2]*Departments of Anesthesiology and Medicine, Duke University Medical Center, Durham, NC, USA*

DECOMPRESSION SICKNESS

Decompression sickness (DCS) occurs when inert gas (usually nitrogen or helium) comes out of solution, forming bubbles following a reduction in ambient pressure (decompression). This commonly occurs after breathing compressed gas while diving. As the diver descends, and is exposed to elevated environmental pressure, increased amounts of inert gas dissolve in the tissues. This is in accordance with Henry's Law, which states that the amount of gas dissolved in a fluid is directly proportional to the partial pressure of that gas. The amount of inert gas dissolved depends on the depth and the duration of the dive. If, during ascent, tissue gas is not washed out of tissues by the circulation, the partial pressure of the inert gas taken up during the dive may exceed ambient pressure (supersaturation) and come out of solution, forming bubbles in tissues and in venous blood. Procedures have been developed to minimize the risk of bubble formation, which include limits on dive time and staged ascent, in which the diver makes "decompression stops" in the water at prescribed depths in order to allow extra time for re-equilibration of tissue tensions. Inert gas supersaturation and DCS can also occur during rapid ascent to altitude.

The extent of bubble formation depends on the depth, the duration of the dive, and the rate of the ascent. DCS can occur due to a procedural error on the part of the diver, where maximum bottom time or ascent rate is exceeded, or appropriate decompression stops are not made ("deserved"). It can also occur even when appropriate dive time and decompression procedures are followed ("undeserved"). DCS after diving is not generally experienced unless the dive depth exceeds 20–25 feet (Van Liew and Flynn, 2005). *De novo* altitude DCS only occurs during rapid (over several minutes or an hour or two) decompression to an ambient pressure of 0.5 atmospheres or lower (380 mmHg, 18 000 feet). It can be precipitated at more modest altitudes (8000 feet or less) if there has been a preceding dive (Freiberger et al., 2002).

Once bubbles develop, they induce a cascade of events within the circulation tissues and in tissues probably including secondary effects described in other types of CNS injury such as oxidative stress, excitatory amino acid release and inflammation. Vascular injury results in extravasation of plasma into the interstitium, hypovolemia and hemoconcentration (Malette et al., 1962; Brunner et al., 1964; Boussuges et al., 1996a). Animal experiments have revealed neutrophil margination (Martin and Thom, 2002; Nossum et al., 2002) and loss of vasoreactivity due to endothelial damage (Nossum et al., 2002).

ARTERIAL GAS EMBOLISM

Arterial gas embolism (AGE) occurs when a diver breathing compressed gas at depth ascends without exhaling air from the lungs. During a breath-holding ascent, due to the reduction in ambient pressure lung volume will progressively increase (Boyle's Law), and may eventually exceed the alveolar/capillary elastic limit, causing tissue disruption. When alveoli rupture, air escapes or dissects into the surrounding spaces. Regional overinflation can also occur due to lung conditions such as obstructive disease (e.g., asthma) (Weiss and Van Meter, 1995), where local gas trapping can occur. In order for DCS to occur there must be a significant depth-time exposure, while AGE can occur after a brief compressed gas dive to a depth as shallow as 1 meter (Benton et al., 1996). AGE has also been described during commercial aircraft flight in a person due to expansion and rupture of a bulla (Closon et al., 2004).

Air entering the pleural cavity results in pneumothorax, air escaping into the mediastinum causes

*Correspondence to: E. Wayne Massey, M.D., FAAN, FACP, Professor of Medicine (Neurology), Box 3909, Duke University Medical Center, Durham, NC 27710, USA. Tel: +1-919 684-5816, Fax: +1-919- 681-7936, E-mail: masse010@mc.duke.edu

subcutaneous or mediastinal emphysema, and air dissecting into the pericardium causes pneumopericardium. More dangerous yet, air may enter the pulmonary capillaries, and hence the arterial circulation. Emboli that enter the cerebral vessels cause stroke-like events that typically occur within minutes of surfacing.

Pulmonary overpressure accidents often occur in inexperienced divers, who may simply forget to exhale during ascent. More commonly, this may occur during an emergency ascent, perhaps from an out of air situation or equipment failure.

AGE can also occur when otherwise asymptomatic venous bubbles, which can be detected by ultrasound in a large fraction of divers (Dunford et al., 2002), cross into the systemic circulation via either a patent foramen ovale (PFO) or by overwhelming the pulmonary capillary filter. The presence of a PFO is a risk factor for serious neurologic DCS (Lairez et al., 2009).

EPIDEMIOLOGY

The probability of DCI during a dive depends on a number of factors, including the depth-time exposure, breathing gas, exertion level of the diver, and environmental conditions (e.g., water temperature). Exertion and warm conditions while the diver is in the bottom both increase the uptake of inert gas, while warm conditions and mild exertion during decompression facilitate inert gas washout, and reduce DCS (Gerth et al., 2007). If appropriate decompression procedures are observed, DCS is uncommon, typically 0.015% for scientific divers, 0.01–0.019% for recreational divers, 0.030% for US Navy divers, and 0.095% for commercial divers (Ladd et al., 2002; Vann, 2004). The Divers Alert Network (DAN) collected a sample of 135000 dives by 9000 recreational divers in which the DCS incidence was 0.03%, with a higher prevalence during cold water wreck dives than during warm water

live-aboard dives (Pollock, 2008). Of 441 confirmed or possible DCI incidents in recreational divers reported to the Divers Alert Network (DAN), 3.9% were classified as possible AGE (Pollock, 2008).

The annual number of injury (non-fatal AGE, DCS) in North America is approximately 1000. The mean age of divers in the DAN injury population was 39 years (Pollock, 2008). Interestingly, divers with advanced certification had the highest percentage of injuries, possibly due to greater exposure among more qualified divers.

The annual number of diving fatalities in the US typically ranges from 80 to 120 (Fig. 63.1). The general diving population seems to be aging with a larger percentage of divers more than a decade out since certification. The aging of the diving population may account for an increase in the mean age of diving fatalities from 33 to 39 years in recent years (Pollock, 2008).

Medical history was available in 40% of the fatality cases and the most frequently reported medical conditions were heart disease and hypertension. Most of the fatalities in the DAN report had open water or advanced certification, and 25% had been certified 10 years or greater versus 45% who had 1 year or less (Pollock, 2008). The most common causes of death in the judgment of the pathologist reviewing each case were, in descending order, drowning, an acute heart condition, and arterial gas embolism. The cause of death was not determined in 10% of the cases, either because the body was not found or because the cause was not specified by the local medical examiner.

CLINICAL MANIFESTATIONS AND DIAGNOSIS

Manifestations of DCS can vary in severity, from mild (typically paresthesias, joint pains, fatigue) to manifestations involving the inner ear (vertigo, hearing loss) and

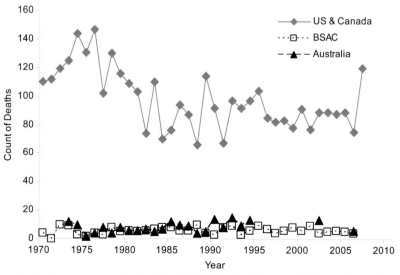

Fig. 63.1. Annual record of North American diving fatalities. BSAC, British Sub Aqua Club data. (Reproduced from Pollock, 2008.)

spinal cord (paraplegia, quadriplegia). Frequency of DCS manifestations in recreational divers is shown in Fig. 63.2. The most common neurologic manifestation is paresthesia, often without objective hypesthesia. When hypesthesia is present it is often nondermatomal. Occasionally hypesthesia is present in a peripheral nerve distribution (Butler and Pinto, 1986). More serious manifestations include weakness or paralysis, disturbance of vision, bowel and bladder dysfunction, and vertigo. Most often, the target organ is the thoracic spinal cord, probably due to the vascular anatomy of the spinal cord. The paravertebral veins allow for nitrogen bubbles to collect due to a stagnant flow resulting in venous infarction in the spinal cord. Cerebral involvement occurs in 30% of cases of

type II decompression sickness (Francis et al., 1988). Divers with cerebral involvement may complain of confusion, lethargy, "mental cloudiness," difficulty with concentration, and visual disturbances. Serious neurologic manifestations usually occur shortly after surfacing, while milder symptoms may be delayed for several hours (Fig. 63.3). A retrospective review of 1070 cases of neurologic DCS reported that 90% of cerebral manifestations occurred within 30 minutes after surfacing, while 90% of spinal cord manifestations occurred within 4 hours (Francis et al., 1988). In a US Navy database that contains data on several thousand air dives, 98% of all DCS cases (neurologic and non-neurologic) became symptomatic within 24 hours (Navy Department, 2008).

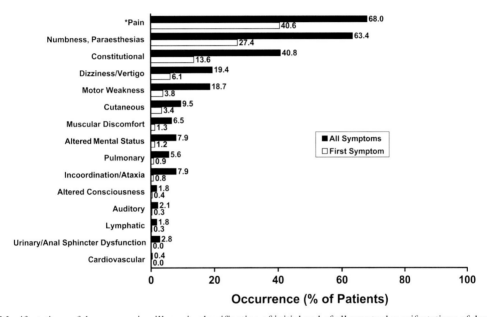

Fig. 63.2. Manifestations of decompression illness in classification of initial and of all eventual manifestations of decompression illness in 2346 recreational diving accidents reported to the Divers Alert Network from 1998 to 2004. *For all instances of pain, 58% consisted of joint pain, 35% muscle pain, and 7% girdle pain. Girdle pain often portends spinal cord involvement. [†]Constitutional symptoms included headache, lightheadedness, inappropriate fatigue, malaise, nausea/vomiting, and anorexia. [‡]Muscular discomfort included stiffness, "pressure," cramps, and spasm, but excluded pain. [§]Pulmonary manifestations included dyspnea and cough. (Reproduced from Vann et al., 2011.)

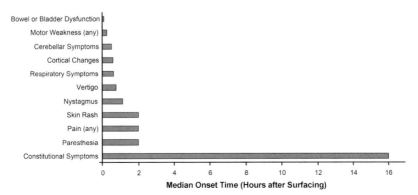

Fig. 63.3. Median symptom onset time in hours in 363 cases of decompression illness. (Reproduced from Pollock NW (2007). Annual Diving Report. 2007 edn. Divers Alert Network, Durham, NC).

Individuals experiencing AGE or pulmonary overinflation can experience pain and respiratory distress, coughing, hemoptysis, headache, but also cortical symptoms of unconsciousness, seizures, hemiparesis, quadriparesis, and cortical blindness. When AGE occurs following ascent from a dive in which there has been a significant depth-time exposure, where inert gases in some tissues may be close to supersaturation, the clinical manifestations often resemble those seen with DCS, such as spinal cord involvement (Neuman and Bove, 1990).

The diagnosis of both DCS and AGE is based almost exclusively on the clinical examination, including the neurologic examination, and the dive history. Laboratory and imaging studies rarely add to the diagnosis. Freiberger and colleagues, using simulated diving injury cases, identified important diagnostic factors for DCS: (1) a neurologic symptom as the primary presenting symptom; (2) onset time to symptoms; (3) joint pain as a presenting symptom; (4) any relief after recompression treatment; (5) maximum depth of the last dive (Freiberger et al., 2004). Age, gender, or physical characteristics were not statistically important. The top five diagnostic factors for AGE in this study were: (1) the onset time of symptoms; (2) altered consciousness; (3) any neurologic symptoms as a presenting symptom; (4) motor weakness; (5) seizure as the primary presenting symptom.

Often, when a diver develops neurologic manifestations shortly after surfacing from a dive it is impossible to differentiate between DCS and AGE. The two often occur together in the same patient. Furthermore, the differentiation is rarely of clinical importance as the treatment for both conditions is essentially the same. Therefore the term *decompression illness* (DCI) is often used to indicate either DCS or AGE, or both (Francis, 1990).

The original and most widely used classification of DCS divides manifestations into type I (originally defined as symptoms without signs) and type II (physical signs present, usually neurologic) (Golding et al., 1960). The definitions have changed slightly since then. Type I DCS is now defined in the US Navy Diving Manual as including joint pain (musculoskeletal or pain-only symptoms) and symptoms involving the skin (cutaneous symptoms), or swelling and pain in lymph nodes. Type II DCS includes neurologic, inner ear ("staggers"), and cardiopulmonary ("chokes") (Navy Department, 2008). Several more detailed DCI severity scores have since been proposed for use as prognosticators (Dick and Massey, 1985; Bond et al., 1990; Boussuges et al., 1996b; Kelleher et al., 1996; Mitchell et al., 1998; Holley, 2000; Gempp and Blatteau, 2010). Also included is the National Institute of Health Stroke Scale (NIHSS); when applied to cerebral neurologic diving injuries, this

is a tool for severity stratification and has adequate predictive ability while providing a more standardized scale (Holck and Hunter, 2006).

PREVENTION

Divers can reduce the risk of decompression sickness by adhering to decompression procedures ("dive tables"). Diving tables were designed by the US Navy and other agencies based on theoretical and empirical data. The tables were created from the theoretical picture of the body consisting of different tissues that accept and relieve gas at different rates, and the decompression tables are designed to allow the diver to surface at a rate compatible with the slowest tissue for the depth and duration of the dive. Computers worn on the diver's wrist, which provide real time simulation of body uptake and washout of inert gas using continuous input from a pressure gauge, have now largely replaced tables. Neither decompression tables nor decompression computer algorithms have eliminated decompression illness. Temperature, breathing gas, sea conditions, and rate of ascent can all affect inert gas uptake and washout, and hence the probability of decompression illness.

Some medical illnesses increase the risk of decompression illness, such as asthma, where bronchospasm can lead to air trapping and pulmonary barotrauma during ascent (Weiss and Van Meter, 1995). Diving candidates with pulmonary dysfunction should be evaluated by a physician. Several neurologic diseases could affect the diver and may increase the risk of diving. Seizures are the most obvious, and when a seizure occurs underwater the outcome is likely to be fatal. Assessing the risk of seizure predive is the same as with any environmental situation with these individuals: driving, work situations, sport activities, and other activities where sudden loss of consciousness could cause injury or death. The risk of subsequent seizures is increased above that of the general population after a single seizure as an adult (Hauser et al., 1990). Requirements for driving, for example, vary between states but are only guidelines (Beghi and Sander, 2005), although there are no federal or state guidelines that apply to diving. The implication of a seizure occurring while driving is serious for the individual and others; likewise, it is serious while diving, primarily for the individual, but also for dive partners. Although the dive itself, under pressure, is not known to increase risk, when the seizure occurs the outcome can be fatal. Thus, a seizure disorder is considered to be a contraindication to diving.

Other neurologic diseases adding risk to divers include complicated migraine, spasticity from multiple sclerosis (MS) or other spinal disease, muscle weakness (i.e., muscular dystrophies) or any problems altering strength or perception. For example, previous brachial plexopathy in a young person could alter function/risks in certain situations of temperature, pressure, or currents.

It is generally accepted that inert gas bubbles in the tissue and venous system cause decompression sickness and the greater the bubble load, the higher risk of developing decompression sickness. Factors that augment inert gas uptake during a dive, including exercise during the dive and warm environment, can increase bubble formation after decompression. Similarly, bubble formation is more likely if there is impaired inert gas washout, such as cold conditions during decompression or dehydration. Most experts recommend avoidance of strenuous exercise after diving as this can increase bubble formation. The use of alcohol could increase the risk of dysbaric illness in divers as it may induce dehydration and adversely affect judgment, making adherence to decompression procedures more difficult.

DIAGNOSIS

No serum assay, imaging or electrophysiologic test has yet been identified that provides an acceptable sensitivity or specificity for the diagnosis of decompression illness. Thus, DCI diagnosis is entirely based on clinical evaluation. This includes the depth-time profile(s), the onset and symptoms and signs (see Fig. 63.2). The lone exception to date is audiometry and vestibular testing, the sensitivity of which for inner ear DCS (IEDCS) exceeds clinical assessment. While these techniques are not required before initiating treatment of IEDCS based on clinical examination, they are especially useful in the recovery phase of vestibular involvement, where clinical manifestations routinely resolve even when pathology remains. Brain imaging studies can detect abnormalities in neurologic DCS, although magnetic resonance imaging (MRI) studies of either the brain or spinal cord are often normal even in the presence of clinical abnormalities (Warren et al., 1988; Benson et al., 2003; Gronning et al., 2005; Yoshiyama et al., 2007; Gempp et al., 2008). Similarly, positron emission tomography (PET) is less sensitive than clinical evaluation in finding abnormalities (Lowe et al., 1994). Attempting to visualize air in cases of AGE with brain imaging is particularly wasteful, as air is seen in only a minority of cases (Benson et al., 2003), and imaging delays treatment. The only role for imaging studies in the acute management of DCI is to exclude other pathologies such as hemorrhage when there is uncertainty about the diagnosis of DCI or, in the event of a rapid or suspected breath-hold ascent, to detect pneumothorax, for which a chest tube may be required before hyperbaric treatment.

Neuropsychological testing has been studied in commercial and recreational divers with conflicting results, but generally adds little to the clinical examination. Computed tomography (CT) scanning has not been found to be sensitive in detecting structural abnormalities associated with cerebral decompression sickness or arterial gas embolism. Although lesions are sometimes detected by MRI (Gronning et al., 2005), this imaging modality is relatively insensitive to spinal cord lesions caused by decompression sickness and is not recommended for routine use in DCS evaluation. Similarly, MRI often fails to identify cerebral lesions (Gronning et al., 2005). Cerebral perfusion studies (single-photon emission computed tomography (SPECT) and PET) have not been found to be helpful in the diagnosis of dysbaric illness (Lowe et al., 1994).

In the setting of dysbaric illness, electroencephalography (EEG) demonstrates nonspecific abnormalities in some divers, typically 30–50% (Gorman et al., 1987; Gronning et al., 2005). The value of electronystagmography is in cases of vestibular DCS. Evoked potential studies have limited value.

Some coincidental neurologic events could be confused with decompression illness, such as multiple sclerosis, complicated migraine, fish poisoning such as ciguatera, and other conditions (Table 63.1). Carotid or vertebral artery dissection has been reported in multiple cases during or around a dive (Nelson, 1995; Konno et al., 2001; Gibbs et al., 2002; Skurnik and Sthoeger, 2005; Bartsch et al., 2009; Kocyigit et al., 2010), perhaps from pressure related to the diving apparatus or extension of the neck during swimming in the horizontal direction. Peripheral nerve symptoms from median neuropathy or lateral femoral nerve entrapment may lead to misdiagnosis as DCS.

TREATMENT

Scuba divers breathing from a compressed air source are subject to trauma, hypothermia, asphyxiation, and water aspiration, but may also have decompression sickness or arterial gas embolism. The neurologic outcome of dysbaric illness is greatly influenced by effective management. Typically, the diagnosis must be suspected and made in the field by a companion or dive supervisor.

Prompt recognition within the diving party is essential to begin on-site treatment. Development of pulmonary or cerebral symptoms on reaching the surface or immediately after leaving the water suggests pulmonary overpressure injury. If cerebral symptoms such as convulsion, cortical blindness, hemiplegia, or aphasia are present, air embolism is likely. Symptoms delayed minutes to hours after surfacing and localizing to the spinal cord implicate decompression sickness. Recompression treatment is recommended in either case.

First aid

Once the presumptive diagnosis of dysbaric illness is established, the most important on-site treatment is

Table 63.1

Differential diagnosis of decompression illness

Condition	Description
Ciguatera poisoning (Bagnis et al., 1979; Eastaugh and Shepherd, 1989; Swift and Swift, 1993)	Due to ingestion of heat-stable toxin in large fish, such as barracuda, grouper, red snapper, amber jack, king fish. Vomiting and diarrhea usually precede paresthesias, altered thermal sensation, occasionally weakness, vertigo, ataxia
Puffer fish poisoning (Eastaugh and Shepherd, 1989; Mines et al., 1997)	Due to tetrodotoxin. Mild poisoning is similar to ciguatera poisoning; severe poisoning can cause paralysis and death
Paralytic shellfish poisoning (Eastaugh and Shepherd, 1989; Mines et al., 1997)	Due to saxitoxin or brevetoxin. Paresthesias, and burning around the lips, tongue and face occur within 30 minutes of ingestion. Ataxia, aphonia and death due to respiratory muscle paralysis have been reported
Guillain-Barré syndrome (AIDP)	Sensory symptoms usually minor or absent, and progression usually slower than in decompression illness
Porphyria	History of the disease usually present
Multiple sclerosis (MS)	Vertigo, visual loss, focal sensory, motor or cerebellar symptoms due to MS may mimic decompression illness when temporally related to a dive. Heat stress in tropical conditions may exacerbate symptoms in demyelinating diseases. MRI, CSF evaluation may help
Spinal cord compression/myelopathy	Hemorrhage, disc protrusion or epidural infection. Diagnosis usually confirmed by MRI, which is commonly negative in decompression illness. Spinal fluid analysis may help
Inner ear barotrauma (Farmer, 1977; Money et al., 1985; Shupak et al., 1991; Klingmann et al., 2007)	Inadequate equalization of middle ear pressure during descent can cause rupture of the round or oval windows, resulting in sudden onset of tinnitus, vertigo and unilateral deafness
Facial baroparesis (FB) (Molvaer and Eidsvik, 1987; Basnyat, 2001; Grossman et al., 2004) or other facial palsies	FB is due to facial nerve compression as a result of inadequate decompression of the middle ear cavity during decompression from a dive or aircraft flight. Differentiated from gas embolism as it presents with both upper and lower facial weakness. Manifestations of FB are usually transient, relieved by equalization of middle ear pressure
Paranasal sinus overpressurization (Garges, 1985; Idicula, 1972; Murrison et al., 1991; Neuman et al., 1975; Shepherd et al., 1983)	Compression of trigeminal nerve within the maxillary sinus due to over-pressurization in the same manner as in facial baroparesis (above)
Seizures	Spontaneous seizures immediately after a dive may be difficult to differentiate from arterial gas embolism
Thromboembolic or hemorrhagic stroke	Age and risk factors help differentiate. MRI will reveal hemorrhage or ischemia. If doubt exists, recompression therapy will not worsen outcome after stroke
Migraine (Engel et al., 1944; Ferris et al., 1951; Flinn and Womack, 1963; Lieppman, 1981; Ostachowicz, 1987; Butler, 1991)	Visual manifestations, including scintillating scotomata, have been described in altitude-related DCS. Migraine history may help differentiate from decompression illness. No adverse effect of recompression therapy in migraine
Carotid or vertebral artery dissection (Nelson, 1995; Kocyigit et al., 2010; Bartsch et al., 2009; Skurnik and Sthoeger, 2005; Gibbs et al., 2002; Konno et al., 2001)	Neck pain is usual

MRI, magnetic resonance imaging; CNS, central nervous system; DCS, decompression sickness.

administration of 100% oxygen. Most sport dive boats do carry oxygen and ideally this includes a close-fitting mask and reservoir that will provide a high fraction of inspired oxygen and a large oxygen supply to allow for treatment until the patient is delivered to a recompression chamber.

The purpose of oxygen is to facilitate oxygenation of tissues rendered hypoxic due to bubble-related ischemia and to increase the rate of nitrogen removal. The basis of oxygen treatment for dysbaric illness was termed "the oxygen window" by Behnke (Behnke, 1967; Van Liew et al., 1993), and describes the changing pressure of nitrogen in the alveoli. The administration of 100% oxygen creates a nitrogen gradient that tends to eliminate nitrogen bubbles from tissue. When the patient breathes pure oxygen, the nitrogen partial pressure in alveoli (and eventually blood and tissue) becomes 0 mmHg and the gradient for diffusion of inert gas (usually nitrogen) from bubble into tissue is then increased to 713 mmHg, accelerating bubble resolution. This is an important component of treatment of both DCS and AGE.

In the field, the next crucial step is timely transportation to a recompression chamber. If air evacuation is required, to avoid bubble expansion it is best done with aircraft that can be flown at low altitude or with sea level cabin altitude. If this is not possible, supplemental oxygen is recommended during flight.

Recompression

The definitive treatment for DCI is recompression with oxygen (usually to an ambient pressure of 2.8 atmospheres absolute (ATA)), preferably as soon as possible after symptom onset. This achieves a nitrogen diffusion gradient that may exceed 2000 mmHg. In addition to the efflux of inert gas from the bubble by diffusion, bubble volume is also reduced due to the increase in ambient pressure (Boyle's Law). Hyperbaric oxygen may also have other ameliorative effects on ischemia, tissue edema, and other factors that may be important in DCI pathophysiology such as leukocyte adhesion and inflammation (Vann et al., 2011).

The pressure generally used for treatment of neurologic DCI is 2.8 ATA, although pressures up to 6.0 ATA are sometimes used. The most commonly used treatment schedules were established by the US Navy in the late 1960s; in these the diver is compressed initially to 2.8 ATA, where 100% oxygen is breathed for 25 minute periods interspersed with 5 minute air breaks. Air breaks reduce oxygen toxicity, which can affect the lung (tracheobronchitis, edema) and CNS (seizures). After up to 125 minutes, there is a 30 minute decompression to 1.9 ATA, where additional oxygen/air cycles are administered. The length of each treatment ranges between 5 and 8 hours, depending on the clinical response of the patient. Additional details of recompression treatment can be found in the US Navy Diving Manual (http://www.supsalv.org/pdf/DiveMan_rev6.pdf (accessed 9/19/2010)). Shorted oxygen schedules that are more suitable for monoplace chambers have also been found to be effective in the treatment of decompression sickness (Cianci and Slade, 2006). In a randomized trial, use of helium-oxygen (heliox 50–50) instead of 100% oxygen was found to reduce the requirement for multiple compressions: nine of 25 divers receiving heliox versus 20 of receiving 100% oxygen (Drewry and Gorman, 1994; Bennett et al., 2007). However, details of the trial have not been fully published, and heliox is not routinely used.

Adjunctive therapy

In addition to recompression, some agents may be helpful as adjuncts. Use of tenoxicam (a nonselective COX inhibitor) has been studied in a randomized controlled trial. Although it did not change the clinical outcome, its use was associated with a reduced number of recompressions required to achieve a clinical endpoint (Bennett et al., 2003). Because endothelial leak can result in hypovolemia and hemoconcentration due to extravasated plasma, vigorous fluid resuscitation may be required to normalize organ perfusion. Intravenous lidocaine bolus and infusion to achieve standard antiarrhythmic serum levels has improved short-term outcome in animal models of AGE. No human trials in AGE have been published. Avoidance of hyperthermia and hyperglycemia are recommended as for other CNS insults. For divers with paraplegia or paraparesis, low molecular weight heparin is recommended for thromboembolism prophylaxis.

Perfluorocarbon emulsions (PFCs) are promising adjunctive agents, which have a high solubility for both oxygen and inert gases. In animal models these agents reduce the probability and severity of DCS (Dromsky et al., 2004; Mahon et al., 2006; Dainer et al., 2007; Spiess, 2009). Human trials await the availability of a PFC approved for human use. Further details of adjunctive therapies can be found in a consensus workshop report (Moon, 2003) and a review article (Vann et al., 2011).

LONG-TERM NEUROLOGIC CONSEQUENCES

Fortunately, most divers achieve a complete recovery from dysbaric illness. In contrast, when there are excessively long delays to treatment or negligent diving profiles, outcomes may not be as good. The latter is supported by the 2008 Divers Alert Network Report, where only 70% of the divers obtained complete relief at discharge and 29.7% had residual symptoms (Pollock, 2008). In a series of divers unable to walk due to spinal cord DCS, at long-term follow-up one-half had no residual symptoms, and only one-third had manifestations that impaired daily activities (Vann et al., 2011). The most common residual symptoms are peripheral paresthesias. In a small proportion of divers who have experienced significant spinal cord DCS residual symptoms may be obvious and debilitating, and include spasticity, urinary incontinence, impotence, or weakness.

Similarly, divers who survive arterial gas embolism typically make a full recovery. Of 307 patients with diving-related or iatrogenic AGE reported in two case series (van Hulst et al., 2003; Trytko and Bennett, 2008), 60% experienced full recovery. The fact that most divers are young and have healthy circulatory and neurologic systems is likely responsible for their favorable prognosis. Formal neuropsychological testing can reveal abnormalities that are not obvious on clinical examination (Curley et al., 1988); however, most divers who do not fully return to normal after arterial gas embolism experience minor symptoms that do not affect quality of life (Trytko and Bennett, 2008).

The question of cumulative neurologic damage from asymptomatic diving is unclear. A Norwegian 1990 multivariate analysis demonstrated that professional divers had more neurologic symptoms and neurologic findings than nondivers (Todnem et al., 1990). These divers most commonly complained of difficulties with concentration, and short- and long-term memory. The most prominent abnormal finding was distal spinal cord and nerve root dysfunction. The incidence of symptoms and abnormal findings was higher in divers having had recognized decompression sickness. Other studies have not supported the notion of subclinical long-term effects (Elliott and Moon, 1993).

APPENDIX: CASE EXAMPLES

Decompression sickness (1)

A 32-year-old sport diver with several years experience was in the fifth day of a diving vacation trip to the South Pacific. On each of the previous days, he had made two or three dives, and at least one dive each day had exceeded 100 feet. He was using a decompression computer and was quite sure that he had stayed within the parameters required by the computer throughout his trip. On the fifth day, he made dives to 150 feet, 90 feet, and 90 feet, each separated by surface intervals that met the requirements of his computer. About 5 minutes after surfacing from his third dive, he had an aching pressure-like pain around his flanks and into his groin. The right side was somewhat worse than the left, but as the pain became more intense, both sides were equally affected. He was sitting on the bench at the time of the onset. A few minutes later, he got to his feet and was unable to walk without assistance. His companions and the boat captain helped him to the bench, where he lay down and was treated with oxygen. Symptoms did not improve. Arrangements were made to evacuate him to a recompression chamber on an island several hundred miles distant. The flight was delayed by darkness, and when he arrived at the chamber the next day, about 10 hours after symptom onset, he had moderate weakness in both thighs and virtually no strength in his left foot and lower leg. The right foot was less affected. He had altered sensation and patchy loss of sensation from the umbilicus downward, although he could feel pressure in his feet. He was unable to void without pressing on his abdomen. On urinary catheterization, he had 1500 mL residual urine. Reflexes were hyperactive.

He was treated according to US Navy Table 6 (Navy Department, 2008). He made some improvement during the first 2 hours and treatment was extended to a full 10 hours. At the conclusion of treatment, his quadriceps and thigh strength had largely returned, his left foot was still nearly flaccid, but his right was only slightly weak. Sensation was improved, and pain resolved. The indwelling catheter was removed on the second day, and he was able to void with a Credé maneuver.

For each of the following 3 days he was retreated with Table 5 (Navy Department, 2008), but made no further improvement after the first treatment.

A week after completion of treatment, he returned to the US by commercial aircraft. There was no change in his symptoms. In the ensuing year, he reported slow improvement in his mobility and in bladder control. One year after the event, he had persistent spastic paraparesis. He was able to ambulate without a cane or crutches, but with moderate discernable weakness and bilateral hyperreflexia. Sensation about the perineum was decreased and in the feet nearly normal.

This case typifies serious decompression sickness with delayed treatment and with partial response. This patient had severe DCS manifestations despite diving within accepted guidelines.

Decompression sickness (2)

A 46-year-old woman, an experienced diver, surfaced after an uneventful dive to 110 feet for 27 minutes, conservatively decompressing for 13 minutes at 10 feet (only 7 minutes normally required). On climbing into the boat, about 10 minutes after the dive, her right foot felt hot, then tingly (as if it were going to sleep); the limb became progressively numb from foot to thigh over 20 minutes while the left leg also became warm and tingly, and she had low back pain. Reaching the shore after 30 minutes, she could not walk. She recovered sensation and strength while breathing pure oxygen for 60 minutes. For several days, her left leg felt unusual, and there was some loss of feeling in the left foot, but she felt normal after 1 week. This represents a case of decompression sickness with resolution after breathing first aid oxygen. Had she sought medical evaluation in the acute phase recompression treatment would have been recommended.

Arterial gas embolism

A 28-year-old man made a certification dive in a fresh water lake as part of a primary scuba course. The students were carrying out an emergency drill, in which they made a free ascent from 30 feet simulating an out of air situation. They were instructed to take a full breath and then swim to the surface while exhaling constantly.

The man reached the surface, had a generalized convulsion, and lost consciousness. He was towed to shore by his companions and carried to the truck. Oxygen was not available and the patient was transported about 60 miles in the back of a pick-up truck to an emergency medical facility. During this transit, he was conscious, but stuporous and uncommunicative. The emergency department physician found that he had a right hemiparesis and was aphasic and recommended the likelihood of arterial gas embolism. The patient was treated with oxygen and transported by helicopter to a recompression chamber 200 miles away. Dysphagia and paresis persisted. He was treated in a monoplace oxygen chamber for 90 minutes, at a depth equivalent to 50 feet of sea water. Directly after removal from the chamber, he had a generalized and largely right-sided seizure. Oxygen treatment was continued without further recompression. Over the next several hours, the paresis improved and he began to utter simple words. Oxygen was continued. The next morning, he had a minimal persisting paresis and a moderate dysphagia. He was discharged after 3 days, substantially improved, with minimum persisting findings. Two months after the event, his hemiparesis was no longer apparent, his speech had improved to normal, and he was functioning at near his normal level.

This case typifies cerebral arterial gas embolism, illustrating a good prognosis in patients who survive the initial insult.

REFERENCES

Bagnis R, Kuberski T, Laugier S (1979). Clinical observations on 3,009 cases of ciguatera (fish poisoning) in the South Pacific. Am J Trop Med Hyg 28: 1067–1073.

Bartsch T, Palaschewski M, Thilo B et al. (2009). Internal carotid artery dissection and stroke after SCUBA diving: a case report and review of the literature. J Neurol 256: 1916–1919.

Basnyat B (2001). Isolated facial and hypoglossal nerve palsies at high altitude. High Alt Med Biol 2: 301–303.

Beghi E, Sander JW (2005). Epilepsy and driving. BMJ 331: 60–61.

Behnke AR (1967). The isobaric (oxygen window) principle of decompression. The New Thrust Seaward. Transactions of the Third Marine Technology Society Conference, Marine Technology Society, San Diego.

Bennett M, Mitchell S, Dominguez A (2003). Adjunctive treatment of decompression illness with a non-steroidal anti-inflammatory drug (tenoxicam) reduces compression requirement. Undersea Hyperb Med 30: 195–205.

Bennett MH, Lehm JP, Mitchell SJ et al. (2007). Recompression and adjunctive therapy for decompression illness. Cochrane Database Syst Rev: CD005277.

Benson J, Adkinson C, Collier R (2003). Hyperbaric oxygen therapy of iatrogenic cerebral arterial gas embolism. Undersea Hyperb Med 30: 117–126.

Benton PJ, Woodfine JD, Westwook PR (1996). Arterial gas embolism following a 1-meter ascent during helicopter escape training: a case report. Aviat Space Environ Med 67: 63–64.

Bond JG, Moon RE, Morris DL (1990). Initial table treatment of decompression sickness and arterial gas embolism. Aviat Space Environ Med 61: 738–743.

Boussuges A, Blanc P, Molenat F et al. (1996a). Haemoconcentration in neurological decompression illness. Int J Sports Med 17: 351–355.

Boussuges A, Thirion X, Blanc P et al. (1996b). Neurologic decompression illness: a gravity score. Undersea Hyperb Med 23: 151–155.

Brunner F, Frick P, Bühlmann A (1964). Post-decompression shock due to extravasation of plasma. Lancet 1: 1071–1073.

Butler FK (1991). Decompression sickness presenting as optic neuropathy. Aviat Space Environ Med 62: 346–350.

Butler FK Jr, Pinto CV (1986). Progressive ulnar palsy as a late complication of decompression sickness. Ann Emerg Med 15: 738–741.

Cianci P, Slade JB Jr (2006). Delayed treatment of decompression sickness with short, no-air-break tables: review of 140 cases. Aviat Space Environ Med 77: 1003–1008.

Closon M, Vivier E, Breynaert C et al. (2004). Air embolism during an aircraft flight in a passenger with a pulmonary cyst: a favorable outcome with hyperbaric therapy. Anesthesiology 101: 539–542.

Curley MD, Schwartz HJ, Zwingelberg KM (1988). Neuropsychologic assessment of cerebral decompression sickness and gas embolism. Undersea Biomed Res 15: 223–236.

Dainer H, Nelson J, Brass K et al. (2007). Short oxygen prebreathing and intravenous perfluorocarbon emulsion reduces morbidity and mortality in a swine saturation model of decompression sickness. J Appl Physiol 102: 1099–1104.

Dick AP, Massey EW (1985). Neurologic presentation of decompression sickness and air embolism in sport divers. Neurology 35: 667–671.

Drewry A, Gorman DF (1994). A progress report on the prospective, randomised, double-blind controlled study of oxygen and oxygen-helium in the treatment of air-diving decompression illness (DCI). Undersea Hyperb Med 21 (Suppl): 98.

Dromsky DM, Spiess BD, Fahlman A (2004). Treatment of decompression sickness in swine with intravenous perfluorocarbon emulsion. Aviat Space Environ Med 75: 301–305.

Dunford RG, Vann RD, Gerth WA et al. (2002). The incidence of venous gas emboli in recreational diving. Undersea Hyperb Med 29: 247–259.

Eastaugh J, Shepherd S (1989). Infectious and toxic syndromes from fish and shellfish consumption A review. Arch Intern Med 149: 1735–1740.

Elliott DH, Moon RE (1993). Long term health effects of diving. In: PB Bennett, DH Elliott (Eds.), The Physiology and Medicine of Diving. WB Saunders, Philadelphia, pp. 585–604.

Engel GL, Webb JP, Ferris EB Jr et al. (1944). A migraine-like syndrome complicating decompression sickness. War Med 5: 304–314.

Farmer JC Jr (1977). Diving injuries to the inner ear. Ann Otol Rhinol Laryngol Suppl 86: 1–20.

Ferris EB, Engel GL, Romano J (1951). The clinical nature of high altitude decompression sickness. In: JF Fulton (Ed.), Decompression Sickness. WB Saunders, Philadelphia, pp. 4–52.

Flinn DE, Womack GJ (1963). Neurological manifestations of dysbarism: a review and report of a case with multiple episodes. Aerosp Med 34: 956–962.

Francis T (1990). Describing decompression illness. Paper read at Describing Decompression Illness: Forty-second Undersea and Hyperbaric Medical Society Workshop, at Institute of Naval Medicine Alverstoke, Gosport, Hampshire, UK.

Francis TJ, Pearson RR, Robertson AG et al. (1988). Central nervous system decompression sickness: latency of 1070 human cases. Undersea Biomed Res 15: 403–417.

Freiberger JJ, Denoble PJ, Pieper CF et al. (2002). The relative risk of decompression sickness during and after air travel following diving. Aviat Space Environ Med 73: 980–984.

Freiberger JJ, Lyman SJ, Denoble PJ et al. (2004). Consensus factors used by experts in the diagnosis of decompression illness. Aviat Space Environ Med 75: 1023–1028.

Garges LM (1985). Maxillary sinus barotrauma-case report and review. Aviat Space Environ Med 56: 796–802.

Gempp E, Blatteau JE (2010). Risk factors and treatment outcome in scuba divers with spinal cord decompression sickness. J Crit Care 25: 236–242.

Gempp E, Blatteau JE, Stephant E et al. (2008). MRI findings and clinical outcome in 45 divers with spinal cord decompression sickness. Aviat Space Environ Med 79: 1112–1116.

Gerth WA, Ruterbusch VL, Long ET (2007). The Influence of Thermal Exposure on Diver Susceptibility to Decompression Sickness. NEDU Technical Report 06-07, Navy Experimental Diving Unit, Panama City, FL.

Gibbs JW, 3rd, Piantadosi CA, Massey EW (2002). Internal carotid artery dissection in stroke from SCUBA diving: a case report. Undersea Hyperb Med 29: 167–171.

Golding F, Griffiths P, Hempleman HV et al. (1960). Decompression sickness during construction of the Dartford Tunnel. Br J Ind Med 17: 167–180.

Gorman DF, Edmonds CW, Parsons DW et al. (1987). Neurologic sequelae of decompression sickness: a clinical report. In: AA Bove, AJ Bachrach, LJ Greenbaum Jr. (Eds.), Underwater and Hyperbaric Physiology IX Proceedings of the Ninth International Symposium on Underwater and Hyperbaric Physiology. Undersea and Hyperbaric Medical Society, Bethesda, pp. 993–998.

Gronning M, Risberg J, Skeidsvoll H et al. (2005). Electroencephalography and magnetic resonance imaging in neurological decompression sickness. Undersea Hyperb Med 32: 397–402.

Grossman A, Ulanovski D, Barenboim E et al. (2004). Facial nerve palsy aboard a commercial aircraft. Aviat Space Environ Med 75: 1075–1076.

Hauser WA, Rich SS, Annegers JF et al. (1990). Seizure recurrence after a 1st unprovoked seizure: an extended follow-up. Neurology 40: 1163–1170.

Holck P, Hunter RW (2006). NIHSS applied to cerebral neurological dive injuries as a tool for dive injury severity stratification. Undersea Hyperb Med 33: 271–280.

Holley T (2000). Validation of the RNZN system for scoring severity and measuring recovery in decompression illness. SPUMS J 30: 75–80.

Idicula J (1972). Perplexing case of maxillary sinus barotrauma. Aerosp Med 43: 891–892.

Kelleher PC, Pethybridge RJ, Francis TJ (1996). Outcome of neurological decompression illness: development of a manifestation-based model. Aviat Space Environ Med 67: 654–658, erratum Aviat Space Environ Med 1997; 68: 246.

Klingmann C, Praetorius M, Baumann I et al. (2007). Barotrauma and decompression illness of the inner ear: 46 cases during treatment and follow-up. Otol Neurotol 28: 447–454.

Kocyigit A, Cinar C, Kitis O et al. (2010). Isolated PICA dissection: an unusual complication of scuba diving: case report and review of the literature. Clin Neuroradiol 20: 171–173.

Konno K, Kurita H, Ito N et al. (2001). Extracranial vertebral artery dissection caused by scuba diving. J Neurol 248: 816–817.

Ladd G, Stepan V, Stevens L (2002). The Abacus Project: establishing the risk of recreational scuba death and decompression illness. SPUMS J 32: 124–128.

Lairez O, Cournot M, Minville V et al. (2009). Risk of neurological decompression sickness in the diver with a right-to-left shunt: literature review and meta-analysis. Clin J Sport Med 19: 231–235.

Lieppman ME (1981). Accommodative and convergence insufficiency after decompression sickness. Arch Ophthalmol 99: 453–456.

Lowe VJ, Hoffman JM, Hanson MW et al. (1994). Cerebral imaging of decompression injury patients with

^{18}F-2-fluoro-2-deoxyglucose positron emission tomography. Undersea Hyperb Med 21: 103–113.

Mahon RT, Dainer HM, Nelson JW (2006). Decompression sickness in a swine model: isobaric denitrogenation and perfluorocarbon at depth. Aviat Space Environ Med 77: 8–12.

Malette WG, Fitzgerald JB, Cockett AT (1962). Dysbarism A review of thirty-five cases with suggestion for therapy. Aerosp Med 33: 1132–1139.

Martin JD, Thom SR (2002). Vascular leukocyte sequestration in decompression sickness and prophylactic hyperbaric oxygen therapy in rats. Aviat Space Environ Med 73: 565–569.

Mines D, Stahmer S, Shepherd SM (1997). Poisonings: food, fish, shellfish. Emerg Med Clin North Am 15: 157–177.

Mitchell SJ, Holley T, Gorman DF (1998). A new system for scoring severity and measuring recovery in decompression illness. SPUMS J 28: 89–94.

Molvaer OI, Eidsvik S (1987). Facial baroparesis: a review. Undersea Biomed Res 14: 277–295.

Money KE, Buckingham IP, Calder IM et al. (1985). Damage to the middle ear and the inner ear in underwater divers. Undersea Biomed Res 12: 77–84.

Moon RE (2003). Adjunctive Therapy for Decompression Illness. Undersea and Hyperbaric Medical Society, Kensington, MD.

Murrison AW, Smith DJ, Francis TJR et al. (1991). Maxillary sinus barotrauma with fifth cranial nerve involvement. J Laryngol Otol 105: 217–219.

Navy Department (2008). US Navy Diving Manual Revision 6, vol 5 Diving Medicine and Recompression Chamber Operations. NAVSEA 0910-LP-106-0957, Naval Sea Systems Command, Washington, DC.

Nelson EE (1995). Internal carotid artery dissection associated with scuba diving. Ann Emerg Med 25: 103–106.

Neuman TS, Bove AA (1990). Combined arterial gas embolism and decompression sickness following no-stop dives. Undersea Biomed Res 17: 429–436.

Neuman T, Settle H, Beaver G et al. (1975). Maxillary sinus barotrauma with cranial nerve involvement: case report. Aviat Space Environ Med 46: 314–315.

Nossum V, Hjelde A, Brubakk AO (2002). Small amounts of venous gas embolism cause delayed impairment of endothelial function and increase polymorphonuclear neutrophil infiltration. Eur J Appl Physiol 86: 209–214.

Ostachowicz MZ (1987). History of the ophthalmological investigations in decompression sickness. Bull Inst Marit Trop Med Gdynia 38: 207–209.

Pollock NW (2008). Annual Diving Report. 2008 edn. Divers Alert Network, Durham, NC.

Shepherd TH, Sykes JJW, Pearson RR (1983). Case reports: peripheral cranial nerve injuries resulting from hyperbaric exposure. J R Nav Med Serv 69: 154–155.

Shupak A, Doweck I, Greenberg E et al. (1991). Diving-related inner ear injuries. Laryngoscope 101: 173–179.

Skurnik YD, Sthoeger Z (2005). Carotid artery dissection after scuba diving. Isr Med Assoc J 7: 406–407.

Spiess BD (2009). Perfluorocarbon emulsions as a promising technology: a review of tissue and vascular gas dynamics. J Appl Physiol 106: 1444–1452.

Swift AE, Swift TR (1993). Ciguatera. J Toxicol Clin Toxicol 31: 1–29.

Todnem K, Nyland H, Kambestad BK et al. (1990). Influence of occupational diving upon the nervous system: an epidemiological study. Br J Ind Med 47: 708–714.

Trytko BE, Bennett MH (2008). Arterial gas embolism: a review of cases at Prince of Wales Hospital, Sydney, 1996 to 2006. Anaesth Intensive Care 36: 60–64.

van Hulst RA, Klein J, Lachmann B (2003). Gas embolism: pathophysiology and treatment. Clin Physiol Funct Imaging 23: 237–246.

Van Liew HD, Flynn ET (2005). Direct ascent from air and N$_2$-O$_2$ saturation dives in humans: DCS risk and evidence of a threshold. Undersea Hyperb Med 32: 409–419.

Van Liew HD, Conkin J, Burkard ME (1993). The oxygen window and decompression bubbles: estimates and significance. Aviat Space Environ Med 64: 859–865.

Vann RD (2004). Mechanisms and risks of decompression. In: AA Bove (Ed.), Bove and Davis' Diving Medicine. Saunders, Philadelphia, pp. 127–164.

Vann RD, Butler FK, Mitchell SJ et al. (2011). Decompression illness. Lancet 377: 153–164.

Warren LP, Djang WT, Moon RE et al. (1988). Neuroimaging of scuba diving injuries to the CNS. AJNR Am J Neuroradiol 9: 933–938.

Weiss LD, Van Meter KW (1995). Cerebral air embolism in asthmatic scuba divers in a swimming pool. Chest 107: 1653–1654.

Yoshiyama M, Asamoto S, Kobayashi N et al. (2007). Spinal cord decompression sickness associated with scuba diving: correlation of immediate and delayed magnetic resonance imaging findings with severity of neurologic impairment – a report on 3 cases. Surg Neurol 67: 283–287.

Handbook of Clinical Neurology, Vol. 120 (3rd series)
Neurologic Aspects of Systemic Disease Part II
Jose Biller and Jose M. Ferro, Editors

Chapter 64

Neurologic complications of carbon monoxide intoxication

KERSTIN BETTERMAN[1]* AND SURJU PATEL[2]

[1]*Department of Neurology, Penn State College of Medicine, Hershey, PA, USA*

[2]*Department of Internal Medicine, Conemaugh Health System, Jonestown, PA, USA*

INTRODUCTION

French physiologist Claude Bernard was one of the first to describe the pathophysiology of carbon monoxide (CO) poisoning during the mid 19th century (Bernard, 1857). He observed that CO causes tissue hypoxia by interaction with red blood cells requiring him to develop a new method to measure blood-gas transfer. He performed many experiments which showed that CO prevented red blood cells from taking up oxygen and delivering it to the tissues, and described the cherry red appearance of the blood following CO intoxication (Bernard, 1858, 1870). Carbon monoxide poisoning is still the leading cause of poison-related morbidity and mortality worldwide. In the US it results in more than 50 000 emergency visits yearly (Weaver, 2009).

Carbon monoxide is an odorless, colorless gas that can be found at toxic levels in homes with gas heating furnaces. It is a product of incomplete combustion of fuels from multiple sources and is found in motor vehicle exhausts or indoor heating units with burning of oil, coal, wood, or kerosene. Frequently chronic intoxication occurs in settings of chimney malfunction or dysfunctional ventilation. Deadly CO poisoning often occurs in the setting of a building fire or from exposure to fuel powered generators and heaters used during natural disasters or with suicide using motor vehicle exhaust gas (Prockop and Chichkova, 2007; Studdert et al., 2010).

PATHOPHYSIOLOGY

Endogenous CO production occurs during normal heme metabolism at concentrations not interfering with normal blood- or tissue-oxygen exchange. However, increased CO concentrations following intoxication impact the transport of oxygen to the tissues. Normally, oxygen diffuses across the alveolar-capillary membrane and binds to hemoglobin. Carbon monoxide interferes with this process by diffusing rapidly through the alveolar-capillary membrane and binding to hemoglobin more than 200 times faster than oxygen. Carboxyhemoglobin (COHb) is formed which causes a left-shift in the oxyhemoglobin dissociation curve (Hardy and Thom, 1994). The tetrameric structure of the hemoglobin molecule goes through a conformational change where the sigmoidal curve is no longer maintained. COHb is unable to transport as much oxygen as normal hemoglobin leading to decreased oxygen delivery to the tissues and subsequent tissue hypoxia.

Moreover the allosteric property of hemoglobin induced by CO binding causes other CO molecules to bind more rapidly. Carbon monoxide binds to hemoglobin at such high rate that partial pressures of CO in the capillaries stay relatively low. Carbon monoxide is not perfusion limited meaning it will not be affected by the rate of blood flow or the amount of hemoglobin in the blood. As long as there is hemoglobin, it will bind. Although COHb is a completely reversible complex, the release of oxygen from COHb is relatively slow and depends on the inhaled oxygen concentration. The higher the inhaled oxygen concentration, the faster the CO elimination rate, which is the rationale to treat CO intoxication victims with 100% oxygen or to consider hyperbaric oxygen (HBO) therapy. After COHb levels decrease, tissue oxygenation, mitochondrial function, and cellular energy metabolism are restored, but even transient exposure to high concentrations of CO may cause brain injury acutely or within days to weeks (Okeda et al., 1982; Piantadosi et al., 1997).

Carbon monoxide causes tissue hypoxia, ischemia and secondary injury through multiple mechanisms of

---

*Correspondence to: Kerstin Bettermann, M.D., Ph.D., Department of Neurology, Penn State College of Medicine, 500 University Drive, P.O. Box 850, Hershey, PA 17033, USA. Tel: +1-717-531-1803, Fax: +1-717-531-0963, E-mail: kbettermann@hmc.psu.edu

Table 64.1

Summary of the cerebral pathology and pathophysiology associated with CO poisoning

Carbon monoxide causes acute cerebral ischemia and hypoxia as well as secondary injury via multiple mechanisms of action	
Brain pathology	Injury of neurons of cortical layers III and V
	Decreased volume of the hippocampus
	Globus pallidus injury
	Demyelination of the white matter
	Loss of Purkinje cells in the cerebellum
	Cerebral edema
	Necrosis and apoptosis
Cerebral pathophysiology	Interruption of cellular respiration
	Decreased glucose metabolism
	Increase in lactid acid
	Production of reactive oxygen species
	Endothelial peroxynitrite deposition
	Decreased dopamine turnover in caudate nucleus
	Activation of the inflammatory cascade
	Modification of myelin basic protein and malonyaldehyde
	Increased intracellular iron deposition
	Increased nitric oxide levels
	P450 inhibition
	Lipid peroxidation
	Increase of cytosol heme concentration
	Activation of genes mediating apoptosis

action (Table 64.1). Highly metabolic organs such as the heart and the brain are especially vulnerable.

Carbon monoxide binds to platelet heme-protein and cytochrome C oxydase, interrupting cellular respiration in the mitochondria with subsequent tissue acidosis and production of reactive oxygen species (Miro et al., 1998). As a result, the cells shift to anaerobic metabolism and toxic lactic acids and nitrates build up. Oxidative stress results in neuronal necrosis, apoptosis, and activation of hypoxia-induced factors mediating secondary injury. Carbon monoxide also activates the inflammatory cascade, causes peroxidation of lipids and deposition of peroxynitrate in blood vessel endothelium, causing vascular damage that can potentiate tissue ischemia soon after or even during exposure to CO and at relatively low concentrations (Alonso et al., 2003; Cronje et al., 2004; Thom et al., 2006; Thom, 2008).

In the heart CO binds to myoglobin about 60 times faster than oxygen, causing myocardial hypoxia. It causes coronary vasodilation and increased coronary flow which can result in additional hypoxic-ischemic damage to the myocardium and decreased cardiac output. Low cardiac output and hypotension in turn can decrease cerebral perfusion and contribute to hypoxic-ischemic brain injury (Prockop and Chichkova, 2007). Studies in mice have shown that cerebral flow increases within minutes of CO exposure which is caused by guanylyl cyclase-mediated relaxation of the cerebral arteries (Komuro et al., 2001; Kanu et al., 2006). Cerebral blood flow remains elevated until cardiac compromise causes decrease in blood pressure and cardiac output, at which point cerebral autoregulation fails and asphyxia and apnea start, all contributing to the hypoxic-ischemic brain injury (Thom, 1990; Thom et al., 2006).

Carbon monoxide is a naturally occurring signaling molecule in the brain, but following exposure to high CO concentrations during an acute or chronic intoxication CO has detrimental effects on the central nervous system (CNS). Cytosol heme concentrations in the brain increase about tenfold after CO poisoning, adding to its toxicity (Cronje et al., 2004). There are acute as well as delayed neurologic effects following CO intoxication. Acute CO poisoning often causes damage to brain areas with great susceptibility to hypoxic injury, including the second and third cortical layers, watershed areas within the white matter, the basal ganglia and the Purkinje cells of the cerebellum. The nature and distribution of brain lesions depend on the acuteness, the severity, and the duration of exposure to CO.

Furthermore CO poisoning causes lipid peroxidation with degradation of unsaturated fatty acids leading to demyelination of CNS lipids and damage to myelin and axons. This process is to some extent reversible and can be observed acutely or with delayed brain injury. Many of the delayed neurologic complications may be mediated by inflammatory and immune responses (Thom et al., 2004). In experimental studies CO causes over-reactivity of neuronal nitric oxide synthase which produces nitrous oxygen (NO). NO is released from platelets and causes changes in cerebral blood flow and aggregation with neutrophils. Neutropohils and platelets interact, producing reactive oxygen species that mediate lipid peroxidation in the brain (Thom et al., 2006). Additionally the peroxidation product malonlylaldehyde (MDA) alters the ionic charge and configuration of myelin basic protein inducing change in its antigenic nature. In experimental studies this causes an increase in macrophages and CD4 lymphocytes with subsequent activation of brain microglia that is associated with learning difficulties, not present in rats without an altered myelin basic protein structure (Thom et al., 2004).

PATHOLOGY

The neuropathology of CO intoxication has been well described (Lapresle and Fardeau, 1967; O'Donnell et al., 2000; Chu et al., 2004). Postmortem studies have shown petechial hemorrhages in the white matter, particularly in the corpus callosum, and multifocal necrosis within the globus pallidus, the hippocampus, and the pars reticularis of the substantia nigra. Other findings include laminar necrosis of the cortex and loss of Purkinje cells in the cerebellum. White matter lesions are frequently observed which can be asymmetrical. The typical pallidal lesions are well defined involving the globus pallidus with microscopic infarctions extending anteriorly, superiorly, and into the internal capsules. Often a small linear focus of necrosis is found at the junction of the internal capsule and the internal nucleus of the globus pallidus. The hypothalamus, the thalamus, the third ventricle, and the brainstem are often spared (Lapresle and Fardeau, 1967).

In comatose patients who die soon after CO intoxication there is frequently myelin damage with perivascular lesions in the corpus callosum, the internal and external capsules, and the optic tracts. Demyelinating plaques, extensive periventricular demyelination and axonal destruction can be observed in postmortem studies of patients who died from chronic CO intoxication or in comatose patients who survive for longer periods of time after an acute CO intoxication. Demyelination of the subcortical and periventricular white matter is often associated with a delayed neuropsychiatric syndrome following CO intoxication which will be described in the following section (O'Donnell et al., 2000).

Because of their increased metabolic rate, both brain and myocardium are especially vulnerable to hypoxic injury associated with CO poisoning. Findings related to brain hypoxia include laminar necrosis of the cortex. Here neurons of layers III and V are greatly affected, as is the hippocampus and the Purkinje cells of the cerebellum.

Globus pallidus injury is the hallmark of carbon monoxide intoxication (Kumar et al., 2005). The predilection for the globus pallidus remains unclear but may be related to the high iron affinity of CO. The globus pallidus is iron rich, resulting in greater concentration of CO in this area. Additionally the globus pallidus receives blood supply from blood vessels belonging to one of the watershed areas of the brain, making it more susceptible to ischemic injury from cardiac and hypotensive effects which are typically associated with CO poisoning (Lo Ping et al., 2007). If the globus pallidus and basal ganglia are damaged by injury and necrosis, movement disorders such as Parkinsonism can develop. Although globus pallidus lesions are considered to be pathognomonic of CO intoxication, they may not occur even in survivors suffering Parkinsonism (Choi, 1983). In these patients white matter lesions, present on magnetic resonance imaging (MRI), are often responsible for the clinical picture of parkinsonism (Sohn et al., 2000).

CLINICAL FINDINGS

Carbon monoxide poisoning can cause acute and delayed signs and symptoms which can be specific (see Table 64.2). However, at times the clinical picture can

Table 64.2

Associations between clinical presentation, carbon monoxide concentration, and exposure times (modified from Struttmann et al., 1998)

Carbon monoxide concentration (in parts per million)	COHb level	Symptoms, CO exposure time
35 ppm	<10%	Headache and dizziness, within 6–8 h
100 ppm	>10%	Slight headache, in 2–3 h
200 ppm	20%	Slight headache and loss of judgment, within 2–3 h
400 ppm	25%	Headache, within 1–2 h
800 ppm	30%	Dizziness, nausea, and seizures, within 45 min
1600 ppm	40%	Headache, tachycardia, dizziness, and nausea within 20 min; death in less than 2 h
3200 ppm	50%	Headache, dizziness, and nausea in 5–10 min; death within 30 min
6400 ppm	60%	Headache and dizziness in 1–2 min; seizures, respiratory arrest, and death in less than 20 min
12 800 ppm	>70%	Death in less than 3 min

be rather vague and a high level of clinical suspicion is therefore crucial. The CO concentration and the exposure time are associated with specific symptoms which are summarized in Table 64.2. Depending on the duration of CO exposure symptoms are typically first noted with measured blood COHb concentrations of about 10%. Patients with underlying chronic heart and lung disease may present earlier at lower CO concentrations and with more severe symptoms. In a healthy person, the average carboxyhemoglobin levels are approximately 1–2%. In anemic patients the COHb levels are about 5% and in non-symptomatic smokers the levels are as high as 15%. The most common symptoms of CO poisoning include nausea, vomiting, dizziness, and generalized weakness (Ginsberg, 1985; Prockop, 2005). COHb levels below 40% are not typically associated with coma or death.

Acute intoxication

Acute CO poisoning is rarely detected until the patient becomes ill. The so-called classic cherry red discoloration of the skin and cyanosis are very rare. Headache is one of the most common presenting features of CO poisoning, occurring in over 80% of victims. It is typically dull, frontally located, and continuous, or it can mimic migraine headaches (Handa and Tai, 2005). In mild cases only mild flu-like symptoms can be observed. About half of the victims with CO intoxication complain about generalized weakness, nausea, confusion, and shortness of breath. Sometimes abdominal pain, vision changes, chest pain, and other vague symptoms are present (Prockop, 2005). Hypoxia leading to increased intracranial pressure from cytotoxic cerebral edema causes not only headaches, but also confusion, seizures, coma, and death. Transient cerebral edema can develop followed by widespread tissue necrosis and can be diagnosed early by diffusion-weighted brain MRI. Other neurologic findings include tinnitus, central hearing loss, nystagmus, and ataxia, visual disturbances, and syncope (Llano and Raffin, 1990; Blumenthal, 2001). Varying degrees of cognitive impairment have been observed following chronic and acute CO intoxication, and are pathognomonic for the delayed neurologic sequelae following CO intoxication.

Cardiac symptoms are ischemic in nature and consist of chest pain, myocardial infarct, cardiac dysrhythmias, hypotension, and tachycardia. Frequently ischemic EKG changes are present and cardiac enzymes are elevated. Patients with underlying chronic heart and lung disease are especially at risk of dying from cardiac complications and myocardial infarct. The mortality rate is higher in patients with moderate to severe CO poisoning, which also causes respiratory depression and pulmonary edema (Ginsberg, 1985).

Chronic intoxication

Chronic carbon monoxide poisoning occurs when low levels of CO are inhaled over a prolonged period of time, for instance in the setting of an undetected gas leak. This can mimic flu-like symptoms and frequently causes nausea, lethargy, and headaches. Depression, vomiting, gastrointestinal problems, weight loss, short-term memory difficulties, and confusion can develop. A high level of suspicion is essential to make the diagnosis.

Delayed neuropsychiatric syndrome

Cognitive deficits develop within 2–240 days following CO intoxication (Tibbles and Perrotta, 1994). Severe dementia, psychosis, anxiety, and other neuropsychological symptoms suddenly start after an initially excellent functional recovery period. Carbon monoxide encephalopathy can also present with alterations in attention, executive function, visuomotor skills, learning, short-term memory, mood, and social behavior. The delayed neuropsychiatric syndrome occurs in about 3% of CO intoxication cases and personality changes, urinary and fecal incontinence, and parkinsonism may develop (Mimura et al., 1999). The incidence is higher in the elderly and in those being exposed to CO for at least 12–48 hours. After an initial recovery phase, patients rapidly deteriorate, developing some or all of the neuropsychiatric symptoms above (Ernst and Zibrak, 1998). On neurologic examination frontal release and extrapyramidal signs are frequently present. In 57% of cases, the EEG will show delta range slowing and neuroimaging studies are abnormal (Tibbles and Perrotta, 1994). Head CT shows hypodensities in the basal ganglia in half of the patients. MRI usually shows hyperintensities in the globus pallidus and white matter changes in the frontal lobes. Neuropathology often shows extensive lesions in the brain including the globus pallidum, caudate, putamen, substantia nigra, hippocampus, hypothalamus, periventricular white matter, corona radiata, cerebellum, and hippocampus (Brucher, 1967; Lapresle and Fardeau, 1967) (Figs 64.1 and 64.2). About 60–75% of patients with delayed neuropsychiatric syndrome recover within a year. About 15% continue to suffer from dementia and parkinsonism (Bhatia et al., 2007).

DIAGNOSIS

The diffuse symptoms and the absence of specific laboratory tests makes it difficult to suspect CO intoxication; especially chronic poisoning. History of exposure to fire, presence of a fireplace, indoor compression appliances, or occupational exposure can be indicative of CO intoxication. Following intoxication, ambient air CO levels at

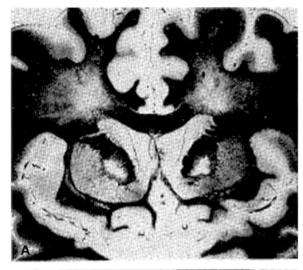

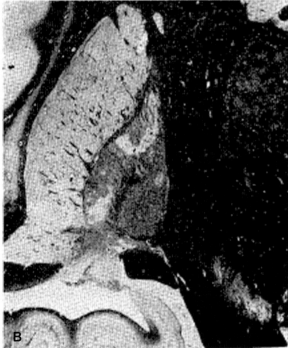

Fig. 64.1. Carbon monoxide intoxication. (**A**) Symmetrical necrosis in oral pallidum and diffuse leukoencephalopathy in intermittent form. (**B**) Multiple focal necroses in posterior and lateral parts of the globus pallidus and in the reticular zone of the substantia nigra. Heidenhein stain. (Reproduce from Jellinger, 1986.)

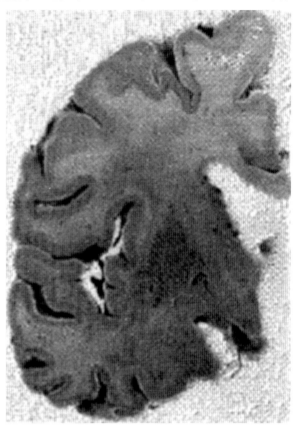

Fig. 64.2. Small cystic necrosis in internal pallidal segment and laminary cortical necroses after coal gas poisoning. The patient survived many years in a rigid-akinetic state with severe dementia. (Reproduce from Jellinger, 1986.)

LABORATORY TESTS

The COHb concentration in blood depends on the amount of CO in the inhaled air, the ventilation rate and the exposure time. Often the clinical outcome correlates poorly with measured blood COHb concentrations which may be due to the fact that blood samples are often obtained after a significant amount of time has passed following CO exposure. Another reason for the poor correlation is delayed neurologic injury which can develop independently of measured HbCO levels. Pulse CO oximetry can be used at the bedside to detect increased levels of HbCO in the blood. If it is elevated the value is significant. However, if the value is low carbon monoxide poisoning cannot be completely ruled out as inhalation of low levels of oxygen can also cause low HbCO levels. Pulse oximeters frequently overestimate the arterial oxygenation in patients with severe CO poisoning. Automated spectrophotometers or oximeter devices are now available and are increasingly recommended to assess victims of CO intoxication (Prockop and Chichkova, 2007).

the scene of exposure should be measured as soon as possible. The half-life of CO is only 4–5 hours so that blood COHb levels are rather unreliable to determine the severity of an intoxication. Only CO levels measured at the scene of an acute exposure may have potential to assess the degree of intoxication.

Lactic acid levels, basic metabolic panels with glucose levels, electrolytes and arterial blood gases should also be closely monitored as patients with CO intoxication frequently develop lactate acidosis. Renal function can be diminished due to myoglobinuria and hypokalemia and hyperglycemia can occur with severe intoxication. Cardiac function must be closely monitored by serial EKGs, echocardiograms and measurements of cardiac enzymes for the development of brady- or tachycardia, atrial or ventricular fibrillation, premature ventricular contractions, conduction abnormalities, or myocardial infarct.

NEUROIMAGING STUDIES

One of the most sensitive measures of cerebral injury following CO intoxication is brain MRI, which shows variable findings. Most comatose patients show abnormalities within the globus pallidus, lentiform nucleus, caudate nuclei, thalamus, periventricular and subcortical white matter, especially of the frontal and temporal lobes. Hippocampal and cerebellar lesions can be present. Diffuse high signal abnormalities within the bilateral centrum semiovale are also common (Tuchman et al., 1990).

T1-weighted MRI sequences show typically low signal intensity bilaterally in the globus pallidus. This corresponds to high signal intensities on T2-weighted and fluid attenuated inversion recovery (FLAIR) imaging. Pathognomonic pallidal lesions are well visualized by contrast-enhanced MRI (see Fig. 64.1). In the acute intoxication phase contrast enhanced T2-weighted MRI may show patchy or peripheral enhancement of necrotic areas. Diffusion-weighted MRI often shows restriction of water diffusion due to cytotoxic edema within the white matter or diffusely within the brain (Sener, 2003). These changes can develop early after CO exposure. Most acute stages also show restricted water diffusion in the globus pallidus and in the substantia nigra.

White matter changes are often reversible. However, following severe CO intoxication persistent changes on MRI can be found for years following the exposure even without clinical deficits (O'Donnell et al., 2000; Durak et al., 2005). T2 and FLAIR sequences often show bilateral symmetric hyperintensities in the white matter of the centrum semiovale with relative sparing of the brainstem (see Fig. 64.2). Clinical status and outcome often correlate with diffuse white matter changes. MR spectroscopy can now be used to help assess prognosis. N-acetylaspartate (NAA) decreases in demyelinated white matter regions representing most likely axonal and neuronal loss (Van Zijl and Barker, 1997). This can often be observed in the basal ganglia or in the white matter. Proton magnetic resonance spectroscopy may show increased choline peak which indicated progressive demyelination in early CO poisoning cases (Murata et al., 1995). Kamada and coworkers (Kamada et al., 1994) have shown that a marked lowering of the NAA/Cr ratio and a slight increase in the Cho/Cr ratio with subsequent normalization can parallel clinical improvement. MR spectroscopy is currently mainly investigational but may become useful as prognostic indicator in CO poisoning.

Cranial CT typically reveals unilateral or bilateral low attenuation areas in the globus pallidus but is less sensitive than MRI. Hemorrhagic infarctions have been described on both CT and brain MRI. Positron emission tomography (PET) and SPECT can also provide additional information showing decreased glucose metabolism and hypoperfusion that parallel the development of focal and diffuse lesions after CO intoxication.

DIFFERENTIAL DIAGNOSIS

Carbon monoxide poisoning can present in a similar way to many other disease states. The symptoms are nonspecific and therefore CO poisoning can easily be mistaken for other conditions such as the flu, gastrointestinal disorders, chronic fatigue syndrome, depression, hypothyroidism, anemia, or chronic migraine headaches. Neurologic and neuropsychiatric signs and symptoms may suggest a neurodegenerative disorder such as dementia, Parkinson disease, other movement disorders, or may mimic psychiatric conditions such as schizoaffective disorder or depression.

TREATMENT

Oxygen should be administered to all patients with suspected CO intoxication via face mask with 100% oxygen flow (Elkharrat, 1998). This must be initiated immediately and independently of blood COHb levels as measured COHb levels may underestimate the true intoxication level. The airway needs to be secured and adequate ventilation needs to be maintained. Following inhalation of 100% oxygen at normobaric pressure, the half-life of COHb is reduced from 4–5 hours to 1 hour. Patients should be on strict bed rest and every measure should be taken to decrease oxygen demand and to lower metabolic needs. Patients with respiratory distress and a decreased level of consciousness must be intubated and mechanically ventilated. Chest X-rays and arterial blood gases should be assessed periodically. Cardiac function needs to be closely monitored. Serum pH and lactid acid levels should be closely monitored since aerobic metabolism generates lactate acidosis. Acidosis with pH below levels of 7.15 should be treated with sodium bicarbonate.

The use of hyperbaric oxygen therapy remains controversial for the treatment of victims with CO intoxication (Weaver et al., 1995; Juurlink et al., 2000; Stoller, 2007). HBO therapy consists of inhalation of 100% oxygen at higher than normal ambient pressures. It significantly increases the amount of oxygen that is physically dissolved in blood and becomes available for delivery to hypoxic tissues. At pressures of 2.5 atmospheres absolute (ATA) HBO reduces the half-life of COHb from 4 hours to 20 minutes. A single treatment at pressures of 2.5–3.0 ATA given over a duration of 90–120 minutes is commonly considered for treatment of patients with syncope, coma, seizures, and focal neurologic deficits who present with COHb levels of more than 25% (and of more than 15% in pregnant women) (Tibbles and Perotta, 1994; Van Meter et al., 1994; Thom et al., 1995; Weaver et al., 1995; Tibbles and Edelsberg, 1996). However, in clinical practice it is difficult to make a decision on when to use hyperbaric oxygen as COHb levels might underestimate the degree of intoxication and do not necessarily correlate with clinical severity. Hyperbaric oxygen treatment is also sometimes considered for victims of CO intoxication who are at risk of developing the delayed neuropsychological sequelae (Weaver et al., 2007). In one study, patients aged 36 years and older who had been exposed to CO for at least 24 hours and who did not receive HBO treatment had an increased risk of cognitive sequelae at 6 weeks compared with those without these characteristics (Weaver et al., 2007).

Pregnant women should probably be treated with hyperbaric oxygen as the fetus is especially vulnerable after CO intoxication, with high rates of fetal mortality and morbidity (Prockop and Chichkova, 2007). The treatment of patients who remain in coma with HBO remains controversial.

HBO therapy can increase tissue oxygen concentrations, promoting CO elimination. It increases ATP, and reduces oxidative stress and inflammatory responses. Animal studies suggest that HBO also has additional benefits such as inhibition of neutrophil adherence to the wall of ischemic vessels, decrease in free radical production, vasoconstriction and tissue destruction, but data from clinical trials remain controversial (Juurlink et al., 2000). Subsequently there are no guidelines available which are based on high-level evidence regarding the use of HBO in CO intoxication.

Several authors noted that the unselected use of HBO for acute CO poisoning does not reduce the frequency of neurologic symptoms at 1 month, but that further research is necessary to comment on the benefit of HBO use (Juurlink et al., 2000). There are several randomized controlled trials but only one of the trials follows standardization guidelines for the reporting of clinical trials (Juurlink et al., 2000). Four of six clinical trials did not find any evidence that HBO reduces neurologic sequelae and two studies showed benefit. However, these studies have methodological limitations, are heterogenous, and have different selection criteria of patients, follow-up protocols, and outcome measures. The methodologies are difficult to compare as different study designs and treatment protocols were used (for details that are beyond the scope of this text see Raphael et al., 1989; Ducasse et al., 1995; Thom et al., 1995; Scheinkestel et al., 1999; Juurlink et al., 2000). One trial showed that cognitive impairment was significantly lower in patients receiving initial treatment with HBO within 24 hours of an intoxication (Weaver et al., 1995). However, the study did not clearly identify subgroups of patients in whom HBO was less beneficial. A Cochrane review of six clinical trials does not support the use of HBO for treatment of patients with CO intoxication (Weaver et al., 2002). It remains currently unknown which patient should receive HBO treatment, if any. Additionally, if HBO is used, the dose, number and duration of treatments remain controversial. Usually a single treatment at 2.5–3 ATA for a duration of 90 minutes has been advocated by some (Prockop and Chichkova, 2007). The effectiveness of different protocols using more frequent treatments or different pressures and treatment durations has not been compared in a systematic fashion.

The Undersea and Hyperbaric Medical Society recommends treatment of the following patients with HBO after CO intoxication: patients with transient or prolonged episodes of loss of consciousness, abnormal neurologic signs, cardiovascular dysfunction or severe acidosis, patients who are 36 years or older when exposed for more than 24 hours, or those who have COHb levels of 25% or more, as well as pregnant women (Gesell, 2008). The clinical policy subcommittee of the American College of Emergency Physicians states that the use of HBO therapy is still controversial and advocates randomized controlled trials to assess its effectiveness (Wolf et al., 2008).

PROGNOSIS

Clinical outcome in patients after CO exposure is highly variable. Patients with CO poisoning need follow-up after discharge as they may develop the delayed neuropsychological syndrome. There is no specific therapy for this sequela, but usually empirical treatment with various medications, physical, occupational and vocational therapy, and potentially, rehabilitation. The incidence of the delayed neuropsychological syndrome following CO intoxication is not precisely known. In one study 46% of patients had abnormal neuropsychological findings and symptoms at 6 weeks (Weaver et al., 2002). Information about neuropsychological outcome beyond the first year after CO intoxication is limited (Weaver et al., 2002, 2007; Jasper et al., 2005). In a cohort study which followed patients for 6 years, 19% had cognitive impairment and 37% had abnormal neurologic findings on examination (Weaver et al., 2008). Patients with white matter lesions or hippocampal atrophy on brain MRI were at higher risk to show delayed cognitive abnormalities (den Heijer et al., 2006; Smith et al., 2008).

The initial clinical presentation does not predict the outcome but several factors indicate poor outcomes such as severity and duration of CO exposure. Given the role of inflammation in CO intoxication associated injury, inflammatory biomarkers may help in the future to predict the risk of neuropsychological symptoms. Children are often symptomatic earlier, but can also recover faster than adults (Weaver et al., 2002). The fetus is especially susceptible to the adverse effects of CO poisoning. Fetal mortality exceeds 50% in case of severe CO intoxication (Koren et al., 1991). Patients with underlying cardiopulmonary disease, the elderly, and patients with multiple comorbidities are at increased risk for poor outcome after CO poisoning. Because treatment is often ineffective, emphasis is on prevention by close environmental monitoring.

REFERENCES

Alonso JR, Cardellach F, Lopez S et al. (2003). Carbon monoxide specifically inhibits cytochrome c oxidase of human mitochondrial respiratory chain. Pharmacol Toxicol 93: 142–146.

Bernard C (1857). Leçons sur les effets des substances toxiques et médicamenteuses. Baillière et Fils, Paris.

Bernard C (1858). Sur la quantité d'oxygène que contient le sang veineux des organes glandulaires à l'état de conction et à l'état de repos, et sur l'emploi de l'oxyde de carbone pour déterminer les proportions d'oxygène du sang. C R Hebd Acad Sci 47: 393–400.

Bernard C (1870). Sur l'asphyxie par le charbon. J Pharm 12: 125–133.

Bhatia R, Chacko F, Lal V et al. (2007). Reversible delayed neurophsychiatric syndrome following acute carbon monoxide exposure. Indian J Occu Environ Med 11: 80–82.

Blumenthal I (2001). Carbon monoxide poisoning. J Royal Soc Med 94: 270–272.

Brucher JM (1967). Neuropathological problems posed by carbon monoxide poisoning and anoxia. Prog Brain Res 24: 75–100.

Choi S (1983). Delayed neurological sequelae in carbon monoxide intoxication. Arch Neurol 40: 433–435.

Chu KC, Jung KH, Kim HJ et al. (2004). Diffusion-weighted MRI and 99mTc-HMPAO SPECT in delayed relapsing type of carbon monoxide poisoning: evidence of delayed cytotoxic edema. Eur Neurol 51: 98–103.

Cronje FJ, Carraway MS, Freiberger JJ et al. (2004). Carbon monoxide actuates O(2)-limited heme degradation in the rat brain. Free Radic Biol Med 37: 1802–1812.

den Heijer T, Sijens PE, Prins ND et al. (2006). MR spectroscopy of brain white matter in the prediction of dementia. Neurology 66: 540–544.

Ducasse JL, Celsis P, Marc-Vergnes JP (1995). Non-comatose patients with acute carbon monoxide poisoning: hyperbaric or normobaric oxygenation? Undersea Hyperb Med 22: 9–15.

Durak AC, Coskun A, Yikilmaz A et al. (2005). Magnetic resonance imaging findings in chronic carbon monoxide intoxication. Acta Radiol 46: 322–327.

Elkharrat D (1998). Indications of normobaric and hyperbaric oxygen therapy in acute CO intoxication. In: Proceedings satellite meeting IUTOX, VIIIth International Congress of Toxicology, Dijon, France, July 3–4, 1998.

Ernst A, Zibrak JD (1998). Carbon monoxide poisoning. N Engl J Med 339: 1603–1608.

Gesell LB (Ed.), (2008). Hyperbaric Oxygen 2009: Indications and Results: The Hyperbaric Oxygen Therapy Committee Report. Undersea and Hyperbaric Medical Society, Durham, NC.

Ginsberg MD (1985). Carbon monoxide intoxication: clinical features, neuropathology and mechanisms of injury. Clin Toxicol 23: 281–288.

Handa PK, Tai DY (2005). Carbon monoxide poisoning: a five year review at Tan Tock Seng Hospital, Singapore. Ann Acad Med Singapore 34: 611–614.

Hardy K, Thom S (1994). Pathophysiology and treatment of carbon monoxide poisoning. Clin Toxicol 32: 613–629.

Jasper BW, Hopkins RO, Duker HV et al. (2005). Affective outcome following carbon monoxide poisoning: a prospective longitudinal study. Cogn Behav Neurol 18: 127–134.

Jellinger K (1986). Exogenous lesions of the pallidum. In: PJ Vinken, GW Bruyn, HL Klawans (Eds.), Handbook of Clinical Neurology, vol. 49. Elsevier Science, Amsterdam, pp. 465–491.

Juurlink DN, Stanbrook MB, McGuigan MA (2000). Hyperbaric oxygen for carbon monoxide poisoning. Cochrane Database Syst Rev CD002041.

Kamada K, Houkin K, Aoki T et al. (1994). Cerebral metabolic changed in delayed carbon monoxide sequelae studied by proton MR spectroscopy. Neuroradiology 36: 104–106.

Kanu A, Whitfield J, Leffler A (2006). Carbon monoixde contributes to hypotension- induced cerebrovascular vasodilation in piglets. Am J Physiol Heart Circ Physiol 291: H2409–H2414.

Komuro T, Borsody M, Ono S et al. (2001). The vasorelaxation of cerebral arteries by carbon monoxide. Exp Biol Med 226: 860–865.

Koren G, Sharav T, Pastuszak A et al. (1991). A multicenter, prospective study of fetal outcome following accidental carbon monoxide poisoning in pregnancy. Reprod Toxicol 5: 397–403.

Kumar V, Abbas A, Fausto N (2005). Robins and Cotran: Pathologic Basis of Disease. 7th edn. Elsevier Saunders, Philadelphia.

Lapresle J, Fardeau M (1967). The central nervous system and carbon monoxide poisoning II. Anatomical study of brain lesions following intoxication with carbon monoxide (22 cases). In: H Bour, IM Ledingham (Eds.), Carbon Monoxide Poisoning. Prog Brain Res 24: 31–74.

Llano A, Raffin T (1990). Management of carbon monoxide poisoning. Chest 97: 165–169.

Lo Ping C, Chen S, Lee K et al. (2007). Brain injury after acute carbon monoxide poisoning early and late complications. Neuroradiology 189: 205–211.

Mimura K, Harada M, Sumiyoshi S et al. (1999). Long-terms follow-up study on sequelae of carbon monoxide poisoning: serial investigation 33 years after poisoning. Seishin Shinkeigaku Zasshi 101: 592–618.

Miro O, Casademont J, Barrientos A et al. (1998). Mitochondrial cytochrome c oxidase inhibition during acute carbon monoxide poisoning. Pharmacol Toxicol 82: 199–202.

Murata T, Itoh S, Koshino Y et al. (1995). Serial proton magnetic resonance spectroscopy in a patient with the interval form of carbon monoxide poisoning. J Neurol Neurosurg Psychiatry 58: 100–103.

O'Donnell P, Buxton PJ, Pitkin A et al. (2000). The magnetic resonance imaging appearances of the brain in acute carbon monoxide poisoning. Clin Radiol 55: 273–280.

Okeda R, Funata N, Song SJ et al. (1982). Comparative study pathogenesis of selective cerebral lesions in carbon monoxide poisoning and nitrogen hypoxia in cats. Acta Neuropathol (Berl) 56: 265–272.

Piantadosi CA, Zhang J, Levin ED et al. (1997). Apoptosis and delayed neuronal damage after carbon monoxide poisoning in the rat. Exp Neurol 147: 103–114.

Prockop LD (2005). Carbon monoxide brain toxicity: clinical, magnetic resonance imaging, magnetic resonance spectroscopy, and neuropsychological effects in 9 people. J Neuroimaging 15: 144–149.

Prockop LD, Chichkova RI (2007). Carbon monoxide intoxication: an updated review. J Neurol Sci 262: 122–130.

Raphael JC, Elkharrat D, Jars-Guincestre MC et al. (1989). Trial of normobaric and hyperbaric oxygen for acute carbon monoxide intoxication. Lancet 2: 414–419.

Scheinkestel CD, Bailey M, Myles PS et al. (1999). Hyperbaric or normobaric oxygen for acute carbon monoxide poisoning: a randomized controlled clinical trial. Med J Aust 170: 203–210.

Sener RN (2003). Acute carbon monoxide poisoning: diffusion MR imaging findings. AJNR Am J Neuroradiol. 24: 1475–1477.

Smith EE, Egorova S, Blacker D et al. (2008). Magnetic resonance imaging white matter hyperintensities and brain volume in the prediction of mild cognitive impairmentand dementia. Arch Neurol 65: 94–100.

Sohn YH, Jeong Y, Kim HS et al. (2000). The brain lesion responsible for parkinsonism after carbon monoxide poisoning. Arch Neurol 57: 1214–1218.

Stoller KP (2007). Hyperbaric oxygen and carbon monoxide poisoning: a critical review. Neurol Res 29: 147–155.

Struttmann T, Scheerer A, Prince S et al. (1998). Unintentional carbon monoxide poisoning from an unlikely source. J Am Board Fam Pract 11: 481–484.

Studdert DM, Gurrin LC, Jatkar U et al. (2010). Relationship between vehicle emissions laws and incidence of suicide by motor vehicle exhaust gas in Australia, 2001–06: an ecological analysis. PLoS Med 7: e1000210.

Thom SR (1990). Carbon monoxide-mediated brain lipid peroxidation in the rat. J Appl Physiol 68: 997–1003.

Thom SR (2008). Carbon monoxide pathophysiology and treatment. In: TS Neuman, SR Thom (Eds.), Physiology and Medicine of Hyperbaric Oxygen Therapy. Saunders Elsevier, Philadelphia, pp. 321–347.

Thom SR, Taber RI, Mediguren II et al. (1995). Delayed neuropsychological sequelae after carbon monoxide poisoning: prevention by treatment with hyperbaric oxygen. Ann Emerg Med 25: 479–486.

Thom S, Bhopale V, Fisher D et al. (2004). Delayed neuropathology after carbon monoxide poisoning is immune-mediated. Proc Natl Acad Sci U S A 101: 13660–13665.

Thom SR, Bhopale VM, Fisher D (2006a). Hyperbaric oxygen reduces delayed immune-mediated neuropathology in experimental carbon monoxide toxicity. Toxicol Appl Pharmacol 213: 152–159.

Thom SR, Bhopale VM, Han ST et al. (2006b). Intravascular neutrophil activation due to carbon monoxide poisoning. Am J Respir Crit Care Med 174: 1239–1248.

Tibbles PM, Edelsberg JS (1996). Hyperbaric-oxygen therapy. N Engl J Med 334: 1642–1648.

Tibbles PM, Perrotta PL (1994). Treatment of carbon monoxide poisoning: a critical review of human outcome studies comparing normobaric oxygen with hyperbaric oxygen. Ann Emerg Med 24: 269–276.

Tuchman RF, Moser FG, Moshe SL (1990). Carbon monoxide poisoning: bilateral lesions in the thalamus on MR imaging of the brain. Pediatr Radiol 20: 478–479.

Van Meter KW, Weiss L, Harch PE et al. (1994). Should the pressure be off or on with use of oxygen in the treatment of carbon monoxide poisoned patients. Ann Emerg Med 24: 283–288.

Van Zijl PCM, Barker PB (1997). Magnetic resonance spectroscopy and spectroscopic imaging for the study of brain metabolism. Ann N Y Acad Sci 820: 75–96.

Weaver L (2009). Carbon monoxide poisoning. N Engl J Med 360: 1217–1225.

Weaver LK, Hopkins RO, Larson-Lorh V et al. (1995). Double blind, controlled, prospective, randomized clinical trial (RCT) in patients with acute carbon monoxide (CO) poisoning: outcome of patients tested with normobaric oxygen or hyperbaric oxygen (HBO2), an interim report. Undersea Hyperb Med 22 (Suppl): 14.

Weaver LK, Hopkins RO, Chan KJ et al. (2002). Hyperbaric oxygen for acute carbon monoxide poisoning. N Engl J Med 347: 1057–1067.

Weaver LK, Valentine KJ, Hopkins RO (2007). Carbon monoxide poisoning: risk factors for cognitive sequelae and the role of hyperbaric oxygen. Am J Respir Crit Care Med 176: 491–497.

Weaver LK, Hopkins RO, Churchill S et al. (2008). Neurological outcomes 6 years after acute carbon monoxide poisoning. Undersea Hyperb Med 35: 258–259.

Wolf SJ, Lavonas EJ, Sloan EP et al. (2008). American College of Emergency Physicians. Critical issues in the management of adult patients presenting to the emergency department with acute carbon monoxide poisoning. Ann Emerg Med 51: 138–152.

Handbook of Clinical Neurology, Vol. 120 (3rd series)
Neurologic Aspects of Systemic Disease Part II
Jose Biller and Jose M. Ferro, Editors

Chapter 65

Lightning and thermal injuries

ARTHUR SANFORD AND RICHARD L. GAMELLI*
Department of Surgery, Loyola University Medical Center, Maywood, IL, USA

HISTORY (INCLUDING TERMINOLOGY)

Electrical injuries have become a more common problem in a society where we have come to depend on electricity for our everyday lives. Over 2 million burn injuries occur each year in the US; fortunately only 3% of these injuries are due to electricity or lightning. Most devastating are the electrical injuries from workplace accidents, because the victims are usually young, productive people with resulting significant functional losses. Areas of social disparity and "pirating" of electricity can cause even more unsafe conditions as amateurs try to steal electricity.

"Electrocution" is commonly used, incorrectly, to describe all electrical injuries. It actually means the stopping of life (determined by a stopped heart) by any type of electric shock. The term used throughout this chapter, "electrical injuries," describes both fatal and nonfatal consequences of conduction of electricity.

Electrical burns are classified as either high voltage (1000 volts and higher) or low voltage (<1000 volts). Most injuries in North America are caused by low voltage (110–240 volt), 60 cycles per second household alternating current electricity. High voltage injuries are usually only seen in industrial accidents or electrical company line workers.

Alternating current does not have a continuous flow of electrons from positive to negative terminals, so the terms entrance and exit wounds are not appropriate. A more precise term is contact point.

CLINICAL FINDINGS

The surface appearance of wounds is used to identify depth and subsequent need for further intervention. First-degree wounds are superficial, and reddened. They do not require surgical intervention and are generally treated with topical moisturizers and avoidance of recurrent injury. These would typically be from prolonged sun exposure without blisters. Their presence is not significant for ongoing fluid loss of a burn, but may represent an area requiring investigation for underlying electrical injury. Second-degree burns are deeper, causing a superficial edema deposition between deeper viable tissues and more superficial, injured tissues. The surface appearance is moist with blisters in various degrees of rupture. Treatment involves debridement of intact blisters at risk for rupture to remove the fluid, which contain high concentrations of thromboxanes and coverage with topical antimicrobial agents or synthetic wound dressings. The deeper elements of the skin remain intact and can regenerate the epithelial layer. Third-degree wounds are deeper and appear as whitened, black, or dry, leather-like skin. They require surgical debridement and skin grafting if larger than 2 cm. The term sometimes used to describe the massive destruction of soft tissue deep to the skin is a fourth-degree burn, one where subcutaneous fat, muscles, and even bones are injured. This is the typical injury with a high voltage electrical contact.

Evaluation of burn extent is an essential step in appropriate treatment of these injuries. Clinical examination and repeated operative intervention to debride devitalized tissue remains the most effective way to evaluate electrical burns.

There are reports of development of ocular cataracts over time following electrical injury, with incidence rates between 0.03% and 20% (Saffle et al., 1985; Boozalis et al., 1991). These are typically bilateral, and underscore the need for early examination and documentation at the time of injury to monitor development. The changes can be associated with burns even long periods of time after injury, mandating prolonged follow-up.

There are approximately 100 000 thunderstorms in the US each year, with more than 80 fatalities annually. Texas and Florida are the states with the most deaths,

*Correspondence to: Richard L. Gamelli, M.D., FACS, Dean, Stritch School of Medicine, Loyola University Chicago, 2160 South First Avenue, Maywood, IL 60153, USA. Tel: +1-708-216-8881, E-mail: rgamell@lumc.edu

resulting from a combination of the high frequency of storm and outdoor lifestyle exposing victims to risk of strike (Tribble et al., 1984; Hiestand and Colice, 1988; Centers for Disease Control and Prevention, 1998). Lightning strikes may conduct millions of volts of electricity, yet the effects can range from minimal cutaneous injuries to significant injury comparable to a high voltage industrial accident. Large surface area skin burns are unusual unless the strike involves a nearby object becoming incandescent with a flash/flame injury. A characteristic fern-like skin pattern on the skin (Lichtenberg figure) (ten Duis et al., 1987) that appears within an hour of strike injury and fades rapidly may be present as well as on the tips of toes (Fahmy et al., 1999). Lightning strikes commonly result in cardiorespiratory arrest, for which cardiopulmonary resuscitation (CPR) is effective when begun promptly (Moran et al., 1986). The ears of a lightning strike victim also need to be examined carefully as they can suffer from ruptured tympanic membranes or even middle and inner ear destruction (Bergstrom et al., 1974).

Neurologic complications of lightning injuries are also common and include unconsciousness, seizures, paresthesias, and paralysis which may not be present initially, but develop over several days postinjury. "Keraunoparalysis" is the term used to describe this delayed paralysis with vasomotor disorders. Some mood and personality changes can be seen as well. All of these effects are usually self-limiting and resolve spontaneously. Surgically treatable lesions including epidural, subdural, and intracerebral hematomas may occur, and should be investigated in a persistently altered patient (Hiestand and Colice, 1988). The prognosis for lightning-related neurologic injuries is generally better than for other types of traumatic causes, although subtle neurologic changes may persist, suggesting a conservative approach with serial neurologic examinations after an initial computed tomography (CT) scan to rule out correctable causes. Long-term follow-up for 12.3 years after injury showed no patients out of the 10 followed had long-term neurologic or psychological deficits (Muehlberger et al., 2001). The differences in long-term outcomes may better reflect the effectiveness of initial CPR than the sequelae of the injury itself (Purdue et al., 2007).

NATURAL HISTORY

Neurologic complications from electrical and lightning injuries are highly variable and may present early or late (up to 2 years) after the injury. Neuromuscular defects including paralysis, Guillain–Barré syndrome, transverse myelitis, or amyotrophic lateral sclerosis can be caused by electrical injury (Petty and Parkin, 1986). Review of 64 high-voltage electrical injury patients revealed 67% with immediate central or peripheral neurologic symptoms. One-third had peripheral neuropathies with one-third of

those persistent. Some 12% had delayed onset of peripheral neuropathy with 50% of those resolving. They reported no late onset, central neuropathies. Ko reported on 13 patients with delayed onset of spinal cord injuries, postulating a vascular cause of the deficit (Ko et al., 2004). The most common peripheral deficit is a peripheral neuropathy, with weakness being the most common clinical finding (Haberal et al., 1996). Typically, recovery from electrical injury neurologic symptoms is associated with a better prognosis if it is an early-onset lesion. There is more likely to be spasticity than flaccidity and function is more affected than sensation. Sympathetic overactivity is predominant with changes in bowel habits, and urinary and sexual dysfunction.

LABORATORY INVESTIGATIONS

Electrocardiographic monitoring of cardiac complications

Because of the potential to override the normal cardiac electrical activity, there is particular concern for cardiac dysrythmias. One of the most common complications of electrical injury is a cardiac dysrythmia. Ventricular fibrillation is the most common cause of death at the scene of an electrical injury. Resuscitation and treatment of dysrythmias are treated using the same algorithms as for medical causes. This can only reinforce the need for widespread education of the principles of CPR and use of defibrillators.

Direct myocardial injury may also result from electrical injury. This injury behaves more like a myocardial contusion than a true myocardial infarction, not having the hemodynamic or recurrence consequences of atherosclerotic myocardial infarctions. Housinger et al. have shown that creatine kinase (CK) and MB fraction creatine kinase (MB-CK) levels are poor indicators of myocardial injury in the absence of EKG findings of myocardial damage, especially in the presence of significant skeletal muscle injury (Housinger et al., 1985; McBride et al., 1986; Dilworth et al., 1998). Myocardial damage and arrhythmias are manifested very soon after injury (Purdue and Hunt, 1986). All patients should be monitored during transport and in the emergency room. Selective monitoring of those with early signs of cardiac involvement is the most effective use of resources (Purdue and Hunt, 1986; Arnoldo et al., 2004) (Table 65.1).

Myoglobinuria

Because of the potential for large volumes of muscle loss and the release of myoglobin, the presence of heme pigments in the urine must be evaluated promptly. Presence of these products of breakdown of myoglobin and hemoglobin puts the injured at risk for acute renal

Table 65.1

Indications for cardiac monitoring

- Documented cardiac arrest
- Cardiac dysrhythmia during transport or in the emergency room
- Abnormal EKG upon arrival to emergency room (other than sinus bradycardia or tachycardia)
- Burn size, patient age or other indications for monitoring

Table 65.2

Tissue resistance (lowest to highest)

- Nerve
- Blood vessels
- Muscle
- Skin
- Tendon
- Fat
- Bone

failure and must be cleared promptly. Urine dipsticks will pick up both free pigments and intact red blood cells (RBCs) in the urine, so confirmation with either a microscopic exam to exclude intact RBCs or serum electrophoresis to quantify and follow levels may be necessary. Once urine is grossly cleared, it can be assumed the pigments have been eliminated.

NEUROIMAGING INVESTIGATIONS

Radionuclide scanning with xenon-133 and technetium pyrophosphate has been shown to be accurate in predicting extent of tissue damage (Clayton et al., 1977; Hunt et al., 1979; Hammond and Ward, 1994). Hammond showed that scanning did not change the number of procedures or hospital length of stay using these techniques. Magnetic resonance imaging provides poor sensitivity for evaluation of injury in areas with compromised perfusion. Gadolinium-enhanced MR imaging demonstrates potential viability in zones of tissue edema and good correlation with histopathology (Fleckenstein et al., 1993; Lee, 1997; Ohashi et al., 1998). Imaging of electrical injuries is generally not productive, other than to follow progression of gross neurologic injuries in the central nervous system. Clinical examination best directs further workup, including neurologic imaging. In general, delays in treatment of obvious corporal injuries are not indicated while other studies are obtained.

PATHOLOGY

Severity of electrical injury and its consequences are determined by the properties of electricity and relative orientation of the victim. Voltage, current (amperage), type of current (alternating or direct), path of current flow across the body, resistance at the point of contact, duration of contact, and individual susceptibility all determine what final injury will occur. The amount of current flowing is related to both the voltage and the resistance of the body by Ohm's Law:

Current (I) = Voltage (E)/Resistance (R)

Animal experiments have shown that resistance varies continuously with time, initially dropping slowly, then much more rapidly until arcing occurs at contact points.

Resistance then rises to infinity and current flow ceases (Hunt et al., 1976). Tissue temperature rise is proportional to current flow. The electrical injury has the potential to injure via three mechanisms: injury caused by current flow, an arc injury as the current passes from source to an object, and a flame injury caused by ignition of material in the local environment. Different tissues have different resistance to the conduction of electricity (Table 65.2), but in an animal model, the body acts as a single uniform resistance.

Normal action potentials for cells and nerves are on the order of -80 to -120 millivolts (mV). When presented with significantly higher external voltages, these action potentials can become overwhelmed, resulting in loss of chemical gradients and ultimate cellular death as the cell is no longer able to release neurotransmitters or make adenosine triphosphate (ATP). Breakdown of cell membranes is one of the mechanisms by which cell damage can occur (Lee and Kolodney, 1987). As vascular endothelium injured along the path of the original current flow dies, there is a progressive vascular thrombosis and tissue loss that can progress for up to 1 week postinjury. This process of electroporation of cellular membranes may explain the injury not directly caused by heat (Lee et al., 1993).

The exact mechanism of nerve injury has not been explained, but both direct injury by electrical current overload or a vascular cause receive the most attention.

MANAGEMENT

Fluid resuscitation

Because electrical injuries carry both externally visible cutaneous injuries and possible hidden musculoskeletal damage, conventional burn resuscitation formulas based on body surface area injured may not provide enough fluid to maintain urine output. Venous access is best obtained via two large bore peripheral IVs, although alternate methods are sometime necessary, such as central access, venous cutdowns, or interosseous infusions. Delay in administration of resuscitation has been shown to have a direct negative correlation with survival (Rockwall and Ehrlich, 1992). In the absence of gross myoglobinuria, the goal of fluid resuscitation is to maintain normal vital signs and urine output of 30–50 cc/hour. This is done with Lactated Ringer's solution at rates adjusted hourly.

Evaluation of peripheral circulation after circumferential or electrical burns to the extremities is an often overlooked aspect of the successful resuscitative efforts. Damaged muscle resulting in swelling within the investing fascia of an extremity may increase the compartmental pressures to where perfusion of the muscle is compromised. Initially restriction of venous outflow due to edema leads to increased compartmental pressures and collapse of the capillaries with ultimate loss of arterial pulse, which can only be relieved by escharotomy or fasciotomy. An extremity that does not seem tight on first evaluation is still at risk of becoming compromised as edema accumulates with resuscitation. Previously, aggressive fasciotomies have been advocated, but some studies suggest that a more conservative approach, waiting for development of clinical signs of deterioration, has been proposed (Mann et al., 1996).

Myoglobinuria clearance

Once myoglobin has been detected in the urine, treatment is aggressively initiated. Aggressive volume loading to increase urine outputs above 1–2 cc/kg/hour is the first step. Protocols where 12.5–25 g mannitol is given IV push are common. Consideration is also given to administration of sodium bicarbonate in the intravenous fluids. The rationale is to create a rapid, osmotic diuresis with possible alkalinization of the urine to minimize pigment precipitation in the renal tubules. Loop diuretics are not as efficient as mannitol in clearing the myoglobin from the urine.

Associated trauma

The initial step in any burn resuscitation follows the ABCs of trauma management. First the airway must be secured, depending on the patient's level of ability to protect his or her airway. Then the caregiver must ascertain pulmonary and circulatory competence. It is possible to suffer phrenic nerve damage with an electrical injury, raising concern for loss of function in one or both hemidiaphragms. Approximately 15% of electrical burn victims also sustain traumatic injuries. This is because of falls from height or being thrown against an object. The tetanic contractions that result from exposure to electrical injury cause imbalance in flexor versus extensor muscles, with the flexor groups being stronger. Not only is the victim unable to release from the electrical contact, but they are at risk for fracture of bones from this prolonged muscular contracture (Layton et al.,

1984). A thorough history and physical examination will identify those who need a full trauma evaluation.

Abdominal wounds provide the potential for internal injuries both directly under contact points and as a result of later ischemic necrosis (Newsome et al., 1972; Reilley et al., 1985). Depending on the current path, the bowel may be injured, so caution is warranted in the usual aggressive pattern of enteral feeding common to isolated cutaneous burns. Any deterioration in clinical examination mandates laparotomy. Once deemed appropriate, the provision of adequate calories and the replacement of large protein losses are the central tenets of support. Parenteral nutrition is to be avoided in burn patients secondary to metabolic and immunologic complications (Herndon et al., 1987; Herndon et al., 1989). Current recommendations are to have 20–40% of the calories as protein, 10–20% of the calories as fat, and 40–70% of the calories as carbohydrate (Waymack and Herndon, 1992), with supplementation of arginine, glutamine, and general vitamins and minerals (Currei et al., 1974).

Early excision and wound care

Assessment of the burn wound to determine what areas will require excision is the first step in planning for early excision or conservative treatment. If initial attempts at clearing gross myoglobinuria are unsuccessful, or with a persistent metabolic acidosis, then immediate operative debridement is needed. It is also possible that swelling of an extremity has induced a compartment syndrome that requires fasciotomy. Symptoms of median nerve dysfunction also merit immediate carpal tunnel and possibly Guyton's tunnel release. In general, serial explorations and repeat debridements are performed starting at post-injury day 3–5 and repeated at 24–48 hour intervals to try and preserve as much viable tissue as possible. Wound excision can be done either with electrocautery to fascia, and the resulting cosmetic deformity, or tangentially with serial "shavings" of the wound using dermatomes or covered blades (and increased blood loss if a tourniquet cannot be used). Muscle compartments should be opened if there is any concern clinically about involvement, keeping in mind that muscle groups closest to bone carry the highest risk of injury as the adjacent bone heats when current passes through an extremity. In order to minimize operating time and blood loss at initial operations, primary amputations are not performed, except in the presence of a mummified extremity. Grossly infected wounds, or with persistent nonviable tissue at time of presentation, require special treatment, with early excision still stressed, but complete coverage is first done with cadaver allograft to prepare the wound bed and not risk the loss of autograft to infection. Cadaveric allograft skin is an effective biological dressing, shown to prevent evaporative water loss, reduce pain, and reduce the density of bacteria on a wound (Shuck et al., 1969). Porcine and amphibian xenografts are also proposed biological dressings, but their application is limited by inability to control bacterial proliferation (Ersek and Denton, 1984).

Topical antimicrobials are used to control bacterial overgrowth and prevent invasive infection in contaminated wounds until autografting can be completed. The three commonly used agents are silver sulfadiazine (Silvadine®), mafenide acetate (Sulfamylon®), and 0.5% silver nitrate solution. Unexcised eschar is usually over deeper injury at contact points, so the penetration ability of mafenide acetate makes it the most useful agent.

Low-voltage, high-amperage electricity, as found in automotive electrical systems, can result in both direct injury and thermal injury. The electricity can turn a ring, wristwatch, bracelet, or necklace incandescent, resulting in a deep circumferential thermal burn. These are treated in the same manner as a thermal burn (Manstein et al., 1987). Low-voltage alternating current injury is usually localized to the points of contact, although deeper structures may be damaged with prolonged contact. These wounds are treated by excision to viable tissue and covered with skin grafts based on wound depth and location. An exception is burns to the oral commisure that result typically from young children chewing on an electrical cord. These injuries are treated conservatively (D'Italia and Hunlick, 1984; Leake and Curtin, 1984), but carry the risk of significant bleeding from the labial artery when the eschar separates at 5–10 days postinjury. Nonoperative treatment is usually adequate, but the scars are hard to splint with only one side of the mouth injured and the other supple and unable to support cross-mouth splinting.

Wound care and surgical debridement is best done using general anesthetic agents and intravenous analgesia because of the risk of developing later neurologic symptoms that cannot be differentiated from the original injury in origin.

Rehabilitation

An ongoing program of physical therapy and functional splinting is begun upon arrival and continued throughout the hospitalization. Early splinting combined with pressure garments reduces the formation of joint contractures. Frequent and vigorous physical therapy is important to maintain joint mobility, but has also been implicated in the formation of heterotopic ossification where the trauma to tendons can lead to scarring and abnormal bone formation. Pressure garments appear to cause the collagen in a wound to orient in such a way as to become smoother, flatter, and mature more

quickly, and studies are underway to evaluate how much pressure is needed, and for how long.

While the effects of a high-voltage electrical injury may be obvious with massive soft tissue loss, there are still a significant number of problems associated with low-voltage injuries. In a long-term follow-up of 38 patients, neurologic (81.6%) and psychological (71%) symptoms were the most common sequelae. The most frequent neurologic symptoms were numbness (42%), weakness (32%), memory problems (32%), paresthesias (24%), and chronic pain (24%). The most common psychological symptoms were anxiety (50%), nightmares (45%), insomnia (37%), and flashbacks (37%) of the event. Patients with more neurologic symptoms were found to have more psychological symptoms. Many of these symptoms are nonspecific, and they often do not appear until several months after the injury (Singerman et al., 2008).

Psychologically, these patients have varied responses to electrical injuries. In a study comparing electrical injury patients to noninjured electricians, Pliskin showed significantly higher cognitive, physical, and emotional complaints not related to injury or litigation status (Pliskin et al., 1998). A full neurologic examination must be performed on admission, documenting initial presentation, and at any change in symptoms. Consistent long-term follow-up with repeated examinations by the same practitioner becomes important. Electrodiagnostic examination may be helpful to determine the extent of persistent deficits. Early involvement of a physiatrist and therapy team to formulate a plan of rehabilitation facilitates long-term recovery. Despite optimal medical management, only about 50% of even low voltage electrical injury patients will return to their own preinjury occupation (Theman et al., 2008).

CONCLUSIONS (INCLUDING FUTURE DIRECTIONS)

Electrical injuries can have devastating consequences, particularly among the populations at risk, productive and vigorous workers, but also among increasing populations as our world comes to depend more and more on electricity. Prevention of electrical injuries is clearly the preferred strategy for treatment. Once the initial damage is done, the potential for rehabilitation and recovery is possible with support and through follow-up.

REFERENCES

Arnoldo BD, Purdue GF, Kowalske K et al. (2004). Electrical injuries: a 20-year review. J Burn Care Rehabil 25: 479–484.
Bergstrom L, Neblet LM, Sando I et al. (1974). The lightning damaged ear. Arch Otolaryngol 100: 117–121.

Boozalis GT, Purdue GF, Hunt JL et al. (1991). Ocular changes from electrical burn injuries A literature review and report of cases. J Burn Care Rehabil 12: 458–462.

Centers for Disease Control and Prevention (CDC) (1998). Lightning associated deaths – United States, 1980–1995. MMWR Morb Mortal Wkly Rep 19: 391–394.

Clayton JM, Hayes AC, Hammel J et al. (1977). Xenon-133 determination of muscle blood flow in electrical injury. J Trauma 17: 293–298.

Currei PW, Richmond D, Marvin J et al. (1974). Dietary requirements of patients with major burns. J Am Diet Assoc 65: 415.

D'Italia JG, Hunlick SJ (1984). Outpatient management of electric burns of the lip. J Burn Care Rehabil 5: 465–466.

Dilworth D, Hasan D, Alford P et al. (1998). Evaluation of myocardial injury in electrical burn patients. J Burn Care Rehabil 19: S239.

Ersek RA, Denton DR (1984). Silver-impregnated porcine xenografts for treatment of meshed autografts. Ann Plast Surg 13: 482.

Fahmy FS, Brinsden MD, Smith J et al. (1999). Lightning: the multisystem group injuries. J Trauma 46: 937–940.

Fleckenstein JL, Chason DP, Bonte FJ et al. (1993). High voltage electric injury: assessment of muscle viability with MR imaging and Tc-99 m pyrophosphate scintigraphy. Radiology 195: 205–210.

Haberal MA, Gureu S, Akman N et al. (1996). Persistent peripheral nerve pathologies in patients with electric burns. J Burn Care Rehabil 17: 147–149.

Hammond J, Ward CG (1994). The use of technetium-99 pyrophosphate scanning in management of high voltage electrical injuries. Am Surg 68: 886–888.

Herndon DN, Stein MD, Rutan TC et al. (1987). Failure of TPN supplementation to improve liver function, immunity, and mortality in thermally injured patients. J Trauma 27: 195.

Herndon DN, Barrow RE, Stein M et al. (1989). Increased mortality with intravenous supplemental feeding in severely burned patients. J Burn Care Rehabil 10: 309.

Hiestand D, Colice GL (1988). Lightning strike injury. J Intensive Care 3: 303–314.

Housinger TA, Green L, Shahangian S et al. (1985). A prospective study of myocardial damage in electrical injuries. J Trauma 25: 122–124.

Hunt JL, Mason AD, Masterson TS et al. (1976). The pathophysiology of acute electrical burns. J Trauma 16: 335–340.

Hunt J, Lewis S, Parkey R et al. (1979). The use of technetium-^{99m} stannous pyrophosphate scintigraphy to identify muscle damage in acute electric burns. J Trauma 19: 409–413.

Ko SH, Chun W, Kim HC (2004). Delayed spinal cord injury following electrical burns: a 7-year experience. Burns 30: 691–695.

Layton TR, McMurtry JM, McClain EJ et al. (1984). Multiple spine fractures from electric injury. J Burn Care Rehabil 5: 373–375.

Leake JE, Curtin JW (1984). Electrical burns of the mouth in children. Clin Plast Surg 11: 669–683.

Lee RC (1997). Injury by electrical forces: pathophysiology, manifestations, and therapy. Curr Probl Surg 34: 738–740.

Lee RC, Kolodney SB (1987). Electrical injury mechanisms: electrical breakdown of cell membranes. Plast Reconstr Surg 80: 672–680.

Lee RC, Canaday DJ, Hammer SM (1993). Transient and stable ionic permeabilization of isolated skeletal muscle cells after electrical shock. J Burn Care Rehabil 14: 528–540.

Mann R, Gibran N, Engrav L et al. (1996). Is immediate decompression of high voltage electrical injuries to the upper extremity always necessary? J Trauma 40: 584–589.

Manstein CM, Manstein ME, Manstein G (1987). Circumferential electric burns of the ring finger. J Hand Surg 12A: 808.

McBride JW, Labrosse KR, McCoy HG et al. (1986). Is serum creatine kinase MB in electrically injured patients predictive of myocardial injury? JAMA 255: 764–768.

Moran KT, Thupari JN, Munster AM (1986). Electric- and lightning-induced cardiac arrest reversed by prompt cardiopulmonary resuscitation. JAMA 255: 2157.

Muehlberger T, Vogt PM, Munster AM (2001). The long-term consequences of lightning injuries. Burns 27: 829–833.

Newsome TW, Currei PW, Kurenius K (1972). Visceral injuries – an unusual complication of an electrical burn. Arch Surg 105: 494–497.

Ohashi M, Kozumi J, Hosoda Y et al. (1998). Correlation between magnetic resonance imaging and histopathology of an amputated forearm after electrical injury. Burns 24: 362–368.

Petty PG, Parkin G (1986). Electrical injury to the central nervous system. Neurosurgery 19: 282–284.

Pliskin NH, Capelli-Schellpfeffer M, Law RT et al. (1998). Neuropsychological symptom presentation after electrical injury. J Trauma 44: 709–715.

Purdue GF, Hunt JL (1986). Electrocardiographic monitoring after electrical injury: necessity or luxury. J Trauma 26: 166–167.

Purdue GF, Arnoldo BD, Hunt JL (2007). Electrical injuries. In: DN Herndon (Ed.), Total Burn Care. Saunders Elsevier, Philadelphia, pp. 513–520.

Reilley AF, Rees R, Kelton P et al. (1985). Abdominal aortic occlusion following electric injury. J Burn Care Rehabil 6: 226–229.

Rockwall WB, Ehrlich HP (1992). Reversible burn injury. J Burn Care Rehabil 13: 403–406.

Saffle JR, Crandall A, Warden GD (1985). Cataracts: a long-term complication of electrical injury. J Trauma 25: 17–21.

Shuck JM, Pruitt BA Jr, Moncrief JA (1969). Homograft skin for wound coverage. Arch Surg 98: 472.

Singerman J, Gomez M, Fish JS (2008). Long-term sequelae of low-voltage electrical injury. J Burn Care Res 29: 773–777.

ten Duis HJ, Klasen HJ, Nijsten MWN (1987). Superficial lightning injuries – their "fractal" shape origin. Burns 13: 141–146.

Theman K, Singerman J, Gomez M et al. (2008). Return to work after low voltage electrical injury. J Burn Care Res 29: 959–964.

Tribble CG, Pershing JA, Morgan RF et al. (1984). Lightning injury. Curr Concept Trauma Care Spring 5–10.

Waymack JP, Herndon DN (1992). Nutritional support of the burn patient. World J Surg 16: 80.

Handbook of Clinical Neurology, Vol. 120 (3rd series)
Neurologic Aspects of Systemic Disease Part II
Jose Biller and Jose M. Ferro, Editors

Chapter 66

Venomous snake bites, scorpions, and spiders

S.A.M. KULARATNE* AND NIMAL SENANAYAKE

Department of Medicine, Faculty of Medicine, University of Peradeniya, Kandy, Sri Lanka

INTRODUCTION

Historical background

Of approximately 2700 described species of snakes in the world, 500 are venomous, mainly distributed in warm tropical regions (Chippaux, 2006). Species of scorpions and spiders number 600 and 30 000, respectively (Senanayake and Roman, 1992). Many other venomous creatures potentially dangerous to people exist in the environment, including insects (Hymenoptera), paralytic ticks, centipedes (Chilopoda), caterpillars, cone snails, shellfish, puffer fish, jellyfish, fish with ciguatoxins, and poisonous frogs. The destructive power of snakes caused serpents to be associated with the divine in most ancient cultures, and the neuroparalysis caused by the venom of the Egyptian cobra (*Naja haje*) was believed to have brought about the instantaneous death of queen Cleopatra (Chippaux, 2006). From the Middle Ages and Renaissance onwards, scientific thinking began to come to the fore, and Leoniceno Nicolo (1428–1524), a Greek scholar and Italian physician, studied herpetology and the toxicology of snake bites (Adler and Louis, 2007). At the end of the 19th century, Albert Calmette developed the concept of antivenom, which remains the treatment for envenomation by the bite or sting of venomous creatures (Calmette, 1907). Evolutionarily, snakes (the Squamata) can be traced to the middle of the Cretaceous period more than 100 million years ago. They originated in the ancient southern continent of Gondwana and their dispersal to the north could be explained by continental drift and ice ages that created land bridges (Holman, 2000; Ivanov et al., 2000; Pook et al., 2009).

Venom apparatus

Snakes can be classified into more than 15 families, with venomous snakes belonging to the Viperidae, Elapidae, Colubridae, and Atractaspididae families (Wuster and McCarthy, 1996; Chippaux, 2006). The venomous snakes posses a venom apparatus which is a complex device consisting of a specialized gland that synthesizes venom and a fang which injects the venom on bite. Depending on the position of the fang on the maxilla and the dentition, the snakes are further classified into four groups: aglyphous (fangless), opisthoglyphous (back-fanged), proteroglyphous (front-fanged), and solenoglyphous (mobile front-fanged) (De Silva, 1980; Chippaux, 2006). The terminal segment of a scorpion's tail, called the telson, contains two venom glands connecting with a curved, needle-sharp sting, whilst spiders have a pair of horny fangs (chelicerae) among their mouth parts (Brownell and Polis, 2001; Sutherland and Tibballs, 2001; White, 2008). Among the insects, bees inject venom through a barbed sting which gets embedded and remains in the skin of the victim, but wasps and hornets carry modified ovipositors used for repeated stinging (Imms, 1939; Fitzgerald and Flood, 2006).

Venom

Snake venom is a complex mixture of proteins that can be divided into two groups, the enzymes and the toxins. The enzymes are proteins which are generally high in molecular weight. These most often act on blood coagulation, compliment activation, and cause cytolysis and activation of metabolism. The venoms of the Viperidae are particularly rich in enzymes. Examples of enzymes that act on the nervous system are phospholipase A2 and acetylcholinesterase (AChE) (Ahmed et al., 2009; Robin et al., 2010). The toxins, on the other hand, have variable molecular weights, generally less than 30 kDa. These have the ability to bind to specific receptors on membranes of different anatomical sites including the nervous system, the cardiovascular system,

*Correspondence to: S.A.M. Kularatne, Professor, Department of Medicine, Faculty of Medicine, University of Peradeniya, Kandy, Sri Lanka. E-mail: samkul@sltnet.lk

and muscle. The venoms of Elapidae are particularly rich in toxins (Chippaux, 2006; Mebs, 2008). Scorpion venom contains peptides capable of a variety of actions, whilst spider venoms are usually complex mixtures of substances, with the most potent neuroexcitatory toxins (White, 2008). The venom of the Hymenoptera contains mainly biogenic amines (histamine, 5-hydroxytryptamine, dopamine, noradrenaline, and acetylcholine (ACh)) and also some enzymes and toxins (Schmidt, 1995). The toxins in venom affecting the functions of the nervous system are referred to as neurotoxins (Table 66.1).

PATHOPHYSIOLOGY OF ENVENOMING

Effects of venom on the nervous system

From an evolutionary point of view, neurotoxins would be considered a hunting device, used in rapid immobilization of a prey. However, in clinical situations of envenoming, onset and progression of neurotoxicity is highly variable. A good knowledge of the structure and function of the nervous system is required to understand the mechanism of neurotoxic manifestations. The nervous signal is propagated along the nerve by means of

Table 66.1

Neurotoxins, their sources and mechanisms of action

Source	Toxin	Action
Snake venom		
Elapidae		
Cobra	α-toxin, cobrotoxin	Postsynaptic
Krait		Presynaptic, except *Bungarus multicinctus* which has both α- and
	β-bungarotoxin	κ-bungarotoxin
Mamba	*Dendrotoxin, [†]fasciculins, muscarines	*Presynaptic, increases ACh, [†]ACh-esterase, muscarine receptors
Coral snake	α- neurotoxin	Postsynaptic
Australian elapids	Taipoxin, notexin, both α- and β-bungarotoxins	Presynaptic and postsynaptic
Sea snakes	Erabutoxins, phospholipase A2	Presynaptic, myotoxic
Viperidae	Vipoxin, phospholipase A2	Pre- and postsynaptic
Daboia russelii		? adrenergic receptor
Rattlesnake	Crotoxin, crotamine	Postsynaptic, myotoxic
Scorpion venom		
All scorpions	More toxins and less enzymes	Increase autonomic activity
Tityus	Tityustoxin	Pre-/postsynaptic, increases Na$^+$ permeability
Mesobuthus tamulus	α and β scorpion toxins, mixture	Na$^+$/K$^+$ channels, autonomic storm
Hemiscorpion lepturus		Autonomic storm
Centruroides	Toxins on Na$^+$ channels	Presynaptic and axonal membrane
Spider venom		
All venomous spiders	Neuroexcitotory toxins	Increase autonomic/somatic transmission
Latrodectus	α-latrotoxin	Presynaptic – increase neurotransmission
Australian funnel-web	Atracotoxins	Voltage-gated Na^{++} channels
Hymenoptera venom		
Apidae	Apitoxins, mellitin, apamin, etc.	Mild effect
Vespidae	Mandaratoxins	?Pre- and postsynaptic
Tick venom		
Ixodidae	Salivary toxins	Presynaptic (terminal part of motor nerve fiber)
Argasidae		
Ciguatera		
Barracuda, grouper, red snapper, amber jack	Ciguatoxin from *Gambierdiscus toxicus*	Presynaptic (Na$^+$ channels of axonal membrane) and ?postsynaptic

Table 66.1

Continued

Source	Toxin	Action
Shellfish	Saxitoxin	Presynaptic (Na^+ channels of axonal
	Brevitoxin	membrane)
Pufferfish, porcupinefish, king crab, goby, newt, octopus, frog venom, etc.	Tetrodotoxin	Presynaptic (Na^+ channels of axonal membrane)
Frog venom	Batrachotoxin, histrionicotoxin, pumiliotoxin B	Presynaptic (Na^+ channels of axonal membrane), postsynaptic
Cone snail venom	Conotoxin	Postsynaptic, presynaptic (Na^+ channels of axonal membrane)
Bacterial toxins		
Clostridium botulinum	Botulinum toxin	Presynaptic
C. tetani	Tetanus toxin	Presynaptic

depolarization of the cell membrane. The depolarization travels from one nerve to another or from nerve to muscle across a synapse resulting in contraction of the muscle. The synapse in the neuromuscular junction (NMJ) is a complex structure in which a fine balance exists between the release of the chemical neuromediator ACh and its inactivating enzyme AChE (Estable, 1959).

The neuron, at rest, has a difference in the electrical potential on the two sides of the cell membrane. A stimulus causes depolarization of the nerve by means of releasing potassium out of the cell and an inward flux of sodium through specific voltage-dependent ion channels. The resultant nervous signal propagates along the axon in the form of a wave called the action potential. The synapse presents itself as an interruption between two neurons or between a neuron and the muscle. Thus, synapse consists of presynaptic terminal/membrane, synaptic cleft/gap and postsynaptic terminal/membrane. On arrival of an impulse, ACh is released from the vesicles of presynaptic terminal to the synaptic cleft, establishing contact with the cholinergic receptors on the postsynaptic membrane. The receptor in turn activates the sodium and potassium ion channels allowing propagation of the action potential. Two types of cholinergic receptors have been identified by their response to transmitter substances. Of these, nicotinic receptors are found in the ganglia, the NMJ of skeletal muscles, medulla of the adrenal gland, and some areas of the brain and the spinal cord. Muscarinic receptors are widely distributed in the brain and in the ganglia of the parasympathetic nervous system. After activation of the cholinergic receptor, ACh is hydrolyzed by the enzyme AChE in the synaptic gap, making the receptor free for the next action. Certain other neurotransmitters, such as GABA, noradrenaline,

adrenaline, dopamine and γ-aminobutyrate, also exist in the nervous system, but their involvement in neurotoxic snake envenoming is poorly understood. However, these neurotransmitters are thought to play an important role in scorpion, spider and mollusc envenomation (Ganong, 1999; Chippaux, 2006).

Neurotoxins

Neurotoxins are classified into four groups according to their site and mode of action (Fig. 66.1).

POSTSYNAPTIC TOXINS (α-TOXINS AND κ-TOXINS)

Examples of postsynaptic neurotoxins are α-bungarotoxins in Chinese krait (*Bungarus multicinctus*), cobrotoxins in many cobra species such as *Naja haja, N. kaouthia, N. naja, N. nigrecollis*, and sea snake venom, for example, laticotoxin in *L. laticaudata* and hydrophitoxin in *Hydrophis cyanocinctus.* They comprise of 60–62 or 66–74 amino acids (Chippaux, 2006).

α-Toxins are three-finger protein complexes and act in the same way as curare, an alkaloid extracted from strychnous, a Central and South American plant used as arrow-poisons by the native inhabitants (Senanayake and Roman, 1992; Chippaux, 2006; Del Brutto and Del Brutto, 2011). Nearly 150 years ago, Claude Bernard's experiments showed that the crude extracts of curare were highly specific in interruption of electrical signals between nerve and muscle. Subsequent investigations have used curare as a ligand for binding studies on the nicotine ACh receptor (AChR) (Estable, 1959; Senanayake and Roman, 1992). The α-neurotoxins have a stronger affinity to the nicotinic ACh in the NMJ than others. Irditoxins are the best characterized α-neurotoxins (Del Brutto and Del Brutto, 2011).

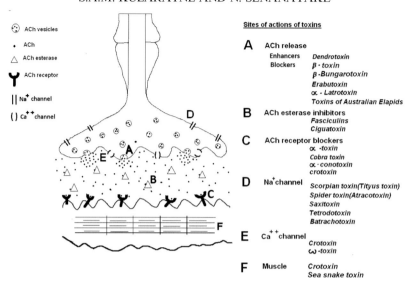

Fig. 66.1. Site of action of toxins in neuromuscular transmission.

In contrast, κ- neurotoxins have a high affinity to the cells of the parasympathetic (ciliary ganglia) and sympathetic lumbar ganglia. They have less pronounced effects on the central nicotinic receptors such as cervical ganglia, retinal ganglia, cerebellum, and corpus striatum (Grant and Chiappinelli, 1985; Dewan et al., 1994). The venom of many banded kraits, particularly Chinese krait (*Bungarus multicinctus*), contains both α- and κ-bungarotoxins (Lee, 1972; Dewan et al., 1994).

Other postsynaptic neurotoxins are adrenergic toxins and muscarinic toxins, the latter being found in African mamba venom. The first protein toxins that bind to muscarinic ACh receptors (mAChRs) were isolated from the venom of African green mamba (*Dendroaspis angusticeps*) (Adem et al., 1988). Some unclassifiable toxins, such as vipoxin from *Daboia russelii,* which do not act on either nicotinic or muscarinic receptors, but may be on adrenergic receptors, have also been isolated (Chippaux, 2006).

PRESYNAPTIC TOXINS (β-TOXIN)

These toxins, present in the venom of many elapids and certain viperids, act by inhibiting the release of ACh from the presynaptic nerve terminal, e.g., β-bungarotoxin, crotoxin, taipoxin, paradoxyn, trimucrotoxin, viperotoxin, pseudocerastes, and textilotoxin, which contains 120–140 amino acids and phospholipase A subunit. These toxins consist of one, two, or four subunits and have in common a phospholipase-like action that is necessary for their toxic activity (Chippaux, 2006; Robin et al., 2010; Del Brutto and Del Brutto, 2011). Of these, β-bungarotoxin (e.g., venom of kraits) acts on the voltage-dependent potassium channel, while crotoxin (venom of South American rattlesnakes, e.g.,

Crotalus durissus terrificus) binds to a not yet identified protein membrane (Chippaux, 2006; Doley et al., 2010). The progressive blockage of ACh release under the action of β-toxins occurs in three stages. The first stage is independent of phospholipase action, but in the third stage catalytic activity of phopholipase causes definitive arrest of ion exchange and damage to nerve terminal (Seu et al., 1976). The phospholipase activity is high in marine and Australian elapids that cause muscle necrosis and myoglobinuria (Doley et al., 2010). The venoms of *Dendroaspis* have calciseptin and calcicludin acting on calcium channels that can be included in this group (Chippaux, 2006; Hedge et al., 2009).

PRESYNAPTIC FACILITATING TOXINS AND FASCICULINS

These facilitate the release of ACh from presynaptic terminal and are extremely potent, causing paralysis. Dendrotoxins that fall into this category have an elevated affinity to certain voltage-dependent potassium channels. The victim develops convulsions leading to respiratory paralysis (Chippaux, 2006). Fasciculins are small proteins found in the venoms of mambas (*Dendroaspis*; family Elapidae) which inhibit acetylcholinesterase and prevent destruction of ACh in the synaptic gap leading to repeated depolarization of the postsynaptic membrane. The victim develops muscle fasciculation and contraction. This effect is somewhat reversible with atropine (Chippaux, 2006; Harvey, 2010).

SNAKE ENVENOMING

Epidemiology

Snake envenoming is an important problem worldwide, mainly in Southeast Asia, sub-Saharan Africa, Central and South America, Australia and even in the US (Kasturiratne et al., 2008). In 1998, an appraisal of the global situation regarding snake bites estimated that worldwide there were 5 million snake bites with 125 000 deaths (Chippaux, 1998), and in 2008, a similar attempt estimated that the global burden of snake envenoming was, at a minimum, 421 000 envenomings and 20 000 deaths (Kasturiratne et al., 2008). Being a neglected tropical problem, lack of accurate data from many regions has made these estimates questionable. Australia records approximately 1000–1500 snake bites, 150 envenomings, and two to four deaths annually (White, 2010). Conversely, sub-Saharan Africa estimates that there are more than 1 million bites and 25,000 deaths per year (Chippaux, 2010). The estimates from South Asia record the highest burden of snake envenoming, ranging from 121 333 to 463 550 annually (Kasturiratne et al., 2008). In Sri Lanka, hospital records show approximately 40 000 snake bites and 100 deaths annually (Kularatne, 2001).

Elapidae

Among the venomous snake families, the Elapidae family consists of cobras, kraits, mambas, coral snakes, and Australian elapids, whose venom is rich in neurotoxins. They have unfoldable anterior fangs (proteroglyphous).

COBRAS

In cobras, the genus *Naja* has 18 species spread over Africa and Asia. The principal African species are *N. haje* in deserts, *N. nigricollis* in savannas, *N. melanoleuca* in forests, and *N. mossambica* (Chippaux, 2010). Over the whole of Asia, 10 subspecies of *Naja* are recognized; of these, four are found in India (Wuster, 1998b). The *Naja naja* or spectacled cobra is found in India, Pakistan, Sri Lanka, and Bangladesh (Wuster, 1998b; Kularatne, 2009). *N. kaouthia* or the monocellate cobra, is found in northeastern India, Bangladesh, Malaysia, southern Vietnam, and China. Other Indian *Naja* include *N. oxiana* (northern India) and *N. sagittifera* (Andaman cobra) (Wuster, 1998b). The spitting cobras include the Indo-Chinese spitting cobra (*N. siamensis*), the Sumatran spitting cobra (*N. sumatrana*), *N. sputatrix*, and *N. mandalayensis* (Warrell, 2010b). The king cobra (*Ophiophagus hannah*) is found in Myanmar, Thailand, and India and the venom is strongly neurotoxic (Warrell, 2010b). Most cobras are generally diurnal and they live close to human dwellings, in agricultural fields and water courses where prey is easy to find. Postsynaptic toxins are the main lethal principle in cobra venom. The clinical manifestations vary with the species, *Naja philippinensis* being an example causing severe neurotoxicty with mild local reactions. The muscle paralysis is typical of the myasthenic syndrome and repetitive nerve

stimulation shows a decrement abolished by edrophonium (Watt et al., 1998). The bite of the spectacled cobra (*Naja naja*), on the other hand, causes severe local reaction leading to spreading necrosis and gangrene; only 36% of victims developed neurotoxicity which had rapid onset leading to respiratory failure in 2 hours (Kularatne, 2009). Spitting cobras spit venom into eyes of victims causing venom ophthalmia manifested as keratoconjuctivitis and occasional cranial nerve palsies (Chu et al., 2010).

KRAITS

Kraits (*Bungarus*) are distributed through Asia and they consist of 12 species of which the principal ones are *B. candidus* or Malayan krait, *B. fasciatus* or banded krait, *B. caeruleus* or common krait, *B. multicinctus* or Chinese krait, and *B. niger* or greater black krait (Chippaux, 2006; Warrell, 2010b). Of these, the common krait, *B. caeruleus*, is found in Sri Lanka, Bangladesh, India, and Pakistan. It is reputed to be the deadliest in Sri Lanka (Kularatne, 2001). Krait venom contains β-bungarotoxin, a presynaptic blocker which causes muscle paralysis as the sole clinical manifestation. The common krait is a nocturnal terrestrial snake living close to human dwellings and the bites happen mostly at night where people sleep on the floor in mud huts. Very often the victims are unaware of the bite. Abdominal pain and progressive muscle paralysis occurs, causing respiratory failure in about 50% of cases. The level of consciousness deteriorates and some patients develop a deep comatose state similar to brain death. They may still recover with the help of assisted ventilation (Kularatne, 2001; Gawarammana, 2010). The observation of GABA release and production of deep coma in animal experiments with β-bungarotoxins (Wernicke, 1975), and binding of α-bungarotoxins to hippocampal interneurons in experimental studies (Freedman, 1993) are some explanations to support the mechanism of changing sensorium in krait bite. Hypokalemia is yet another problem (Kularatne, 2001; Gawarammana, 2010). Even after recovery from the effects of acute envenoming, a few patients develop lasting neurologic deficits such as peripheral neuropathy with delayed nerve conduction, ulnar nerve palsies, sensory deficits at the local site, and even cerebellar ataxia (Kularatne, 2001). The damaging effects of neurotoxins and their effects on nicotinic receptors in the brain and the involvement κ-toxins and receptors should be considered to explain these wide arrays of neurologic problems. In krait envenoming the mortality can be high when intensive care facilities are limited and anticholinesterases showed no benefit in reversing the paralysis (Sethi and Rastogi, 1981; Theakston et al., 1990). Similar to common kraits, *B. candidus* also bites victims in their sleep and *B. fasciatus* frequents rice paddies at night and inflicts bites (Chippaux, 2006).

MAMBAS

The mamba (*Dendroaspis*) is an arboreal snake in Africa and the genus consists of four species: the green mambas (*D. angusticeps, D. jamesoni, D. viridis*) and the black mamba (*D. polylepis*). The venom contains phospholipases, dendrotoxins, fasciculins, and α-neurotoxins commonly enhancing nervous transmission (Chippaux, 2006, 2010). The mamba bite causes painful local inflammation. Neurologic manifestations include muscarine-like features such as sweating, lacrimation, disturbed vision, abdominal pain, diarrhea and vomiting. Rapid onset of respiratory paralysis can kill the victim (Harvey and Anderson, 1985; Chippaux, 2006).

CORAL SNAKES

The genus *Micrurus* (coral snake) consists of 64 species distributed in Central and South America. The species responsible for the majority of coral snake bites is *M. nigrocinctus* which often bites fingers of the victim during handling (Gutierrez, 1995; Chippaux, 2010). The bites are not frequent and the venom contains postsynaptic α-neurotoxins which have a high affinity to the cholinergic receptors at the motor endplate (Chippaux, 2010; Gutierrez, 2010). Muscle paralysis sets in within several hours and it can last up to 2 weeks. This postsynaptic defect is not corrected by edrophonium (Pettigrew and Glass, 1985; Gutierrez, 2010).

AUSTRALIAN ELAPIDS

Australia contains a diverse array of snakes, with a predominance of elapids, and their bite causes neurotoxic paralysis, myolysis, coagulopathy, renal failure, and microangiopathic hemolytic anemia. These snakes are classified under five major groups: brown snake (*Pseudonaja* spp.), tiger snake (*Notechis* spp.), black snake (*Pseudechis* spp.), death adder (*Acanthophis* spp.), and taipan (*Oxyuranus* spp.) consisting 29 species of snakes (White, 2010).). Of these, brown snake bite is the commonest in both the rural and the urban environment, and the inland taipan is the deadliest. Neurotoxicity of the venom of many Australian elapids is responsible for deaths. The venom contains both presynaptic and postsynaptic neurotoxins belonging to high molecular weight β-bungarotoxin types and smaller molecular weight α-bungarotoxin types. The first sign of flaccid paralysis may appear from 1 hour after envenoming to as late as 24 hours, leading to progressive respiratory paralysis requiring ventilatory support. The first signs to appear are cranial nerve palsies with ptosis, external

opthalmoplegia, and fixed dilated pupils, followed by paralysis of limbs (Jamieson and Pearn, 1989; White, 2010).

SEA SNAKES

Sea snakes represent a diverse lineage of elapid snakes that have adopted a marine lifestyle. They are distributed in the Australasian region, across the Indian Ocean, and in the Western Pacific region. The Hydrophiinae or true sea snakes comprise 16 genera and as many as 53 species whilst the partially terrestrial *Laticauda* or sea kraits comprise five species (Lukoschek and Keogh, 2006). The important species include beaked sea snake (*Enhydrina schistose*), blue spotted sea snake (*Hydrophis cyanocinctus*), banded sea snake (*Hydrophis fasciatus atriceps*), Hardwick's sea snake (*Lapemis curtus*), yellow-bellied sea snake (*Pelamis platurus*), and sea krait (*Laticauda colubrine*) (Warrell, 2010b). The erabutoxins a and b are the major neurotoxins in the venom of *Laticauda semifasciatus* (Guinea et al., 1983; Tamiya and Arai., 1966). The venoms of *E. schistose, H. cyanocinctus* and *Microcephalophis gracifis gracilis* are rich in 5′-nucleotidase and phospholipase A2 activity (Alam et al., 1996; Tamiya et al., 1983). The myotoxic activity causes myalgia and passage of dark urine indicating myoglobinuria. The myasthenic manifestations become superimposed on the myotoxic syndrome and produce ptosis, external opthalmoplegia, dysphagia, and even respiratory paralysis. Recovery occurs within 1 week, but respiratory failure may cause death (Reid, 1975a, b).

Viperidae

The family Viperidae has relatively long upper jaw fangs which are kept folded but erected upon strike (solenoglyph). Viperidae consists of two subfamiles: Viperinae or "old world vipers" (*Atheris*, African bush vipers; *Bitis*, African vipers; *Cerastes*, horned vipers; *Daboia russelii*, Russell's viper; *Echis*, saw-scaled or carpet vipers) and Crotalinae or "pit vipers" (*Cerrophidion*, Central American mountain pit vipers, *Bothrops*, lanceheads; *Crotalus*, rattlesnakes; *Calloselasma rhodostoma*, Malayan pit viper; *Trimeresurus* complex, Asiatic arboreal pit vipers; *Agkistrodon, Deinagkistrodon, Hypnale*). Viperidae are relatively short, thick-bodied snakes, having a triangular head and characteristic patterns of colored markings on the dorsal surface of the body. The subfamily Crotalinae has a sense organ, the loreal pit organ, situated between the nostril and the eye, which is heat-sensitive to detect warm-blooded prey. A few species of Viperidae, notably Palla's pit viper (*Agkistrodon halys*), Sri Lankan and South Indian *Daboia russelii*; South American rattlesnake *Crotalus durissus terrificus*, Mamushi or Fu-she *Gloydius* from China, cause neurotoxic manifestations in man (Mascarenas and Wuster, 2010; Warell, 2010b). Recent clinical, laboratory and neurophysiologic evidence supports neurotoxic envenoming in the Sri Lankan hump-nosed pit viper (*Hypnale*) bite (Kularatne and Ratnatunga, 1999).

RUSSELL'S VIPER (*DABOIA RUSSELII*)

The genus *Daboia* has two species, the Eastern Russell's viper (*D. siamensis*) distributed in far eastern countries such as Thailand, Indonesia, and Myanmar, and the Western Russell's viper (*D. russelii*), mainly found in Sri Lanka and southern India (Wuster, 1998a; Warrell, 2010b). Envenoming by *D. russelii* produces frequent neurotoxic manifestations similar to elapid bites. Studies in Sri Lanka showed an incidence of neuroparalytic manifestations exceeding 70%, predominantly involving cranial nerves, manifesting as ptosis and external ophthalmoplegia and lasting up to 5 days. Weakness of limb muscles and respiratory muscles, however, is extremely rare (Phillips, 1988; Kularatne, 2003). Only the comorbidities such as bronchial asthma, allergies, anaphylactic reactions to antivenom, or intracranial problems demand artificial ventilatory support in managing these patients. In Sri Lanka, *D. russelii* is responsible for frequent bites causing high morbidity and mortality among rural paddy farmers. It is a nocturnal snake, but day biting is frequent during harvest time as the snake prefers to rest in the paddy fields during daytime. Envenoming causes severe coagulopathy, acute renal failure, and multiorgan dysfunction. The procoagulant and anticoagulant components of the venom cause acute cerebrovascular accidents such as intracerebral hemorrhages and acute ischemic strokes, and in rare situations, ischemia to the pituitary gland causing chronic pituitary insufficiency similar to Sheehan's syndrome (Ameratunga, 1972; Kularatne, 2003; Gawarammana et al., 2009; Antonypillai et al., 2011). *D. siamensis* envenoming, on the other hand, is free of neurotoxic manifestations, but there are many reports of pituitary insufficiency following its bites (Tun pe et al., 1987; Antonypillai et al., 2011). The mechanism of neurotoxicity in *D. russelii* is less clear, but may be attributed to phospholipase A2 acting presynaptically and also postsynaptic toxins (Shelke et al., 2002; Gopalan et al., 2007). A study on the molecular diversity in venom protein of *D. russelii* has shown that its phospholipase A2 is of "S" type in contrast to *D. siamensis* which has phospholipase A2 of "N" type to support the differences in clinical manifestations in these two species (Suzuki et al., 2010). The venom of *D. palaestinae* is also known to contain a phospholipase A2 that can provoke neurotoxic manifestations (Chippaux, 2010).

RATTLESNAKES (*CROTALUS*)

The rattlesnake venom contains mainly enzymes that cause severe local inflammation, necrosis, and severe hemorrhagic syndromes. Several North American species, namely *C. atros, C. horridu, C. scutulatus,* cause neurologic manifestations. The South American species *C. durissus durissus* and *C. d. terrificus* also have myotoxic and neurotoxic venoms (Chippaux, 2010). The neurotoxins are crotamine and crotoxin that block the NMT by competitively, antagonised by edrophonium and succinylcholine (Vital-Brazil et al., 1979). Reduced release of ACh due to interference with calcium entry or other mechanisms has also been suggested (Howard and Gundersen, 1980). The envenoming manifests as cranial nerve palsies, myalgia, and muscle weakness. Myokymia responding to antivenin and calcium has been observed following envenoming by the timber rattlesnake (Brick et al., 1987).

SCORPIONS

Scorpion envenoming is a serious public health problem in some regions in the world. In Tunisia, 30 000–45 000 cases are reported per year with 10–100 fatalities (Krifi et al., 2005). A similar situation prevails in Mexico, Iran, Algeria, and even in India. *Hottentotta tamulus* (Scorpiones: Buthidae), the Indian red scorpion (according to the most recent taxonomic revision) has recently been found in Sri Lanka too (Ranawana et al., 2013). Scorpions belong to the group *Scorpionida* and the most dangerous species to man are *Centruroides* (southern United States, Central America), *Tityus* (South America), *Androctonus* (Africa), *Leiurus* (Africa and the Middle East), and *Buthus* (Asia). Scorpion venom is a complex mixture consisting of low molecular weight basic proteins, neurotoxins, mucus oligopeptidases, nucleotides, and amino acids. Unlike most spider or snake venoms, many scorpion venoms generally lack enzymes or possess low levels of enzymes with the exception of *Heterometrus scaber*. 5-Hydroxytryptanine, proteases, angiotensinase, and succinate-dehydrogenase are found in the venoms of *Mesobuthus tamulus, Centruroides exilicauda*, and *Heterometrus fulvipes* (Gwee et al., 2002).

The main molecular targets of scorpion neurotoxins are the voltage-gated sodium channels and the voltage-gated potassium channels. There are α- and β-scorpion toxins acting at different receptor sites. Venom from the Israeli scorpion (*Leiurus quinquestriatus quinquestriatus*) has the most lethal of scorpion venoms. Other scorpions, including the Indian red scorpion (*Mesobuthus tamulus*) and the Chinese scorpion (*Buthus matensi Karsch*), can cause lethal envenoming to humans (Gwee et al., 2002). *Tityus* toxins (TsTx) of the Brazilian scorpion *Tityus serrulatus* have pre- and postsynaptic actions at the NMJ by increasing sodium permeability (Meves et al., 1982). The Asian black scorpions *Heterometrus longimanus* and *Heterometrus spinifer* of the family Scorpionidae are the largest in the Southeast Asian region. However, there has been no documentation of the black scorpion causing lethal envenoming in humans.

Clinical manifestations

As a result of venom action on the voltage-gated channels, massive release of autonomic neurotransmitters leading to an autonomic storm is a major contributor to the pathophysiology of scorpion envenoming. The clinical manifestations of envenoming by the Buthidae family include sympathetic excitatory effects such as tachycardia, hypertension, arrhythmia, and mydriasis. Parasympathetic effects manifest as excessive salivation, lacrimation, bradycardia, and hypotension. Death is related to cardiac failure and pulmonary edema as a result of massive release of catecholamines from the adrenals and noradrenergic nerve terminals (Bawaskar and Bawaskar, 1982, 2011; Gwee et al., 2002). Envenoming by *Hemiscorpion lepturus*, the Iranian scorpion, produces dry mouth, thirst, dizziness, vomiting, fever, confusion, convulsions, hypoglycemia, leukocytosis, thrombocytopenia, ST depression in ECG, and severe local envenoming. *Centruroides* stings produce fasciculations and spasms; *Tityus* sting may cause acute pancreatitis.

Management of scorpion envenoming

The local pain could be alleviated by local infiltration or digital block with 1% lidocaine or peripheral nerve block with 0.25% bupivacaine. Opiates may relieve the symptoms. Severe envenoming may need intensive care. Scorpion antivenoms are available for specific species. α_1-Adrenergic receptor blockers, e.g., prazosin, are effective in controlling the autonomic storm. An Indian study used oral prazosin 250 µg for children and 500 µg for adults in repeated doses 3 hourly until the peripheries were cold. The same study found that a combination of prazosin and antivenom was superior to prazosin alone in treating *Mesobuthus tamulus* envenoming (Bawaskar and Bawaskar, 2011). Management of complications such as arrhythmias, pulmonary edema, and convulsions is also required.

SPIDERS

Spiders (Araneae) are an enormous group, comprising ubiquitous arthropod predators found in many environments. They act as biological controls for pests and insects to maintain natural balance. The Order Aranea, suborder Mygalomorphae and Arneamorphae contain the vast majority of spiders, and about 12 species of spiders stand out as clinically important. These include widow spiders, recluse spiders, banana spiders, and Australian funnel web spiders. The most dangerous are the female widow spiders of the genus *Latrodectus*, e.g., black widow (*L. mactans*), grey widow (*L. geometricus*), American *Loxosceles* causing cytotoxin-mediated local cutaneous damage, and world's most toxic, Australian funnel web spiders. In Brazil, three groups of spiders are found: banana spiders (genus *Phoneutria*; phoneutrism), recluse or violin spiders (genus *Loxosceles*; loxoscelism), and widow spiders (genus *Latrodectus*; lactrodectism). Widow spiders are widely distributed in all continents including Australia (Senanayake and Roman, 1992; White, 2008). The subfamilies Ornithoctoninae, Poecilotheriinae, and Selenocosmiinae are found in India and Sri Lanka, but their envenoming does not cause fatalities despite high morbidity due to muscle spasms (Ahmed et al., 2009). Spider venoms are usually a complex mixture of substances containing peptides falling within neuroexcitatory toxins and necrotoxins in recluse spider venom.

Clinical effects of spider bites

The dry bite rate could exceed 80% and both neuroexcitatory envenoming and necrotic envenoming do not coexist in the same spider. Most species cause local effects such as pain, mild swelling, and erythema. Systemic symptoms include headache, malaise, nausea, abdominal pain lasting a few days. The toxins responsible for such symptoms are not characterized. Fang marks, if present, lie close together depending on the size of the spider. A few species will cause notable local effects such as distinct lumps or even blistering. The recluse spider venom contains a number of toxins that cause tissue necrosis, directly or indirectly. The necrosis sets in gradually taking days to become established.

The widow spiders, banana spiders, and Australian funnel web spiders are known to cause neuroexcitatory effects of envenoming. A subset of recluse spiders can induce hemolysis, DIC, renal failure, shock, liver failure, and multiple organ dysfunction.

The widow spider bite causes progressive severe local pain, often with swelling. The pain and swelling migrate proximally associated with sweating, nausea, and hypertension. The clinical picture could mimic acute abdomen or myocardial ischemia. On many occasions, the bites are nonlethal. In contrast, the Australian funnel web spider bite causes immediate pain and rapid onset of systemic manifestations. In 2–5 minutes, the victim develops tingling around the lips and tongue followed by catecholamine storm with piloerection, hypersalivation, lacrimation, hypertension, abdominal pain, nausea, pulmonary edema, and impaired conscious state. Without adequate antivenom therapy, death is likely (White, 2008). The "facies lactrodectismica" is characterized by the flushed, sweating face with painful grimace present in *Lactrodectus* envenoming. The patient may develop opisthotonus, cogwheel neck movements, and "pavor mortis"(fear of death). In the untreated patient, the duration of illness varies from 1 to 21 days. The management may demand assisted ventilation (Maretic, 1983). In recent literature, two clinical syndromes are described, "latrodectism and loxoscelism," caused by widow spiders (*Latrodectus* spp.) and *Loxosceles* spp., respectively, where latrodectism causes pain and autonomic effects while loxoscelism is characterized by formation of necrotic ulcer (Isbister and Fan, 2011).

Treatment of spider bite

Reassurance is important. Where available, antivenom is the most effective treatment for systemic envenoming, particularly in Australian funnel web spider bite, to prevent deaths. The antivenoms are available in Australia and Brazil (White, 2008). However, the effectiveness of antivenom against recluse spiders in Brazil in preventing tissue necrosis is contestable (White, 2008).

ANT, BEE, HORNET, AND WASP (INSECTA, HYMENOPTERA) STINGS

Ants, bees and wasps constitute a stinging hazard to humans. The commonest and most severe Hymenoptera stings are caused by members of the family Apidae (Giant Asian honeybee or *Apis dorsata*, Africanized honey bees or killer bee or *Apis mellifera scutellata*), Vespidae (e.g., wasp, *Vespula vulgaris*), American yellow jackets (genus *Dolichovespula*) and hornets (genus *Vespa*). Only females of Hymenoptera are able to sting, the sting being a modified ovipositor found at the posterior tip of the body. Associated with the sting is the venom gland. Venom glands of bees produce a mixture of various enzymes, peptides, and amines, sometime labeled apitoxin; and those of wasps contain a mixture of histamine-releasing factors, enzymes, hemolysins, neurotoxins, vasodilators, and vasospastic amines. Stings are used for both offense and defense. Of practical significance is the fact that the stings of bees are barbed and therefore left embedded at the sting sites together with their associated structures. The sting apparatus has its own musculature and ganglion which keeps delivering venom even after detachment. Wasps have barbless stings, leaving behind only a puncture wound (Franca et al., 1994; Fitzgerald and Flood, 2006; Ciszowski and Mietka-Ciszowska, 2007).

Clinical manifestations and treatments

The commonest manifestations of envenoming following bee stings are allergy and anaphylaxis; rarely, myocardial infarction and ischemia to visceral organs (bowel infarction) can occur. Wasp stings rarely cause myasthenia gravis, allergic encephalomyelopolyradiculoneuritis, mastocytosis and reversible optic neuropathy (Kularatne et al., 2003; Budagoda., 2010). Bee venom can induce a weak muscle contracture followed by abolition of indirect excitability. The block is irreversible and not antagonized by neostigmine. The respiratory paralysis is probably peripheral in origin (Vital-Brazil, 1972). Hornet venom probably has both pre- and postsynaptic actions causing NMJ blockage (Kawai and Hori, 1975).

Management includes immobilization of the patient and, if retained, stings should be removed carefully to prevent continuous delivery of venom. Attention should be given to all vital signs as anaphylaxis may cause bronchospasm and hypotension.

TICK PARALYSIS

In human and veterinary medicine, ticks are important reservoirs and vectors of numerous viruses, bacteria, and protozoa. Certain tick species cause pathologic and pathophysiologic changes in their hosts after inoculating noninfectious noxious substances, which are generally considered to be toxins which could cause neuromuscular paralysis. Some 43 tick species in 10 genera including both hard ticks (Ixodidae) and soft ticks (Argasidae) have been incriminated as causing tick paralysis (Gothe et al., 1979). A tick embeds itself in the victim's skin with its barbed hypostome introducing the salivary toxins to the host. The toxins appear to be rapidly excreted or metabolized once the tick is removed. The early experiments suggested action of the toxins at the NMJ causing a presynaptic failure to liberate acetylcholine (Rose and Gregson, 1956). Subsequent studies showed reduction of both amplitude and conduction velocities of mixed motor and sensory nerves (Emmons and McLennan, 1960). The *Dermacentor* and *Argas* paralysis are generally defined essentially as motor polyneuropathies with only limited participation of the afferent pathways. However, *Ixodes holocyclus* paralysis is of a different mechanism and has been implicated in intra-aural infestation and facial nerve palsy (Gothe et al., 1979; Indudharan et al., 1996).

Weakness usually begins about 5 days after attachment of the tick. A prodromal phase is often present, consisting of fatigue, irritability, distal paresthesias, and ataxia. An ascending flaccid paralysis develops over a period of hours to a day, involving bulbar and respiratory muscles. Muscle stretch reflexes are either diminished or absent. Although diplopia is common, extraocular palsy is not a usual finding. The clinical features may be mistaken for Guillain–Barré syndrome. However, finding a tick, usually hidden by hair in the neck or scalp, provides the clue to the diagnosis. Removal of the tick leads to recovery within 24 hours (Senanayake and Roman, 1992).

OTHER NATURAL TOXINS

Ciguatoxin is the commonest form of fish poisoning in the tropics. It is produced by a dinoflagellate, *Gambierdiscus toxicus*, loosely attached to algae on coral reefs. Ingestion of the flagellate by small fish and maintaining it in the food chain has resulted in more than 400 species of fish harboring the toxins. Clinical features include gastrointestinal and neurologic manifestations, sometimes even causing paralysis of respiratory muscles (Craig, 1980). The view is that ciguatoxin enhances quantal transmitter release at the NMJ due to an abnormally prolonged sodium channel opening in nerve membranes (Molgo et al., 1990).

Paralytic shellfish poisoning (PSP) may cause similar manifestations due to saxitoxins produced by dinoflagellates belonging to the *Porotogonyaulax* species causing high mortality (Rodrigue et al., 1990). The consumption of bivalve molluscs such as mussels, clams, scallops, and oysters that have ingested the dinoflagellate cause acute paralytic illness worldwide. PSP is one of the most severe forms of food poisoning with a high mortality rate, as high as 50% in children (Rodrigue et al., 1990). Within minutes of ingestion of the contaminated shellfish intraoral and circumoral paresthesias occur, which soon spread to the trunk and distal parts of the limbs. Pupils may remain dilated and nonreactive. Respiratory paralysis may cause death.

Some crab species, particularly king crab in Southeast Asia, also contain saxitoxins and tetrodotoxins, and their flesh causes poisoning resembling that caused by PSP (Yasumura et al., 1986). Puffer fish and porcupine fish also contain tetrodotoxins which act as sodium channel blockers. Poisoning occurs when the highly toxic liver is used in the preparation of fugu which is consumed to achieve a state of exhilaration. In severe poisoning, the patient develops descending paralysis and respiratory failure; risk of fatality is high. Tetrodotoxin has also been discovered in some species of goby, newt, skin, and eggs of frogs, octopus, shellfish, and starfish (Mosher and Fuhrman, 1984).

Ingestion of the flesh of the hawksbill turtle had caused poisoning in India and Sri Lanka. Toxic algae ingested by the turtle is supposed to make its flesh poisonous, and the poisoning causes flaccid paralysis of muscles (Senanayake and Roman, 1992). Conotoxins are a group of neurotoxic peptides found in the venom of fish-hunting marine snails of the genus *Conus*. Careless handling of the cone shell has resulted in human fatalities (Cruz et al., 1985). The sting causes numbness at the site which spreads to the rest of the body followed by blurred vision, impaired speech and paralysis of respiratory muscles.

The skin secretion of certain frogs which live in the humid rain forests of South America and southern Central America belonging to the family *Dendrobatidae* are used as dart poisons by Amerindians. It has alkaloids such as batrachotoxin and histrionicotoxin which act on ion channels at the NMJ causing paralysis (Myers and Dally, 1983).

The venom of centipedes (Chilopoda) contain neurotoxins which are potent enough to paralyze its prey, but insignificant clinically. These nerotoxins involve G-protein-coupled receptors (Undheim and King, 2011).

Bacterial exotoxins such as botulinum toxins and tetanus toxins are known neurotoxins of importance. Botulism commonly results from consumption of canned foods contaminated with *Clostridium botulinum* which produces toxins that block the release of Ach from cholinergic nerve terminals (Brown, 1981).

MANAGEMENT OF SNAKE BITE

Immediate management

First aid is important to retard venom absorption. Reassurance of the victim and the immobilization of the bitten limb by using a splint or sling are the important first steps until arrangements are made to take the patient to the nearest medical facility. Tampering with the bite wound or applying a constriction band above it should be avoided (Warrell, 1990; Cheng and Currie, 2004). Pressure immobilization using a crepe bandage has proved effective in animal experiments, but it has not been subjected to formal clinical trials (Sutherland et al., 1979).

Distressing and life-threatening manifestations of envenoming may appear before the patient reaches hospital. For severe local pain, oral paracetamol is preferable to aspirin or nonsteroidal anti-inflammatory drugs, which carry a risk of bleeding. Avoiding anything orally is prudent as the patient has a risk of vomiting, and of aspiration and choking due to neuromuscular paralysis. The patient should be laid in the left lateral position with head down to avoid aspiration. The venom could induce anaphylaxis, which should be treated with adrenaline by intramuscular injection followed by antihistamine and hydrocortisone. If cyanosed, or if the respiratory movements are weak, oxygen should be given. If respiratory effort is significantly compromised and the tidal volume is falling, a cuffed endotracheal tube should be introduced using a laryngoscope (Warrell, 2010a, b).

Treatment in the hospital

Any snake bite needs immediate attention. The history, symptoms, and signs must be assessed rapidly to decide appropriate management. The airway, breathing and circulation should be monitored, and if compromised, resuscitation should begin immediately. In the case of neuromuscular paralysis, the patient builds up hypoxemia gradually, but it remains undetected as the patient remains still due to weakness of muscles. Thus, careful monitoring of breathing, paradoxical abdominal breathing, and measurement of tidal volume is essential. The earliest symptoms and signs of neurotoxicity after elapid bites are often blurring of vision, a feeling of heaviness in the eyelids, drowsiness and contraction of the frontalis muscle to keep eyes open. Subsequently, ptosis and double vision can be demonstrated. Patients with generalized rhabdomyolysis may have trismus, stiff tender muscles resistant to passive stretching (Warrell, 2010a, b). The level of consciousness may decline for many reasons. In common krait bite, some patients develop a progressive deep comatose state lasing days that may mimic brain death. However, gradual improvement can be anticipated with sustained life support (Kularatne, 2001).

Antivenom is the only specific treatment available that has proved effective against snake envenoming. Antivenom neutralizes the venom antigens in the blood and significantly reverses the coagulopathy. However, its ability to penetrate and neutralize the bound toxins in the NMJ is limited. Thus, reversal of established neurotoxicity is unlikely to happen with antivenom. Ativenom is a refined γ immunoglobulin or a fragment of it raised in horses or sheep. The antivenom could be either monovalent or polyvalent, depending on the spectrum of species of snakes. Monovalent antivenom is raised against the venom of a single species and is effective for treating envenoming by that species of snake only. Polyvalent antivenom is raised against the venom of more than one species of snake in a particular geographical region. As antivenom contains foreign proteins, severe allergic reactions can develop. Thus, it should be used only for specific indications. These include hemostatic abnormalities such as incoagulable blood, spontaneous bleeding, thrombocytopenia; cardiovascular abnormalities such as hypotension, arrhythmias; neurotoxic paralysis, rhabdomyolysis, and severe local envenoming. However, depending on the species of snake and type of anivenom available, the indications for therapy may differ from region to region. Antivenom is given as an infusion over 30–60 minutes. The dose regimen and repeated administration should depend on the local guidelines.

Supportive treatment in neurotoxic envenoming

Assisted ventilation is the most important life-saving management measure. With the onset of bulbar and respiratory muscle paralysis, the patient needs assisted ventilation in an intensive care unit. Neurotoxic effects are fully reversible with time, and the duration of ventilation depends on the species of snake. Neurotoxic paralysis is faster in onset lasting about 24 hours in cobra bite, but in common krait bite the onset could be slow and the duration extend a few days (Kularatne, 2001; Kularatne et al., 2009). The anticholinesterase drugs may produce a rapid improvement in neuromuscular transmission in patients envenomed by some species of Asian and African cobras, mambas, death adders, and Malayan krait (Warrell et al., 1983; Watt et al., 1986). The edrophonium test will be useful to detect response, and in positive cases, anticholinesterase drugs can be used to treat the patient. However, there is a risk of acute cholinergic crisis in overdosing. Snake venom ophthalmia should be managed initially by irrigation of the eyes with a large volume of water followed by specific ophthalmologic management.

CONCLUSION

Natural neurotoxins continue to be an important health hazard to man, particularly in tropical countries. In the limited space in the globe, with rapid expansion of the human population, a conflict exists between humans and other creatures in nature. This has resulted in an imbalance in ecology and even the extinction of some species from the earth. On the other hand, the identification of neurotoxins from these biological sources has helped in the study of neurophysiology. The use of purified toxins from Elapidae snakes constituted a crucial event in the understanding of the pathophysiology of myasthenia gravis and the myasthenic syndrome. The use of purified AChRs from the electric organ of the electric ray *Torpedo californica* and the electric eel provided the first quantifiable laboratory diagnostic test for myasthenia gravis. Neurotoxins have already led to the development of several groups of pharmacologic and therapeutic agents, and there is vast potential in the future in this sphere. A testimony to this is provided by the results obtained by the use of botulinum toxin in the treatment of dystonic disorders (Kraft and Lang, 1988; Cohen et al., 1989). Similarly, μ-conotoxins have been used to develop new analgesics (Nortan, 2010) and a toxin called "ancrod," a serine protease derived from the venom of the Malayan pit viper, has been used to treat acute ischemic strokes (Del Brutto and Del Brutto, 2011). However, many unanswered questions remain. Observations made in good clinical studies need neurophysiologic and biochemical explanations. For example, the deep comatose state with EEG changes and retrograde memory loss in common krait envenoming has so far remained unexplained. Bridging these gaps in knowledge is necessary. For most of the toxins there are no antidotes. This has hampered the management. Toxinology is a neglected field, and there is lack of enthusiasm in manufacturing good quality antivenoms. Even the available antivenoms seriously lack efficacy and cause severe anaphylaxis upon administration (Warrell, 2008). Neurotoxic paralysis results in death within minutes or hours. Shortage of ventilators and intensive care beds in affected regions in the globe hamper its effective management. Making Ambu bags available in the field, training of volunteers in resuscitation, and transportation of victims are important. In Nepal, an attempt has been made to introduce motor bikes to transport victims of snake bite (Sharma et al., 2004). Finally, a concerted effort should be made to enhance research interests in toxinology and to develop good quality antivenoms to salvage the lives which otherwise would be lost from fatal envenoming.

ACKNOWLEDGMENTS

The authors are grateful to Dr. Kalana Maduwage for his assistance in preparation of references and the figure.

REFERENCES

Adem A, Asblom A, Johansson et al. (1998). Toxins from the venom of the green mamba (*Dendroaspis anguaticeps*) that inhibit the binding of quinuchidinyl benzilate to muscarinic acetylcholine receptors. Biochem Biophys Acta 968: 340–345.

Adler K, Louis S (2007). Leoniceno N (1428–1524) Italian physician/Greek scholar toxicology of snake bite (volume II) Missouri, USA, Society for the Study of Amphibians and Reptiles "contributions to the history of Herpetology", pp. 11–12.

Ahmed M, Rocha JBT, Morsch VM, Schetinger MRC (2009). Snake venom acetylcholinesterase. In: SP Mackessy (Ed.), Handbook of venoms and toxins of reptiles. Taylor and Francis, New York, USA, pp. 207–220.

Alam JM, Qasim R, Alam SM (1996). Enzymatic activities of some snake venoms from families of Elapidae and Viperidae. Pak J Pharm Sci 9: 37–41.

Ameratunga B (1972). Middle cerebral occlusion following Russell's viper bite. J Trop Med Hyg 75: 95–97.

Antonypillai CN, Wass JAH, Warrell DA et al. (2011). Hypopitiutarism following envenoming by Russell's viper (*Daboia siamensis* and *D russellii*) resembling Sheehan's syndrome: first case report from Sri Lanka A review of the literature and recommendations for management. QJM 104: 97–108.

Bawaskar HS, Bawaskar HS (1982). Diagnostic cardiac premonitory signs and symptoms of red scorpion sting. Lancet 2: 552–554.

Bawaskar HS, Bawaskar HS (2011). Efficacy and safety of scorpion antivenom plus prazosin compared with prazosin alone for venomous scorpion (*Mesobuthus tamulus*) sting: randomised open label clinical trial. BMJ 342: c7136.

Brick FJ, Gutmann L, Brick J et al. (1987). Timber rattlesnake venom induced myokymia: evidence for peripheral nerve origin. Neurology 37: 1545–1546.

Brown LW (1981). Infant botulism. Adv Pediatr 28: 141–157.

Brownell P, Polis G (Eds.), (2001). Scorpian biology and research. Oxford University Press, New York, p. 431.

Budagoda BDSS, Kodikara KAS, Kularatne WKS et al. (2010). Giant Asian honeybee or Bambara stings causing myocardial infarction, bowel gangrene and fatal anaphylaxis in Sri Lanka: a case series. Asian Pac J Trop Med 3: 586–588.

Calmette A (1907). Les venins, les animaux venimeux et la sérothérapie antivenimeuse. La Press MW dicale, Paris, pp. xxvii, 165.

Cheng AC, Currie BJ (2004). Venomous snakebites worldwide with a focus on the Australia-Pacific region: current management and controversies. J Intensive Care Med 19: 259–269.

Chippaux JP (1998). Snake bite: appraisal of the global situation. Bull WHO 76: 515–524.

Chippaux JP (2006). Snake venoms and envenomations. Krieger, Florida, pp. 3–88.

Chippaux JP (2010). Snake bite in Africa: current situation and urgent needs. In: SP Mackessy (Ed.), Handbook of Venoms and Toxins of Reptiles. Taylor and Francis, New York, USA, pp. 452–474.

Chu ER, Weinstein SA, White J et al. (2010). Venom ophthalmia caused by venoms of spitting elapid and other snakes: report of ten cases with review of epidemiology, clinical features, pathophysiology and management. Toxicon 56: 259–272.

Ciszowski K, Mietka-Ciszowska A (2007). Hymenoptera stings. Przegl Lek 64: 282–289.

Cohen LG, Hallett M, Geller BD et al. (1989). Treatment of local dystonias of the hand with botulinum toxin injections. J Neurol Neurosurg Psychiatry 52: 355–363.

Craig CP (1980). It's always the big ones that should get away. JAMA 244: 272–273.

Cruz LJ, Gray WR, Yoshikami D et al. (1985). Conus venoms: a rich source of neuroactive peptides. J Toxicol Toxin Rev 4: 107–132.

De Silva PHDH (1980). Snake Fauna of Sri Lanka with Special References to Skull, Dentition and Venom in Snake. National Museum of Sri Lanka, Sri Lanka, pp. 102–106.

Del Brutto OH, Del Brutto VJ (2011). Neurological complications of venomous snake bites: a review. Acta Neurol Scand 125: 363–372.

Dewan JC, Grant GA, Sacchettini JC (1994). Crystal structure of kappa bungarutoxin at 23A0 resolution. Biochemistry 33: 13147–13154.

Doley R, Shou X, Kini RM (2010). Snake venom phospholipase A$_2$ enzymes. In: SP Mackessy (Ed.), Handbook of venoms and toxins of reptiles. Taylor and Francis, New York, USA, pp. 173–206.

Emmons P, McLennan H (1960). Some observations on tick paralysis in marmots. J Exp Biol 37: 355–362.

Estable A (1959). Curare and synapse. In: D Bovet (Ed.), Curare and Curare-like Agents. Elsevier, Amsterdam, p. 357.

Fitzgerald KT, Flood AA (2006). Hymenoptera stings. Clin Tech Small Anim Pract 21: 194–204.

Franca FO, Benvenuti LA, Fan HW et al. (1994). Severe and fatal mass attacks by "killer" bees (Africanized honey bees – Apis mellifera scutellata) in Brazil: clinicopathological studies with measurement of serum venom concentrations. QJM 87: 269–282.

Freedman R, Wetmore C, Stromberg I et al. (1993). Alpha-bungarutoxin binding to hippocample interneuron, immounocyts chemical characterization and effects on growth feature expression. J Neurosci 13: 1965–1975.

Ganong WF (1999). Synaptic and junctional transmission. In: Review of medical physiology, 19th edn Prentice-Hall International, London, pp. 80–112.

Gawarammana I, Mendis S, Jeganathan K (2009). Acute ischemic stroke due to the bite by Dabioa russelli in Sri Lanka – first authenticates case series. Toxicon 54: 421–428.

Gawarammana IB, Kularatne SAM, Kularatne K et al. (2010). Deep coma and hypokalaemia of unknown etiology following Bungarus caeruleus bites: exploration of pathophysiological mechanisms with two case studies. J Venom Res 1: 71–75.

Gopalan G, Thowrn MM, Gopalakrishnakone P et al. (2007). Structural and pharmacological comparison of dabioatoxin from Daboia russelli siamensis with Viperotoxin F and Vipoxin from other vipers. Acta Crystallogr D Biol Crystallogr 63: 722–729.

Gothe R, Kunze K, Hoogastraol H (1979). The mechanism of pharmacology in the tick paralysis. N Engl J Med 16: 357–369.

Grant GA, Chiappinelli VA (1985). Kappa-Bungarotixin complete amino acid sequence of a neuronal nicotinic receptor. Biochemistry 24: 1532–1537.

Guinea M, Tamiya N, Cogger HG (1983). The neurotoxins of the sea snakes Laticauda schistorhynchus. Biochem J 213: 39–41.

Gutierrez JM (1995). Clinical toxicology of snake bite in Central America. In: J Meier, J White (Eds.), Handbook of Clinical Toxicology of Animal Venom and Poisons. CRC Press, Boca Raton, Florida, pp. 164–165.

Gutierrez JM (2010). Snake bite envenomation in Central America. In: SP Mackessy (Ed.), Handbook of Venoms and Toxins of Reptiles. Taylor and Francis, New York, USA, pp. 491–508.

Gwee MC, Nirthanan S, Khoo HE et al. (2002). Autonomic effects of some scorpion venoms and toxins. Clin Exp Pharmacol Physiol 29: 795–801.

Harvey AL (2010). Fasciculins: toxins from mamba venoms that inhibit acetylcholinesterase. In: SP Mackessy (Ed.), Handbook of Venoms and Toxins of Reptiles. Taylor and Francis, New York, USA, pp. 317–324.

Harvey AC, Anderson AJ (1985). Dendrotoxins: snake toxins that block potassium channels and facilitate neurotransmitter release. Pharmacol Ther 31: 33–55.

Hedge RP, Rajagopalan N, Doley R et al. (2009). Snake venom three finger toxins. In: SP Mackessy (Ed.), Handbook of Venoms and Toxins of Reptiles. Taylor and Francis, New York, USA, pp. 287–302.

Holman JA (2000). Fossil Snake of North America Origin, Evolution, Distribution, Paleoecology. Indiana University Press, Bloomington, p. 357.

Howard BD, Gundersen CB Jr (1980). Effects and mechanisms of polypeptide neurotoxins that act presynaptically. Annu Rev Pharmacol Toxicol 20: 307–336.

Imms AD (1939). Hymenoptera Text Book of Entomology Vol. 684, 730–732.

Indudharan R, Dharap AS, Ho AB (1996). Intra-aural tick causing facial palsy. Lancet 348: 613.

Isbister GK, Fan HW (2011). Spider bite. Lancet 378: 2039–2047.

Ivanov M, Ragi JC, Szyndlar Z et al. (2000). Histoire et origine géographique des faunes de serpents en Europe. Bull Soc Herp Fr 96: 15–24.

Jamieson R, Pearn J (1989). An epidemiological and clinical study of snake bite in chilehood. Med J Aust 150: 698–702.

Kasturiratne A, Wickremasinghe AR, de Silva N et al. (2008). The global burden of snakebite: a literature analysis and modelling based on regional estimates of envenoming and deaths. PLoS Med 5: e218.

Kawai N, Hori S (1975). Effects of hornet venom on crustacean neuromuscular junction. Toxicon 13: 103–104.

Kraft SP, Lang AE (1988). Cranial dystonia, blepharospasm and hemifacial spasm: clinical features and treatment Including the use of botulinum toxin. Can Med Assoc J 139: 837–844.

Krifi MN, Savin S, Debray M et al. (2005). Pharmacokinetic studies of scorpion venom before and after immunotherapy. Toxicon 45: 187–198.

Kularatne SAM (2001). Clinical profile of snake envenoming: a study in North Central Province of Sri Lanka The 23rd Bibile Memorial Oration in 2001. Sri Lanka Journal of Medicine 10: 4–12.

Kularatne SAM (2003). Epidemiology and clinical picture of the Russell's viper (Daboia russellii russellii) bite in Anuradhapura, Sri Lanka: a prospective study of 336 patients. Southeast Asian J Trop Med Public Health 34: 855–862.

Kularatne SAM, Ratnatunga N (1999). Severe systemic effects of Merrem's hump-nosed viper bite. Ceylon Med J 44: 169–170.

Kularatne SAM, Gawarammana IB, De Silva PHJU (2003). Severe multi-organ dysfunction following multiple wasp (Vespa affinis) stings. Ceylon Med J 48: 146–147.

Kularatne SAM, Budagoda BDSS, Gawarammana IB et al. (2009). Epidemiology, clinical profile and management of cobra (Naja naja) bites in Sri Lanka: first authentic case series. Trans R Soc Trop Med Hyg 103: 924–930.

Lee CY (1972). Chemistry and pharmacology of polypetic toxins in snake venom. Annu Rev Pharmacol 12: 265–286.

Lukoschek V, Keogh JS (2006). Molecular phylogeny of sea snakes a rapidly developed adaptive radiation. Biol J Linn Soc 89: 523–539.

Maretic Z (1983). Latrodectism: variations in clinical manifestions provoked by *Latrodectus* species of spider. Toxicon 21: 457–466.

Mascarenas AQ, Wuster W (2010). Recent advances in venomous snake systematics. In: SP Mackessy (Ed.), Handbook of Venoms and Toxins of Reptiles. Taylor and Francis, New York, USA, pp. 25–64.

Mebs D (2008). Overview of venomous and poisonous animals. In: J White (Ed.), Handbook of Clinical Toxinology Short Course. University of Adelaide, Australia, pp. 5–7.

Meves H, Rubly N, Watt DD (1982). Effect of toxin isolated from the venom of the scorpion *Centruroides sculpturatus* on the Na currents of node of Ranvier. Pflugers Arch 393: 56–62.

Molgo J, Comella JX, Legrand AM (1990). Ciguatoxin enhances quantal transmitter release from frog nerve terminals. Br J Pharmacol 90: 695–700.

Mosher HS, Fuhrman FA (1984). Occurrence and origin of tetrodotoxin. In: EP Regelis (Ed.), ACS symposium series No 262 Seafood Toxins. American Chemicals Society, USA, pp. 333–344.

Myers CW, Dally JW (1983). Dart-poison frogs. Sci Am 248: 120–133.

Nortan RS (2010). Mu-conotoxins as leads in the development of new analgesics. Molecules 15: 2825–2844.

Pettigrew LC, Glass JP (1985). Neurologic complications of a coral snake bite. Neurology 35: 589–592.

Phillips RE, Theakston RDG, Warrell DA et al. (1988). Paralysis, rhabdomyolysis and haemolysis caused by bites of Russell's viper (*Vipera russelli pulchella*) in Sri Lanka: failure of Indian (Haffkine) antivenom. QJM New Series 68: 691–716.

Pook CE, Joger U, Stumpel N et al. (2009). When continents collide: phylogeny, historical biogeography and systematic of the medically important viper genus Echis (Squamata: Serpentes: Viperidae). Mol Phylogenet Evol 53: 792–807.

Ranawana KB, Dinamithra NP, Sivansuthan S, Nagasena II, Kovarik F, Kularatne SAM. First report on Hottentotta tumulus (Scopiones: Buthidae) from Sri Lanka, and its medical importance. Euscorpius: 155; 4th March 2013. http://www.science.marshall.edu/fet/euscorpius/.

Reid HA (1975a). Epidemiological and clinical aspect of sea snake bites. In: WA Dunson (Ed.), The Biology of Sea Snakes. University Park Press, Baltimore, pp. 417–462.

Reid HA (1975b). Antivenom in sea snakes poisoning. Lancet I: 622–627.

Robin D, Zhou X, Kini M (2010). Snake venom phospholipase A2 enzymes. In: SP Mackessy (Ed.), Handbook of Venoms and Toxins of Reptiles. Taylor and Francis, New York, USA, pp. 173–206.

Rodrigue DC, Etzel RA, Hall S et al. (1990). Lethal paralytic shelfish poisoning in Guatemala. Am J Trop Med Hyg 42: 267–271.

Rose I, Gregson JD (1956). Evidence of a neuromuscular block in tick paralysis. Nature 178: 95–96.

Schmidt JO (1995). Toxinology of venoms from the honeybee genus *Apis*. Toxicon 33: 917–927.

Senanayake N, Roman GC (1992). Disorders of neuromuscular transmission due to natural environmental toxins. J Neurol Sci 107: 1–13.

Sethi PK, Rastogi JK (1981). Neurological aspects of ophitoxemia (Indian Krait) – a clinico-electromyographic study. Indian J Med Res 73: 269–276.

Seu I, Grantham PA, Cooper JR (1976). Mechanism of action A beta bungarotoxin in synaptosomal preparation. Proc Natl Acad Sci U S A 73: 2664–2668.

Shama SK, Chappuis F, Jha N (2004). Impact of snake bites and determinants of fatal outcomes in southeastern Nepal. Am J Trop Med Hyg 7: 234–238.

Shelke RR, Sathosh S, Godwa TV (2002). Isolation and characterization of a novel postsynaptic/cytotoxic neurotoxin from *Dabioa russelli russelli* venom. J Pept Res 59: 257–263.

Sutherland SK, Tibballs J (2001). Australian animal toxins The creatures, their toxins and care of the poisoned patient. 2nd edn Oxford University Press, Melbourne.

Sutherland SK, Coulter AR, Harris RD (1979). Rationalization of first-aid measures for elapid snake bite. Lancet i: 183–186.

Suzuki M, Itoh T, Bandaranayake BMAIK et al. (2010). Molecular diversity of venom proteins of Russell's viper (*Dabioa russellii russellii*) and Indian cobra (*Naja naja*) in Sri Lanka. Biomed Res 31: 71–81.

Tamiya N, Arai H (1966). Studies on sea snake venom Crystallization of erabutoxins a and b from *Laticauda semifasciata* venom. Biochem J 99: 624–630.

Tamiya N, Maeda N, Cogger G (1983). Neurotoxins from the venom of the sea snake *Hydrophis arnatus* and *Hydrophis lapemaides*. Biochem J 213: 31–38.

Theakston RDG, Phillips RE, Warrell DA et al. (1990). Envenoming by the common krait (*Bungarus caeruleus*) and Sri Lankan cobra (*Naja naja naja*): efficacy and complications of therapy with Haffkine antivenom. Trans R Soc Trop Med Hyg 84: 301–308.

Tun pe, Phillips RE, Warrell DA et al. (1987). Acute and chronic pituitary failure resembling Sheehan's syndrome following bite by Russell's viper in Burma. Lancet 2: 763–767.

Undheim EAB, King GF (2011). On the venom system of centipedes(Chilopoda), a neglected group of venomous animals. Toxicon 57: 512–534.

Vital-Brazil O (1972). Venoms: their inhibitory action on neuromuscular transmission. In: C Radouco-Thomas (Ed.), International Encyclopedia of Pharmacology and Therapeutics Section 14: Neuromuscular Blocking and Stimulating Agents. Vol. I. Pergamon Press, Oxford, pp. 145–167.

Vital-Brazil O, Prado-Franceschi J, Laure CJ (1979). Repetitive muscle responses induced by crotamine. Toxicon 17: 61–67.

Warrell DA (1990). Treatment of snake bite in the Asia-Pacific region: a personal view. In: P Gopalakrishnakone, LM Chou (Eds.), Snakes of Medical Importance (Asia-Pacific Region). National University of Singapore, Singapore, pp. 641–670.

Warrell DA (2008). Unscrupulous marketing of snake bite antivenoms in Africa and Papua New Guinea: choosing the right product—'what's in a name?'. Trans R Soc Trop Med Hyg 102 (5): 397–399.

Warrell DA (2010a). Guidelines for the Management of Snake Bite Treatment of Neurotoxic Envenoming. World Health Organization, India, pp. 95–106.

Warrell DA (2010b). Guideline for the Management of Snake Bites. World Health Organization, India, pp. 11–15.

Warrell DA, Looareesuwan S, White NJ (1983). Severe neurotoxic envenoming by the Malayan krait *Bungarus candidus* (Linnaeus): response to antivenom and anticholinesterase. Br Med J 286: 678–680.

Watt G, Theakston RDG, Hayes CG (1986). Positive response to edrophonium in patients with neurotoxic envenoming by cobras (*Naja naja philippinensis*). A placebo-controlled study. N Engl J Med 315: 1444–1448.

Watt G, Patrick L, Tuazon MAL et al. (1998). Bites by the Philippine cobra (*Naja naja philippinus*) Prominent neurotoxicity with minimal local signs. Am J Trop Med Hyg 39: 306–311.

Wernicke JF, Vanker AD, Howard BD (1975). Mechanism of action of beta bungarutoxin. J Neurochem 25: 483–496.

White J (2008). Overview of spider bite. In: J White (Ed.), Handbook of Clinical Toxinology Short Course. University of Adelaide, Australia, pp. 185–188.

White J (2010). Envenomation, prevention and treatment in Australia. In: SP Mackessy (Ed.), Handbook of Venoms and Toxins of Reptiles. Taylor and Francis, USA, pp. 424–449.

Wuster W (1998a). The genus *Daboia* (Serpentes: Viperidae): Russell's viper. Hamadryad 23: 33–40.

Wuster W (1998b). The cobra of the genus *Naja* in India. Hamadryad 23: 15–32.

Wuster W, McCarthy CJ (1996). Venomous snake systematics: implications for snake bite treatment and toxinology. In: C Bon, M Goytton (Eds.), Envenoming and Their Treatment. Foundation Marcel Merieux, USA, pp. 13–21.

Yasumura D, Oshima Y, Yasumoto T et al. (1986). Tetrodotoxin and paralytic shellfish toxins in Philippine crabs. Agric Biol Chem 50: 593–598.

Section 10

Neurologic aspects of hematologic disorders

Handbook of Clinical Neurology, Vol. 120 (3rd series)
Neurologic Aspects of Systemic Disease Part II
Jose Biller and Jose M. Ferro, Editors

Chapter 67

Anemias excluding cobalamin and folate deficiencies

STEPHANIE DUBLIS[1], SHEFALI SHAH, SUCHA NAND*, AND ELISE ANDERES

[1]*Division of Hematology and Oncology, Department of Medicine, Loyola University Chicago, Stritch School of Medicine, Maywood, IL, USA*

INTRODUCTION

Across the world, anemias constitute one of the commonest disorders to affect humans. The types and causes of anemia change with the geography and socioeconomic status of the affected population. In developing countries, iron deficiency anemia is common and results from lack of dietary intake or parasitic infestation of the bowel. In developed nations, the main causes of anemia are gastrointestinal blood loss, heavy uterine bleeding, and pregnancy. The impact of anemia extends beyond a subnormal hemoglobin level. It can affect performance status of the patient, lowering work output. In patients with compromised cardiac and pulmonary functions, it can lead to decompensation of the affected organs. Neurologic consequences can be nonspecific, such as fatigue and lack of interest, or specific, such as neuropathy. Certain microangiopathic anemias, such as thrombotic thrombocytopenic purpura (TTP), are associated with fluctuating central nervous system (CNS) symptoms that can include aphasia, focal sensory and motor deficits, and seizures.

In this chapter, we discuss anemias other than those caused by cobalamin or folate deficiency. Wherever appropriate, neurologic complications associated with a particular type of anemia, or its treatment, have been discussed.

Definition and pathophysiology of anemias

The term "anemia" indicates a reduction in the absolute number of red cells or a reduced red cell mass. It is defined as a reduction of hemoglobin concentration, hematocrit, or red blood cell (RBC) count by more than two standard deviations below the mean for the patient's age and gender. Hemoglobin (HGB) measures the

concentration of this major oxygen-carrying pigment in whole blood. Hematocrit (HCT) is the percentage of a sample of whole blood occupied by intact red blood cells. RBC count is the number of red blood cells contained in a specified volume of whole blood. By using the range of two standard deviations below the mean, HGB < 13.5 g/dL or HCT < 41.0% represents anemia in men and HGB < 12.0 g/dL or HCT < 36.0% represents anemia in women. Other authors have proposed different lower limits of normal, ranging from 13 g/dL to 14.2 g/dL for men and from 11.6 g/dL to 12.3 g/dL for women (Beutler and Waalen, 2006). However, there are limitations in the ranges considered within normal limits as they may not be appropriate for all populations. For example, patients living at high altitude have higher HGB and HCT values than those living at sea level. A study of American blood donors who smoke found a direct correlation between the patient's blood carboxyhemoglobin and HGB values. The same study also found a relationship between HGB values and the degree of environmental air pollution with carbon dioxide in nonsmoking blood donors. Therefore, patients who smoke or who have a significant exposure to secondary smoke or other sources of carbon monoxide may have hematocrits higher than normal (Stewart et al., 1974; Nordenberg et al., 1990). Also, values for HGB in African Americans are 0.5–1.0 g/dL lower than values in comparable Caucasian populations. Some, but not all, of these differences may be attributable to coexisting α-thalassemia (Beutler and Waalen, 2006). It is also important to remember that HGB, HCT, and RBC counts are concentrations and are therefore dependent on the red blood cell mass as well as the plasma volume. For example, a patient with volume depletion may present with normal values for HGB and HCT, and the anemia may not be apparent until the

---

*Correspondence to: Sucha A. Nand, M.D., Loyola University Medical Center, Cancer Center, Room 345, 2160 S. First Avenue, Maywood, IL 60153, USA. E-mail: SNAND@lumc.edu

volume deficit is replaced. In contrast, in the third trimester of pregnancy, the RBC mass and plasma volume expand by 25% and 50%, respectively, resulting in reductions in HGB, HCT, and RBC count, often to anemic levels, when, in fact, according to the RBC mass, they may be polycythemic. The terms physiologic or dilutional anemia have been applied in this setting.

RBCs normally survive 90–120 days. Approximately 1% of RBCs die per day and are replaced, therefore a normal reticulocyte count is also 1%. A senescence antigen appears on the membrane of old RBCs. The antigen is recognized by the reticuloendothelial system and old RBCs are removed from the circulation by macrophages in the marrow, liver, and spleen. A normal bone marrow can increase RBC production to a great extent. For example, in hemolytic anemias, the RBC survival has to be < 20 days for the patient to become anemic.

Erythropoietin is one of the main agents responsible for RBC production and maturation. It is secreted by specialized cells in deep cortex and outer medulla of the kidneys in response to hypoxia. There are no stores of erythropoietin. Less than 10% erythropoietin is produced in the liver.

Etiologies of anemia are diverse and often multifactorial, and range from external blood loss, underproduction of RBCs, to increased destruction of developing or mature red blood cells. An approach using reticulocyte count and red cell indices, as a rule, leads to the diagnosis, which may require specific tests to determine the etiology.

Diagnostic approach

In some cases the cause of anemia is evident, e.g., a patient with a known history of sickle cell disease or thalassemia, GI bleeding, or surgical blood loss. When the cause is not obvious, a systematic diagnostic approach often leads to the correct diagnosis. The hallmarks of such an approach are reticulocyte count and red cell indices. The reticulocyte count, which is a reflection of the bone marrow output for the previous 24 hour period, is used to differentiate hypoproliferative from hyperproliferative anemias. In hyperproliferative anemias, the absolute reticulocyte count is elevated to 100 000/µL or higher. This indicates that the bone marrow is functioning normally, and that the cause of the anemia is outside the bone marrow. Examples include hemolytic anemias, either immune or nonimmune, and acute blood loss. In underproduction or hypoproliferative anemias, the reticulocyte count is typically low or inappropriately low. This indicates that the bone marrow is unable to produce the required number of RBCs. Therefore, the cause of the anemia is within the bone marrow. Examples of hypoproliferative anemias include nutrient deficiencies, endocrinopathies, infiltrative processes, or stem cell pathology. The most useful red cell indices are the mean

red blood cell volume (mean corpuscular volume or MCV) and the red blood cell distribution width (RDW). The MCV is used to subclassify the anemic process as microcytic, normocytic, or macrocytic. Etiologies of microcytic anemias include iron deficiency and thalassemias. Normocytic anemia is often found in anemia of chronic disease or endocrinopathies. Macrocytic anemias are seen in B_{12} or folate deficiencies, hemolytic anemias, and myelodysplastic syndromes. The RDW is a quantitative measure of the variation in red cell size, and is expressed as a percentage. Higher than normal RDW values are seen in iron deficiency, B_{12} deficiency, and folate deficiency. Significantly, RDW is usually normal in thalassemias and anemia of chronic disorders. Thus a low MCV with a high RDW indicates presence of iron deficiency with a sensitivity of over 90%. Low MCV with a normal RDW usually suggests a minor or major thalassemia. High MCV with an elevated RDW indicates a megaloblastic anemia. Once an anemia is classified as hyper- or hypoproliferative, additional workup is usually necessary to find the underlying cause. Laboratory studies such as iron and ferritin levels, vitamin levels, direct antigen test, osmotic fragility, and HGB electrophoresis are examples of such investigations. Examination of the blood smear and bone marrow biopsy are often helpful in establishing the diagnosis.

Clinical (including neurologic) consequences of anemia

Symptoms of anemia result from decreased oxygen delivery to tissues. Generally speaking, the signs and symptoms of anemia are dependent on the degree of anemia and the rate at which it has developed, as well as the oxygen requirement of the patient. Symptoms tend to be less severe with anemia that evolves slowly, because there is time for multiple homeostatic mechanisms to adjust to a reduced oxygen carrying capacity of blood. The extraction of oxygen by the tissues can increase as well as compensatory increases in stroke volume and heart rate and, therefore, cardiac output. Oxygen delivery can be maintained at rest at a hemoglobin concentration as low as 5 g/dL, assuming intravascular volume is maintained. However, symptoms develop when hemoglobin falls below this level at rest, or at higher hemoglobin concentrations with exertion or due to cardiac disease.

In a slowly progressing anemia, initial symptoms are fatigue, lethargy and muscle cramps. Other symptoms include dyspnea on exertion or even at rest. More severe anemia may lead to confusion and potentially life-threatening complications such as congestive heart failure, angina, cardiac arrhythmias, or myocardial infarction. Anemia from acute bleeding is associated with volume depletion, which can be associated with fatigue, dizziness, syncope, hypotension, and shock.

Pica, which is the habit of eating unusual substances such as ice, clay, cardboard, or raw starch, can indicate iron deficiency. Other symptoms may include mental confusion, loss of sexual drive, irritability, and other mood disturbances. On physical examination, mucous membrane changes such as smooth tongue and cheilitis, and flattening or spooning of the nails (koilonychia) are signs of chronic iron deficiency. Signs of advanced anemia include pallor, tachypnea, tachycardia, and cardiac flow murmurs. Megaloblastic anemias from vitamin B_{12} or folic acid deficiencies may also cause psychiatric and neurologic problems. Vitamin B_{12} deficiency produces abnormal muscle stretch reflexes and impaired vibration and position sense, as well as paresthesias, depression, memory loss, and irritability. Folate deficiency may result in depression and dementia in severe cases. These anemias are discussed elsewhere.

IRON DEFICIENCY ANEMIA

Causes of iron deficiency

Iron deficiency is the most common nutritional deficiency in the US. It has the highest prevalence among women and young children (Looker et al., 1997). Data from the NHANES III survey estimated the prevalence of iron deficiency was approximately 7% in toddlers aged 1–2 years. In women aged 12–49 years the prevalence of iron deficiency was 9–16%, while the prevalence of iron deficiency anemia was 3–5%. Worldwide, the problem is even greater, with as many as 49% of children under the age of 5 and 25% of adult women being iron deficient (Umbreit, 2005). Typically, iron deficiency is a secondary outcome due to an underlying medical condition. In developing countries, parasitic infection leading to chronic intestinal blood loss is the most common cause of iron deficiency. In the developed world, noninfectious GI blood loss and uterine menstrual blood loss in premenopausal females are the most common etiologies of iron deficiency. Other causes of GI blood loss include peptic ulcer disease, esophageal varices, gastritis, and angiodysplasia. GI malignancy should also be considered in all adults with unexplained iron deficiency (Rockey and Cello, 1993; Ho et al., 2005). Iron deficiency can also develop after chronic blood donation or be iatrogenic in hospitalized patients due to frequent laboratory tests. Erythropoietin use in renal failure has also been noted to lead to depletion of iron stores when iron is not administered concurrently. Uncommonly, iron deficiency anemia may be due to chronic intravascular hemolysis by way of urinary loss or pulmonary hemosiderosis.

Inadequate iron supply can also lead to iron deficiency anemia. Iron deficiency from inadequate intake is most often noted in infants and children, and is rare in adults. Pregnancy and lactation, however, can increase the demand for iron by threefold, leading to deficiency. Gastric malabsorption of iron often occurs in patients with celiac disease or after gastric bypass surgery. Finally, achlorhydria, may be a common cause of iron deficiency in the elderly. This is because gastric acid is necessary to maintain the common ferric form of inorganic iron soluble. *Helicobacter pylori* infection is known to affect both iron and ferritin levels independent of active GI bleeding; this may be due to altered pH of the stomach (Umbreit, 2005).

Clinical findings

Patients with iron deficiency anemia may be asymptomatic, or develop excessive fatigue, pallor, and other findings of anemia with progressive fall in the hemoglobin levels. Pica in the form of pagophagia or ice eating, as well as eating clay, cardboard, or raw starch, is a recognized symptom of iron deficiency. Patients may also have leg cramping. Physical examination may, although rarely, demonstrate stomatitis, glossitis, and koilonychias. These findings are specific to iron deficiency anemia and are caused by the effect of iron deficiency on rapidly dividing epithelial cells. Dysphagia due to esophageal webs (Plummer–Vinson syndrome) is a rare complication of iron deficiency and may reverse with replacement therapy (Umbreit, 2005). In infants and children, iron deficiency anemia can lead to a multitude of neurodevelopmental abnormalities including behavioral problems, decreased motor activity, and poor cognitive development (Pollitt, 1993; Grantham-McGregor and Ani, 2001). Restless legs syndrome is associated with lower iron content of the brain and a low ferritin level. Iron deficiency has deleterious effects on brain function by affecting neurotransmission. Therefore, it can lead to cognitive dysfunction and can cause significant decrease in work output.

Severe iron deficiency has been associated with carotid artery thrombosis in patients both with and without reactive thrombocytosis. Akins et al. reported three patients with identifiable thrombus in the carotid artery but without underlying atherosclerosis (Akins et al., 1996). All patients had severe anemia and significant reactive thrombocytosis. Medical management included anticoagulation and correction of iron deficiency with subsequent normalization of platelet counts. Keung and Owen reported 26 cases of cerebral thrombosis in patients with iron deficiency (Keung and Owen, 2004). Nine patients had normal platelet counts, suggesting that thrombocytosis is not required for thrombus formation.

Thrombosis in severe iron deficiency may be related to increased blood flow associated with severe anemia (Akins et al., 1996). Turbulent blood flow could damage the endothelium and lead to platelet activation and thrombus formation. This effect is more likely to be seen in the cerebral circulation where maintaining oxygen delivery is critical.

Kikuchi et al. recognized the association between cerebrovascular disease and anemia in a cohort of elderly patients (Kikuchi et al., 2001). They reported 5 year survival rates in nursing home patients to be significantly less when anemia was present (48% versus 67% in matched controls). Cardiovascular disease, including stroke, was the main cause of death in patients with anemia.

The association between iron deficiency anemia and stroke in healthy young children was reported by Maguire et al. in a prospective case control study conducted in Canada. They demonstrated that previously healthy children with vaso-occlusive stroke were 10 times more likely to have iron deficiency anemia compared with healthy controls. In addition, children with iron deficiency anemia accounted for more than 50% of all stroke cases in children without an underlying medical illness. The authors were able to demonstrate that iron deficiency anemia was a more common finding than other prothrombotic risk factors in young children with stroke, identifying iron deficiency anemia as a significant risk factor for stroke in otherwise healthy young children (Maguire et al., 2007). The mechanism underlying this documented association is incompletely defined; however, the presence of underlying congenital heart disease is thought to be a confounding factor (Lanthier et al., 2000).

Laboratory findings

Laboratory findings in iron deficiency follow an expected course. First, iron stores in the bone marrow, liver, and spleen are depleted. Bone marrow biopsy for evaluation of iron stores to establish the diagnosis has been regarded as the gold standard; however, it is not routinely performed due to the expense, discomfort, and technical sampling variability (Barron et al., 2001; Cook, 2004). Once iron stores are depleted, the total iron binding capacity (TIBC) begins to rise and serum iron saturation begins to fall. The definitive test involves measurement of serum ferritin, and a low serum ferritin is diagnostic of an iron-deficient state (Guyatt et al., 1992). Although ferritin is an acute phase reactant and can be elevated in an inflammatory state, a serum ferritin > 100 μg/L is rare in an iron-deficient state. Other clues for diagnosis include a microcytic anemia associated with increased RDW. The peripheral blood smear in iron deficiency anemia usually shows anisocytosis and poikilocytosis, or red blood cells of variable size and shape, respectively. In severe cases, cigar-shaped red blood cells and elliptocytes are present. Iron deficiency anemia may also be associated with a reactive thrombocytosis.

Treatment

Treatment of iron deficiency anemia includes oral iron replacement in addition to determining and correcting the underlying cause of iron loss. Oral ferrous iron salts are preferred due to improved solubility at the pH of the duodenum and jejunum. The typical replacement dose of oral iron is 325 mg of ferrous sulfate (66 mg of elemental iron) three times daily in adults and 3–6 mg of elemental iron/kg/day in children. Side-effects of oral iron tablets include epigastric pain, nausea, and vomiting. Taking iron tablets with food can reduce these symptoms, though it also decreases bioavailability. Indications for parenteral iron therapy include malabsorptive states (e.g., bowel resection or celiac disease), high iron requirements due to chronic ongoing blood loss or failure of oral therapy. Patients should respond to oral iron replacement with an increase in HGB apparent within 4 weeks of initiation of oral iron. The anemia then usually resolves in 4–6 months. Iron therapy should be continued for several months following correction of the anemia in order to adequately replete iron stores.

ANEMIA OF CHRONIC INFLAMMATION/DISEASE

Anemia of chronic disease (AOCD) is the most frequent anemia among hospitalized patients. The common disorders that cause such anemias are infections, inflammatory processes such as rheumatoid arthritis, and malignancies. AOCD is a hypoproliferative state with a normocytic or microcytic anemia. The disorder is mediated through various cytokines, the most prominent of which are interleukin 1, interleukin 6, and tumor necrosis factor α. The anemia is mild and frequently not severe enough to require transfusions. Iron studies demonstrate decreased serum iron, TIBC, and serum iron saturation. Serum ferritin is often normal or elevated. An elevated ESR or C-reactive protein may provide a clue to the diagnosis of AOCD. In most patients, AOCD does not require therapy and corrects itself in a few weeks after the underlying cause has been corrected. Even though erythropoietin therapy has been used in the management of AOCD, this therapy is not recommended in view of recently reported toxicities such as hypertension and increased risk of myocardial ischemia and stroke.

MEGALOBLASTIC ANEMIAS EXCLUDING FOLATE AND COBALAMIN DEFICIENCIES

The most common causes of macrocytic anemias in adults include alcoholism, liver disease, hemolysis, hypothyroidism, folate or vitamin B_{12} deficiency, exposure to chemotherapy and other drugs, and myelodysplasia. Drugs commonly associated with macrocytosis include hydroxyurea, methotrexate, trimethoprim, zidovudine, and 5-fluorouracil (Colon-Otero et al., 1992). Diagnostic evaluation for megaloblastic anemia includes serum measurements of cobalamin and folate, TSH, liver function tests, and a careful history to include alcohol intake, medication profile, and risk factors for hepatitis C. If these blood tests are normal, and in the absence of identifiable drugs or a history of alcohol abuse, further evaluation with a bone marrow biopsy is indicated to exclude myelodysplasia.

Myelodysplastic syndromes

Myelodysplastic syndromes (MDS) are clonal, preleukemic disorders that arise due to accumulated somatic mutations of the hematopoietic stem cell. In primary cases, they are a disease of the elderly, usually presenting in the sixth or seventh decade of life. MDS can also result from prior chemotherapy (alkylating agents and topoisomerase inhibitors) and ionizing radiation therapy. Clinical features are related to ineffective hematopoiesis and include peripheral cytopenias in the setting of a hypercellular bone marrow. A common presentation is macrocytic anemia without lymphadenopathy or splenomegaly.

MDS is classified according to bone marrow morphology as well as cytogenetic and molecular features of the affected hematopoietic cells. Prognostic factors include the percentage of myeloblasts in the bone marrow, karyotype, and number of peripheral cytopenias. Low risk MDS, as defined by the International Prognostic Scoring System (IPSS), has a median survival of 5.7 years, whereas patients with a high IPSS score have a median survival of 5 months. The clinical course of the myelodysplastic syndromes is highly variable, ranging from chronic mild anemia, to transfusion-dependent anemia, to rapid progression to acute myeloid leukemia.

Therapeutic strategies range from supportive care to curative attempts with hematopoietic stem cell transplantation (SCT). Goals of therapy depend on the age of the patient and the subtype of the myelodysplastic syndrome. In younger patients, allogeneic SCT should be considered with a curative intent. In others, therapy is directed at symptom control and slowing progression to acute myeloid leukemia. In patients with endogenous erythropoietin levels < 500, epoietin α or darbepoetin may increase the hemoglobin level and decrease the need for red cell transfusions. Newer novel therapies include epigenetic modifiers such as DNA hypomethylators (azacitidine (Vidaza)), immunomodulators (lenalidomide (Revlimid)), and histone deacetylase inhibitors (vorinostat). Azacitidine is currently approved for use in patients with all FAB subtypes, and lenalidomide is approved for use especially in patients with deletion 5q cytogenetic abnormality. Azacitidine induces hematologic responses in a substantial number of patients and prolongs survival in patients with high-risk MDS. In those who are candidates for SCT, long-term remission rates are 40–50%.

Toxicities associated with the use of the erythropoiesis-stimulating agents (ESAs) erythropoietin and darbepoietin include arthralgias (11%), hypertension (5–21%) and venous thromboembolism (11%). Neurologic toxicities include dizziness (5–21%), insomnia (13%), headache (10%), paresthesias (11%), seizures (1–3%), and CVA in < 1% of patients. In the US, ESAs carry a boxed warning regarding the risk of cardiovascular and thromboembolic events, stroke, and increased mortality in cancer patients. Use of ESAs for treatment of chemotherapy-associated anemia has largely been abandoned due to side-effects and adverse effects on patient survival. Major indications for the use of ESAs are anemia of chronic kidney disease and MDS (Singh et al., 2006; National Kidney Foundation Clinical Practice Guidelines, 2007; Phronmmintikul et al., 2007; Rizzo et al., 2008).

BONE MARROW FAILURE SYNDROMES

Background

In the case of bone marrow failure syndromes, anemia is a part of a more global disorder resulting in inadequate hematopoiesis. The fall in hemoglobin is usually accompanied by other cytopenias including leukopenia and thrombocytopenia, as underproduction can affect all three cell lines. In the setting of a hypercellular marrow, the cytopenias are due to ineffective hematopoiesis. Disorders resulting in bone marrow failure include aplastic anemia, acute leukemia, myelodysplastic syndrome, Fanconi's anemia, and paroxysmal nocturnal hemoglobinuria (PNH). Unique among bone marrow failure syndromes is red cell aplasia, where only the erythroid cell line is affected. There is significant clinical and pathophysiologic overlap with many of these diseases. In this section, we will focus on aplastic anemia, Fanconi's anemia, and pure red cell aplasia. PNH, myelodysplastic syndromes, and acute leukemia are discussed separately.

Pure red cell aplasia

Pure red cell aplasia (PRCA) can be inherited, as in Diamond–Blackfan anemia (DFA), or acquired. It is diagnosed when patient has anemia in the absence of circulating reticulocytes and marrow erythroid precursor cells. It can result from autoimmune, viral, or chemical inhibition of erythoblastic hematopoiesis. Acquired PRCA is often immunologically mediated secondary to thymomas, collagen-vascular syndromes, myasthenia gravis, and lymphoproliferative disorders such as chronic lymphocytic leukemia and large granular lymphocytic leukemia. PRCA can also be secondary to various viral infections including parvovirus B19 or a serious complication from certain drugs such as erythropoietin, phenytoin, and isoniazid. Therapy for acquired PRCA is directed at the underlying disorder and usually involves corticosteroids, followed by other immunosuppressives such as ciclosporin, antithymocyte globulin, rituximab, or sometimes cytotoxic therapies for refractory or relapsed disease (Djaldetti et al., 2003). Persistent parvovirus B19 infection responds to intravenous immunoglobulin therapy. Supportive care with transfusional therapy and attention to the complications of chronic transfusion is also necessary. With the appropriate treatment, prognosis is generally favorable with a median survival of greater than 10 years (Raghavachar, 1990).

Aplastic anemia

Acquired aplastic anemia arises when normal hematopoietic tissue is replaced by fat, resulting in pancytopenia and bone marrow hypocellularity. It has traditionally been associated with occupational and environment-specific toxins such as benzene or drugs such as chloramphenicol, NSAIDS, allopurinol, and gold. More recently, it has been shown to also result from infection with the hepatitis viruses. However, most cases of aplastic anemia are idiopathic, and no definitive causal agent is identified. The incidence of aplastic anemia is bimodal in distribution with a peak between 15 and 25 years of age and another in patients over the age of 60. It is an uncommon disease in the West, with a three to four times higher incidence in East Asia and the developing world (Brodsky and Jones, 2005).

Clinical features include anemia-related fatigue and weakness, thrombocytopenia-related petechiae and mucosal bleeding, and neutropenia-related infections. Constitutional symptoms (fever, night sweats, and weight loss) are usually absent. Specifically, cachexia, lymphadenopathy, and splenomegaly are not seen, and if present usually suggest an alternative diagnosis. In the setting of pancytopenia, the diagnostic test of choice is a bone marrow biopsy. In aplastic anemia, hematopoietic elements are significantly decreased with bone marrow cellularity of less than 30% in the absence of malignant or markedly dysplastic cells.

There is some evidence to suggest an immune-mediated pathogenesis of aplastic anemia, and many patients respond to immunosuppressant therapies such as antithymocyte globulin and ciclosporin. However, definitive curative therapy involves allogeneic hematopoietic stem cell transplantation (HSCT). Immunosupression is preferred in elderly patients and HSCT is almost always preferred in children if an appropriate donor is available. Prognosis is correlated with hematologic response to therapy at 3 months, with 5 year survival of 75% with either immunosuppressant or HSCT therapy (Bacigalupo et al., 2000).

Fanconi's anemia

Fanconi's anemia (FA), although rare, is the most common inherited bone marrow failure syndrome. The inheritance pattern is autosomal or X-linked, and occurs in patients from a variety of ethnic backgrounds, with a mean age at diagnosis of 8–9 years (Heimpel, 2004). In addition to pancytopenia, patients generally have characteristic physical findings involving cutaneous, musculoskeletal, and urogenital systems. These physical findings including hyper- or hypopigmented skin lesions, microcephaly, short stature, male hypogonadism, and malformations of the thumb and kidneys. In the setting of this constellation of physical findings and hematologic abnormalities, the diagnosis can be made by identification of certain well-described gene mutations. These are demonstrated by a chromosome breakage test with either standard diepoxybutane (DEB) or mitomycin C (MMC) (Kennedy and D'Andrea, 2005).

Some 80% of patients will develop signs of bone marrow failure by the age of 20 years. FA is also complicated by an increased incidence of malignancies including acute myeloid leukemia (AML), MDS, liver tumors, and squamous cell carcinomas. Given this association, regular tumor surveillance beginning in the second decade of life is recommended (Heimpel, 2004). The only curative therapy for FA is allogeneic stem cell transplantation. Patients in whom a suitable donor is not available or who cannot tolerate stem cell transplantation should be treated palliatively with androgens and hematopoietic growth factors to improve hematopoiesis.

Anemia associated with lead poisoning

Lead poisoning has been known since antiquity and some believe lead poisoning contributed to the fall of the Roman Empire (Klein et al., 1970). In children, anemia is an important part of the clinical syndrome that results from lead toxicity. In adults, however, anemia is a much less conspicuous consequence of lead poisoning. Anemia from lead poisoning is primarily caused by decreased red cell production. Red cell destruction (hemolysis) contributes to anemia (Beutler, 2006).

With improved awareness and preventive measures to eliminate the danger of lead poisoning, its incidence has fallen significantly in the US in the past 30 years. At present, its prevalence in adults is estimated to be 6.3 per 100 000 (Centers for Disease Control, 2009).

In children, symptoms and signs associated with lead poisoning vary greatly according to the level of exposure. The spectrum of neurologic toxicity varies from inattentiveness, irritability, and hyperactivity to learning disabilities, delayed growth, hearing loss, motor paralysis, and encephalopathy (Mendelsohn et al., 1998). At high levels, lead can cause permanent brain damage and even death. In adults, the clinical picture includes abdominal pain or colic, arthralgias, headaches, anorexia, decrease in memory, and Fanconi-type nephropathy.

HEMOLYTIC ANEMIAS

Background

Hemolytic anemia is defined as decreased levels of erythrocytes in circulating blood due to their premature destruction. It can be acute, chronic, or episodic. Destruction and removal of erythrocytes occurs via the reticuloendothelial system (extravascular hemolysis) or lysis within the circulation (intravascular hemolysis). When the bone marrow can no longer compensate for the shortened RBC lifespan, anemia develops.

The causes of hemolytic anemia are numerous, but can generally be divided into disorders intrinsic or extrinsic to the red blood cell. Most intrinsic causes of hemolysis are inherited, while extrinsic causes are typically acquired (Rodgers and Young, 2010). Careful diagnostic investigation to determine the underlying cause of the hemolytic syndrome is necessary in order to develop an effective treatment plan. Intrinsic pathologies include: congenital and acquired RBC membrane disorders such as hereditary spherocytosis and paroxysmal nocturnal hemoglobinuria (PNH), respectively; disorders of RBC metabolism such as pyruvate kinase and glucose-6-phosphate dehydrogenase (G6PD) deficiency; and disorders of hemoglobin synthesis such as the thalassemias and sickle cell disease. Extrinsic causes of hemolysis include: immunologic abnormalities such as autoimmune syndromes and alloantibodies; a hyperactive reticuloendothelial system such as is seen with splenomegaly; mechanical injury such as the shear stress associated with defective mechanical heart valves and microangiopathy; and certain infections. Infectious causes of hemolysis are either toxin-mediated or by direct organism invasion of the red blood cell. The causes of intravascular hemolysis are almost exclusively extrinsic to the red blood cell.

Diagnosis and clinical findings

The hallmark of hemolytic anemia is reticulocytosis, or an elevated number of immature erythrocytes. An increased number of reticulocytes is present in hemolysis unless erythropoiesis is inadequate or suppressed. In adults without anemia, reticulocytes comprise 0.5–1.5% of circulating erythrocytes. If the reticulocyte percentage is above this normal range, compensatory erythropoiesis due to either blood loss or hemolysis is suspected. Other diagnostic tests include examination of the peripheral blood smear and measurement of serum lactate dehydrogenase (LDH), bilirubin, and haptoglobin. Suggestive findings of hemolysis include an elevated LDH and indirect bilirubin, and low haptoglobin. Reduced levels of haptoglobin and increased levels of LDH provide 96% specificity for predicting hemolytic anemia (Rodgers and Young, 2010). Intravascular hemolysis can also be associated with RBC fragmentation manifested by schistocytes on the peripheral smear and urinary hemosiderin excretion.

A useful and commonly used laboratory test to discern the cause of hemolysis is the indirect and direct antigen test, also known as the Coombs' test. In immune-mediated hemolysis, the direct antigen test can detect the presence of autoantibodies. The test is performed by incubating a patient's red blood cells with antibodies to human IgG. If IgG or complement is present on the red blood cell membrane, agglutination occurs and the test is positive. The indirect antigen test involves incubation of patient serum with reagent RBCs, followed by addition of human anti-IgG antibodies. If agglutination occurs, autoantibodies against red blood cells are present in the patient's serum and the test is positive. Systemic manifestations of hemolytic anemia can be a result of the anemia itself or the consequences of increased red cell destruction. The severity of clinical presentation is determined by the rate of red cell destruction and the host's ability to compensate with increased erythropoiesis. Symptoms may be mild and include pallor, fatigue, and dizziness. Acute severe hemolysis (hemolytic crisis) causes severe symptoms such as chills, fever, back and abdominal pain, prostration, and even hemodynamic compromise. Chronic hemolysis can be associated with jaundice and splenomegaly. Patients can also report reddish-brown or "coca-cola"-colored urine caused by hemoglobinuria.

Treatment

Therapeutic strategies should be designed based on both the severity of clinical symptoms and the underlying etiology of hemolysis. A broad range of inherited and acquired diseases are manifested by hemolysis, and many require a different therapeutic approach. Immune-mediated causes of hemolytic anemia are generally treated with corticosteroids, immunoglobulin infusion, or other immunosuppressant therapies. The treatment of choice for microangiopathic hemolytic anemia associated with thrombotic thrombocytopenic purpura is plasma exchange (Szczepiorkowski et al., 2007). Treatment of hemolysis due to infection involves treatment of the underlying disorder with antimicrobial therapy. Avoidance of certain medications is imperative to prevent G6PD deficiency-associated hemolysis. Splenectomy is generally not first-line therapy for the hemolytic anemias, and is reserved for severe or refractory disease. In addition to treatment of the underlying cause of the hemolysis, supportive care, especially in patients with chronic hemolysis, is necessary. This includes red blood cell transfusion if bone marrow compensation is inadequate and the patient's cardiopulmonary status is compromised. In the case of the need for long-term transfusion therapy, iron overload may develop and may necessitate chelation therapy. Folate supplementation at a dose of 1 mg/day is needed for patients with chronic hemolysis because of the nutritional needs associated with accelerated erythropoiesis.

Autoimmune hemolytic anemia

Autoimmune hemolytic anemia (AIHA) is characterized by the presence of antibodies against the patient's own red blood cells (autoantibodies), resulting in accelerated destruction and subsequent clinical and laboratory findings of hemolytic anemia. Autoimmune hemolytic anemias are classified according to the subtype of immunoglobulin responsible for red cell destruction and the temperature at which they react and agglutinate. In the case of warm AIHA, the implicated antibody is usually IgG that reacts optimally at 37°C *in vitro*. It is usually associated with an underlying systemic disease such as systemic lupus erythematous (SLE) or a lymphoproliferative disorder. The hemolysis from warm AIHA is mainly extravascular and symptoms are often mild. In addition to those described above, characteristic laboratory findings include a positive direct antigen test and spherocytes on the peripheral smear. Treatment with oral corticosteroids at a dose of 1 mg/kg/day is effective in more than half of patients, and splenectomy is effective in approximately half of those who are steroid refractory (Rodgers and Young, 2010). Intravenous immunoglobulin and rituximab, a monoclonal antibody targeting the B lymphocyte CD20 antigen, may also benefit a select group of patients (Gehrs and Freidberg, 2002).

In cold agglutination syndrome the implicated antibody is usually IgM, reacting at temperatures lower than 30°C. The syndrome may be primary or secondary to an underlying viral illness such as mycoplasma pneumonia and infectious mononucleosis or a lymphoproliferative disorder. Patients may present with cold-induced acrocyanosis, hematuria, and acral dysthesias. Treatment is primarily preventative, and patients are advised to avoid exposure to cold temperatures. If necessary, immunosuppressant therapy such as corticosteroids or rituximab can be used.

G6PD deficiency

Deficiency of glucose 6-phosphate deaminase is the most frequently encountered abnormality of red cell metabolism resulting in hemolytic anemia. It is an inherited, X-linked disorder with significant polymorphism . Enzyme-deficient red blood cells cause inadequate NADPH production and reduced glutathione levels, rendering them susceptible to oxidation and HGB denaturation. The formation of Heinz bodies, or intraerythrocytic denatured HGB aggregates, heralds the diagnosis, and results in extravascular hemolysis in the spleen. Prevention of hemolysis requires avoidance of "oxidant challenges" such as certain drugs, foods, and infections (Beutler, 1994).

Hereditary spherocytosis

Hereditary spherocytosis is an inherited cause of hemolytic anemia. It is the most common inherited hemolytic anemia in northern Europeans and is characterized by a defect in the red cell membrane resulting in spherocytic, osmotically fragile red cells. In addition to the usual laboratory abnormalities indicative of hemolysis previously described, the hallmark of diagnosis is the identification of spherocytes on the peripheral blood smear. A positive osmotic fragility test verifies the diagnosis. In addition to supportive care with folate supplementation and attention to gallstone formation, definitive treatment with splenectomy may be necessary in some patients (Bolton-Magge et al., 2004).

Paroxysmal nocturnal hemoglobinuria

Paroxysmal nocturnal hemoglobinuria (PNH) is an acquired clonal disorder of hematopoietic stem cells resulting in the absence of glycosyl phophatidylinositol (GPI)-linked proteins on the red cell membrane surface. The lack of GPI proteins subjects the red cell to complement activation and subsequent intravascular hemolysis. Specific mutations in the *PIGA* gene have been identified in individuals with PNH (Chen et al., 2005). In addition to hemolytic anemia, the PNH syndrome is associated with a coagulopathy leading to thrombotic complications. The thromboembolism seen in PNH is primarily venous involving mesenteric veins, but can involve other parts of the body including the central nervous system (Donhowe and Lazaro, 1984; Ziakas et al., 2008). Classically, hepatic venous thrombosis (Budd–Chiari syndrome) is associated with PNH. Even though uncommon, intracranial thromboembolism in PNH can have devastating consequences. In most of the cases the thrombosis involves the major venous sinuses but individual veins can also be affected. Arterial thrombi are rare but frequently result in cerebral infarctions (Audebert et al., 2005). Renal, splenic, iliac, and coronary arteries can also be involved. Diagnosis of PNH is made via peripheral blood flow cytometry with the identification of cells deficient in GPI anchored proteins. In addition to supportive care including anticoagulation when clinically warranted, treatment with a humanized monoclonal antibody to the C5 terminal complement component, eculizumab, has shown some benefit in terms of decreasing hemolysis and the need for transfusion in some patients (Hill et al., 2005).

Hemoglobinopathies

Inherited abnormalities of hemoglobin synthesis and structure such as the thalassemias and sickle cell anemia are common causes of hemolysis. They are discussed separately in another chapter.

CONCLUSIONS

In anemic patients, a systematic approach, based on pathophysiology is likely to yield the diagnosis. Many patients have multiple causes of anemia. The treatment should be aimed at the underlying etiology, and red cell transfusions should be used conservatively.

REFERENCES

Akins PT, Glenn S, Nemeth PM et al. (1996). Carotid artery thrombus associated with severe iron deficiency anemia and thrombocytosis. Stroke 27: 1002–1005.

Audebert HJ, Planck J, Eisenburg M et al. (2005). Cerebral ischemic infarction in paroxysmal nocturnal hemoglobinuria. Report of 2 cases and updated review of 7 previously reported cases. J Neurol 252: 1379–1383.

Bacigalupo A, Brand R, Oneto R et al. (2000). Treatment of acquired severe aplastic anemia: bone marrow transplantation compared with immunosuppressive therapy – the European Group for Blood and Marrow Transplantation experience. Semin Hematol 37: 69–80.

Barron B, Hoyer J, Tefferi A (2001). A bone marrow report of absent stainable iron is not diagnostic of iron deficiency. Ann Hematol 80: 166–169.

Beutler E (1994). G6PD deficiency. Blood 84: 3613–3636.

Beutler E (2006). Hemolytic anemia resulting from chemical and physical agents. In: E Beutler, K Kaushansky, TJ Kipps, MA Lichtman, JT Prchal, U Selighsohn (Eds.),

Williams Hematology. McGraw-Hill, United States, pp. 717–719.

Beutler E, Waalen J (2006). The definition of anemia: what is the lower limit of normal of the blood hemoglobin concentration? Blood 107: 1747–1750.

Bolton-Magge PH, Stevens RF, Dodd NJ et al. (2004). Guidelines for the diagnosis and treatment of hereditary spherocytosis. Br J Haematol 126: 455–474.

Brodsky RA, Jones RJ (2005). Aplastic anemia. Lancet 365: 1647–1656.

Centers for Disease Control (2009). Adult blood lead epidemiology and surveillance–United States, 2005–2007. Morb Mortal Wkly Rep. 58: 365.

Chen G, Zeng W, Maciejewski JP et al. (2005). Differential gene expression in hematopoietic progenitors from paroxysmal nocturnal hemoglobinuria patients reveals an apoptosis/immune response in "normal" phenotype cells. Leukemia 19: 862–868.

Colon-Otero G, Menke D, Hook CC (1992). A practical approach to the differential diagnosis and evaluation of the adult patient with macrocytic anemia. Med Clin North Am 76: 581–597.

Cook J (2004). Diagnosis and management of iron-deficiency anemia. Best Pract Res Clin Haematol 18: 319–332.

Djaldetti M, Blay A, Bergman M et al. (2003). Pure red cell aplasia – a rare disease with multiple causes. Biomed Pharmacother 57: 326–332.

Donhowe SP, Lazaro RP (1984). Dural sinus thrombosis in paroxysmal nocturnal hemoglobinuria. Clin Neurol Neurosurg 86: 149–154.

Gehrs BC, Freidberg RC (2002). Autoimmune hemolytic anemia. Am J Hematol 69: 258–271.

Grantham-McGregor S, Ani C (2001). A review of studies on the effect of iron deficiency on cognitive development in children. J Nutr 131: 649S–668S.

Guyatt G, Oxman A, Ali M et al. (1992). Laboratory diagnosis of iron-deficiency anemia: an overview. J Gen Intern Med 7: 145–153.

Heimpel H (2004). Congenital dyserythropoietic anemias: epidemiology, clinical significance, and progress in understanding their pathogenesis. Ann Hematol 83: 613–621.

Hill A, Hillmen P, Richards SJ et al. (2005). Sustained response and long-term safety of eculizumab in paroxysmal nocturnal hemoglobinuria. Blood 106: 2559–2565.

Ho C, Chau W, Hsu H et al. (2005). Predictive risk factors and prevalence of malignancy in patients with iron deficiency anemia in Taiwan. Am J Hematol 78: 108–112.

Kennedy RD, D'Andrea AD (2005). The Fanconi anemia/BRCA pathway: new faces in the crowd. Genes Dev 19: 2925–2940.

Keung YK, Owen J (2004). Iron deficiency and thrombosis: literature review. Clin Appl Thromb Hemost 10: 387–391.

Kikuchi M, Inagaki T, Shinagawa N (2001). Five-year survival of older people with anemia: variation with hemoglobin concentration. J Am Geriatr Soc 49: 1226–1228.

Klein M, Namer R, Harpur E et al. (1970). Earthenware containers as a source of fatal lead poisoning. N Engl J Med 283: 669–672.

Lanthier S, Carmant L, David M et al. (2000). Stroke in children: the coexistence of multiple risk factors predicts poor outcome. Neurology 54: 371–378.

Looker A, Dallman P, Carrol M et al. (1997). Prevalence of iron deficiency in the United States. JAMA 227: 973–976.

Maguire J, deVeber G, Parkin P (2007). Association between iron-deficiency anemia and stroke in young children. Pediatrics 120: 1053–1057.

Mendelsohn AL, Dreyer BP, Fierman AH et al. (1998). Low-level lead exposure and behavior in early childhood. Pediatrics. 101:E10.

National Kidney Foundation KDOQI (2007). Clinical practice guidelines and recommendations in chronic kidney disease. Am J Kidney Dis 50: 529–530.

Nordenberg D, Yip R, Binkin N (1990). The effect of cigarette smoking on hemoglobin levels and anemia screening. JAMA 264: 1556–1599.

Phronmmintikul A, Haas SJ, Elsik M et al. (2007). Mortality and target hemoglobin concentrations in anaemic patients with chronic kidney disease treated with erythropoietin. A meta-analysis. Lancet 369: 381–388.

Pollitt E (1993). Iron deficiency and cognitive function. Annu Rev Nutr 13: 521–537.

Raghavachar A (1990). Pure red cell aplasia: review of treatment and proposal for treatment strategy. Blut 61: 47–51.

Rizzo JD, Somerfield MR, Hegarty LK et al. (2008). Use of epoietin and darbepoietin in patients with cancer: 2007 American Society of Hematology/American Society of Clinical Oncology clinical practice guidelines. Blood 111: 25–41.

Rockey D, Cello J (1993). Evaluation of the gastrointestinal tract in patients with iron-deficiency anemia. N Engl J Med 329: 1691–1695.

Rodgers G, Young N (2010). The Bethesda Handbook of Clinical Hematology. Lipincott Williams and Wilkins.

Singh AJ, Szczech L, Tang KI et al. (2006). Correction of anemia with epoetin alfa in chronic kidney disease. N Engl J Med 355: 2085–2098.

Stewart R, Baretta E, Platte L et al. (1974). Carboxyhemoglobin levels in American blood donors. JAMA 229: 1187–1195.

Szczepiorkowski ZM, Bandarenko N, Kim HC et al. (2007). Guidelines on the use of therapeutic apheresis in clinical practice – evidence based approach from the apheresis applications committee of the American Society for Apheresis. J Clin Apher 22: 106–175.

Umbreit J (2005). Iron deficiency: a concise review. Am J Hematol 78: 225–231.

Ziakas PD, Poulou LS, Pomoni A (2008). Thrombosis in paroxysmal nocturnal hemoglobinuria at a glance: a clinical review. Curr Vasc Pharmacol 6: 347–354.

Handbook of Clinical Neurology, Vol. 120 (3rd series)
Neurologic Aspects of Systemic Disease Part II
Jose Biller and Jose M. Ferro, Editors

Chapter 68

Neurologic complications of sickle cell disease

AKILA VENKATARAMAN[1] AND ROBERT J. ADAMS[2*]

[1]*Pediatric Neurology and Epilepsy Division, Lutheran Medical Center, Brooklyn, NY, USA*

[2]*South Carolina Stroke Center of Economic Excellence and Medical University of South Carolina Stroke Center,
Charleston, SC, USA*

HISTORY

Sickle cell anemia and related hemoglobinopathies are disorders of the red cell, in particular the hemoglobin. This group of blood disorders includes sickle cell disease (SCD), sickle C disease, and sickle-β thalassemia. Those afflicted with these hemoglobinopathies commonly suffer damage to vital organs, especially to the central nervous system, the spleen, the kidney, the lung, and the heart, as a result of microvascular vaso-occlusion by the sickled erythrocytes.

The genes responsible for the transmission of sickle cell syndromes from one generation to the next were recognized during the 17th century. Herrick (1910) first recorded this disease in the medical literature in the US in 1910. The neurologic complications of SCD were first reported in 1923, when Sydenstricker (Sydenstricker et al., 1923) detailed the case of a 5-year-old sickle cell patient with hemiparesis and seizures. Following this, additional case reports of SCD and stroke were soon published (Arena, 1935). In 1972, Stockman and colleagues published the cerebral angiographic results of a series of SCD children with neurologic deficits, documenting the vasculopathy that is seen in the large vessels of the central nervous system (Stockman et al., 1972).

Sickle cell disease, usually presenting in childhood, occurs more commonly in people (or their descendants) from parts of tropical and subtropical regions. One-third of all indigenous inhabitants of Sub-Saharan Africa carry the gene (Platt et al., 1994). The prevalence of the disease in the US is approximately 1 in 5000, mostly affecting Americans of Sub-Saharan African descent, according to the National Institutes of Health (NIH). In the US, about 1 in 500 black births have sickle cell anemia. Life expectancy is shortened, with studies reporting an average life expectancy of 42 in males and 48 in females (http://www.nhlbi.nih.gov/health/dci/Diseases/Sca/SCA_Summary.html).

Numerous breakthroughs in the diagnosis and management of central nervous system complications of SCD have been made since. There have been several seminal studies and trials establishing guidelines for investigation and prevention of the neurologic complications of SCD. These studies have laid the foundation for the extensive research that is needed for the development of optimal prevention and curative treatment of the cerebrovascular complications of SCD.

CLINICAL FINDINGS

The clinical course of patients with SCD is highly variable, with much diversity in the expression of the clinical phenotype.

Central nervous system complications are unfortunately common in sickle cell disease. The neurologic complications associated with SCD are related to vaso-occlusive phenomena and hemolysis and are manifest as cerebral infarction, transient ischemic attacks, intracranial hemorrhage, subsequent cognitive and behavioral changes, and seizures. Occasionally aneurysms and arteriovenous malformations are also seen in these patients.

Stroke is clinically characterized by focal symptoms, such as hemiparesis or hemisensory deficits. Symptoms depend on both the location and size of the lesions involved. The underlying vasculopathy varies from extensive, clinically devastating infarcts involving the entire territory of a large artery to smaller, subtler lacunar infarcts that may only present with more diffuse symptoms such as neurocognitive dysfunction. (Pavlakis et al., 1989).

---

*Correspondence to: Robert J. Adams, M.S., M.D., Professor of Neuroscience, Medical University of South Carolina, 19 Hagood Avenue - Suite 501 HOT, Charleston, SC 29425, USA. Tel: +1-843-792-7058, Fax: +1-843-792-2484, E-mail: adamsrj@musc.edu

Stroke is one of the major complications of SCD and can affect ~11% of affected individuals by age 20 (Ohene-Frempong et al., 1998).

Intracranial hemorrhage represents a smaller stroke phenotype in SCD, often manifesting with dramatic and nonfocal symptoms, including severe headache or coma. Hemorrhagic stroke is usually caused by hemorrhagic conversion of a large brain infarction, friable moyamoya vessels, or ruptured aneurysms (Oyesiku et al., 1991).

One cerebrovascular phenomenon recognized in SCD is the "silent cerebral infarct." With advanced neuroimaging techniques and more widespread screening, clinically asymptomatic ischemic lesions suggestive of small vessel occlusion, usually occurring in the arterial border zones, have been detected in almost 25% of children with SCD (Armstrong et al., 1996). Silent infarct white matter lesions and atrophy are more common in neurologically asymptomatic adults compared to community controls without SCD (Vichinsky et al., 2010). Children with silent infarcts identified by MRI may appear asymptomatic, but perform significantly lower on neuropsychological tests than their counterparts with a normal MRI (Armstrong et al., 1996). Cognitive deficits are associated with frontal lobe infarction in children with sickle cell disease. Compared with healthy controls, adults with SCD had poorer cognitive performance, which was associated with anemia and age (Vichinsky et al., 2010). Neurocognitive dysfunction has been implicated as an important contributor to the poor social, economic, and quality-of-life factors reported in adult SCD (Watkins et al., 1998; Noll et al., 2001; Powars et al., 2001). Patients who had silent infarcts were significantly more likely to have a history of seizure.

Peripheral nervous system involvement is rare in sickle cell disease. Mononeuropathy resulting from peripheral nerve infarction, as a complication of sickle vaso-occlusive crisis, is uncommon. Reports of patients with SCD who developed acute mononeuropathy multiplex in the setting of sickle cell pain crisis suggests a multifocal nerve disorder resulting from an ischemic process caused by a sickle cell vaso-occlusive crisis (Roohi et al., 2001).

NATURAL HISTORY

Much progress has been made during the past several decades in understanding the natural history of sickle cell disease and its complications, particularly those affecting the central nervous system.

The Cooperative Study of Sickle Cell Disease (CSSCD), one of the landmark population studies, has provided the best evidence for risk factors leading to brain infarction and hemorrhage.

The overall age-specific incidence of first stroke in SCD is 0.13% at ages younger than 24 months, increasing to just over 1% at ages 2–5 years, with only a slight decrement to 0.79% at ages 6–9 years. The risk of brain infarction declines until a second peak is seen at ages older than 50 years, when the incidence again increases to nearly 1.3% (Ohene-Frempong et al., 1998b). Children with SCD carry a 200-fold increased risk for cerebral infarction.

The CSSCD observed that the incidence of ischemic stroke was highest in children between 2 and 10 years and again in adults older than 30 years, while hemorrhagic stroke peaks among patients 20–29 years (Powars et al., 2001, 2005). Prior transient ischemic attack, a low steady-state hemoglobin level, hypertension, and a history of acute chest syndrome were the only risk factors found to be significantly associated with brain infarction (Powars et al., 2001) Risk factors for intracranial hemorrhage included low steady-state hemoglobin values and a high leukocyte count (Ohene-Frempong et al., 1998c). In patients who develop symptomatic stroke, the risk of recurrent stroke approaches 70% (Powars et al., 2001).

Silent infarct recognized at age 6 years or older is associated with increased stroke risk (Miller et al., 2001). Lower hemoglobin level, increased leukocyte count, and β^S-globin gene haplotype were associated also with the presence of silent infarcts (Kinney et al., 1999). Data from the CSSCD revealed a strong association between silent infarcts and future stroke risk, suggesting that these lesions are progressive and may occur with increased frequency in older patients.

Despite substantial advances in the understanding of the pathophysiology and clinical course of sickle cell disease, management of morbidity and mortality remains a challenge for adult patients. However, childhood mortality has improved considerably as the consequence of advances in stroke management (Powars et al., 2005). Recognition of risk factors, prevention of primary and recurrent strokes, and treatment of neurologic complications with novel therapies all contribute to a shift in the natural history of sickle cell disease, with better overall outcomes.

LABORATORY INVESTIGATIONS

The majority of initial laboratory investigations are directed toward the establishment of the specific hemoglobinopathy.

Diagnostic recommendations set forth by the 1975 International Committee for Standardization in Hematology expert panel on abnormal HbS and thalassemias include an initial panel of a complete blood count (CBC), electrophoresis at pH 9.2, tests for solubility and sickling, and quantification of Hb A2 and Hb F. Further tests such as electrophoresis at pH 6.0–6.2, globin chain separation, and isoelectric focusing (IEF) were recommended if an abnormal hemoglobin is identified on initial testing (Clarke and Higgins, 2000). Cation-exchange high performance light chromatography (HPLC) (Fisher et al., 1997; Rioux et al., 1997) is now touted as the method of choice for quantification of Hb A2 and Hb F and identification of Hb variants (British Committee for Standards in Haematology, 1988; International Committee for Standardization in Haematology, 1988). Diagnosis of sickle cell trait and disease depends on a typical HPLC and Hb electrophoretic pattern. The %HbS is also an important value to obtain as it guides transfusion protocols to afford primary prevention against strokes.

Further laboratory tests may then be conducted to evaluate the coagulation profile and propensity toward hypercoaguability, to consider differential diagnoses for the etiology of strokes. These tests include PT, PTT, INR, protein C and S, factor V Leiden mutation, anticardiolipin antibody, antithrombin, and serum homocysteine, to name a few.

Liver biopsy is considered the most accurate and sensitive method to assess the iron burden after long-term transfusion therapy in patients with SCD. However, this is an invasive technique and hepatic iron measurements from a liver biopsy specimen may be confounded by hepatic fibrosis and uneven tissue distribution of iron (Bonkovsky et al., 1990).

The most promising newer methods to noninvasively measure iron are based on measurement of hepatic magnetic susceptibility, either using superconducting quantum interference device susceptometry (SQUID) or magnetic resonance susceptometry (MRS) (Brittenham and Badman, 2003; Fischer et al., 2003; Carneiro et al., 2005). At present, biomagnetic susceptometry is possibly the most reliable noninvasive method for measurement of tissue iron stores (Fischer et al., 1999). Special imaging software with MRI has now become available for reliable noninvasive liver iron results (St Pierre et al., 2005).

NEUROIMAGING

Almost all modalities of neuroimaging are useful in sickle cell disease, considering the extent of cerebrovascular disease that is seen in this condition.

Cranial computed tomography (CT) is typically the initial study performed in situations where clinically a stroke, hemorrhagic or infarct, is suspected. However, CT has limitations in detecting very early brain ischemia.

Conventional MRI is much more sensitive and specific for parenchymal lesions. Diffusion-weighted imaging (DWI) detects brain ischemia within an hour after stroke onset and is able to distinguish ischemic stroke from other conditions.

MRI is also useful in detecting silent cerebral infarcts. Silent cerebral infarcts are diagnosed on the basis of an abnormal MRI of the brain and a normal neurologic examination. Some studies using brain MR imaging have showed infarction/ischemia in the absence of a recognized cerebrovascular accident in 13% of patients (Moser et al., 1996). It is twice as common as clinical infarction and may occur in up to 22% of children with sickle cell disease by 12 years of age (Moritania et al., 2004). A silent cerebral infarct has been defined as an area of abnormally increased signal intensity on the intermediate and T2-weighted pulse sequences of MRI. The area of abnormal signal must have an appearance consistent with infarction and include a focal 3 mm or larger area of abnormally increased signal intensity on the T2-weighted image in more than one view (Armstrong et al., 1996).

Another common finding on MRI in patients with sickle cell disease is cerebral atrophy. This is a nonspecific finding that serves as a marker for disease severity in the brain.

Based on MR studies, cortical infarction is often seen to be unilateral and in the frontoparietal location, and related to large vessel disease. White matter infarction is often bilateral and in the frontoparietal location and this appears to be related to small vessel vasculopathy (Moritania et al., 2004).

The neurologic complications of sickle cell disease occur mainly as a result of the vasculopathy of the central nervous system (Stockman et al., 1972). It is therefore most logical to investigate the disease process with neuroimaging that is primarily based on evaluating the vasculature of the nervous system. Magnetic resonance angiography (MRA) provides critical information on the status of the cerebral vasculature, and has replaced intra-arterial catheter angiography as an accurate and noninvasive technique to detect cerebral artery lesions (Kandeel et al., 1996). Moyamoya, a description that comes from the Japanese for "puff of smoke" because of the angiographic appearance of secondary extensive collateral formation, is a secondary complication of the cerebral vasculopathy of SCD. It is seen in 35% of sickle cell disease patients at conventional angiography. In comparison, moyamoya vessels were seen in 20% at MRI/MRA (Moritania et al., 2004).

Brain imaging abnormalities were reported in up to 44% of children with sickle cell disease. The frequency of brain imaging abnormalities detected by MRI/MRA in adults with sickle cell disease was higher than that described for children (Silva et al., 2009).

The prevention of stroke in children with SCD has been markedly advanced by the introduction and testing of transcranial Doppler (TCD) as a noninvasive diagnostic test indicating high risk of first stroke. TCD uses pulsed Doppler to measure the velocity and pulsatility of blood flow within the major intracranial arteries of the circle of Willis. In children with sickle cell disease, there is involvement of the distal intracranial internal carotid artery (ICA) and the proximal portions of the middle (MCA) and anterior (ACA) cerebral arteries (Jeffries et al., 1980). The risk of stroke increases dramatically as TCD flow velocity increases in these basal arteries, first probably on the basis of increased flow velocity generally, and due to stenosis in the later stages. The risk of stroke rises about 30% for each 10 cm/second increase above the median velocity for children with SCD (Adams et al., 2004). A large single center prospective study demonstrated the likelihood of stroke in children with sickle cell anemia was predicted by TCD in the absence of regular transfusion (Adams et al., 1992, 1997).

Using TCD, a multicenter randomized controlled trial, the Stroke Prevention Trial in Sickle Cell Anemia (STOP trial) confirmed that TCD, using a cutoff of 200 cm/second velocity or higher, was associated with a 10% risk of stroke in the untreated group for the 2 years that the trial was allowed to continue. In those children who were randomized to regular transfusions (every 4 weeks or so), however, the stroke risk was less than 1% (p < 0.001). The STOP study confirmed both the remarkable predictive power of TCD (10–20 times the background risk of stroke for unselected children with SCD) and the striking reduction of stroke with regular transfusions (Adams et al., 1998). The STOP study led to a clinical alert, issued by the National Heart, Lung, and Blood Institute (NLBHI), recommending TCD screening of children with sickle cell disease between the ages of 2 and 16 years as effective for assessing stroke risk.

TCD screening, followed by regular transfusion in cases with high risk TCD, has now become the standard of care for children with SCD and is recommended by the NHLBI (http://www.nhlbi.nih.gov/health/dci/Diseases/Sca/SCA_Treatments.html) and the American Stroke Association (Goldstein et al., 2011).

Transcranial Doppler velocities in adult patients with intracranial stenoses have been shown to be lower than those described for the pediatric population with sickle cell disease and it is not clear how predictive TCD is for adults with SCD and stroke risk (Valadi et al., 2006; Silva et al., 2009).

Sibling studies have been conducted with TCD to investigate the possibility of a familial predisposition to elevated cerebral blood flow velocity. The presence of a sibling with a positive TCD result was significantly associated with an elevated cerebral blood flow velocity in other siblings with SCD, consistent with a familial predisposition to cerebral vasculopathy in SCD (Kwiatkowski et al., 2003).

Other tests indicate abnormalities in glucose metabolism and microvascular blood flow, particularly in the frontal lobes, demonstrated in SCD patients using positron emission tomography (PET). The addition of PET to MRI identifies a greater proportion of children with sickle cell disease with neuroimaging abnormalities, particularly in those who had no history of overt neurologic events (Rodgers et al., 1988; Powars et al., 1999; Reed et al., 1999).

Perfusion magnetic resonance (dynamic susceptibility contrast MRI) and blood oxygen level-dependent (BOLD) MRI are additional imaging modalities to assess cerebral blood flow and perfusion. Perfusion abnormalities are associated with neurologic symptoms in patients with SCD, whether or not MRI, MRA, and TCD are abnormal (Kirkham et al., 2001a). Voxel-based morphometry analysis of MRI images is a sensitive method to detect widespread white matter injury in SCD patients in border zones between arterial territories even in the absence of evidence of infarction (Baldeweg et al., 2006).

GENETICS

Sickle cell disease (SCD) and β-thalassemia, caused by lesions that affect the β-globin gene, form the most common human genetic disorders worldwide. The autosomal recessive genetic mutation producing sickle hemoglobin is a single nucleotide substitution (GTG for GAG) at codon 6 of the β-globin gene on chromosome 11 that results in the substitution of valine for glutamic acid in the β-globin peptide. In an environment of hypoxia, this causes HbS to polymerize and form stiff bundles that distort the red cell, which in turn are less compliant through the microcirculation and result in vascular occlusion and the eventual chronic end organ damage. These RBCs are also prematurely removed from the circulation, resulting in a chronic hemolytic anemia.

Sickle cell disease is phenotypically complex, with different clinical courses ranging from early childhood mortality to a virtually unrecognized condition. Considering the well characterized molecular details of HbS polymerization, the explanation for the broad phenotypic heterogeneity in patients with identical genetic mutations is still under investigation. If the primary mutation is the same, variations in disease severity generally are due to genetic modifiers. In most genetic diseases involving β-globin, the most clear-cut influence on phenotype results from elevated fetal hemoglobin levels (Rund and Fucharoen, 2008). Other factors include β-globin cluster haplotypes, α-globin gene number, and fetal hemoglobin expression. The β-globin haplotypes are associated with different severities in sickle cell disease probably due to the variation in fetal hemoglobin concentration, which is protective against the stroke risk. The α-globin gene also influences the risk and protection against different complications of sickle cell anemia (Ashley-Koch et al., 2000).

Studies of sickle cell disease have drawn attention to the importance of modifier genes and of gene–gene interactions in determining stroke risk (Dichgans, 2007). Modifier genes might interact to determine the susceptibility to stroke. To find additional genetic modulators of disease, genotype-phenotype association studies, where single nucleotide polymorphisms (SNPs) in candidate genes are linked with a particular phenotype, have been informative (Steinberg, 2009).

A candidate gene study involving the analysis of 28 genetic polymorphisms in 20 candidate genes, including mutations in coagulation factor genes (factor V, prothrombin, fibrinogen, factor VII, factor XIII, PAI-1), platelet activation/function (GpIIb/IIIa, GpIb IX-V, GpIa/IIa), vascular reactivity (ACE), endothelial cell function (MTHFR, thrombomodulin, VCAM-1, E-selectin, L-selectin, P-selectin, ICAM-1), inflammation (TNF-α), lipid metabolism (Apo A1, Apo E), and cell adhesion (VCAM-1, E-selectin, L-selectin, P-selectin, ICAM-1) has been proposed. A genome-wide screen of validated single nucleotide polymorphisms (SNPs) to study the possible association of additional polymorphisms with the high-risk phenotype has also been designed (Adams et al., 2003).

Studies of genetic risk factors for stroke in SCD (in addition to the sickle mutation) have included association studies of predisposition genes for thrombosis and human leukocyte antigen (HLA) loci. Both class I HLA-B and class II HLA-DRBI (DR3) and DQBI (DQ2) alleles were associated with stroke risk in patients with clinical stroke and silent infarction on MRI (Zimmerman and Ware, 1998; Driscoll and Prauner, 1999; Styles et al., 2000; Hoppe et al., 2004). VCAM-1 is a cell adhesion molecule postulated to play a critical role in the pathogenesis of SS disease. In a study of single nucleotide polymorphisms (SNPs) within the *VCAM1* gene locus, Taylor identified a variant that appears to be protective (Taylor et al., 2002).

There is also a familial predisposition to stroke noted in sickle cell disease (Driscoll et al., 2003). This should prompt studies to identify genetic modifiers with family-based studies.

PATHOLOGY

The events clinically recognized as sickle cell disease are set off by a cascade of pathophysiological processes triggered by red cell injury secondary to the sickled hemoglobin polymer. These include general cellular and tissue damage caused by hypoxia, oxidant damage, and inflammation and reduced nitric oxide bioavailability (Steinberg, 2008).

Recurrent inflammation and vasculopathy occur in sickle cell disease, during crises, and in steady state. During the inflammatory process, leukocytes and vascular endothelial cells are activated and increase their expression of adhesion molecules. Adhesion of leukocytes to other blood cells and endothelium contributes to vaso-occlusion in sickle cell disease. High-level expression of adhesion molecules by leukocytes is associated with clinically severe disease (Anyaegbu et al., 1998; Awogu, 2000). Pancellular membrane lipid abnormalities, including reduced proportions of v-3 fatty acids, also occur in sickle cell disease. These lipid abnormalities are more severe in patients with disease complications and in those with a greater degree of anemia (Okpala, 2006). Other markers of inflammation seen in sickle cell disease include platelets (Okpala, 2002), C-reactive protein, α_2-macroglobulin, transferrin (Hedo et al., 1993), interleukin (IL)-2, IL-4, IL-6, IL-8, fibrinogen, and activated circulating vascular endothelial cells (Hebbel et al., 2004).

On a cellular membrane level in the erythrocyte, after recurrent episodes of sickling, membrane damage occurs and the cells are no longer capable of resuming the biconcave shape upon reoxygenation. Thus, they become irreversibly sickled. When erythrocytes sickle, they gain Na^+ and lose K^+. Membrane permeability to Ca^{++} increases, possibly due, in part, to impairment in the Ca^{++} pump that is dependent on adenosine triphosphatase (ATPase). The membrane becomes more rigid, possibly due to changes in cytoskeletal protein interactions.

The pathophysiology of cerebrovascular disease in sickle cell anemia may involve stenosis of large arteries of the circle of Willis, intracranial hemorrhage, and/or microvascular disease (Stockman et al., 1972; Moser et al., 1996) Cerebral infarction, a common complication of sickle cell disease, usually occurs in the distribution of the large vessels comprising the anterior circle of Willis, most often as a result of stenosis or occlusion in the area of the bifurcation of the carotid artery (Pavlakis et al., 1989). Vascular neuroimaging of patients with sickle cell anemia often demonstrates progressive narrowing of the large vessels with collateral vessel development in a pattern very similar to moyamoya disease (Dobson et al., 2002). Patients with this moyamoya-like vasculature are at a higher risk for strokes. Histology of these narrowed vessels is suggestive of intimal hyperplasia and proliferation of the internal elastic lamina, consistent with endothelial damage (Rothman et al., 1986).

Presumably, stroke is caused by perfusion failure in areas of stenosis or to arterial embolization. Factors that have been implicated in the development of the vascular lesions in the brain include the above mentioned inflammatory processes such as leukocyte-mediated injury to the endothelium, damage caused directly by the sickled red cells, inflammation mediated by cytokines, and quantitative and qualitative platelet abnormalities (Francis, 1991; Hebbel and Vercellotti, 1997). The disease also involves enhanced angiogenic propensity, activation of coagulation, disordered vasoregulation, and a component of chronic vasculopathy (Hebbel et al., 2004b).

In conjunction with diminished NO bioavailability, these processes likely underlie the chronic vasculopathy component of sickle disease. Endothelium-derived nitric oxide (NO) plays a major role in the regulation of vasomotor tone. These results suggest that endothelial dysfunction may prevent vasoregulation, which may also contribute to the pathophysiology of vaso-occlusive crisis in patients with sickle cell disease (Belhassen et al., 2001). Reduced activity of naturally occurring anticoagulants protein C and protein S may contribute to vaso-occlusion in sickle cell disease (Schnog et al., 2004).

A growing body of evidence supports the existence of a novel mechanism of human disease, namely, hemolysis-associated smooth muscle dystonia, vasculopathy, and endothelial dysfunction (Rother et al., 2005). Given the pathophysiological processes mentioned above, it is a possibility that this mechanism of disease is essentially the hallmark of the pathology of sickle cell disease.

MANAGEMENT

When contemplating management of the neurologic complications of SCD, one must take into account treatment of acute cerebrovascular accidents and its sequelae, while also considering prophylactic methods for long-term better outcomes.

In the acute setting, stroke, particularly hemorrhagic, may initially require intensive monitoring of intracranial pressures, treatment of vasospasm with volume expansion and/or nimodipine, and aggressive treatment of seizures if any. Craniotomy may be necessary to prevent herniation or for clipping or wrapping of the cerebral aneurysm. Other strategies such as adequate hydration, normothermia, and euglycemia should be maintained and hypotension should be avoided in the setting of acute stroke.

Antiplatelet therapy is generally recommended in adults after ischemic stroke, and there are no apparent reasons why this should not be advocated in adults with ischemic stroke who have SCD. Other options are discussed in the American Stroke Association Guidelines on Secondary Stroke Prevention (Furie et al., 2011). There are no specific recommendations regarding the use of antiplatelet agents or anticoagulants in stroke in children with SCD either acutely or long term. Antiplatelet agents (e.g., aspirin) and heparins (e.g., low molecular weight heparin) have been used on an individual patient basis in children with arterial ischemic strokes (Nowak-Gottl et al., 2003; Soman et al., 2006). There have been no randomized controlled clinical trials with thrombolytics in the treatment of acute ischemic stroke in children and although the risk of hemorrhage may be higher, SCD does not represent a known contraindication to tPA use in adults.

Physical, occupational, and speech therapy are important and should be initiated early in the children who have suffered a stroke. Early rehabilitation has a more favorable prognosis for recovery of function.

One of the essential interventions in the management of acute ischemic stroke in children with SCD is emergent blood transfusion to reduce the HbS level below 30%. The multicenter STOP trial demonstrated that transfusion to maintain HbS < 30% decreased the incidence of first stroke in high-risk pediatric patients, identified by transcranial Doppler (TCD). This is the only proven paradigm with class I evidence for primary stroke prevention in SCD (Adams et al., 1998b). Transfusion should be continued at least until age 18; HbS may be allowed to rise to approximately 50% in older adolescents and young adults by reducing either the intensity or frequency of transfusions. The STOP II study showed that discontinuing chronic transfusions after 30 months, even though the TCD values had dropped from above 200 to < 170 cm/second (considered low risk or normal at that point), nonetheless resulted in a high rate of reversion to abnormal TCD values and stroke (class I) (Adams and Brambilla, 2005).

The role of chronic transfusion for the prevention of recurrent events has not been defined for patients with their initial stroke as an adult.

It has also been shown that the incidence of silent infarcts (radiologically detected) were decreased in patients receiving chronic transfusion as compared to standard care showing that chronic transfusion therapy may also prevent silent infarcts in children with SCD (Pegelow et al., 2001). However, chronic transfusion therapy is associated with complications such as iron overload, alloimmunization, and infections. Erythrocytapheresis, an automated method of red blood cell exchange, is a safe method of controlling HbS levels and limiting or preventing iron load in chronically transfused SCD patients (Kim et al., 1994; Marques Junior et al., 1995; Adams et al., 1996).

Hemosiderosis is well known consequence of intensive and long-term transfusion therapy. Although both SCD and thalassemia patients suffer from iron-induced organ injury, the onset of clinical manifestations due to iron overload appears to be more gradual in SCD patients, suggesting a relative protection from iron-related organ injury (Finch, 1982). Exchange transfusions and chelation therapy are two methods to manage transfusion-related iron overload. Iron chelation therapy is done with deferoxamine at a dose of 25 mg/kg/day as a subcutaneous or intravenous infusion. Complications of this chelation method include ototoxicity, rash, and growth retardation in young children. The US Food and Drug Administration (FDA) recently approved deferasirox for treatment of chronic iron overload due to blood transfusions in patients aged 2 years and older. The drug is taken orally once daily which may improve compliance over deferoxamine. Chelation therapy with more than one agent offers the possibility of more effective removal of iron without compromising safety or compliance.

Recent studies have documented alloimmunization rates as high as 47% in adult and 27% in pediatric transfused SCD patients, respectively (Rosse et al., 1990; Vichinsky et al., 1990; Tahhan et al., 1994; Aygun et al., 2002). One method to decrease the rates of alloimmunization and hemolytic transfusion reactions is using leuko-depleted red cells matched for E, C, and Kell antigens. Other strategies to minimize alloimmunization include PEG-coating of red cells to mask red cell antigens from antibodies (Fisher, 2000), as well as artificial blood substitutes, such as perfluorocarbon emulsions and hemoglobin-based substitutes (Lowe, 2003; Habler et al., 2005; Maevsky et al., 2005).

The use of leukocyte-depleted red cell transfusions has had a significant effect on reducing the transmission of intracellular viruses such as cytomegalovirus (CMV), human lymphotrophic virus, Epstein–Barr virus (EBV), and human herpes virus 6, 7, 8 infectious complications (Fergusson et al., 2003). Transmission of HIV, hepatitis B and C, and human T cell leukemia/lymphoma virus-1 has dramatically decreased with improved donor selection criteria and screening of banked units (AuBuchon et al., 1997).

For adult patients who decide to discontinue transfusions, or those with problematic alloimmunization, iron overload, or other impediments to chronic red blood cell administration, hydroxyurea (HU) therapy should be considered to prevent recurrent events. Based on results from the double blind, placebo-controlled Multicenter Study of Hydroxyurea (MSH), HU was approved in adults with SCD to decrease the frequency of vaso-occlusive episodes and blood transfusion requirements (Charache et al., 1995). Follow-up data from the MSH have confirmed a reduced mortality after 9 years of HU therapy (Steinberg et al., 2003). Hydroxyurea therapy is started at a dose of 15 mg/kg/day and increased by 5 mg/kg/day every 8–12 weeks with monthly

monitoring of the platelets, reticulocytes, and neutrophils. Hydroxyurea was tested for secondary stroke prevention in children with SCD based on a single center study by Ware et al. (2004). They discontinued chronic transfusion (after more than 2 years of treatment) in 35 children and put them on hydroxyurea. These patients also received phlebotomies for iron overload. Although these phase II results showed a promising trend, the randomized controlled trial called SWiTCH was terminated early due to futility.

The results are not yet published but the following information was available from the sponsor's website on NHLBI (http://www.nih.gov/news/health/jun2010/nhlbi-03.htm):

> The 26-site trial, Stroke With Transfusions Changing to Hydroxyurea, or SWiTCH, studied 133 participants between the ages of 5 and 18 who had already experienced a stroke. All had been receiving the standard treatment of blood transfusions for at least 18 months and high levels of iron before entering the study. Without further preventive measures, these children were at high risk of another stroke as well as life-threatening conditions due to iron overload.
>
> The study tested whether the drug hydroxyurea, known to prevent complications of sickle cell disease in adults, was as effective as transfusions, the standard therapy, in reducing the risk of recurrent strokes. Hydroxyurea is the only FDA-approved drug for treating sickle cell anemia.
>
> The study also compared two approaches to remove excess iron, a consequence of regular blood transfusions. Participants who continued to receive transfusion therapy were given the standard oral iron-removal drug deferasirox, and participants who were switched to hydroxyurea underwent regular phlebotomy (blood removal) to eliminate excess iron that had accumulated from their earlier transfusions.
>
> Phlebotomy did not reduce liver iron better than deferasirox therapy. Analysis of the available data indicated that continuing the trial was unlikely to show that phlebotomy would provide a greater benefit than deferasirox to control iron accumulation. Without the ability to provide benefits for the management of liver iron, the potential risks of continuing study treatments were no longer warranted.
>
> . . . The DSMB noted that no strokes occurred in the 66 participants who received the standard therapy of blood transfusions and deferasirox. In contrast, seven strokes occurred in the group of 67 participants who received hydroxyurea with

phlebotomy. Study participants and their families have been contacted, and they will discuss future care options with their health care providers.

(http://www.nih.gov/news/health/jun2010/nhlbi-03.htm, 2010)

A study of similar design called TWiTCH, comparing hydroxyurea to regular blood transfusion for primary stroke prevention (based on the STOP protocol), will begin enrolling patients in 2011 (http://ccct.sph.uth.tmc.edu/twitch/, 2009).

Allogeneic bone marrow transplantation (BMT) from HLA-identical siblings is an accepted treatment for both thalassemia and sickle cell disease. Related cord blood transplantation for hemoglobinopathies is reported to offer a good probability of success (Locatelli et al., 2003). Bone marrow transplantation (BMT) is potentially curative alternative for secondary stroke prevention (Walters et al., 2004). Lack of an eligible HLA-compatible sibling donor and potential transplant-related complications remain substantial barriers to BMT in SCD. Novel conditioning regimens that minimize transplant-associated toxicity and alternative stem cell sources show promise for the wider application of BMT in SCD.

Moyamoya patients with ischemic symptoms and poor perfusion on a cerebral blood flow study are good candidates for direct or indirect bypass procedures. Encephaloduroarteriosynangiosis (EDAS) permits neovascularization to develop over a larger area of the brain than observed with direct anastomosis and has been revealed to cause cessation of symptomatic attacks much sooner than the natural course of the disease. The EDAS procedure is a safe and effective treatment option in patients with sickle cell anemia who develop moyamoya disease (Fryer et al., 2003). Operative treatment of moyamoya syndrome using pial synangiosis appears to be safe and confers long-lasting protection against further stroke in this population, and provides an alternative for failure of optimal medical therapy in patients (Smith et al., 2009).

Emerging novel primary prophylaxis regimens being tested include citrulline and arginine, aspirin, short-chain fatty acids, lovastatin, decitibine, and overnight oxygen supplementation. Screening for, and appropriate management of, nocturnal hypoxemia might be a safe and effective alternative to prophylactic blood transfusion for primary prevention of central nervous events in sickle cell disease (Kirkham et al., 2001b). Antioxidant therapy using a stable and long-acting molecule such as an intravascular superoxide dismutase mimetic polynitroxyl albumin may have a potential in ameliorating SS red cell adhesion and related vaso-occlusion (Kaul et al., 2006).

There are several studies underway to investigate the promise of some of the above-mentioned therapies in primary prevention and prevention of recurrent strokes in patients with SCD, and possibly even curative in this condition.

CONCLUSIONS

Sickle cell disease and related hemoglobinopathies are complex conditions, with patients exhibiting a vast variety of neurologic complications. The health burden for children with SCD and their families is profound and may be exacerbated by barriers to accessing comprehensive medical care (Boulet et al., 2010). SCD patients are reported to experience health-related quality of life worse than the general population. Greater public awareness of the neurocognitive effects of SCD and their impact on child outcomes is a critical step toward improved treatment, adaptation to illness, and quality of life (Schatz and McClellan, 2006).

In spite of all the progress in the understanding of the complicated nature of neurologic sequelae of SCD, there remains much work to be done in this field to aid in the prevention and cure of this disease. For now, prevention of first stroke is one important step that can be taken to lower the stroke burden in SCD.

REFERENCES

Adams RJ, Brambilla D (2005). Discontinuing prophylactic transfusions used to prevent stroke in sickle cell disease. N Engl J Med 353: 2769–2778.

Adams RJ, McKie VC, Nichols FT et al. (1992). The use of transcranial ultrasonography to predict stroke in sickle cell disease. N Engl J Med 326: 605–610.

Adams DM, Schultz WH, Ware RE et al. (1996). Erythrocytapheresis can reduce iron overload and prevent the need for chelation therapy in chronically transfused pediatric patients. J Pediatr Hematol Oncol 18: 46–50.

Adams RJ, McKie VC, Carl EM et al. (1997). Long-term stroke risk in children with sickle cell disease screened with transcranial Doppler. Ann Neurol 43: 699–704.

Adams RJ, McKie VC, Hsu L et al. (1998). Prevention of a first stroke by transfusions in children with sickle cell anemia and abnormal results on transcranial Doppler ultrasonography. N Engl J Med 339: 5–11.

Adams GT, Snieder H, McKie VC et al. (2003). Genetic risk factors for cerebrovascular disease in children with sickle cell disease: design of a case-control association study and genomewide screen. BMC Med Genet 4: 6.

Adams RJ, Brambilla DJ, Granger S et al. (2004). Stroke and conversion to high risk in children screened with transcranial Doppler ultrasound during the STOP study. Blood 103: 3689–3694.

Anyaegbu CC, Okpala IE, Aken'Ova AY et al. (1998). Peripheral blood neutrophil count and candidacidal activity correlate with the clinical severity of sickle cell anaemia. Eur J Haematol 60: 267–268.

Arena JM (1935). Vascular accident and acute hemiplegia in sickle cell anemia. Am J Dis Child 49: 722–723.

Armstrong FD, Thompson RJ Jr, Wang W et al. (1996). Cognitive functioning and brain magnetic resonance imaging in children with sickle cell disease. Neuropsychology Committee of the Cooperative Study of Sickle Cell Disease. Pediatrics 97: 864–870.

Ashley-Koch A, Yang Q, Olney RS (2000). Sickle hemoglobin (HbS) allele and sickle cell disease: a HuGE review. Am J Epidemiol 151: 839–845.

AuBuchon JP, Birkmeyer JD, Busch MP (1997). Safety of the blood supply in the United States: opportunities and controversies. Ann Intern Med 127: 904–909.

Awogu AU (2000). Leucocyte counts in children with sickle cell anaemia: usefulness of stable state values during infections. West Afr J Med 19: 55–58.

Aygun B, Padmanabhan S, Paley C et al. (2002). Clinical significance of RBC alloantibodies and autoantibodies in sickle cell patients who received transfusions. Transfusion 42: 37–43.

Baldeweg T, Hogan AM, Saunders DE et al. (2006). Detecting white matter injury in sickle cell disease using voxel-based morphometry. Ann Neurol 59: 662–672.

Belhassen L, Pelle G, Sediame S et al. (2001). Endothelial dysfunction in patients with sickle cell disease is related to selective impairment of shear stress-mediated vasodilation. Blood 97: 1584–1589.

Bonkovsky HL, Slaker DP, Bills EB et al. (1990). Usefulness and limitations of laboratory and hepatic imaging studies in iron-storage disease. Gastroenterology 99: 1079–1091.

Boulet SL, Yanni EA, Creary MS et al. (2010). Health status and healthcare use in a national sample of children with sickle cell disease. Am J Prev Med 38 (4 Suppl): S528–S535.

British Committee for Standards in Haematology (1988). Guidelines for haemoglobinopathy screening. Clin Lab Haematol 10: 87–94.

Brittenham GM, Badman DG (2003). Noninvasive measurement of iron: report of an NIDDK workshop. Blood 101: 15–19.

Carneiro AA, Fernandes JP, de Araujo DB et al. (2005). Liver iron concentration evaluated by two magnetic methods: magnetic resonance imaging and magnetic susceptometry. Magn Reson Med 54: 122–128.

Charache S, Terrin ML, Moore RD et al. (1995). Effect of hydroxyurea on the frequency of painful crises in sickle cell anemia. N Engl J Med 332: 1317–1322.

Clarke GM, Higgins TN (2000). Laboratory investigation of hemoglobinopathies and thalassemias: review and update. Clin Chem 46: 1284–1290.

Dichgans M (2007). Genetics of ischaemic stroke. Lancet Neurol 6: 149–161.

Dobson SR, Holden KR, Nietert PJ et al. (2002). Moyamoya syndrome in childhood sickle cell disease: a predictive factor for recurrent cerebrovascular events. Blood 99: 3144–3150.

Driscoll MC, Prauner R (1999). The methylenetetrahydrofolate reductase gene C677T mutant and ischemic stroke in sickle cell disease. Thromb Haemost 82: 1780–1781.

Driscoll MC, Hurlet A, Styles L et al. (2003). Stroke risk in siblings with sickle cell anemia. Blood 101: 2401–2404.

Fergusson D, Hebert PC, Lee SK et al. (2003). Clinical outcomes following institution of universal leukoreduction of blood transfusions for premature infants. JAMA 289: 1950–1956.

Finch CA (1982). The detection of iron overload. N Engl J Med 307: 1702–1704.

Fischer R, Tiemann CD, Engelhardt R et al. (1999). Assessment of iron stores in children with transfusion siderosis by biomagnetic liver susceptometry. Am J Hematol 60: 289–299.

Fischer R, Longo F, Nielsen P et al. (2003). Monitoring long-term efficacy of iron chelation therapy by deferiprone and desferrioxamine in patients with beta-thalassaemia major: application of SQUID biomagnetic liver susceptometry. Br J Haematol 121: 938–948.

Fisher TC (2000). PEG-coated red blood cells – simplifying blood transfusion in the new millennium? Immunohematol 16: 37–48.

Fisher SI, Haga JA, Castleberry SM et al. (1997). Validation of an automated HPLC method for quantification of HbS. Clin Chem 43: 1667–1668.

Francis RB (1991). Large-vessel occlusion in sickle cell disease: pathogenesis, clinical consequences, and therapeutic implications. Med Hypotheses 35: 88–95.

Fryer RH, Anderson RC, Chiriboga CA et al. (2003). Sickle cell anemia with moyamoya disease: outcomes after EDAS procedure. Pediatr Neurol 29: 124–130.

Furie KL, Kasner SE, Adams RJ et al. (2011). Guidelines for the prevention of stroke in patients with stroke or transient ischemic attack. Stroke 42: 227–276.

Goldstein LB, Bushnell CD, Adams RJ et al. (2011). Guidelines for the primary prevention of stroke: a guideline for healthcare professionals from the American Heart Association/American Stroke Association. Stroke 42: 517–584.

Habler O, Pape A, Meier J et al. (2005). Artificial oxygen carriers as an alternative to red blood cell transfusion. Anaesthesist 54: 741–754.

Hebbel RP, Vercellotti GM (1997). The endothelial biology of sickle cell disease. J Lab Clin Med 129: 288–293.

Hebbel RP, Osarogiagbon R, Kaul D (2004). The endothelial biology of sickle cell disease: inflammation and a chronic vasculopathy. Microcirculation 11: 129–151.

Hedo CC, Aken'Ova AY, Okpala IE et al. (1993). Acute phase reactants and the severity of homozygous sickle cell anaemia. J Intern Med 233: 467–470.

Herrick JB (1910). Peculiar elongated and sickle-shaped red blood corpuscles in a case of severe anemia. Arch Intern Med 6: 517–521.

Hoppe C, Klitz W, Cheng S et al. (2004). Gene interactions and stroke risk in children with sickle cell anemia. Blood 103: 2391–2396.

International Committee for Standardization in Haematology (1988). ICSH Expert Panel on Abnormal Haemoglobins.

Recommendations for neonatal screening of haemoglobi- nopathies. Clin Lab Haematol 10: 335–345.

Jeffries BF, Lipper MH, Kishore PR (1980). Major intracerebral arterial involvement in sickle cell disease. Surg Neurol 14: 291–295.

Kandeel AY, Zimmerman RA, Ohene-Frempong K (1996). Comparison of magnetic resonance angiography and conventional angiography in sickle cell disease: clinical significance and reliability. Neuroradiology 38: 409–416.

Kaul DK, Liu XD, Zhang X et al. (2006). Inhibition of sickle red cell adhesion and vaso-occlusion in the microcirculation by antioxidants. Am J Physiol Heart Circ Physiol 291: H167–H175.

Kim HC, Dugan NP, Silber JH et al. (1994). Erythrocytapheresis therapy to reduce iron overload in chronically transfused patients with sickle cell disease. Blood 83: 1136–1142.

Kinney TR, Sleeper LA, Wang WC et al. (1999). Silent cerebral infarcts in sickle cell anemia: a risk factor analysis. The Cooperative Study of Sickle Cell Disease. Pediatrics 3: 640–645.

Kirkham FJ, Calamante F, Bynevelt M et al. (2001a). Perfusion magnetic resonance abnormalities in patients with sickle cell disease. Ann Neurol 49: 477–485.

Kirkham FJ, Hewes DK, Prengler M et al. (2001b). Nocturnal hypoxaemia and central-nervous-system events in sicklecell disease. Lancet 357: 1656–1659.

Kwiatkowski JL, Hunter JV, Smith-Whitley K et al. (2003). Transcranial Doppler ultrasonography in siblings with sickle cell disease. Br J Haematol 121: 932–937.

Locatelli F, Rocha V, Reed W et al. (2003). Related umbilical cord blood transplantation in patients with thalassemia and sickle cell disease. Blood 101: 2137–2143.

Lowe KC (2003). Engineering blood: synthetic substitutes from fluorinated compounds. Tissue Eng 9: 389–399.

Maevsky E, Ivanitsky G, Bogdanova L et al. (2005). Clinical results of Perftoran application: present and future. Artif Cells Blood Substit Immobil Biotechnol 33: 37–46.

Marques Junior JF, Saad ST, Costa FF et al. (1995). Automated erythrocytapheresis in sickle cell anaemia. Int J Artif Organs 18: 345–346.

Miller ST, Macklin EA, Pegelow CH et al. (2001). Silent infarction as a risk factor for overt stroke in children with sickle cell anemia: a report from the Cooperative Study of Sickle Cell Disease. J Pediatr 3: 385–390.

Moritania T, Numaguchia Y, Lemerb NB et al. (2004). Sickle cell cerebrovascular disease: usual and unusual findings on MR imaging and MR angiography. Clin Imaging 28: 173–186.

Moser FG, Miller ST, Bello JA et al. (1996). The spectrum of brain MR abnormalities in sickle-cell disease: a report from the Cooperative Study of Sickle Cell Disease. AJNR Am J Neuroradiol 17: 965–972.

Noll RB, Stith L, Gartstein MA et al. (2001). Neuropsychological functioning of youths with sickle cell disease: comparison with non-chronically ill peers. J Pediatr Psychol 26: 69–78.

Nowak-Gottl U, Straeter R, Sebire G et al. (2003). Antithrombotic drug treatment of pediatric patients with ischemic stroke. Paediatr Drugs 5: 167–175.

Ohene-Frempong K, Weiner SJ, Sleeper LA et al. (1998). Cerebrovascular accidents in sickle cell disease: rates and risk factors. Blood 91: 288–294.

Okpala IE (2002). Steady state platelet count and complications of sickle cell disease. Hematol J 3: 214–215.

Okpala IE (2006). Leukocyte adhesion and the pathophysiology of sickle cell disease. Curr Opin Hematol 13: 40–44.

Oyesiku NM, Barrow DL, Eckman JR et al. (1991). Intracranial aneurysms in sickle-cell anemia: clinical features and pathogenesis. J Neurosurg 75: 356–363.

Pavlakis SG, Prohovnik I, Piomelli S et al. (1989). Neurologic complications of sickle cell disease. Adv Pediatr 36: 247–276.

Pegelow CH, Wang W, Granger S et al. (2001). STOP trial. Silent infarcts in children with sickle cell anemia and abnormal cerebral artery velocity. Arch Neurol 58: 2017–2021.

Platt OS, Brambilla DJ, Rosse WF et al. (1994). Mortality in sickle cell disease. Life expectancy and risk factors for early death. N Engl J Med 330: 1639–1644.

Powars DR, Conti PS, Wong WY et al. (1999). Cerebral vasculopathy in sickle cell anemia: diagnostic contribution of positron emission tomography. Blood 93: 71–79.

Powars DR, Wong WY, Vachon LA (2001). Incomplete cerebral infarctions are not silent. J Pediatr Hematol Oncol 23: 79–83.

Powars DR, Chan LS, Hiti A et al. (2005). Outcome of sickle cell anemia: a 4-decade observational study of 1056 patients. Medicine 84: 363–376.

Reed W, Jagust W, Al-Mateen M et al. (1999). Role of positron emission tomography in determining the extent of CNS ischemia in patients with sickle cell disease. Am J Hematol 60: 268–272.

Rioux J, Godart C, Hurtrel D et al. (1997). Cation-exchange HPLC evaluated for presumptive identification of hemoglobin variants. Clin Chem 43: 34–39.

Rodgers GP, Clark CM, Larson SM et al. (1988). Brain glucose metabolism in neurologically normal patients with sickle cell disease. Regional alterations. Arch Neurol 45: 78–82.

Roohi F, Gowda RM, Goel N et al. (2001). Mononeuropathy multiplex in sickle cell disease: a complication in need of recognition. J Clin Neuromuscul Dis 2: 63–69.

Rosse WF, Gallagher D, Kinney TR et al. (1990). Transfusion and alloimmunization in sickle cell disease. The Cooperative Study of Sickle Cell Disease. Blood 76: 1431–1437.

Rother RP, Bell L, Hillmen P et al. (2005). The clinical sequelae of intravascular hemolysis and extracellular plasma hemoglobin: a novel mechanism of human disease. JAMA 293: 1653–1662.

Rothman SM, Fulling KH, Nelson JS (1986). Sickle cell anemia and central nervous system infarction: a neuropathological study. Ann Neurol 20: 684–690.

Rund D, Fucharoen S (2008). Genetic modifiers in hemoglobinopathies. Curr Mol Med 8: 600–608.

Schatz J, McClellan CB (2006). Sickle cell disease as a neurodevelopmental disorder. Ment Retard Dev Disabil Res Rev 12: 200–207.

Schnog JB, Mac Gillavry MR, van Zanten AP et al. (2004). Protein C and S and inflammation in sickle cell disease. Am J Hematol 76: 26–32.

Silva GS, Vicari P, Figueiredo MS et al. (2009). Brain magnetic resonance imaging abnormalities in adult patients with sickle cell disease: correlation with transcranial Doppler findings. Stroke 40: 2408–2412.

Smith ER, McClain CD, Heeney M et al. (2009). Pial synangiosis in patients with moyamoya syndrome and sickle cell anemia: perioperative management and surgical outcome. Neurosurg Focus 26: E10.

Soman T, Rafay MF, Hune S et al. (2006). The risks and safety of clopidogrel in pediatric areterial ischemic stroke. Stroke 37: 1120–1122.

St Pierre TG, Clark PR, Chua-anusorn W et al. (2005). Noninvasive measurement and imaging of liver iron concentrations using proton magnetic resonance. Blood 105: 855–861.

Steinberg MH (2008). Sickle cell anemia, the first molecular disease: overview of molecular etiology, pathophysiology, and therapeutic approaches. ScientificWorldJournal 8: 1295–1324.

Steinberg MH (2009). Genetic etiologies for phenotypic diversity in sickle cell anemia. ScientificWorldJournal 9: 46–67.

Steinberg MH, Barton F, Castro O et al. (2003). Effect of hydroxyurea on mortality and morbidity in adult sickle cell anemia: risks and benefits up to 9 years of treatment. JAMA 289: 1645–1651.

Stockman JA, Nigro MA, Mishkin MM et al. (1972). Occlusion of large cerebral vessels in sickle-cell anemia. N Engl J Med 287: 846–849.

Styles LA, Hoppe C, Klitz W et al. (2000). Evidence for HLA-related susceptibility for stroke in children with sickle cell anemia. Blood 95: 3563–3567.

Sydenstricker VP, Mulherin WA, Houseal RW (1923). Sickle cell anemia. Am J Dis Child 26: 132–154.

Tahhan HR, Holbrook CT, Braddy LR et al. (1994). Antigen-matched donor blood in the transfusion management of patients with sickle cell disease. Transfusion 34: 562–569.

Taylor JG, 6th, Tang DC, Savage SA et al. (2002). Variants in the VCAM1 gene and risk for symptomatic stroke in sickle cell disease. Blood 100: 4303–4309.

Valadi N, Silva GS, Bowman LS et al. (2006). Transcranial Doppler ultrasonography in adults with sickle cell disease. Neurology 67: 572–574.

Vichinsky EP, Earles A, Johnson RA et al. (1990). Alloimmunization in sickle cell anemia and transfusion of racially unmatched blood. N Engl J Med 322: 1617–1621.

Vichinsky EP, Neumayr LD, Gold JI et al. (2010). Neuropsychological dysfunction and neuroimaging abnormalities in neurologically intact adults with sickle cell anemia. JAMA 303: 1823–1831.

Walters MC, Patience M, Edwards S et al. (2004). Hematopoietic cell transplantation for sickle cell disease: updated results of the multicenter trial. Blood 104: 105a.

Ware RF, Zimmerman SA, Sylvestre PB et al. (2004). Prevention of secondary stroke and resolution of transfusional iron overload in children with sickle cell anemia using hydroxyurea and phlebotomy. J Pediatr 145: 346–352.

Watkins KE, Hewes DK, Connelly A et al. (1998). Cognitive deficits associated with frontal-lobe infarction in children with sickle cell disease. Dev Med Child Neurol 40: 536–543.

Zimmerman SA, Ware RE (1998). Inherited DNA mutations contributing to thrombotic complications in patients with sickle cell disease. Am J Hematol 59: 267–272.

Handbook of Clinical Neurology, Vol. 120 (3rd series)
Neurologic Aspects of Systemic Disease Part II
Jose Biller and Jose M. Ferro, Editors
© 2014 Elsevier B.V. All rights reserved

Chapter 69

Neurologic aspects of lymphoma and leukemias

MATTHEW McCOYD[1]*, GREGORY GRUENER[1,2], AND PATRICK FOY[3]

[1]*Department of Neurology, Loyola University Medical Center, Maywood, IL, USA*

[2]*Leischner Institute for Medical Education, Loyola University Medical Center, Maywood, IL, USA*

[3]*Department of Hematology, Medical College of Wisconsin, Milwaukee, WI, USA*

INTRODUCTION

Lymphoma and leukemia include a heterogenous group of blood malignancies arising from hematopoietic stem cells (Fig. 69.1). Historically, the two entities have been considered separately. Leukemia has been used to describe a cancerous change in the hemopoietic stem cells and their progenitors, usually with widespread involvement of the bone marrow and peripheral blood (Mughal et al., 2006; Kumar et al., 2009a). Lymphoma has been used for proliferations of lymphoid cells that arise as discrete tissue masses, most commonly within lymphoid tissue including nodes (Kumar et al., 2009a). However, with improved diagnostic tools including immunophenotyping, genetics, and cytochemistry, the juxtaposition of leukemia and lymphoma has blurred as the same entity can present in either fashion (Ottensmeier, 2001).

Multiple classification systems for the leukemias and lymphomas have been proposed since Thomas Hodgkin's paper "On some morbid experiences of the absorbent glands and spleen," published in 1832 (Jaffe et al., 2008), and the first description of leukemia in 1845 (Goldman and Velo, 2003). The leukemias can be considered neoplasms of myeloid and lymphoid precursors (Glass, 2006). They are broadly considered as "acute" or "chronic" and are classified by the salient features of the aberrant hematopoietic cell populations (Mughal et al., 2006). The lymphomas are lymphoid tissue tumors and historically were divided into Hodgkin lymphoma or the larger, non-Hodgkin group (Glass, 2006). However, the current and most broadly accepted classification is the World Health Organization (WHO) classification of myeloid and lymphoid neoplasms. Under constant revision, it is a consensus classification based not only on morphology, genetics, and immunophenotype, but

clinical features. Table 69.1 is representative of the current classification of lymphoid neoplasms (Ottensmeier, 2001; Vardiman et al., 2009; Vardiman, 2010).

Early and late neurologic complications of leukemia and lymphoma have long been recognized as both a result of the disease and its treatment. This review will highlight the most frequent lymphomas and leukemias, or those with the greatest neurologic significance. Complications of treatment are considered within separate contributions of this handbook and elsewhere (Dropcho, 2011). This review should begin to address delays in referral when patients with hematologic disorders present first to a neurologist (Abel et al., 2008).

LYMPHOMAS

The lymphomas can be conceptualized as two broad categories of disorders: non-Hodgkin lymphoma (NHL) and Hodgkin lymphoma (HL) (Fig. 69.2). Further classification relies on clinical features and histopathology that is further defined by immunophenotype and cytogenetic characterization. While the clinical presentation can hint at classification, tissue characterization is always necessary as symptoms cannot be relied on accurately to identify the specific type of lymphoma.

The vast majority of lymphomas are of B cell origin with the remainder T cell. Non-Hodgkin lymphoma cells tend to circulate within the vascular system and are often widely dispersed at the time of diagnosis, while Hodgkin lymphoma tends to spread contiguously from their site of origin. Lymphomas arise from a clonal expansion of a malignant lymphoid hematopoietic stem cell. Each malignant cell expresses a conserved set of aberrant genes, transcription products, and proteins that can be detected through morphologic, immunohistochemistry,

---

*Corresponding author: Matthew McCoyd, M.D., Loyola University Medical Center, Building 105, room 2700, 2160 South First Ave; Maywood, IL 60153, USA. Tel: +1-708-216-2127, Fax: +1-708-216-5617, E-mail: mmcoyd@lumc.edu

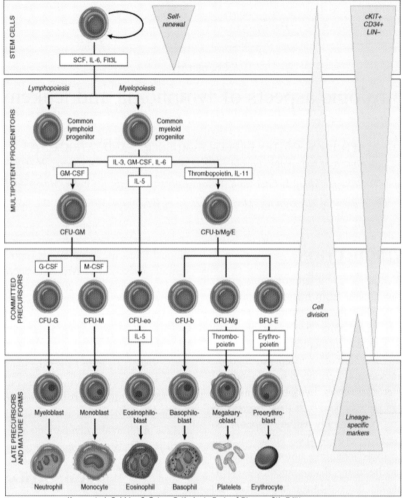

Kumar et al: Robbins & Cotran Pathologic Basis of Disease, 8th Edition.
Copyright © 2009 by Saunders, an imprint of Elsevier, Inc. All rights reserved.

Fig. 69.1. Differentiation of hematopoietic cells.

chromosomal, and cytometric methods to prove origination from a primary malignant stem. These markers can help to identify these cells as an abnormal monoclonal population, rather than the expected polyclonal expansion of hematologic and immunologic cells seen in a reactive lymphoid process.

Non-Hodgkin's lymphomas

This group comprises up to two-thirds of lymphomas and is classified based on pathologic, immunophenotypic, and clinical presentation. Many subtypes exist (Table 69.1). This discussion will first focus on two subtypes of peripheral B cell lymphoma, primary CNS lymphoma (PCL) and Burkitt lymphoma, because of their high rate of involvement and relapse within the central nervous system (CNS). Multiple myeloma, its variants, and Waldenström's macroglobulinemia will be described as a group. Finally, we will also discuss complications

of an infrequent extranodal subtype of peripheral B cell lymphoma, intravascular large B cell lymphoma, because of its frequent presentation with CNS or skin manifestations and delay in diagnosis.

PRIMARY CENTRAL NERVOUS SYSTEM LYMPHOMA

Perhaps 90% of the cases of primary CNS lymphoma (PCL) demonstrate diffuse large B cell lymphoma morphology that while confined, can involve any level of the neuraxis, brain, spinal cord, leptomeninges, or eyes. Upon diagnosis, searching for evidence of occult systemic disease is recommended. The remaining 10% of cases of PCL represent Burkitt lymphoma, T cell lymphoma, or poorly characterized low-grade lymphomas and is more often identified in younger patients (Kim et al., 2011). As a group, PCL comprise between 1% and 6% of primary brain tumors, but are much more common in immunodeficiency syndromes including

Table 69.1

World Health Organization classification of lymphoid neoplasms (representative)

Precursor lymphoid neoplasms
B lymphoblastic leukemia/lymphoma
T lymphoblastic leukemia/lymphoma
Mature B cell neoplasms
Chronic lymphocytic leukemia/small lymphocytic lymphoma
B cell prolymphocytic leukemia
Hairy cell leukemia
Lymphoplasmacytic lymphoma
Heavy chain disease
Plasma cell myeloma
Solitary plasmacytoma of bone
Extranodal marginal zone lymphoma of mucosa-associated
    lymphoid tissue (MALT lymphoma)
Nodal marginal zone lymphoma
Mantle cell lymphoma
Diffuse large B cell lymphoma
Intravascular large B cell lymphoma
Burkitt lymphoma
Mature T cell and NK cell neoplasms
T-cell prolymphocytic leukemia
Chronic lymphoproliferative disorder of NK cells
Aggressive NK cell leukemia
Adult T cell leukemia/lymphoma
Enteropathy-associated T cell lymphoma
Mycosis fungoides
Sézary syndrome
Primary cutaneous T cell lymphoproliferative disorders
Primary cutaneous anaplastic large cell lymphoma
Primary cutaneous CD4 positive small/medium T cell
    lymphoma
Angioimmunoblastic T cell lymphoma
Hodgkin lymphoma
Histiocytic lymphoma
Langerhans cell sarcoma
Follicular dendritic cell sarcoma
Fibroblastic reticular cell tumor
Histiocytic and dendritic cell neoplasm
Classic subtypes
Nodular sclerosis
Mixed cellularity
Lymphocyte-rich
Lymphocyte depletion
Post-transplant lymphoproliferative disorders (PTLD)

human immune deficiency (HIV) infection and post-transplant settings, and the frequency of PCL increased at the same time as the appearance of individuals with HIV infection. While the institution of more effective therapy for HIV has been associated with a concomitant decline in the incidence of PCNSL their prognosis remains worse than HIV-negative patients and HIV testing is still recommended in all cases of PCL (Gerstner and Batchelor, 2010; Bayraktar et al., 2011).

In non-HIV-related cases of PCL it is just as likely at presentation to suggest a focal CNS lesion as a more diffuse neurologic process, with clinical signs at presentation including focal deficit (70%), neuropsychiatric symptoms (43%), increased intracranial pressure (33%), seizures (14%), and vitreous involvement (4%). Systemic symptoms such as weight loss, night sweats, or fever are less common at presentation (Bataille et al., 2000).

Contrast-enhanced magnetic resonance (MR) imaging of the brain is the preferred diagnostic imaging study. Spinal cord involvement is rare so empiric spinal cord neuroimaging is not routinely recommended. Cerebrospinal fluid (CSF) examination is the most sensitive technique to evaluate for leptomeningeal disease. Characteristic radiologic features include a superficial location, contrast enhancement, and absence of necrosis. In the majority of immunocompetent cases a single uniformly enhancing lesion is identified. The most common sites of involvement include cerebral hemisphere (38%), thalamus/basal ganglia (16%), corpus callosum (14%; bulky infiltration of the corpus callosum is considered the most characteristic sign of PCL), periventricular (12%), and cerebellum (9%) (Haldorsen et al., 2011). In HIV-related PCL the lesion may appear ring enhancing. New imaging modalities that include fludeoxyglucose (18 F) (FDG), positron emission tomography (PET), and single-photon emission computed tomography (SPECT) are increasingly used to aid in differential diagnosis, but as of yet no imaging modality is diagnostic and histology is still required (Tang et al., 2011).

There is no clear consensus in regard to treatment protocols for PCL, but methotrexate appears to be the most effective chemotherapeutic drug. However, it necessitates high doses in order to penetrate the blood–brain barrier (BBB) and the eyes (which can be a potential reservoir for partly treated lymphoma) as well as treat leptomeningeal involvement (perhaps in up to 42% of people at diagnosis), and often part of a multidrug regimen. Rituximab, a monoclonal antibody targeted against CD20, is incorporated into most treatment regimens as most PCL express CD20, but data suggesting benefit are limited to case series. Whole-brain radiation therapy produces an initial radiographic response and control of disease in 90% of patients, relapse occurs within the first few months, and delayed neurotoxicity in those older than 60 years is common. If possible, corticosteroid administration should be withheld until diagnosis since its direct lymphocytolytic effect may impair histologic diagnosis. Like radiation therapy, corticosteroids can also produce a sudden response, but relapse also occurs quickly and alternative therapies are required (Gerstner and Batchelor, 2010; Roth et al., 2012).

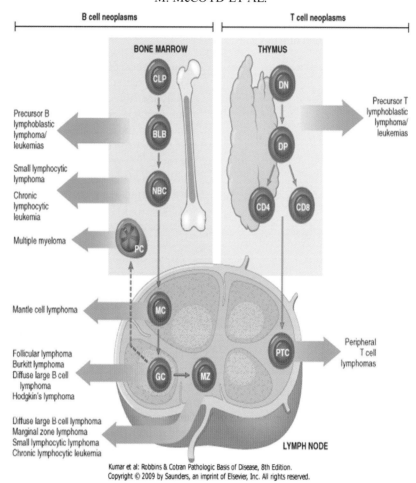

Fig. 69.2. Origin of lymphoid neoplasms.

The location of PCL and associated treatments are accompanied by significant delayed neurotoxicity, more common in those older than 60 years. Typically there are signs of cognitive impairment and when more severe, subcortical dementia, gait impairment, and incontinence develop. The clinical presentation can be accompanied by MRI changes consistent with periventricular demyelination and cerebral atrophy, while pathologically there is evidence of demyelination, neuronal loss, and gliosis (Gerstner and Batchelor, 2010).

One unique and rare manifestation of PCL is a diffuse infiltrating form without evidence of a mass lesion, referred to as *lymphomatosis cerebri*. Clinically it presents as a rapidly progressive dementia and gait disorder that is accompanied by a characteristic MRI finding of patchy T2-hyperintense areas that do not demonstrate contrast enhancement and are suggestive of a diffuse leukoencephalopathy. These MRI changes are felt to reflect infiltration of the white matter by lymphoma cells. The infrequency of the disorder has not allowed specific recommendations in regards to treatment, but

empirically has been the same as those for typical PCL (Kanai et al., 2008).

BURKITT LYMPHOMA

It is convenient to consider three variants of Burkitt lymphoma (BL) distinguished by their geographic distribution, epidemiology, and pathogenesis: endemic, sporadic, and immunodeficiency-associated BL (Perkins and Friedberg, 2008; de Leval and Hasserjian, 2009). All cases share a common characteristic of frequent involvement of the CNS and often are "driven" by Epstein–Barr virus (EBV) viral DNA incorporation into the genome. EBV-associated BL is highest in endemic cases (>90%) and immunodeficiency cases (25–40%), and lowest in sporadic BL (15–30%). Endemic BL occurs with a peak incidence in children (4–7 years), male:female ratio of 2:1, a geographic distribution within equatorial Africa, and Papua, New Guinea, and is commonly extranodal, with jaw and facial bone involvement in 50% of cases. Immunodeficiency-associated BL is encountered within HIV-infected individuals as well as those with a congenital or iatrogenic immunodeficiency and is more frequently nodal or involving bone marrow (de Leval and Hasserjian, 2009). The terms endemic or sporadic BL are epidemiologic terms and neither predict the clinical course nor are currently used within a clinical, pathologic, molecular, or pathologic classification scheme.

Essentially all cases of BL share a translocation of the c-myc gene on the long arm of chromosome 8 with one of the immunoglobulin heavy or light (κ or λ) chain loci on chromosome 14, 2 or 22. This translocation brings the c-myc gene, an oncogene that enhances cell proliferation and apoptosis, under the transcriptional control of an immunoglobulin locus. How EBV then contributes or facilitates the development of BL as well as the process where cell proliferation remains enhanced with respect to apoptosis is currently not entirely explained (Bornkamm, 2009).

In the US, the sporadic variant of BL is more typically encountered, mainly within adult patients who present with an abdominal mass, B symptoms (fever, weight loss, night sweats) and laboratory evidence of tumor lysis. Extranodal involvement is frequent with bone marrow involvement in 70% and leptomeningeal involvement in 40% of adults at the time of diagnosis. BL exhibits a high rate of mitosis as well as apoptosis with phagocytic, pale-appearing histiocytes on microscopy, dispersed throughout the tumor, taking up the debris and resulting in a "starry-sky" (nonspecific) appearance on low power magnification.

The potentially rapid rate of progression necessitates that treatment be instituted as soon as a diagnosis is confirmed. Optimal therapy for an adult patient is not established, although CNS prophylaxis with either high-dose systemic therapy, intrathecal therapy or both is part of all regimens. Treatment regimens used in adults are adapted from treatment protocols that are used in children. In general these include intensive high-dose chemotherapy, similar to those used in ALL with initial "induction therapy" followed by a high-dose chemotherapy consolidation therapy. Both autologous and allogenic hematopoietic stem cell transplantation has been used either as part of a consolidation strategy or upon relapse of disease. Radiation therapy is not part of the therapeutic regimen in BL since the response to chemotherapy is near universal. Prophylaxis against tumor lysis syndrome is essential given the high rate of chemotherapy-associated tumor cell death. Prognosis of BL is excellent when the disease is limited to a single site, and when it occurs in children (5 year survival rates can exceed 90%). There are fewer trials of treatment in adults over the age of 40 years, but outcomes are currently inferior to those reached with children (Perkins and Friedberg, 2008).

MULTIPLE MYELOMA, PLASMACYTOMA, AND AMYLOIDOSIS

Multiple myeloma (MM) comprises 13% of all hematologic malignances and is second in frequency after non-Hodgkin lymphomas. The median age at diagnosis is 70 years with only 2% of cases younger than 40. The frequency of occurrence increases from 1% at age 50 up to 10% in those older than 80 years, and is two- to three-fold more common in African-Americans versus whites (Turesson et al., 2010). The typical presentation is with symptoms of fatigue and weakness, anemia, renal failure, or lytic bone lesions; less frequently it presents with a hyperviscosity syndrome, hypercalcemia, or spinal cord compression from epidural tumor or vertebral body collapse. Diagnosis of MM is based on serum and urine electrophoresis (identifies and quantifies M protein), bone marrow evaluation (enumeration and genetic assessment of plasma cells), and skeletal survey (staging of MM, and may identify the characteristic "punched-out" lytic lesions) (Table 69.2) (Lin, 2009; Raab et al., 2009).

MM is almost always preceded by a *monoclonal gammopathy of undetermined significance (MGUS)* of which there is a 1% per year risk of progression to MM and the necessity for long-term follow-up. At times an intervening stage to MM, *smoldering myeloma*, may be identified. "Smoldering myeloma" is defined by the

Table 69.2

World Health Organization diagnostic criteria for MGUS, SM, and MM*

Monoclonal gammopathy of undetermined significance (MGUS)
Serum monoclonal protein ($<$30 g/L)
Bone marrow $<$ 10% plasma cells
No evidence of other B cell proliferative disorders
No related organ or tissue impairment†
Smoldering multiple myeloma (SM) (asymptomatic)
Serum monoclonal protein ($\geq$ 30 g/L) and/or
Bone marrow clonal plasma cells $\geq$ 10%
No related organ or tissue impairment†
Multiple myeloma (MM)
Bone marrow clonal plasma cells $\geq$ 10%
Monoclonal protein present in serum and/or urine
Clonal bone marrow plasma cells or plasmacytoma
Related organ or tissue impairment†

*(Modified from Kumar et al., 2009b.)
†CRAB: Calcium elevation ($>$1 mg/dL above the upper limit of normal)
  Renal dysfunction (creatinine $>$ 2 g/dL)
  Anemia (hemoglobin 2 g/dL below lower limit of normal)
Bone lesions (lytic lesions or osteoporosis with compression fracture) attributable to the plasma cell disorder
Other features include symptomatic hyperviscosity, amyloidosis, and recurrent bacterial infection.

presence of a monoclonal paraprotein greater than 3 g/dL or bone marrow involvement by atypical plasma cells > 10%, in the absence of clinical symptoms of multiple myeloma (hypercalcemia, renal failure, anemia, or lytic bone lesions). The majority of patients will evolve into MM; median time to progression is 4.8 years and the probability of progression to MM (or AL amyloidosis) is 54% at 5 years, 66% at 10 years. The percent of clonal bone marrow plasma cells is the strongest predictor of progression; M protein size, free light chain immunoglobulin ratio, immunophenotype and an evolving type (increasing M protein level over time) are all predictors of progression MM and both of these disorders are associated with a monoclonal protein, but distinguished by extent and evidence of end-organ effects (Table 69.2) (Kumar et al., 2009b).

MGUS is usually an incidental discovery from routine laboratory screening or discovered during the evaluation of an individual with a polyneuropathy. The M protein is usually IgG (~70%) or IgM (~17%) and κ light chains are detected more frequently than λ (urinary Bence Jones protein is usually absent). While MGUS can evolve into a malignant plasma cell proliferative disorder with approximately a 30% actuarial and 11% real (accounting for other causes of death) probability at 25 years of follow-up, but 75–90% of MGUS will not progress. At time of detection it is unclear whether the abnormal plasma cells in MGUS will proliferate and lead to systemic disease or will remain stable. The combination of a non-IgG MGUS, abnormal free chain ratio, and an M protein level $\geq$ 1.5 g/dL identify the greatest risk of progression (Madan and Greipp, 2009). Routine laboratory follow-up helps to confirm diagnosis, identify progression or evidence of end-organ damage. There is no evidence that immediate treatment will alter long-term outcome (Bladé et al., 2009).

MM demonstrates variable clinical outcomes, primarily related to the genetic characteristics of the tumor cells, and that information can be used to reinforce the current risk stratification guidelines that further guide treatment decisions. The genetic profile is primarily established from the results of three tests; fluorescence in situ hybridization (FISH), cytogenetics, and plasma cell labeling index (measures the synthesis of DNA). Using these techniques two broad groups are recognized, those where MM cells are hyperdiploid (usually trisomies) carrying a better outcome, and the non-hyperdiploid group, usually having translocations that involve chromosome 14 immunoglobulin heavy chain locus with other chromosomes that lead to activation of their oncogenes (Zhou et al., 2009).

Initial therapy for MM has historically included steroids and combination chemotherapy in anticipation of high-dose melphalan and stem cell transplant. Over the past decade, thalidomide, lenalidomide, pomalidomide, and bortezomib are increasingly used in initial protocols or regimens for a relapse. These drugs exert their effect by disrupting the microenvironment of the MM cells and also demonstrate characteristic patterns of toxicity, with neuropathy (often painful) a frequent component (Kumar et al., 2009b). Survival of MM patients has historically averaged 3–5 years, but has dramatically improved with development of new pharmacologic therapies and improvement in transplantation techniques.

There are several clinical variants of MM that include a *primary plasma cell leukemia*, diagnosed by absolute blood plasma cell count and representing an aggressive disease with a poor prognosis comprising 5% of newly diagnosed MM cases. *Solitary extramedullary plasmacytoma* usually develops within the head and neck. While associated with a good prognosis, 15% will later develop into a typical MM. Solitary plasmacytoma usually develops within the axial skeleton causing local bone pain or spinal cord/root compression. Accompanied by low levels of M protein, most eventually develop into systemic disease. A *nonsecretory myeloma* is present in 3% of MM cases. Cmposed of plasma cells, confirmatory diagnosis requires immunophenotyping, immunochemistry and detection of cytogenetic alterations.

Polyneuropathy, organomegaly, endocrinopathy, monoclonal gammopathy, and skin changes (POEMS) syndrome (Crow–Fukase syndrome, Takatsuki disease, PEP syndrome, or osteosclerotic myeloma) is a rare variant of MM (< 1%) where an osteosclerotic rather than a lytic bone lesion is discovered; polyneuropathy, organomegaly, endocrinopathy, monoclonal gammopathy, and skin lesions comprise the syndrome. It is associated with low levels of M protein (usually an IgA λ). The median age at presentation is 51 years with a monoclonal gammopathy and a predominantly chronic inflammatory demyelinative motor polyneuropathy. This is accompanied by varying degrees of other associated organ system involvement including organomegaly, endocrinopathy (excluding diabetes mellitus and hypothyroidism) as well as various skin lesions, but all having some temporal relationship to one another and no other explanation. The pathogenesis remains unclear, but may be cytokine-mediated, and elevated levels of vascular endothelial growth factor are also found. It is distinct from MM in that anemia and bone pain are uncommon and renal failure, when present, is not related to light chain deposition. Radiation therapy to the bone lesion can improve clinical symptoms and signs, but therapy, when instituted, is similar to MM, including the use of autologous stem cell transplant. Untreated the neuropathy progresses, as does anasarca and inanition; pulmonary dysfunction leads to death (Rajkumar et al., 2006).

Amyloid light chain (AL) amyloidosis (primary amyloidosis) is the most common type of systemic amyloidosis and the amyloidogenic protein is an Ig light chain or fragment of a light chain (usually λ isotype) that is produced by a clonal population of plasma cells in the bone marrow. The plasma cell burden is typically low, but 10–15% of cases of AL amyloidosis are associated with MM although conversion of MM to AL amyloidosis is infrequent and possibly a reflection of shorter survival in AL amyloidosis (Madan et al., 2010). It is the aggregation of these proteins followed by their tissue disposition and direct cytotoxic effects that disrupts normal tissue architecture and leads to organ dysfunction. The median age at diagnosis of AL is 65 years and the clinical presentation reflects organ dysfunction and includes nephrotic syndrome, restrictive cardiomyopathy, peripheral/autonomic neuropathy or soft tissue deposition, but cardiac involvement is the most important negative prognostic factor (Rajkumar et al., 2006).

Diagnosis of AL amyloidosis includes the need to demonstrate a monoclonal plasma cell dyscrasia (either by serum protein electrophoresis (SPEP) with immunofixation, urine protein electrophoresis (UPEP) with immunofixation, free light chain analysis, or bone marrow biopsy) and identify amyloid fibrils by their appearance histologically (birefringence when viewed under polarized light microscopy following Congo red staining). Amyloid can usually be detected histologically on rectal biopsy, on abdominal fat pad aspirate, or on bone marrow aspirate (Sanchorawala, 2006). Peripheral neuropathy has been reported in up to 17% of patients with AL, usually sensorimotor in type, but concomitant autonomic nervous system involvement occurs in up to 65% and ANS dysfunction carries a poorer prognosis. Treatment protocols have included high-dose chemotherapy (usually including melphalan) and autologous stem cell transplantation; improvement in free light chain (FLC) assay correlates with improvement in neuropathy score and neuropathic symptoms (Katoh et al., 2010). Prognosis reflects organ involvement and indirectly treatments that are used; there is a median survival of 18 months for those ineligible and 40 months for those eligible for autologous bone marrow transplantation (Székely et al., 2008).

Waldenström's macroglobulinemia (WM), or lymphoplasmacytic lymphoma, is manifested by infiltration of bone marrow (≥ 10% lymphoplasmacytic infiltration), lymph nodes, and spleen but uncommonly extranodal sites and an IgM monoclonal gammopathy. CNS involvement is a very rare complication of WM and referred to as *Bing–Neel syndrome.* Clinical manifestations reflect site of involvement, but include stroke, subarachnoid hemorrhage (SAH), other focal or multifocal syndromes as well as a diffuse encephalopathy.

Symptoms include headache, confusion/cognitive dysfunction, motor or sensory deficits, pain and psychiatric manifestations. Laboratory tests are those that are consistent with WM. MRI can show isointense T1 lesions that may enhance, hyperintense on T2 with FLAIR hyperintensities and edema. CSF exam shows lymphocytosis and cytology/cell flow cytometry may identify the abnormal cells; protein levels are elevated, glucose normal or decreased; immunofixation may demonstrate an IgM κ or λ band. Biopsy is usually necessary for a confirmatory diagnosis. Treatment recommendations are based on the results of individual case reports, but are essentially the same as those currently employed in the treatment of WM (Rajkumar et al., 2006; Malkani et al., 2010).

Intravascular large B cell lymphoma is a rare extranodal subtype of diffuse large B cell lymphoma, usually of a B cell immunophenotype, and is the preferred name for a disorder that was first described by Pfleger and Tappeiner in 1959 as "Angioendotheliomatosis proliferans systemisata" (Ferreri et al., 2004; Zuckerman et al., 2006). As a rare disorder (estimated incidence is one per million) most clinical information is gathered from individual case reports; treatment regimens tend to be extrapolations from more frequent lymphoma protocols. The histologic appearance is of large malignant lymphocytes filling small vascular lumina, "sparing" surrounding tissue and demonstrating the predilection of these cells for capillary endothelium.

Typically affected patients are elderly (median age of 70 years, range 34–90), without gender preference (women may be more frequently affected by the "cutaneous variant" with a better outcome) and present with a poor performance status, B symptoms, fever, anemia and a high serum lactate dehydrogenase (LDH). The clinical presentation is heterogenous, but lymphadenopathy, hepatosplenomegaly, or circulating tumor cells are uncommon. Neurologic symptoms or findings may be the exclusive or prominent presentation manifesting as sensory or motor deficits, altered sensorium, rapidly progressive dementia, seizures, ataxia or vertigo. Clinical diagnoses have included stroke, encephalomyelitis, Guillain–Barré syndrome, vasculitis, and multiple sclerosis. There are no pathognomonic findings on brain MRI, but abnormalities can be interpreted as suggestive of small vessel ischemia or demyelination. Hence the most common alternative diagnosis in these cases is CNS vasculitis. Recently two individuals presenting with presumed atherosclerotic stroke underwent FDG-PET (and in one case IMP-SPECT) that demonstrated areas of increased uptake within the infarction. One case had a brain biopsy and intravascular lymphoma was diagnosed, the other assumed from its responsiveness to chemotherapy. This unexpected pattern of enhancement may be useful in supporting the diagnosis in selected cases (Yamada et al., 2010). CSF analysis may identify a lymphocytosis, but CSF cytopathology is typically not diagnostic. When intravascular lymphoma is suspected, any skin lesion that is present should then be biopsied and biopsy of a CNS lesion considered. The value of a random skin biopsy remains uncertain (Zuckerman et al., 2006).

There is another presentation of intravascular lymphoma reported within the Japanese literature (*Asian variant*, often with hemophagocytic syndrome) with a presentation consisting of fever, anemia, thrombocytopenia and hepatosplenomegaly. The course is aggressive, rapidly progressive, and it has a poor median survival (Ferreri et al., 2004).

Whether there is a true predilection or it is only a manifestation of vascular "vulnerability," brain and skin are the most commonly involved areas, but bone marrow infiltration (32%) and hepatosplenic involvement (26%) occur. Nodal disease is rare (11%). At the time of diagnosis, all patients should be considered to have disseminated disease and bone marrow biopsy should be performed as part of initial staging evaluation of both systemic and cutaneous intravascular lymphoma (Roglin and Boer, 2007). The prognosis is poor in intravascular lymphoma and most cases are rapidly progressive. Half of the cases are only diagnosed at postmortem. Aggressive treatment of intravascular lymphoma includes non-Hodgkin lymphoma chemotherapy regimens (typically R-CHOP chemotherapy with rituximab, cyclophosphamide, doxorubicin, vincristine and prednisone), plus high-dose systemic methotrexate when there is evidence of disease within the CSF, are standard (Ferreri et al., 2004).

Hodgkin lymphoma

Hodgkin lymphoma (HL) is now recognized as a distinct form of lymphoma characterized by the presence of multinucleated giant neoplastic Reed–Sternberg (RS) cells derived from B-lineage lymphocytes that induce an inflammatory background of small lymphocytes. Individuals typically present between the ages of 20 and 60 years with persistent, painless lymphadenopathy, usually within the neck, supraclavicular or axillary locations. Some lymphadenopathy, particularly when confined to the mediastinum, may not be clinically apparent without imaging, and may be present as chest pain, cough, or dyspnea. Infradiaphragmatic lymphadenopathy, which occurs in approximately 10% of patients, is more common in those above the age of 60 years. Presenting symptoms include abdominal or back pain, abdominal mass, or may be discovered during the evaluation of constitutional or systemic symptoms (Connors, 2009; Küppers, 2009).

There is a 5–10-fold increase in the incidence of HL in patients with HIV infection, often associated with Epstein–Barr virus. In more than 80% of cases the presentation is an advanced stage with a higher incidence of involvement of multiple extranodal sites (often without first involving the spleen), and B symptoms including fever, night sweats and weight loss when compared to HIV-negative HL. The recent concomitant use of highly active antiretroviral therapy (HAART) with judicious use of standard treatment protocols for HL have improved survival with 5 year overall survival, in selected patients, approaching 60—70% (Berenguer et al., 2008).

On the basis of the histologic picture, 95% of the cases of HL are of the classic type, which can be further subdivided into nodular sclerosis, mixed cellularity, lymphocyte-rich and lymphocyte depletion based on the histologic picture. The tumor cells are designated Hodgkin Reed–Sternberg cells (HRS). The remaining 5% of cases are of the nodular lymphocyte predominant type and their tumor cells are designated LP (lymphocyte predominant). In addition to morphology the two types of HL differ in regards to immunophenotype of the lymphoma cells, cellular microenvironment, genetic pathogenesis and the origin of the tumor cells (HRS derive from germinal center B cells with immunoglobulin V gene mutations while the LP cells derive from antigen selected germinal center B cells). HL is unusual in that the clonal neoplastic tumor cells (HRS and LP cells) comprise only 0.1–10% of the cells observed in tissue samples which have impeded molecular analysis until recently (Küppers, 2009). Greater than 90% of the cells within affected tissue are part of a reactive inflammatory milieu composed of small B and T lymphocytes with abundant collagen fibrosis. Latent infection by the Epstein–Barr virus is identified in about 40% of HRS cells and felt to play an important role in the development of the disease as well as its pathogenesis by assisting the survival of the HRS cells.

HL typically spreads from one set of lymph nodes to an adjacent group, but at the time of initial diagnosis the majority (75%) of individuals will show no evidence of extranodal extension. In those with evidence of extranodal extension there are two primary categories to consider; direct involvement of structures contiguous to the involved lymph nodes, e.g., thyroid or pleura, but not signifying evidence of widespread metastasis and can be addressed with local therapy. The other extranodal extension is to distant organs, including the spleen, liver, lung, bone and bone marrow. In less than 1% of cases are the extranodal sites skin, brain, gastrointestinal, or musculoskeletal tissue.

While the usual manifestation of HL at the time of diagnosis is an observable mass lesion or localized symptoms from one, B symptoms (night sweats, fever, or weight loss) are frequently reported (35%). Presentation with nonspecific constitutional symptoms, organ-related dysfunction or laboratory abnormalities (e.g., elevated ESR, anemia, hypoalbuminemia) is diagnostically more challenging. This provides the rationale for including HL within a broad set of differential diagnoses and necessitates radiologic imaging studies to identify tissue/lymph node involvement. Less specific is the occurrence of pruritus, often precipitated by alcohol use, and eosinophilia. Finally, there are infrequent reports of paraneoplastic syndromes, neurologic (e.g., cerebellar) or renal attributed to HL and at times arrested with its treatment.

The natural history of HL with the current chemotherapy and radiation techniques is curative in greater than 80% of patients. In North America, the standard of care for advanced HL is combination chemotherapy of ABVD (doxorubicin, bleomycin, vinblastine, dacarbazine), IFRT (involved-field radiotherapy) therapy and autologous hematopoietic stem cell transplantation that can rescue approximately 50% of those who failed primary therapy. The rate of recurrences (50% do so within 1–2 years of their initial treatment and 80–90% within 5 years) has led to trials of new regimens to improve efficacy and reduce toxicity (Advani, 2011). Lymphocyte-predominant HL is more frequently associated with later recurrences greater than 5 years from the time of diagnosis. Recurrences usually develop at the sites of initial involvement, and typically are of the same histologic subtype. Mortality is the result of organ involvement, infection, nutritional compromise, and generalized weakness. By the time of death there is usually evidence of extensive extranodal involvement, including the CNS. Despite what has been an impressive rate of cure of classic HL, markers that predict response to therapy as well as ways to limit unnecessary "overtreatment" are under investigation.

The current staging system of classic HL makes use of clinical presentation to determine management and predict prognosis, but none of the current prognostic systems are successful in identifying cases where current treatments will be ineffective. A clearer understanding of the biology and behavior of the HRS cells is clarifying the picture, but their infrequent occurrence makes such efforts difficult. They are known to activate numerous signaling pathways and secrete numerous cytokines, surrounding themselves with normal appearing cells that are necessary for their survival, but also initiating the migration of macrophages into the tumors. While it was once believed that the presence of macrophages signaled an immune response occurring against the tumor, their presence is actually linked to a poor prognosis. These tumor-associated macrophages behave in a trophic manner by mediating blood vessel formation through the secretion of growth factors. Recently a single immunohistochemical marker used on tissue samples, CD68, associated with normal macrophages was shown to be associated with clinical outcome. Although the functional link between the number of macrophages and outcome is unclear, an increased number of CD68+ macrophages in lymph node samples were correlated with a shortened progression-free survival. In limited stage disease the absence of CD68+ cells identified a subgroup of patients with a rate of long-term disease-specific survival of 100% with current treatments (Steidl et al., 2010).

As treatment has become more successful so have the late complications and the necessity for screening for secondary neoplasms (e.g., breast, head and neck, thyroid, skin, pleura), cardiovascular disease, thyroid dysfunction, infertility, dental disease, and other infectious complications.

Clinical presentations of lymphomas

CENTRAL NERVOUS SYSTEM

Lymphoma cells enter into the CNS via a hematogenous route, contiguous from adjacent bones or along neurovascular structures. Typically, when CNS dissemination occurs it is within 14 months from lymphoma diagnosis and usually associated with systemic recurrence. In these circumstances it is often isolated, involving brain, spinal cord, leptomeninges, or eyes in nearly half of the cases, and carries a poor prognosis, with a median survival of 4–5 months in NHL (Ferreri et al., 2009).

Involvement of the CNS varies with the lymphoma type. In lymphomas considered to be low grade, CNS involvement occurs clinically in less than 3% of cases (Hodgkin's is 0.2–0.6%), but in aggressive types, such as diffuse large B cell or T cell lymphoma, it may be 30%. Signs and symptoms are related to site, but in 6–11% of patients they may be asymptomatic at the time of discovery.

SPINAL CORD

Myelopathy can occur in patients with lymphoma and consist of epidural spinal cord compression, intramedullary metastases, paraneoplastic or adverse effects of treatment. While epidural spinal cord compression is of greatest concern and accompanied by back pain (80%) or weakness (35–75%) at the time of diagnosis it is uncommon in malignant lymphoma with an occurrence of 0.8–2.8% (Székely et al., 2008). Evaluation is urgent and currently MRI with contrast of the entire spine is recommended to exclude multiple sites of involvement. Compression occurs through direct involvement of the vertebral body or extension of a paravertebral mass through the neural foramina. The thoracic spine is the most likely site to be involved, followed by lumbar and then cervical (Graber and Nolan, 2010).

Steroid therapy is considered the initial form of intervention, but subsequent chemotherapy, radiation or surgery may be undertaken (Székely et al., 2008). Which course to follow is decided by (1) neurologic status, (2) nature of the tumor, (3) mechanical stability of the spine and, (4) clinical or performance status of the patient. Primary intramedullary spinal cord involvement is rare, diagnosis is often delayed and with a presumptive diagnosis of CNS demyelinative disease. Spinal cord MRI demonstrates multifocal, persistently enhancing gadolinium lesions, often with conus medullaris or cauda equina involvement. While diagnosis may be confirmed through CSF cytologic evaluation, spinal cord biopsy may be necessary for confirmatory diagnosis (Flanagan et al., 2011).

Ischemic spinal cord lesions are uncommon, but intravascular lymphoma may present in such a way. Intravascular lymphoma can produce direct vascular occlusion resulting in ischemic injury to neural tissue. Angiotropic large cell lymphoma has a predilection for tumor cells to aggregate inside vascular lumina (Glass, 2006). Sudden onset may also reflect hemorrhage within the spinal cord or an epidural hematoma.

A dysfunctional immune system is common in patients with hematologic malignancy and a result of the cancer as well as treatment. Epstein–Barr virus, as well as varicella zoster, CMV and others in addition to fungal and parasitic infections, can result in myelitis. While MRI may show increased signal on T2-weighted images and enhancement, CSF studies could be normal or demonstrate lymphocytosis, but polymerase chain reaction (PCR) studies can provide further diagnostic information. Direct compression by an epidural abscess or osteomyelitis is less common, but a possible occurrence, and provides further rationale for obtaining an MRI to assist in diagnosis of an individual presenting with spinal cord dysfunction.

LEPTOMENINGEAL

The increasingly successful control of malignancies will likely contribute to an increasing incidence of CNS metastases. While new antineoplastic agents result in more successful disease control, these new agents show limited CSF penetration and increasingly the CNS may become a protected site. In addition, these treatments may result in the selection of more chemoresistant tumor cells resulting in greater resistance to therapy (Wu et al., 2009; Groves, 2010).

Leptomeningeal (LM) metastasis may be associated with 24% of hematologic malignancies. In general, median survival ranges from 8 to 16 weeks and in 24–34% of cases death is a result of these metastases.

Strategies are directed at prevention or identification of individuals who have a higher propensity for their development. Current intrathecal treatment protocols for LM include methotrexate, cytarabine and thiotepa. Systemic therapies are based on tumor histology and their penetration into the CSF and prior drug exposure. The BBB and the blood–CSF barrier (BCSFB) are not equivalent so that these differences may be exploited and guide future treatment paradigms, lessen unnecessary interventions, and limit neurotoxicity.

Clinical suspicion of LM is considered when neurologic signs and symptoms are generalized (headache), focal cerebral, cranial nerve, radicular, neck/back pain, or suggest spinal cord dysfunction. Confirmatory diagnosis can be assisted by CSF cytopathology examination, but malignancy based on morphology alone is difficult (Wu et al., 2009). Contrast-enhanced MRI as well as PCR are not only useful but should be considered complementary. The role for tumor markers continues to be defined.

There is some controversy in regards to the frequency of meningeal involvement in PCL and the sensitivity of the evaluations used to substantiate its presence. Using cytomorphometry, PCR and MRI, the relative frequency of meningeal dissemination was 17.4% (higher in other series). The discordance between PCR and cytomorphometry is high so the tests should be considered as complementary. In regards to routine studies, CSF pleocytosis has predictive value, but elevated CSF protein does not. While clinically presenting with similar manifestations as other forms of leptomeningeal involvement, cauda equina involvement in PCL may result in a clinical syndrome suggestive of an inflammatory polyradiculoneuropathy (Fischer et al., 2008).

Primary dural lymphoma represents a rare presentation and typically an extranodal manifestation of a marginal zone lymphoma that arose from the dura. It is more frequent in middle-aged women and symptoms reflect localization. Neuroimaging reveals an extracranial mass that enhances diffusely, usually over the cerebral convexity, and in 50% of the cases more than one lesion is discovered. The primary differential is meningoma and both share similar imaging features. The limited number of cases does not allow specific treatment recommendations, but complete surgical resection is difficult, while low-dose RT, in light of this tumor's radiosensitivity, may provide excellent immediate results. The role of other chemotherapeutic regimens is not clear and recurrence necessitates long-term monitoring (Iwamoto and Abrey, 2006).

Cranial vault lymphomas are another rare presentation of lymphoma and more often reported as a large B cell lymphoma type (39%). Presentation is usually at the age of 60 years, no sex predominance is evident, and the presenting sign is that of a focal skull deformity or scalp swelling. The parietal area is more frequently involved. Radiologic imaging demonstrates an expansive lesion that involves the scalp, skull bone, and pachymeninges, in the absence of osteolysis; brain involvement may also occur. This particular radiologic pattern may have some diagnostic sensitivity in the appropriate clinical setting (da Rocha et al., 2010).

PERIPHERAL NERVOUS SYSTEM

Neurolymphomatosis is a rare metastatic complication of lymphoma (usually a diffuse B cell lymphoma in the majority of cases, but PCL in up to 25%) that histopathologically is manifested as lymphomatous infiltration of all components of the peripheral nerve including endoneurium. The clinical presentation consists of painful nerve or root involvement (31%), cranial neuropathy (25%), painless involvement of peripheral nerves (30%), or painful/painless involvement of a peripheral nerve (15%). A painful, asymmetric syndrome of peripheral nerve involvement of all the limbs with rapid evolution is suggestive of this etiology (a mononeuritis multiplex presentation) (Chamberlain et al., 2009).

Diagnosis is delayed because of the infrequency of this disorder and this presentation, but contrast-enhanced MRI has been helpful (contrast enhancement and enlargement/nodularity). Biopsy is less frequently performed of involved sites so diagnosis is clinical with radiologic findings providing support. Leptomeningeal metastases may be present in 20–25% of cases.

Peripheral neuropathy is a common occurrence in those NHLs which are associated with paraproteinemia. These include multiple myeloma (3–48%), monoclonal gammopathy of undetermined significance (MGUS) (8–37%), Waldenström's macroglobulinemia (lymphoplasmacytic lymphoma) (5–10%), systemic amyloidosis (15–20%) and POEMS syndrome (50–85%). A particular paraprotein is felt to be responsible for each observed clinical syndrome. IgM monoclonal paraproteins are more commonly associated with neuropathy (50%) than IgG and IgA monoclonal paraprotein neuropathy is uncommon. IgM monoclonal paraproteins are identified in nearly all cases of Waldenström's macroglobulinemia (lymphoplasmacytic lymphoma). Monoclonal paraproteins can be indentified in > 94% of cases of multiple myeloma and in all cases of MGUS. The most common monoclonal paraprotein in myeloma is IgG (52%), IgA (21%) and light chain only (κ or λ, 16%). POEMS syndrome is typically seen in patients with IgG λ or IgA λ monoclonal paraproteins.

Clinical syndromes typically are slowly progressive distal sensory polyneuropathies and usually axonal in character. However, POEMS produces a more prominent/disabling sensorimotor polyneuropathy with ataxia that clinically resembles a chronic inflammatory demyelinating polyneuropathy (CIDP)-like sensorimotor polyneuropathy. Amyloidosis can present as a neuropathy in 15–20% of cases. Characteristically it is a painful, progressive distal sensorimotor process and accompanied by autonomic dysfunction. Prognostic factors for an IgM MGUS includes older age and evidence of demyelination on neurophysiologic studies as negative predictors while the presence of an anti-MAG antibody may decrease the risk of future disability. However, these factors were not clearly shown to be associated with responsiveness to treatments (Niermeijer et al., 2010).

INFECTIOUS DISEASE

While infectious complications are too broad an area to completely address, they are important to mention. In general, patients with cancer have a greater tendency to develop infections, and their illness as well as their treatment places them at a higher probability for complications (Thirumala et al., 2010).

Patients with hematologic malignances carry a higher probability of developing severe sepsis (66.4/1000) than those individuals with solid tumors (7.6/1000) and carry a higher mortality. The appearance of neutropenic fever necessitates urgent evaluation and antibiotic administration (half of cases have bacteremia), lack of a clinical response may necessitate consideration of a fungal infection and empiric treatment during evaluation. Treatment is increasingly complicated as the responsible organism is more often Gram positive and resistant nosocomial isolates have begun to restrict treatment options. Most often the source is respiratory and gastrointestinal tract, while genitourinary infections are a less frequent complication.

CNS infections often present in a nondescript way and more prominent focal findings or nuchal rigidity can be lacking. In the setting of unexplained malaise, headache, fever, personality change, delirium or seizures a CNS infection must be considered as well as the possibility of CNS metastases (necessitating neuroimaging) or a metabolic abnormality. Lymphoma and stem cell transplantation are risk factors for a CNS infection and an indication for empiric treatment during evaluation. Antimicrobial agents are selected for the clinical setting and in light of underlying immune disorder (T cell dysfunction may necessitate the inclusion of sulfadiazine or TMP/SMZ to cover *Nocardia asteroides*). In addition, ventricular shunts or Ommaya reservoirs may need to be externalized or removed.

VASCULAR/HEMATOLOGIC

The usual risk factors for stroke in patients with or without cancer are the same and can be addressed in a similar fashion. Chemotherapy-induced risk of stroke appears to be small. Cerebral hemorrhage does occur more often in patients with hematologic (and lung) malignancy (25% versus 14% in one review). The pathophysiologic mechanism is attributed to a coagulopathy and typically occurs in acute disseminated intravascular coagulation (DIC), thrombocytopenia or hyperviscosity. Management of cancer patients with stroke follows general recommendations. However, comorbidity and prior treatments may limit some interventions (Fain et al., 2007; Oberndorfer et al., 2009).

Malignancies can be associated with vasculitides, more frequently hematologic (myelodysplastic or lymphoid). The NHL are more often associated with some disorders (leukocytoclastic vasculitis, lymphocytic cutaneous granulomatous, polyarteritis nodosa, and Henoch–Schönlein purpura) than HL. Cryoglobulins were found in 22% of patients with vasculitic NHL and assumed to be the etiology. Vasculitis and lymphoma are diagnosed simultaneously > 70% of the time, but response to treatment may differ. Of the disorders associated with monoclonal gammopathies, cutaneous vasculitides (leukocytoclastic, erythema elevatum diutinum) are mostly monoclonal IgA in type.

PARANEOPLASTIC

Although rare disorders in patients with cancer (< 1%), such neurologic syndromes present unique insights into dysfunction and similar frustrations when they present as the initial manifestation of a cancer. As a group they can affect any level of the nervous system, grouped by presentations that tend to be associated with specific cancers as well as paraneoplastic antibodies. While the pathophysiology has not been identified for each, in general they are believed to be immune-mediated (Ko et al., 2008; Graber and Nolan, 2010; Briani et al., 2011).

Paraneoplastic cerebellar degeneration is a pancerebellar disorder that develops over days to weeks and results in truncal/limb ataxia, dysarthria, dysphagia, and nystagmus. At times there can be additional symptoms (i.e., optic neuritis or encephalopathy). The disorder stabilizes but the deficit, usually severe, often persists. It is most commonly associated with lung and breast cancer and Hodgkin disease. Of the approximately nine antibodies identified, anti-Yo and anti-Tr, described in Hodgkin disease, are most prevalent. The MRI usually appears normal at onset (later cerebellar atrophy develops) and the CSF may demonstrate a mild lymphocytic pleocytosis, elevated protein and oligoclonal bands, but cytology is negative. In Hodgkin disease the median age is 54 years and the median survival from time of diagnosis is longer than compared to a similar syndrome occurring with anti-Yo, but likely related to the underlying tumor prognosis.

The deficit does not improve with treatment of the Hodgkin disease, but in some studies with early immune therapy (IVIg or plasmapheresis) there may be improvement in the cerebellar deficit and the anti-Tr may disappear in successful treatment. A similar dramatic change in anti-Yo antibody titers has not been noted.

LEUKEMIAS

Patients with leukemia often present with signs and symptoms arising from bone marrow failure and organ infiltration by leukemic cells. The symptoms of bone marrow failure include those arising from anemia, infections (due lack of white blood cells), bleeding (due to lack of platelets and coagulopathy), and organomegaly (especially liver and spleen) (Mughal et al., 2006). The diagnosis may be suspected on blood studies as patients with leukemia frequently have increased white blood cells (usually in the range of $20–200 \times 10^9/L$).

Leukemia refers to hematologic neoplasms of myeloid or lymphoid precursors that present with widespread involvement of the bone marrow and, usually, the peripheral blood (Fig. 69.2) (Kumar et al., 2009a). Myeloid precursors give rise to cells of granulocytic (neutrophil, eosinophil, basophil), monocytic/macrophage, erythroid, megakaryocytic and mast cell lineages (Vardiman et al., 2009). Lymphoid precursors give rise to B cells, T cells, NK cells and plasma cells. The term "lymphocytic leukemia" can lead to some confusion. Though considered separate entities, the distinction between lymphocytic leukemia and lymphoma has become increasingly blurred. The leukemias are broadly classified as "acute" or "chronic" and by the salient features of the abnormal excessive blast cell (lymphoid or myeloid) (Mughal et al., 2006; Kumar et al., 2009a). Classification as "acute" or "chronic" does not reflect the severity of the disease.

Acute leukemias are often of short duration or rapid onset (symptoms of a few weeks or months). Acute leukemia rarely presents as an incidental finding on routine blood work. Most of the white blood cells will be of the immature (blast cell) variety due to maturation arrest within the normal hematopoietic progression. "Blast cells" represent the immature precursors of lymphocytes or granulocytes. The two major subtypes of acute leukemia are acute lymphoblastic leukemia (ALL) and acute myeloid leukemia (AML). ALL is the predominant acute leukemia of childhood, while AML is more common in adulthood (median age at onset of 63 years) (Kolitz, 2008).

Myeloid neoplasms with 20% or more blasts in the peripheral blood or bone marrow are considered to be AML when they occur de novo; evolution to AML can also occur in the setting of previously diagnosed myelodysplastic syndrome (MDS) or myeloproliferative neoplasm (MPN), or blast transformation in a previously diagnosed MPN. Exposure to previous chemotherapy treatments and radiation increase the risk of AML. The standard treatment for AML includes induction therapy with 7 days of continuous infusion of cytarabine and 3 days of anthracycline chemotherapy (doxorubicin, idarubarin, or daungrubacin) ("7 and 3"). Repeat courses of induction chemotherapy are frequently required to achieve disease remission (Shipley and Butera, 2009). Postremission therapy includes consolidation chemotherapy (often with cytarabine) in patients less than 60, autologous stem cell transplant or allogenic stem cell transplant (Bosch et al., 2005).

Treatment for ALL includes high intensity multiagent chemotherapy regimens, frequently with weekly doses of vincristine combined with prednisone or dexamethasone. As improved treatments have extended life expectancy, it has become increasingly clear that the CNS is a major sanctuary site in ALL, with meningeal leukemia appearing in upwards of 50% of patients. This has led to standard CNS prophylactic therapies including intrathecal methotrexate and/or cytarabine in all cases. Whole brain radiotherapy is often also given with evidence of established CNS disease (Kolitz, 2008).

Chronic leukemias are of long duration or evolve gradually. Chronic lymphocytic leukemia is the most common adult leukemia in the Western world, with a median age of presentation of 65–70 years of age. Nearly 50% of patients are asymptomatic at presentation with the diagnosis being suggested incidentally on routine blood studies (the white blood cell can be over 50×10^9/L) (Enright and Bond, 2008). The disease course is highly variable and a proportion of patients never require treatment ("watchful waiting"). Chronic myelogenous leukemia (CML) is a myeloproliferative disorder characterized by a specific chromosomal translocation (t (9;22)(q34;q11) (the Philadelphia chromosome) (Goldman and Velo, 2003). This translocation induces a fusion of bcr/abl genes and chronic activation of a tyrosine kinase gene product causing increased cell signaling. Imatinib, dasatinib, and nilotinib represent a set of molecular targeted therapies which inactivate the bcr/abl tyrosine kinase. Since their introduction, survival of CML has increased with patients routinely living over a decade without evidence of relapse.

Clinical presentations of leukemias

LEPTOMENINGEAL

The most common "direct" CNS involvement of hematologic malignancies is leptomeningeal (LM) metastasis (Walker, 1991). Leukemic meningitis can occur without systemic disease or during remission, and even occasionally

as the initial presentation (Gieron et al., 1987). The peak incidence of clinically detectable meningeal leukemia is 3-6 months after bone marrow diagnosis (Wiernik, 2001). Leukemic cells likely invade the meninges via the arachnoid veins, with subsequent involvement of CSF spaces. Acute leukemias, especially ALL, have a higher propensity to invade the meninges than the chronic leukemias, which only rarely invade the meninges (Chamberlain and Marc, 2008). Prior to the introduction of CNS prophylaxis, 70% of autopsied ALL patients had postmortem evidence of leukemic meningitis. With current induction protocols, only 5-10% of adult patients with acute leukemia develop CNS disease (Kolitz, 2008). *Acute myelomonocytic leukemia* (*AMML*), a subtype of AML (FAB classification M4), and acute monocytic leukemia (FAB classification M5), also carries a high risk for leukemic meningitis, occurring in upwards of 20% of patients (Chamberlain et al., 2005). The occurrence of leukemic meningitis is a predictor of systemic disease and carries with it a poor prognosis, with a median survival of 2-6 months (Chamberlain et al., 2005; Chamberlain and Marc, 2008).

Risk of relapse of leukemic meningitis is associated with several prognostic factors, including young age, leukocytosis, the presence of extramedullary disease, high leukemia cell proliferation rate, elevated serum LDH, mature B cell immunophenotype, Philadelphia chromosome positivity, CD56 expression by leukemia cells, and an elevated β2-microglobulin level. Patients with one of three risk factors (elevated serum LDH, elevated serum β2-microglobulin, high leukemia cell proliferation rate) had a 13% risk of leukemic meningitis at 1 year. Risk increased to 20% if two or more risk factors were present (Kantarjian et al., 1992).

Leukemic meningitis can affect the cerebral hemispheres, the cranial nerves or the spinal cord and roots. Hemispheric dysfunction is often characterized by headache (possibly due to increased intracranial pressure) and mental status changes. Meningitis due to leukemia is usually associated with headache; photophobia may occasionally be present (Ballen and Hasserjian, 2005). Cranial nerve dysfunction occurs more frequently in patients with hematologic malignancies than with solid tissue tumors due to nerve compression or infiltration. Cranial neuropathies are usually unilateral and often involve the longer cranial nerves (Wiernik, 2001). Abducens palsies are more common than oculomotor palsies, which are more common than trochlear palsies. Trigeminal sensory/motor dysfunction, particularly the "numb chin" phenomenon seen with mental nerve involvement, hearing loss and optic neuropathy have also been described. Optic neuropathy may be a particularly common presentation of leukemic meningitis and warrants emergent radiotherapy to preserve vision (Chamberlain and Marc, 2008). Spinal cord and nerve root dysfunction findings are associated with the level of involvement. Leg weakness is more common than upper extremity weakness (Chamberlain et al., 2005). Hypothalamic involvement is rare but distinct when it occurs, clinically presenting with hyperphagia, obesity and somnolence, more commonly in children (Pochedly, 1975).

The diagnosis of leukemic meningitis can be difficult to ascertain, but diagnostic inquiries include cerebral spinal fluid analysis including flow cytometry, radiographic imaging and meningeal biopsy. CSF protein is usually mildly elevated (Glass, 2006). CSF cytology has a specificity of >95% but a sensitivity of less than 50% (Cheng et al., 1994). In one study, 41% of patients with autopsy proven leukemic meningitis had negative CSF cytology (Glass et al., 1979). CSF flow cytometry may increase the diagnostic yield. Immunohistochemistry studies can be used to distinguish between reactive and neoplastic lymphocytes in the CSF. The finding of CSF lymphocytes of all B cell lineages is highly suggestive as reactive lymphocytes in the CSF are of T cell lineage (Chamberlain and Marc, 2008). Contrast enhanced brain magnetic resonance imaging is superior to contrast enhanced computerized tomography. Abnormalities include parenchymal volume loss and enhancement; however, both carry a high false positive rate (30% by MRI, 58% by CT) (Chamberlain et al., 2005). MRI findings consistent with leptomeningeal disease are detected in fewer than 50% of patients. Several candidate CSF biomarkers have been identified, but none have been reliably been shown to be diagnostic to date (Chamberlain and Fink, 2009). Early detection may not improve survival. Neither MRI nor CSF analysis is sensitive enough to stand alone as a diagnostic method for leptomeningeal metastases (Clarke et al., 2010). Meningeal biopsy can also be employed in patients in whom there is a high clinical index of suspicion. Biopsy is more likely to be revealing if taken from an area that enhances on MR imaging (Bosch et al., 2005).

CENTRAL NERVOUS SYSTEM

Mass lesions can occur in the brain or spinal cord, though their occurrence is uncommon in the leukemias (Walker, 1991). The cerebral hemispheres are more frequently involved, usually with parenchymal involvement adjacent to blood vessels. Spinal cord compression is rare (1% occurrence) and fortunately highly radiosensitive. There is some controversy as to whether leukemic infiltrates within the brain and spinal cord may represent an extension of meningeal disease rather than a distinct entity. They are rarely hemorrhagic and are more common in ALL than in AML (Glass, 2006).

Chloromas (or *granulocytic sarcomas*) represent a subset of leukemia-associated solid tumors consisting of myeloid leukemic blast cells (Glass, 2006). The name derives from *chloros*, the Greek word for green, due to the tumor's greenish color. Chloromas may be more common in younger patients (mean age 38), though they are uncommon in children (in part due to their association with the myeloid leukemias, AML and CML, which are rare in childhood). The only chloroma more frequently associated with children is the granulocytic sarcoma of the orbit, for unclear reasons. Chloromas are commonly found adjacent to the skull or facial bones, usually with a dural attachment. They are rarely found within the brain parenchyma (accounting for only 1–4% of all chloromas) and spinal canal (they account for 3% of all spinal tumors). The thoracic and lumbar spine are the most commonly involved, with the cauda equina less so (Wiernik, 2001). They can be found in several other non-CNS sites, including the skin, bone, lymph nodes or the liver. There are rare reports of chloromas arising in peripheral nerves (such as the sciatic) and nerve roots. They are usually clinically silent, but are readily apparent on contrast-enhanced imaging studies, appearing similar to meningiomas. Though the tumors themselves are highly radiosensitive, their presence is associated with aggressive systemic disease (Chamberlain and Marc, 2008).

SPINAL CORD

Isolated spinal cord disorders are rare in the leukemias. They can be seen in the setting of leptomeningeal disease or with focal masses, as stated above. A more distinct myelopathy syndrome is seen as a complication of treatment. Myelopathic symptoms can arise within 2 days to 2 weeks of injection of intrathecal methotrexate, characterized by typical symptoms including back pain, sensory loss, and weakness. There are no specific predictors of occurrence, no treatment, and variable recovery (Glass, 2006).

A *paraneoplastic progressive necrotizing myelopathy* due to leukemias, and not due to antileukemic agents, has been described in limited case reports. The findings may be nonspecific, including elevated CSF white blood cell count and protein with negative cytology and increased T2 signal changes on MRI (Gieron et al., 1987).

VASCULAR/HEMATOLOGIC

CNS leukemic vascular disorders consist of hemorrhagic lesions, arterial and venous thromboses. CNS hemorrhage represents 70% of all cerebrovascular disease in patients with leukemia. It occurs in 20% of all patients with acute leukemia and accounts for 10–20% of leukemic deaths. Hemorrhage is particularly common in *acute promyelocytic leukemia (APL)*, and patients are increasingly treated with arsenic trioxide and/or all-trans retinoic acid (ATRA) to limit DIC complications associated with APL. Intraparenchymal hemorrhage is the most common while subdural hematoma is relatively uncommon. Predisposing factors include disseminated intravascular coagulation (DIC), disseminated aspergillosis or mucormycosis in the setting of neutropenia, vasculopathy due to leukemic cell invasion of the blood vessel walls, severe thrombocytopenia ($<25000/mm^3$) and sepsis. Hemorrhage may also be seen in the setting of blast crisis and extreme leukocytosis (WBC count > 100 K). Extreme leukocytosis can lead to blood hyperviscosity and sludging of blast cells at the venous end of a capillary bed, causing aneurysmal dilatation of blocked vessels and vessel destruction (Paleologos, 1993). This complication can be prevented by lowering the circulating blast count with oral hydroxyurea or leukapheresis, as well as whole brain radiation. Leukostasis is rarely seen in CLL, ALL, or the chronic phase of CML because the leukemic cells in these disorders do not increase blood viscosity (Wiernik, 2001). Solitary, often massive, ICH is typically seen in the setting of DIC and thrombocytopenia (Chamberlain and Marc, 2008). Multiple hemorrhages are associated with extreme leukocytosis.

The most common cause of cerebral infarction at or shortly after diagnosis is venous sinus thrombosis (VST). VST can be due to leukemic infiltration of the superior sagittal sinus, and in children receiving L-asparaginase chemotherapy for ALL (L-asparaginase interferes with fibrinogen). Multiple arterial microinfarcts can lead to a global encephalopathy syndrome, and may be associated with DIC (Glass, 2006). Evaluation for DIC is warranted in any patient with leukemia and encephalopathy. Septic emboli, particularly *Aspergillus* fungal infarcts, are frequently seen in patients with advanced disease.

A *mineralizing microangiopathy* associated with dystrophic calcifications of the gray matter, basal ganglia, and cerebral cortex following cranial radiation has been well described (Glass, 2006). Symptoms include focal seizures, ataxia, incoordination and behavioral disorders occurring 1 or more years after cranial radiotherapy, particularly in young children.

PERIPHERAL NERVOUS SYSTEM

Peripheral nervous system complications are less common than the CNS complications of leukemia (Bosch et al., 2005). One of the more common PNS complications is herpes zoster-related radiculopathies. It is most common in CLL where 7% of patients have at least one infection during the course of their disease (Chamberlain and Marc, 2008).

Neuropathy due to direct leukemic infiltration is rare, lagging far behind therapy-related neuropathy, even more so if cranial neuropathies associated with leukemic meningitis are excluded. The PNS blood–nerve barrier can theoretically provide a pharmacologic sanctuary for leukemic cells. However, many direct PNS manifestations of leukemia are limited to case reports. Peripheral neuropathy, usually an axonal sensorimotor polyneuropathy, is most commonly seen in CLL, but still occurs in less than 1% of patients (Walker, 1991). By comparison, nerve conduction abnormalities were seen in nearly 30% of children 2 or more years after therapy for ALL. Leukemic infiltration of peripheral nerves and roots may result in an axonal polyradiculoneuropathy or severe sensory ataxic neuropathy. A monoclonal protein is detected in 8% of patients with CLL, and can be associated with chronic demyelinating neuropathies.

CONCLUSION

Neurologic complications of the leukemias and lymphomas are multifold. Symptoms can range from generalized, nonspecific features that may not raise the suspicion of a clinician, to readily apparent focal disturbances. While neurologic symptoms are rarely the presenting feature of the hematologic malignancies, the neurologist must be familiar with the common neurologic presentation of these disorders and their treatments.

REFERENCES

Abel GA, Friese CR, Magazu LS et al. (2008). Delays in referral and diagnosis for chronic hematologic malignances: literature review. Leuk Lymphoma 49: 1352–1359.

Advani R (2011). Optimal therapy of advanced Hodgkin lymphoma. Hematology Am Soc Hematol Educ Program 2011: 447–450.

Ballen KK, Hasserjian RP (2005). Case 2-2005: A 39-year-old woman with headache, stiff neck, and photophobia. N Engl J Med 352: 274–283.

Bataille B, Delwail V, Ment E et al. (2000). Primary intracerebral lymphoma: report of 248 cases. J Neurosurg 92: 261–266.

Bayraktar S, Bayraktar UD, Ramos JC et al. (2011). Primary CNS lymphoma in HIV positive and negative patients: comparison of clinical characteristics, outcome and prognostic factors. J Neurooncol 101: 257–265.

Berenguer J, Miralles P, Ribera JM et al. (2008). Characteristics and outcome of AIDS-related Hodgkin lymphoma before and after the introduction of highly active antiviral therapy. J Acquir Immune Defic Syndr 47: 422–428.

Bladé J, Dimopoulos M, Rosiňol L et al. (2009). Smoldering (asymptomatic) multiple myeloma: current diagnostic criteria, new predictors of outcome, and follow-up recommendations. J Clin Oncol 28: 690–697.

Bornkamm GW (2009). Epstein–Barr virus and its role in the pathogenesis of Burkitt's lymphoma: an unresolved issue. Semin Cancer Biol 19: 351–365.

Bosch EP, Habermann TM, Tefferi A (2005). Peripheral neuropathy associated with lymphoma, leukemia and myeloproliferative disorders. In: PJ Dyck, PK Thomas (Eds.), Peripheral Neuropathy. 4th edn. Elsevier Saunders, Philadelphia, pp. 2489–2504.

Briani C, Vitaliani R, Grisold W et al. (2011). Spectrum of paraneoplastic disease associated with lymphoma. Neurology 76: 705–710.

Chamberlain MC, Fink J (2009). Neurolymphomatosis: a rare metastatic complication of diffuse large B-cell lymphoma. J Neurooncol 95: 285–288.

Chamberlain MC, Marc C (2008). Neurologic complications of leukemia. In: D Schiff, S Kesari, PY Wen (Eds.), Cancer Neurology in Clinical Practice: Neurologic Complications of Cancer and its Treatment. 2nd edn. Humana Press, Totowa NJ, pp. 555–565.

Chamberlain MC, Nolan C, Abrey LE (2005). Leukemic and lymphomatous meningitis: incidence, prognosis and treatment. J Neurooncol 75: 71–83.

Chamberlain MC, Glantz M, Groves MD et al. (2009). Diagnostic tools for neoplastic meningitis: detecting disease, identifying patient risk, and determining benefit of treatment. Semin Oncol 36 (Supplement 2): S35–S45.

Cheng TM, O'Neill BP, Sheithauer BW (1994). Chronic meningitis: the role of meningeal or cortical biopsy. Neurosurg 34: 590–595.

Clarke JL, Perez HR, Jacks LM et al. (2010). Leptomeningeal metastases in the MRI era. Neurology 74: 1449–1454.

Connors JM (2009). Clinical manifestations and natural history of Hodgkin's lymphoma. Cancer J 15: 124–128.

da Rocha AJ, da Rocha TM, da Silva CJ et al. (2010). Cranial vault lymphoma: a systematic review of five patients. J Neurooncol 100: 9–15.

de Leval L, Hasserjian RP (2009). Diffuse large B-cell lymphomas and Burkitt lymphoma. Hematol Oncol Clin North Am 23: 791–827.

Dropcho EJ (2011). The neurologic side effects of chemotherapeutic agents. Continuum 17: 95–112.

Enright H, Bond J (2008). Chronic leukemias. Dis Mon 54: 242–255.

Fain O, Hamidou M, Laloub P et al. (2007). Vasculitides associated with malignancies: analysis of sixty patients. Arthritis Rheum 57: 1473–1480.

Ferreri AJ, Campo E, Seymour JF et al. (2004). Intravascular lymphoma: clinical presentation, natural history, management and prognostic factors in a series of 38 cases, with special emphasis on the "cutaneous variant. Br J Haematol 127: 173–183.

Ferreri AJM, Assanelli A, Crocchiolo R et al. (2009). Central nervous system dissemination in immunocompetent patients with aggressive lymphomas: incidence, risk factors and therapeutic options. Hematol Oncol 27: 61–70.

Fischer L, Martus P, Weller M et al. (2008). Meningeal dissemination in primary CNS lymphoma: prospective evaluation of 282 patients. Neurology 71: 1102–1108.

Flanagan EP, O'Neill BP, Porter AB et al. (2011). Primary intramedullary spinal cord lymphoma. Neurology 77: 784–791.

Gerstner ER, Batchelor TT (2010). Primary central nervous system lymphoma. Arch Neurol 67: 291–297.

Gieron MA, Margraf LR, Korthals JK et al. (1987). Progressive necrotizing myelopathy associated with leukemia: clinical, pathologic, and MRI correlation. J Child Neurol 2: 44–49.

Glass J (2006). Neurologic complications of lymphoma and leukemia. Semin Oncol 33: 342–347.

Glass J, Melamed M, Chernik N (1979). Malignant cells in cerebrospinal fluid (CSF). The meaning of a positive CSF cytology. Neurology 29: 1369–1375.

Goldman JM, Velo JV (2003). Chronic myeloid leukemia – advances in biology and new approaches to treatment. N Engl J Med 349: 1451–1464.

Graber JJ, Nolan CP (2010). Myelopathies in patients with cancer. Arch Neurol 67: 298–304.

Groves MD (2010). New strategies in the management of leptomeningeal metastases. Arch Neurol 67: 305–312.

Haldorsen IS, Espeland A, Larsson EM (2011). Central nervous system lymphoma: characteristic findings on traditional and advanced imaging. AJNR Am J Neuroradiol 32: 984–992.

Iwamoto FM, Abrey LE (2006). Primary dural lymphomas: a review. Neurosurg Focus 21: 1–5.

Jaffe ES, Harris NL, Stein H et al. (2008). Classification of lymphoid neoplasms: the microscope as a tool for disease discovery. Blood 112: 4384–4399.

Kanai R, Shibuya M, Hata T et al. (2008). A case of "lymphomatosis cerebri" diagnosed in an early phase and treated by whole brain radiation: case report and literature review. J Neurooncol 86: 83–88.

Kantarjian HM, Smith T, Estey E et al. (1992). Prognostic significance of elevated serum beta 2-microglobulin levels in adult acute lymphocytic leukemia. Am J Med 93: 599–604.

Katoh N, Matsuda M, Yoshida T et al. (2010). Primary AL amyloid polyneuropathy treated with high-dose melphalan followed by autologous stem cell transplantation. Muscle Nerve 41: 138–143.

Kim T, Kim SJ, Kim E et al. (2011). Primary CNS lymphoma other than DLBCL: a descriptive analysis of clinical features and treatment outcomes. Ann Neurol 90: 1391–1398.

Ko MW, Dalmau J, Galetta SL (2008). Neuro-ophthalmologic manifestations of paraneoplastic syndrome. J Neuroophthalmol 28: 58–68.

Kolitz JE (2008). Acute leukemias in adults. Dis Mon 54: 226–241.

Kumar V, Abbas AK, Fausto N et al. (2009a). Diseases of white blood cells, lymph nodes, spleen and thymus. In: V Kumar, AK Abbas, N Fausto et al. (Eds.), Robbins and Cotram Pathologic Basis of Disease. 8th edn. Saunders Elsevier, Philadelphia, pp. 589–638.

Kumar SK, Mikhael JR, Buadi FK et al. (2009b). Management of newly diagnosed symptomatic multiple myeloma: updated Mayo stratification of myeloma and risk-adapted therapy (mSMART) consensus guidelines. Mayo Clin Proc 84: 1095–1110.

Küppers R (2009). The biology of Hodgkin's lymphoma. Nat Rev Cancer 9: 15.

Lin P (2009). Plasma cell myeloma. Hematol Oncol Clin North Am 23: 709–727.

Madan S, Greipp PR (2009). The incidental monoclonal protein: current approach to management of monoclonal gammopathy of undetermined significance (MGUS). Blood Rev 23: 257–265.

Madan S, Dispenzieri A, Lacy MQ et al. (2010). Clinical features and treatment response of light chain (AL) amyloidosis diagnosed in patients with previous diagnosis of multiple myeloma. Mayo Clin Proc 85: 232–238.

Malkani RG, Tallman M, Gottardi-Littell N et al. (2010). Bing–Neel syndrome: an illustrative case and a comprehensive review of the literature. J Neurooncol 96: 301–312.

Mughal TI, Goldman JM, Mughal ST (2006). Understanding Leukemias, Lymphomas and Myelomas. Taylor and Francis Group, Boca Faton, FL.

Niermeijer JMF, Fisher K, Eurelings M et al. (2010). Prognosis of polyneuropathy due to IgM monoclonal gammopathy: a prospective cohort study. Neurology 74: 406–412.

Oberndorfer S, Nussgruber V, Berger O et al. (2009). Stroke in cancer patients: a risk factor analysis. J Neurooncol 94: 221–226.

Ottensmeier C (2001). The classification of lymphomas and leukemias. Chem Biol Interact 135–136: 653–654.

Paleologos NA (1993). Neurologic complications of disorders of white blood cells. In: CG Goetz, CM Tanner, MJ Aminoff (Eds.), Handbook of Clinical Neurology. Elsevier Science Publishers, Amsterdam, pp. 339–354.

Perkins AS, Friedberg JW (2008). Burkitt lymphoma in adults. Hematology Am Soc Hematol Educ Program 2008: 341–348.

Pochedly C (1975). Neurologic manifestations in acute leukemia: involvement of cranial nerves and hypothalamus. N Y State J Med 75: 715–721.

Raab MA, Podar K, Breitkreutz I et al. (2009). Multiple myeloma. Lancet 374: 324–339.

Rajkumar SV, Dispenzieri A, Kyle RA (2006). Monoclonal gammopathy of undetermined significance, Waldenstrom macroglobulinemia, Al amyloidosis, and related plasma cell disorders: diagnosis and treatment. Mayo Clin Proc 81: 693–703.

Roglin J, Boer A (2007). Skin manifestations of intravascular lymphoma mimic inflammatory disease of the skin. Br J Dermatol 157: 16–25.

Roth P, Korfel A, Martus P et al. (2012). Pathogenesis and management of primary CNS lymphoma. Expert Rev Anticancer Ther 12: 623–633.

Sanchorawala V (2006). Light-chain (AL) amyloidosis: diagnosis and treatment. Clin J Am Soc Nephrol 1: 1331–1341.

Shipley JL, Butera JN (2009). Acute myelogenous leukemia. Exp Hematol 37: 649–658.

Steidl C, Lee T, Shah SP et al. (2010). Tumor-associated macrophages and survival in classic Hodgkin's lymphoma. N Engl J Med 362: 875–885.

Székely G, Miltényi Z, Mezey G et al. (2008). Epidural malignant lymphoma of the spine: collected experiences with epidural malignant lymphoma of the spinal canal and their treatment. Spinal Cord 46: 278–281.

Tang YZ, Booth TC, Bhogal P et al. (2011). Imaging of primary central nervous system lymphoma. Clin Radiol 66: 768–777.

Thirumala R, Ramaswamy M, Chawla S (2010). Diagnosis and management of infectious complications in critically ill patients with cancer. Crit Care Clin 26: 59–91.

Turesson I, Velez R, Kristinsson SY et al. (2010). Patterns of multiple myeloma during the past 5 decades: stable incidence rates for all age groups in the population but rapidly changing age distribution in the clinic. Mayo Clin Proc 85: 225–230.

Vardiman JW (2010). The World Health Organization (WHO) classification of tumors of the hematopoietic and lymphoid tissues: an overview with emphasis on the myeloid neoplasms. Chem Biol Interact 184: 16–20.

Vardiman JW, Thiele J, Arber DA et al. (2009). The 2008 revision of the World Health Organization (WHO) classification of myeloid neoplasms and acute leukemia: rationale and important changes. Blood 114: 937–951.

Walker RW (1991). Neurologic complications of leukemia. Neurol Clin 9: 989–997.

Wiernik PH (2001). Extramedullary manifestations of adult leukemia. In: PH Wiernik (Ed.), Adult Leukemias. BC Decker, Hamilton, pp. 275–306.

Wu JM, Georgy MF, Burroughs FH et al. (2009). Lymphoma, leukemia, and pleocytosis in cerebrospinal fluid: is accurate cytopathologic diagnosis possible based on morphology alone. Diagn Cytopathol 27: 8204.

Yamada S, Nishii R, Oka S et al. (2010). FDG-PET a pivotal imaging modality for diagnosis of stroke-onset intravascular lymphoma. Arch Neurol 67: 366–367.

Zhou Y, Barlogie B, Shaughnessy JD Jr (2009). The molecular characterization and clinical management of multiple myeloma in the post-genome era. Leukemia 23: 1941–1956.

Zuckerman D, Seliem R, Hochberg E (2006). Intravascular lymphoma: the oncologist's "Great Imitator. Oncologist 11: 496–502.

Handbook of Clinical Neurology, Vol. 120 (3rd series)
Neurologic Aspects of Systemic Disease Part II
Jose Biller and Jose M. Ferro, Editors

Chapter 70

Bleeding diathesis and hemophilias

CHIRAG AMIN[1], ANJALI SHARATHKUMAR[1,2], AND ANNE GRIEST[1,3]*

[1]*Indiana Hemophilia and Thrombosis Centre, Indianapolis, IN, USA*

[2]*Department of Pediatrics, Riley Whitcomb Hospital for Children, Indiana University School of Medicine, Indianapolis, IN, USA*

[3]*Department of Medicine, Indiana University School of Medicine, Indianapolis, IN, USA*

INTRODUCTION

Hemophilia and other congenital bleeding disorders are caused by quantitative or qualitative deficiencies of components of hemostasis such as coagulation proteins, or platelets. These patients can present with a wide spectrum of clinical symptoms ranging from being asymptomatic to presenting with severe central nervous system (CNS) bleeding. Accurate diagnosis and appropriate clinical intervention such as infusion of specific factor (F) concentrates is of paramount importance to control the bleeding diathesis. Diagnosis of a bleeding disorder requires a personal history of bleeding, family history of bleeding, examination of potential bleeding sites, and appropriate laboratory testing. Understanding the physiology of hemostasis and its relationship with the clinical symptoms of bleeding is critical to suspect and diagnose an underlying bleeding disorder in order to offer appropriate clinical management.

Pathophysiology of hemostasis

Hemostasis refers to the process whereby bleeding is halted in a closed circulatory system, and in human physiology, involves two phases (Fig. 70.1): primary hemostasis and secondary hemostasis.

Primary hemostasis is characterized by vascular contraction, platelet adhesion and formation of a soft platelet plug. Primary hemostasis is activated immediately after endothelial disruption. In response to an injury, local vasoconstriction reduces the blood flow to prevent bleeding from the injured vessel. This is followed by platelet adhesion which occurs when circulating Von Willebrand factor (VWF) attaches to the exposed subendothelium. Next, glycoprotein receptors on the platelet surface adhere to the "sticky" VWF. These platelets are then "activated" by contact with collagen within the vascular endothelium. Collagen-activated platelets form pseudopods which stretch out to cover the injured surface and bridge the exposed fibers. The collagen-activated platelet membranes expose receptors which bind with circulating fibrinogen. Fibrinogen has many platelet binding sites and it is required for platelet aggregation. Aggregation of platelets through fibrinogen leads to a formation of a soft plug. The platelet plug contributes to cessation of bleeding but is unstable. Thus, for stability, the platelet plug must be reinforced by the formation of an organized fibrin clot through the activation of the blood coagulation system.

This process of activation of the coagulation system is referred to as secondary hemostasis. Blood coagulation involves a cascade of activation reactions. At each stage, a precursor protein (e.g., factor VII) is converted to an active protease (e.g., factor VIIa); some of these proteins require the presence of calcium and a phospholipid surface. Activated platelets and damaged endothelium provide a phospholipid surface upon which the coagulation cascade is assembled. Physiologically, coagulation is initiated through the "extrinsic pathway or tissue factor pathway" which involves formation of activated factor VII (FVIIa) by tissue factor (TF). TF binds to FVIIa and forms the TF/FVIIa complex which activates FX. The TF/FVIIa complex also activates factors XI, IX, and X from the intrinsic pathway which continues propagation of the coagulation cascade. FVIIIa and FVa act as cofactors for FIXa and FXa respectively. Additionally, the intrinsic pathway is activated through

---

*Correspondence to: Dr. Anne Greist, M.D., Indiana Hemophilia and Thrombosis Center, 8402 Harcourt Rd., Ste. 500, Indianapolis, IN 46260, USA. Tel: +1-317-871-0000, Fax: +1-317-871-0010, E-mail: agreist@ihtc.org

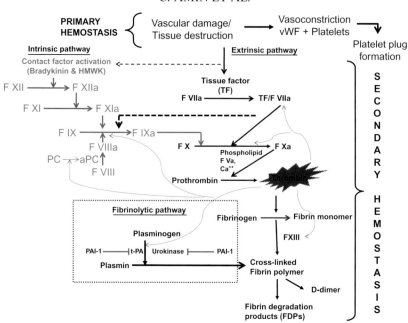

Fig. 70.1. Tissue factor-based coagulation cascade. Dashed arrows show the amplification loops created by thrombin. PAI-1, plasminogen activator inhibitor-1; F, factor; PC, protein C; aPC, activated protein C; a, activated; tPA tissue plasminogen activator.

contact factors that convert FXI to FXIa; FXIa activates FIX which in turn activates FX. Since both the intrinsic and extrinsic pathways merge at the activation of FX, it is known as the "common pathway." FXa activates prothrombin to thrombin. Generation of thrombin is the critical step in coagulation as the thrombin-mediated feedback loop in turn activates FIX and two cofactors of coagulation, FVIII and FV, which in turn enhances and amplifies both extrinsic and intrinsic pathways. This ultimately leads to a "thrombin burst" which is sufficient for effective hemostasis. The prime function of coagulation is to convert soluble fibrinogen into insoluble fibrin. These fibrin monomers polymerize in the vicinity of the primary platelet plug. These fibrin polymers are further strengthened through cross-linking by FXIII to form a fibrin clot. Simultaneously, the fibrinolytic pathway is activated to prevent the pathologic propagation of fibrin clot. Plasminogen is the key protein in the fibrinolytic pathway. It is converted to plasmin by tissue plasminogen activator (tPA) and urokinase. The function of plasmin is to dissolve the fibrin clot and restore the normal vascular architecture. The activation of plasminogen is kept in check by inhibitors of plasmin: plasminogen activator inhibitor-1 (PAI-1) and α_2-antiplasmin.

Thus, for all practical purposes any quantitative or qualitative deficiency of platelets, VWF, and the coagulation proteins could potentially lead to a bleeding tendency. Additionally formation of excess plasmin due to the deficiency of PAI-1 or α_2-antiplasmin can cause bleeding symptoms due to hyperfibrinolysis. Table 70.1 provides the overview of bleeding symptoms of various

bleeding disorders. In general patients with disorders of primary hemostasis present with mucocutaneous bleeding and/or bleeding after hemostatic challenge such as surgical procedures or menstrual periods while disorders of secondary hemostasis present with deep tissue bleeds such as musculoskeletal bleeds.

The following section elaborates the disorders of various coagulation proteins that are involved in primary and secondary hemostasis. Additionally inherited platelet abnormalities and miscellaneous bleeding disorders such as deficiencies of antifibrinolytic proteins are discussed briefly.

HEMOPHILIA

Conventionally, hemophilia refers to deficiencies of coagulation proteins, factor VIII and factor IX. Factor VIII deficiency is known as hemophilia A or classic hemophilia while factor IX deficiency is known as hemophilia B or Christmas disease.

Epidemiology of hemophilia

The incidence of hemophilia A is approximately 1 in 5000 live male births while the incidence of hemophilia B is 1 in 30 000 live male births. Hemophilia has no racial predilection, and is present in all ethnic and racial groups.

Genetics of hemophilia

Hemophilia A and B are transmitted as X-linked recessive disorders, hence males are typically clinically affected and

Table 70.1

Overview of congenital bleeding disorders

Type of hemostatic defect	Characteristic bleeding pattern	Commonly encountered Bleeding disorder	CNS bleeding	Diagnostic test	Specific treatment
Disorders of primary hemostasis	Mucocutaneous bleeding: Patechial rash, Ecchymoses, Subcutaneous hematoma formation, Epistaxis, Gum bleeding, Menorrhagia, Prolonged bleeding after a minor trauma, Hemorrhagic ovarian cysts, Bleeding after hemostatic challenge: Bleeding after T & A procedure, Bleeding after wisdom tooth extraction	Von Willebrand's disease (Types 1,2,3)	Spontaneous CNS bleeding uncommon; Reported in Type 2B & Type 3 VWD either in newborn period or after trauma	Platelet function test (PFA-1-l00 CT); VWF Ag, activity, FVIII levels; VWF multimer pattern; Ristocetin induced platelet aggregation	DDAVP/Stimate, Antifibrinolytics: Tranexamic acid, EACA, topical hemostatic agents, Humate-P: Plasma derived VWF containing product
		Platelet function disorders: Bernard-Soulier Syndrome, Glanzmann's thrombasthenia, Dense granule deficiency, Gray platelet syndrome, Scott syndrome, Cyclooxigenase deficiency, Quebec platelet disorder	Rare	Platelet count, Evaluation of blood smear, Platelet function test, Platelet aggregation test, Platelet EM studies, Flow cytometry for platelet receptor expression, Genetic mutation analysis e.g. *MYH9*, History of drug consumption	DDAVP/Stimate, Antifibrinolytics: Tranexamic acid, EACA, topical hemostatic agents, Platelet transfusions
		Disorders associated with thrombocytopenia: Bone marrow failure syndromes: Amegakaryocytic thrombocytopenia, Fanconi's anemia; *MYH9* disorders: May-Hegglin anomaly, Fletchner syndrome, Epstein syndrome	Rare	Complete blood count, Platelet count, Evaluation of blood smear, Platelet autoantibody test, Bone marrow evaluation, *MYH9* gene mutation analysis	DDAVP/Stimate, Antifibrinolytics: Tranexamic acid, EACA, topical hemostatic agents, Platelet transfusions, NovoSeven for Glanzmann's thrombasthenia

Continued

Table 70.1

Continued

Type of hemostatic defect	Characteristic bleeding pattern	Commonly encountered Bleeding disorder	CNS bleeding	Diagnostic test	Specific treatment
Disorders of secondary hemostasis	Mucocutaneous bleeding Joint bleeding Muscle bleeding and deep tissue hematoma Bleeding within the internal organs	Hemophilia A (FVIII deficiency) Hemophilia B (FIX deficiency)	Spontaneous CNS bleeding reported	Prolongation of PTT FVIII levels FIX levels	Recombinant FVIII products Recombinant FIX products Plasma derived FVIII & IX products FFP (only if specific concentrates are unavailable) DDAVP: only for mild FVIII deficiency Hemophilia with inhibitors: Recombinant FVIIa FEIBA, PCCs
	Variable bleeding phenotype: Mucocutaneous bleeding Bleeding after hemostatic challenge Joint bleeding Musculoskeletal bleeding Deep muscle hematoma	Other clotting factors deficiencies: FII, FVII, FIX, FX, FXI, fibrinogen	Spontaneous CNS bleeding reported in FII, FVII, FX and FXI deficiency	Prolongation of PT only: FVII deficiency Prolongation of PTT only: FXI Prolongation of PT and PTT: FII, FV,FX deficiency Quantitation of coagulation factors: FII, FV, FX, FXI level Mixing studies: Correction of prolonged screening tests	FVII deficiency: Recombinant FVII (NovoSeven) FV deficiency: Platelet transfusion or FFP, NovoSeven FXI deficiency: FFP, NovoSeven Other factor deficiencies: FFP
	Mucocutanous bleeding Joint bleeding Muscle bleeding and deep tissue hematoma Bleeding within the internal organs: CNS Miscarriages	Disorders of fibrinogen: Dysfibrinogenemia Afibrinogenemia	Spontaneous CNS bleeding reported	Prolongation of screening coagulation tests: PT,PTT, TT Fibrinogen antigen Fibrinogen activity Mixing studies: Correction of prolonged screening tests	Cryoprecipitate Fibrinogen concentrates FFP
	Neonatal intracranial bleeding Bleeding from umbilical cord stump Deep muscle hematoma Bleeding from surgical wounds & delayed wound healing Recurrent miscarriages	Severe FXIII deficiency	Spontaneous CNS bleeding common. Lifetime prevalence of CNS bleeding is ~23%	Urea clot solubility test	FXIII concentrates (FibroGamin) FFP
Disorders of fibrinolysis	Mucocutaneous bleeding, Bleeding after hemostatic challenge, Rarely musculoskeletal bleeding	Homozygous PAI-1 deficiency α₁-antitrypsin deficiency	Spontaneous CNS bleeding uncommon	PAI-1 activity and antigen levels Clot lysis time	Antifibrinolytic agents: EACA Tranexamic acid FFP

F, factor; CNS, central nervous system; T&A, tonsillectomy and adenoidectomy; FFP, fresh frozen plasma; PT, prothrombin time; PTT, partial thromboplastin time; TT, thrombin time; PAI, plasminogen activator inhibitor-1; FEIBA, factor VIII inhibitor bypassing agent; PCC, prothrombin complex concentrates; EACA, ε-aminocaproic acid; ICH, intracranial hemorrhage.

females are carriers of the disease. The genes for both hemophilia A and B are located near the terminus of the long arm of X-chromosome, at *Xq28* (OMIM#306700) and *Xq27.1-q27.2* (OMIM#300746) locus, respectively. Although the majority of cases of hemophilia are inherited, approximately 30% of cases arise from a spontaneous mutation with no family history of hemophilia (Goodeve and Peake, 2003; Oldenburg et al., 2004). The type of mutation within the FVIII or FIX gene predicts the disease severity. Mutations that result in significant disruption of the FVIII or FIX protein or alter the important functional site within FVIII or FIX protein will result in severe disease, while mutations that alter the minor regions of the protein result in mild to moderate disease. The majority of patients with hemophilia A have severe disease and 40% of patients with severe hemophilia A carry an intron 22 mutation. An additional inversion of intron 1 of the FVIII gene is found in 5% of patients with severe hemophilia A. Unlike hemophilia A, the majority of patients with hemophilia B have mild disease and up to 25% of Caucasian patients have one of three founder mutations (Gly60Ser, Ile397Thr, and Thr296Met) (Ketterling et al., 1991). Besides these common mutations, the list of numerous mutations causing hemophilia A is available from the UK mutation database (Kemball-Cook and Tuddenham, 1997).

Although hemophilia primarily affects males, some female carriers of hemophilia A and B have sufficient reduction of their FVIII and FIX through skewed lyonization of the normal X chromosome to produce mild bleeding disorders. These females are known as "symptomatic carriers." Rarely hemophilia has been described in women with Turner's syndrome and after a mating between a carrier female and hemophilia male patient.

Clinical classification of hemophilia

Hemophilia is classified on the basis of the patient's baseline FVIII or FIX level and factor levels usually correlate with the severity of bleeding symptoms. By convention, 1 unit of factor is defined as the amount of that factor present in 1 mL of normal plasma. Thus 100 mL of normal plasma contains 100 U/dL of each coagulation factor (100% activity). The hemostatic level, the minimal amount required for cessation of bleeding, for factor VIII is greater than or equal to 30–40 U/dL, and for FIX is greater than or equal to 25–30 U/dL. Hemophilia is classified as mild, moderate, or severe (corresponding to plasma coagulation factor levels of > 5% to 50%, ≥ 1% to 5%, and < 1% of normal, respectively) (White et al., 2001).

Clinical manifestations of hemophilia

Bleeding in patients with hemophilia depends upon the severity of hemophilia and the type of hemophilia.

In general, patients with severe disease bleed more often than the patients with mild and moderate disease. For every level of severity, patients with hemophilia A bleed more often than patients with hemophilia B, despite carrying the same factor level.

FREQUENCY OF BLEEDING

Patients with severe hemophilia (factor levels < 1%) experience an annual average of 20–30 episodes of spontaneous or excessive bleeding after incidental injury, particularly into joints and muscles. In some patients the episodes are more frequent, occurring approximately once weekly. Patients with mild hemophilia do not experience spontaneous bleeding. They can experience excessive bleeding only after trauma or surgery. Patients with moderate hemophilia exhibit an intermediate pattern. They may experience 4–6 bleeding events in a year. Although the majority of bleeding events occur after trivial trauma, spontaneous bleeding events are also reported in these patients.

BLEEDING SYMPTOMS

Depending on the severity of the factor deficiency, the clinical spectrum of bleeding varies from easy bruising, subcutaneous hematomas, hemarthoses, and soft tissue hemorrhage to bleeding within an internal organ. Although bleeding may occur in any area of the body, the hallmark of hemophilia is hemarthrosis. Bleeding within the joint space causes joint damage leading to debilitating hemophilic arthropathy. Life-threatening bleeding in the hemophilic patients is caused by bleeding into vital structures (central nervous system, upper airway) or by exsanguination (external, gastrointestinal, or iliopsoas hemorrhage). Due to the fact that the primary hemostasis is intact in patients with hemophilia, bleeding may not occur immediately after tissue injury, but after some time interval. Since clot formation is delayed and the clot is friable, these patients have a tendency to rebleed during physiologic clot lysis or with minimal new trauma.

Patients with mild hemophilia who have FVIII or FIX levels greater than or equal to 5 U/dL are usually asymptomatic. These individuals may experience excessive bruising, prolonged bleeding after exposure to hemostatic stress such as dental extractions, surgery, or traumatic injuries. The clinical spectrum of patients with moderate hemophilia ranges from being asymptomatic to occurrence of spontaneous joint bleeding. Similar to mild hemophilia, these patients usually bruise easily and tend to experience bleeding episodes after trivial injuries or surgical procedures.

Neither factor VIII nor factor IX crosses the placenta; thus, bleeding symptoms may be present from birth. The majority of bleeding symptoms in the newborn period are related either to trauma during labor and delivery, or interventions and procedures, such as injections, heel sticks, and/or circumcision. Neonates with hemophilia may develop intracranial hemorrhage (ICH) (Ljung et al., 1994; Kulkarni and Lusher, 1999). Nearly 18% of newborns with hemophilia who are born to those women not known to be carriers of hemophilia develop ICH. Surprisingly, only 30% of affected male infants with hemophilia bleed with circumcision. Thus, if the family history does not alert the physician to be suspicious for these disorders, hemophilia may go undiagnosed in the newborn period and the diagnosis is often delayed until the infant is more mobile when bruising and hemarthrosis develops. Quite often these infants are diagnosed after minor traumatic lacerations of the mouth as this bleeding may persist for hours or days.

Diagnosis of hemophilia

COAGULATION TESTS

The laboratory screening test that is affected by a reduced level of FVIII or FIX is the activated partial thromboplastin time (aPTT). In severe hemophilia, this aPTT is usually two to three times the upper limits of normal. Prolongation of the aPTT is usually investigated by performing mixing studies. The mixing studies try to evaluate if the aPTT is corrected in 1:1 concentration of a patient's plasma and pooled plasma from healthy donors. Correction of the aPTT with mixing studies implies a factor deficiency while failure to correct the aPTT with mixing studies indicates the presence of an inhibitor, acquired antibodies against a coagulation protein. Specific assays for factor VIII or factor IX are required to confirm the diagnosis and severity of hemophilia. The other screening tests of hemostasis (platelet count, bleeding time, prothrombin time, and thrombin time) are normal in patients with hemophilia.

GENETIC TESTING FOR HEMOPHILIA

Direct DNA-based analysis of FVIII (Xq28) and FIX (Xq27.3) gene to identify the mutations within these genes is available for clinical use. Therefore, genetic testing for families with hemophilia is rapidly becoming part of routine care (Pruthi, 2005). Identification of a mutation in a proband is particularly useful in carrier detection and prenatal diagnosis of hemophilia. Because of the substantial costs of these tests, the utilization of these tests should be performed in conjunction with healthcare practitioners who are experts in hemophilia care.

Management of hemophilia

Currently there is no cure for hemophilia. The principles of management of patients with hemophilia include two simple main principles: prevention of bleeding events and treatment of acute bleeding events.

Although prevention of trauma is important to the care of the patients with hemophilia, hemorrhages often occur in the absence of trauma, especially in patients with severe disease. These bleeding episodes can be controlled with regular infusions of the deficient clotting factor, i.e., FVIII in hemophilia A or FIX in hemophilia B. These clotting factors are derived from either plasma or recombinant technology, the latter being the most widely used in the US. In Western countries, common standards of care fall into one of two infusion regimens, an on-demand or a prophylaxis regimen:

- On-demand treatment regimen: on-demand treatment involves treating bleeding episodes once they arise.
- Prophylaxis treatment regimen: prophylaxis involves the infusion of clotting factor on a regular schedule in order to keep clotting factor levels sufficiently high (>1%) to convert a severely deficient patient into a moderately deficient state and hence prevent spontaneous bleeding episodes.

Recent studies have suggested that long-term outcome of joint disease in patients with hemophilia is superior and best prevented with prophylactic regimens rather than with on-demand therapy (Manco-Johnson et al., 2007). In North America, children with severe hemophilia are treated with "prophylaxis" treatment regimens.

In the event of an acute bleeding episode, it is critical to raise the levels of FVIII or FIX to hemostatic levels. The following criteria determine the dose of exogenously administered factor concentrates: (1) severity of hemophilia, and (2) severity of bleeding . In general, for minor bleeding episodes, it is recommended to raise the factor level up to 30–50 U/dL (~30% to 50%). Usually one or two doses are enough to control minor bleeding events. For life-threatening or major hemorrhages the factor levels should be raised up to 80–100 U/dL (~80% to 100%) until the bleeding is arrested. Subsequent maintenance of hemostatic levels will depend upon the severity of bleeding episode and its response to treatment. In patients with suspected CNS bleeding it is recommended to maintain the factor levels above 100% until the bleeding is completely arrested and to maintain factor levels above 50% for at least 2–3 weeks. In order to maintain a constant hemostatic level, factor concentrate should be administered as a continuous infusion rather than giving it as a bolus infusion.

Table 70.2

Treatment of hemophilia and factor replacement dosing for the treatment and prevention of CNS bleeding

	Hemophilia A	Hemophilia B
Underlying deficiency	Factor VIII deficiency	Factor IX deficiency
Subtypes according to severity	Severe : <1%; Moderate: 1–5%; Mild: >5–40%	Severe : <1%; Moderate: 1–5% Mild: >5–40%
Recombinant products	Recombinant FVIII (Advate, Kogenate FS, Xyntha, Recombinate, Helixate FS)	Recombinant FIX (BeneFIX), RIXUBIS
Plasma derived products	Fresh frozen plasma (FFP), cryoprecipitate, Humate-P, Hemofil-M, Monoclate-P	FFP, Mononine, Profilnine, Konyne-HT
Dose increment	1 Unit of exogenous F VIII will increase in vivo plasma FVIII levels by 2 %	1 Unit of exogenous FIX will increase in vivo plasma FVIII levels by 0.8 %
Dose calculation	Units required to raise blood levels (%) =0.5 Units/kg × body weight (Kg) × desired increase (%)	Units required to raise blood levels (%) =1.2 Units/kg × body weight (Kg) × desired increase (%)
Half-life of exogenously infused product	8–12 hours	~24 hours
Frequency of administration	8–12 hours	24 hours
Mode of administration	Intravenous bolus or continuous infusion	Intravenous bolus or continuous infusion
Recommended factor infusion for treatment & prevention of CNS bleeding		
Major CNS bleeding* **(ICH*, compartment syndrome, surgical procedure around head and neck area, subarachnoid/ subdural bleeding)**	100% correction until bleeding is controlled & patient is stable; 50–100% correction × 2–3 weeks Continuous infusion preferred over bolus	100% correction until bleeding is controlled & patient is stable; 50–100% correction × 2-3 weeks Continuous infusion preferred over bolus
Minor CNS bleeding (minor surgery, extracranial trauma)	30–50% correction × 1–7 days	30–50% correction × 1–7 days
Lumbar puncture (LP)	100% correction × 1 dose within an hour prior to LP. Repeat dose after 12 hours if traumatic LP or patient continues to have headache	100% correction × 1 dose within an hour prior to LP. Repeat dose after 24 hours if traumatic LP or patient continues to have headache
Special consideration: Hemophilia with inhibitor*	NovoSeven (90–270 g/kg/dose, q2–4 hourly) FEIBA: 100 IU/kg every 12 hours PCC: 50–100 IU/kg, q12 hourly Porcine FVIII:50–100 IU/kg,q12 hourly Humate-P: 100 IU/kg q daily	Novoseven (90–270 g/kg/dose, q2–4 hourly) FEIBA: 90 IU/kg, q 12 hourly PCC: 50–100 IU/kg, q12 hourly

*Indicates consider hematology consultation for the management of these bleeding episodes.
CNS, central nervous system; FEIBA, factor eight inhibitor bypassing agent; PCC, prothrombin complex concentrates; LP, lumbar puncture.

Table 70.2 provides the brief overview of clinical classification and management of CNS bleeding in patients with hemophilia.

In mild hemophilia A, an important alternative to factor concentrates is desmopressin acetate (1-desamino-8-D-arginine vasopressin, DDAVP), a vasopressin analog (Mannucci et al., 1977; Mannucci, 1997). DDAVP raises the FVIII levels through the endogenous release of FVIII and VWF. DDAVP can be administered via intranasal route and intravenous/subcutaneous route, Stimate 1.5 mg/mL. The dose of Stimate is based on the weight of the patient; 150 µg or one nasal spray for patients weighing 20–50 kg and 300 µg or two nasal sprays for ≥ 50 kg. The dose of intravenous/subcutaneous

DDAVP (4 µg/mL) is 0.3 µg/kg/dose. Since the rise in FVIII is quite variable between patients (but reproducible from time to time), a "DDAVP challenge test" should be done in each patient to evaluate the response. Generally older patients with a higher baseline factor level tend to respond better (Revel-Vilk et al., 2002). Therefore depending on the baseline factor VIII levels and a DDAVP response, DDAVP can be used to prevent and to treat bleeding in patients with mild hemophilia A. The common side-effects of DDAVP include tachycardia, flushing, fluid retention, and hyponatremia. Due to the concerns about hyponatremia, the intravenous or subcutaneous route is preferred in young children (age < 3 years) who weigh less than 20 kg. The dose of DDAVP is preferably given 1 hour before the procedure and may have to be repeated every 24 hours (maximum three doses), depending on the bleeding risk. However, repeated doses may cause fluid retention with severe hyponatremia, and in sensitive subjects (children and women at the time of delivery) seizures. *It is important to underscore that in a patient with suspected ICH, treatment with DDAVP is not an option, irrespective of the severity of the disease.* These patients should be treated with factor concentrate therapy.

Other nontransfusional adjuvant therapy includes use of antifibrinolytic agents such as tranexamic acid (20 mg/kg/dose every 6 hours) and ε-aminocaproic acid (EACA; dose: 50–100 mg/kg/dose every 6 hours) (Mannucci, 1998). Both drugs bind reversibly to plasminogen and thereby block the binding of plasminogen to fibrin and its transformation to plasmin. Decreased production of plasmin prevents fibrinolysis and clot survival is enhanced. Additionally, use of topical hemostatic agents such as bovine thrombin (Thrombin-JMI) and fibrin sealant (Tisseel VH®, consisting of human thrombin, fibrinogen concentrate, and bovine aprotinin), is helpful to control local bleeding such as epistaxis or bleeding after dental extractions.

Inhibitors of coagulation factor VIII and factor IX

Development of allo-antibodies, conventionally known as "inhibitors," against exogenously administered factor (FVIII or FIX) is one of the most serious complications in hemophilia. About 30% of patients with severe hemophilia A develop inhibitors to exogenously administered FVIII while 3–5% of patients with severe hemophilia B develop inhibitors against exogenously administered FIX. These antibodies are directed against the active clotting site; hence they neutralize the functional activity of exogenously administered clotting factor making the treatment ineffective. The quantitative Bethesda assay is performed to assess the level of inhibitor titer. One

Bethesda unit (BU) is the amount of antibody that will neutralize 50% of FVIII or FIX in a 1:1 mixture of the patient's plasma and normal plasma (after 2 hour incubation at 37°C). Any patient who does not show an appropriate response to the treatment regimen should be screened for the presence of an inhibitor. Management of inhibitors depends upon the inhibitor titer and bleeding episode.

The principles of management of an inhibitor are twofold: treatment of an acute bleeding episode and eradication of the inhibitor. Treatment of acute bleeding episodes includes use of bypassing agents such as activated prothrombin complex concentrates (APCC), factor eight inhibitor bypassing activity (FEIBA), recombinant factor VIIa (rFVIIa) or NovoSeven (Dimichele, 2007). For eradication of the inhibitor, immune tolerance induction regimens are used (Mariani et al., 1994). These regimens include daily infusions of high doses of factor concentrates (100–200 IU/kg) with or without immunosuppressive drugs including steroids or cyclophosphamide, immunoglobulins, and rituximab. Patients with inhibitors should be treated at a specialized center.

ACQUIRED HEMOPHILIA

Acquired deficiency of FVIII due to development of autoantibodies or inhibitors to FVIII in normal individuals is known as "acquired hemophilia." This should be considered in the differential diagnosis of patients presenting with intracerebral hemorrhage, especially the elderly and postpartum women. The median age at presentation is somewhere between 60 and 67 years, but a wide range of 2 through 89 years has been reported, including a small series of six children (Ma and Carrizosa, 2006). The age of presentation has two peaks, one occurring between 20 and 30 years of age that represents postpartum inhibitors, and one greater than 60–70 years of age representing the elderly population. Acquired hemophilia classically presents with purpura or soft tissue bleeding. Severe muscle bleeding, hematuria, epistaxis, gastrointestinal bleeding, and even intracranial hemorrhage are seen more frequently than are hemarthroses. The diagnosis of acquired hemophilia requires both clinical acumen and sophisticated laboratory evaluation including PT/aPTT assay, mixing studies, measurement of residual activity of clotting proteins, and measurement of an inhibitor titer or Bethesda assay. Patients with acquired hemophilia typically have residual factor activity despite the presence of the inhibitor and exhibit type 2 pharmacokinetics (Jacquemin and Saint-Remy, 1998). Therapies such as DDAVP, high doses of rFVIII are effective if the inhibitor titer is low (<5 BU), but in patients with severe bleeding and or an inhibitor titer greater than 5 BU, it is prudent to use rFVIIa and or FEIBA, as factor VIII products, even in very high doses, may not achieve adequate hemostasis. Recently rituximab (monoclonal chimeric antibody to the CD20 antigen) has shown success in eradicating inhibitors in patients with acquired hemophilia (Franchini, 2007). Hematologic management of patients with inhibitors to FVIII or FIX should not be done without the involvement of a hematologist with specific expertise in this area.

The subsequent sections briefly describe the remaining bleeding disorders such as rare deficiencies of coagulation factors, the deficiencies of fibrinolytic proteins, Von Willebrand disease(VWD), and platelet function disorders.

NEUROLOGIC MANIFESTATIONS IN PATIENTS WITH HEMOPHILIA

Hemophilia in and of itself is not a condition that is associated with neurologic symptoms but it may lead to neurologic sequelae due to bleeding events within the central nervous system or entrapment/compression of peripheral nerves from a regional hemorrhage.

Neurologic complications in patients with hemophilia can be classified as:

1. central nervous system manifestations: these patients present due to intracranial or intraspinal hemorrhage
2. peripheral nervous system manifestations: these patients present with compression or entrapment of peripheral nerves due to compartment syndrome and pseudotumor, respectively
3. neurologic comorbidities due to aging: these patients present with ischemic stroke or transient ischemic attacks due to cerebrovascular disease.

Central nervous system manifestations

Neurologic symptoms due to intracranial or intraspinal bleeding may be the first clinical presentation in neonates and older children with hemophilia (Klinge et al., 1999; Kulkarni and Lusher, 1999). Identified risk factors associated with intracranial hemorrhage that require a high index of suspicion include: (1) severe disease; (2) presence of inhibitors; (3) history of injury; (4) patients not treated on prophylactic regimens; (5) young age (Traivaree et al., 2007). With the exception of subdural hematoma, the majority of patients with CNS bleeding present within first 24 hours after the injury and the mean symptom-free interval following head trauma is 4 ± 2.2 days (Eyster et al., 1978). Depending on the age of the patient, location, and amount of bleeding, the neurologic manifestations vary from signs of irritability, headache, or vomiting to those associated with elevated intracranial pressure, including seizures and coma. Spinal cord hemorrhage can result in significant impairment of motor, sensory, or autonomic function including sudden onset of quadriparesis with or without respiratory distress, paraparesis, loss of bowel and/or bladder control, sexual dysfunction, or symptoms of neurogenic shock such as lightheadedness, diaphoresis, and bradycardia. Imaging studies such as cranial ultrasound, CT scan and/or MRI studies are required to define the location and the extent of bleeding prior to appropriate surgical intervention. *It is important to underscore that, if clinical suspicion for CNS bleeding is sufficient to require radiologic evaluation, factor replacement must precede the radiographic studies.* Treatment of these events is focused on aggressive replacement with factor concentrates with or without surgical decompression.

Peripheral nervous system manifestations

COMPARTMENT SYNDROME

Since muscle bleeding is the second most common type of bleeding in patients with hemophilia, quite often these patients present with symptoms of compartment syndrome. Compartment syndrome is caused by regional hemorrhage within a confined fascial compartment. This leads to pressure on the neurovascular bundle leading to impairment of its function. The most commonly affected muscle compartments include the flexor groups of the arms and gastrocnemius of the legs. Intramuscular hemorrhages within the closed compartments, such as volar aspect of the wrist, deep palmar compartments of the hand, anterior or posterior tibial compartments, can cause significant morbidity due to compression of neurovascular bundle. Iliopsoas hemorrhage can be life-threatening as large volumes of blood can be lost within a retroperitoneal space prior to its diagnosis. These patients present with symptoms of severe pain and paresthesias and signs of pallor and absence of pulses in the extremities. Untreated compartment syndrome leads to permanent neurologic deficit due to peripheral nerve damage. CT and MRI evaluation and direct measurement of intracompartmental pressure is required to evaluate the extent of bleeding. The treatment of compartment syndrome involves aggressive replacement with coagulation factor concentrates, decompression of intracompartmental pressure and pain control. In hemophilia patients with inhibitors, surgical decompression should be deferred due to the risk of excessive bleeding after the surgery.

PSEUDOTUMORS

Rarely, patients with hemophilia may present with neuropathic pain or neurologic deficit due to compression caused by a pseudotumor. A hemophilic pseudotumor is an encapsulated, chronic, slowly expanding hematoma seen most often in patients with a severe coagulation disorder. Pseudotumors are an uncommon complication of hemophilia in developed countries, occurring in 1–2% of patients with severe disease (Jaovisidha et al., 1997). The diagnosis and extent of a pseudotumor can be visualized by ultrasound and CT or MRI. Therapy for a hemophilic pseudotumor is aimed at preserving function of the affected bone and soft tissue. Conservative treatment with immobilization and intensive clotting factor replacement therapy may be efficacious for pseudotumors resulting from more recent hemorrhage, whereas surgical management yields the best results for pseudotumors that have been present for years or for those in which conservative measures have failed. Radiation therapy with doses of 10–20 Gy has been used only in patients who do not respond to conservative treatment and in whom surgery is contraindicated.

Neurologic comorbidites due to aging

Age-related comorbidities such as occurrence of cardiovascular disease, peripheral vascular disease, and cerebrovascular accidents (CVAs) including ischemic and hemorrhagic strokes are increasingly being reported in patients with hemophilia (Konkle et al., 2009). Neurologists will encounter these patients due to CVAs, peripheral neuropathy, issues due to balance and coordination or Alzheimer's disease. These patients pose a therapeutic challenge to a treating physician as conventional therapeutic modalities for the treatment of these diseases such as antiplatelet agents, anticoagulants, and thrombolytic agents are contraindicated in patients. Since age-related comorbidities in patients with hemophilia are an emerging problem, evidence-based guidelines for the acute management and secondary prophylaxis of these diseases are currently lacking. In general, expert recommendations suggest treating patients with hemophilia like their age-group peers without hemophilia, provided their replacement therapy is adapted according to the baseline plasma factor deficiency (Mannucci et al., 2009).

RARE BLEEDING DISORDERS

Besides hemophilia, qualitative and quantitative deficiencies of remaining coagulation factors such as fibrinogen, FII, FV, FV + FVIII, FVII, FX, FXI, FXIII, and multiple deficiencies of vitamin K-dependent factors can present with CNS bleeding and need to be considered in the differential diagnosis of bleeding disorders that present with CNS bleeding (Peyvandi and Spreafico, 2008; Peyvandi and Favaloro, 2009). These disorders are collectively known as rare bleeding disorders

(RBD), as their prevalence in the general population is low. For example, the prevalence of homozygous or double heterozygous deficiencies varies from 1:500 000 for FVII deficiency to 1:2 000 000 for prothrombin and FXIII deficiencies (Mannucci et al., 2004; Peyvandi et al., 2008). These disorders are usually transmitted in an autosomal recessive manner. Therefore they can affect both males and females equally. The prevalence of RBDs is also strongly influenced by the ethnicity and is significantly increased by a high rate of consanguinity in the population, such as Middle Eastern communities (Mannucci et al., 2004). Due to their rarity and a lack of awareness, RBD pose significant difficulties in diagnosis and treatment.

Bleeding symptoms

In general, the bleeding patterns among patients with RBDs are quite variable, and unlike hemophilia the coagulation factor levels do not necessarily correlate with the severity of the bleeding. Patients with severe deficiencies (factor levels < 10%) tend to have relatively severe symptoms. The majority of these patients are diagnosed either due to the positive family history or history of unexpected bleeding when exposed to hemostatic challenge such as menstruation, labor, and delivery and surgical procedures. On the whole, life-threatening bleeding events, such as CNS and musculoskeletal bleeding, appear to be less frequent than in hemophilia, except in patients with FXIII deficiency. Patients with severe FXIII deficiency (FXIII < 1%) present with ICH in the newborn period. Review of the literature suggests that the rate of spontaneous ICH in newborn patients with FXIII deficiency is about 23.9% (95% CI; 16.2–31.7%) (Burrows et al., 2000). Hence, these patients are commenced on lifelong prophylaxis with plasma-derived FXIII concentrates such as Fibrogamin® once every 3–4 weeks.

Diagnosis of rare bleeding disorders

A detailed clinical history and high index of suspicion are the key to the diagnosis of RBDs. Screening coagulation tests such as PT and aPTT are usually sensitive enough to detect FV, FV + FVIII, FVII, FX, or FXI deficiencies. Specific assays are necessary to quantitate the activity of these coagulation proteins and therefore the severity of these deficiencies. Since the PT and aPTT can be normal in fibrinogen, FII, and FXIII deficiencies, specific assays are required to further delineate the deficiencies of these proteins:

- Fibrinogen deficiency: the thrombin time (TT) is required for the diagnosis of fibrinogen deficiency in addition to the PT and aPTT. The diagnosis of dysfibrinogenemia requires an immunoreactive fibrinogen assay to quantify the antigen levels in addition to an activity or functional assay, as the disease is expressed by a discrepancy between activity (clottable fibrinogen) and antigen (immunoreactive fibrinogen).

- Prothrombin deficiency: the prothrombin time is often prolonged in patients with hypoprothrombinemia. The diagnosis of dysprothrombinemia requires an immunologic assay to quantitate the antigen level, and without obtaining prothrombin antigen levels, patients with prothrombin deficiency cannot be properly classified.
- Factor XIII deficiency: screening tests for factor XIII deficiency are based upon the observation that there is an increased solubility of the clot because of the failure to cross-link the fibrin monomers (Fig. 70.1). The normal clot remains insoluble in the presence of 5 M urea, whereas the clot formed from a patient with factor XIII deficiency dissolves rapidly within hours. It is important to underscore that this method detects only very severe FXIII deficiency (with activity below 0.5–3%) and carries a risk of underdiagnosing this deficiency. More specific immunologic assays for factor XIII quantitation are also available in specialized laboratories to further delineate the severity of factor XIII deficiency.

Scope of genetic testing for the diagnosis of rare bleeding disorders

Unlike hemophilia, the molecular pathology of RBDs is not well understood. Therefore genetic testing for the diagnosis of RBDs is not available for clinical use. These tests, however, may be obtained by enrolling patients in specific research studies for RBDs.

Management of rare bleeding disorders

Similar to hemophilia, the treatment of RBDs focuses on prevention of bleeding, and treatment of acute bleeding using replacement therapy and or nontransfusional adjuvant therapies (Bolton-Maggs et al., 2004; Mannucci et al., 2004). Due to the unavailability of specific factor concentrates for the majority of these disorders, the use of non-transfusional adjuvant therapies is the primary therapeutic option such as antifibrinolytics (tranexamic acid, etc), estrogens, and topical hemostatic agents.

As for hemophilia, replacement of the deficient coagulation factor is the mainstay of treatment for RBDs. Unfortunately, a recombinant factor concentrate is available only for FVII deficiency. Plasma-derived concentrates of fibrinogen, FVII, FXI, and FXIII are currently available, but they are licensed only in some European countries. Unlike hemophilia, information on the safety and efficacy of the few available products for RBDs is scarce, and experience with their optimal use is much more limited. Table 70.3 provides the list of available blood products for the treatment of RBDs.

Table 70.3

Available factor concentrates and pharmacological agents used for the treatment of congenital bleeding disorders

Hemophilia A
- Recombinate® [r]
- Advate® [r]
- Xyntha® [r]
- Kogenate FS® [r]
- Helixate FS® [r]
- Hemofil-M® [pd]
- Monoclate-P® [pd]
- Desmopressin or Stimate® [drug]: Used only in mild hemophilia

Hemophilia B (Factor IX products)
- BeneFIX® [r]
- Mononine® [pd]
- Profilnine® [pd]
- Konyne-HT® [pd]
- RIXUBIS®[r]

Congenital hemophilia with inhibitors, acquired factor inhibitors against coagulation factors, and other rare bleeding disorders
- Recombinant Factor VIIa (Novo Seven®)
- Porcine factor VIII (pd)
- Factor VIII inhibitor Bypassing activity or FEIBA® [pd]
- Prothrombin complex concentrates or PCC [pd]

Von Willebrand's Disease
- Desmopressin or Stimate® [drug]
- Humate-P® [pd]
- Alphanate® [pd]

Platelet function disorders
- Desmopressin or Stimate® [drug]
- ε-Aminocaproic Acid (Amicar®)
- Tranexamic Acid (Cyklokapron®)
- Platelet transfusions
- Recombinant Factor VIIa (Novo Seven®)

Other rare bleeding disorders
- Factor VII deficiency: Recombinant Factor VIIa (Novo Seven®), FFP
- Afibrinogenemia/Dysfibrinogenemia: Cryoprecipitate [pd]
- FXI deficiency: FFP [pd]
- FV deficiency: FFP and platelets [pd]
- FXIII: Fibrogamin® [pd]

Other supportive therapies:
Antifibrinolytics (used for the treatment of multiple bleeding disorders, including hemophilia A and B, von Willebrand's disease, and dysfibrinogenemias)
- ε-Aminocaproic Acid (Amicar®)
- Tranexamic Acid (Lysteda®, Cyklokapron®)

r, recombinant product; pd, plasma-derived product.

The commonly used products include fresh frozen plasma, prothrombin complex concentrates (PCC), cryoprecipitate, and recombinant factor VIIa (rFVIIa).

Although replacement therapy is an effective treatment of the bleeding episodes, due to the lack of accurate pharmacokinetics studies, the effectiveness of treatment could be highly variable among patients, and it is important to individually adjust treatment, particularly in children.

Role of prophylaxis therapy in patients rare bleeding disorders

Currently primary prophylaxis is recommended for FXIII deficiency. Patients with severe FXIII deficiency are maintained on primary or secondary prophylaxis with FXIII concentrates given every 3-4 weeks (Todd T, J Perry D. Haemophilia. 2009 Nov). Secondary prophylaxis might be appropriate in cases with potential life-threatening hemorrhages such as CNS bleeding because of the risk of recurrences, particularly in FXIII, FX, FVIII, FV and fibrinogen deficiencies.

DEFICIENCIES OF FIBRINOLYTIC PATHWAY: α_2-ANTIPLASMIN AND PLASMINOGEN ACTIVATOR INHIBITOR-1 (PAI-1) DEFICIENCY

Deficiency of either of these two fibrinolytic pathway proteins results in increased plasmin generation and premature lysis of fibrin clots. These patients can experience mucocutaneous bleeding but rarely have joint hemorrhages. *Because the usual hemostatic tests are normal*, specific factor analysis is required in a patient with a suspicious bleeding history and should include the euglobulin clot lysis time that measures fibrinolytic activity and is shortened in the presence of these deficiencies. Specific assays for alpha-2-antiplasmin and PAI-1 are available. Antifibrinolytic drugs such as epsilon aminocaproic acid and tranexamic acid are the cornerstones of management of bleeding in these patients. Rarely FFP is used as a source of these proteins to control severe bleeding.

VON WILLEBRAND DISEASE

Von Willebrand Disease (VWD) is the most common bleeding disorder with an autosomal dominant or recessive inheritance and has a prevalence of about 1% in the general population (Rodeghiero et al., 1987). Von Willebrand factor (VWF) is a multimeric glycoprotein that facilitates adhesion between platelets and the vessel wall and acts as a carrier protein for Factor VIII.

Types of Von Willebrand disease

Von Willebrand disease is classified into three subtypes: Type 1, type 2 and type 3. It can be essentially understood as quantitative deficiency of VWF (Type 1 or Type 3) or a qualitative disorder of VWF (Type 2A, 2B, 2 N, 2 M) (Sadler, 1994; Rodeghiero et al., 2009). Most cases appear to have a partial quantitative deficiency of VWF (type 1 VWD) with variable bleeding tendency, whereas qualitative variants (type 2 VWD), due to a dysfunctional VWF, are clinically more homogeneous. Type 3 VWD is rare and the patients have a moderate to severe bleeding diathesis because of the virtual absence of VWF.

Clinical presentation

In general, VWD is a mild bleeding disorder. Since VWF plays an important role in primary hemostasis, the primary clinical presentation in patients with VWD is mucocutaneous bleeding such as bruising, subcutaneous hematoma formation, epistaxis and bleeding after exposure to hemostatic stress such as menstrual cycles, wisdom tooth extraction, tonsillectomy and adenoidectomy and post-partum period (Table 70.1). Spontaneous bleeding symptoms are extremely rare in patients with VWD. Type 3 VWD is the most severe and is associated with absence of VWF. Since VWF is a carrier molecule of FVIII, absence of VWF leads to faster clearance of FVIII from the circulation leading to lower levels of FVIII. Therefore, patients with Type 3 VWD can present like mild to moderate hemophilia. Regardless, the rate of spontaneous or trauma related CNS hemorrhage is considered to be extremely low.

Diagnosis of Von Willebrand disease

Clinical history including personal history of bleeding, family history of bleeding and abnormal laboratory testing for VWD are critical components for the diagnosis of VWD. Prolongation of in vivo bleeding time or PFA-100 closure time is an important screening test for the diagnosis of VWD. Screening coagulation tests, PT and aPTT are usually normal; occasionally the aPTT may be prolonged due to low FVIII levels. Special assays including VWF antigen, VWF coagulant activity (ristocetin cofactor activity), FVIII levels and VWF multimer evaluation are required to confirm the diagnosis of VWD. These tests are available in specialized coagulation laboratories. In patients with Type 1 VWD, the VWF antigen and VWF activity are proportionately decreased with decrease in concentration of VWF multimers while in patients with Type 3 VWD, there is complete absence of VWF. In patients with Type 2 VWD, there is a discrepancy between VWF antigen and activity and the VWF multimer pattern may be abnormal. Specialized assays such as binding assays to evaluate the affinity between VWF with platelets and VWF with FVIII are required to accurately diagnose Type 2B and Type 2 N VWD respectively. Usually patients with Type 2B VWD develop thrombocytopenia and can be suspected based on blood count evaluation.

Treatment of Von Willebrand disease

The principles of treatment of VWD include: 1) treatment of bleeding episodes and 2) prevention of bleeding episodes during a period of hemostatic stress. (Mannucci, 2004) DDAVP and VWF concentrates (Humate-P® or Alphanate SD/HT®) are the specific treatment options to increase VWF levels.

In the majority of instances, use of adjuvant therapies such as antifibrinolytic agents (EACA and tranexamic acid) and topical hemostatic agents - such as topical bovine thrombin (Thrombin-JMI) or fibrin sealant (Tisseel VH®) - is enough to control bleeding episodes such as epistaxis or bleeding after dental extractions. Topical collagen sponges are also approved for the control of bleeding wounds or epistaxis.

DDAVP is used for treating mild to moderate bleeding in patients with Type 1, Type 2A Type 2 N and Type 2 M patients. DDAVP is contraindicated in Type 2B VWD, Type 3 VWD and is often not the choice of treatment for patients with severe Type 1 VWD.

Plasma derived VWF concentrates (Humate-P, Alphanate) are usually recommended for the treatment of bleeding in Type 3 VWD, Type 2B VWD and severe Type 1 VWD. They are also used for any other bleeding episodes which are unresponsive to medical therapy and for the treatment of major bleeding episodes such as CNS bleeding. VWF concentrates contain the large multimers of VWF, which are more hemostatic and the dose of VWF concentrates is calculated based on the ristocetin cofactor units. One unit of ristocetin cofactor activity per kilogram body weight raises the hemostatic activity of VWF by 1%. Similar to hemophilia, for major bleeding episodes the levels of VWF (calculated by ristocetin cofactor units) should be raised up to 80-100% and for minor bleeding events the level should be raised up to 30-50%. The half-life of VWF is ~12-24 hours. Hence, the VWF containing products can be infused as once daily regimen until the bleeding is well controlled.

PLATELET FUNCTION DISORDERS

Overview of anatomy and physiology of platelets

Platelets are produced as the fragments of bone marrow megakaryocytes and circulate in blood as disc-shaped anucleate organelles. Platelets are limited by a trilaminar membrane with an outer glycoprotein (GP) coat that mediates platelet activation; GP Ib/IX mediates adhesion of platelets with VWF while GP IIb/IIIa mediates binding of platelets to fibrinogen. Platelet cytoplasm contains 2 unique types of granules, the alpha granules and the dense granules. The alpha granules contain hemostatic proteins such as fibrinogen, FV, FVIII, VWF, albumin, fibronectin, and growth factors (eg, platelet-derived growth factor). The dense granules contain chemical substances such as ADP, ATP, calcium, and 5-hydroxytryptamine (serotonin). During platelet activation, the granules are centralized and their contents are discharged into the lumen of the open canalicular system, from which they are then released to the exterior (the release reaction). Platelets are metabolically active and platelet activation initiates arachidonic acid pathway to produce thromboxane A2 (TXA2). TXA2 is an important chemical mediator of platelet aggregation (Nurden and Nurden, 2008; Salles et al., 2008).

To form a hemostatic plug, platelets undergo a series of morphologically identifiable events: adhesion, secretion, aggregation, and clot retraction. A defect in any of these steps could lead to platelet function abnormalities. For example, a deficiency of GPIb/IX and GPIIb/IIIa produces Bernard-Soulier syndrome and Glanzmann thrombasthenia respectively. In grey platelet syndrome, there is a deficiency of alpha-granules. Additionally, conditions associated with inherited thrombocytopenia such as *MYH9* (Myosine Heavy Chain-9) disorders are associated with bleeding tendencies. With improvement in our understanding of platelets, the list of these disorders is increasing. Due to the rarity of these disorders, the precise prevalence of platelet function abnormalities is not known. The mode of inheritance is either autosomal recessive or autosomal dominant (Nurden and Nurden, 2008; Salles et al., 2008).

Bleeding symptoms

The clinical spectrum of platelet function disorders overlaps with VWD. It is predominated by mucocutaneous bleeding and bleeding after hemostatic challenges such as menstruation, wisdom tooth extraction and tonsillectomy and adenoidectomy (Table 70.1). Patients with *MYH9* disorders are associated with other systemic manifestations such as cataracts, deafness, and nephritis. *CNS bleeding is extremely rare in patients with platelet function disorder.*

Diagnosis of platelet function disorders

A complete blood count and evaluation of the peripheral blood smear are essential to diagnose platelet function disorders. If the platelet count is low then further evaluation should be focused on conditions associated with thrombocytopenia. In *MYH9* disorders one can see giant platelets on the blood smear. Additionally, neutrophils show inclusion bodies. In grey platelet disorder, platelets look pale colored. Bleeding time or PFA-100 closure time test are helpful screening tests for platelet function disorders. Prolongation of the bleeding time favors the diagnosis of VWD or platelet function disorders. Platelet aggregation studies using platelet agonists such as epinephrine, collagen, thrombin, arachidonic acid and ristocetin are helpful to diagnose the disorders of adhesion and aggregation. Flow cytometry can be performed to diagnose the deficiency of glycoprotein receptors such as GPIb/IX and GPIIb/IIIa expression to diagnose Bernard-Soulier syndrome and Glanzmann thrombasthenia. Electron microscopy of platelets is also often helpful to diagnose granular abnormalities of platelets. Overall, genetic testing is currently not applicable for most platelet disorders but can be used in *MYH9* disorders.

Treatment of platelet function disorders

Although platelet transfusion is the specific therapeutic option for patients with platelet function disorders, in the majority of instances these disorders are primarily managed by non-transfusional adjuvant therapies such as DDAVP, antifibrinolytic medications and topical hemostatic agents. Platelet transfusions are reserved for major bleeding episodes such as CNS bleeding or bleeding within vital organs or for any bleeding episode which is unresponsive to adjuvant therapy. The usual dose of platelets for children is about 10-15 ml/kg, while for adults about 6-12 Units of random donor platelets or 1-2 units of single donor platelet units are used. Similar to FFP, platelet transfusions are associated with concerns about blood borne viral infection. In patients with GP receptor deficiency such as Glanzmann thrombasthenia and Bernard-Soulier syndrome, antibodies against the absent receptor, GPIIb/IIIa and GPIb/IX respectively, have been reported. Therefore, if possible platelet transfusions should be avoided in these patients. Recombinant factor VIIa has been used in patients with Glanzmann thrombasthenia with inhibitors to GPIIb/IIIa (White, 2006).

ROLE OF HEMOPHILIA TREATMENT CENTERS IN THE MANAGEMENT OF BLEEDING DISORDERS

Overall management of patients with bleeding disorders is complex. Therefore these patients should be managed in conjunction with physicians from a nearby hemophilia treatment center who are experts in treating patients with bleeding disorders. Hemophilia treatment centers are federally recognized specialized clinics where a team of doctors, nurses, social workers, and physical therapists work together to deliver comprehensive care to people with bleeding disorders. These centers have been shown to significantly decrease the morbidity and mortality for patients with bleeding disorders, specifically hemophilia (Soucie et al., 2000). The list of these centers is available on the Centers for Disease Control and Prevention website (http://www.cdc.gov/ncbddd/hbd/htc_list.htm).

SUMMARY

Patients with bleeding disorders are at risk for development of CNS hemorrhage and can present with acute or chronic neurologic symptoms. Availability of clotting factor concentrates and adjuvant therapies such as DDAVP, EACA and transexamic acid has revolutionized the management of patients with bleeding disorders. Therefore accurate diagnosis and immediate intervention with administration of specific treatment such as infusion of specific clotting factor concentrate or adjuvant therapy are the key to prevent the morbidity associated with a bleeding diathesis. A multi-disciplinary comprehensive treatment approach with the involvement of hemophilia treatment centers is required to improve the long-term outcome of patients with hemophilia and other bleeding disorders.

REFERENCES

Bolton-Maggs PH, Perry DJ, Chalmers EA et al. (2004). The rare coagulation disorders – review with guidelines for management from the United Kingdom Haemophilia Centre doctors' organisation. Haemophilia 10: 593–628.

Burrows RF, Ray JG, Burrows EA (2000). Bleeding risk and reproductive capacity among patients with factor XIII deficiency: a case presentation and review of the literature. Obstet Gynecol Surv 55: 103–108.

Dimichele D (2007). Immune tolerance therapy for factor VIII inhibitors: moving from empiricism to an evidence-based approach. J Thromb Haemost 5(Suppl 1): 143–150.

Eyster ME, Gill FM, Blatt P et al. (1978). Central nervous system bleeding in hemophiliacs. Blood 51: 1179–1188.

Franchini M (2007). Rituximab in the treatment of adult acquired hemophilia A: a systematic review. Crit Rev Oncol Hematol 63: 47–52.

Goodeve AC, Peake IR (2003). The molecular basis of hemophilia A: genotype-phenotype relationships and inhibitor development. Semin Thromb Hemost 29: 23–30.

Jacquemin MG, Saint-Remy JM (1998). Factor VIII immunogenicity. Haemophilia 4: 552–557.

Jaovisidha S, Ryu KN, Hodler J et al. (1997). Hemophilic pseudotumor: spectrum of MR findings. Skeletal Radiol 26: 468–474.

Kemball-Cook G, Tuddenham EG (1997). The factor VIII mutation database on the world wide web: the haemophilia

A mutation search test and resource site. HAMSTeRS update (version 30). Nucleic Acids Res 25: 128–132.

Ketterling RP, Bottema CD, Phillips JA 3rd et al. (1991). Evidence that descendants of three founders constitute about 25% of hemophilia B in the United States. Genomics 10: 1093–1096.

Klinge J, Auberger K, Auerswald G et al. (1999). Prevalence and outcome of intracranial haemorrhage in haemophiliacs – a survey of the paediatric group of the German Society of Thrombosis and Haemostasis (GTH). Eur J Pediatr 158 (Suppl 3): S162–S165.

Konkle BA, Kessler C, Aledort L et al. (2009). Emerging clinical concerns in the ageing haemophilia patient. Haemophilia 15: 1197–1209.

Kulkarni R, Lusher JM (1999). Intracranial and extracranial hemorrhages in newborns with hemophilia: a review of the literature. J Pediatr Hematol Oncol 21: 289–295.

Ljung R, Lindgren AC, Petrini P et al. (1994). Normal vaginal delivery is to be recommended for haemophilia carrier gravidae. Acta Paediatr 83: 609–611.

Ma AD, Carrizosa D (2006). Acquired factor VIII inhibitors: pathophysiology and treatment. Hematology Am Soc Hematol Educ Program 2006: 432–437.

Manco-Johnson MJ, Abshire TC, Shapiro AD et al. (2007). Prophylaxis versus episodic treatment to prevent joint disease in boys with severe hemophilia. N Engl J Med 357: 535–544.

Mannucci PM (1997). Desmopressin (DDAVP) in the treatment of bleeding disorders: the first 20 years. Blood 90: 2515–2521.

Mannucci PM (1998). Hemostatic drugs. N Engl J Med 339: 245–253.

Mannucci PM (2004). Treatment of Von Willebrand's disease. N Engl J Med 351: 683–694.

Mannucci PM, Ruggeri ZM, Pareti FI et al. (1977). 1-Deamino-8-d-arginine vasopressin: a new pharmacological approach to the management of haemophilia and Von Willebrand's diseases. Lancet 1: 869–872.

Mannucci PM, Duga S, Peyvandi F (2004). Recessively inherited coagulation disorders. Blood 104: 1243–1252.

Mannucci PM, Schutgens RE, Santagostino E et al. (2009). How I treat age-related morbidities in elderly persons with hemophilia. Blood 114: 5256–5263.

Mariani G, Scheibel E, Nogao T et al. (1994). Immunetolerance as treatment of alloantibodies to factor VIII in hemophilia. The international registry of immune-tolerance protocols. Semin Hematol 31: 62–64.

Nurden P, Nurden AT (2008). Congenital disorders associated with platelet dysfunctions. Thromb Haemost 99: 253–263.

Oldenburg J, Ananyeva NM, Saenko EL (2004). Molecular basis of haemophilia A. Haemophilia 10 (Suppl 4): 133–139.

Peyvandi F, Favaloro EJ (2009). Rare bleeding disorders. Semin Thromb Hemost 35: 345–347.

Peyvandi F, Spreafico M (2008). National and international registries of rare bleeding disorders. Blood Transfus 6 (Suppl 2): S45–S48.

Peyvandi F, Cattaneo M, Inbal A et al. (2008). Rare bleeding disorders. Haemophilia 14 (Suppl 3): 202–210.

Pruthi RK (2005). Hemophilia: a practical approach to genetic testing. Mayo Clin Proc 80: 1485–1499.

Revel-Vilk S, Blanchette VS, Sparling C et al. (2002). DDAVP challenge tests in boys with mild/moderate haemophilia A. Br J Haematol 117: 947–951.

Rodeghiero F, Castaman G, Dini E (1987). Epidemiological investigation of the prevalence of Von Willebrand's disease. Blood 69: 454–459.

Rodeghiero F, Castaman G, Tosetto A (2009). How I treat Von Willebrand disease. Blood 114: 1158–1165.

Sadler JE (1994). A revised classification of Von Willebrand disease. For the Subcommittee on Von Willebrand factor of the Scientific and Standardization Committee of the International Society on Thrombosis and Haemostasis. Thromb Haemost 71: 520–525.

Salles II, Feys HB, Iserbyt BF et al. (2008). Inherited traits affecting platelet function. Blood Rev 22: 155–172.

Soucie JM, Nuss R, Evatt B et al. (2000). Mortality among males with hemophilia: relations with source of medical care. The hemophilia surveillance system project investigators. Blood 96: 437–442.

Traivaree C, Blanchette V, Armstrong D et al. (2007). Intracranial bleeding in haemophilia beyond the neonatal period – the role of CT imaging in suspected intracranial bleeding. Haemophilia 13: 552–559.

White GC 2nd (2006). Congenital and acquired platelet disorders: current dilemmas and treatment strategies. Semin Hematol 43: S37–S41.

White GC 2nd, Rosendaal F, Aledort LM et al. (2001). Definitions in hemophilia. Recommendation of the Scientific Subcommittee on Factor VIII and Factor IX of the Scientific and Standardization Committee of the International Society on Thrombosis and Haemostasis. Thromb Haemost 85: 560.

Handbook of Clinical Neurology, Vol. 120 (3rd series)
Neurologic Aspects of Systemic Disease Part II
Jose Biller and Jose M. Ferro, Editors
© 2014 Elsevier B.V. All rights reserved

Chapter 71

Thrombophilic states

IDA MARTINELLI*, SERENA MARIA PASSAMONTI, AND PAOLO BUCCIARELLI
*A. Bianchi Bonomi Hemophilia and Thrombosis Center, Department of Internal Medicine and
Medical Specialties, Fondazione IRCCS Ca' Granda, Ospedale Maggiore Policlinico, University of Milan, Milan, Italy*

THROMBOPHILIC STATES

Definition

Thrombophilia is defined as a hypercoagulable state leading to a thrombotic tendency. Thrombophilic abnormalities can be inherited, acquired, or "mixed" (both congenital and acquired) and the risk of thrombosis is different according to each abnormality (Lane et al., 1996) (Table 71.1).

Inherited thrombophilias include deficiencies of the natural anticoagulant proteins antithrombin (AT), protein C (PC), and protein S (PS), as well as the gain-of-function mutations in the factor V gene (factor V Leiden (FVL)) and prothrombin gene (PT G20210A). The anticoagulant effect of AT, PC, and PS on various procoagulant factors is shown in Figure 71.1. Acquired thrombophilia is mainly represented by the presence of antiphospholipid antibodies; the most frequently investigated mixed abnormality is mild to moderate hyperhomocysteinemia.

Inherited thrombophilia

Deficiencies of the natural anticoagulant proteins AT, PC, and PS are rare but strong risk factors for venous thromboembolism (VTE) and are generally found in young patients with positive family history and frequent recurrences (De Stefano et al., 1994; Martinelli et al., 1998).

AT is a glycoprotein synthesized by the liver and is the major inhibitor of the coagulation serine proteases, in particular thrombin and activated factor X (Xa), other than factors IXa, XIa and XIIa; its inhibition is amplified by the presence of heparin and the endogenous sulphated glycosaminoglycans that lie on the endothelial surface. Two functional domains are recognized: the reactive site domain (which interacts with the serine residue of the protease) and the heparin-binding domain. The antithrombin gene (*SERPIN*1), located at chromosome 1q 23-25, has been cloned and its entire nucleotide sequence determined; currently, more than 80 different mutations have been identified (Lane and Caso, 1989). AT deficiency has a dominant autosomal transmission and was firstly identified in 1964 in a Norwegian family (Egeberg, 1965). Its prevalence is 1:3000 in the general population and 3–5% in nonselected and selected patients with VTE, respectively (Tait et al., 1994; De Stefano et al., 1996). The risk of VTE in carriers of AT deficiency is 50-fold higher than in noncarriers (Rosendaal, 1999). On the basis of functional and immunologic assays, AT deficiency is classified into types I and II. Type I is due to a wide variety of heterogeneous DNA mutations and is a quantitative defect characterized by reduced functional and antigen AT levels; type II is due to missense mutations (leading to single amino acid substitutions) and is a qualitative defect in which antigenic level are normal with an impaired plasma activity due to the production of a variant protein (Lane and Caso, 1989). Clinically, type I is associated with recurrent juvenile VTE, whereas in type II the risk of thrombosis is closely related to the position of the mutation within the protein. Thus, heterozygous mutations within the heparin binding domain of AT have a relatively low risk of thrombosis compared to those with mutations at or close to the reactive site of the molecule.

PC, described for the first time in 1979 (Kisiel, 1979), is a vitamin K-dependent glycoprotein synthesized in the liver in an inactive form. It is activated by thrombin (after its binding to thrombomodulin on endothelial cell surfaces) through the binding with the endothelial cell protein C receptor), a type I transmembrane protein highly expressed on the endothelium of large blood

*Correspondence to: Ida Martinelli, M.D., Ph.D., Hemophilia and Thrombosis Center, Fondazione IRCCS Ca' Granda, Ospedale Maggiore Policlinico, University of Milan, Via Pace, 9, 20122 Milan, Italy. Tel: +39-02-55-03-54-68, Fax: +39-02-55-03-44-39, E-mail: martin@policlinico.mi.it

Table 71.1

Prevalence of thrombophilia abnormalities and relative risk of venous thromboembolism

Thrombophilia abnormality	Prevalence in the general population (%)	Prevalence in patients with VTE (%)	Relative risk of VTE
Antithrombin deficiency	0.02–0.17	1.1	50
Protein C deficiency	0.14–0.5	3.2	15
Protein S deficiency	?	2.2	6–10
Factor V Leiden*	2–10	20–50	7
Prothrombin G20210A*	1–4	6–18	3–4
Antiphospholipid antibodies	1–2	5–15	11
Hyperhomocysteinemia	5	10–15	1.5

VTE, venous thromboembolism.
*Heterozygous.

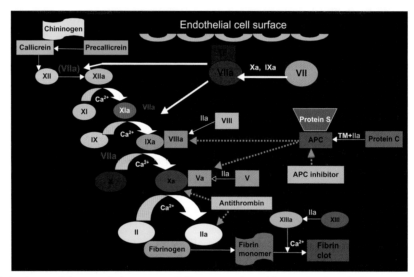

Fig. 71.1. Simplified scheme of the coagulation system. "a" means activated factor. On the left side are the procoagulant factors leading to thrombin activation and fibrin production, essential in venous thrombi. On the right side are the anticoagulant mechanisms of antithrombin, protein C, and its cofactor protein S. Dotted lines indicate inhibition. TF, tissue factor; APC, activated protein C.

vessels that enhances protein C activation more than 10-fold (Fukudome et al., 1996). Upon activation, activated PC has an important natural anticoagulant activity and, together with its cofactor PS, suppresses thrombin generation by inhibition of coagulation factors Va and VIIIa. PC gene (*PROC*) lies on 2q13-q14 chromosome; numerous loss-of-function mutations can cause the deficiency. PC deficiency has a dominant autosomal transmission and is very rare in the general population (around 0.2%), while its frequency in nonselected and selected patients with VTE is 3% and 8%, respectively (Tait et al., 1995; De Stefano et al., 1996). The risk of VTE is approximately 15-fold higher in carriers than in noncarriers (Rosendaal, 1999). PC deficiency is defined on the basis of PC plasma level activity and antigen measurements. As for AT deficiency, there are two types of

PC deficiency: type I is a quantitative defect (plasma reduction of antigen and function) and type II is a qualitative defect (reduction of activity with normal plasma antigen) (Griffin et al., 1981). Type I deficiency is the most common PC defect, and it is due to a reduced synthesis or stability of PC.

PS is the PC cofactor and derives its name from Seattle, the town where it was discovered in 1984 (Comp and Esmon, 1984). Like PC, it is a vitamin K-dependent glycoprotein of liver synthesis that circulates in a free form (~40%) and in a form bound with the acute phase C4b-binding protein (~60%), the latter having no anticoagulant activity. Together with PC cofactor activity, free PS can inhibit the prothrombinase and tenase complex independently (Dahlbäck, 1991). Its gene (*PROS1*) lies on chromosome 3q11.2 and more than 130 loss-of-function genetic mutations have been described. The deficiency has a dominant autosomal transmission and its frequency in the general population is difficult to establish, particularly because of the absence of laboratory standardized criteria. The prevalence in patients with VTE is similar to that of PC deficiency, ranging from 2% to 7% (De Stefano et al., 1996). The risk of VTE is 6–10-fold higher in carriers than in noncarriers (Rosendaal, 1999). Three types of PS defects have been described: type I is a quantitative deficiency with decreased plasma levels of functional and antigenic total and free PS; type II is a qualitative deficiency with decreased cofactor activity but normal total and free PS levels; type III is a quantitative deficiency with reduced functional activity and free PS antigen levels and normal total PS levels.

The two most common genetic risk factors for VTE are FVL (a G to A substitution at position 1691 in exon 10 of the factor V gene) and PT G20210A (a G to A substitution in the 3'-untranslated region of the prothrombin (factor II) gene). In 1993 a poor anticoagulant response to activated PC was associated with an increased risk of VTE (Dahlbäck et al., 1993; Koster et al., 1993). The so-called activated PC resistance is mainly caused by the G1691A mutation (chromosome 1q23) in the Arg506 cleavage site of FVa, described first in Leiden in 1994 (Bertina et al., 1994; Voorberg et al., 1994). FVL is inactivated by activated PC more slowly than wild type factor Va, thus promoting a hypercoagulable state and an increased susceptibility to VTE. The abnormality has a dominant autosomal transmission and, in its heterozygous form, is the most common prothrombotic mutation in the Caucasian population, with a prevalence of about 3%, ranging from 2% to 10% from Southern to Northern Europe (Rees et al., 1995) that rises to 20% and 50% in nonselected and selected patients with VTE, respectively. FVL is very rare in Africans and in Asian populations. The risk of VTE is increased approximately sevenfold in heterozygous and 80-fold in homozygous carriers compared to noncarriers (Rosendaal et al., 1995; Rosendaal, 1999).

PT G20210A was discovered in 1996 by the Leiden group, and is associated with an approximately 20% increase of prothrombin plasma levels (Poort et al., 1996). As for FVL, this mutation has a dominant autosomal transmission and it is the second most common coagulation abnormality, with a prevalence of the heterozygous form in populations of Caucasian descent ranging from 1% to 4% from Northern to Southern Europe. PT G20210A is found in 6% of unselected and 18% of selected patients with VTE (Rosendaal et al., 1998). The risk of VTE is three- to fourfold higher in heterozygous carriers than in noncarriers. Homozygous PT G20210A is extremely rare in the general population and therefore the risk of VTE associated with this abnormality remains unknown.

Acquired thrombophilia

Antiphospholipid antibodies are a strong acquired risk factor for thrombosis (Ginsburg et al., 1992; Runchey et al., 2002; De Groot et al., 2005; Naess et al., 2006). The corresponding syndrome is characterized by the presence of circulating antiphospholipid antibodies in plasma and either arterial and/or venous thrombosis, or pregnancy complications, particularly fetal loss (Wilson et al., 1999; Miyakis et al., 2006). The clinically relevant antiphospolipid antibodies include lupus anticoagulant, anticardiolipin, and anti-β_2-glycoprotein I antibodies. The term "antiphospholipid antibodies" derives from the previous opinion that they acted against negatively charged endothelial and cellular membrane phospholipids. Now we know that these autoantibodies are directed towards a wide variety of protein cofactors that exert their role on phospholipid membrane surfaces (β_2-glycoprotein I, prothrombin, PC, PS, annexin V, coagulation factor XII, and others) (Galli et al., 2003). The resulting complexes interact with several cell types, including endothelial cells, monocytes and platelets, all of which play an important role in hemostasis and thrombogenesis. The indirect activation of these cells results in the release of prothrombotic and proinflammatory mediators (e.g., tissue factor-bearing microparticles, interleukin-6, proteins of the complement system), leading to the activation of platelet and coagulation pathways (Urbanus et al., 2008). Recently, it has been shown that antiphospholipid antibodies interact directly with the vessel wall and cause alterations of plasma lipoprotein (i.e., high-density lipoprotein) function increasing the atherotrombotic risk (Charakida et al., 2009). The antiphospholipid antibodies can be isolated, or drug-related, or associated with autoimmune (e.g., systemic lupus erythematosus or rheumatoid arthritis), lymphoproliferative or inflammatory diseases (Harris et al., 1985). The prevalence of thrombosis in the presence of antiphospholipid antibodies is around 15% in the general population, with an incidence of 7.5 patient-years (Galli and Barbui, 2003). The relative risk of thrombosis varies depending on the type of antibody and is higher in the presence of lupus anticoagulant with or without anticardiolipin antibodies (OR 11.0 (95%CI 3.81–32.3)) and lower if only anticardiolipin antibodies are present at a clinically significant titration (>40 IU) (OR 3.21 (95%CI 1.11–9.28)), or at a titer < 40 IU (OR 1.56 (95%CI 1.10–2.24)) (Wahl et al., 1998).

Mixed thrombophilia

Mild to moderate hyperhomocysteinemia (HHcy) is a weak risk factor for both venous and arterial thrombosis (Falcon et al., 1994; den Heijer et al., 1996; Ortel, 1999). Homocysteine is an intermediate degradation product in the metabolic pathway in which the aminoacid methionine is converted into cysteine. An impairment of this metabolic pathway leads to increased plasma homocysteine levels. The possible mechanisms by which HHcy promotes thrombosis are different and still under investigation; they include a toxic effect on endothelial cells, smooth muscle cell proliferation and intimal thickening, impaired generation of nitric oxide and prostacyclin, increased platelet adhesion, activation of factor V, interference with PC activation and thrombomodulin expression, induction of tissue factor activity and inhibition of tissue-type plasminogen activator (D'Angelo and Selhub, 1997). Both genetic (e.g., mutations in methylenetetrahydrofolate reductase (MTHFR) and cystathionine-β-synthase genes) and acquired factors (e.g., deficiencies of folate, vitamin B_{12} and vitamin B_6, renal impairment, the use of antifolic drugs, and older age) interact to determine plasma homocysteine concentrations. Hence, HHcy is considered a "mixed" risk factor for thrombosis (Cattaneo, 1999).

Lipoprotein(a)

Since the homology between apoliproprotein(a) (apo(a)) and plasminogen was described in 1987, the role of lipoprotein(a) (Lp(a)) as an inhibitor of normal fibrinolytic activity of plasminogen was hypothesized. It has recently been reported that the inhibition of plasminogen activation by apo(a) results from the interaction of apo(a) with the ternary complex that includes tissue-type plasminogen activator, plasminogen and fibrin, rather than competition of apo(a) and plasminogen for binding site of fibrin, and that Lp(a) types containing smaller apo(a) isoforms bind more avidly to fibrin and are better inhibitors of plasminogen activation (Anglés-Cano et al., 2001). Recent clinical studies showed that Lp(a), either alone or in synergy with other thrombophilic risk factors (Nowak-Göttl et al., 2008), significantly increases the risk of arterial (Danesh et al., 2000; Smolders et al., 2007) and venous thrombosis, the latter particularly in childhood (Nowak-Göttl et al., 1999). Individuals with smaller apo(a) isoforms have an approximately twofold higher risk of coronary heart disease or ischemic stroke than those with larger proteins (Erqou et al., 2010). To date, whether or not smaller apo(a) isoforms are independent from Lp(a) concentration and other risk factors is not clarified.

THROMBOPHILIC STATES AND CEREBRAL VENOUS SINUS THROMBOSIS

Epidemiology and clinical symptoms

The incidence of cerebral venous sinus thrombosis (CVST) is uncertain, because of the absence of epidemiologic studies. At variance with arterial stroke, CVST affects mainly young adults and children, with an estimated annual incidence of three to four cases per million adults and seven cases per million neonates and children (deVeber et al., 2001; Stam, 2005). Symptoms are varied and related to the involved venous structure. When thrombosis involves the cortical veins, localized edema and parenchymal infarction generally develop (Stam, 2005). Intracranial hemorrhage complicates 14–39% of CVST (Ferro et al., 2004; Wasay et al., 2008). The most common symptoms and signs are headache and papilledema due to intracranial hypertension, seizures, focal neurologic deficits, and altered consciousness. Headache occurs in 90% or more of patients and papilledema (30% of patients) may cause visual loss and, if the sixth cranial nerve is compressed, diplopia. Seizures (focal or generalized) develop in up to 40% of patients, as well as motor deficits, whereas symptoms such as dysarthria and aphasia are uncommon. The onset of symptoms is subacute, developing from 2 days to 1 month in 50–80% of patients, and can be even longer in the 10–20% of patients with isolated intracranial hypertension.

Prognosis of CVST is favorable in more than 80% of cases (Dentali et al., 2006a) and recurrence occurs in only 2.2% of patients (Ferro et al., 2004). Death is mainly caused by cerebral herniation in the acute phase and to underlying illnesses, e.g., cancer, during follow-up.

Inherited thrombophilia

Inherited thrombophilia is an established risk factor for CVST (Table 71.2). Due to the rarity of the disease, only few studies with a relatively small sample size are

Table 71.2

Prevalence of thrombophilia abnormalities and relative risk of cerebral venous sinus thrombosis*

Thrombophilia abnormality	Prevalence in patients with CVST (%)	Relative risk of CVST
Antithrombin deficiency	1–7	3
Protein C deficiency	3–6	11
Protein S deficiency	3–8	12
Factor V Leiden[†]	3–12	4
Prothrombin G20210A[†]	11–21	9
Antiphospholipid antibodies	4–17	9[‡]
Hyperhomocysteinemia	4–29	4

CVST, cerebral venous sinus thrombosis.
*Percentage ranges derive from single studies (Martinelli et al., 2003; Ferro et al., 2004; deVeber et al., 2001; Stam, 2005) and risks from a revision paper (Dentali et al., 2006a).
[†]Heterozygous.
[‡]From Christopher et al. (1999).

available in the literature. The largest study investigating the risk of a first episode of CVST associated with thrombophilia included 121 patients and 242 controls and showed that by far the most common thrombophilia abnormality was PT G20210A, present in 22% of patients and 2% of controls, for an 11-fold increased risk of the disease (Martinelli et al., 2003). These data have been consistently reported in the literature, as well as the strong association of CVST with the use of oral contraceptives. Indeed, CVST affects predominantly women of childbearing age (Stam, 2005) because of the use of oral contraceptives. A meta-analysis of eight case-control studies showed a sixfold increased risk of CVST in oral contraceptive users and a ninefold increased risk in heterozygous carriers of PT G20210A (Dentali et al., 2006b). Both PT G20210A and oral contraceptive use are independent risk factors for CVST, and their combined presence increases the risk of CVST in multiplicative terms, up to 79-fold (Martinelli et al., 2003; Gadelha et al., 2005). The same is true for heterozygous FVL, which increases the risk of a first CVST fivefold when present alone and up to 30-fold when associated with oral contraceptive use. The relationship between the risk of CVST and the lack-of-function deficiencies of AT, PC, and PS is less established because of the relatively small number of patients investigated so far and the low prevalence of these coagulation abnormalities in patients and controls. Taken together, AT, PC, and PS deficiencies increase sixfold the risk of a first CVST (Martinelli et al., 2003).

When inherited thrombophilia is investigated in relation to the risk of recurrent venous thrombosis after a first CVST, it appears that only "severe" abnormalities (AT, PC, PS deficiencies, antiphopsholipid antibodies, or combined abnormalities) are associated with an increased risk of VTE, mainly deep vein thrombosis of the lower limbs (hazard ratio 4.71 (95%CI 1.34–16.5)), and not of CVST, whereas PT G20210A and FVL are not. Therefore, only patients with severe thrombophilia have an indication for anticoagulant therapy of indefinite duration (Martinelli et al., 2010).

Acquired thrombophilia

Antiphopsholipid antibodies are associated with an increased risk of both arterial and venous thrombosis. Among the latter, the association is demonstrated with the most common manifestation by far, namely, deep vein thrombosis of the lower limbs. The magnitude of the risk of CVST associated with antiphospholipid antibodies is not well established due to both the rarity of the disease (leading to studies of small sample sizes) and the rarity of acquired thrombophilia among controls. A case-control study on 31 patients and the same number

of controls showed an approximately ninefold increased risk of CVST associated with anticardiolipin antibodies, with wide confidence intervals that skimmed statistical significance (Christopher et al., 1999). A larger case-control study showed the presence of antiphospholipid antibodies in 4% of patients but in no controls, thus rendering it unfeasible to estimate the relative risk of the disease (Martinelli et al., 2003). As for the more common thrombotic manifestations, venous or arterial, the presence of antiphospholipid antibodies is an indication for the maintenance of anticoagulant therapy.

Mixed thrombophilia

The first observation of mild to moderate HHcy as a risk factor for deep vein thrombosis of the lower limbs was done in 1994 (Falcon et al., 1994). Some years later, the same group reported a fourfold (OR 4.2 (95%CI 2.3–7.6)) increased risk of CVST associated with fasting or postmethionine load homocysteine plasma levels (Martinelli et al., 2003), which was confirmed by other smaller subsequent studies of fewer than 50 patients (Boncoraglio et al., 2004; Cantu et al., 2004; Ventura et al., 2004). The concomitant use of oral contraceptives, as for FVL and PT G20210A, leads to a synergistic interaction with HHcy relating to the risk of CVST, which rises to almost 20-fold (OR 18.3 (95%CI 4.9–68.1)) (Martinelli et al., 2003).

Cerebral venous sinus thrombosis in children

In children and neonates the main risk factors for CVST are gestational or perinatal complications (24% of cases), dehydration (25%), head infections (18%), and thrombophilia (32%). Concerning the latter, a recent meta-analysis showed a statistically significant association between CVST and AT (OR 18.4 (95%CI 3.3–104.3)), PC (OR 6.3 (95%CI 1.6–25.4)), PS (OR 5.3 (95%CI 1.5–18.3)) deficiency and FVL (OR 2.7 (95%CI 1.7–4.3)), and a trend toward an association with PT G20210A (OR 2.0 (95%CI 0.9–4.1)) and combined inherited thrombophilic abnormalities (OR 6.1 (95%CI 0.9–43.1)) (Kenet et al., 2010). A previous multicenter study by the same authors as the meta-analysis showed a role for thrombophilia in idiopathic CVST and not in CVST associated with comorbid conditions (such as head/neck trauma, systemic illnesses, and infections) (Kenet et al., 2004). It has to be noted that laboratory investigation of inherited thrombophilia based on plasma measurements, such as AT, PC, and PS testing, is difficult to interpret in neonates and children because of the lack of specific normal ranges. Common concomitant liver or kidney diseases or sepsis are often responsible for an acquired deficiency of one or more of these proteins. Whether or not elevated Lp(a), that is associated with an increased risk for VTE in children, is also a risk factor for CVST has not yet been properly investigated (Young et al., 2008).

THROMBOPHILIC STATES AND ISCHEMIC STROKE

Inherited thrombophilia

In the pathogenesis of arterial ischemic stroke (AIS) and of arterial thrombosis in general, a major role is played by such well-established risk factors as diabetes, high blood pressure, dyslipidemia, obesity, smoking, and family history. Inherited thrombophilia has long been recognized as contributing to VTE, but its association with arterial thrombosis is controversial (de Moerloose and Boehlen, 2007). A few cases of arterial thrombosis, including cerebral thromboembolic events, associated with a deficiency of AT (Vomberg et al., 1987; Ueyama et al., 1989; Johnson et al., 1990), PC or PS (Israels and Seshia, 1987; Girolami et al., 1989; Sacco et al., 1989; Camerlingo et al., 1991; Green et al., 1992) have been reported, mainly in children, but the association between these inherited coagulation abnormalities and AIS is very uncommon. Few studies have specifically addressed such a relationship in large populations, and prospective studies have given conflicting results. An early prospective study (Finazzi and Barbui, 1994) with more than 160 patient-years of follow-up found no cases of AIS among nine patients with AT deficiency, 36 patients with PC deficiency, and 36 patients with PS deficiency. Two other prospective studies found that low PC (but not AT) levels had a borderline significant association with the risk of AIS over a 6–9-year follow-up, and were also associated with cerebral infarctions as identified by MRI imaging (Folsom et al., 1999; Knuiman et al., 2001). However, baseline MRI was not performed for comparison, and no distinction was made between inherited and acquired PC and AT deficiencies. A case-control study of 219 patients with a first episode of AIS and 205 healthy controls failed to find an association between AIS (all pathogenic subtypes) and AT, PC, or PS deficiency (Hankey et al., 2001). A retrospective cohort family study of 150 families with inherited thrombophilia found that 0% of AT-, 1.6% of PC-, and 4.8% of PS-deficient relatives experienced an AIS, compared to 0.6% of relatives without deficiencies, but the overall rate of arterial thrombotic events (either AIS or myocardial infarction) was not significantly different between deficient and nondeficient relatives (Martinelli et al., 1998). Finally, Brouwer et al. (2005) investigated the risk of venous and arterial thrombosis in 156 and 268 first-degree relatives from type I- and type III-deficient PS probands, finding no association with arterial thrombosis.

The possible association between AIS and the two gain-of-function mutations FVL and PT G20210A has been addressed by several studies reviewed in meta-analyses. One of these, published as part of the Copenaghen City Heart Study, included eight studies for a total of 1270 adult patients with AIS and 2269 healthy controls, and did not find any significant association between FVL and AIS (OR 1.1 (95%CI 0.7–1.5)) (Juul et al., 2002). A small but not statistically significant association between AIS and FVL was found in a second meta-analysis of 15 case-control studies for a total of 3039 patients and 12 200 controls (OR 1.3 (95%CI 0.9–1.9)) (Kim and Becker, 2003). Ten case-control studies from the same meta-analysis (1625 patients and 5050 controls) also investigated the impact of PT G20210A on AIS, finding a similar weak association (OR 1.3 (95%CI 0.9–1.9)). Combining AIS and myocardial infarction, and considering individuals younger than 55 years, the association was significantly stronger for PT G20210A (OR 1.7 (95%CI 1.1–2.5)) than for FVL (OR 1.4 (95%CI 1.0–2.0)). A third meta-analysis of 26 case-control studies for a total of 4588 patients and 13 798 controls (Casas et al., 2004) found a moderate and statistically significant association between FVL and AIS (OR 1.3 (95%CI 1.1–1.6)) which disappeared when one study (mainly responsible of the high heterogeneity observed) was excluded (OR 1.2 (95%CI 1.0–1.4)). In this meta-analysis, 19 case-control studies (3028 patients and 7131 controls) evaluated the contribution of PT G20201A on the risk of AIS, finding a statistically significant association (OR 1.44 (95%CI 1.11–1.86)) without any significant inter-study heterogeneity. After these three meta-analyses, a few studies have been published focusing on the effect of the two gain-of-function mutations on the risk of AIS. In a study of 49 young patients with cryptogenic stroke, Aznar et al. (2004) found a significant association with PT G20210A (OR 3.8 (95%CI 1.1–13.3)) but not with FVL (OR 2.6 (95%CI 0.5–14.0)), perhaps because the study was underpowered. The same study highlighted the effect of inherited thrombophilia in enhancing the risk of AIS in oral contraceptive users (OR 14.3 (95%CI 0.7–31.0) for carriers of both risk factors). In another case-control study (294 patients and 286 controls) carried out in a population from Sardinia, an Italian island with a well-known elevated genetic homogeneity, no association between AIS and either FVL or PT G20210A was observed (Rubattu et al., 2005).

Other coagulation abnormalities or genetic variants in genes coding for proteins involved in primary hemostasis, coagulation, and fibrinolysis have been recently associated with the risk of AIS, but their role as potential risk factors is still under investigation. These include: high plasma levels of factor VIII and von Willebrand factor, dysfibrinogenemia, β-fibrinogen G/A -455 and 448 gene polymorphisms (Ortel, 1999), platelet glycoprotein Ib-α Thr→Met and plasminogen activator inhibitor 1 (PAI1) 4G/5G polymorphism (Casas et al., 2004), two haplotypes in factor VIII and one haplotype in factor XIIIA1 carrying minor alleles for V35L and P565L variants (Smith et al., 2008), the factor XIIIA1 Tyr204Phe variant (Pruissen et al., 2008).

The presence of inherited thrombophilia does not change the normal attitude towards therapy after an episode of AIS. The standard therapy is represented by antiplatelet agents (either aspirin 100 mg per day or clopidogrel 75 mg per day), unless a cardioembolic origin of the stroke is demonstrated (atrial fibrillation or patent foramen ovale with paradoxical embolism), that requires an anticoagulant therapy with vitamin K antagonists.

Acquired thrombophilia

A number of studies demonstrated that antiphospholipid antibodies are an independent risk factor for first and possibly recurrent AIS in young adults (Brey, 2005). Among these are one cohort and four case-control studies (Brey et al., 1990; Nencini et al., 1992; Toschi et al., 1998; Blohorn et al., 2002; Brey et al., 2002). All but one showed an increased risk of incident AIS in young people. The negative study tested only anticardiolipin antibodies, whereas the others tested both lupus anticoagulant and anticardiolipin antibodies. Lupus anticoagulant is associated with a higher risk of AIS than isolated anticardiolipin antibodies. In the elderly the contribution of antiphospholipid antibodies to the risk of AIS is less evident, likely because other major systemic risk factors (such as diabetes, hypertension, dyslipidemia) play a major role in the pathogenesis of the disease.

The best therapeutic strategy for preventing antiphospholipid antibody-related recurrent stroke in patients with a first episode of AIS is not completely clear. A randomized double-blind controlled trial comparing the risk of recurrent stroke and other thromboembolic diseases over a 2 year period in patients with a first episode of AIS who were randomized to either aspirin therapy (325 mg per day) or warfarin therapy (target INR 2.0) showed that in patients with antiphospholipid antibodies at the time of the first AIS and without atrial fibrillation or high-grade carotid stenosis, aspirin and warfarin therapy (at a mean INR target of 2.0) were equally effective (APASS Investigators, 2004). The WAPS study showed that high-intensity warfarin therapy (INR range 3.0–4.5) was not clearly superior to standard therapy (warfarin with INR range of 2.0–3.0 or aspirin 100 mg per day) in preventing recurrent thrombosis in patients with antiphospholipid antibody syndrome, and was associated with an increased rate of minor hemorrhagic events (Finazzi et al., 2005).

Mixed thrombophilia

HHcy is associated with a mild increased risk of arterial thrombosis (den Heijer et al., 1996; Ortel, 1999). Although the risk factor is represented by HHcy independently of its genetic or acquired origin, the effect of the mutated homozygous MTHFR 677TT polymorphism on AIS was investigated in two meta-analyses (Kim and Becker, 2003; Casas et al., 2004) that showed a mild increased risk (OR 1.2 (95%CI 1.1–1.4)) (Casas et al., 2004). Patients with HHCy can be treated with folic acid, cobalamin, and pyridoxine in order to lower plasma homocysteine levels and thereby potentially decreasing the risk of thrombosis. Previous randomized clinical trials and meta-analyses of these trials on the efficacy of vitamin supplementation either in primary or in secondary prevention of arterial thrombosis gave conflicting results. It is likely that the possible benefit of reducing the smaller effect of HHcy on the risk of arterial thrombosis was masked by the effect of such stronger risk factors as arterial hypertension, diabetes, smoking, and dyslipidemia. A recent meta-analysis showed that folic acid supplementation was not effective in secondary prevention of AIS, but there might be a mild benefit in primary prevention, especially in males and in combination with B vitamins (Lee et al., 2010).

Stroke in children

The meta-analysis by Juul et al. (2002) included seven studies on infants and children with AIS (453 patients and 1180 controls), and the pooled analysis demonstrated a fivefold increased risk of AIS in carriers of FVL (OR 4.8 (95%CI 3.3–7.0)). A systematic review of 18 case-control studies (3235 patients and 9019 controls) assessed the risk of first AIS associated with thrombophilia in children, finding a pooled OR of 1.2 (95%CI 0.8–1.9) for FVL, 1.1 (95%CI 0.5–2.3) for PT G20210A, 1.0 (95%CI 0.3–3.7) for AT, 6.5 (95%CI 3.0–14.3) for PC, and 1.1 (95%CI 0.3–3.8) for PS deficiency (Haywood et al., 2005). A 5 year prospective follow-up study of 301 children with AIS and an objectively demonstrated inherited thrombophilia abnormality confirmed the association between the risk of recurrent AIS and PC deficiency (relative risk 3.5 (95%CI 1.1–10.9)), but not AT or PS deficiency, FVL or PT G20210A, and found that also Lp(a) was an independent risk factor for stroke (relative risk 4.4 (95%CI 1.9–10.5)) (Strater et al., 2002).

A recent meta-analysis of 22 observational studies (1526 patients with AIS and 2799 controls) showed a significant association between a first AIS and PC deficiency (OR 11.0 (95%CI 5.1–23.6)), FVL (OR 3.7 (95%CI 2.8–4.9)), PT G20210A (OR 2.6 (95%CI 1.7–4.1)), combined genetic defects (OR 18.8 (95%CI 6.5–54.1)), antiphospholipid antibodies (OR 7.0 (95%CI 3.7–13.1)), Lp(a) (OR 6.5 (95%CI 4.5–9.6)), and, to a lesser extent, MTHFR 677 TT (OR 1.6 (95%CI 1.2–2.1)), whereas no statistically significant association was found for AT (OR 3.3 (95%CI 0.7–15.5)) and PS deficiencies (OR 1.5 (95%CI 0.3–6.9)) (Kenet et al., 2010).

Concerning neonates, a case-control study of 91 neonates found an association between AIS and FVL (OR 4.0 (95%CI 1.7–9.0)) or Lp(a) (OR 4.8 (95%CI 2.2–10.9)) (Gunther et al., 2000). A high prevalence of FVL (21%) has also been found in a case series of 24 neonates with cerebral infarction (Mercuri et al., 2001). The follow-up of these patients showed that all five patients with FVL had hemiplegia (100%), compared to only 21% of patients without FVL.

Stroke related to paradoxical embolism

Studies investigating the role of thrombophilia in AIS secondary to paradoxical embolism (i.e., in the presence of patent foramen ovale) gave conflicting results. Some of them showed that either FVL or PT G20210A (Karttunen et al., 2003; Pezzini et al., 2003) was significantly and independently associated with the occurrence of AIS in patients with patent foramen ovale. The Young Adult Myocardial Infarction and Ischemic Stroke (YAMIS) study investigated the frequency of venous-to-arterial circulation shunts, usually caused by patent foramen ovale, and thrombophilia (AT, PC, and PS deficiency, FVL, PT G20210A, antiphospholipid antibodies) in young adults with AIS and in matched healthy controls (Sastry et al., 2006), finding a higher prevalence of venous-to-arterial shunts in the former but no association between thrombophilia and AIS. Anticoagulant therapy with vitamin K antagonists is the best choice when the cardioembolic origin of AIS is demonstrated.

CONCLUSIONS

Thrombophilia abnormalities are well recognized risk factors for CVST, especially in those cases not related to such strong risk factors as tumors in the brain or other sites, cerebral infections, or traumas. In most patients, thrombophilia interacts with environmental risk factors, the most frequent being oral contraceptive use and pregnancy/puerperium, leading to CVST. This explains, at least in part, the higher prevalence of women than men with a first CVST. Thrombophilia seems to be also a risk factor for CVST recurrence, but only in its severe form (AT, PC, PS deficiencies, antiphospholipid antibodies, or combined abnormalities). A complete thrombophilia screening (AT, PC, PS, FVL, PT G20210A, antiphospholipid antibodies, FVIII, homocysteine) should be considered for all patients in which CVST is not related to cancer, brain infections, or traumas. Testing for thrombophilia is rarely urgent, so careful consideration is required concerning the timing as well as the need for assessment.

The role of thrombophilia in the pathogenesis of AIS and, in general, of arterial thrombosis, is less important than its role in VTE, and it is still debated. The two thrombophilic defects recognized as risk factors for both VTE and arterial thrombosis are antiphospholipid antibodies and HHcy, while the risk associated with the two common mutations, FVL and PT G20210A, is of little value, and limited to particular subsets of patients (e.g., young patients with AIS in the absence of classic risk factors, such as arterial hypertension, diabetes, smoking, dyslipidemia, or patients with cryptogenic AIS). Deficiencies of naturally occurring inhibitors AT, PC, and PS do not play a significant role in the etiopathogenesis of AIS. Hence, thrombophilia screening should be reserved for patients with AIS at a young age (i.e. <50 years) and with no other risk factors, and it should be limited to antiphospholipid antibodies, HHcy, FVL, and PT G20210A. An exception is AIS during childhood, which seems to also be associated with PC deficiency and high levels of Lp(a), which should be searched for.

REFERENCES

Anglés-Cano E, de La Pena Diaz A, Loyau S (2001). Inhibition of fibrinolysis by lipoprotein(a). Ann N Y Acad Sci 936: 261–275.

APASS Investigators (2004). Antiphospholipid antibodies and subsequent thrombo-occlusive events in patients with ischemic stroke. JAMA 291: 576–584.

Aznar J, Mira Y, Vaya A et al. (2004). Factor V Leiden and prothrombin G20210A mutations in young adults with cryptogenic ischemic stroke. Thromb Haemost 91: 1031–1034.

Bertina RM, Koeleman BPC, Koster T et al. (1994). Mutation in blood coagulation factor V associated with resistance to activated protein C. Nature 369: 64–67.

Blohorn A, Guegan-Massardier E, Triquenot A et al. (2002). Antiphospholipid antibodies in the acute phase of cerebral ischemia in young adults: a descriptive study of 139 patients. Cerebrovasc Dis 13: 156–162.

Boncoraglio G, Carriero MR, Chiapparini L et al. (2004). Hyperhomocysteinemia and other thrombophilic risk factors in 26 patients with cerebral venous thrombosis. Eur J Neurol 11: 405–409.

Brey RL (2005). Antiphospholipid antibodies in young adults with stroke. J Thromb Thrombolysis 20: 105–112.

Brey RL, Hart RG, Sherman DG et al. (1990). Antiphospholipid antibodies and cerebral ischemia in young people. Neurology 40: 1190–1196.

Brey RL, Stallworth CL, McGlasson DL et al. (2002). Antiphospholipid antibodies and stroke in young women. Stroke 33: 2396–2400.

Brouwer JL, Veeger NJ, van der Schaaf W et al. (2005). Difference in absolute risk of venous and arterial thrombosis between familial protein S deficiency type I and type III. Results from a family cohort study to assess the clinical impact of a laboratory test-based classification. Br J Haematol 128: 703–710.

Camerlingo M, Finazzi G, Casto L et al. (1991). Inherited protein C deficiency and nonhemorrhagic arterial stroke in young adults. Neurology 41: 1371–1373.

Cantu C, Alonso E, Jara A et al. (2004). Hyperhomocysteinemia, low folate and vitamin B12 concentrations, and methylene tetrahydrofolate reductase mutation in cerebral venous thrombosis. Stroke 35: 1790–1794.

Casas JP, Hingorani AD, Bautista LE et al. (2004). Meta-analysis of genetic studies in ischemic stroke: thirty-two genes involving approximately 18,000 cases and 58,000 controls. Arch Neurol 61: 1652–1661.

Cattaneo M (1999). Hyperhomocysteinemia, atherosclerosis and thrombosis. Thromb Haemost 81: 165–176.

Charakida M, Besler C, Batuca JR et al. (2009). Vascular abnormalities, paraoxonase activity, and dysfunctional HDL in primary antiphospholipid syndrome. JAMA 302: 1210–1217.

Christopher R, Nagaraja D, Dixit NS et al. (1999). Anticardiolipin antibodies: a study in cerebral venous thrombosis. Acta Neurol Scand 99: 121–124.

Comp PC, Esmon CT (1984). Recurrent venous thromboembolism in patients with partial deficiency of protein S. N Engl J Med 311: 1525–1528.

D'Angelo A, Selhub J (1997). Homocysteine and thrombotic disease. Blood 90: 1–11.

Dahlbäck B (1991). Protein S and the C4b-binding protein: components involved in the regulation of the protein C anticoagulation system. Thromb Haemost 66: 49–61.

Dahlbäck B, Carlsson M, Svesson PJ (1993). Familial thrombophilia due to a previously unrecognized mechanism characterized by poor anticoagulant response to activated protein C. Proc Natl Acad Sci USA 90: 1004–1008.

Danesh J, Collins R, Peto R (2000). Lipoprotein (a) and coronary heart disease: a meta-analysis of prospective studies. Circulation 102: 1082–1085.

De Groot PG, Lutters B, Derksen RH et al. (2005). Lupus anticoagulants and the risk of a first episode deep vein thrombosis. J Thromb Haemost 3: 1993–1997.

de Moerloose P, Boehlen F (2007). Inherited thrombophilia in arterial disease: a selective review. Semin Hematol 44: 106–113.

De Stefano V, Leone G, Mastrangelo S et al. (1994). Clinical manifestation and management of inherited thrombophilia: retrospective analysis and follow-up after diagnosis of 238 patients with congenital deficiency of antithrombin III, protein C, protein S. Thromb Haemost 72: 352–358.

De Stefano V, Finazzi G, Mannucci PM (1996). Inherited thrombophilia: pathogenesis, clinical syndrome and management. Blood 87: 3531–3544.

deVeber G, Andrew M, Adams C for the Canadian Pediatric Ischemic Stroke Study Group (2001). Cerebral sinousvenous thrombosis in children. N Engl J Med 345: 417–423.

den Heijer M, Koster T, Blom HJ et al. (1996). Hyperhomocysteinemia as a risk factor for venous thromboembolism. N Engl J Med 334: 759–762.

Dentali F, Gianni M, Crowther MA et al. (2006a). Natural history of cerebral vein thrombosis: a systematic review. Blood 108: 1129–1134.

Dentali F, Crowther MA, Ageno W (2006b). Thrombophilic abnormalities, oral contraceptives, and risk of cerebral vein thrombosis: a meta-analysis. Blood 107: 2766–2773.

Egeberg O (1965). Inherited antithombin deficiency causing thrombophilia. Thromb Diath Haemorrh 13: 516–530.

Erqou S, Thompson A, Di Angelantonio E et al. (2010). Apolipoprotein(a) isoforms and the risk of vascular disease: systematic review of 40 studies involving 58,000 participants. J Am Coll Cardiol 55: 22160–22167.

Falcon CR, Cattaneo M, Panzeri D et al. (1994). High prevalence of hyperhomocysteinemia in patients with juvenile venous thromboembosis. Arterioscler Thromb 14: 1080–1083.

Ferro J, Canhão P, Stam J et al. for the ISCVT Investigators (2004). Prognosis of cerebral vein and dural sinus thrombosis. Stroke 35: 664–670.

Finazzi G, Barbui T (1994). Different incidence of venous thrombosis in patients with inherited deficiencies of antithrombin III, protein C, and protein S. Thromb Haemost 71: 15–18.

Finazzi G, Marchioli R, Brancaccio V et al. (2005). A randomized clinical trial of high-intensity warfarin vs. conventional antithrombotic therapy for the prevention of recurrent thrombosis in patients with the antiphospholipid syndrome (WAPS). J Thromb Haemost 3: 848–853.

Folsom AR, Rosamond WD, Shahar E et al. (1999). Prospective study of markers of hemostatic function with risk of ischemic stroke. The Atherosclerosis Risk in Communities (ARIC) Study Investigators. Circulation 100: 736–742.

Fukudome K, Kurosawa S, Stearns-Kurosawa DJ et al. (1996). The endothelial cell protein C receptor. Cell surface expression and direct ligand binding by the soluble receptor. Biol Chem 271: 17491–17498.

Gadelha T, André C, Jucá et al. (2005). Prothrombin 20210A and oral contraceptive use as risk factors for cerebral venous thrombosis. Cerebrovasc Dis 19: 49–52.

Galli M, Barbui T (2003). Antiphospholipid antibodies and thrombosis: strength of association. Hematol J 4: 180–186.

Galli M, Luciani D, Bertolini G et al. (2003). Lupus anticoagulants are stronger risk factors for thrombosis than anticardiolipin antibodies in the antiphospholipids syndrome: a systematic review of the literature. Blood 101: 1827–1832.

Ginsburg KS, Liang MH, Newcomer L et al. (1992). Anticardiolipin antibodies and the risk for ischemic stroke and venous thrombosis. Ann Intern Med 117: 997–1002.

Girolami A, Simioni P, Lazzaro AR et al. (1989). Severe arterial cerebral thrombosis in a patient with protein S deficiency (moderately reduced total and markedly reduced free protein S): a family study. Thromb Haemost 61: 144–147.

Green D, Otoya J, Oriba H et al. (1992). Protein S deficiency in middle-aged women with stroke. Neurology 42: 1029–1033.

Griffin JH, Evatt B, Zimmerman T et al. (1981). Deficiency of congenital protein C in congenital thrombotic disease. J Clin Invest 68: 1370–1373.

Gunther G, Junker R, Strater R et al. (2000). Childhood Stroke Study Group. Symptomatic ischemic stroke in full-term neonates: role of acquired and genetic prothrombotic risk factors. Stroke 31: 2437–2441.

Hankey GJ, Eikelboom JW, van Bockxmeer FM et al. (2001). Inherited thrombophilia in ischemic stroke and its pathogenic subtypes. Stroke 32: 1793–1799.

Harris EN, Gharavi AE, Hughes GRV (1985). Antiphospholipid antibodies. Clin Rheum Dis 11: 591–609.

Haywood S, Liesner R, Pindora S et al. (2005). Thrombophilia and first arterial ischaemic stroke: a systematic review. Arch Dis Child 90: 402–405.

Israels SJ, Seshia SS (1987). Childhood stroke associated with protein C or S deficiency. J Pediatr 111: 562–564.

Johnson EJ, Prentice CRM, Parapia LA (1990). Premature arterial disease associated with familial antithrombin III deficiency. Thromb Haemost 63: 13–15.

Juul K, Tybjaerg-Hansen A, Steffensen R et al. (2002). Factor V Leiden: the Copenaghen City Heart Study and 2 meta-analyses. Blood 100: 3–10.

Karttunen V, Hiltunen L, Rasi V et al. (2003). Factor V Leiden and prothrombin gene mutation may predispose to paradoxical embolism in subjects with patent foramen ovale. Blood Coagul Fibrinolysis 14: 261–268.

Kenet G, Waldman D, Lubetsky A et al. (2004). Paediatric cerebral sinus vein thrombosis. A multi-center, case controlled study. Thromb Haemost 92: 713–718.

Kenet G, Lütkhoff LK, Albisetti M et al. (2010). Impact of thrombophilia on risk of arterial ischemic stroke or cerebral sinovenous thrombosis in neonates and children: a systematic review and meta-analysis of observational studies. Circulation 121: 1838–1847.

Kim RJ, Becker RC (2003). Association between factor V Leiden, prothrombin G20210A, and methylenetetrahydrofolate reductase C677T mutations and events of the arterial circulatory system: a meta-analysis of published studies. Am Heart J 146: 948–957.

Kisiel W (1979). Human plasma protein C. Isolation, characterization and mechanism of activation by alpha-thrombin. J Clin Invest 64: 761–769.

Knuiman MW, Folsom AR, Chambless LE et al. (2001). Association of hemostatic variables with MRI-detected cerebral abnormalities: the Atherosclerosis Risk in Communities Study. Neuroepidemiology 20: 96–104.

Koster T, Rosendaal FR, Bertina RM (1993). Venous thrombosis due to poor anticoagulant response to activated protein C: Leiden Thrombophilia Study. Lancet 342: 1503–1506.

Lane DA, Caso R (1989). Antithrombin: structure, genomic organization, function and inherited deficiency. In: EGD Tuddenham (Ed.), The Molecular Biology of Coagulation. Baillière's Clinical Haematology. Baillière Tindall, London p. 961.

Lane DA, Mannucci PM, Bauer KA et al. (1996). Inherited thrombophilia: part 1. Thromb Haemost 76: 651–662.

Lee M, Hong KS, Chang SC et al. (2010). Efficacy of homocysteine-lowering therapy with folic acid in stroke prevention – a meta-analysis. Stroke 41: 1205–1212.

Martinelli I, Mannucci PM, De Stefano V et al. (1998). Different risk of thrombosis in four coagulation defects associated with inheredited thrombophilia. A study of 150 families. Blood 92: 2353–2358.

Martinelli I, Battaglioli T, Pedotti P et al. (2003). Hyperhomocysteinemia in cerebral vein thrombosis. Blood 102: 1363–1366.

Martinelli I, Bucciarelli P, Passamonti SM et al. (2010). Long-term evaluation of the risk of recurrence after cerebral sinus-venous thrombosis. Circulation 121: 2740–2746.

Mercuri E, Cowan F, Gupte G et al. (2001). Prothrombotic disorders and abnormal neurodevelopmental outcome in infants with neonatal cerebral infarction. Pediatrics 107: 1400–1404.

Miyakis S, Lockshin MD, Atsumi T et al. (2006). International consensus statement on an update of the classification criteria for definite antiphospholipide syndrome (APS). J Thromb Haemost 4: 295–306.

Naess IA, Christiansen SC, Cannegieter SC et al. (2006). A prospective study of anticardiolipin antibodies as a risk factor for venous thrombosis in a general population (the HUNT study). J Thromb Haemost 4: 44–49.

Nencini P, Baruffi MC, Abbate R et al. (1992). Lupus anticoagulant and anticardiolipin antibodies in young adults with cerebral ischemia. Stroke 23: 189–193.

Nowak-Göttl U, Junker R, Hartmeier M et al. (1999). Increased lipoprotein (a) is an important risk factor for venous thromboembolism in childhood. Circulation 100: 743–748.

Nowak-Göttl U, Kurnik K, Krumpel A et al. (2008). Thrombophilia in the young. Hamostaseologie 20: 16–20.

Ortel TL (1999). Genetics of coagulation disorders. In: MJ Alberts (Ed.), Genetics of Cerebrovascular Disease. Futura Publishing, Armonk, NY, pp. 129–156.

Pezzini A, Del Zotto E, Magoni M et al. (2003). Inherited thrombophilic disorders in young adults with ischemic stroke and patent forame ovale. Stroke 34: 28–33.

Poort SR, Rosendaal FR, Reitsma PM et al. (1996). A common genetic variation in the 3′-untranslated region of the prothrombin gene is associated with elevated plasma prothrombin levels and an increase in venous thrombosis. Blood 88: 3698–3703.

Pruissen DMO, Slooter AJC, Rosendaal FR et al. (2008). Coagulation factor XIII gene variation, oral contraceptives, and risk of ischemic stroke. Blood 111: 1282–1286.

Rees DC, Cox M, Clegg JB (1995). World distribution of factor V Leiden. Lancet 346: 1133–1134.

Rosendaal FR (1999). Risk factor for venous thromboembolism. Thromb Haemost 82: 610–619.

Rosendaal FR, Koster T, Vandenbroucke JP et al. (1995). High risk of thrombosis in patients homozygous for factor V Leiden (activated protein C resistance). Blood 85: 1504–1508.

Rosendaal FR, Doggen CJM, Zivelin A et al. (1998). Geographic distribution of the 20210G to A prothrombin variant. Thromb Haemost 79: 706–709.

Rubattu S, Di Angelantonio E, Nitsch D et al. (2005). Polymorphisms in prothrombotic genes and their impact on ischemic stroke in a Sardinian population. Thromb Haemost 93: 1095–1100.

Runchey SS, Folsom AR, Tsa MY et al. (2002). Anticardiolipin antibodies as a risk factor for venous thromboembolism in a population-based prospective study. Br J Haematol 119: 1005–1010.

Sacco RL, Owen J, Mohr JP et al. (1989). Free protein S deficiency: a possible association with cerebrovascular occlusion. Stroke 20: 1657–1661.

Sastry S, Riding G, Morris J et al. (2006). Young Adult Myocardial Infarction and Ischemic Stroke: the role of paradoxical embolism and thrombophilia (The YAMIS Study). J Am Coll Cardiol 48: 686–691.

Smith NL, Bis JC, Biagiotti S et al. (2008). Variation in 24 hemostatic genes and associations with non-fatal myocardial infarction and ischemic stroke. J Thromb Haemost 6: 45–53.

Smolders B, Lemmens R, Thijs V (2007). Lipoprotein (a) and stroke: a meta-analysis of observational studies. Stroke 38: 1959–1966.

Stam J (2005). Thrombosis of the cerebral vein and sinuses. N Engl J Med 352: 1791–1798.

Strater R, Becker S, von Eckardstein A et al. (2002). Prospective assessment of risk factors for recurrent stroke during childood – a 5-year follow-up study. Lancet 360: 1540–1545.

Tait RC, Walker ID, Perry DJ et al. (1994). Prevalence of antithrombin deficiency in the healthy population. Br J Haematol 87: 106–111.

Tait RC, Walker ID, Reitsma PH et al. (1995). Prevalence of protein C deficiency in the healthy population. Thromb Haemost 73: 87–93.

Toschi V, Motta A, Castelli C et al. (1998). High prevalence of antiphospholipid antibodies in young patients with cerebral ischemia of undetermined cause. Stroke 29: 1759–1764.

Ueyama H, Hashimoto Y, Uchino M (1989). Progressing ischemic stroke in a homozygote with variant antithrombin III. Stroke 20: 815–818.

Urbanus RT, Derksen RH, de Groot PG (2008). Current insight into diagnostics and pathophysiology of the antiphospholipid syndrome. Blood Rev 22: 93–105.

Ventura P, Cobelli M, Marietta M et al. (2004). Hyperhomocysteinemia and other newly recognized inherited coagulation disorders (factor V Leiden and prothrombin gene mutation) in patients with idiopathic cerebral vein thrombosis. Cerebrovasc Dis 17: 153–159.

Vomberg PP, Breederveld C, Fleury P (1987). Cerebral thromboembolism due to antithrombin III deficiency in two children. Neuropediatrics 18: 42–44.

Voorberg J, Roelse J, Koopman R et al. (1994). Association of idiopathic venous thromboembolism with a single point-mutation at Arg506 of factor V. Lancet 343: 1535–1536.

Wahl DG, Guillemin F, de Maistre E et al. (1998). Meta-analysis of the risk of venous thrombosis in individuals with antiphospholipid antibodies without underlying autoimmune disease or previous thrombosis. Lupus 7: 15–22.

Wasay M, Bakshi R, Bobustuc G et al. (2008). Cerebral venous thrombosis: analysis of a multicentre cohort from the United States. J Stroke Cerebrovascular Dis 17: 49–54.

Wilson WA, Gharavi AE, Koile T et al. (1999). International consensus statement on preliminary classification criteria for definite antiphospholipid syndrome: report of an international workshop. Arthritis Rheum 42: 1309–1311.

Young G, Albisetti M, Boundel M et al. (2008). Impact of inherited thrombophilia on venous thromboembolism in children: a systematic review and meta-analysis of observational studies. Circulation 118: 1373–1382.

Handbook of Clinical Neurology, Vol. 120 (3rd series)
Neurologic Aspects of Systemic Disease Part II
Jose Biller and Jose M. Ferro, Editors

Chapter 72

Chronic myeloproliferative diseases

JOÃO FORJAZ DE LACERDA[1], SOFIA N. OLIVEIRA[2], AND JOSÉ M. FERRO[3]*

[1]*Department of Hematology and Bone Marrow Transplantation, Hospital de Santa Maria, Lisbon, Portugal*

[2]*Department of Neurology, Hospital da Luz, Lisbon, Portugal*

[3]*Neurology Service, Department of Neurosciences, Hospital de Santa Maria, University of Lisbon, Lisbon, Portugal*

INTRODUCTION AND DEFINITIONS

The chronic myeloproliferative disorders, also referred to as myeloproliferative neoplasms, are a group of diseases in which there is an increased proliferation of one or more subtypes of myeloid cells. The myeloid compartment comprises myeloid leukocytes, red blood cells, and platelets. In 1951, William Dameshek grouped together chronic myeloid leukemia, where there is an increased proliferation of myeloid leukocytes, essential thrombocythemia (ET), which has significant thrombocytosis, polycythemia vera (PV), characterized by considerable erythrocytosis, and primary myelofibrosis (PMF), where bone marrow reticulin and collagen deposition is dominant (Dameshek, 1951). Later, the discovery of the Philadelphia chromosome in chronic myeloid leukemia, which is the result of reciprocal translocation between the chromosomes 9 and 22 (Baikie et al., 1960), raised the question as to whether all of these diseases should be considered as part of the same family. More recently, the identification of the new mutation in the *JAK2* gene in PV, PMF, and ET has directed the division of these syndromes into two main categories: chronic myeloid leukemia and the other three chronic myeloproliferative disorders (James et al., 2005). These diseases have an incidence ranging from 0.5 to 2.8 per 100 000 individuals (Anía et al., 1994; Mesa et al., 1999). This chapter will review the main characteristics and neurologic complications of PV, PMF, and ET.

The *JAK2* mutation and the relationship between polycythemia vera, primary myelofibrosis, and essential thrombocythemia

The *JAK2* V617F mutation is present in the vast majority of patients with PV and in approximately 50% of those

with PMF and ET. This observation raises a question regarding the role of the mutation in the emergence of three diseases with apparently different clinical phenotypes (Beer and Green, 2009). There is now some consensus around the concept that attempts to explain the role of *JAK2* mutations in chronic myeloproliferative disorders (Beer and Green, 2009; Harrison, 2010). Compared to patients with ET that are negative for *JAK2*, those with the *JAK2* mutation have higher red and white blood cell counts, lower erythropoietin levels, and increased propensity for venous thrombosis (Scott et al., 2006). These ET patients are heterozygous for *JAK2* mutation, whereas the majority of patients with PV are homozygous for *JAK2* mutation (Beer and Green, 2009). The rare PV patient lacking the V617F mutation in the *JAK2* gene is usually found to bear an exon 12 mutation, which is associated with a stronger intracellular activation and is only found in patients with PV (Scott et al., 2007). Therefore, it is tempting to speculate that the increasing expression of *JAK2* mutations leads to a PV-like phenotype. There is also significant overlap between ET and PV with PMF. The prevalence of *JAK2* and *MPL* mutations is identical in ET and PMF. Clinically, PMF is indistinguishable from myelofibrosis secondary to ET or PV, and many patients with ET have increased marrow reticulin but lack anemia and splenomegaly, which are a hallmark of PMF. However, over time, these features may develop and, in these cases, it is unclear whether the initial thrombocytosis was, in fact, a cellular manifestation of PMF. While karyotype abnormalities are rare in patients with ET, they are present in at least 50% of patients with PMF (Tefferi et al., 2001). Moreover, PMF has higher levels of ineffective erythropoiesis and increased progression to acute myeloid

---

*Correspondence to: Prof. José M. Ferro, Serviço de Neurologia, 6th floor, Hospital de Santa Maria, 1649-028 Lisbon, Portugal. Fax: +351-21-795-7474, E-mail: jmferro@fm.ul.pt

leukemia (Cervantes et al., 1997). All these factors suggest that PMF is a clinically accelerated myeloproliferative disorder, while ET and PV have a more chronic behavior. It is still not known whether the JAK2 mutation is the initiating event in the disease or if it is preceded by other genetic abnormalities (Beer and Green, 2009). In any case, the expression of a mutant JAK2 eliminates cytokine requirement in cytokine-dependent cell lines and promotes the activation of signaling pathways, ultimately leading to the development of a myeloproliferative disorder *in vivo* (Levine et al., 2007), suggesting that it plays a central role in the pathogenesis of the disease.

POLYCYTHEMIA VERA

Main clinical characteristics

Vaquez described in 1892 an unknown entity in a patient with persistent erythrocytosis and cyanosis, likely to be the first description of PV (Vaquez, 1892). Approximately one decade later, Osler would present the first series of patients with the new syndrome (Osler, 1903).

PV usually has an insidious onset, more frequently in the 6th decade of life (Berlin, 1975). Many patients are led to diagnosis after the initial identification of erythrocytosis in a routine blood test. Patients who refer symptoms may have headaches, weakness, pruritus, dizziness, sweating, plethora, thrombosis and gastrointestinal bleeding (Berlin, 1975). Approximately one third of the patients have thrombotic complications. Arterial events, predominantly ischemic strokes and transient ischemic attacks (TIA), account for approximately 30% of such thrombotic complications, followed in frequency by myocardial infarction, deep vein thrombosis and pulmonary embolism (Berk et al., 1986; Gruppo Italiano Studio Policitemia, 1995). Up to 25% of the patients have mucosal bleeding and bruising, which are usually not severe (Wehmeier et al., 1991). Approximately 10% of the patients have erythromelalgia, a burning sensation and erythema of the fingers, which is related to thrombocytosis and usually responds to low dose aspirin. In the brain an increase in the hematocrit above 45% is associated with a decrease in cerebral blood flow conductive to stasis and endothelial damage, interfering with nitrous oxide vasodilatory effects and therefore increasing the thrombotic tendency, even without associated thrombocytosis (Thomas et al., 1977; Fiermonte et al., 1993). Platelet counts $> 1000 \times 10^9$/L are associated with hemorrhagic diathesis due to an acquired von Willebrand syndrome (Spivak, 2002).

Later in the course of the disease, patients may evolve to a spent phase, which is a form of secondary myelofibrosis with anemia and splenomegaly. It is usually a terminal complication of PV. Finally, patients with PV have a 5–6% risk of developing secondary acute myeloid leukemia at 10 years, which is lower in patients treated only with phlebotomy and higher in those receiving ^{32}P and chlorambucil (Spivak et al., 2003). Interestingly, the leukemic clone more frequently arises from a hematopoietic cell not bearing the *JAK2* mutation (Theocharides et al., 2007).

Diagnostic criteria and risk assessment

The distinction between PV and secondary polycythemias may be cumbersome. The 2008 World Health Organization (WHO) criteria help to differentiate between these entities. Polycythemias can be primary, due to clonal proliferation of bone marrow precursors, or secondary, due to reactive erythrocytosis. Secondary polycythemias include congenital and acquired syndromes, mostly erythropoietin mediated, due to hypoxia, erythropoietin-producing tumors or drug-associated (McMullin et al., 2005).

Patients must have either both major and one minor criteria or the first major and two minor criteria in order to fulfill the diagnostic requirements for PV (Vardiman et al., 2009). Briefly, the major criteria are significant erythrocytosis and *JAK2* mutations and the minor criteria are marrow trilineage myeloproliferation, subnormal serum erythropoietin levels, and endogenous erythroid colony growth.

High-risk patients are defined by any one of the following: age above 60 years, previous documented thrombosis, aspirin-resistant erythromelalgia, platelet count above 1000×10^9/L, diabetes, or hypertension requiring pharmacologic therapy, significant or symptomatic splenomegaly. Low-risk patients should not have any of these risk factors (Harrison, 2010).

Frequent neurologic symptoms

Neurologic symptoms are common in PV and their importance was first recognized in 1892 by Vaquez, who described a case of a PV patient with vertigo and tinnitus.

The most frequent neurologic symptoms in PV are headache and dizziness. The PV-related headache has no defining characteristic and varies from a generalized headache to a unilateral intermittent throbbing migraine-like pain (Silverstein et al., 1962). Other neurologic symptoms resulting from microvascular circulation disturbances due to spontaneous activation and aggregation of platelets in the endarterial circulation can occur even with normal hematocrit values and include: paresthesias, erythromelalgia, episodic neurologic symptoms such as atypical transient ischemic attack (TIA) preceded by migraine-like headache, scotomata, blurred vision, and transient ocular ischemic attacks. Most of these symptoms can be relieved with aspirin (Silverstein et al., 1962; Michiels et al., 2004, 2006a, b).

Thrombosis and hemorrhage

In 1213 PV patients followed for 20 years, 14% had a thrombotic event prior to the diagnosis and 20% as the presenting symptom of the disease. Of these, ischemic stroke and TIA accounted for 70% of arterial thrombosis at diagnosis and 30% before diagnosis. On follow-up, TIA were the most common nonfatal event followed by myocardial infarction and ischemic stroke (9.5%) (Gruppo Italiano Studio Policitemia, 1995).

The central nervous system (CNS) is the most frequent site of thrombosis, more common than coronary artery complications (Michiels et al., 2004). CNS thrombosis can be arterial or venous. Thrombosis can precede the diagnosis by up to 2 years in 14–15% of patients; it can be a presenting feature in 12–57% and occur in follow-up in up to 40% of patients. It is the cause of death in 20–40% of PV patients. The rate of thrombotic events increases with age and a history of previous thrombotic event.

Cerebral venous thrombosis (CVT) is a frequent complication of PV and PV is listed among the possible causes of CVT (Ferro et al., 2004). CVT can present as headache, papilledema, seizures, or a focal deficit, or a combination of the above, and in severe forms as encephalopathy or coma. Usually several sinuses or veins are occluded simultaneously. PV should be searched for in cases of cryptogenic CVT, as venous occlusion can antedate laboratory and clinical manifestations of PV by several months.

PV is an independent risk factor for the recurrence of CVT and other thrombotic events (Miranda et al., 2010).

Hemorrhage is less frequent than thrombosis and primarily involves the CNS or gastrointestinal tract. It can be a presenting feature in 6–58% of PV patients and the cause death in up to 30% of the patients (Perkins et al., 1964; Berk et al., 1995; Gruppo Italiano Studio Policitemia, 1995; Passamonti et al., 2003, 2004; De Stefano et al., 2008b).

Other neurologic symptoms

Neurologic deficits in PV, such as headache and focal deficits, may present as a progressive syndrome mimicking a brain tumor, which would explain several craniotomies performed before modern imaging techniques were available (Kremer et al., 1972).

Although paresthesias and limb pain are common in PV, peripheral neuropathy is rare. A sensory neuropathy affecting all sensory modalities due to chronic axonal degeneration with loss of large diameter myelinated fibers has been described in three PV patients with symptoms suggesting peripheral nerve involvement (Yiannikas et al., 1983).

Chorea is a rare symptom in PV. Polycythemic chorea manifests predominantly in women after the age of 50 and should therefore be considered in the differential diagnosis of late-onset chorea. It is generalized involving the brachial and faciolingual muscles with associated muscular hypotonia (Bryn and Padberg, 1984). The pathophysiology remains unclear, but since it is not seen in secondary polycythemia, an underlying molecular abnormality is suggested (Silverstein et al, 1962; Nazabal et al., 2000; Cao et al., 2006). Magnetic resonance imaging (MRI) and single photon emission computed tomography (SPECT) have failed to demonstrate definite perfusion or structural changes that could clarify this issue (Kim et al., 2008).

Rarely, in advanced PV progressing to myelofibrosis, spinal epidural extramedullary hematopoiesis can cause spinal cord compression (Rice et al., 1980; De Morais et al., 1996; Scott and Poynton, 2008).

General treatment recommendations

The current guidelines for all patients involve the careful assessment of cardiovascular risk and the use of low-dose aspirin, unless contraindicated. Erythrocytosis should be controlled by phlebotomy to maintain a hematocrit lower than 45% (Harrison, 2010).

Pharmacologic therapy may be needed not only to control the red blood cell count, but also to lower the platelet count in patients with thrombocytosis. Hydroxycarbamide and busulfan are usually reserved for high-risk patients above the age of 60 years, whereas younger patients should receive interferon and/or anagrelide (Harrison, 2010). Low-risk patients may be managed with low-dose aspirin and phlebotomy alone.

ESSENTIAL THROMBOCYTHEMIA
Main clinical characteristics

Essential thrombocythemia (ET) is a chronic myeloproliferative syndrome characterized by sustained (>1 month) high platelet counts ($>450 \times 10^9$/L) and increased number of mature large megakaryocytes in the bone marrow. ET has to be distinguished from other causes of high platelet count (thrombocytosis). The most common reactive causes of thrombocytosis are acute and chronic blood loss and anemia, chronic infections and inflammation, malignancy, and splenectomy (Brière, 2007; Miller and Farquharson, 2010; Tefferi, 2011). ET was first described in 1934, in a patient with hemorrhage (Epstein and Goedel, 1934). It is frequently diagnosed after the incidental finding of an elevated platelet count. Only 10% of the patients have splenomegaly at diagnosis

(Harrison et al., 2005). A significant number of patients have coagulation abnormalities and approximately one quarter of high-risk patients not receiving myelosuppressive drugs have thrombosis (Cortelazzo et al., 1995). The main predictive factors for thrombosis are age above 60 years and a history of previous thrombosis (Passamonti et al., 2008). Arterial thrombosis predominates, affecting the CNS (ischemic stroke, TIA) and the cardiovascular system (myocardial infarction, unstable angina, peripheral arterial occlusion) (Cortelazzo et al., 1995; Harrison et al., 2005). Venous events comprise primarily deep venous thrombosis and pulmonary embolism. Significant hemorrhage is less frequent than thrombosis and it affects primarily the nasal, buccal, and gastrointestinal mucosae (Cortelazzo et al., 1995; Harrison et al., 2005). It is typical for ET patients to have abnormalities in platelet aggregation and loss of large von Willebrand factor multimers, determining an increased hemorrhage time. However, these laboratory findings do not necessarily correlate with clinical bleeding (Elliott and Tefferi, 2005). Although it has been reported that 15% of the patients with ET may evolve to secondary myelofibrosis at 15 years (Cervantes et al., 2002), it is unclear whether these cases are true evolutions or if they represent misdiagnosed cellular phases of PMF. The risk of progression to acute myeloid leukemia is low and it may be in the order of 5–8% in the second decade after the diagnosis (Wolanskyj et al., 2006).

Diagnostic criteria and risk assessment

The 2008 WHO criteria for the diagnosis of ET considers five main factors: platelet count above 450×10^9/L; mutation in *JAK2* or *MPL* genes; no other myeloid malignancy, especially myelodysplastic syndromes or other chronic myeloproliferative disorder; no reactive cause for thrombocytosis and normal marrow iron stores; marrow studies showing increased megakaryocytes with hyperlobulated forms and absence of increased reticulin. For the diagnosis of ET, the first criterion must always be present together with the second plus the third or, in the absence of mutations, in conjunction with the remaining three criteria (Vardiman et al., 2009).

High-risk ET is defined by the presence of at least one of the following criteria: age above 60 years, platelet count above 1500×10^9/L, previous thrombosis and aspirin-refractory erythromelalgia, previous hemorrhage related to ET, diabetes, or hypertension requiring pharmacologic treatment. Intermediate and low risk applies to patients lacking all these risk factors but with an age between 40 and 60 years, and below 40 years, respectively (Harrison, 2010).

Neurologic manifestations

Neurologic manifestations in ET are also due to large artery and vein thrombosis, microvascular ischemia, and thrombosis (Jabaily et al., 1983; Kesler et al., 2000; Miller and Farquharson, 2010). Strokes (Arboix et al., 1995) and CVT (Haan et al., 1988) are often the inaugural presentation of ET and may even antedate the diagnosis of ET by months.

The most common neurologic symptom is headache, sometimes resembling migraine. Migrainous aura-like episodes are also common. Atypical TIA (isolated dysarthria, diplopia or unsteadiness, hearing loss, transient focal deficits with prominent headache, very brief or sequential) or typical TIA (amaurosis fugax, aphasia, motor deficits) are frequent, but seizures have rarely been reported. Erythromelalgia is a burning or painful sensation of the palms and soles and sometimes also of the toes and fingertips accompanied by a red-cyanotic skin discoloration of the affected skin areas, which is highly characteristic and prevalent in both ET and PV. All these symptoms are attributed to microvascular ischemia and thrombosis, induced by activated platelets and by products released by the platelets (Michiels et al., 1993, 1996a, b).

Other arterial cerebrovascular complications include ischemic strokes due to large artery and small vessel disease (Jabaily et al., 1983; Arboix et al., 1995; Kesler et al., 2000; Gonthier and Bogousslavsky, 2004; Mallada-Frechin et al., 2004). Nevertheless, ET (and also PV) are infrequent causes of ischemic stroke: two cases in 4697 strokes in the Lausanne Registry and six out of 1099 in L'Aliança Registry.

Two unusual cases of progressive occlusive disease of the internal carotid with recurrent strokes or TIA (Mosso et al., 2004; Kornblihtt et al., 2005) have been reported. One of these patients had a moyamoya angiographic pattern and was successfully treated with an internal carotid stent (Kornblihtt et al., 2005).

Thrombosis of the dural sinus and cerebral veins are frequent in ET and can be the inaugural clinical manifestation (Fig. 72.1) (Haan et al., 1988). The frequency of venous sinus thrombosis in ET is estimated to be 2%. In a cohort of 624 patients with CVT, five (0.8%) had ET (Ferro et al., 2004). Although the *JAK2* mutation is rare in unselected cases of cerebral venous thrombosis (1–6%) (Bellucci et al., 2008; De Stefano et al., 2008a; Shetty et al., 2010), this mutation is more frequent (RR 2.26) in ET patients with CVT (De Stefano et al., 2011). ET and also PV are risk factors for the occurrence of further venous thrombotic events after CVT (Miranda et al., 2010).

Faivre et al. (2009) described a patient with ET who sustained a spinal cord infarct. However, the patient also had aortic atheroma. Unusual neurologic complications

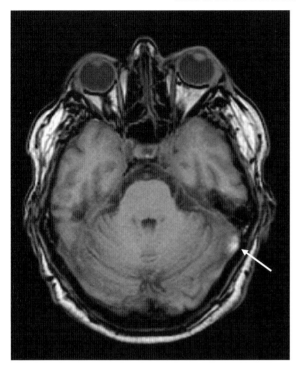

Fig. 72.1. A 57-year-old male with essential thrombocythemia. Headache for 2 weeks and transient bilateral visual scotomata. Bilateral papilledema. Platelet count on admission 400.000 UL. Brain MR: thrombosis of the left lateral sinus (arrow).

include hemichorea with MRI showing a area of T1 high signal in the contralateral basal ganglia (Ito et al., 2011), third nerve palsy (Prabhakaran et al., 2006), and neuromyotonia (Benito-León et al., 2000).

General treatment recommendations

Similarly to PV, the current guidelines for all patients involve the careful assessment of cardiovascular risk and the use of low-dose aspirin, unless contraindicated. High-risk patients above 60 years should receive hydroxycarbamide, whereas younger patients may receive interferon or anagrelide instead as first-line treatment (Harrison, 2010). UK guidelines currently recommend regular monitoring of patients treated with anagrelide for the eventual emergence of marrow fibrosis (Harrison, 2010).

The treatment of cerebrovascular complications of ET should follow the general recommendation for the treatment of the different types of stroke. In general, therapies to reduce platelet count are added. For thrombosis of the dural sinus and cerebral veins, anticoagulation is used in the acute phase. Platelet counts should be monitored frequently during unfractionated heparin treatment, to detect heparin-induced thrombocytopenia, which can have a deleterious influence in the clinical course.

PRIMARY MYELOFIBROSIS

Main clinical characteristics

PMF was first described by Heuck in 1879. The disease is characterized by the association of anemia, splenomegaly, increased immature granulocytes, progenitor cells, erythroblasts, and teardrop-shaped red blood cells in the peripheral blood, and prominent bone marrow reticulin and collagen deposition and osteosclerosis (Barosi, 2003; Hoffman and Rondelli, 2007). Thrombocytosis is also very frequent. Approximately one quarter of the patients are asymptomatic at the time of the diagnosis. More frequently, patients complain of fatigue, weakness, shortness of breath, pruritus, weight loss, and early satiety due to splenic enlargement (Ward and Block, 1971; Barosi and Hoffman, 2003). Later in the course of the disease, patients may present with fever, night sweats, and bone pain. Hepatomegaly is present in the majority of patients and splenomegaly is detected in virtually all patients at the time of diagnosis. The spleen is significantly enlarged in over two-thirds of the patients (Ward and Block, 1971). The massive increase in splenoportal blood flow, the decrease in hepatic vascular compliance, and the development of hepatic vein thrombosis may lead to portal hypertension, ascites, esophageal and gastric varices (Rosenbaum et al., 1966; Dubois et al., 1993). PMF is not infrequently associated with extramedullary hematopoiesis, primarily in the gastrointestinal, central nervous, pulmonary, and genitourinary systems, which may result in symptoms due to enlarging masses or reduction in organ function. The risk of arterial and venous thrombosis is also increased in patients with PMF, albeit to a lesser degree than that observed in PV and ET. It is estimated that 12% of the patients may develop a thrombotic event in the first 4 years after diagnosis (Cervantes et al., 2006). Patients with PMF are also at increased risk for developing secondary acute myeloid leukemia and is estimated that 8–23% of the patients may develop this complication in the first decade after the diagnosis (Cervantes et al., 1991; Mesa et al., 2005).

Diagnostic criteria and risk assessment

The WHO recently updated the diagnostic criteria of PMF (Vardiman et al., 2009). The diagnosis requires the presence of all three major criteria (megakaryocyte proliferation and atypia accompanied by either reticulin/collagen fibrosis or increased marrow cellularity characterized by granulocyte proliferation and decreased erythropoiesis; not meeting WHO criteria for other myeloproliferative disorders; presence of *JAK2* or *MPL* mutations) and two of the four minor criteria (leukoerythroblastosis; increased lactate dehydrogenase serum levels; anemia; palpable splenomegaly).

The Lille scoring system is particularly useful for selecting intermediate and high-risk patients for allogeneic transplantation of hematopoietic progenitors based on three poor prognostic factors: hemoglobin < 10 g/dL, leukocytes < 4000 × 10⁶/L or > 30 000 × 10⁶/L (Dupriez et al., 1996). Low-risk patients have none of these risk factors. More recently, adding low platelet count to the other three variables further strengthens this index (Dingli et al., 2006).

Neurologic manifestations

Neurologic complications of PMF are very rare. The most common neurologic manifestations are due to spinal cord compression by extramedullary hematopoietic masses (Appleby et al., 1964; Oustwani et al., 1980; De Klippel et al., 1993; Horwood et al., 2003; Di Leva et al., 2007). There are also isolated reports of compression of the cerebral hemispheres (Rutman et al., 1972) or of the cauda equina (Goh et al., 2007).

In the Mayo Clinic series of 205 patients with PMF, 13% experienced a vaso-occlusive event at or prior to their diagnosis, including four strokes, two TIA, and one CVT (Elliot and Tefferi, 2005). There is a single case report of spinal cord ischemia in PMF (Periad et al., 2009).

Concerning neuromuscular complications there are single case reports describing the co-occurrence of PMF and lower motor neuron disease (Bir et al., 2000) and dermatomyositis (Ito et al., 2006).

General treatment recommendations

The treatment of PMF is largely palliative. The anemia and thrombocytopenia are frequently treated with transfusions. Many agents have been used, primarily in uncontrolled trials, including danazol, erythropoietin, thalidomide, lenalidomide, hydroxyurea, anagrelide, among others. These agents occasionally improved cytopenias but had no effect on the natural history of the disease (Hoffman and Rondelli, 2007). There is no consensus regarding the use of splenectomy, which may be indicated in patients with portal hypertension, anemia, thrombocytopenia, or splenic pain. However, this procedure has significant morbidity and mortality and is difficult to recommend in a generalized way (Mesa et al., 2006). Allogeneic transplantation of hematopoietic progenitors is the only curative treatment for PMF and should be offered to fit high- and intermediate-risk younger patients (Guardiola et al., 1999). A number of experimental treatments, including inhibitors of *JAK2*-V617F mutation are currently under investigation.

Treatment of CNS compression, namely the spinal cord, by extramedullary haematopoietic tissue is better managed by a combined approach of surgical decompression by laminectomy and irradiation and/or chemotherapy, with 75% of the patients showing neurologic improvement and 100% survival with this strategy (Scott and Poynton, 2008).

REFERENCES

Anía BJ, Suman VJ, Sobell JL et al. (1994). Trends in the incidence of polycythemia vera among Olmsted County, Minnesota residents, 1935–1989. Am J Hematol 47: 89–93.

Appleby A, Batson GA, Lassman LP et al. (1964). Spinal cord compression by extramedullary haematopoiesis in myelosclerosis. J Neurol Neurosurg Psychiatry 27: 313–316.

Arboix A, Besses C, Acin P et al. (1995). Ischemic stroke as first manifestation of essential thrombocythemia. Report of six cases. Stroke 26: 1463–1466.

Baikie AG, Court-Brown WM, Buckton KE et al. (1960). A possible specific chromosome abnormality in human chronic myeloid leukaemia. Nature 188: 1165–1166.

Barosi G (2003). Myelofibrosis with myeloid metaplasia. Hematol Oncol Clin North Am 17: 1211–1226.

Barosi G, Hoffman R (2003). Idiopathic myelofibrosis. Semin Hematol 42: 248–258.

Beer PA, Green AR (2009). Pathogenesis and management of essential thrombocythemia. Hematology Am Soc Hematol Educ Program 2009: 621–628.

Bellucci S, Cassinat B, Bonnin N et al. (2008). The V617F JAK2 mutation is not a frequent event in patients with cerebral venous thrombosis without overt chronic myeloproliferative disorder. Thromb Haemost 99: 1119–1120.

Benito-León J, Martín E, Vincent A et al. (2000). Neuromyotonia in association with essential thrombocythemia. J Neurol Sci 173: 78–79.

Berk PD, Goldberg JD, Donovan PB et al. (1986). Therapeutic recommendations in polycythemia vera based on Polycythemia Vera Study Group protocols. Semin Hematol 23: 132–143.

Berk PD, Wasserman LR, Fruchtman SM et al. (1995). Treatment of polycythemia vera: a summary of clinical trials conducted by the Polycythemia Vera Study Group. In: LR Wasserman, PD Berk, NI Berlin (Eds.), Polycythemia Vera and the Myeloproliferative Disorders. WB Saunders, Philadelphia, pp. 166–194.

Berlin NI (1975). Diagnosis and classification of the polycythemias. Semin Hematol 12: 339–351.

Bir LS, Keskin A, Yaren A et al. (2000). Lower motor neuron disease associated with myelofibrosis. Clin Neurol Neurosurg 102: 109–112.

Brière JB (2007). Essential thrombocythemia. Orphanet J Rare Dis 2: 3.

Bryn GW, Padberg G (1984). Chorea and polycythaemia. Eur Neurol 23: 26–33.

Cao M, Olsen RJ, Zu Y (2006). Polycythemia vera: new clinicopathologic perspectives. Arch Pathol Lab Med 130: 1126–1132.

Cervantes F, Tassies D, Salgado C et al. (1991). Acute transformation in nonleukemic chronic myeloproliferative disorders: actuarial probability and main characteristics in a series of 218 patients. Acta Haematol 85: 124–127.

Cervantes F, Pereira A, Esteve J et al. (1997). Identification of "short-lived" and "long-lived" patients at presentation of idiopathic myelofibrosis. Br J Haematol 97: 635–640.

Cervantes F, Alvarez-Larrán A, Talarn C et al. (2002). Myelofibrosis with myeloid metaplasia following essential thrombocythaemia: actuarial probability, presenting characteristics and evolution in a series of 195 patients. Br J Haematol 118: 786–790.

Cervantes F, Alvarez-Larrán A, Arellano-Rodrigo E et al. (2006). Frequency and risk factors for thrombosis in idiopathic myelofibrosis: analysis in a series of 155 patients from a single institution. Leukemia 20: 55–60.

Cortelazzo S, Finazzi G, Ruggeri M et al. (1995). Hydroxyurea for patients with essential thrombocythemia and a high risk of thrombosis. N Engl J Med 332: 1132–1136.

Dameshek W (1951). Some speculations on the myeloproliferative syndromes. Blood 4: 372–375.

De Klippel N, Dehou MF, Bourgain C et al. (1993). Progressive paraparesis due to thoracic extramedullary hematopoiesis in myelofibrosis. J Neurosurg 79: 125–127.

De Morais JC, Spector N, Lavrado FP et al. (1996). Spinal cord compression due to extramedullary hematopoiesis in the proliferative phase of polycythemia vera. Acta Heamatol 96: 242–244.

De Stefano V, Rossi E, Za T et al. (2008a). The JAK2 V617F mutation in patients with cerebral venous thrombosis: a rebuttal. Thromb Haemost 99: 1121.

De Stefano V, Za T, Rossi E et al. (2008b). Recurrent thrombosis in patients with polycythemia vera and essential thrombocythemia: incidence, risk factors, and effect of treatments. Haematologica 93: 372–380.

De Stefano V, Rossi E, Za T et al. (2011). The JAK2 V617F mutational frequency in essential thrombocythemia associated with splanchnic or cerebral vein thrombosis. Am J Hematol 86: 526–528.

Di Leva A, Aimar E, Tancioni F et al. (2007). Focal extra-axial hemorrhagic mass with subdural hemorrhage secondary to extramedullary haematopoiesis in idiopathic myelodysplasic syndrome. J Neurosurg Sci 51: 29–32.

Dingli D, Schwager SM, Mesa RA et al. (2006). Prognosis in transplant-eligible patients with agnogenic myeloid metaplasia: a simple CBC-based scoring system. Cancer 106: 623–630.

Dubois A, Dauzat M, Pignodel C et al. (1993). Portal hypertension in lymphoproliferative and myeloproliferative disorders: hemodynamic and histological correlations. Hepatology 17: 246–250.

Dupriez B, Morel P, Demory JL et al. (1996). Prognostic factors in agnogenic myeloid metaplasia: a report on 195 cases with a new scoring system. Blood 88: 1013–1018.

Elliott MA, Tefferi A (2005). Thrombosis and haemorrhage in polycythaemia vera and essential thrombocythaemia. Br J Haematol 128: 275–290.

Epstein E, Goedel A (1934). Haemorrhagische thrombocythamie bei vascularer schrumpfmilz. Virchov's Archiv Abteilung 293: 233.

Faivre A, Bonnel S, Leyral G et al. (2009). Infarctus médullaire révélant une thrombocytémie essentielle. Presse Med 38: 1180–1183.

Ferro JM, Canhão P, Stam J et al. (2004). Prognosis of cerebral vein and dural sinus thrombosis: results of the International Study on Cerebral Vein and Dural Sinus Thrombosis (ISCVT). Stroke 35: 664–670.

Fiermonte G, Aloe Spiriti MA, Latagliata R et al. (1993). Polycythemia vera and cerebral blood flow: a preliminary study with transcranial doppler. J Intern Med 234: 599–602.

Goh DH, Lee SH, Cho DC et al. (2007). Chronic idiopathic myelofibrosis presenting as cauda equina compression due to extramedullary hematopoiesis: a case report. Korean Med Sci 22: 1090–1093.

Gonthier A, Bogousslavsky J (2004). Infarctus cérébraux artériels d'origine hématologique: expérience lausannoise et revue de la littérature. Rev Neurol (Paris) 160: 1029–1039.

Gruppo Italiano Studio Policitemia (1995). Polycythemia vera: the natural history of 1213 patients followed for 20 years. Ann Intern Med 123: 656–664.

Guardiola P, Anderson JE, Bandini G et al. (1999). Allogeneic stem cell transplantation for agnogenic myeloid metaplasia: a European Group for Blood and Marrow Transplantation, Société Française de Greffe de Moelle, Gruppo Italiano per il Trapianto del Midollo Osseo, and Fred Hutchinson Cancer Research Center Collaborative Study. Blood 93: 2831–2838.

Haan J, Caekebeke JFV, Van Der Meer FJM et al. (1988). Cerebral venous thrombosis as presenting sign of myeloproliferative disorders. J Neurol Neurosurg Psychiatry 51: 1219–1220.

Harrison C (2010). Rethinking disease definitions and therapeutic strategies in essential thrombocythemia and polycythemia vera. Hematology Am Soc Hematol Educ Program 2010: 129–134.

Harrison CN, Campbell PJ, Buck G et al. (2005). Hydroxyurea compared with anagrelide in high-risk essential thrombocythemia. N Engl J Med 353: 33–45.

Heuck G (1879). Zwei Fälle von Leukämie mit eigenthümlichem Blut-resp Knochenmarksbefund. Virchows Arch (Pathol Anat) 78: 475.

Hoffman R, Rondelli D (2007). Biology and treatment of primary myelofibrosis. Hematology Am Soc Hematol Educ Program 2007: 346–354.

Horwood E, Dowson H, Gupta R et al. (2003). Myelofibrosis presenting as spinal cord compression. J Clin Pathol 56: 154–156.

Ito A, Umeda M, Koike T et al. (2006). A case of dermatomyositis associated with chronic idiopathic myelofibrosis. Rinsho Shinkeigaku 46: 210–213.

Ito H, Kinoshita I, Joh T et al. (2011). Case report of essential thrombocythemia with sudden onset of hemichorea. Rinsho Shinkeigaku 51: 211–214.

Jabaily J, Iland HJ, Laszlo J et al. (1983). Neurologic manifestations of essential thrombocythemia. Ann Intern Med 99: 513–518.

James C, Ugo V, Le Couédic JP et al. (2005). A unique clonal JAK2 mutation leading to constitutive signalling causes polycythaemia vera. Nature 434: 1144–1148.

Kesler A, Ellis MH, Manor Y et al. (2000). Neurological complications of essential thrombocytosis (ET). Acta Neurol Scand 102: 299–302.

Kim W, Kim JS, Lee KS et al. (2008). No evidence of perfusion abnormalities in the basal ganglia of a patient with generalized chorea-ballism and polycythaemia vera: analysis using subtraction SPECT co-registered to MRI. Neurol Sci 29: 351–354.

Kornblihtt LI, Cocorullo S, Miranda C et al. (2005). Moyamoya syndrome in an adolescent with essential thrombocythemia. Successful intracranial carotid stent placement. Stroke 36: e71–e73.

Kremer M, Lambert CD, Lawton N (1972). Progressive Neurological deficits in primary polycythemia. BMJ 3: 216–218.

Levine RL, Pardanani A, Tefferi A et al. (2007). Role of JAK2 in the pathogenesis and therapy of myeloproliferative disorders. Nat Rev Cancer 7: 673–683.

Mallada-Frechin J, Abellán-Miralles I, Medrano V et al. (2004). Ischemic stroke as a presentation of essential thrombocythemia. Four case reports. Rev Neurol (Paris) 38: 1032–1034.

McMullin M, Bareford D, Campbell P et al. (2005). Guidelines for the diagnosis, investigation and management of polycythemia/erythrocytosis. Br J Haematol 130: 174–195.

Mesa RA, Silverstein MN, Jacobsen SJ et al. (1999). Population-based incidence and survival figures in essential thrombocythemia and agnogenic myeloid metaplasia: an Olmsted County Study, 1976–1995. Am J Hematol 61: 10–15.

Mesa RA, Li CY, Ketterling RP et al. (2005). Leukemic transformation in myelofibrosis with myeloid metaplasia: a single institution experience with 91 cases. Blood 105: 973–977.

Mesa RA, Nagorney DS, Schwager S et al. (2006). Palliative goals, patient selection, and perioperative platelet management: outcomes and lessons from 3 decades of splenectomy for myelofibrosis with myeloid metaplasia at the Mayo Clinic. Cancer 107: 361–370.

Michiels JJ, Koudstaal PJ, Mulder AH et al. (1993). Transient neurologic and ocular manifestations in primary thrombocythemia. Neurology 43: 1107–1110.

Michiels JJ, van Genderen PJ, Jansen PH et al. (1996a). Atypical transient ischemic attacks in thrombocythemia of various myeloproliferative disorders. Leuk Lymphoma 22 (Suppl 1): 65–70.

Michiels JJ, van Genderen PJ, Lindemans J et al. (1996b). Erythromelalgic, thrombotic and hemorrhagic manifestations in 50 cases of thrombocythemia. Leuk Lymphoma 22 (Suppl 1): 47–56.

Michiels JJ, Berneman ZN, Schroyens W et al. (2004). Pathophysiology and treatment of platelet-mediated microvascular disturbances, major thrombosis and bleeding complications in essential thrombocythaemia and polycythemia vera. Platelets 15: 67–84.

Michiels JJ, Berneman Z, Schroyens W et al. (2006a). Platelet-mediated erythromelalgic, cerebral, ocular and coronary microvascular ischemic and thrombotic manifestations in patients with essential thrombocythemia and polycythemia vera: a distinct aspirin-responsive and Coumadin-resistant arterial thrombophilia. Platelets 17: 528–544.

Michiels JJ, Berneman Z, Van Bockstaele D et al. (2006b). Clinical and laboratory features, pathobiology of platelet-mediated thrombosis and bleeding complications, and the molecular etiology of essential thrombocythemia and polycythemia vera: therapeutic implications. Semin Thromb Hemost 32: 174–207.

Miller TD, Farquharson MH (2010). Essential thrombocythaemia and its neurological complications. Pract Neurol 10: 195–201.

Miranda B, Ferro JM, Canhão P et al. (2010). Venous thromboembolic events after cerebral vein thrombosis. Stroke 41: 1901–1906.

Mosso M, Georgiadis D, Baumgartner RW (2004). Progressive occlusive disease of large cerebral arteries and ischemic events in a patient with essential thrombocythemia. Neurol Res 26: 702–703.

Nazabal ER, Lopez JM, Perez et al. (2000). Chorea disclosing deterioration of polycythemia vera. Postgrad Med J 76: 658–659.

Osler W (1903). Chronic cyanosis, with polycythaemia and enlarged spleen: a new clinical entity. Am J Med Sci 126: 187.

Oustwani MB, Kurtidis ES, Christ M et al. (1980). Spinal cord compression with paraplegia in myelofibrosis. Arch Neurol 37: 389–390.

Passamonti F, Malabarba L, Orlandi E et al. (2003). Polycythemia vera in young patients: a study on the long-term risk of thrombosis, myelofibrosis and leukemia. Haematologica 88: 13–18.

Passamonti F, Rumi E, Pungolino E et al. (2004). Life expectancy and prognostic factors for survival in patients with polycythemia vera and essential thrombocythemia. Am J Med 117: 755–761.

Passamonti F, Rumi E, Arcaini L et al. (2008). Prognostic factors for thrombosis, myelofibrosis, and leukemia in essential thrombocythemia: a study of 605 patients. Haematologica 93: 1645–1651.

Periad D, Currat M, Qanadli SD et al. (2009). Myelofibrosis and spinal cord ischemia. Thromb Haemost 101: 584–585.

Perkins J, Israels MCG, Wilkinson JF (1964). Polycythemia vera: clinical studies on a series of 127 patients managed without radiation therapy. Q J Med 33: 499–518.

Prabhakaran VC, Chohan A, Husain R et al. (2006). Third nerve paralysis as a presenting sign of essential thrombocythaemia. Eye (Lond) 20: 1483–1484.

Rice GP, Assis LJ, Barr RM et al. (1980). Extramedullary hematopoiesis and spinal cord compression complicating polycythemia rubra vera. Ann Neurol 7: 81–84.

Rosenbaum DL, Murphy GW, Swisher SN (1966). Hemodynamic studies of the portal circulation in myeloid metaplasia. Am J Med 41: 360–368.

Rutman JY, Meidinger R, Keith JL (1972). Unusual radiologic and neurologic findings in a case of myelofibrsis with extramedullary hematopoiesis. Neurology 22: 567–570.

Scott IC, Poynton CH (2008). Polycythaemia rubra vera and myelofibrosis with spinal cord compression. J Clin Pathol 61: 681–683.

Scott LM, Scott MA, Campbell PJ et al. (2006). Progenitors homozygous for the V617F mutation occur in most patients with polycythemia vera, but not essential thrombocythemia. Blood 108: 2435–2437.

Scott LM, Tong W, Levine RL et al. (2007). JAK2 exon 12 mutations in polycythemia vera and idiopathic erythrocytosis. N Engl J Med 356: 459–468.

Shetty S, Kulkarni B, Pai N et al. (2010). JAK2 mutations across a spectrum of venous thrombosis cases. Am J Clin Pathol 134: 82–85.

Silverstein A, Gilbert H, Wasserman LR (1962). Neurologic complications of polycythemia. Ann Intern Med 57: 909–916.

Spivak JL (2002). Polycythemia vera: myths, mechanisms and management. Blood 100: 4272–4290.

Spivak JL, Barosi G, Tognoni G et al. (2003). Chronic myeloproliferative disorders. Hematology Am Soc Hematol Educ Program 2003: 200–224.

Tefferi A (2011). Annual Clinical Updates in Hematological Malignancies: a continuing medical education series: polycythemia vera and essential thrombocythemia: 2011 update on diagnosis, risk-stratification, and management. Am J Hematol 86: 292–301.

Tefferi A, Mesa RA, Schroeder G et al. (2001). Cytogenetic findings and their clinical relevance in myelofibrosis with myeloid metaplasia. Br J Haematol 113: 763–771.

Theocharides A, Boissinot M, Girodon F et al. (2007). Leukemic blasts in transformed JAK2-V617F-positive myeloproliferative disorders are frequently negative for the JAK2-V617F mutation. Blood 110: 375–379.

Thomas DJ, du Boulay GH, Marshall J et al. (1977). Cerebral blood-flow in polycythemia. Lancet 2: 161–163.

Vardiman JW, Thiele J, Arber DA et al. (2009). The 2008 revision of the World Health Organization (WHO) classification of myeloid neoplasms and acute leukemia: rationale and important changes. Blood 114: 937–951.

Vaquez H (1892). Sur une forme spéciale de cyanose s'acccompagnant d'hyperglobulie excessive et persistant. CR Soc Biol (Paris) 44: 384–388.

Ward HP, Block MH (1971). The natural history of agnogenic myeloid metaplasia (AMM) and a critical evaluation of its relationship with the myeloproliferative syndrome. Medicine (Baltimore) 50: 357–420.

Wehmeier A, Daum I, Jamin H et al. (1991). Incidence and clinical risk factors for bleeding and thrombotic complications in myeloproliferative disorders. A retrospective analysis of 260 patients. Ann Hematol 63: 101–106.

Wolanskyj AP, Schwager SM, McClure RF et al. (2006). Essential thrombocythemia beyond the first decade: life expectancy, long-term complication rates, and prognostic factors. Mayo Clin Proc 81: 159–166.

Yiannikas C, McLeod JG, Walsh JC (1983). Peripheral neuropathy associated with polycythemia vera. Neurology 33: 139–143.

Handbook of Clinical Neurology, Vol. 120 (3rd series)
Neurologic Aspects of Systemic Disease Part II
Jose Biller and Jose M. Ferro, Editors

Chapter 73

Neurologic aspects of plasma cell disorders

URSZULA SOBOL* AND PATRICK STIFF

*Department of Hematology and Oncology, Cardinal Bernardin Cancer Center, Loyola University Medical Center,
Maywood, IL, USA*

INTRODUCTION

Plasma cell disorders, also known as plasma cell dyscrasias, are a group of malignant diseases arising from proliferation of a single clone of plasma cells which often produce a homogenous (monoclonal) immunoglobulin protein (M protein) (Drappatz and Batchelor, 2004). This M protein can be easily identified as a spike on serum and/or urine protein electrophoresis (SPEP, UPEP, respectively) and further characterized by immunofixation as immunoglobulin (Ig) G, IgA, IgM, IgD, which represents the two heavy chains of the immunoglobulin, and κ (kappa) or λ (lambda), which represents the type of light chain. The secreted immunoglobulin can react with or deposit in various tissues resulting in organ dysfunction and damage.

Plasma cells disorders cover a wide spectrum of clinical manifestations, ranging from clinically aggressive and treatment requiring to more indolent and benign illnesses that can be monitored. Plasma cell disorders include: monoclonal gammopathy of undetermined significance (MGUS), multiple myeloma (MM), Waldenström macroglobulinemia (WM, also known as lymphoplasmacytic lymphoma), solitary plasmacytoma, plasma cell leukemia, POEMS syndrome (*polyneuropathy, organomegaly, endocrinopathy, monoclonal gammopathy, and skin changes*), immunoglobulin-related amyloidosis and immunoglobulin-related cryoglobulinemia. Within this group, multiple myeloma can be further subclassified into symptomatic MM requiring treatment due to associated end organ damage and smoldering (asymptomatic) MM with no associated end organ damage and not requiring treatment. Rarely MM can be nonsecretory, where neoplastic plasma cells do not secrete the monoclonal immunoglobulin.

Neurologic complications arising from these plasma cell disorders primarily affect the peripheral nervous system, with peripheral neuropathy (PN) being the predominant manifestation of the underlying disease or its treatment. The central nervous system (CNS) is less likely to be affected but clinically more significant. Tables 73.1 and 73.2 summarize the major neurologic complications of plasma cell disorders. A detailed discussion of the various plasma cell disorders and their specific neurologic implications follows below.

MONOCLONAL GAMMOPATHY OF UNDETERMINED SIGNIFICANCE

The majority, 50–75%, of all monoclonal immunoglobulins (monoclonal gammopathy) fall into the category of monoclonal gammopathy of undetermined significance (MGUS) (Kyle et al., 2006). MGUS is more common in men and can be identified in 1–3% of the population over the age of 50 years and 3–5% over the age of 70 years (Kyle et al., 2006). The diagnosis of MGUS is defined by the presence of serum M protein of less than 3 g/dL (as detected by SPEP), with less than 10% plasma cells on bone marrow examination, and no related organ or tissue impairment (Table 73.3) (International Myeloma Working Group, 2003). MGUS is a premalignant state and can progress to MM, with a risk of progression of 1% per year (Kyle et al., 2002). MGUS can also progress to other related plasma cell disorder (WM or amyloidosis) (Fig. 73.1). Main risk factors for progression include concentration of serum M protein > 1.5 g/dL and an abnormal serum free light chain ratio (κ:λ light chain ratio). Also, patients with IgM and IgA are at higher risk as compared to patients with IgG gammopathy (Kyle et al., 2002). MGUS does not require treatment

---

*Correspondence to: Urszula Sobol, M.D., Loyola University Medical Center, Cardinal Bernardin Cancer Center, Department of Hematology/Oncology, 2160 S. First Ave., Maywood, IL 60153, USA. Tel: +1-708-327-1248, Fax: +1-708-216-3319, E-mail: usobol@lumc.edu

Table 73.1

Plasma cell disorders and peripheral neuropathy

Peripheral neuropathy	Associated disease	Ig	Incidence of PN	Symptoms	Treatment
Sensory > motor demyelinating neuropathy	MGUS – anti-MAG positive WM – anti-MAG positive	IgM	8–37% in MGUS 5–10% in WM	Slowly progressive gait ataxia, tremor, loss of joint position, Romberg sign. Usually men > 50 years, favorable course	Observation/supportive; in severe cases steroids, plasma exchange, chemotherapy, IVIg, rituximab can be considered
	MGUS – anti-MAG negative	IgG, IgA		Chronic, symmetric, progressive, distal sensory or sensorimotor (CIDP-like)	Supportive
	WM – anti-MAG negative	IgM		CIDP-like	Treat underlying disorder
Sensory > motor axonal neuropathy	Cryoglobulinemia	IgG (or IgM)	~70%	Painful, progressive, symmetric distal sensorimotor, ± multiple mononeuritis	Plasma exchange, steroids, cyclophosphamide
	Treatment-related	n/a	40–75%	Primarily sensory neuropathy	Drug holiday, complete cessation or dose reduction
Motor > sensory demyelinating neuropathy	MM	IgG (or IgM)	5–50%	CIDP-like	MM therapy, which may actually exacerbate PN
	POEMS	IgG, IgA	>90%	Proximal and distal sensorimotor, loss of vibration and proprioception	Treat the underlying disorder
Sensory > motor neuropathy ± autonomic dysfunction	Amyloidosis	IgG, IgA	15–20%	Painful, progressive, symmetric distal sensorimotor. Autonomic dysfunction with orthostatic hypotension, bladder or bowel dysfunction	Treat the underlying disorder but PN may not improve

MGUS, monoclonal gammopathy of undetermined significance; MM, multiple myeloma; WM, Waldenström macroglobulinemia; Ig, immunoglobulin; PN, peripheral neuropathy; CIDP, chronic inflammatory demyelinating polyneuropathy.
(Modified from Drappatz and Batchelor, 2004.)

Table 73.2

Plasma cell disorders and central nervous system

Pathology	Plasma cell disorder	Symptoms
Spinal cord compression	MM/pathologic fracture Plasmacytoma	Back pain, paralysis, sensory loss, loss of bowel and bladder function, Lerhmitte's sign
Leptomeningeal Infiltration	MM	Multiple cranial neuropathies, HA, confusion, obstructive hydrocephalus
Hyperviscosity syndrome	WM MM	HA, vertigo, ataxia, confusion, hearing loss, strokes
Bing–Neel syndrome	WM	Leukoencephalopathy with seizures, altered mental status, paralysis
Hypercalcemia	MM	HA, weakness, seizures, lethargy, confusion, coma Cognitive decline, dementia
Amyloidoma	AL amyloidosis	CVA, symptoms due to mass effect
Cerebral amyloid angiopathy	AL amyloidosis	Cognitive decline, dementia, CVA, hemorrhage

MM, multiple myeloma; WM, Waldenström macroglobulinemia; HA, headache; CVA, cerebrovascular accident
(Modified from Drappatz and Batchelor, 2004.).

but does require indefinite monitoring at periodic intervals for evidence of progression to a malignant condition.

MGUS and peripheral neuropathy

Peripheral neuropathy (PN) is the only clinically significant neurologic complication of MGUS. It can be seen in 8–37% of MGUS patients and is often the only clinical manifestation of the underlying hematologic process (Vrethem et al., 1993). Of all patients with idiopathic neuropathy approximately 10% have an underlying monoclonal gammopathy, prevalence six to ten times that in the general population (Kelly et al., 1981). The most common type of MGUS is IgG; however, it is IgM gammopathy that is responsible for most cases of symptomatic neuropathy (typically with κ light chain). This is likely due to the fact that IgM is the most likely antibody to cross-react with neural antigens (60%), followed by IgG (30%), and IgA (10%) (Yeung et al., 1991). In general, PN due to MGUS appears insidiously and progresses slowly over months to years. Most common presentation is distal, symmetric, sensorimotor neuropathy. Less frequent presentation is predominantly sensory neuropathy, about 20% of patients (Katirji and Koontz, 2012). Lower extremities are affected earlier and to a greater extent than upper extremities. Muscle stretch reflexes are universally decreased or absent. Electrodiagnostic studies commonly show evidence of both demyelination and axonal degeneration. Sural nerve biopsies show nerve fiber loss, segmental

demyelination, and axonal atrophy and degeneration (Katirji and Koontz, 2012).

There are several distinct groups that patients with M protein-associated PN may be categorized into based on unique clinical features, type of immunoglobulin, and the underlying disease process (Table 73.1).

IgM-RELATED PERIPHERAL NEUROPATHY, ANTI-MAG POSITIVE

IgM MGUS neuropathy represents a distinct homogenous group. Approximately 50% of patients with IgM gammopathy and PN will have detectable IgM autoantibodies directed at myelin-associated glycoprotein (MAG) (Silberman and Lonial, 2008). MAG acts as an adhesion molecule for Schwann cells and axons, and the intercalation of anti-MAG antibodies between layers of myelin appears to explain the wide spacing between myelin lamellae (as seen on peripheral nerve biopsies) and consequent demyelination (Ritz et al., 1999; Vital, 2001). This immune-mediated destruction of nerve fibers may be the pathogenesis of neuropathy yet there has been a lack of correlation between the deposition of anti-MAG and amount of M protein with the degree of pathologic nerve damage (Katirji and Koontz, 2012).

Patients with high anti-MAG antibodies are clinically unique, typically men in their sixties to seventies, with slowly progressive sensory gait ataxia, with loss of proprioception, vibration, and Romberg's sign (features of large-fiber sensory dysfunction) (Drappatz and Batchelor, 2004). Tremor and paresthesias may be prominent. Patients have absent deep tendon reflexes and little

Table 73.3

Diagnostic criteria for common plasma cell disorders*

	MGUS	Smoldering MM	MM	Nonsecretory MM	Waldenström macroglobulinemia
Bone marrow plasma cells (%)	<10%	≥ 10%	≥ 10%	≥ 10%	>10%[‡]
	and	and/or	and		and
Serum monoclonal protein (M protein, g/dL)	<3	≥ 3	Any serum/urine M protein	None	Any serum M protein (IgM type)
Clinical manifestations	No end-organ damage[†]	No end-organ damage[†]	One or more symptoms of end-organ damage[†]	One or more symptoms of end-organ damage[†]	Anemia, constitutional symptoms, hyperviscosity, LAD, HSM

*(Modified from Rajkumar, 2012.)

[†]End-organ damage defined as (1) renal failure, (2) hypercalcemia, (3) anemia, (4) lytic bone lesions that can be attributed to a plasma cell disorder.

[‡]>10% lymphoplasmacytic cells.

MGUS, monoclonal gammopathy of undetermined significance; MM, multiple myeloma; HSM, hepatosplenomegaly; LAD, lymphadenopathy.

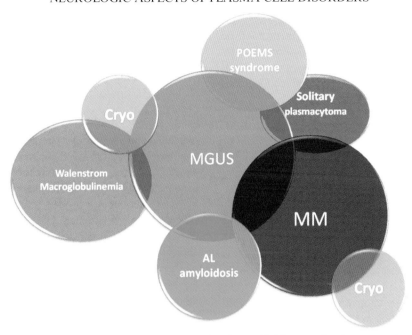

Fig. 73.1. Overlap and relationship of the different plasma cell disorders. MGUS, monoclonal gammopathy of undetermined significance; MM, multiple myeloma; POEMS syndrome, polyneuropathy, organomegaly, endocrinopathy, M-protein, skin changes; Cryo, cryoglobulinemia.

to no weakness. Fortunately the majority of patients have a favorable course with respect to neuropathy-related disability.

A number of therapies directed at the underlying IgM monoclonal gammopathy have been investigated: plasma exchange (Gertz, 2006), steroids, chemotherapy (Blume et al., 1995; Notermans et al., 1996), intravenous immunoglobulins (IVIg) (Lunn and Nobile-Orazio, 2006) and rituximab (Benedetti et al., 2008; Dalakas et al., 2009; Leger et al., 2010). However, due to very mixed and transient responses along with substantial side-effects of such therapies, treatment of the underlying hematologic condition cannot be routinely recommended and has to be considered on a case by case basis. Severity and rate of objective functional decline should guide any attempts at treatment and consideration of treatment should be given only to patients with progressive deficits. Patients with mild deficits should be observed. This is especially important as patients with anti-MAG neuropathy typically have a benign course with long-term favorable prognosis and little functional deterioration.

IgM-RELATED PERIPHERAL NEUROPATHY, ANTI-MAG NEGATIVE AND/OR NO DETECTABLE AUTOANTIBODY

Additional antineuronal antibodies have been identified, although they are less common than anti-MAG antibodies (of all patients with detectable antibodies, 70% have anti-MAG antibodies and 30% have other

antibodies) (Silberman and Lonial, 2008). They include antibodies against sulfate-3-glucuronyl paragloboside (SGPG), sulfoglucuronyl lactosaminyl paragloboside, neurofilaments, sufatides, gangliosides (anti GM1, GD1a, GD1b, GM2, GQ1b), P0 (a myelin-associated protein), and chondroitin sulfate (Drappatz and Batchelor, 2004). The specific antimyelin or other nerve component antibodies can produce distinct clinical syndromes. For example, the antiganglioside antibody GM1 tends to be purely motor neuropathy (known as multifocal motor neuropathy, with clinical symptoms similar to ALS but without upper motor neuron findings), while the antiganglioside antibody GD1b and GQ1b tends to be purely sensory neuropathy (Sadiq et al., 1990). Lastly, patients who have disialosyl-ganglioside antibodies present with a rare clinical syndrome, CANOMAD (chronic ataxic neuropathy, ophthalmoplegia, IgM monoclonal protein, cold agglutinins, and disialosyl antibodies) (Willison et al., 2001; Arbogast et al., 2007). It is important to note that anti-MAG antibodies can cross-react with some of these neural components as well (P0 for example) (Katirji and Koontz, 2012).

The clinical implications of detecting these antibodies remain controversial as no clear prognostic or therapeutic value has been identified (Eurelings et al., 2001); nevertheless, some argue that the more favorable disease course in anti-MAG PN justifies its identification.

About one-third of IgM MGUS and two-thirds of WM patients will not have identifiable antineural antibodies (Silberman and Lonial, 2008). Proposed pathogenesis in these cases includes direct infiltration of nerves, microangiopathy, hyperviscosity, and vascular precipitation of immunoglobulins. Clinical manifestations may vary from mononeuropathy and mononeuritis multiplex to symmetric polyneuropathy.

IgG- AND IgA-RELATED NEUROPATHY

PN associated with IgG or IgA gammopathies are less common and not well described. The underlying diseases may include not only MGUS but also MM, POEMS syndrome, amyloidosis and cryoglobulinemia. The majority of patients with IgG gammopathy do not have symptoms of neuropathy, even in circumstances where an anti-neural antibody is detected (Hadden et al., 2010). However, if neuropathy is present it can be sensory, motor, or mixed.

Patients with IgG gammopathy and rarely IgA or IgM gammopathy can present with polyradiculoneuropathy that closely resembles chronic inflammatory demyelinating polyneuropathy (CIDP). CIDP is an autoimmune inflammatory disorder of the peripheral nerves with demyelination resulting in proximal and distal symmetric muscle weakness, typically with motor greater than sensory symptoms. Although weakness is a characteristic feature of CIDP, and not MGUS neuropathy, a primary sensory variant of CIDP has been recognized, making the distinction rather difficult (Simmons and Tivakaran, 1996). Patients with MGUS and symptoms of CIDP tend to be older and have worse long-term functional outcome than patients with CIDP without MGUS (Simmons et al., 1995).

Treatment of IgG or IgA neuropathy is not routinely recommended, similarly to IgM PN. If it is treated it tends to respond better than IgM-driven neuropathy. Also, the closer it resembles CIDP the better, as patients are more likely to respond to immunomodulatory treatments (IVIg, plasma exchange, steroids). In fact, patients with IgG MGUS resembling CIDP should be treated like patients with CIDP without the gammopathy (Katirji and Koontz, 2012). Nevertheless, the distinction between the two (CIDP with or without M protein) is important as the underlying hematologic condition, if present, requires appropriate diagnostic evaluation and indefinite monitoring.

MGUS and the central nervous system

MGUS does not have any clinical manifestation in the central nervous system but cerebral spinal fluid (CSF) protein elevation (>100 mg/dL) can be seen in 80% of cases (Yeung et al., 1991; Rajabally, 2011). Cellularity is normal.

SMOLDERING MULTIPLE MYELOMA

As stated above, MM can be divided into smoldering (asymptomatic, with no associated end organ damage) or symptomatic MM due to end organ dysfunction (Table 73.3). End organ damage is defined as presence of any one or more of the following features: hypercalcemia, renal failure, anemia, and lytic bone lesions (which can be diagnosed on bone radiographs). Without the associated end organ damage smoldering MM, just like MGUS, does not require treatment but can progress to symptomatic MM, with a higher progression risk than in MGUS (1% per year in MGUS versus 10% per year for the first 5 years in smoldering MM) and a median time to progression of 2–3 years (Kyle et al., 2007). Randomized clinical trials are ongoing to determine if early institution of therapy can delay progression, and until the results are known, the standard of care remains observation alone with close follow-up. Neurologic complications of smoldering MM, if any, are similar to those of MM and described in the following section.

MULTIPLE MYELOMA

Monoclonal gammopathy with $>10\%$ plasma cells in the bone marrow along with associated end organ dysfunction is diagnostic of symptomatic MM (Table 73.3). Median age at diagnosis is 70 years (Altekruse et al., 2007). MM is the second most prevalent hematologic neoplasm, with a higher incidence in men and African Americans (Altekruse et al., 2007). With autologous stem cell transplantation, availability of immunomodulatory agents (lenolidomide, thalidomide) and proteasome inhibitors (bortezomib, carfilzomib) survival is increasing but cure has not been realized. Patients with MM are staged using the International Staging System, which takes into account levels of β_2-microglobulin and albumin (Table 73.4). Prognosis and risk can be further classified with chromosomal assessment using cytogenetic and FISH (fluorescent in situ hybridization) data (Table 73.5) (Kyle and Rajkumar, 2009).

Treatment of MM consists of induction therapy, intensification with autologous stem cell transplantation

Table 73.4

International staging system for multiple myeloma

Stage	β_2-microglobulin	Albumin
1	<3.5 mg/dL	>3.5 g/dL
2	Neither stage 1 or 2	
3	>5.5 mg/dL	Any

(Modified from Kyle and Rajkumar, 2009.)

Table 73.5

Classification of active multiple myeloma based
on cytogenetic abnormalities

High risk	Intermediate risk	Standard risk
Deletion 17p	t(4;14)	t(11;14)
t(14;16)	Hypodiploidy	t(6;14)
t(14;20)	Deletion 13	Hyperdiploidy

(Modified from Rajkumar, 2012.)

in transplant-eligible patients, followed by consolidation and maintenance therapy in the majority of patients. After this prolonged treatment, if and when relapse occurs additional active therapy is indicated. The various agents used at different times during MM therapy typically include cytotoxic chemotherapy such as melphalan, cyclophosphamide, and doxorubicin (liposomal) as well as newer agents, such as lenolidomide, thalidomide, bortezomib and carfilzomid. These drugs are typically given with dexamethasone to form two or three drug combinations which can be administered together.

Neurologic complications can stem from MM itself or its therapy. Both peripheral and central nervous systems can be affected.

Multiple myeloma and peripheral neuropathy

Incidence of PN and untreated MM can be variable, with estimates ranging from 5% (Katirji and Koontz, 2012) to 50% (Silberman and Lonial, 2008). Neuropathy in these patients can be clinically heterogeneous but most patients present with mild distal sensorimotor polyneuropathy. Pure sensory neuropathy is possible but not as frequent. Pathogenesis is thought to be due to perineurial or perivascular IgG (and IgM κ) deposition (Ramchandren and Lewis, 2012), due to nutritional and metabolic factors, and/or due to treatment-related toxicity. Patients may also have symptoms of radiculopathy, sometimes associated with myelopathy, due to epidural spinal compression. Electrophysiology reveals axonal damage but sural nerve biopsies can show demyelination as well (Katirji and Koontz, 2012; Ramchandren and Lewis, 2012). Unfortunately treatment of MM does not reverse the neuropathy and can actually cause or exacerbate existing PN.

About 30–40% of MM patients have related AL amyloidosis with amyloid deposits consisting of light or heavy chain immunoglobulins (Drapppatz and Batchelor, 2004). In these patients the sensorimotor neuropathy tends to be more painful and severe with an overall poor prognosis. This is discussed in greater detail below under AL amyloidosis.

Multiple myeloma and treatment-related neuropathy

Treatment emergent PN and exacerbation of existing PN is a real concern in MM treatment. About 30–75% of patients experience treatment-related PN (O'Connor et al., 2009; Richardson et al., 2012). The incidence, symptoms, reversibility and etiology varies across the MM treatment spectrum. Treatment-related PN can be sensory, motor, sensorimotor, and autonomic. Clinical assessment by a neurologist may be helpful in distinguishing between MM-related and treatment-related PN. Electomyogram (EMG) may help, as MM-associated PN is primarily demyelinating while treatment-related PN is largely axonal (Richardson et al., 2012). Also, treatment-related PN needs to be distinguished from myopathy, which can be steroid-induced in many MM patients. Medications most likely to cause neuropathy include bortezomib, thalidomide, vinca alkaloids (vincristine), and cisplatin.

Bortezomib-induced peripheral neuropathy (BiPN) preferentially induces sensory neuropathy, typically mild (Sonneveld and Jongen, 2010). Bortezomib is a reversible proteasome inhibitor which prevents degradation of ubiquitinated proteins (Orlowski and Kuhn, 2008). Potential mechanisms for BiPN include: (1) accumulation of proteins in neuronal (dorsal root ganglia) and supportive cells; (2) mitochondrial-mediated neural apoptosis (as seen in *in vitro* studies when bortezomib was combined with calcium modulators); (3) blockade of transcription (of nerve growth factor); (4) increased tubulin polymerization and microtubule stabilization (Landowski et al., 2005; Poruchynsky et al., 2008). Incidence of BiPN can range between 44% and 70% (Jagannath et al., 2004; Richardson et al., 2012). Early recognition is of the greatest importance, with appropriate dose modification to prevent progression and severe symptoms. Symptomatic neuropathy, once present, can improve or completely resolve, in about 60–64% of patients, after completion or interruption in bortezomib therapy (Richardson et al., 2009b; Dimopoulos et al., 2011). Bortezomib administration via subcutaneous route (as opposed to intravenous) results in a significantly lower rate of BiPN with no loss in efficacy (Moreau et al., 2011). Weekly as opposed to twice-weekly bortezomib also results in significantly decreased rates of PN with equal efficacy (Bringhen et al., 2010).

A newer, irreversible proteasome inhibitor, carfilzomib, was recently (July 2012) FDA approved for patients with relapsed MM. The incidence of PN with carfilzomib appears to be lower than in bortezomib-treated patients, estimated at 10–15% (in contrast to 44–70% with bortezomib), with only 1.1% being grade 3 or higher (O'Connor et al., 2009; Siegel et al., 2012). Another similar agent in development, marizomib, is also showing promising low incidences of PN (Richardson et al., 2009a).

Thalidomide, as described above, is an immuno-modulatory agent used in the treatment of MM with neuropathy being a major side-effect. Incidence of thalidomide-induced peripheral neuropathy (TiPN) increases with duration of therapy, with an overall estimate of 40–75% (Richardson et al., 2012). Pathogenesis has been proposed to include dorsal root ganglia degeneration, wallerian degeneration and demyelination through downregulation of tumor necrosis factor-α (TNF-α) (Chaudhry et al., 2002; Giannini et al., 2003). Neuropathy is sensorimotor with preferential degeneration of the longest axons. Unlike BiPN, TiPN can be permanent and emerge even after therapy has been stopped. Newer agents in this class, lenalidomide (FDA approved) and pomalidomide (not yet FDA approved) have been associated with substantially lower rates and much less severe PN (Richardson et al., 2012).

Cisplatin and vincristine are other agents that are occasionally used in MM treatment. The neuropathy with these agents tends to be distal symmetric sensorimotor. About 10–13% of MM patients develop PN with vincristine but no specific data on cisplatin and MM patients are available; in other malignancies cisplatin has been shown to cause long-term peripheral sensory nerve damage (Cavaletti et al., 1994; Dimopoulos et al., 2003).

Careful monitoring for treatment-related PN, early recognition of symptoms, and early intervention are necessary to prevent progression to more severe, debilitating, neuropathy. Appropriate guideline-driven dose adjustment and discontinuation of the offending medication(s) is indicated. Early dose modification may allow for ongoing use of the drug and its therapeutic effect, while possibly improving existing neurologic symptoms and more importantly preventing further damage. If needed, symptomatic treatment with antiepileptics, antidepressants, calcium channel α2-δ ligands (gabapentin, pregabalin), and opioids can be tried, as long as the underlying cause of neuropathy has been addressed. α-Lipoic acid and antidepressant venlafaxine have appeared promising in patients with colorectal cancer and treatment-related neuropathy (Gedlicka et al., 2002; Barton et al., 2011). Other agents including acetyl-L-carnitine, topical baclofen, amitriptyline, ketamine, and topical methanol creams appear effective as well (Richardson et al., 2012). Unfortunately there is no proven porphylaxis for treatment-related PN but multivitamis (vitamins B, E, B_{12}, folic acid), magnesium, amino acid, omega-3 fatty acids and fish oil supplements can be tried; however, this is based on anecdotal evidence alone (Richardson et al., 2012). Of note, pre-existing neuropathy or the use of combination therapy with both drugs being neurotoxic (e.g., bortezomib-thalidomide), are not contraindications to initiation (or retreatment) with bortezomib-containing regimens, but more vigilant monitoring is required in such instances.

Multiple myeloma and the central nervous system

EPIDURAL DISEASE IN MULTIPLE MYELOMA

Spinal cord compression occurs in approximately 20% of patients with MM (Colak et al., 1989). Most commonly it results from vertebral body collapse due to myeloma bone involvement (Byrne, 1992) (Fig. 73.2). Less frequently, plasma cell tumors (also known as plasmacytoma(s)) can extend into the epidural space causing spinal cord compression (Blumenthal and Glenn, 2002) (Fig. 73.3). A majority (60%) of epidural metastases arise in the thoracic spine while 30% arise in the lumbosacral spine (Drappatz and Batchelor, 2004).

Symptoms of spinal cord compression can include back pain, weakness (present in 60–85% of patients), sensory deficits (with a sensory level usually 1–5 segments below the anatomic level of cord compression), Lhermitte's sign (characterized by electric shock-like sensation upon neck flexion), as well as bowel and bladder disturbances (which tend to occur late in the disease process) (Drappatz and Batchelor, 2004). Early recognition of these symptoms is important as neurologic status

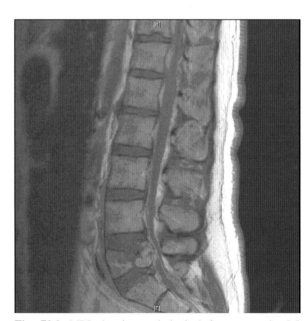

Fig. 73.2. MRI showing pathological fracture at the L5 vertebral body with retropulsion of the bony fragments causing central canal stenosis and mass effect on the lumbar nerve roots. Pathology confirmed plasma cell infiltration (plasmacytoma). (Figure courtesy of Edward Melian, M.D., Loyola University Medical Center.)

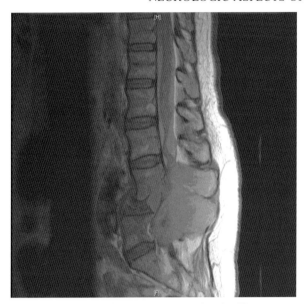

Fig. 73.3. MRI showing a large mass with significant retrolisthesis of L4 and L5 with almost complete destruction of the L4 and L5 vertebral bodies and posterior elements. There is near complete effacement of the central spinal canal. Mass was biopsy proven plasmacytoma. (Figure courtesy of Edward Melian, M.D., Loyola University Medical Center.)

at the time of diagnosis predicts outcome after treatment (Maranzano and Latini, 1995). Spinal cord compression requires immediate diagnosis and appropriate emergent treatment to prevent permanent motor and sensory damage. Corticosteroids with urgent radiation therapy are appropriate. Occasionally decompressive surgery is required, especially when the diagnosis is uncertain, the bulk of tumor is located posteriorly, or there is associated spine instability. Bisphosphonate therapy in MM can reduce pain associated with lytic lesions and significantly reduce skeletal-related events (such as vertebral pathologic fractures) (Morgan et al., 2010).

LEPTOMENINGEAL INVOLVEMENT

Involvement of leptomeninges by clonal plasma cells of MM is very rare, estimated at about 1% (Mendez et al., 2010). Pathogenesis is thought to be due to hematogenous spread (as opposed to direct extension from bone). Leptomeningeal infiltration can be focal, multifocal, or diffuse. Diffuse involvement of the leptomeninges is also referred to as CNS myelomatosis (Mendez et al., 2010). Patients can present with cranial nerve palsies, paraparesis, seizures, or confusion. Obstructive hydrocephalus from leptomeningeal infiltration has been described (Dennis and Chu, 2000). Primary dural involvement is rare but has been described primarily in case reports (Mendez et al., 2010). Cerebrospinal fluid (CSF) analysis in patients with meningeal involvement

shows plasma cells within the CSF, significantly increased protein with detectable M protein on protein electrophoresis of the CSF.

Treatment of leptomeningeal disease includes intrathecal chemotherapy, systemic chemotherapy, and cranial irradiation (Mendez et al., 2010). Prognosis is poor with a median survival of only 1.5–3 months (Mendez et al., 2010).

INTRACRANIAL PLASMACYTOMA

Plasmacytomas can be found in the vertebral column, as described above, as well as intracranially. Solitary intracranial plasmacytomas have been described in the pituitary, typically with preserved pituitary function and associated cranial nerve neuropathies (McLaughlin et al., 2004). They have also been described to involve the orbit and base of skull with involvement of the neural foramina or distortion of nerves by tumor masses (Cerase et al., 2008). Metastatic involvement of the mandible can lead to unilateral chin hypoesthesia ("numb chin syndrome"), which can be present in about 10–15% of MM patients (Hogan et al., 2002). Treatment for intracranial plasmacytomas is typically surgery followed by radiation therapy, or radiation therapy alone if the tumor is unresectable (Cerase et al., 2008). Solitary plasmacytomas (outside of the CNS) are described in greater detail below.

METABOLIC DISTURBANCES

Encephalopathy and cranial nerve palsies can also result from metabolic derangements including hypercalcemia, uremia, and hyperviscosity. Hypercalcemia of malignancy is common in MM patients, estimated to occur in about 30% of MM patients at some point during the course of the disease (Mundy, 1998) and in 13% of newly diagnosed patients (Kyle et al., 2003). Hypercalcemia is caused by increased bone resorption by osteoclasts which is driven by a variety of mediators including interleukin (IL)-6, IL-1, tumor necrosis factor-β and macrophage inflammatory protein (Drappatz and Batchelor, 2004). Increased bone resorption can be appreciated as lytic lesions on plain radiographs. Neurologic symptoms of hypercalcemia include weakness, confusion, headache, even coma and seizures. Other symptoms include nausea, vomiting, anorexia, constipation, abdominal pain, increased thirst and urination (from hypercalcemia-induced nephrogenic diabetes insipidus). Treatment consists of immediate lowering of the serum calcium with aggressive hydration (with or without loop diuretics) or hemodialysis in severe cases or in patients who cannot tolerate hydration. Equally important is decreasing bone resorption and calcium release into the bloodstream by inhibiting osteoclast activity with bisophosphonates (and/or calcitonin).

Hyperviscosity due to hypergammaglobulinemia can occur in MM; however, it is much more common in Waldenström macroglobulinemia (10–30% in WM and 2–6% in MM) (Mehta and Singhal, 2003). Hyperviscosity syndrome is discussed in greater detail below under Waldenström macroglobulinemia.

NONSECRETORY MYELOMA

Rarely, patients with symptomatic MM do not have a detectable M protein in the serum or urine (Table 73.3). These patients are categorized as having nonsecretory MM, estimated to occur in only 3% of MM patients (International Myeloma Working Group, 2003). With more sensitive testing, including free light chain assays (to identify patients with light chain only MM) the incidence of true nonsecretory MM may actually be lower. Renal insufficiency is less common in these patients. Neurologic complications in patients with nonsecretory MM have not been well described, likely due to the rarity of the disorder. Treatment and prognosis of nonsecretory MM are similar to symptomatic MM.

SOLITARY PLASMACYTOMA

Solitary plasmacytoma (plasma cell tumor) is the only known potentially curable plasma cell disorder. It can arise in bone or soft tissue. When it is confined to bone it is categorized as solitary bone plasmacytoma (also known as intramedullary plasmacytoma or osteosclerotic myeloma); when it occurs in soft tissue sites (most commonly the upper respiratory tract but also CNS, gastrointestinal tract, bladder, thyroid, breast, testes, parotid gland, and lymph nodes) it is called extramedullary plasmacytoma (Rajkumar et al., 2006). In patients with plasma cell disorders, the incidence of solitary plasmacytoma is only 3–5% (International Myeloma Working Group, 2003). The diagnosis is confirmed by biopsy-proven solitary lesion of bone or soft tissue with clonal plasma cells but normal bone marrow with no clonal plasma cells, normal skeletal survey, and MRI of spine/pelvis and no evidence of end organ damage (anemia, hypercalcemia, renal failure, or additional lytic bone lesion) (Rajkumar et al., 2006). Patients with solitary plasmacytoma are at risk of progression to multiple myeloma (with higher progression rate in patients with solitary bone plasmacytoma as opposed to extramedullary plasmacytoma). Patients with solitary bone plasmacytomas may also have systemic manifestations such as POEMS syndrome (described below).

Solitary plasmacytoma, a potentially curable plasma cell disorder, is in contrast to multiple plasmacytomas, which tend to occur in late stages of the disease and in high-risk MM (as defined by Table 73.5). Radiation therapy alone may be a treatment option for solitary plasmacytoma but systemic therapy is indicated in patients with multiple plasmacytomas and MM.

Neurologic complications from plasmacytomas can vary depending on the location of mass effect (spinal cord versus intracranial), as described above.

POEMS SYNDROME

POEMS syndrome is a rare paraneoplastic syndrome due to an underlying plasma cell disorder (Dispenzieri, 2012). POEMS syndrome can have multisystem manifestations as represented by the acronym, which refers to the constellation of salient signs and symptoms: polyneuropathy, organomegaly, endocrinopathy, M protein, and skin changes. It is also known as osteosclerotic myeloma, Crow–Fukase syndrome and Takatsuki syndrome (Rajkumar et al., 2006). Diagnostic criteria required for POEMS syndrome are listed in Table 73.6. Patients with

Table 73.6

POEMS syndrome diagnostic criteria

Mandatory major criteria (both required):
1. Monoclonal plasma cell disorder
2. Peripheral neuropathy
Other major criteria (at least one is required):
1. Sclerotic bone lesions (single or multiple plasmacytoma(s))
2. Castleman disease (angiofollicular lymph node hyperplasia)
3. Vascular endothelial growth factor (VEGF) elevation
Minor criteria (at least one is required):
1. Organomegaly (hepatomegaly, splenomegaly, lymphadenopathy)
2. Endocrinopathy (adrenal, thyroid, pituitary, gonadal, parathyroid, pancreatic)[†]
3. Edema (anasarca, pleural effusion, ascites)
4. Typical skin changes (hyperpigmentation, hypertrichpsis, plethora, hemangioma, white nails, acrocyanosis, thickening)
5. Papilledema
6. Thrombocytosis/erythrocytosis
Other signs and symptoms:
Clubbing, weight loss, hyperhidrosis, pulmonary hypertension/restrictive lung disease, thrombotic diatheses, diarrhea, low vitamin B_{12} values

Note: not every patient who meets these criteria will have POEMS syndrome; features should be in temporal relationship with no other attributable cause. Absence of osteoclerotic lesions or Castleman disease should make the diagnosis suspect. Elevations in plasma or serum levels of VEGF (vascular endothelial growth factor) and thrombocytosis are commonly present and may help with the diagnosis.
[†]Hypothyroidism and diabetes mellitus alone are not sufficient to meet this criteria.
(Modified from Rajkumar, 2012.)

POEMS syndrome tend to be younger (median 51 years), usually men, and can have an indolent or a fulminant disease course (Rajkumar et al., 2006). Typical monoclonal protein is IgG or IgA with almost exclusively λ light chain restriction (Katirji and Koontz, 2012). The prognosis for patients with POEMS syndrome is poor but clinical improvement can occur after the disappearance of the monoclonal protein. If a solitary bone plasmacytoma or < 3 plasmacytomas are detected in a patient with POEMS syndrome, treatment with radiation therapy may be effective in controlling the symptoms (Dispenzieri, 2012). Patients with more diffuse bone lesions or clonal plasma cells on bone marrow biopsies should be treated with systemic chemotherapy, resembling that of MM and light chain amyloidosis.

POEMS syndrome and peripheral neuropathy

Neuropathy is the main feature in these patients and actually a requirement for the diagnosis of POEMS syndrome (Table 73.6). Patients have symmetric distal, ascending, motor neuropathy with variable sensory loss (Katirji and Koontz, 2012). Neuropathy can be progressive, debilitating, and painful. Electrophysiologic testing reveals demyelinating neuropathy with superimposed or secondary axonal loss (Ramchandren and Lewis, 2012; Rajabally, 2011). Nerve biopsy can show endoneurial deposits and uncompacted myelin lamellae (Vital, 2001). Neuropathy may improve (although slowly) with successful treatment of the underlying plasma cell disorder.

WALDENSTRÖM MACROGLOBULINEMIA

Waldenström macroglobulinemia (WM), also known as lymphoplasmacytic lymphoma, is a low-grade IgM producing lymphoid and plasma cell disorder. Median age at diagnosis is 65 years with a slight male predominance (Rajkumar et al., 2006). Diagnosis is confirmed by the presence of monoclonal IgM, >10% bone marrow lymphoplasmacytic infiltration with a characteristic immunophenotype (Rajkumar et al., 2006). Treatment for patients with WM is indicated if they have disease-associated anemia, thrombocytopenia, constitutional symptoms (weakness/fatigue, weight loss, night sweats), hyperviscosity, symptomatic cryoglobulinemia, significant hepatosplenomegaly, or lymphadenopathy.

Waldenström macroglobulinemia and peripheral neuropathy

PN occurs in about one-third of patients with WM (Katirji and Koontz, 2012). Typically it is chronic, symmetric, predominantly sensory neuropathy, similar to IgM-MGUS PN. Anti-MAG antibodies can be found in about 50% of WM patients (Katirji and Koontz, 2012). Electrophysiologic studies demonstrate demyelination, similar to IgM-MGUS. Treatment is geared at the underlying disease process with some responses in neuropathy symptoms. WM can also produce cryoglobulinemia (described below), which may manifest with an immune-mediated vasculitis, leading to painful, distal symmetric sensorimotor neuropathy (Drappatz and Batchelor, 2004).

Waldenström macroglobulinemia and the central nervous system

HYPERVISCOSITY SYNDROME

The IgM antibody that is secreted by the malignant lymphoplasmacytic cells is a multivalent molecule that has the tendency to aggregate, leading to slowing of the cerebral and retinal circulation resulting in symptoms due to transient ischemia (Drappatz and Batchelor, 2004). Symptoms usually occur when IgM levels are > 3 g/dL and/or serum viscosity is ≥ 4.0 centipoise (normal 1.4–1.8 centipoise), although this may vary among individual patients (Mehta and Singhal, 2003). The clinical triad of hyperviscosity syndrome includes neurologic symptoms, vision changes, and mucosal bleeding (Ghobrial et al., 2003). Neurologic symptoms include dizziness, headache, vertigo, ataxia, confusion, syncope, and stroke. Vision changes include blurry vision and diplopia with fundoscopic examination revealing papilledema, tortuosity of veins and thrombosis (Ghobrial et al., 2003). Mucosal bleeding in the oropharynx, gastrointestinal tract, ureter, or vagina can occur as the monoclonal IgM interferes with platelet function. Rarely patients can have retinal and intracranial hemorrhage. As a result of increased plasma volume patients may experience dyspnea, chest pain, pulmonary edema, or congestive heart failure.

Treatment is aimed at emergently decreasing the IgM level in order to provide rapid relief of symptoms and avoid long-term complications. In severe situations this can be quickly achieved with aggressive intravenous hydration and plasmapheresis. Long-term management consists of systemic chemotherapy in order to decrease the IgM production.

Much less frequently, MM can result in hyperviscosity syndrome. This can be seen when IgG levels are > 4 g/dL and IgA levels > 6 g/dL along with increased serum viscosity (Mehta and Singhal, 2003).

BING–NEEL SYNDROME

Bing–Neel syndrome is an extremely rare neurologic complication of WM and usually presents late in the disease course. It occurs when the neoplastic lymphoplasmacytic or plasma cells infiltrate the perivascular spaces, leptomeninges, and/or brain parenchyma in the CNS. These infiltrates can be found in other organs as well, including bone marrow, lymph nodes, spleen, and liver. The infiltrate may be diffuse in the CNS, causing symptoms of confusion and lethargy. Alternatively, the cells may coalesce into tumors with symptoms mainly from mass effect including paralysis and seizures (Malkani et al., 2009). Additional symptoms can include headache, blurry vision, psychiatric manifestations, numbness, paresthesias, hearing loss, and weakness. CSF analysis can show leukocytosis (WBC 100–500 cells/mm^3), elevated total protein (>100 mg/dL), normal or decreased glucose, and hypergammaglobulinemia with detectable M protein on protein electrophoresis and IgM confirmation on immunofixation of the CSF (Malkani et al., 2009). These CSF abnormalities are more common in diffuse rather than coalescent CNS disease. Brain imaging can be normal or show regions of enhancement on T2-weighted MRI images and occasionally tumoral or nodular masses on CT scans (Grewal et al., 2009).

Treatment includes intrathecal chemotherapy and radiation therapy (focal or cariospinal radiation therapy),

along with systemic chemotherapy. Preliminary data suggest a role for intrathecal rituximab; however, additional studies are needed to evaluate dosing and potential toxicities before it can be recommended as a treatment option (Rubenstein et al., 2007). Due to the rarity of the disease, randomized controlled studies which establish the treatment recommendations in this disease have been difficult to do and will continue to be a challenge. Fortunately, with treatment, patients can have an improvement in their quality of life and remission can be achieved, with some patients having a sustained, long-lasting remission (Grewal et al., 2009).

AL AMYLOIDOSIS (IMMUNOGLOBULIN LIGHT CHAIN AMYLOIDOSIS)

Amyloidosis refers to the deposition of insoluble fibrillar proteins in various tissues (Kyle et al., 2005). The deposited protein is detected by Congo red staining based on characteristic apple-green birefringence under polarized light (Gertz et al., 2005). Amyloidosis consists of several distinct types, based on the protein composition of the amyloid fibril, as seen in Table 73.7. Only one

Table 73.7

Classification of amyloidosis

Type of amyloidosis	Precursor protein component	Symptoms
AL amyloidosis*	λ or κ immunoglobulin light chain (λ is more common; λ to κ ratio, 3:1)	Systemic: nephrotic syndrome, restrictive cardiomyopathy, neuropathy Localized: isolated organ involvement (e.g., carpal tunnel syndrome, isolated lesions in ureter, urethra, bladder, lung, bronchus or trachea)
AA amyloidosis[†]	Serum amyloid A protein	Renal presentation most common, associated with chronic inflammatory conditions
ATTR amyloidosis		
Mutant TTR[‡]	Mutated transthyretin	Hereditary; peripheral neuropathy and/or cardiomyopathy (commonly referred to as familial amyloid polyneuropathy)
Normal TTR[‡]	Normal transthyretin	Restrictive cardiomyopathy; carpal tunnel syndrome (commonly referred to as senile amyloidosis)
β$_2$-microglobulin amyloidosis	β$_2$-microglobulin	Carpal tunnel syndrome (associated with long-term dialysis)
Aβ amyloidosis	Aβ protein precursor	Alzheimer's syndrome
Other hereditary amyloidosis		
A fibrinogen	Fibrinogen α-chain	Renal presentation (also called familial renal amyloidosis)
Lysozyme	Lysozyme	Renal presentation most common
Apolipoprotein A-I	Apolipoprotein A-I	Renal presentation most common

*Previously referred to as primary amyloidosis; the only amyloidosis secondary to a plasma cell disorder.
[†]Previously referred to as secondary amyloidosis.
[‡]TTR, transthyretin (prealbumin).
(Modified from Rajkumar et al., 2006.)

form of amyloidosis is secondary to a clonal plasma cell disorder, AL amyloidosis (also referred to as immunoglobulin light chain amyloidosis and previously known as primary systemic amyloidosis). Diagnostic criteria for AL amyloidosis are listed in Table 73.8. Potential areas to biopsy for tissue confirmation of amyloid deposition include the affected organ (e.g., heart, kidney, peripheral nerve, rectum), bone marrow, or abdominal fat. In clinical practice the diagnosis can be quite challenging and often delayed given the vague constellation of symptoms, which mimic more common diseases.

AL amyloidosis may be localized or systemic. Localized AL amyloidosis is often benign, can affect isolated organ systems (e.g., carpal tunnel syndrome) and treatment consists primarily of symptom relief. Systemic AL amyloidosis, on the other hand, can have profound multisystem involvement and requires treatment with chemotherapy and stem cell transplantation in transplant-eligible patients. Presentation may be variable depending on dominant organ involvement, with nephrotic syndrome, restrictive cardiomyopathy, peripheral and autonomic neuropathy being most common. Patients may also have macroglossia, carpal tunnel syndrome, organomegaly, weight loss, and periorbital and face purpura ("raccoon eyes sign") (Rajkumar et al., 2006). AL amyloidosis can coexist with MM in 10% of patients but typically one of the two disorders dominates the clinical picture (Rajkumar et al., 2006). Improvement in organ dysfunction can be seen in about 50% of responding patients and prolonged organ remission can be achieved with stem cell transplantation (Rajkumar et al., 2006). Overall prognosis is poor but improving over the years thanks to the advances in therapy, stem cell transplantation and supportive care. Patients with confirmed amyloidosis need to be referred to tertiary medical center for a thorough evaluation and appropriate management.

AL amyloidosis and peripheral neuropathy

Amyloid neuropathy can be present in about 17–35% of patients with AL amyloidosis and is the presenting manifestation in 10% (Kyle and Gertz, 1995; Matsuda et al., 2011). It is a progressive, usually painful sensory polyneuropathy, with or without autonomic dysfunction. Neuropathy may be asymmetric, worse distally than proximal, with lower limbs being affected earlier than upper limbs (i.e., length-dependent neuropathy). Pain and temperature sensation are lost before light touch or vibratory sense and motor neuropathy tends to appear after sensory loss (Drappatz and Batchelor, 2004). Patients typically complain of burning, painful electrical sensations as well as symptoms of carpal tunnel syndrome, which may be present in up to 25% of patients and is due to amyloid deposition in the flexor retinaculum (Katirji and Koontz, 2012). Electrophysiologic studies show an axonal, sensory greater than motor neuropathy (Ramchandren and Lewis, 2012). Nerve biopsy can confirm the diagnosis by identifying endoneurial amyloid deposits. This direct toxin effect and amyloid-induced vascular insufficiency have been proposed as possible mechanisms in the pathogenesis of neuropathy. Unfortunately there is no clear evidence that treatment directed at the underlying plasma cell disorder improves symptoms of PN.

Autonomic neuropathy is frequently present. It may present with symptoms due to orthostatic hypotension, impotence, bladder dysfunction, or gastrointestinal dysfunction. Symptomatic treatment with elastic stockings, fluorinated steroids, or dihydroergotamine may be helpful in patients with orthostatic hypotension.

AL amyloidosis and the central nervous system

A subset of amyloid fibrils can deposit in the CNS; examples include amyloid β (Aβ, responsible for some cases of Alzheimer's disease), transthyretin (TTR), and British amyloid protein (BR12) (Lee and Picken, 2012). Common symptoms include cognitive decline, dementia, stroke, and less frequently, symptoms due to mass effect. AL amyloidosis is extremely rare in the CNS but has been reported in the literature with clinical manifestations related to amyloidoma and leptomeningeal cerebral amyloid angiopathy.

CNS amyloidoma contains light chain amyloid which can form nodules or space-occupying lesions within the brain parenchyma or vertebral spinal axis (Tabatabai et al., 2005; Lee and Picken, 2012). CNS amyloidoma can occur in patients with or without evidence of

Table 73.8

Diagnostic criteria for AL amyloidosis

Diagnosis (all four required)	Signs and symptoms
1. Amyloid related systemic syndrome*	Fatigue, weight loss, proteinuria (nephrotic range), CHF, hepatomegaly, peripheral and autonomic neuropathy
2. Positive Congo red staining in any tissue	
3. Light chain confirmation†	
4. Clonal plasma cell disorder‡	

*Nephrotic syndrome, restrictive cardiomyopathy, hepatomegaly, malabsorption, peripheral or autonomic neuropathy (axonal neuropathy).
†By direct examination of the amyloid using mass spectrometry.
‡M-protein, abnormal free light chain ratio, or clonal plasma cells.
CHF, congestive heart failure.
(Modified from Rajkumar, 2012.)

systemic amyloidosis or plasma cell dyscrasia. Leptomeningeal cerebral amyloid angiopathy occurs when light chain amyloid fibrils deposit in small- and medium-sized blood vessels, similarly to the more common amyloid angiopathy in Alzheimer's disease with amyloid β deposition (Lee and Picken, 2012). Focal intracranial hemorrhages have been reported as a complication of amyloid angiopathy. Unfortunately there is no effective treatment for this complication; supportive care and symptom relief are recommended.

CRYOGLOBULINEMIA

Cryoglobulins are immunoglobulins that precipitate when cooled and dissolve when heated. Cryoglobulins are classified into three types: type I is monoclonal, type II is mixed (one monoclonal immunoglobulin the other polyclonal, most commonly associated with hepatitis C infection), and type III is strictly polyclonal (without monoclonal immunoglobulins). Type I cryoglobulinemia is most commonly of the IgM or IgG class and is associated with Waldenström macroglobulinemia, MM, or MGUS (Drappatz and Batchelor, 2004). It is estimated that 5–7% of patients with MM and 20% of patients with WM have an associated cryoglobulinemia (Bloch and Franklin, 1982).

Patients with cryoglobulinemia can be asymptomatic or can present with Raynaud's phenomenon, purpura, acrocyanosis, and skin ulceration. Other manifestations can include arthralgias, renal disease, and neuropathy. Treatment usually consists of rewarming and decreasing the immunoglobulin concentration by plasma exchange, with systemic chemotherapy if cryoglobulinemia is driven by underlying MM or WM (type I cryoglobulinemia). Therapy in type II should be directed at the underlying hepatitis C infection, if present.

Cryoglobulinemia and peripheral neuropathy

Peripheral neuropathy has been reported in 17–56% of patients with cryoglobulinemia (Hoffman-Snyder and Smith, 2008). Neuropathy in type I (monoclonal) cryoglobulinemia is infrequent but a lot more common in type II and III cryoglobulinemia. Presentations of neuropathy can range from subacute mononeuritis multiplex to a chronic distal symmetric sensorimotor polyneuropathy, with sensory symptoms usually preceding motor dysfunction (Garcia-Bragado et al., 1988). Neuropathy is most often characterized by axonal degeneration with some reports of demyelination, either primary demyelination or secondary to axonal damage (Ropper and Gorson, 1998). Nerve biopsy can show epineurial vasculitis and epineurial cryoglobulin deposits (which have been described in MM and WM) (Vital

et al., 1991). Improvement in symptoms of neuropathy, even with treatment of the underlying cause, may be slow and very limited.

CONCLUSION

Plasma cell disorders range from benign and indolent to malignant and aggressive disease processes. Clinical manifestations are variable and an array of neurologic complications can be present. Although the impact on the peripheral central nervous system is far more common, the clinical implications are typically greater with central nervous system involvement. Peripheral neuropathy is the most common complication and symptoms may vary from mild to debilitating, pure sensory to sensorimotor. Treatment of the underlying plasma cell disorder is often ineffective at controlling or improving neuropathy and, in fact, treatment of the underlying malignancy may cause or exacerbate the neuropathy. Symptomatic relief is necessary, though not always successful or adequate. Central nervous system involvement is rare, can have variable etiologies and symptoms, and usually carries a poor prognosis with limited treatment options. Recognition of the underlying plasma cell disorder is of great importance as it requires a proper diagnostic evaluation, surveillance, and treatment, if indicated.

REFERENCES

Altekruse SF, Kosary CL, Krapcho M et al. (Eds.), (2007). SEER Cancer Statistics Review, 1975–2007. National Cancer Institute, Bethesda, MD, http://seer.cancer.gov/csr/1975_2007/, based on November 2009 SEER data submission, posted to the SEER website, 2010.

Arbogast SD, Khanna S, Koontz DW et al. (2007). Chronic ataxic neuropathy mimicking dorsal midbrain syndrome. J Neurol Neurosurg Psychiatry 78: 1276–1277.

Barton DL, Wos EJ, Qin R et al. (2011). A double-blind, placebo-controlled trial of a topical treatment for chemotherapy-induced peripheral neuropathy: NCCTG trial N06CA. Support Care Cancer 19: 833–841.

Benedetti L, Briani C, Franciotta D et al. (2008). Long-term effect of rituximab in anti-MAG polyneuropathy. Neurology 71: 1742–1744.

Bloch KJ, Franklin E (1982). Plasma cell dyscrasias and cryoglobulins. JAMA 248: 2670–2676.

Blume G, Pestronk A, Goodnough LT (1995). Anti-MAG antibody-associated polyneuropathies: improvement following immunotherapy with monthly plasma exchange and IV cyclophosphamide. Neurology 45: 1577–1580.

Blumenthal DT, Glenn MJ (2002). Neurologic manifestations of hematologic disorders. Neurol Clin 20: 265–281.

Bringhen S, Larocca A, Rossi D et al. (2010). Efficacy and safety of once-weekly bortezomib in multiple myeloma. Blood 116: 4745–4753.

Byrne TN (1992). Spinal cord compression from epidural metastases. N Engl J Med 327: 614–649.

Cavaletti G, Bogliun G, Marzorati L et al. (1994). Long-term peripheral neurotoxicity of cisplatin in patients with successfully treated epithelial ovarian cancer. Anticancer Res 14: 1287–1292.

Cerase A, Tarantino A, Gozzetti A et al. (2008). Intracranial involvement in plasmacytomas and multiple myeloma: a pictorial essay. Neuroradiology 50: 665–674.

Chaudhry V, Cornblath DR, Corse A et al. (2002). Thalidomide-induced neuropathy. Neurology 59: 877–878.

Colak A, Cataltepe O, Erbengi A (1989). Spinal cord compression caused by plasmacytomas: a retrospective series of 14 cases. Neurosurg Rev 12: 305–308.

Dalakas MC, Rakocevic G, Salajegheh M et al. (2009). Placebo-controlled trial of rituximab in IgM anti-myelin-associated glycoprotein antibody demyelinating neuropathy. Ann Neurol 65: 286–293.

Dennis M, Chu P (2000). A case of meningeal myeloma presenting as obstructive hydrocephalus – a therapeutic challenge. Leuk Lymphoma 40: 219–220.

Dimopoulos MA, Pouli A, Zervas K et al. (2003). Propsective randomized comparison of vincristine, doxorubicin and dexamethasone (VAD) administered as intravenous bolus injection and VAD with liposomal doxorubicin as first-line treatment in multiple myeloma. Ann Oncol 14: 1039–1044.

Dimopoulos MA, Mateos MV, Richardson PG et al. (2011). Risk factors for, and reversibility of, peripheral neuropathy associated with bortezomib-melphalan-prednisone in newly diagnosed patients with multiple myeloma: subanalysis of the phase 3 VISTA study. Eur J Haematol 86: 23–31.

Dispenzieri A (2012). POEMS syndrome: update on diagnosis, risk-stratification, and management. Am J Hematol 87: 805–814.

Drappatz J, Batchelor T (2004). Neurologic compications of plasma cell disorders. Clin Lymphoma 5: 163–171.

Eurelings M, Moons KGM, Notermans NC et al. (2001). Neuropathy and IgM M proteins: prognostic value of antibodies to MAG, SGPD, and sulfatide. Neurology 56: 228–233.

Garcia-Bragado F, Fernandez JM, Navarro C et al. (1988). Peripheral neuropathy in essential mixed cryoglobulinemia. Arch Neurol 45: 1210–1214.

Gedlicka C, Scheithauer W, Schull B et al. (2002). Effective treatment of oxaliplatin-induced cumulative polyneuropathy with alpha-lipoic acid. J Clin Oncol 20: 3359–3361.

Gertz MA (2006). Managing monoclonal gammopathy-associated neuropathy. Leuk Lymphoma 47: 785–786.

Gertz MA, Lacy MQ, Dispenzieri A et al. (2005). Amyloidosis. Best Pract Res Clin Haematol 18: 709–727.

Ghobrial IM, Gertz MA, Fonseca R (2003). Waldenström macroglobulinaemia. Lancet Oncol 4: 679–685.

Giannini F, Volpi N, Rossi S et al. (2003). Thalidomide-induced neuropathy: a gangliopathy? Neurology 60: 877–878.

Grewal JS, Preetkanwal KB, Sahijdak WM et al. (2009). Bing–Neel syndrome: a case report and systematic review of clinical manifestations, diagnosis, and treatment options. Clin Lymphoma Myeloma 9: 462–466.

Hadden RD, Nobile-Orazio E, Sommer CL et al. (2010). European Federation of Neurological Societies/Peripheral Nerve Society Guideline on management of paraproteinemic demyelinating neuropathies. Report of a Joint Task Force of the European Federation of Neurological Societies and the Peripheral Nerve Society – first revision. J Peripher Nerv Syst 15: 185–195.

Hoffman-Snyder C, Smith BE (2008). Neuromuscular disorders associated with paraproteinemia. Phys Med Rehabil Clin N Am 19: 61–79.

Hogan MC, Lee A, Solberg LA et al. (2002). Unusual presentation of multiple myeloma with unilateral visual loss and numb chin syndrome in a young adult. Am J Hematol 70: 55–59.

International Myeloma Working Group (2003). Criteria for the classification of monoclonal gammopathies, multiple myeloma and related disorders: a report of the International Myeloma Working Group. Br J Haematol 121: 749–757.

Jagannath S, Barlogie B, Berenson J et al. (2004). A phase 2 study of two doses of bortezomib in relapse or refractory myeloma. Br J Haematol 127: 165–172.

Katirji B, Koontz D (2012). Disorders of peripheral nerves. In: RB Daroff, GM Fenichel, J Jankovic et al. (Eds.), Bradley's Neurology in Clinical Practice. Vol. II. Elsevier, Philadelphia, pp. 1971–1976.

Kelly JJ, Kyle RA, O'Brien PC et al. (1981). Prevalence of monoclonal protein in peripheral neuropathy. Neurology 31: 1480–1483.

Kyle RA, Gertz MA (1995). Primary systemic amyloidosis: clinical and laboratory features in 474 cases. Semin Hematol 32: 45–49.

Kyle RA, Rajkumar SV (2009). Treatment of multiple myeloma: a comprehensive review. Clin Lymphoma Myeloma 9: 278–288.

Kyle RA, Therneau TM, Rajkumar SV et al. (2002). A long term study of prognosis in monoclonal gammopathy of undetermined significance. N Engl J Med 346: 564–569.

Kyle RA, Gertz MA, Witzig TE et al. (2003). Review of 1027 patients with newly diagnosed multiple myeloma. Mayo Clin Proc 78: 21–33.

Kyle RA, Kelly JJ, Dyck PJ (2005). Amyloidosis and neuropathy. In: PJ Dyck, PK Thomas (Eds.), Peripheral Neuropathy. 4th edn. Elsevier Saunders, Philadelphia, pp. 2427–2451.

Kyle RA, Therneau TM, Rajkumar SV et al. (2006). Prevelance of monoclonal gammopathy of undetermined significance. N Engl J Med 354: 1362–1369.

Kyle RA, Remstein ED, Therneau TM et al. (2007). Clinical course and prognosis of smoldering (asymptomatic) multiple myeloma. N Engl J Med 356: 2582–2590.

Landowski TH, Megli CJ, Nullmeyer KD et al. (2005). Mitochondrial-mediated disregulation of Ca2 + is a critical determinant of Velcade (PS-34/bortezomib) cytotoxicity in myeloma cell lines. Cancer Res 65: 3828–3836.

Lee JM, Picken MM (2012). Cerebrovascular amyloidosis. In: MM Picken, A Dogan, GA Herrera (Eds.), Amyloid and Related Disorders, Surgical Pathology and Clinical Correlations. Springer Science + Business Media, New York, pp. 106–109.

Leger J-M, Viala K, Bombelli F et al. (2010). For the RIMAG trial group (France and Switzerland): randomized controlled trial of rituximab in demyelinating neuropathy associated with anti-MAG IgM gammopathy (RIMAG study). J Peripher Nerv Syst 15: 269.

Lunn MP, Nobile-Orazio E (2006). Immunotherapy for IgM anti-myelin associated glycoprotein paraprotein associated neuropathy. Cochrane Database Syst Rev (2): CD002827.

Malkani RG, Tallman M, Gottardi-Littell N et al. (2009). Bing–Neel syndrome: an illustrative case and a comprehensive review of the published literature. J Neurooncol 96: 301–312.

Maranzano E, Latini P (1995). Effectiveness of radiation therapy without surgery in metastatic spinal cord compression: final results from a prospective trial. Int J Radiat Oncol Biol Phys 32: 959–967.

Matsuda M, Gono T, Morita H et al. (2011). Peripheral nerve involvement in primary systemic AL amyloidosis. Eur J Neurol 18: 604–610.

McLaughlin DM, Gray WJ, Jones FGC et al. (2004). Plasmacytoma: an unusual cause of a pituitary mass lesion. A case report and review of the literature. Pituitary 7: 179–181.

Mehta J, Singhal S (2003). Hyperviscosity syndrome in plasma cell dyscrasias. Semin Thromb Hemost 29: 467–471.

Mendez CE, Hwang BJ, Destian S et al. (2010). Intracranial multifocal dural involvement in multiple myeloma: case report and review of the literature. Clin Lymphoma Myeloma Leuk 10: 220–223.

Moreau P, Pylypenko H, Grosicki S et al. (2011). Subcuteous versus intravenous administration of bortezomib in patients with relapsed multiple myeloma: a randomised-phase 3 non-inferiority study. Lancet Oncol 12: 431–440.

Morgan GJ, Davies FE, Gregory WM et al. (2010). First-line treatment with zoledronic acid as compared with clodronic acid in multiple myeloma (MRC Myeloma IX): a randomised controlled trial. Lancet 376: 1989–1999.

Mundy GR (1998). Myeloma bone disease. Eur J Cancer 34: 246–251.

Notermans NC, Lokhorst HM, Franssen H et al. (1996). Intermittent cyclophosphamide and prednisone treatment or polyneuropathy associated with monoclonal gammopathy of undetermined significance. Neurology 47: 1227–1233.

O'Connor OA, Stewart AK, Vallone M et al. (2009). A phase I dose escalation study of the safety and pharmacokinetics of the novel proteasome inhibitor carfilzomib (PR-171) in patients with hematologic malignancies. Clin Cancer Res 15: 7085–7091.

Orlowski RZ, Kuhn DJ (2008). Proteasome inhibitors in cancer therapy: lessons from the first decade. Clin Cancer Res 14: 1649–1657.

Poruchynsky MS, Sackett DL, Robey RW et al. (2008). Proteasome inhibitors increase tubulin polymerization and stabilization in tissue culture cells: a possible mechanism contributing to peripheral neuropathy and cellular toxicity following proteasome inhibition. Cell Cycle 7: 940–949.

Rajabally YA (2011). Neuropathy and paraproteins: review of a complex association. Eur J Neurol 18: 1291–1298.

Rajkumar SV (2012). Multiple myeloma : 2012 update on diagnosis, risk-stratification, and management. Am J Hematol 87: 78–88.

Rajkumar SV, Dispenzieri A, Kyle RA (2006). Monoclonal gammopathy of undetermined significance, Waldenström macroglobulinemia, AL amyloidosis, and related plasma cell disorders: diagnosis and treatment. Mayo Clin Proc 81: 693–703.

Ramchandren S, Lewis RA (2012). An update on monoclonal gammopathy and neuropathy. Curr Neurol Neurosci Rep 12: 102–110.

Richardson PG, Sonneveld P, Schuster MW et al. (2009a). Reversibility of symptomatic peripheral neuropathy with bortezomib in the phase III APEX trial in relapsed multiple myeloma: impact of a dose-modification guideline. Br J Haematol 144: 895–903.

Richardson P, Hofmeister C, Jakubowiak A et al. (2009b). Phase 1 clinical trial of the novel structure proteasome inhibitor NPI-0052 in patients with relapsed and relapsed/refractory multiple myeloma. Blood (ASH Annual Meeting Abstracts), 114. Abstract 431.

Richardson PG, Delforge M, Beksac M et al. (2012). Management of treatment-emergent peripheral neuropathy in multiple myeloma. Leukemia 26: 595–608.

Ritz MF, Erne B, Ferracin F et al. (1999). Anti MAG IgM penetration into myelinated fibers correlates with the extent of myelin widening. Muscle Nerve 22: 1030–1037.

Ropper AH, Gorson KC (1998). Neuropathies associated with paraproteinemia. N Engl J Med 338: 1601–1607.

Rubenstein JL, Fridlyand J, Abrey L et al. (2007). Phase I study of intraventricular administration of rituximab in patients with recurrent CNS and intraocular lymphoma. J Clin Oncol 25: 1350–1356.

Sadiq SA, Thomas FP, Kilidireas K et al. (1990). The spectrum of neurologic disease associated with anti-DM1 antibodies. Neurology 40: 1067–1072.

Siegel DS, Martin T, Wang M et al. (2012). A phase 2 study of single-agent carfilzomib (PX-171-003-A1) in patients with relapsed and refractory multiple myeloma. Blood 120: 2817–2825.

Silberman J, Lonial S (2008). Review of peripheral neuropathy in plasma cell disorders. Hematol Oncol 26: 55–65.

Simmons Z, Tivakaran S (1996). Acquired demyelinating polyneuropathy presenting as a clinical sensory syndrome. Muscle Nerve 19: 1174–1176.

Simmons Z, Albers JW, Bromberg M et al. (1995). Long-term follow-up of patients with chronic inflammatory demyelinating polyradiculoneuropathy, without and with monoclonal gammopathy. Brain 118: 359–368.

Sonneveld P, Jongen JLM (2010). Dealing with neuropathy in plasma-cell dyscrasias. Hematology 423–430.

Tabatabai G, Boehring J, Hochberg FH (2005). Primary amyloidoma of the brain parenchyma. Arch Neurol 62: 477–480.

Vital A (2001). Paraproteinemic neuropathies. Brain Pathol 11: 399–407.

Vital A, Vital C, Ragnaud JM et al. (1991). IgM cryoglobulin deposits in the peripheral nerve. Virchows Arch A Pathol Anat Histopathol 418: 83–85.

Vrethem M, Cruz M, Wen Xin H et al. (1993). Clinical neurophysiological, and immunological evidence of polyneuropathy in patients with monoclonal gammopathies. J Neurol Sci 114: 193–199.

Willison HJ, O'Leary CP, Veitch J et al. (2001). The clinical and laboratory features of chronic sensory ataxic neuropathy with anti-disialosyl IgM antibodies. Brain 124: 1968–1977.

Yeung KB, Thomas PK, King RHM (1991). The clinical spectrum of peripheral neuropathies associated with benign monoclonal IgM, IgG and IgA paraproteinemia: comparative clinical immunological and nerve biopsy findings. J Neurol 238: 383–391.

Handbook of Clinical Neurology, Vol. 120 (3rd series)
Neurologic Aspects of Systemic Disease Part II
Jose Biller and Jose M. Ferro, Editors

Chapter 74

Neurologic manifestations of Henoch–Schönlein purpura

MAXIME D. BÉRUBÉ[1], NORMAND BLAIS[2], AND SYLVAIN LANTHIER[1]*

[1]*Department of Neurology, Centre Hospitalier de l'Université de Montréal, and Faculty of Medicine,
Université de Montréal, Montreal, QC, Canada*

[2]*Department of Haematology, Centre Hospitalier de l'Université de Montréal, and Faculty of Medicine,
Université de Montréal, Montreal, QC, Canada*

Henoch–Schönlein purpura (HSP) is a systemic small vessel vasculitis seen predominantly in children. It usually affects the skin, joints, gastrointestinal tract, and kidneys. While often underappreciated, neurologic complications may occur in one of every 14 patients with the disease. Up to 20% of these patients are left with persistent deficits, highlighting the importance of early recognition and treatment.

GENERAL ASPECTS

Historical aspects

The first description of the disease is generally credited to the English physician William Heberden, who published his princeps observation in 1801. It was Johann Lukas Schönlein, though, who established the association of joint symptoms and rash as a distinct clinical entity, which he named "peliosis rheumatica." Abdominal pain and nephritis were later recognized as part of the clinical picture by his former student, Eduard Heinrich Henoch. In 1914, Sir William Osler described the first case of neurologic involvement (Osler, 1914). In the same paper, he also made the initial suggestion that the disease might be caused by an allergic or immunologic derangement (Gairdner, 1948; Roberts et al., 2007). This hypothesis would be confirmed decades later with the demonstration of the essential pathologic feature of the disease, vascular IgA deposition (Urizar et al., 1968).

Systemic disease

HSP is largely a disease of childhood, with over 75% of patients having their onset before age 10 (Gedalia, 2004).

Estimates of its annual incidence range from 13.5 to 20.4 per 100 000 children. While rarely affected, adults often have a more severe disease course, especially regarding renal involvement. The male to female ratio is approximately 1.5 to 1.

The distribution of vasculitic involvement gives rise to the characteristic association of purpuric rash, arthralgias, abdominal pain, and nephritis. While these manifestations may appear in any order, purpura is usually the first, and its presence at some point in the evolution is mandatory for diagnosis (Ozen et al., 2010). It consists of small (2–10 mm in diameter), palpable, nonblanching lesions found predominantly over buttocks, ankles, and extensor surfaces. Arthralgias affect close to 75% of patients and involve especially the large joints such as knees and ankles (Saulsbury, 2007). Gastrointestinal involvement takes the form of colicky abdominal pain in 60% of patients. It is usually moderate in intensity but occasionally so severe as to mimic an acute abdomen. It may be complicated by bleeding in 30% and, rarely, intussusception. Renal impairment remains by far the main contributor to the long-term morbidity and mortality of this disease (Fervenza, 2003). It is seldom present at onset and may even be delayed for weeks. Its earliest manifestation is usually microscopic hematuria, which can eventually be accompanied by proteinuria in two-thirds of patients (Saulsbury, 1999). The risk of end-stage renal failure in an unselected patient population is around 1–3%, but rises to 50% in those with a nephritic-nephrotic syndrome.

Other infrequent complications that have been described include carditis, pulmonary hemorrhage, pancreatitis, cholecystitis, pseudomembranous colitis, orchitis, and urethritis (Gedalia, 2004; Saulsbury, 2007).

---

*Correspondence to: Sylvain Lanthier, Department of Neurology, Centre Hospitalier de l'Université de Montréal, CHUM - Hôpital Notre-Dame, 1560 est Sherbrooke, Suite GR-1159, Montréal (Qué), H2L 4 M1, Canada. Tel: +1-514-890-8000 × 26268, E-mail: sylanthier@gmail.com

Diagnostic criteria

The first set of formal diagnostic criteria established by the American College of Rheumatology in 1990 required the patient to meet at least two of the following criteria: (1) palpable purpura, not related to thrombocytopenia; (2) age 20 years or younger; (3) abdominal pain usually with gastrointestinal bleeding; (4) biopsy showing granulocytes in the vessel wall (arterioles or venules) (Mills et al., 1990). These criteria yielded a sensitivity of 87.1% and a specificity of 87.7%. However, they did not account for occurrence of the disease in adults or require demonstration of the signature presence of IgA deposits. These issues were addressed in a new set of criteria proposed by the European League Against Rheumatism (EULAR), Paediatric Rheumatology International Trials Organization (PRINTO), and Paediatric Rheumatology European Society (PRES) consensus conference (see Table 74.1) (Ozen et al., 2010). These criteria have now been validated, and were found to have a sensitivity and specificity of 100% and 87%, respectively (Ozen et al., 2010).

Pathology

HSP is classified according to the modified Chapel Hill Consensus Criteria in the group of nongranulomatous small vessel vasculitides. In the skin, the histopathologic pattern is that of a nonspecific leukocytoclastic vasculitis characterized by necrosis of the vessel wall and infiltration of inflammatory cells (mostly polymorphonuclear and mononuclear cells) within the capillaries and postcapillary venules (Mills et al., 1990). Delineation of the disease requires demonstration of perivascular IgA deposition, which can be seen by immunofluorescence along with C3, fibrin, and occasional IgG or IgM (Davin et al., 2001). In the kidney, the main site of IgA deposition is the mesangium, where it forms granular deposits. Renal lesions are diverse in type and severity, but in children are most commonly consistent with a focal and segmental glomerulonephritis (Pillebout and Niaudet, 2008).

Etiology and pathogenesis

As in most primary vasculitides, the inciting event in HSP remains unknown. Its predilection for onset in autumn and winter months and the presence of preceding respiratory infections in many cases has led some to suspect a role for infectious agents, although no single pathogen has been consistently identified (Yang et al., 2008). Evidence of group A β-hemolytic streptococcus infection can be found in 20–50% of HSP children. A host of "secondary causes" including exposure to medications such as L-dopa or chlorpromazine and medical conditions such as cancer have been linked to HSP, but in many cases their

Table 74.1

EULAR/PRINTO/PRES diagnostic criteria for Henoch–Schönlein purpura (Ozen et al., 2010)

Criterion	Glossary
Purpura (mandatory criterion)	Purpura (commonly palpable and in crops) or petechiae, with lower limb predominance,* not related to thrombocytopenia
1. Abdominal pain	Diffuse abdominal colicky pain with acute onset assessed by history and physical examination. May include intussusception and gastrointestinal bleeding
2. Histopathology	Typically leukocytoclastic vasculitis with predominant IgA deposit or proliferative glomerulonephritis with predominant IgA deposit
3. Arthritis or arthralgias	Arthritis of acute onset defined as joint swelling or joint pain with limitation on motion Arthralgia of acute onset defined as joint pain without joint swelling or limitation on motion
4. Renal involvement	Proteinuria > 0.3 g/24 h or > 30 mmol/mg of urine albumin/creatinine ratio on a spot morning sample Hematuria or red blood cell casts: >5 red blood cells/high power field or red blood cells casts in the urinary sediment or ≥ 2 + on dipstick
HSP EULAR/ PRINTO/PRES Ankara 2008 classification definition	Purpura or petechiae (mandatory) with lower limb predominance* and at least one of the four following criteria: Abdominal pain Histopathology Arthritis or arthralgia Renal involvement

*For purpura with atypical distribution, demonstration of an IgA deposit in a biopsy is required.

relationship remains uncertain (Aram, 1987; Niedermaier and Briner, 1997; Saulsbury, 1999). Variations in ethnic and geographic distribution also occur and may be related to genetic or environmental specificities of affected populations. For instance, skewing towards Caucasian ethnicity has been reported in North American children (Allen et al., 1960). Certain HLA serotypes, familial Mediterranean fever gene mutations, and specific gene polymorphisms have been suggested to modulate the susceptibility to and clinical expression of the disease (Saulsbury, 1999; Brogan, 2007).

Many lines of evidence point to a pivotal role for humoral immunity, specifically IgA, in the pathophysiology of HSP. In addition to IgA deposition in the vessel walls and mesangium, patients also have evidence of increased serum levels of IgA, circulating IgA-containing immune complexes, and IgA-producing B cells (Davin et al., 2001; Pillebout and Niaudet, 2008; Yang et al., 2008). Immunoglobulin deposits in HSP have been found to be composed exclusively of one of the two subclasses of IgA, IgA1. IgA1 differs from IgA2 by the presence of a hinge region containing N-acetylgalactosamine glycosylation sites. Much attention has been focused on abnormalities in the galactosylation and sialylation of these sites in the genesis of both HSP nephritis and the closely related IgA nephropathy (Davin et al., 2001). However, one study found that these abnormalities were restricted to HSP patients with nephritis, questioning their role in the genesis of the leukocytoclastic vasculitis (Allen et al., 1998).

Antibodies may mediate some of their effect through complement activation. IgA have a known ability to activate the indirect and lectin pathways, and C3 deposits can be seen in biopsy specimens. This, however, contrasts with the generally normal serum complement levels (Saulsbury, 2001; Chen et al., 2010). Some of these antibodies have been shown to directly induce secretion of IL-8 by the endothelial cells that they bind, stimulating recruitment of polymorphonuclear cells and inflammation (Yang et al., 2008).

EPIDEMIOLOGY OF NERVOUS SYSTEM MANIFESTATIONS

Although severe neurologic involvement in HSP is uncommon, milder manifestations may be underappreciated. In one series, seizures or confusion were retrospectively identified in 17 of 244 cases (6.9%) of HSP. More recent studies tend to report lower incidences. For instance, in a review of 100 patients examined over the course of 20 years, Saulsbury (1999) described only two cases of seizures. Similarly, Trapani et al. (2005) found a 3% incidence of headache but no other neurologic manifestations in 150 patients studied over 5 years. Other large series make no mention of neurologic symptoms among their patients (Fischer et al., 1990; Sticca et al., 1999; Calvino et al., 2001; Peru et al., 2008). Whether these discrepancies are due to selection bias, improvement in supportive care or underreporting is hard to ascertain. The latter may be particularly important in the case of headache and subtle behavioral changes which may easily be obscured by or attributed to other manifestations of the disease. In one report, these features were present in a third of HSP patients (Ostergaard and Storm, 1991). Among those with neurologic manifestations, there is a 1.5:1 preponderance of male patients, similar to that of the general HSP population. While no systematic data are available, a seemingly disproportionate number of neurologic cases have been reported in adults (data from Garzoni et al., 2009). This is in line with the previous suggestion that HSP has a more severe expression in this age group.

NERVOUS SYSTEM MANIFESTATIONS

Neurologic manifestations often occur in patients with an unusually severe disease course, comprising frequent renal impairment and unusual multiorgan involvement (Garzoni et al., 2009). When evaluating these complex patients, it is useful to think in terms of the possible pathophysiologic mechanisms that may be responsible of CNS damage, either directly from extension of the vasculitis to the CNS or indirectly from systemic involvement.

Cerebrovascular disease

Vasculitis can extend to cerebral vessels and cause edema, ischemia, infarction and hemorrhage. Pathologically confirmed cases of CNS vasculitis are scarce, however (Gairdner, 1948; Allen et al., 1960; Gilbert and Da Silva, 1966). Foci of vascular fibrinoid necrosis associated with diffuse cortical petechiae and ischemic neuronal changes were described in the brain of an 8-year-old boy with a severe course of HSP (de Montis and Turpin, 1971; Laplane et al., 1973). In another case, IgA deposition could be demonstrated in the cerebral vessels of a patient with intracerebral hematoma, providing some evidence of the identity of the vasculitic process in the brain and other vascular beds (Murakami et al., 2008). Nonetheless, most reports of cerebral vasculitis rely mainly on imaging findings deemed suggestive thereof. Occipital and posterior parietal lobes are preferentially involved, with a predominance of brain edema and infarct in these regions. Frontal, temporal, and cerebellar involvement is rarer. This peculiar topography has led some authors to speculate that hemodynamic characteristics of the posterior circulation might favor preferential IgA deposition in these vessels (Paolini et al., 2003). Brainstem is notably spared but at least one patient was described who presented with an isolated lesion of the medulla oblongata that regressed under corticotherapy (Bulun et al., 2001). The vasculitic process can progress to hemorrhage, with necrosis of the vessel wall leading to rupture and extravasation (Paolini et al., 2003). Coincident zones of putative vasculitic activity and cerebral hemorrhage have been demonstrated in one case on MRI (Wen et al., 2005). Most strikingly, hemorrhages share the same predominantly posterior distribution as vasculitis. They may be life-threatening, and evacuating surgery had to be performed in four of 11 reported cases (Scattarella et al., 1983; Clark and Fitzgerald, 1985; Altinors and Cepoglu, 1991; Ng et al., 1996; Chiaretti et al., 2002; Imai et al., 2002; Paolini et al., 2003; Misra et al., 2004; Wen et al., 2005; Karamadoukis et al., 2008; Murakami et al., 2008).

Subarachnoid bleeding has also been reported as an infrequent complication, mostly in the early series and on the basis of hemorrhagic CSF (Belman et al., 1985). A small aneurysm was found in one case of cerebellar hemorrhage, which was not felt to be related to vasculitis (Paolini et al., 2003). Subdural hematomas have also been described, including two children who needed surgical drainage (Belman et al., 1985). One patient suffered from an extensive venous thrombosis extending to the superior sagittal, straight and transverse sinuses (Abend et al., 2007). His prothombotic workup revealed the presence of a lupus anticoagulant.

Focal neurologic signs occur in 26–32% of patients with neurologic involvement and, in most cases, they are caused by cerebrovascular disease (Belman et al., 1985; Garzoni et al., 2009). Among 79 HSP patients with neurologic manifestations, focal deficits were hemiparesis (n = 11; 14%), aphasia (n = 6; 8%), cortical blindness (n = 4; 5%), ataxia (n = 2; 3%), as well as paraparesis, quadriplegia, and chorea (n = 1 each; 1%) (Belman et al., 1985). Nystagmus, dysarthria, and hemianesthesia were also reported. One case of cerebellar mutism occurred following drainage of a posterior fossa hemorrhage (Paolini et al., 2003).

Hypertensive encephalopathy and posterior reversible encephalopathy syndrome

Hypertension has long been suspected as a cause of neurologic dysfunction in encephalopathic HSP patients (Belman et al., 1985). Posterior reversible encephalopathy syndrome (PRES) cases have provided documented imaging evidence of this association.

PRES is a clinical-radiologic syndrome characterized by the occurrence of headache, visual dysfunction, seizures, and altered consciousness in association with reversible, posteriorly predominant white matter hyperintensities (Hinchey et al., 1996). These hyperintensities are thought to represent vasogenic edema caused by disruption of blood–brain barrier integrity. Although its pathophysiology is complex, loss of cerebral autoregulation from uncontrolled hypertension, volume overload, and endothelial injury from a variety of systemic conditions (including inflammatory disorders, sepsis, or exposure to certain drugs) are believed to be paramount (Bartynski, 2008). Patients with vasculitis often present a combination of these risk factors, making them

especially susceptible (Min et al., 2006). Four HSP patients were described that presented with the typical clinical course of PRES (Woolfenden et al., 1998; Ozcakar et al., 2004; Sasayama et al., 2007; Salloum et al., 2009). Cortical blindness accounts for 5.1% of all focal signs associated with HSP, and may be explained by PRES in many cases (Belman et al., 1985).

Neither the clinical nor the imaging features of PRES are specific, however, and it may be difficult to distinguish these features from those of vasculitic lesions, especially when no clear predisposing factor is present. In fact, among the four cases that were published, only two had hypertension and only one had renal dysfunction. In addition, some authors have pointed out that cases published as "cerebral vasculitis" had an evolution that closely resembled PRES (Woolfenden et al., 1998). Both conditions seemingly affect the same brain regions. Diffusion-weighted imaging (DWI) and apparent diffusion coefficient (ADC) have been advocated as means to distinguish vasogenic edema from ischemic lesions of vasculitis (Mak et al., 2008). Theoretically, ADC is increased in the former and diminished in the latter. However, many vasculitic lesions do not progress to irreversible ischemia and their DWI and ADC signals may sometimes be consistent with vasogenic edema (Moritani et al., 2001, 2004). Presence of inflammatory changes in the CSF has also been proposed as an additional distinguishing feature (Min et al., 2006). However, while data on CSF parameters in these two conditions are scant, it has frequently been reported as normal or noninflammatory in both, and may not permit adequate discrimination. Further compounding the problem is that the two processes may in fact coexist. Absence of hypertension or renal injury in these and other cases suggests that direct vasculitic involvement of cerebral vessels may indeed play a direct causal role in PRES (Bartynski, 2008; Nishio et al., 2008). CSF pleocytosis in one case of PRES was interpreted as indirect evidence of concomitant CNS inflammation (Woolfenden et al., 1998).

Disorders of hemostasis

Brain lesions that result from small vessel CNS vasculitis are frequently reversible, and most patients recover. Nonetheless, vasculitis may be prone to thrombotic complications and thrombosis may be associated with coexistent prothrombotic conditions. A study of 28 HSP and 79 healthy children suggests that markers of hypercoagulability such as fibrinogen, D-dimer, thrombin-antithrombin complex (TAT), prothrombin fragments 1+2 (PF1+2), von Willebrand antigen and activity are significantly elevated in the acute phase of HSP compared with the recovery phase of HSP or in controls (Yilmaz et al., 2006). Transient synthesis of antiphosphatidyl-ethanolamine antibodies was documented in a 17-year-old girl with extensive periopercular ischemic stroke (Sokol et al., 2000). Antiphospholipid antibodies were also uncovered in the one documented case of venous sinus thrombosis (Abend et al., 2007). Antiphospholipid antibodies have been described in association with HSP before, with or without thrombosis. Their relationship remains uncertain, but some have hypothesized that endothelial disruption by IgA antibodies may expose hidden phospholipids and promote synthesis of thrombogenic antiphospholipid antibodies (Abend et al., 2007).

Low levels of factor XIII were found in two patients with intracerebral hemorrhage (ICH) (Imai et al., 2002; Murakami et al., 2008). Factor XIII is an essential hemostasis enzyme that serves to polymerize fibrin. Patients with an inherited deficiency, who usually have serum levels of less than 1%, are prone to severe bleeding complications including spontaneous ICH (Lorand et al., 1980; Hsieh and Nugent, 2008). A somewhat controversial state of acquired deficiency, with levels generally between 50% and 75%, has been described in many inflammatory disorders including HSP (Henriksson et al., 1977). Some authors speculate that such relative deficiency may enhance bleeding in the presence of a pre-existing diathesis such as vasculitis. Administration of factor XIII concentrate in patients with HSP has been suggested to correct the bleeding diathesis (Imai et al., 2002; Prenzel et al., 2006). Another patient with ICH was found to have prolonged prothrombin and partial thromboplastin time suggesting an associated disseminated intravascular coagulation process (Clark and Fitzgerald, 1985). In this regard, mild decreases in factor XIII is more likely a reflection of a mild consumptive coagulopathy (Zajadacz and Juszkiewicz, 2005).

Metabolic abnormalities and infections

The multisystemic nature of HSP exposes patients to many potential disturbances of homeostasis, which may contribute to neurologic dysfunction. In addition to hypertension, renal impairment may lead to uremia, electrolyte disturbances, and volume overload. In two series, hyponatremia was a frequent accompaniment of neurologic symptoms, especially seizures (de Montis and Turpin, 1971; Laplane et al., 1973). Superimposed infections may add to the diagnostic confusion. CMV reactivation was thought to contribute to cerebral vasculitis in one case and concomitant *Staphylococcus aureus* infection was detected in another (Murakami et al., 2008; Temkiatvises et al., 2008). Corticosteroid or cyclophosphamide use may be responsible for opportunistic infections, PRES, and disturbances of electrolytic balance.

Headache and mental status alterations

Headache and mild behavioral alterations are frequently overlooked, and may represent telltale signs of subtle CNS involvement. In the only prospective study documenting neurologic manifestations of HSP, headache accompanied by behavioral changes was found in 31% of patients. Their presence was significantly associated with EEG changes (Ostergaard and Storm, 1991). Severe depression of consciousness may also occur, usually in association with a postictal state, hypertension, hemorrhage, or marked metabolic alterations.

Seizures

Seizures occur in 53% of patients with neurologic manifestations, mostly during the acute phase and occasionally as the initial manifestation of HSP (Belman et al., 1985; Mannenbach et al., 2009). Of these, 17% have partial and 83% have generalized convulsions (Belman et al., 1985; Garzoni et al., 2009). Status epilepticus is reported in 4% (Belman et al., 1985). Postictally, the EEG most often shows slow activity, but an epileptic focus can be seen in a minority of cases. In one study, EEG was reported to be abnormal in 46% of HSP children without seizure or overt neurologic dysfunction (Ostergaard and Storm, 1991). However, the authors could not rule out that these anomalies were benign variants. Seizures rarely recur beyond the acute phase, with only a few cases of epilepsy.

Neuro-ophthalmologic manifestations

Anterior ischemic optic neuropathy attributed to vasculitis was described in a 54-year-old diabetic male with a chronic course of HSP who presented with painless monocular visual loss (Chuah and Meaney, 2005). His vision improved with prednisolone treatment. A case of bilateral central retinal artery occlusion was also reported in a 6-year-old girl with concomitant cerebral vasculitis (Chen et al., 2000; Wu et al., 2002). Other rare ophthalmologic manifestations of HSP include central retinal vein occlusion, episcleritis, scleritis, keratitis, and anterior uveitis (Wu et al., 2002).

Myelopathy

A rare HSP patient was described in whom prolonged treatment with corticosteroids led to epidural lipomatosis and ensuing mild myelopathy (Kano et al., 1998). His symptoms abated completely within 1 month of dose reduction.

Neuromuscular manifestations

In contrast to its high prevalence in other primary small vessel vasculitides, peripheral nervous system involvement in HSP is infrequent. Despite this, a wide spectrum of lesions has been described. Mononeuropathies account for the majority of cases. In 24 HSP patients with peripheral nervous system manifestations, 14 (58%) had mononeuropathies involving the peroneal (n = 4), sciatic (n = 3), posterior tibial (n = 2), femoral (n = 1), and facial nerves (n = 3), four (17%) had Guillain–Barré syndrome, three (13%) had brachial plexopathy, two (8%) had polyradiculopathy, and one (4%) had mononeuritis multiplex (Belman et al., 1985). Interestingly, mononeuritis multiplex, the classic pattern of vasculitic neuropathy, has been reported only rarely (Campbell et al., 1994). The reason is unknown, but may be due to the short course of the disease preventing accumulation of lesions over time. Establishing a causal relationship of vasculitis with these lesions has been hampered by the lack of pathologic confirmation and presence of alternative etiologies in some patients. Temporal association with the onset of HSP and response to corticosteroids have been cited as circumstantial evidence of the presence of a vasculitic process. Other cases have been ascribed to local nerve compression by edema or hematoma (Belman et al., 1985).

Four cases of rapidly progressive polyradiculoneuropathy and ascending paralysis consistent with Guillain–Barré syndrome have been reported in HSP (Sanghvi and Sharma, 1956; Moreau et al., 1988; Goraya et al., 1998; Mutsukura et al., 2007). CSF analysis revealed albuminocytologic dissociation in all cases. Electromyography was performed in two cases and showed an acute motor and sensory neuropathy (AMSAN) pattern in one (Mutsukura et al., 2007) and acute inflammatory demyelinating polyneuropathy (AIDP) in the other (Moreau et al., 1988). This latter patient underwent sural nerve biopsy that revealed demyelination without signs of vasculitis or amyloidosis. In addition, there was evidence of intrathecal formation of IgA-containing immune complexes. On this basis, the authors suggested that IgA may have played a role in the initiation of demyelination in their patient, even though there was no evidence of IgA deposition in the pathologic specimen. Although IgA monoclonal spikes remain controversial as a cause of paraproteinemic neuropathy, recent evidence has borne out the notion that it can sometimes accumulate in and damage nerve fibers (Vital et al., 2008). Cases of Guillain–Barré-like syndrome have been described in patients with IgA MGUS (Ropper and McKee, 1993).

Muscle involvement has been reported in the form of intramuscular hemorrhage. It was present in 2% of patients in one series (Fischer et al., 1990). Pathologic examination in one case uncovered evidence of lymphocytic vasculitis in the hemorrhagic zone (Mahevas et al., 2004). Somekh et al., 2008 attributed severe calf and leg pain in three pediatric patients to muscular hemorrhage, although there was no histological confirmation and muscle enzymes were normal or mildly elevated.

INVESTIGATIONS

Nonspecific laboratory findings

There is no specific marker for HSP and the purpose of laboratory testing is to eliminate alternative diagnoses and to detect complications.

Mild inflammatory changes are commonly seen including anemia, mild leukocytosis, thrombocytosis and slightly elevated erythrocyte sedimentation rate. Elevation in creatinine levels occurs in a minority of patients. Routine coagulation tests are typically unremarkable, but markers of hypercoagulability and inflammation such as fibrinogen, D-dimer, thrombin-antithrombin complex (TAT), prothrombin fragments 1 + 2 (PF1 + 2), von Willebrand antigen and activity may be increased. Factor XIII levels may be slightly decreased in up to 50% of cases (Tizard and Hamilton-Ayres, 2008). Markers of autoimmunity including antinuclear antibody and rheumatoid factor are typically negative. Testing for the lupus anticoagulant, anticardiolipin, and anti-β_2-glycoprotein-I antibodies should be considered in the case of a thrombotic complication in order to rule out a coexistant antiphospholid antibody syndrome.

Antineutrophil cytoplasmic antibodies

Antineutrophil cytoplasmic antibodies (ANCA) are autoantibodies associated with a specific group of small vessel vasculitides that includes Wegener granulomatosis (WG), microscopic polyangiitis (MPA), and Churg–Strauss syndrome. In these conditions, ANCA are usually of the IgG or IgM class. In HSP, systematic series have reported either absence (Robson et al., 1994) or very low rates of IgG ANCA positivity (Ozaltin et al., 2004). The existence of ANCAs of the IgA class in HSP is a contentious issue, with a wide range of reported positivity rates, from 0% to 82% (Ozaltin et al., 2004). Furthermore, it is unclear whether the antibodies that have been detected result from true antigen recognition or from nonspecific interactions attributable for instance to abnormal IgA glycosylation (Coppo et al., 1997). A single HSP patient with cerebral vasculitis and IgA positive and IgG negative ANCA was reported (Fanos, 2009). Another rare case of cerebral vasculitis diagnosed as a "Henoch–Schönlein/MPA overlap syndrome" had mixed IgA predominant and pauci-immune lesions in addition to ANCA positivity (Nagasaka et al., 2009). In general, occurrence of IgG ANCA should lead to a diagnosis of one of the ANCA-positive vasculitides (von Scheven et al., 1998).

Cerebrospinal fluid analysis

Among HSP patients with an imaging study (computed tomography (CT) or magnetic resonance imaging (MRI)) deemed consistent with cerebral vasculitis, lumbar puncture is frequently normal or noninflammatory (Benhamou et al., 1991; Goncalves et al., 2004). Abnormalities that have been reported have included slight proteinorachia (Palesse et al., 1989), raised opening pressure (Elinson et al., 1990), or elevated red blood cells (Chen et al., 2000; Temkiatvises et al., 2008). Results of those with combined HSP and PRES have also been normal (Salloum et al., 2009) or showed mild lymphocytosis with increased red blood cells (Woolfenden et al., 1998). Thus, as already stated, the usefulness of lumbar puncture to differentiate vasculitis from PRES seems limited. Its primary interest lies in excluding vasculitis mimickers and secondary causes of CNS involvement.

Imaging studies

Imaging is indicated in all cases of suspected CNS involvement. CT scan may be normal or show areas of loss of attenuation. MRI is superior to CT in detecting early ischemic changes, hemorrhages and lesions of the posterior fossa. This superiority has been illustrated in many HSP case reports (Chen et al., 2000; Bulun et al., 2001; Fanos, 2009). It should be considered the study of choice. In cases of vasculitis, MRI will most often demonstrate confluent areas of cortical and subcortical T2-hyperintense signal predominant in the parieto-occipital regions. Enhancement with gadolinium can be seen (Eun et al., 2003). One patient with multiple recurrent bouts of HSP over 6 years was found to have moderate cerebral atrophy in addition to multiple periventricular hyperintensities on MRI (Perez et al., 2000). Magnetic resonance angiography was reported to show irregularities on segments of middle and posterior cerebral arteries in a single case of suspected cerebral vasculitis (Eun et al., 2003). These finding should be taken with caution, however, as this technique is subject to artifacts and the nature of the pathology makes it unlikely that anomalies will be seen with the current resolution achieved. Similarly, conventional cerebral angiography has not shown anomalies in patients in whom it was performed (Ng et al., 1996; Paolini et al., 2003; Temkiatvises et al., 2008). Its greater resolution may help identifying alternative diagnoses in selected cases.

DIFFERENTIAL DIAGNOSIS

The hallmark of HSP is purpura. Its palpable nature is a key characteristic that signals inflammation of the small skin vessels and permits distinction from hematological or cutaneous causes, which are associated with nonpalpable lesions (Schreiner, 1989). Though in children its appearance most frequently heralds HSP, palpable purpura may be seen in a number of other inflammatory disorders, some of which also affect the nervous system (Kathiresan et al., 2005). These include chiefly other primary vasculitides, but also infections and embolic phenomena. Wegener's granulomatosis (WG) and microscopic polyangiitis (MPA) in particular are frequently confused with HSP initially (Hall et al., 1985). Unlike HSP, their neurologic manifestations preferentially take the form of peripheral and, in WG, cranial neuropathies; although rarer cases of cerebral vasculitis have been described (von Scheven et al., 1998; Kono et al., 2000; Ulinski et al., 2005). Systemic features unusual for HSP such as rapidly progressive renal failure or pulmonary involvement in the form of upper airway disease (WG), cavitary lung lesions (WG), or pulmonary hemorrhage (WG or MPA) should lead the clinician to suspect these diagnoses. Additional discriminating characteristics include the presence of serum ANCAs and absence of immune complex deposition on biopsy. Necrotizing granulomas may be found in WG. Other vasculitides affecting the small vessels should also be considered, including Churg–Strauss syndrome, the hypersensitivity vasculitides as well as those associated with inflammatory disorders such as systemic lupus erythematosus, Behçet's disease, rheumatoid arthritis, or Sjögren syndrome. Most of these diseases are rarely encountered in children.

Among infectious causes, meningococcemia and Rocky Mountain spotted fever may present with extensive palpable purpura and CNS signs. They should always be kept in mind, especially in cases with a suggestive epidemiological context, septic features, or depressed consciousness. Similarly, the presentation of infectious endocarditis may combine petechiae as well as multifocal CNS signs. Actual cerebral vasculitis from immune complex deposition supervenes in some patients (Johnson and Johnson, 2010).

By definition, the purpura of HSP is nonthrombocytopenic, eliminating such potential etiologies of CNS dysfunction as thrombotic thrombocytopenic purpura and disseminated intravascular coagulation.

The diagnosis of HSP can be difficult when it presents with symptoms other than purpura, as it occurs in 25–50% of cases (Saulsbury, 1999). In one review, CNS manifestations preceded the onset of the rash in 16% (Garzoni et al., 2009). They may even occasionally be the heralding feature of the disorder (Mannenbach et al., 2009). Abdominal presentations are particularly confusing and entail a large differential diagnosis. Among vasculitides, polyarteritis nodosa may present with prominent gastrointestinal complaints. Unlike HSP, however, there is usually a history of prodromal systemic symptoms, cutaneous findings are different, and glomerulonephritis is absent. Again, the PNS is most commonly affected, but focal CNS deficits have been reported in up to 24% of patients (Rosenberg et al., 1990). Abdominal angiography may be required in some case to exclude the diagnosis.

MANAGEMENT

HSP is usually a self-limited disease that requires only supportive care. Steroids are used in patients with refractory abdominal pain, and those with severe nephritis may respond to high-dose methylprednisolone, alone or in combination with cyclophosphamide (Tizard and Hamilton-Ayres, 2008). No controlled data exist in cases of cerebral involvement. Most patients have been treated with corticosteroids, usually as intravenous pulses of methylprednisolone followed by an oral tapering regimen. This is reported to have led to resolution of neurologic manifestations in the majority, but whether this represents true treatment effect or natural evolution of the disease is hard to discern. Cyclophosphamide has also been employed in combination with steroids in a few cases but again, it is unknown if it provides additional benefit for CNS manifestations (Goncalves et al., 2004; Ozkaya et al., 2007; Karamadoukis et al., 2008). Although some have proposed that the combination should be considered as the standard treatment regimen (Garzoni et al., 2009), the literature suggests that most patients do well on steroids alone. Therefore, cyclophosphamide seems best reserved for refractory cases or those with concurrent nephritis. Refractory patients may also benefit from plasma exchange. Several case reports as well as a small retrospective series that included patients with HSP provide some support for its efficacy, either as an initial therapy or as a rescue intervention in those who had failed to improve on steroids (Gianviti et al., 1996; Chen et al., 2000; Eun et al., 2003; Wen et al., 2005; Murakami et al., 2008). An effect for intravenous immunoglobulins was suggested in the case of an adult HSP patient with mild encephalopathy and MR hyperintensities who experienced resolution of his symptoms following their administration (Perez et al., 2000).

It should again be emphasized that distinguishing vasculitis from PRES is difficult and that, when in doubt, one should address the two conditions simultaneously. In PRES, the mainstay of treatment is control of hypertension. Hemodialysis may occasionally be required to reduce fluid overload and uremia. The use of corticosteroids is more controversial. A causal relationship linking high-dose steroids to PRES has been suggested, but not established, in some patients (Hinchey et al., 1996). Others have pointed out that they may be detrimental by amplifying hypertension, volume overload, and hypercoagulability. Nonetheless, steroids have been successfully employed in several cases of PRES attributable to different vasculitides, including those reported in association with HSP (Woolfenden et al., 1998; Ozcakar et al., 2004; Min et al., 2006; Sasayama et al., 2007; Salloum et al., 2009). They may have a role in reducing endothelial injury from systemic inflammation and restoring permeability of the blood–brain barrier (Nishio et al., 2008). Their use may be justified in many cases.

Patients with hemorrhage should be closely monitored and emergent neurosurgical intervention considered in case of deterioration. Attention should be paid to correction of uncontrolled hypertension and metabolic abnormalities. The role of factor XIII replacement has not been firmly established and cannot be recommended at this time.

PNS lesions in HSP generally have a favorable prognosis and most may not warrant immunosuppression (Garzoni et al., 2009). Nonetheless, consideration to treatment should still be given in cases with severe impairment, as illustrated by a report of refractory and persisting brachial plexopathy (Yilmaz et al., 2006).

PROGNOSIS

Most patients with neurologic dysfunction make a good recovery although minor deficits occur with some frequency. In one review, 21% of patients with CNS manifestations were left with sequelae, including visual field defects, verbal disabilities, focal neurologic signs and localization-related epilepsy. Half had previously developed ICH. In 17 patients with a PNS lesion, only one (6%) had residual impairment (Garzoni et al., 2009). While three of 17 patients in the de Montis 1971 series had died, only one death has occurred in the 39 HSP cases with CNS dysfunction (3%) reported since 1983 (Garzoni et al., 2009).

REFERENCES

Abend NS, Licht DJ, Spencer CH (2007). Lupus anticoagulant and thrombosis following Henoch–Schönlein purpura. Pediatr Neurol 36: 345–347.

Allen DM, Diamond LK, Howell DA (1960). Anaphylactoid purpura in children (Schönlein–Henoch syndrome): review with a follow-up of the renal complications. AMA J Dis Child 99: 833–854.

Allen AC, Willis FR, Beattie TJ et al. (1998). Abnormal IgA glycosylation in Henoch–Schönlein purpura restricted to patients with clinical nephritis. Nephrol Dial Transplant 13: 930–934.

Altinors N, Cepoglu C (1991). Surgically treated intracerebral hematoma in a child with Henoch–Schönlein purpura. J Neurosurg Sci 35: 47–49.

Aram H (1987). Henoch–Schönlein purpura induced by chlorpromazine. J Am Acad Dermatol 17: 139–140.

Bartynski WS (2008). Posterior reversible encephalopathy syndrome, part 1: fundamental imaging and clinical features. AJNR Am J Neuroradiol 29: 1036–1042.

Belman AL, Leicher CR, Moshe SL et al. (1985). Neurologic manifestations of Schoenlein–Henoch purpura: report of three cases and review of the literature. Pediatrics 75: 687–692.

Benhamou B, Balafrej A, Jaritz E et al. (1991). Cerebral ischemia and severe digestive manifestations during rheumatoid purpura. Ann Pediatr (Paris) 38: 484–486.

Brogan PA (2007). What's new in the aetiopathogenesis of vasculitis? Pediatr Nephrol 22: 1083–1094.

Bulun A, Topaloglu R, Duzova A et al. (2001). Ataxia and peripheral neuropathy: rare manifestations in Henoch–Schönlein purpura. Pediatr Nephrol 16: 1139–1141.

Calvino MC, Llorca J, Garcia-Porrua C et al. (2001). Henoch–Schönlein purpura in children from northwestern Spain: a 20-year epidemiologic and clinical study. Medicine (Baltimore) 80: 279–290.

Campbell SB, Hawley CM, Staples C (1994). Mononeuritis multiplex complicating Henoch–Schönlein purpura. Aust N Z J Med 24: 580.

Chen CL, Chiou YH, Wu CY et al. (2000). Cerebral vasculitis in Henoch–Schönlein purpura: a case report with sequential magnetic resonance imaging changes and treated with plasmapheresis alone. Pediatr Nephrol 15: 276–278.

Chen M, Daha MR, Kallenberg CG (2010). The complement system in systemic autoimmune disease. J Autoimmun 34: J276–J286.

Chiaretti A, Caresta E, Piastra M et al. (2002). Cerebral hemorrhage in Henoch–Schoenlein syndrome. Childs Nerv Syst 18: 365–367.

Chuah J, Meaney T (2005). Anterior ischaemic optic neuropathy secondary to Henoch–Schönlein purpura. Eye (Lond) 19: 1028.

Clark JH, Fitzgerald JF (1985). Hemorrhagic complications of Henoch–Schönlein syndrome. J Pediatr Gastroenterol Nutr 4: 311–315.

Coppo R, Cirina P, Amore A et al. (1997). Properties of circulating IgA molecules in Henoch–Schönlein purpura nephritis with focus on neutrophil cytoplasmic antigen IgA binding (IgA-ANCA): new insight into a debated issue. Italian Group of Renal Immunopathology Collaborative Study on Henoch–Schönlein purpura in adults and in children. Nephrol Dial Transplant 12: 2269–2276.

Davin JC, Ten Berge IJ, Weening JJ (2001). What is the difference between IgA nephropathy and Henoch–Schönlein purpura nephritis? Kidney Int 59: 823–834.

de Montis G, Turpin JC (1971). Rheumatoid purpura and neurologic manifestations. Ann Med Interne (Paris) 122: 841–848.

Elinson P, Foster KW Jr, Kaufman DB (1990). Magnetic resonance imaging of central nervous system vasculitis. A case report of Henoch–Schönlein purpura. Acta Paediatr Scand 79: 710–713.

Eun SH, Kim SJ, Cho DS et al. (2003). Cerebral vasculitis in Henoch–Schönlein purpura: MRI and MRA findings, treated with plasmapheresis alone. Pediatr Int 45: 484–487.

Fanos V (2009). Cerebral vasculitis and nephritis in a child: complicated Henoch–Schönlein purpura or a rare case of Wegener's granulomatosis? J Paediatr Child Health 45: 163–165.

Fervenza FC (2003). Henoch–Schönlein purpura nephritis. Int J Dermatol 42: 170–177.

Fischer PJ, Hagge W, Hecker W (1990). Schönlein–Henoch purpura. A clinical study of 119 patients with special reference to unusual complications. Monatsschr Kinderheilkd 138: 128–134.

Gairdner D (1948). The Schönlein–Henoch syndrome (anaphylactoid purpura). Q J Med 17: 95–122.

Garzoni L, Vanoni F, Rizzi M et al. (2009). Nervous system dysfunction in Henoch–Schönlein syndrome: systematic review of the literature. Rheumatology (Oxford) 48: 1524–1529.

Gedalia A (2004). Henoch–Schönlein purpura. Curr Rheumatol Rep 6: 195–202.

Gianviti A, Trompeter RS, Barratt TM et al. (1996). Retrospective study of plasma exchange in patients with idiopathic rapidly progressive glomerulonephritis and vasculitis. Arch Dis Child 75: 186–190.

Gilbert EF, Da Silva A (1966). Henoch–Schoenlein purpura. Report of a fatal case with gastrointestinal hemorrhage and necrosis. Clin Pediatr (Phila) 5: 181–186.

Goncalves C, Ferreira G, Mota C et al. (2004). Cerebral vasculitis in Henoch–Schönlein purpura. An Pediatr (Barc) 60: 188–189.

Goraya JS, Jayashree M, Ghosh D et al. (1998). Guillain–Barré syndrome in a child with Henoch–Schönlein purpura. Scand J Rheumatol 27: 310–312.

Hall SL, Miller LC, Duggan E et al. (1985). Wegener granulomatosis in pediatric patients. J Pediatr 106: 739–744.

Henriksson P, Hedner U, Nilsson IM (1977). Factor XIII (fibrin stabilising factor) in Henoch–Schönlein's purpura. Acta Paediatr Scand 66: 273–277.

Hinchey J, Chaves C, Appignani B et al. (1996). A reversible posterior leukoencephalopathy syndrome. N Engl J Med 334: 494–500.

Hsieh L, Nugent D (2008). Factor XIII deficiency. Haemophilia 14: 1190–1200.

Imai T, Okada H, Nanba M et al. (2002). Henoch–Schönlein purpura with intracerebral hemorrhage. Brain Dev 24: 115–117.

Johnson MD, Johnson CD (2010). Neurologic presentations of infective endocarditis. Neurol Clin 28: 311–321.

Kano K, Ozawa T, Kuwashima S et al. (1998). Uncommon multisystemic involvement in a case of Henoch–Schönlein purpura. Acta Paediatr Jpn 40: 159–161.

Karamadoukis L, Ludeman L, Williams AJ (2008). Henoch–Schönlein purpura with intracerebral haemorrhage in an adult patient: a case report. J Med Case Reports 2: 200.

Kathiresan S, Kelsey PB, Steere AC et al. (2005). Case records of the Massachusetts General Hospital. Case 14-2005. A 38-year-old man with fever and blurred vision. N Engl J Med 352: 2003–2012.

Kono H, Inokuma S, Nakayama H et al. (2000). Pachymeningitis in microscopic polyangiitis (MPA): a case report and a review of central nervous system involvement in MPA. Clin Exp Rheumatol 18: 397–400.

Laplane R, Fontaine JL, Escourolle G et al. (1973). The neurological signs of rheumatoid pupura. Pathology and clinical signs in one case. Ann Pediatr (Paris) 20: 525–530.

Lorand L, Losowsky MS, Miloszewski KJ (1980). Human factor XIII: fibrin-stabilizing factor. Prog Hemost Thromb 5: 245–290.

Mahevas M, Makdassi R, Presne C et al. (2004). Muscular haematoma in Henoch–Schönlein purpura. Rev Med Interne 25: 927–930.

Mak A, Chan BP, Yeh IB et al. (2008). Neuropsychiatric lupus and reversible posterior leucoencephalopathy syndrome: a challenging clinical dilemma. Rheumatology (Oxford) 47: 256–262.

Mannenbach MS, Reed AM, Moir C (2009). Atypical presentation of Henoch–Schönlein purpura. Pediatr Emerg Care 25: 513–515.

Mills JA, Michel BA, Bloch DA et al. (1990). The American College of Rheumatology 1990 criteria for the classification of Henoch–Schönlein purpura. Arthritis Rheum 33: 1114–1121.

Min L, Zwerling J, Ocava LC et al. (2006). Reversible posterior leukoencephalopathy in connective tissue diseases. Semin Arthritis Rheum 35: 388–395.

Misra AK, Biswas A, Das SK et al. (2004). Henoch–Schönlein purpura with intracerebral haemorrhage. J Assoc Physicians India 52: 833–834.

Moreau BA, Schuller E, Georges B (1988). Association of Guillain–Barré syndrome and Henoch–Schönlein purpura: is immunoglobulin a responsible for the neurologic syndrome? Am J Med Sci 296: 198–201.

Moritani T, Shrier DA, Numaguchi Y et al. (2001). Diffusion-weighted echo-planar MR imaging of CNS involvement in systemic lupus erythematosus. Acad Radiol 8: 741–753.

Moritani T, Hiwatashi A, Shrier DA et al. (2004). CNS vasculitis and vasculopathy: efficacy and usefulness of diffusion-weighted echoplanar MR imaging. Clin Imaging 28: 261–270.

Murakami H, Takahashi S, Kawakubo Y et al. (2008). Adolescent with Henoch–Schönlein purpura glomerulonephritis and intracranial hemorrhage possibly secondary to the reactivation of latent CMV. Pediatr Int 50: 112–115.

Mutsukura K, Tsuboi Y, Fujiki F et al. (2007). Acute motor sensory axonal neuropathy associated with Henoch–Schönlein purpura. J Neurol Sci 263: 169–173.

Nagasaka T, Miyamoto J, Ishibashi M et al. (2009). MPO-ANCA- and IgA-positive systemic vasculitis: a possibly overlapping syndrome of microscopic polyangiitis and Henoch–Schoenlein purpura. J Cutan Pathol 36: 871–877.

Ng CC, Huang SC, Huang LT (1996). Henoch–Schönlein purpura with intracerebral hemorrhage: case report. Pediatr Radiol 26: 276–277.

Niedermaier G, Briner V (1997). Henoch–Schönlein syndrome induced by carbidopa/levodopa. Lancet 349: 1071–1072.

Nishio M, Yoshioka K, Yamagami K et al. (2008). Reversible posterior leukoencephalopathy syndrome: a possible manifestation of Wegener's granulomatosis-mediated endothelial injury. Mod Rheumatol 18: 309–314.

Osler W (1914). The visceral lesions of purpura and allied conditions. Br Med J Clin Res J 1: 517–525.

Ostergaard JR, Storm K (1991). Neurologic manifestations of Schönlein–Henoch purpura. Acta Paediatr Scand 80: 339–342.

Ozaltin F, Bakkaloglu A, Ozen S et al. (2004). The significance of IgA class of antineutrophil cytoplasmic antibodies (ANCA) in childhood Henoch–Schönlein purpura. Clin Rheumatol 23: 426–429.

Ozcakar ZB, Ekim M, Fitoz S et al. (2004). Hypertension induced reversible posterior leukoencephalopathy syndrome: a report of two cases. Eur J Pediatr 163: 728–730.

Ozen S, Pistorio A, Iusan SM et al. (2010). EULAR/PRINTO/PRES criteria for Henoch–Schönlein pupura, childhood polyarteritis nodosa, childhood Wegener granulomatosis and childhood Takayasu arteritis: Ankara 2008. Part II: Final classification criteria. Ann Rheum Dis 69: 798–806.

Ozkaya O, Bek K, Alaca N et al. (2007). Cerebral vasculitis in a child with Henoch–Schönlein purpura and familial Mediterranean fever. Clin Rheumatol 26: 1729–1732.

Palesse N, Marrelli A, Legge MP et al. (1989). Neurological complications of Schoenlein–Henoch syndrome: contribution of MR to the diagnosis. Case report. Ital J Neurol Sci 10: 351–355.

Paolini S, Ciappetta P, Piattella MC et al. (2003). Henoch–Schönlein syndrome and cerebellar hemorrhage: report of an adolescent case and literature review. Surg Neurol 60: 339–342.

Perez C, Maravi E, Olier J et al. (2000). MR imaging of encephalopathy in adult Henoch–Schönlein purpura. AJR Am J Roentgenol 175: 922–923.

Peru H, Soylemezoglu O, Bakkaloglu SA et al. (2008). Henoch Schönlein purpura in childhood: clinical analysis of 254 cases over a 3-year period. Clin Rheumatol 27: 1087–1092.

Pillebout E, Niaudet P (2008). Henoch–Schönlein purpura. Rev Prat 58: 507–511.

Prenzel F, Pfaffle R, Thiele F et al. (2006). Decreased factor XIII activity during severe Henoch–Schoenlein purpura – does it play a role? Klin Pediatr 218: 174–176.

Roberts PF, Waller TA, Brinker TM et al. (2007). Henoch–Schönlein purpura: a review article. South Med J 100: 821–824.

Robson WL, Leung AK, Woodman RC (1994). The absence of anti-neutrophil cytoplasmic antibodies in patients with Henoch–Schönlein purpura. Pediatr Nephrol 8: 295–298.

Ropper AH, McKee AC (1993). Case records of the Massachusetts General Hospital. Weekly clinicopathological exercises. Case 21-1993. A 71-year-old man with a rash and severe sensorimotor neuropathy. N Engl J Med 328: 1550–1558.

Rosenberg MR, Parshley M, Gibson S et al. (1990). Central nervous system polyarteritis nodosa. West J Med 153: 553–556.

Salloum AC, Cuisset JM, Vermelle M et al. (2009). Posterior reversible encephalopathy as a complication of rheumatoid purpura: a case study. Arch Pediatr 16: 284–286.

Sanghvi LM, Sharma R (1956). Guillain–Barré syndrome and presumed allergic purpura. AMA Arch Neurol Psychiatry 76: 497–499.

Sasayama D, Shimojima Y, Gono T et al. (2007). Henoch–Schönlein purpura nephritis complicated by reversible posterior leukoencephalopathy syndrome. Clin Rheumatol 26: 1761–1763.

Saulsbury FT (1999). Henoch–Schönlein purpura in children. Report of 100 patients and review of the literature. Medicine (Baltimore) 78: 395–409.

Saulsbury FT (2001). Henoch–Schönlein purpura. Curr Opin Rheumatol 13: 35–40.

Saulsbury FT (2007). Clinical update: Henoch–Schönlein purpura. Lancet 369: 976–978.

Scattarella V, Pannarale P, D'Angelo V et al. (1983). Occipital hemorrhage in a child with Schönlein–Henoch syndrome. J Neurosurg Sci 27: 37–39.

Schreiner DT (1989). Purpura. Dermatol Clin 7: 481–490.

Somekh E, Fried D, Hanukoglu A (2008). Muscle involvement in Schönlein-Henoch syndrome. Arch Dis Child 58: 929–930.

Sokol DK, McIntyre JA, Short RA et al. (2000). Henoch–Schönlein purpura and stroke: antiphosphatidylethanolamine antibody in CSF and serum. Neurology 55: 1379–1381.

Sticca M, Barca S, Spallino L et al. (1999). Schönlein–Henoch syndrome: clinical-epidemiological analysis of 98 cases. Pediatr Med Chir 21: 9–12.

Temkiatvises K, Nilanont Y, Poungvarin N (2008). Stroke in Henoch–Schönlein purpura associated with methicillin-resistant Staphylococcus aureus septicemia: report of a case and review of the literature. J Med Assoc Thai 91: 1296–1301.

Tizard EJ, Hamilton-Ayres MJ (2008). Henoch Schönlein purpura. Arch Dis Child Educ Pract Ed 93: 1–8.

Trapani S, Micheli A, Grisolia F et al. (2005). Henoch Schönlein purpura in childhood: epidemiological and clinical analysis of 150 cases over a 5-year period and review of literature. Semin Arthritis Rheum 35: 143–153.

Ulinski T, Martin H, Mac Gregor B et al. (2005). Fatal neurologic involvement in pediatric Wegener's granulomatosis. Pediatr Neurol 32: 278–281.

Urizar RE, Michael A, Sisson S et al. (1968). Anaphylactoid purpura. II. Immunofluorescent and electron microscopic studies of the glomerular lesions. Lab Invest 19: 437–450.

Vital A, Nedelec-Ciceri C, Vital C (2008). Presence of crystalline inclusions in the peripheral nerve of a patient with IgA lambda monoclonal gammopathy of undetermined significance. Neuropathology 28: 526–531.

von Scheven E, Lee C, Berg BO (1998). Pediatric Wegener's granulomatosis complicated by central nervous system vasculitis. Pediatr Neurol 19: 317–319.

Wen YK, Yang Y, Chang CC (2005). Cerebral vasculitis and intracerebral hemorrhage in Henoch–Schönlein purpura treated with plasmapheresis. Pediatr Nephrol 20: 223–225.

Woolfenden AR, Hukin J, Poskitt KJ et al. (1998). Encephalopathy complicating Henoch–Schönlein purpura: reversible MRI changes. Pediatr Neurol 19: 74–77.

Wu TT, Sheu SJ, Chou LC (2002). Henoch–Schönlein purpura with bilateral central retinal artery occlusion. Br J Ophthalmol 86: 351–352.

Yang YH, Chuang YH, Wang LC et al. (2008). The immunobiology of Henoch–Schönlein purpura. Autoimmun Rev 7: 179–184.

Yilmaz C, Caksen H, Arslan S et al. (2006). Bilateral brachial plexopathy complicating Henoch–Schönlein purpura. Brain Dev 28: 326–328.

Zajadacz B, Juszkiewicz A (2005). Increased levels of plasma D-dimer in the course of Henoch–Schönlein purpura. Wiad Lek 58: 581–583.

Handbook of Clinical Neurology, Vol. 120 (3rd series)
Neurologic Aspects of Systemic Disease Part II
Jose Biller and Jose M. Ferro, Editors

Chapter 75

Hemolytic uremic syndrome

KATHLEEN WEBSTER[1]* AND EUGENE SCHNITZLER[2]

[1]*Department of Pediatrics, Loyola University Medical Center, Maywood, IL, USA*

[2]*Department of Neurology, Loyola University Medical Center, Maywood, IL, USA*

INTRODUCTION

The terms "microangiopathic hemolytic anemia" and "thrombotic microangiopathy" have been used to describe disorders consisting of endothelial cell damage, thrombosis, and resulting thrombocytopenia and red cell destruction. Two important causes of these findings are hemolytic uremic syndrome (HUS) and thrombotic thrombocytopenic purpura (TTP). Both disorders can lead to widespread organ damage and predominantly affect the brain and kidney. In TTP, renal disease is less common and neurologic involvement is more pronounced. Although TTP is more commonly reported in adults and HUS in children, there have been reported cases of each disorder occurring outside of the typical age ranges and both should be considered in the appropriate clinical setting (Moake, 2002).

DEFINITION

HUS was first described by Gasser and colleagues in 1955. It is defined by the triad of microangiopathic hemolytic anemia, thrombocytopenia, and acute renal failure (Eriksson et al., 2001; Scheiring et al., 2008; Johnson and Taylor, 2009; Michael et al., 2009). Typical (D+) HUS follows within 2 weeks of an acute diarrheal illness. Atypical (or D−) HUS has also been reported and accounts for 10–20% of reported cases. Potential etiologies of atypical HUS include complement deficiency, inborn errors of metabolism, medications, infectious agents, and autoimmune disease processes (Table 75.1). The distinction between these two types can be important with regards to etiology, pathogenesis, long-term course, and treatment. Atypical HUS (aHUS) is associated with an increased risk of seizures and other neurologic complications (Johnson and Taylor, 2009; Michael et al., 2009; Scheiring et al., 2010).

EPIDEMIOLOGY AND ETIOLOGY

Although HUS is most commonly known as a leading cause of acute renal failure in children (Cerda et al., 2008), other organ systems have also been reported to be affected, particularly the central nervous system (CNS) (Eriksson et al., 2001; Banerjee, 2009; Scheiring et al., 2010). It is reported that up to half of children with HUS will have CNS involvement, most commonly in the form of seizures, altered mental status, or coma. HUS is estimated to occur with a frequency of 0.3–3.3 per 100 000 children worldwide, although it is noted that the incidence has been increasing in the past decade (Eriksson et al., 2001; Pomajzl et al., 2009). The most commonly affected age groups are children less than 5 years old, accounting for 50–70% of cases, and adolescents. Infants have rarely been reported to be affected. Up to 40% of children may require critical care support. Mortality from HUS is 2–7%, with higher risk seen in females, children under 5 years of age, the elderly, and patients with atypical or recurrent HUS (Gould et al., 2009; Rust and Worrel, 2009). In both typical HUS and aHUS, early presentation of CNS symptoms is associated with a less favorable outcome (Rust and Worrel, 2009; Scheiring et al., 2010).

Typical hemolytic uremic syndrome

The typical presentation of HUS occurs following a diarrheal prodrome. Diarrhea is infectious, usually due to Shiga toxin-producing *Escherichia coli* (STEC) (Ruggenenti et al., 2001; Michael et al., 2009). Although the 0157:H7 subtype of *E. coli* is the most commonly identified in the US, other subtypes have been found (Centers for Disease Control, 2009; Melmann et al., 2009). Of

---
*Correspondence to: Kathleen Webster, M.D., Loyola University Medical Center, 2160 S 1st Avenue, Maywood, IL 60153, USA. Tel: +1-708-327-9137, Fax: +1-708-216-5602, E-mail: kwebste@lumc.edu

Table 75.1

Etiologies of atypical hemolytic uremic syndrome

Infectious	Noninfectious
STEC infection	Complement deficiency
Diarrheal	Cobalamin metabolism
	deficiency
Urinary	Malignancy
Other diarrheal infections	Transplant
Shigella	SLE
Citrobacter	Antiphospholipid syndrome
Yersinia	Pregnancy
Clostridium difficile	HELLP syndrome
Giardia	Medication-induced
Viral infections	Quinine
HIV	Oral contraceptives
H1N1 influenza A	Immunosuppressants
CMV	*Tacrolimus*
EBV	*Ciclosporin*
Other infections	*Mycophenolate*
Pertussis	
Malaria	
Pneumococcal	

STEC, Shiga toxin-producing *Escherichia coli*; HIV, human immuno-deficiency virus; CMV, cytomegalovirus; EBV, Epstein–Barr virus; SLE, systemic lupus erythematosus; HELLP, hypertension, elevated liver enzymes, low platelets.

note, although *E. coli* 0157:H7 is well known as the cause of HUS, only 8% of persons with diarrheal illness due to this organism go on to develop HUS. Other infectious causes of diarrhea have been identified in afflicted patients, including *Shigella, Citrobacter, Yersinia, Clostridium difficile* and *Giardia* (Besbas et al., 2006; Pomajzl et al., 2009). STEC associated HUS accounts for up to 90% of cases and follows a seasonal pattern with higher incidence in summer and fall. Food-borne outbreaks have been reported and may be associated with raw ground beef, unpasteurized juice or milk, fresh produce such as lettuce, spinach, and alfalfa sprouts, and contaminated water (Razzaq, 2006; Rivero et al., 2010). The bacteria may be easily spread, and infection may be acquired from contact with animals and their environment, or other infected persons. In cases of multiple family members with symptoms it is important to distinguish concurrent HUS with diarrheal symptoms from asynchronous events, which may be related to genetic causes or complement deficiencies (Centers for Disease Control, 2009; Pomajzl et al., 2009).

Atypical hemolytic uremic syndrome

Atypical HUS (aHUS) is being described in a growing body of literature and is more commonly associated with

neurologic sequelae. In addition to diarrheal infections, HUS may be triggered by STEC infection of the urinary tract. Viral infections may also be associated with HUS. Reported cases have involved human immunodeficiency virus (HIV), novel H1N1 influenza A, cytomegalovirus (CMV), Epstein–Barr virus (EBV), and others (Ariceta et al., 2009; Banerjee, 2009; Printza et al., 2011; Çaltik et al., 2011). There are also several case reports of infants with HUS related to pertussis (Chaturvedi et al., 2010). Sharma et al. (1993) reported HUS following malaria. Another notable infectious cause is bacteremia, meningitis, or empyema due to *Streptococcus pneumoniae*. This particularly virulent form of HUS mainly affects children under 2 years of age and is associated with a much higher mortality (Brandt et al., 2002; Barit and Sakarcan, 2005; Besbas et al., 2006; Lei et al., 2010; Scheiring et al., 2010).

Atypical HUS is most commonly related to noninfectious causes. Over 50% of cases are attributed to congenital or acquired complement deficiency, notably disorders of factor H, factor I, factor B, and membrane cofactor protein (MCP) (Quintrec et al., 2010). Abnormal processing of cobalamin (vitamin B_{12}) leading to severe deficiency is an inborn error of metabolism and well described as an etiology of a particularly severe form of HUS with a high rate of neurologic symptoms (Sharma et al., 2007). Other reported associations with atypical HUS are malignancies, chemotherapy, systemic lupus erythematosis (SLE), antiphospholipid syndrome, pregnancy, and HELLP syndrome, and with medications such as quinine or oral contraceptives (Besbas et al., 2006; Michael et al., 2009; Scheiring et al., 2010). Patients who have had solid organ or bone marrow transplant also seem to be more susceptible to development of HUS. It is unclear whether this is due to the transplant state itself or due to immunosuppressive medications, such as tacrolimus, ciclosporin, and mycophenolate (Ariceta et al., 2009; Banerjee, 2009). In many of the atypical cases of HUS, it has been proposed that both a genetic predisposition and an environmental trigger are required to produce disease (Johnson and Taylor, 2008).

Thrombotic thrombocytopenic purpura

The presentation of HUS is closely related to thrombotic thrombocytopenic purpura (TTP). Like HUS, TTP is associated with microangiopathic hemolytic anemia and thrombocytopenia. The initial description of TTP by Moschowitz in 1925 reported a "pentad" of these two findings in addition to fever, neurologic impairment, and renal dysfunction. As in HUS, platelet aggregation occurs, although the etiology in TTP is deficiency of a protease known as ADAMTS13. This deficiency may be congenital, known as Upshaw–Schulman disease, with presentation occurring early in childhood, even in infancy (Schneppenheim et al., 2004; Lowe and Werner, 2005). Acquired deficiency may be related to autoantibodies against ADAMTS13 and present later in life, triggered by medications, collagen vascular disease, or infection. Untreated, the mortality of TTP is over 90%, although with plasma therapy, the incidence of mortality drops to 10–20%. In the current literature, there is disagreement as to whether TTP is a distinct syndrome from HUS, or whether these two disorders represent a spectrum of disease. HUS is classically thought of as a renal disease with systemic effects, while TTP is considered as a systemic disease with effects on the central nervous system and kidney (Desch and Motto, 2007). Often the two disorders are difficult to distinguish based on clinical presentation alone and further testing of complement and genetic factors is required to make a definitive diagnosis. Many of the same medications and diseases can trigger TTP and atypical HUS (Nolasco et al., 2005; Desch and Motto, 2007). It remains to be seen whether these two disorders will be found to be more similar or more distinct as the pathophysiology continues to be explored.

PATHOPHYSIOLOGY

As described above, a wide range of etiologies of typical and atypical HUS and TTP are reported. Although each of these results in a common clinical picture, the pathophysiology of each is distinct.

Typical hemolytic uremic syndrome

In STEC-associated HUS, the infecting organism enters the gastrointestinal tract and binds to and causes inflammation of the intestinal epithelium (Pomajzl et al., 2009). The bacteria produce a toxin, called Shiga toxin (Stx) or verotoxin. The toxin enters the bloodstream, bound to a carrier such as monocytes, neutrophils, or platelets. The toxin binds to the globotriaosyl ceramide (Gb3) receptor. The toxin results in red cell lysis and damage to vascular endothelium. This in turn leads to a cascade of microthrombosis, platelet activation, and thrombotic injury to the vasculature (Lowe and Werner, 2005; Karpman et al., 2010; Scheiring et al., 2010).

Atypical hemolytic uremic syndrome

Atypical HUS may be caused by a variety of etiologies, each with a different trigger resulting in the final common pathway of inflammatory cascade causing renal endothelial and vascular injury and resultant thrombotic microangiopathy. Up to 50% of patients may have chromosome 1 mutations or autoantibody production leading to deficiency and dysregulation of the complement cascade (Loirat et al., 2008; Banerjee, 2009). Another mutation on chromosome 1 may lead to deficient processing of cobalamin (vitamin B_{12}). This leads to a defect in the processing of cobalamin, with associated homocystinuria and methylmalonic academia (Sharma et al., 2007; Banerjee, 2009; Bouts et al., 2010; Martinelli et al., 2011). This form of aHUS usually presents in infancy and is associated with significant neurologic manifestations including hypotonia, lethargy, feeding difficulties and failure to thrive (Ariceta et al., 2009). Finally, pneumococcal infection may lead to production of neuraminidase, which exposes a protein known as Thomsen-Friedenreich antigen (TF-Ag) on renal endothelial cells, and causing immune activation (Banerjee, 2009; Bouts et al., 2010).

CLINICAL MANIFESTATIONS

In typical HUS, the history may include exposure to contaminated food. Symptoms generally develop 1–8 days following ingestion of the offending agent. Clinically the child usually presents with bloody diarrhea and cramping abdominal pain. Physical examination may show petechiae and/or mucosal bleeding. Diagnostic criteria include anemia, thrombocytopenia, and elevated creatinine. An "incomplete" HUS has been described in children who present with bloody diarrhea, anemia, and thrombocytopenia but have mild or absent elevation of creatinine and do not go on to develop overt renal failure (Lowe and Werner, 2005; Besbas et al., 2006; George, 2009; Scheiring et al., 2010). The differential diagnosis includes sepsis and disseminated intravascular coagulation (DIC), SLE, and TTP. Of note, in both HUS and TTP, other markers of coagulation including PT and aPTT are normal, thus distinguishing these from DIC. Since the anemia is due to hemolysis, the peripheral blood smear will often reveal schistocytes and helmet cells (Lowe and Werner, 2005). Most HUS will have a negative direct Coombs test, with the notable exception of that following *S. pneumoniae* infection, in which up to 90% may be positive (Banerjee, 2009; Scheiring et al., 2010).

NEUROLOGIC FINDINGS AND SEQUELAE

CNS involvement occurs in 20–50% of patients with hemolytic uremic syndrome and is usually seen within the first week of illness (Bale et al., 1980). CNS symptoms may be mild with many patients demonstrating only irritability and lethargy. More severe CNS presentation may be manifested by seizures, stupor, coma, and hemiparesis. Aphasia, ataxia, chorea, dystonia, and visual disturbances may also occur (Hahn et al., 1989). Cerebral edema with headache, vomiting, papilledema, sixth nerve weakness, and altered mental status is commonly observed. HUS presenting with early CNS signs and symptoms is associated with higher rates of mortality as well as neurologic and non-neurologic sequelae (Upadhyahya et al., 1980).

The etiology of CNS pathophysiology in HUS is multifactorial but underlying mechanisms closely parallel those attributed to acute renal failure (ARF). ARF has been known to be associated with altered mental status for more than a century. Although a significant degree of renal failure can be tolerated without neurologic effects, rapid deterioration of kidney function such as occurs in HUS is more likely to result in precipitous alteration of neurologic status (Eriksson et al., 2001).

The neurologic deterioration seen in HUS with ARF relates to uremia, hypertension, and altered fluid and electrolyte metabolism. Water intoxication is seen early in the course of ARF and is accompanied by hyponatremia. Early clinical signs of water intoxication include headache and altered mental status which can progress rapidly to seizures and coma. Uremia in HUS is primarily due to glomerular injury resulting in failure of excretion of toxic catabolites of protein. This is accompanied by acidosis with an increased ion gap, bicarbonate wasting, and elevated serum potassium levels. Early uremic encephalopathy is characterized by subtle changes in mental status including irritability, inattentiveness, confusion, memory lapses, lack of interest, fatigue, speech dyspraxia, and mild cognitive impairment. These symptoms may be followed by movement disorders, particularly tremor, tetany, and asterixis. Primitive reflexes such as snouting and rooting sometimes occur. Hemiparesis and transient loss of vision and hearing have also been noted. Uremia may also produce generalized weakness secondary to neuropathy (Rust and Chun, 1999).

Seizures occur in up to 40% of children with uremia secondary to HUS. These are usually generalized but may also be focal or myoclonic. Hypertension due to ARF also typically results in an encephalopathy characterized by generalized seizures as well as headache and visual changes. Focal findings including aphasia, hemiparesis and particularly sixth nerve palsies have been described. Occipital blindness is common with hypertensive encephalopathy of various etiologies including ARF. This is referred to as "reversible posterior leukoencephalopathy" or "occipital-parietal encephalopathy." Correlating magnetic resonance imaging (MRI) and computed tomography (CT) findings of white matter edema without infarction have been noted to accompany the clinical loss of vision (Sebire et al., 1995; Hinchey et al., 1996).

Early dialysis is effective in prevention and reduction of symptoms of uremic encephalopathy as well as improving outcomes in cases of uremic neuropathy and hearing loss. Dialysis is frequently used as a treatment modality for HUS and is associated with improved survival and prevention of encephalopathy (Stewart and Tina, 1993); however, dialysis itself may cause neurologic abnormalities. Headache is commonly observed during dialysis in adults, adolescents, and older children. Headaches may be migraine variants or secondary to water intoxication or hypertension. Headache is also a component of the dialysis disequilibrium syndrome which also includes mental status changes, fatigue, and muscle cramps. In more severe cases of dialysis disequilibrium syndrome, seizures and coma may develop. Dialysis disequilibrium syndrome tends to occur early in the course of dialysis and as a complication of rapid dialysis. The underlying pathophysiology is incompletely understood but seems to be secondary to cerebral edema produced by osmotic gradients of urea and other osmotically active compounds (Rust and Chun, 1999).

Although hypertension, dialysis equilibrium syndrome, and the metabolic changes of ARF account for a significant proportion of the CNS pathophysiology seen in HUS, other factors appear to be involved. Dhuna et al. (1992) reported a series of 11 children with HUS and seizures. Generalized seizures occurred in four patients and partial seizures in seven patients. The children with generalized seizures had diffuse slowing on EEG and normal CT scans of the brain. All four children had a normal outcome. However, in the patients with partial seizures, there was diffuse slowing, but focal slowing, focal spikes, asynchronous slowing, and burst suppression patterns were also noted. Six of the seven patients with focal seizures had clinical findings of hemiparesis. CT scans in these six patients demonstrated strokes primarily in the basal ganglia and thalamus. All six patients recovered with residual hemiparesis. Thus, partial seizures in HUS were correlated with focal EEG changes and structural pathology. Strokes secondary to infarctions and microinfarctions seemed to account for these structural findings.

Sheth and associates (1986) reviewed 44 children with HUS seen between 1972 and 1984. Fifteen patients had neurologic complications including 12 who had seizures. Statistically significant correlations were noted between CNS involvement and metabolic abnormalities including hypocalcemia, hypocapnia, and elevated serum creatinine levels. CSF protein was elevated in four patients, but there were none with CSF pleocytosis or decreased CSF glucose. Only six patients with CNS involvement recovered completely. Three patients died and six had neurologic and/or renal residuals or hypertension. Postmortem examination of one patient who died showed probable cerebral edema but no findings of any vascular microthrombi. Eriksson et al. (2001) summarized EEG data in 22 patients with HUS. They noted that patients with periodic activity as well as focal and multifocal epi-leptogenic activity had higher rates of mortality, epi-lepsy, and neurologic sequelae. In particular, focal occipital and temporal slowing and epileptiform dis-charges were correlated with residuals of vision impair-ments and complex partial seizures. The majority of patients with only generalized slowing on EEG recovered without neurologic complications.

Rooney et al. (1971) reported a series of postmortem neuropathologic findings in HUS patients and did not describe any unique markers for the disorder. They noted cerebral edema and hypoxic changes. In contrast Upadhyaya and associates (1980) reviewed 15 patients with HUS, three of whom died. Microthrombi were found in the kidneys and lungs in all three patients but also in the brain in two out of the three deceased patients. The authors speculated that nonrenal multiple organ microthrombi formation seemed to correlate with a more fulminant course in patients with HUS.

In a 1980 series, by Bale et al., of 60 patients with HUS, half had encephalopathy and/or seizures. CNS involve-ment was correlated with azotemia, hyponatremia, and the need for dialysis. Coma on admission and elevated CSF protein were associated with subsequent mortality and neurologic morbidity. Only one patient died and was autopsied. No microthrombi were seen in the brain. Only edema and anoxic changes were noted.

Neuroimaging with CT and MRI has proven to be valuable in the diagnosis, treatment, and prognosis of HUS. Hahn and associates (1989) reported 78 children with HUS; 16 had neurologic complications. CT scans showed cerebral edema in four patients, large vessel infarctions in four patients, and multiple hemorrhages in one patient. At autopsy of three patients, cerebral edema was found but no microthrombi or large vessel thrombi were noted. In one patient there was a large hemorrhagic infarction.

In 1987, DiMario et al. first reported a lacunar infarc-tion in the basal ganglia as a complication of HUS in a 5-year-old girl. Following initial presentation with mild encephalopathy, she developed a left hemiparesis. MRI demonstrated increased T1- and T2-weighted images in the consistent with a subacute hemorrhagic infarction in the right caudate and lentiform nuclei. Barnett and associates (1995) presented two additional cases with HUS complicated by coma and dystonic pos-turing. MRI and CT scans showed signal changes in the basal ganglia bilaterally. The authors reviewed the liter-ature on eight other patients with basal ganglia involve-ment. They postulated possible etiologies including microthrombi secondary to endothelial cell damage and/or direct effects of the enteric verotoxin. Since the majority of patients recovered, the authors hypothesized a reversible process. Furthermore they noted that

neurologic involvement does not necessarily imply poor prognosis and that basal ganglia involvement in particu-lar is often associated with full recovery or only mild residuals. Favorable outcome following CNS involve-ment even with thrombotic strokes has also been reported by others (Steinberg et al., 1986; Ogura et al., 1998; Nakahata et al., 2001).

Predilection for basal ganglia involvement in HUS was corroborated by Steinborn et al. (2004). They reviewed MRI and CT scans in 10 patients with HUS who had significant CNS involvement. Some 60% had imaging abnormalities in the basal ganglia. Abnormali-ties were also seen in the brainstem, cerebellum, and thalami. These signal changes were suggestive of micro-infarctions. The authors concluded that the basal ganglia are commonly affected in HUS and a direct toxic effect of verotoxin was again postulated. Furthermore the imaging findings were often reversible and did not necessarily imply an adverse outcome. The presence of hemorrhage in a lesion seemed to correlate with sub-sequent gliotic or cystic MRI findings as well as residual neurologic dysfunction. Two of the MRIs in this series of patients also included diffusion-weighted imaging (DWI). A case with DWI demonstrating basal ganglia lesions was also described by Toldo and associates (2009). DWI may be more sensitive in determining neu-rologic prognosis in that reduced apparent diffusion coefficient (ADC) may correlate with irreversible lesions. A summary of the clinical EEG and neuroimag-ing findings in HUS is found in Table 75.2.

The neuropsychological prognosis of children surviv-ing HUS has generally been favorable even in patients who had coma and seizures. Qamar and associates (1996) reviewed the long-term neurologic and psychoe-ducational outcomes of seven children who had experi-enced at least one seizure during their acute presentation with HUS. Three children had normal neurologic exam-inations but four demonstrated mild neurologic abnor-malities such as clumsiness, fine motor deficits, hyperactivity, and distractibility. However, in-depth psy-chometric studies revealed normal IQ scores and behav-ioral indices in all seven children. In a Canadian multicenter study of 91 case control pairs, Schlieper and associates (1999) found no significant impact on cognitive skills, learning, or academic achievement mea-sured at least 6 months after the acute episode of HUS. A subtle but significant effect of severity of HUS as mea-sured by serum creatinine was correlated with lower scores on subtests of verbal abilities. However, the inci-dence of attention deficit disorder was no higher in sur-vivors of HUS than in age-matched controls.

Cimolai and associates (1992) reviewed the risk fac-tors associated with CNS involvement in HUS in 91 patients. They concluded that younger age and prior

Table 75.2

Clinical EEG and neuroimaging findings in hemolytic uremic syndrome with central nervous system involvement

		Clinical findings
Mild CNS involvement		Irritability, lethargy, headache, altered mental status
	EEG	CT, MRI
Prognosis: favorable for recovery	Normal, mild diffuse slowing	Normal, mild cerebral edema
		Clinical findings
Severe CNS involvement		Seizures, stupor, coma, hemiparesis, aphasia, movement disorders, papilledema, visual disturbances, sixth nerve palsy
	EEG	CT, MRI
Prognosis: variable, increased mortality and neurological sequelae	Diffuse slowing, focal slowing, asynchronous slowing, focal spikes burst suppression	Reversible posterior leukoencephalopathy. Infarction and micro-infarctions, primarily in the basal ganglia and thalamus

treatment with gastrointestinal antimotility drugs led to a higher risk of development of HUS in patients infected with *Escherichia coli* 0157:H7. Using multivariate analysis significant CNS risk factors included female gender, prolonged use of an antimotility drug, and increased hemoglobin levels. Conversely, prior treatment with blood products was associated with a lower risk of neurologic findings. The increased risk factor of female gender applied only to presentation with encephalopathy but not to seizures. The antimotility drugs included opium, codeine, loperamide, diphenoxylate, and anticholinergics. The association of gastrointestinal antimotility agents suggests several possible etiologic mechanisms including more prolonged gastrointestinal absorption of verotoxin. In addition these agents may have direct CNS toxicity which might be further enhanced by impaired renal excretion. It should also be noted that these agents are no longer routinely prescribed by pediatricians for the treatment of diarrhea in infants and young children (Bell et al., 1997).

DIAGNOSIS

Diagnosis of typical HUS is usually made clinically based on history and laboratory findings (Table 75.3) (Levandosky et al., 2008; Johnson and Taylor, 2009). All children with diarrheal HUS should have culture of the stool performed. *E. coli* 0157:H7 is identified by growth on selective agar within 24 hours. Further testing with PCR or EIA may be done. Although these tests are rapid, they are best performed on colonies already isolated on a culture plate, or from enriched broth that has been incubated. Therefore the earliest confirmed diagnosis still requires 24–36 hours to complete (Centers for Disease Control, 2009). In addition to stool, urine culture for STEC has been reported to be positive, even in the absence of diarrhea. Abdominal ultrasound may be useful in diagnosis during the prodromal phase by identifying thickening of large bowel wall and echogenicity of renal parenchyma (Glatstein et al., 2010).

In atypical HUS, a risk factor or deficiency can be identified in approximately 60% of cases (Ariceta et al., 2009). Bacterial culture may help to identify pneumococcal infection as a trigger. For all other causes, serum testing may be of use. Due to the wide range of testing and expense and length of time to diagnosis, a prioritized and stepwise approach to diagnosis is recommended (Table 75.4); however, if therapy with plasma infusion or pheresis is being considered, it is necessary to obtain serum samples prior to initiation of therapy (Banerjee, 2009) or wait a minimum of 2 weeks following plasma infusion (Kavanagh et al., 2007). The most common etiology of atypical HUS is complement deficiency (Besbas et al., 2006; Ariceta et al., 2009). Serum

Table 75.3

Diagnosis of typical hemolytic uremic syndrome

History	Laboratory study	Findings
Diarrhea within past 2 weeks	*Classic features*	
Age > 6 months	Chemistry panel	Elevated BUN
Endemic area		Elevated creatinine
Exposure to contaminated food	CBC	Anemia
Abrupt onset		Thrombocytopenia
Single episode	*Hemolytic studies*	
Concurrent affected contact	Peripheral smear	Schistocytes
		Helmet cells
Etiologic studies		Burr cells
Stool culture	LDH	Elevated
Selective agar for *E. coli* 0157	Haptoglobin	Decreased
Serotyping of isolates		
PCR for Stx1, Stx2	*Coagulation studies*	
	PT, PTT	Normal
	Fibrinogen	Normal
	D-dimer	Elevated
	Red cell production	
	Reticulocyte count	Elevated

PCR, polymerase chain reaction; Stx, Shiga toxin; CBC, complete blood count; LDH, lactate dehydrogenase; PT, prothrombin time; PTT, partial thromboplastin time; BUN, blood urea nitrogen.

Table 75.4

Approach to diagnostic and etiologic work-up in atypical hemolytic uremic syndrome

Clinical factor	Possible etiology	Suggested testing
Meningitis, pneumonia	Pneumococcal infection	Culture of affected site
		Direct Coombs test
Age < 6 months, failure to thrive, neurologic symptoms	Deficient cobalamin metabolism	Urine and serum amino acids
Other atypical HUS	Complement deficiency	C3, C4 levels
		Factor H, B, I levels
		MCP expression
Neurologic symptoms, family history, insidious onset	TTP	ADAMTS13 activity

HUS, hemolytic uremic syndrome; TTP, thrombotic thrombocytopenic purpura; MCP, membrane cofactor protein; ADAMTS13, a disintegrin and metalloproteinase with a thrombospondin type 1 motif, member 13.

assays for levels of C3 along with complement factors H, I and B and MCP should be obtained. If a low level is found, genetic testing or autoantibody assays may also be considered (Kavanagh et al., 2007). In children with coexisting failure to thrive and prominent neurologic symptoms, assessment of urine and serum amino acids may reveal congenital cobalamin deficiency (Ariceta et al., 2009; Banerjee, 2009).

For patients in whom TTP is suspected, activity of the enzyme ADAMTS13 may be analyzed. Activity < 5% is reported to be specific for TTP (George, 2009). Decreased activity < 10% is suggestive but not specific for TTP. Gene mutations versus autoantibodies are still a consideration. Finally, both HUS and TTP can be triggered by autoimmune disease, so evaluation of antinuclear antibody, lupus anticoagulant, and antiphospholipid antibody are also important (Ariceta et al., 2009).

Renal biopsy is not needed for diagnosis; however, it is sometimes undertaken, especially in severe renal failure or patients with recurrent disease. Disctinctive findings on biopsy may help differentiate HUS from TTP (Banerjee, 2009).

TREATMENT

The mainstay of treatment for typical HUS is supportive care. Volume resuscitation, fluid and electrolyte monitoring, and transfusion of blood products are common, as is temporary need for dialysis (Lowe and Werner, 2005; Scheiring et al., 2008; Pomajzl et al., 2009). Treatment of neurologic manifestations is most often associated with control of seizure activity, with care to address any electrolyte imbalance as a potential cause.

Antibiotics

Antibiotic therapy is necessary in infections due to *Shigella* or *S. pneumoniae*. In other causes of diarrheal HUS, there have been reports of worsened outcomes with antibiotic treatment. A meta-analysis of studies in which antibiotics were used was unable to demonstrate conclusively that harm occurs, although wide variation in treatments was observed (Safdar et al., 2002; Banerjee, 2009; Mohsin et al., 2010).

Cobalamin replacement

In cases of cobalamin deficiency, supplementation may help to prevent future episodes (Banerjee, 2009). Unfortunately, despite therapy this disorder is often associated with progression of severe neurologic deficits due to the underlying homocysteine accumulation (Martinielli et al., 2011).

Plasma infusion and plasmapheresis

Plasma infusion has been reported to be of benefit in some patients with atypical HUS or TTP. The goal of plasma infusion is to replace complement factors or ADAMTS13 enzyme that are deficient in the afflicted patient. In patients who have deficiencies, marked improvement is reported (Banerjee, 2009).

Since many of these deficiencies may be caused not only by decreased production but by destruction via autoantibodies, plasma infusion alone may in some cases be harmful. HUS caused by pneumococcal infection (Banerjee, 2009) and by complement antibodies (Boyer et al., 2010) have both been worsened by plasma infusion. Because the underlying etiology is often unknown at the time of presentation, initial empiric therapy should be plasma exchange to remove the offending antibody. Plasma infusion may be useful in preventing recurrence, once the underlying deficiency has been identified (Kohli and Gulati, 2006; Loirat et al., 2010).

Immunotherapy

Plasma exchange is likely to be effective in only 30–50% of patients with atypical HUS (Ariceta et al., 2009; Banerjee, 2009). Some patients may show an initial response but this response is not sustained and/or repeated lifelong prophylactic treatment is needed. In such patients, reports of treatment with corticosteroids, vincristine, azathioprine, and cyclophosphamide have reported anecdotal success (Michael et al., 2009; Boyer et al., 2010). Often a combination of both immunosuppression and intermittent plasma exchange is necessary to sustain remission in severe relapsing forms of the disease.

Inhibition of complement may be effective in aHUS due to complement protein deficiencies. Eculizumab and rituximab have been reported as effective therapies in both atypical HUS (Banerjee, 2009; Mache et al., 2009; Boyer et al., 2010; Köse et al., 2010) and chronic relapsing TTP (Levandovsky et al., 2008).

Currently, investigations are ongoing involving urtoxazumab, a targeted antibody therapy to neutralize Shiga toxin (Lopez et al., 2010). While this may help prevent the cascade of events leading to full HUS, the challenge will be providing therapy within 24–72 hours of exposure (Bitzan et al., 2010). Further investigation of this therapy is needed to provide more conclusive evidence of effect.

Transplantation

Patients with aHUS may progress to renal failure and ultimately require transplantation. Unfortunately, as aHUS is most commonly associated with defective or deficient complement protein, the risk of disease recurrence or graft rejection is high (Cheong, 2009).

Complement therapy

In variations of HUS associated with deficiency of complement regulatory proteins, replacement of these factors would be beneficial and more specific than plasma infusion alone. While no specific factor is currently available, work is ongoing to develop recombinant or concentrate of these important complement factors (Johnson and Taylor, 2008).

Overall, the vast array of etiology and pathophysiology that underlies HUS creates a clinical challenge, with careful attention to presentation, family history, and diagnosis in order to achieve the proper diagnosis and therapy.

REFERENCES

Ariceta G, Besbas N, Johnson S et al. (2009). Guideline for the investigation and initial therapy of diarrhea-negative hemolytic uremic syndrome. Pediatr Nephrol 24: 687–696.

Bale JF Jr, Brasher C, Siegler RL (1980). CNS manifestations of the hemolytic-uremic syndrome. Relationship to metabolic alterations and prognosis. Am J Dis Child 134: 869–872.

Banerjee S (2009). Hemolytic uremic syndrome. Indian Pediatr 46: 1075–1084.

Barit G, Sakarcan A (2005). Antibiotic resistant *Streptococcus pneumoniae* and hemolytic uremic syndrome. Eur J Pediatr 164: 414–416.

Barnett ND, Kaplan AM, Bernes SM et al. (1995). Hemolytic uremic syndrome with particular involvement of basal ganglia and favorable outcome. Pediatr Neurol 12: 155–158.

Bell BP, Griffin PM, Lozano P et al. (1997). Predictors of hemolytic uremic syndrome in children during a large outbreak of *Escherichia coli* O157:H7 infections. Pediatrics 100: E12.

Besbas N, Karpman D, Landau D et al. (2006). A classification of hemolytic uremic syndrome and thrombotic thrombocytopenic purpura and related disorders. Kidney Int 70: 423–431.

Bitzan M, Schaefer F, Reymond D (2010). Treatment of typical (enteropathic) hgemolytic uremic syndrome. Semin Thromb Hemost 36: 594–610.

Bouts AH, Roofthooft MTR, Salomous GS et al. (2010). CD46-associated atypical hemolytic uremic syndrome with uncommon course caused by cblC deficiency. Pediatr Nephrol 25: 2547–2548.

Boyer O, Balzamo E, Charbit M et al. (2010). Pulse cyclophosphamide therapy and clinical remission in atypical hemolytic uremic syndrome with anti-complement factor H autoantibodies. Am J Kidney Dis 55: 923–927.

Brandt J, Wong C, Mihm S et al. (2002). Invasive pneumococcal disease and hemolytic uremic syndrome. Pediatrics 110: 371–376.

Çaltik A, Akyüz SG, Erdogan Ö et al. (2011). Hemolytic uremic syndrome triggered with a new pandemic virus: influenza A (H1N1). Pediatr Nephrol 26: 147–148.

Centers for Disease Control and Prevention (2009). Morbidity and Mortality Weekly Report: Recommendations for diagnosis of Shiga toxin-producing Escherichia coli infections by clinical laboratories. October 16, 2009, Vol. 58, No. RR-12, pp. 1–14.

Cerda J, Lameire N, Eggers P et al. (2008). Epidemiology of acute kidney injury. Clin J Am Soc Nephrol 3: 881–886.

Chaturvedi S, Licht C, Langlois V (2010). Hemolytic uremic syndrome caused by *Bordetella pertussis* infection. Pediatr Nephrol 25: 1351–1364.

Cheong H (2009). Can liver-kidney transplantation cure aHUS? Nephrology 5: 556–557.

Cimolai N, Morrison BJ, Carter JE (1992). Risk factors for the central nervous system manifestations of gastroenteritis-associated hemolytic-uremic syndrome. Pediatrics 90: 616–621.

Desch K, Motto D (2007). Is there a shared pathophysiology for thrombotic thrombocytopenic purpura and hemolytic-uremic syndrome? J Am Soc Nephrol 18: 2457–2460.

Dhuna A, Pascual-Leone A, Talwar D et al. (1992). EEG and seizures in children with hemolytic-uremic syndrome. Epilepsia 33: 482–486.

DiMario FJ Jr, Brönte-Stewart H, Sherbotie J et al. (1987). Lacunar infarction of the basal ganglia as a complication of hemolytic-uremic syndrome: MRI and clinical correlations. Clin Pediatr 25: 586.

Eriksson KJ, Boyd SG, Tasker RC (2001). Acute neurology and neurophysiology of haemolytic-uraemic syndrome. Arch Dis Child 84: 434–435.

Gasser C, Gautier E, Steck A et al. (1955). Hemolytic-uremic syndrome: bilateral necrosis of the renal cortex in acute acquired hemolytic anemia. Schweiz Med Wochenschr 85: 905–909.

George JN (2009). The thrombotic thrombocytopenic purpura and hemolytic uremic syndromes: overview of pathogenesis (experience of the Oklahoma TTP-HUS Registry, 1989–2007). Kidney Int 75 (Suppl 112): S8–S10.

Glatstein M, Miller E, Garcia-Boumissen F et al. (2010). Timing and utility of ultrasound in diarrhea-associated hemolytic uremic syndrome: 7-year experience of a large tertiary care hospital. Clin Pediatr 49: 318.

Gould LH, Demma L, Jones TF et al. (2009). Hemolytic uremic syndrome and death in persons with *Escherichia coli* O157:H7 infection, Foodborne Diseases Active Surveillance Network Sites, 2000–2006. Clin Infect Dis 49: 1480–1485.

Hahn JS, Havens PL, Higgins JJ et al. (1989). Neurological complications of hemolytic-uremic syndrome. J Child Neurol 4: 108–113.

Hinchey J, Chaves C, Appigani B et al. (1996). A reversible posterior leukoencephalopathy syndrome. N Engl J Med 334: 494.

Johnson S, Taylor CM (2008). What's new in haemolytic uraemic syndrome? Eur J Pediatr 167: 965–971.

Johnson S, Taylor CM (2009). In: ED Ainer, D Ellis (Eds.), Pediatric Nephrology. 6th edn. Springer, pp. 1155–1180.

Karpman D, Sartz L, Johnson S (2010). Pathophysiology of typical hemolytic uremic syndrome. Semin Thromb Hemost 36: 575–585.

Kavanagh D, Richards A, Fremeaux-Bacchi V et al. (2007). Screening for complement system abnormalities in patients with atypical hemolytic uremic syndrome. Clin J Am Soc Nephrol 2: 591–596.

Kohli R, Gulati S (2006). Plasma infusion therapy in atypical hemolytic uremic syndrome – long term outcome. Indian Pediatr 43: 164–166.

Köse Ö, Zimmerhackl L-B, Jungraithmayr T et al. (2010). New treatment options for atypical hemolytic uremic syndrome with the complement inhibitor eculizumab. Semin Thromb Hemost 36: 669–672.

Lei T-H, Hsia S-H, Wu C-T et al. (2010). *Streptococcus pneumoniae*-associated haemolytic uremic syndrome following influenza A virus infection. Eur J Pediatr 169: 237–239.

Levandosky M, Harvey D, Lara P et al. (2008). Thrombotic thrombocytopenic purpura-hemolytic uremic syndrome (TTP-HUS): a 24-year clinical experience with 178 patients. J Hematol Oncol 1: 23 http://www.jhoonline.org/content/1/1/23.

Loirat C, Noris M, Fremeaux-Bacchi V (2008). Complement and the atypical hemolytic uremic syndrome in children. Pediatr Nephrol 123: 1957–1972.

Loirat C, Garnier A, Sellier-Leclerc A-L et al. (2010). Plasmatherapy in atypical hemolytic uremic syndrome. Semin Thromb Hemost 36: 673–681.

Lopez EL, Contrini MM, Glatstein E et al. (2010). Safety and pharmacokinetics of urtoxazumab, a humanized monoclonal antibody, against Shiga-like toxin 2 in healthy adults and in pediatric patients infected with Shiga-like toxin-producing *Escherichia coli*. Antimicrob Agents Chemother 54: 239–243.

Lowe EJ, Werner EJ (2005). Thrombotic thrombocytopenic purpura and hemolytic uremic syndrome in children and adolescents. Semin Thromb Hemost 31: 717–729.

Mache CJ, Acham-Roschitz B, Fremeaux-Bacchi V et al. (2009). Complement inhibitor eculizumab in atypical hemolytic uremic syndrome. Clin J Am Soc Nephrol 4: 1312–1316.

Martinelli D, Deodato F, Dionisi-Vici C (2011). Cobalamin C defect: natural history, pathophysiology, and treatment. J Inherit Metab Dis 34: 127–135.

Melmann A, Fruth A, Friedrich AW et al. (2009). Phylogeny and disease association of Shiga toxin-producing *Escherichi coli* O91. Emerg Infect Dis 15: 1474–1477.

Michael M, Elliott EJ, Craig JC et al. (2009). Interventions for hemolytic uremic syndrome and thrombotic thrombocytopenic purpura: a systematic review of randomized controlled trials. Am J Kidney Dis 53: 259–272.

Moake JL (2002). Thrombotic microangiopathies. N Engl J Med 347: 589–600.

Mohsin M, Haque A, Ali A et al. (2010). Effects of ampicillin, gentamicin, and cefotaxime on the release of Shiga toxins from Shiga toxin-producing *Escherichia coli* isolated during a diarrhea episode in Faisalabad, Pakistan. Foodborne Pathog Dis 7: 85–90.

Nakahata T, Tanaka H, Tateyama T et al. (2001). Thrombotic stroke in a child with diarrhea-associated hemolytic-uremic syndrome with a good recovery. Tohoku J Exp Med 193: 73–77.

Nolasco LH, Turner NA, Bernardo A et al. (2005). Hemolytic uremic syndrome-associated Shiga toxins promote endothelial-cell secretion and impair ADAMTS13 cleavage of unusually large von Willebrand factor multimers. Blood 106: 4199–4209.

Ogura H, Takaoka M, Kishi M et al. (1998). Reversible MR findings of hemolytic uremic syndrome with mild encephalopathy. AJNR Am J Neuroradiol 19: 1144–1145.

Pomajzl RJ, Varman M, Holst A et al. (2009). Hemolytic uremic syndrome (HUS) – incidence and etiologies at a regional Children's Hospital in 2001–2006. Eur J Clin Microbiol Infect Dis 28: 1431–1435.

Printza N, Roilides E, Kotsiou M et al. (2011). Pandemic influenza A (H1N1) 2009-associated hemolytic uremic syndrome. Pediatr Nephrol 26: 143–144.

Qamar IU, Ohali M, MacGregor DL et al. (1996). Long-term neurological sequelae of hemolytic-uremic syndrome: a preliminary report. Pediatr Nephrol 10: 504–506.

Quintrec ML, Roumenina L, Noris M et al. (2010). Atypical hemolytic uremic syndrome associated with mutations in complement regulator genes. Semin Thromb Hemost 36: 641–652.

Razzaq S (2006). Hemolytic uremic syndrome: an emerging health risk. Am Fam Physician 74: 991–996.

Rivero MA, Passucci JA, Rodriguez EM et al. (2010). Role and clinical course of verotoxigenic *Escherichia coli* infections in childhood acute diarrhoea in Argentina. J Med Microbiol 59: 345–352.

Rooney JC, Anderson RM, Hopkins IJ (1971). Clinical and pathologic aspects of central nervous system involvement in the haemolytic uraemic syndrome. Proc Aust Assoc Neurol 8: 67–75.

Ruggenenti P, Noris M, Remuzzi G (2001). Thrombotic microangiopathy, hemolytic uremic syndrome, and thrombotic thrombocytopenic purpura. Kidney Int 60: 831–846.

Rust R, Chun R (1999). Interrelationships between renal and neurologic diseases and therapies. In: KF Swaiman, S Ashwal (Eds.), Pediatric Neurology Principles and Practice. 3rd edn. Mosby, St Louis, pp. 1403–1437.

Rust RS, Worrel TE (2009). Hemolytic uremic syndrome. eMedicine Neurology 1–30.

Safdar N, Said A, Gangon RE et al. (2002). Risk of hemolytic uremic syndrome after antibiotic treatment of *Escherichia coli* O157:H7 enteritis: a meta-analysis. JAMA 288: 996–1001.

Scheiring J, Andreoli SP, Zimmerhackl LB (2008). Treatment and outcome of Shiga-toxin-associated hemolytic uremic syndrome. Pediatr Nephrol 23: 1749–1760.

Scheiring J, Rosales A, Zimmerhackl LB (2010). Today's understanding of the haemolytic uraemic syndrome. Eur J Pediatr 169: 7–13.

Schlieper A, Orrbine E, Wells GA et al. (1999). Neuropsychological sequelae of haemolytic uraemic syndrome. Arch Dis Child 80: 214–220.

Schneppenheim R, Budde U, Hassenpflug W et al. (2004). Severe ADAMTS-13 deficiency in childhood. Semin Hematol 41: 83–89.

Sebire G, Husson B, Lasser C et al. (1995). Encephalopathy induced by arterial hypertension: clinical, radiological and therapeutic aspects. Arch Pediatr 2: 513.

Sharma J, Bharadawa K, Shah K et al. (1993). *Plasmodium vivax* malaria presenting as hemolytic-uremic syndrome. Indian Pediatr 30: 369–371.

Sharma AP, Greenberg CR, Prasad AN et al. (2007). Hemolytic uremic syndrome secondary to cobalamin C C (Cb1c) disorder. Pediatr Nephrol 22: 2097–2103.

Sheth KJ, Swick HM, Haworth N (1986). Neurological involvement in hemolytic-uremic syndrome. Ann Neurol 19: 90–93.

Steinberg A, Ish-Horowitcz M, el-Peleg O et al. (1986). Stroke in a patient with hemolytic-uremic syndrome with a good outcome. Brain Dev 8: 70–72.

Steinborn M, Leiz S, Rüdisser K et al. (2004). CT and MRI in haemolytic uraemic syndrome with central nervous system involvement: distribution of lesions and prognostic value of imaging findings. Pediatr Radiol 34: 805–810.

Stewart CL, Tina LU (1993). Hemolytic uremic syndrome. Pediatr Rev 14: 218–224.

Toldo I, Manara R, Cogo P et al. (2009). Diffusion-weighted imaging findings in hemolytic uremic syndrome with central nervous system involvement. J Child Neurol 24: 247–250.

Upadhyahya K, Barwick K, Fishaut M et al. (1980). The importance of non-renal involvement in hemolytic uremic syndrome. Pediatrics 65: 115–120.

Handbook of Clinical Neurology, Vol. 120 (3rd series)
Neurologic Aspects of Systemic Disease Part II
Jose Biller and Jose M. Ferro, Editors

Chapter 76

Commonly used drugs in hematologic disorders

ELISE ANDERES AND SUCHA NAND*

*Division of Hematology and Oncology, Department of Medicine, Loyola University Chicago,
Stritch School of Medicine, Maywood, IL, USA*

AGENTS USED TO TREAT BENIGN HEMATOLOGIC DISORDERS

Replacement therapies

ANEMIAS RESULTING FROM IRON AND VITAMIN DEFICIENCIES

Anemias are commonly encountered in medical practice and are often due to deficiencies of iron and vitamins such as cobalamin (vitamin B_{12}), or folic acid. Iron deficiency is the most common cause of anemia in the US and worldwide (Umbreit, 2005). Iron deficiency can be treated orally, parenterally, or with blood transfusion. Oral iron is the simplest and least expensive option. Ferrous iron salts are preferred due to increased solubility at the pH of the duodenum and jejunum. Approximately 200 mg of elemental iron per day is required to replete iron stores. Each 325 mg tablet of ferrous sulfate contains 66 mg of elemental iron; therefore one tablet three times daily is the recommended replacement dose. The most common side-effects of oral iron sulfate include nausea, heartburn, constipation, or loose stools. Oral iron is best absorbed on an empty stomach, but is best tolerated with foods. The majority of patients will tolerate therapy without significant side-effects. Reducing the frequency of administration or taking iron supplements with meals can alleviate gastrointestinal complaints (Cook, 2005; Killip et al., 2007).

Parenteral iron replacement is indicated in patients with iron malabsorption due to resection or disease of the stomach or bowel, conditions with high iron requirements such as chronic gastrointestinal blood loss or end-stage renal disease, and failure of oral iron replacement due to poor tolerance or compliance (Cook, 2005). Parenteral replacement is best given intravenously, since the intramuscular route has been associated with development of soft tissue sarcomas. Formulations available in the US include iron dextran, iron sucrose, and iron gluconate. All are associated with the risk of life-threatening anaphylaxis, arthralgias, fever, and hypotension. Iron sucrose and iron gluconate have a lower incidence of anaphylaxis and are generally preferred, although they are more expensive (Silverstein, 2004). Headaches and dizziness are associated with intravenous iron preparations. Paresthesias and syncope have also been reported with iron gluconate infusions. Pleocytosis of the cerebrospinal fluid following a febrile reaction to iron dextran has been reported. The patient also developed a peripheral blood leukocytosis (Forristal and Witt, 1968). In another patient, meningismus without increased leukocytes in the spinal fluid but a high spinal fluid iron concentration was documented (Wallerstein, 1968). Iron sucrose and iron gluconate have a lower incidence of anaphylaxis and are generally preferred, although they are more expensive (Silverstein, 2004).

Megaloblastic anemias most commonly result from deficiencies of cobalamin or folic acid. Folate deficiency can occur due to decreased intake secondary to poor nutrition, impaired absorption in the duodenum or jejunum due to tropical or nontropical sprue, or increased requirement due to pregnancy or hemolytic anemia. Various drug interactions can also lead to folate deficiency. Decreased dietary intake is the most common cause of folate deficiency and is often seen in alcoholics or elderly or poor patients. The recommended daily intake of dietary folate is 400 μg daily and inadequate consumption leads to anemia within several months. Folate deficient persons are treated with 1–5 mg daily of oral folate. Changes in mental status, sleep disturbances, irritability, and excitability have been reported with higher

---

*Correspondence to: Sucha A. Nand, MD, Loyola University Medical Center, Cancer Center, Room 345, 2160 S. First Avenue, Maywood, IL 60153, USA. E-mail: snand@lumc.edu

doses of folate such as 15 mg/day (Hunter et al., 1970). Folic acid was also reported to exacerbate seizure activity in a young woman who started supplementation while attempting to become pregnant. She had a history of monthly seizures not controlled by medication, but her seizures became more frequent and more severe after starting folate 0.8 mg/day. Substitution of folinic acid 7.5 mg/day resulted in improvement of her seizure activity (Guidolin et al., 1998).

Concomitant cobalamin deficiency should be excluded prior to beginning treatment with folate, as anemia may improve but neurologic symptoms due to cobalamin deficiency will progress. Folate replacement is inexpensive and effective even in persons with malabsorption (Krishnaswamy and Nair, 2001).

Cobalamin deficiency is most commonly caused by impaired absorption secondary to pernicious anemia. Other causes include gastric or ileal resection, regional enteritis, intestinal lymphoma, bacterial overgrowth in blind intestinal loops, and vegan diet (Babior, 2006). Cobalamin deficiency can result in severe neuropsychiatric complications as well as anemia or pancytopenia. Cobalamin is usually given by intramuscular injections, which saturate tissue stores and compensate for daily losses. Oral and intranasal preparations are also available. In symptomatic patients or those with severe cytopenias, 1000 µg of cobalamin is typically given intramuscularly every day for 2 weeks, then weekly until cytopenias resolve, and then monthly indefinitely. For those with subclinical deficiency (cobalamin levels between 200 and 350 ng/L), replacement with daily injections for 1 week, followed by weekly injections for 4 weeks, then monthly injections indefinitely is acceptable. Oral replacement with 1000–2000 µg daily is equally effective in most cases of cobalamin deficiency (Oh and Brown, 2003), though patients should be monitored closely to ensure that laboratory parameters are correcting and the cobalamin levels are being repleted. For those who respond to oral replacement, lifelong therapy with 1000 µg daily is indicated. For nonresponders, parenteral replacement should be given. Excess cobalamin is excreted in the urine, so toxicity from excess vitamin replacement does not occur. Asthenia, dizziness, and headache have been reported after cobalamin injections in approximately 12% of patients. This may be related to the method of administration.

A summary of the agents used to treat the various hematologic disorders discussed in this chapter is given in Table 76.1.

COAGULOPATHIES

Fresh frozen plasma

Fresh frozen plasma (FFP) is obtained from units of whole blood donation or from plasmapheresis of

Table 76.1

Commonly used drugs in hematologic disorders

1. Agents used to treat benign hematologic disorders
   A. Replacement therapies
      Anemias resulting from iron and vitamin deficiencies
      Coagulopathies
   B. Antifibrinolytic agents
      Lysine analogs
   C. Antiplatelet agents
      Cyclooxygenase inhibitors
      Adenosine diphosphate receptor inhibitors
      Glycoprotein IIb/IIIa antagonists
      Thromboxane synthase inhibitors
   D. Antithrombotic agents
      Unfractionated heparin
      Low molecular weight heparin
      Factor Xa inhibitors
      Warfarin
      Direct thrombin inhibitors
2. Management of hemorrhagic complications of anticoagulation
   A. Intracranial hemorrhages due to
      Warfarin
      Heparin
      Direct thrombin inhibitors
      Antiplatelet agents
3. Agents used to treat hematologic malignancies
   A. Chronic myeloproliferative disorders
      Hydroxyurea (hydroxycarbamide)
      Anagrelide
      BCR-ABL tyrosine kinase inhibitors
   B. Myelodysplasia
      DNA methyltransferase inhibitors
   C. Leukemias, lymphomas and multiple myeloma
      Chemotherapeutic agents
      Targeted therapies
         a. Monoclonal antibodies
         b. Radioimmunotherapy
         c. Immunomodulatory drugs
         d. Proteosome inhibitors

volunteer donors. FFP can be used for replacement of factors II, V, VII, IX, X, or XI, and protein S, since specific factor replacement are often not available. Thus, FFP is most commonly used in the treatment of multiple factor deficiencies, such as in patients with disseminated intravascular coagulation (DIC), patients on warfarin with significant bleeding, those with vitamin K deficiency requiring urgent correction of factor deficiencies, patients with bleeding associated with acute blood loss, or those requiring plasma exchange for treatment of thrombotic thrombocytopenic purpura (TTP) or hyperviscosity syndrome. A typical unit of plasma derived from a collection of whole blood has a volume of nearly 300 mL, and local and national guidelines for usage generally specify a dose of around 10–20 mL/kg (Stanworth, 2007).

Cryoprecipitate

Cryoprecipitate is a relatively concentrated preparation of procoagulant factors, including fibrinogen, factor VIII, von Willebrand factor, factor XIII, and fibronectin. Cryoprecipitate is most commonly used for replacement of acquired or congenital hypofibrinogenemia. An adult dose of around 10 single bags of cryoprecipitate derived from units of whole blood typically raises the plasma fibrinogen level by up to 1 g/L (60–100 mg/dL) (Stanworth, 2007). It can also be used in treatment of von Willebrand disease or hemophilia, though specific replacement with von Willebrand factor or factors VIII and IX are usually preferred. Patients with DIC and low fibrinogen are probably best treated with a combination of FFP and cryoprecipitate, to minimize the risk of inducing thrombosis with transfusion of cryoprecipitate alone. Adequate transfusion should be given to maintain the fibrinogen level above 100 mg/dL. Cryoprecipitate can also be used for treatment of qualitative platelet dysfunction in uremia.

Immunoglobulin

Intravenous immunoglobulin (IVIg) is derived from large pools of human plasma. Most of the immunoglobulin in commercially available preparations of IVIg is IgG, with a subtype distribution of IgG_1–IgG_4 similar to that in normal human plasma. Relatively small amounts of IgA and IgM are also present. IVIg is used to treat a variety of hematologic disorders, including congenital or acquired immunodeficiency syndromes, immune thrombocytopenic purpura (ITP), autoimmune hemolytic anemia (AIHA), autoimmune neutropenia (AIN), and recurrent bacterial infections occurring in association with chronic lymphocytic leukemia (CLL) or multiple myeloma. IVIg is also used to treat a variety of autoimmune disorders. In patients with ITP and AIHA, IVIg is considered the best "emergency" intervention when a rapid, albeit transient, response is required (Knezevic-Maramica and Druskall, 2003). The neurologic indications for the use of IVIg include Guillain–Barré syndrome and myasthenia gravis, among others.

The immediate adverse reactions following IVIg administration are usually mild and transient flu-like symptoms, and include headache, facial flushing, malaise, chest tightness, fever and chills, myalgia, fatigue, dyspnea, nausea, vomiting, diarrhea, change in blood pressure, and tachycardia. These side-effects usually resolve if the infusion rate is decreased (Orbach et al., 2005). Premedication with analgesics, nonsteroidal

anti-inflammatory drugs (NSAIDs), antihistamines, or intravenous glucocorticoids may also be helpful (Reutter and Luger, 2004). Headache is the most common side-effect of IVIg therapy, with reported incidence ranging from 5–80%. Usually the headaches are mild and can be alleviated by slowing the infusion rate and giving analgesics or antihistamines. However, in some patients IVIg therapy must be terminated because of severe headaches (Orbach et al., 2005). Other adverse effects associated with IVIg administration include renal failure, arterial and venous thrombosis, and dermatologic toxicity, such as urticaria, rash, and pruritus (Orbach et al., 2005). Thrombotic events occur in 1–13% of patients, with arterial thromboses (stroke, myocardial infarction) being more common than venous (pulmonary embolism, deep venous thrombosis). Arterial events also tend to occur earlier, with 50% of events occurring within 4 hours of the IVIg infusion. Older age and cardiovascular risk factors increase the risk of arterial thromboses, while obesity and immobility increase the risk of venous thromboses (Paran et al., 2005). Premedication with aspirin may decrease the risk of thromboses in patients with underlying risk factors. Hyperviscosity may also increase the risk of stroke, and a baseline viscosity should be checked in patients at risk for hyperviscosity (e.g., monoclonal gammopathy) (Marie et al., 2006). A significant proportion of patients who receive IVIg develop a positive direct antigobulin test (DAT, or direct Coombs test), due to the presence of anti-A or anti-B derived from type O individuals in the donor pools. Transient hemolysis has been reported (Copelan et al., 1986).

Aseptic meningitis is a rare complication of IVIg treatment, occurring in about 1% of patients. Clinical manifestations include acute severe headache with neck rigidity, fever, lethargy, photophobia, nausea, and vomiting. Cerebrospinal fluid (CSF) examination demonstrates pleocytosis with high protein content and negative culture. Signs and symptoms usually begin 48 hours after the infusion and last for 3–5 days (Orbach et al., 2005). Infusing IVIg at a slow rate and ensuring adequate hydration may prevent or reduce the incidence of aseptic meningitis. In patients with a history of IVIg-induced aseptic meningitis, premedication with acetaminophen or antihistamines may reduce the incidence of recurrence. Corticosteroid treatment is not considered beneficial in IVIg-induced aseptic meningitis (Redman et al., 2002).

Transfusion reactions and risks

Transfusion of plasma and plasma fractions can lead to adverse reactions or events, of which immune-mediated reactions are most common. These include allergic and anaphylactic reactions, transfusion-related acute lung injury (TRALI) and hemolysis, and can range in severity from mild to fatal. TRALI is a leading cause of transfusion-related morbidity and mortality. It is characterized by acute noncardiogenic pulmonary edema and respiratory compromise in the setting of transfusion. TRALI is caused by passive transfusion of antigranulocyte antibodies that interact with recipient neutrophils, resulting in activation and aggregation in pulmonary capillaries, release of local biologic response modifiers causing capillary leak, and lung injury (Triulzi, 2006). Signs and symptoms include hypoxemia, hypotension, dyspnea, fever, and bilateral infiltrates on chest radiograph. Fluid overload and citrate toxicity can occur after rapid or massive transfusion. In developed countries, microbial transmission rates are low because of donor selection and testing. The risk of viral transmission is very low because of the use of two independent viral inactivation steps. The risk of transmission of variant Creutzfeldt–Jakob disease in both plasma components and pooled plasma products is as yet unknown. The low titer of prion infectivity in the blood of an infected individual (approximately 10 infectious units/mL) would be massively diluted by the thousands of units of plasma in the pool, likely making the risk extremely low. Subsequent manufacturing processes also remove prions from the final product (MacLennan and Barbara, 2006).

Recombinant factor VIIa

Recombinant factor VIIa (rfVIIa or NovoSeven®) is a procoagulant protein concentrate that was developed to "bypass" factor VIII or IX inhibitors in patients with hemophilia A or B. It is approved in these patients for the treatment of bleeding episodes, or for prophylaxis prior to invasive procedures or surgery. It is also approved in these settings in patients with congenital factor VII deficiency. RfVIIa is occasionally used off-label in patients with trauma and massive hemorrhage or in patients with platelet disorders or liver disease and uncontrolled bleeding. Recombinant factor VIIa binds directly to activated platelets and activates factor X, which in turn catalyzes the conversion of prothrombin to thrombin. Thrombin generation activates the intrinsic pathway and further promotes thrombin formation. Binding of rfVIIa to activated platelets localizes it to the site of bleeding and helps prevent thrombotic complications (Roberts et al., 2004). The incidence of serious adverse events, including myocardial infarction, stroke and venous thromboembolism, is about 1% in hemophiliacs (Abshire and Kenet, 2004). RfVIIa should be used cautiously in patients with a predisposition to thrombotic complications, such as obesity, cancer, or cardiovascular disease.

Prothrombin complex concentrates

Prothrombin complex concentrates (PCCs) are a source of the vitamin K-dependent coagulation factors, including factors II, VII, IX and X and proteins C and S. They are isolated from the cryoprecipitate supernatant of large plasma pools after removal of antithrombin and factor XI. The PCCs are standardized according to their factor IX content. The concentrates are processed to inactivate the clotting factors and treated to inactivate transfusion-transmitted viruses. PCC administration is indicated for emergent reversal of oral anticoagulant therapy, for example in patients on warfarin with intracerebral hemorrhage. PCCs can also be used in the treatment of hemophilia B or congenital factor VII deficiency when specific factor concentrates are not available. Adverse events associated with PCC use include allergic reactions, heparin-induced thrombocytopenia (when heparin is added to the PCC to inactivate clotting factors), and DIC (Hellstern, 1999).

Antifibrinolytic agents

LYSINE ANALOGS

Fibrinolysis occurs when plasmin that is generated by plasminogen activators digests fibrin clots. Both plasmin and plasminogen bind thrombin through lysine-binding sites. The synthetic lysine analogs ε-aminocaproic acid (EACA, Amicar®) and tranexamic acid (AMCA) compete with plasmin and plasminogen activators at lysine binding sites. Binding of these agents inhibits fibrinolysis and stabilizes the clot. These agents can be administered orally, intravenously or topically, although optimal dosing has not been established in most clinical settings (Verstraete, 1985). They are used in the treatment of severe mucosal hemorrhage (e.g., upper gastrointestinal bleeding, menorrhagia) or other bleeding conditions associated with increased fibrinolysis. EACA and AMCA are also used to control bleeding in thrombocytopenic conditions such as ITP. Both agents are generally well tolerated, although nausea, vomiting, diarrhea, dizziness, malaise, fever, rash, and transient hypotension or cardiac arrhythmias may occur. EACA can also rarely cause rhabdomyolysis, particularly with prolonged use. Headache is a common side-effect of AMCA and can also occur with EACA. Both agents can cause or aggravate cerebral infarction when used in patients with subarachnoid hemorrhage. EACA and AMCA should not be used in patients with DIC, as excessive thrombosis can occur; they are also relatively contraindicated in patients with urologic bleeding conditions.

Antiplatelet agents

CYCLOOXYGENASE INHIBITORS

Aspirin is a nonselective inhibitor of cyclooxygenase (COX), the enzyme that regulates conversion of arachidonic acid to prostaglandins and thromboxane A_2. Aspirin has an irreversible effect on COX-1 that results in inhibition of platelet aggregation and prevention of vasoconstriction. Aspirin has many therapeutic uses, including the prevention and treatment of arterial and venous thromboses. It is most commonly used to prevent or treat coronary or cerebral arterial thromboses. In hematology practice, aspirin is used as thrombosis prophylaxis in patients with primary bone marrow disorders such as multiple myeloma and myeloproliferative disorders. Aspirin can also alleviate microvascular symptoms such as headache, light-headedness, acral paresthesia and erythromelalgia in patients with polycythemia vera (PV) or essential thrombocythemia (ET) (McCarthy et al., 2002; Tefferi, 2003). In patients with arterial thrombophilias such as antiphospholipid antibody syndrome, aspirin is used for prevention of ischemic stroke (APASS Writing Committee, 2004; Albers et al., 2008) and recurrent pregnancy loss (Kutteh, 1996; Rai et al., 1997).

The primary complication of aspirin use is bleeding. Bleeding can occur at any site but most commonly manifests as gastrointestinal bleeding or hemorrhagic stroke. Hypertension, older age and higher doses of aspirin appear to increase the risk of CNS hemorrhage. For most patients the benefits of aspirin in preventing cardiovascular, cerebrovascular, and ischemic events significantly outweigh the risk of a major hemorrhage (Gorelick and Weisman, 2005). Aspirin can also be nephrotoxic, causing acute renal failure from renal vasoconstriction or acute interstitial nephritis. Systemic vasoconstriction can cause exacerbation of congestive heart failure.

ADENOSINE DIPHOSPHATE RECEPTOR INHIBITORS

Adenosine diphosphate (ADP) is a platelet agonist that is stored in platelet-dense granules. When a platelet is activated, ADP is released and binds to platelet surface receptors, thus recruiting additional platelets to form a platelet plug. ADP receptor inhibitors such as clopidogrel (Plavix®) and ticlopidine (Ticlid®) prevent platelet aggregation by selectively and irreversibly binding the platelet surface receptor P2Y12. Platelet aggregation is inhibited for the remainder of the platelet lifespan (7–10 days). Clopidogrel is indicated for treatment of acute ST and non-ST elevation myocardial infarction, peripheral arterial disease, arteriosclerotic vascular disease, and stroke. Ticlopidine is indicated after placement of coronary stents and after thromboembolic stroke (Varon and Spectre, 2009).

A noteworthy side-effect of ticlopidine and clopidogrel is thrombotic thrombocytopenic purpura (TTP). This was first reported with ticlopidine in the late 1990s, and incidence was estimated at 1 case per 1600–5000 patients treated (Bennett et al., 1998). Clopidogrel became the preferred antiplatelet agent after three phase III trials including more than 20 000 patients reported a more favorable safety profile, with less neutropenia, skin and gastrointestinal toxicities, and no cases of TTP. However, in the year 2000 a report of 11 patients who developed TTP while on clopidogrel was published (Bennett et al., 2000). Ten of 11 patients developed TTP within 2 weeks of starting the drug. The mechanism for development of TTP is not known, but is thought to be nonimmunologic given the short time to onset. Patients required a median of eight plasma exchanges (range, 1–30), and were prone to recurrence of TTP. One patient died shortly after the diagnosis of TTP. Treating physicians should be aware of this rare but serious side-effect of clopidogrel.

The newest ADP receptor P2Y12 inhibitors include prasugrel and ticagrelor. Compared to clopidogrel, prasugrel has a more rapid onset of action and its inhibitory effect is stronger (Wallentin et al., 2008). In addition, prasugrel is not affected by genetic variations of cytochrome P450. The effect of prasugrel on platelets is irreversible and appears to be responsible for increased risk of bleeding with this agent (Wiviott et al., 2007). Ticagrelor is different in two respects: Its binding to the P2Y12 is stronger and faster than prasugrel but it is reversible. In a double blind randomized trial, comparing ticagrelor to prasugrel in patients with acute coronary syndromes, ticagrelor was superior in composite death rate, without increasing the risk of major bleeding (Schomig, 2009; Wallentin et al., 2009).

GLYCOPROTEIN IIB/IIIA ANTAGONISTS

The primary use of these agents is in the cardiac catheterization laboratory. The representative agents of this group are abciximab, eptifibatide, and tirofiban. The published trial suggests a 9% reduction in death rate at 30 days in patients with acute coronary syndromes. Oral GPIIb/IIIa blockers (xemilofiban, orbofiban, sibrafiban, and lotrafiban) have been disappointing as they have been shown to be no more effective than aspirin and may even increase the risk of mortality (Chew et al., 2001).

THROMBOXANE SYNTHASE INHIBITORS

A brief mention also must be made of dipyridamole, which inhibits thromboxane synthase. This results in lower uptake of thromboxane A2 and lowered cellular uptake of adenosine. It acts as an antiplatelet agent and is also a vasodilator. Dipyridamole has been studied extensively, frequently in combination with aspirin. A review of over 25 trials suggests that while its effects in coronary syndromes are modest at best, it may reduce the risk of stroke (Diener et al., 1996). Newer formulation of dipyridamole with better bioavailability may confirm such an advantage of this old drug.

Antithrombotic agents

UNFRACTIONATED HEPARIN

Unfractionated heparin is a glycosaminoglycan composed of polysaccharide chains with molecular weights ranging from 5000 to 30 000 kDa (Hirsh et al., 2001). It exerts its anticoagulant effect by binding to antithrombin (AT), causing a conformational change that accelerates the inhibition of thrombin and factor Xa. Inhibition of thrombin and factor Xa prevents the conversion of fibrinogen to fibrin and the activation of other clotting factors, thus minimizing clot formation.

Heparin is effective and indicated for the prevention of venous thromboembolism; for the treatment of venous thrombosis and pulmonary embolism (PE); for the early treatment of patients with unstable angina and acute myocardial infarction (MI); for patients who undergo cardiac surgery using cardiac bypass, vascular surgery, and coronary angioplasty; in patients with coronary stents; and in selected patients with disseminated intravascular coagulation.

Heparin can cause hyperkalemia, osteoporosis after long-term use, and nonimmune-mediated thrombocytopenia due to platelet agglutination. Heparin can cause bleeding at any site, reported to occur in 5–10% of patients receiving heparin (Kelton and Hirsh, 1980). Epidural or spinal hematomas can occur in patients receiving unfractionated or low molecular weight heparin, particularly in patients who undergo lumbar puncture or epidural catheter placement for analgesia. Careful timing of heparin administration, attention to heparin dose, and avoidance of other medications that can cause bleeding are essential to minimize the risk of epidural or spinal hematomas (Wysowski et al., 1998). Heparin can be inactivated by protamine sulfate to prevent or minimize bleeding complications.

The most feared complication of heparin is heparin-inducted thrombocytopenia and thrombosis (HITT), which occurs in about 1% of patients receiving unfractionated heparin. HITT is caused by antibodies directed against heparin-platelet factor 4 complexes, which activate platelets and stimulate thrombin generation. Onset typically occurs 7–10 days after heparin exposure, unless patients have had prior heparin exposure within the past 3 months, in which case onset can occur within 1–2 days. Patients have a drop in platelet count of 50% and about

half of patients develop venous or arterial thrombosis. Thrombosis can occur even after heparin is discontinued, so patients should be placed on anticoagulation with a direct thrombin inhibitor and eventually transitioned to warfarin for a minimum of 2–3 months (longer if thrombosis occurred). Patients presenting with acute thrombosis 1–2 weeks after heparin exposure should be evaluated for HITT (Hirsh et al., 2001).

LOW MOLECULAR WEIGHT HEPARIN

Low molecular weight heparin (LMWH) is derived from depolymerization of unfractionated heparin. It has an average molecular weight of 5000 kDa, with a range of 1000–10 000. The majority of these heparin chains are too short to bind ATIII and thrombin, and the anticoagulant effect is primarily the result of ATIII-mediated inactivation of factor Xa. LMWH has a more predictable pharmacokinetic profile than unfractionated heparin and monitoring is usually not necessary. Anti-factor Xa levels can be measured if anticoagulant monitoring is desired, since LMWH does not reliably prolong the aPTT. LMWH is primarily cleared by the kidneys and it should be used with caution in patients with renal insufficiency. It is prudent to check factor Xa levels periodically in this patient population, though there are few guidelines for dose modifications. Similarly, there are no guidelines for dose adjustments in morbidly obese patients, and factor Xa levels should be checked a few days after therapy is initiated (Hirsh et al., 2001).

LMWH is indicated for prevention of venous thromboembolism (VTE), for treatment of venous thrombosis, for treatment of acute PE, and for the early treatment of patients with unstable angina. Like unfractionated heparin, bleeding can occur with LMWH but is less common. Spinal and epidural hematomas have been reported (see section on unfractionated heparin). HITT can occur with LMWH but the incidence is very low. LMWH is only partially neutralized by protamine sulfate.

FACTOR XA INHIBITORS

Fondaparinux is an indirect factor Xa inhibitor, which acts by catalyzing factor Xa inhibition by antithrombin. It is a synthetic analog of the antithrombin-binding pentasaccharide found in heparin or LMWH (Weitz et al., 2008). Fondaparinux is currently approved for treatment of DVT or PE, and VTE prophylaxis after major orthopedic surgery or abdominal surgery. It was shown to be as effective as LMWH in the treatment of acute DVT (Buller et al., 2004), and as effective as intravenous unfractionated heparin in the treatment of acute PE (Buller et al., 2003). The main complication of therapy is bleeding, and protamine sulfate is not effective at neutralizing fondaparinux (Rosenberg, 2001). As with other heparinoids, spinal and epidural hematomas have been reported. Isolated cases of HITT have also been reported (Warkentin et al., 2007).

WARFARIN

Warfarin (4-hydroxycoumarin) inhibits the synthesis of vitamin K-dependent coagulation factors, including factors II, VII, IX, and X, as well as proteins C and S. It is commonly used for prevention and treatment of VTE, prevention of stroke in atrial fibrillation, anticoagulation for mechanical prosthetic heart valves, and myocardial infarction prevention in coronary artery disease. Hemorrhage is the most common side-effect of anticoagulation with warfarin and can occur at any site. Cases of acute femoral neuropathy have been reported with therapeutic use of warfarin and are secondary to retroperitoneal bleeding (Butterfield et al., 1972). FFP can rapidly, albeit temporarily, reverse the anticoagulant effect in patients with life-threatening bleeding. Otherwise, oral vitamin K should be used to correct the coagulopathy. Warfarin is extensively metabolized by the hepatic cytochrome P450 system and polymorphisms in these enzymes contribute to interpatient variations in dosing (Francis, 2008). Warfarin also interacts with a variety of medications, which can lead to sub- or supratherapeutic INR values in a given patient. Similarly, variations in intake in vitamin K-containing foods can affect warfarin dosing. Warfarin is a teratogen and should not be given to women of child bearing age who may become pregnant. Warfarin-induced skin necrosis and venous gangrene can occur in patients with protein C or S deficiency who start warfarin without prior alternate anticoagulation. Anticoagulation with another medication prior to starting warfarin prevents this rare but serious complication of therapy, but is not uniformly required (Brandjes et al., 1992).

DIRECT THROMBIN INHIBITORS

Direct thrombin inhibitors inactivate thrombin in an antithrombin-independent fashion. Unlike heparin, they can inactivate thrombin that is bound to fibrin. Examples include hirudin (lepirudin), bivalirudin, and argatroban. These agents do not bind to plasma proteins, and therefore have a more predictable anticoagulant response than unfractionated heparin (Bauer, 2006). Also, they do not cause HITT and all three drugs are approved as treatment of patients with HITT. Argatroban does not require dose adjustment in patients with renal failure, but does for patients with liver disease. Lepirudin is renally excreted and should be dose-reduced in patients with decreased glomerular filtration rates. All three agents are given by continuous intravenous infusion and are monitored using the aPTT. Argatroban can also elevate the PT, making the transition to warfarin more complicated. All direct thrombin inhibitors can cause bleeding, including intracranial hemorrhage.

Dabigatran (Pradaxa®) is a reversible oral thrombin inhibitor. Its absorption is pH sensitive and is decreased by approximately 30% in the presence of proton pump inhibitors. Unlike warfarin, its metabolism is not dependent on cytochrome P450 enzymes and there are fewer drug interactions. Dabigatran can accumulate in patients with renal failure. A recent phase III trial of anticoagulation in patients with atrial fibrillation demonstrated rates of stroke and systemic embolism similar to those observed with warfarin, but lower rates of major hemorrhage (Connolly et al., 2009). Another trial (Schulman et al., 2009) shows that dabigatran is as effective as warfarin in the management of acute venous thromboembolism. This drug was recently FDA approved for use in patients with atrial fibrillation. Bleeding is the most common side-effect of dabigatran, including intracranial hemorrhage in 0.3% of patients (Connolly et al., 2009).

MANAGEMENT OF HEMORRHAGIC COMPLICATIONS OF ANTICOAGULATION

(Table 76.2)

Intracranial hemorrhages

WARFARIN

Warfarin use accounts for 10–15% of intracranial hemorrhages (ICH) (SPIRIT Study Group, 1997). The frequency of events is increasing as more elderly patients receive anticoagulation. Warfarin increases the risk of

Table 76.2

Management of coagulopathic intracranial hemorrhage

Anticoagulant	Treatment	Dose
Warfarin	FFP or PCC and Vitamin K	15 mL/kg 15–30 U/kg 10 mg
Heparin (unfractionated or low molecular weight)	Protamine sulfate	1 mg per 100 U of heparin or 1 mg of enoxaparin
Direct thrombin inhibitors	No antidote available	
Antiplatelet agents	Platelet transfusion and/or desmopressin (DDAVP)	Transfuse to > 100 000 platelets 0.3 µg/kg

ICH two to five times, with the risk of bleeding being proportional to the intensity of anticoagulation (Aguilar et al., 2007). There are no randomized trials addressing management of warfarin-induced ICH. Prompt, emergent reversal of anticoagulation is indicated and should be initiated prior to obtaining results of coagulation studies (Rincon et al., 2007). Reversal is usually accomplished with vitamin K and FFP; however, this takes several hours to accomplish. The volume of FFP required to reverse the INR can be > 2 liters, which is problematic in older patient populations. PCCs normalize the INR more rapidly and can be given in smaller volumes than FFP; however, they carry an increased risk of thrombosis and DIC in patients with severe brain injury. There are few data on PCCs in ICH, and different PCCs vary in their coagulation factor components, making comparison between trials difficult. Dosing is dependent on the specific PCC available, but the goal of treatment is reduction of the INR to < 1.2 (Aguilar et al., 2007). Vitamin K should also be administered.

Recombinant FVIIa has been used off-label to reverse anticoagulation in patients with ICH on warfarin. RFVIIa can reverse the INR within minutes, though the effect only lasts several hours and vitamin K and FFP should also be administered (Freeman et al., 2004). The FAST trial investigated two different doses of rFVIIa in ICH. Although rFVIIa reduced growth of the hematoma, there was no survival benefit or improvement in functional outcome at 90 days for either dose compared to placebo. Additionally, treatment increased the frequency of arterial thromboembolic serious adverse events in the high dose arm as compared to placebo (Mayer et al., 2008). Though this trial does not specifically address patients on warfarin with ICH, it does provide safety information and dosing guidelines. RFVIIa is currently not approved for treatment of ICH.

Restarting anticoagulation in patients with atrial fibrillation or mechanical prosthetic valves poses a therapeutic dilemma. There are no large randomized trials, and recommendations in the literature for holding anticoagulation vary from 1–6 weeks. The risk of embolic stroke occurring within 7–14 days after stopping warfarin appears to be low. If the INR is reversed with PCCs, subcutaneous heparin can be considered to reduce the risk of thrombosis. In most patients, warfarin can safely be restarted 7–14 days after the ICH (Aguilar et al., 2007).

UNFRACTIONATED AND LOW MOLECULAR WEIGHT HEPARIN

The anticoagulant effect of unfractionated heparin can be reversed with protamine sulfate. Protamine can partially reverse the effect of low molecular weight heparin.

The recommended dose of protamine is 1 mg per 100 U of heparin, or 1 mg of enoxaparin. Side-effects include flushing, bradycardia, and hypotension.

DIRECT THROMBIN INHIBITORS

The direct thrombin inhibitors lipirudin, argatroban, and bivalirudin directly inhibit thrombin. Unfortunately no direct antidote is available for their reversal.

ANTIPLATELET AGENTS

Aspirin, nonsteroidal anti-inflammatory agents, and ADP receptor inhibitors irreversibly inhibit platelet function. Treatment of hemorrhage associated with these agents involves stopping the drugs and transfusing platelets. Platelet levels should be maintained above 100 000/μL. Desmopressin (DDAVP) 0.3 μg/kg can be considered. This treatment promotes release of von Willebrand factor and enhances platelet function. However, there are few data to support this approach (Rincon et al., 2007).

AGENTS USED TO TREAT HEMATOLOGIC MALIGNANCIES
Chronic myeloproliferative neoplasms

The classic myeloproliferative neoplasms include polycythemia vera (PV), essential thrombocythemia (ET), idiopathic myelofibrosis (IMF), and chronic myeloid leukemia (CML). They are characterized by clonal bone marrow expansion of the myeloid series, with clinical features of hepatosplenomegaly, hypercatabolism, and increased numbers of circulating mature blood cells. The focus of treatment is to reduce cell proliferation and prevent sequelae of thrombosis and hemorrhage. In CML, small molecule tyrosine kinases target the disease defining genetic abnormality, the t(9;22)(q34;q11).

HYDROXYUREA

Hydroxyurea (Hydrea; hydroxycarbamide) is classified as an antimetabolite. It is thought to be cell cycle-specific for the S phase of cell division. Hydrea inhibits the enzyme ribonucleotide reductase, which converts ribonucleotides to deoxyribonucleotides, critical precursors for de novo DNA biosynthesis and DNA repair. There does not appear to be an effect on synthesis of RNA or protein (Chu and DeVita, 2009). In PV and ET, hydroxyurea is used as cytoreductive therapy in patients over the age of 60 years or those with a prior thrombotic event. Treatment with hydroxyurea reduces platelet counts as well as the thrombosis rate in these patients (Cortelazzo et al., 1995; Fruchtman et al., 1997).

The most common side-effect is myelosuppression. Mucocutaneous and skin ulcers, usually in the lower extremities, have been reported. Peripheral neuropathy has been reported in HIV-infected patients who receive hydroxyurea in combination with the antiretroviral agents didanosine (ddI) and stavudine (d4T). ddI and d4T are well known to cause neuropathy, but the addition of hydroxyurea to these medications significantly increases the risk of developing neuropathy. In this setting, hydroxyurea is used to potentiate the effect of these drugs (Moore et al., 2000). The most concerning potential side-effect of hydrea is development of secondary leukemia or myelodysplasia; however, data are not conclusive. Hydrea is teratogenic and is not given to women of child bearing potential. Interferon-α is used in place of hydroxyurea in this patient population.

ANAGRELIDE

Anagrelide is thought to reduce platelet production by decreasing megakaryocyte hypermaturation. It is used as a second-line agent in patients with ET who are intolerant of hydroxyurea. Anagrelide can cause arterial thrombosis including myocardial infarction, stroke, and transient ischemic attack (TIA). Serious hemorrhage, cardiomyopathy, and edema can also occur. Headache is a common side-effect and can lead to drug discontinuation (Harrison et al., 2005). There are no controlled studies on anagrelide in pregnant women, therefore its use is not recommended in this patient population.

BCR-ABL TYROSINE KINASE INHIBITORS

This class of drugs was rationally designed to target the disease-defining genetic abnormality that defines CML: the t(9;22)(q34;q11) or Philadelphia chromosome and its molecular equivalent, the *bcr-abl* fusion tyrosine kinase.

Imatinib mesylate (Gleevec™) was the first drug in this class and is approved for front-line therapy in patients with CML. Imatinib binds to the ATP pocket of the bcr-abl protein and inhibits substrate phosphorylation, thereby inducing apoptosis (Chu and DeVita, 2009). Imatinib also inhibits other receptor tyrosine kinases such as platelet-derived growth factor receptors (PDGFR), stem cell factor (SCF) and c-kit. It is well tolerated and common side-effects include edema and fluid retention, fatigue, rash, nausea and vomiting, diarrhea, myelosuppression, and cough. Congestive heart failure is the most serious reported side-effect. Headaches, insomnia, paresthesias, dizziness and asthenia have been reported in up to approximately 10–20% of patients.

Second-generation bcr-abl tyrosine kinase inhibitors have been developed to overcome resistance to imatinib. These agents were recently approved for first-line treatment of CML and are also used to treat accelerated or blast phase CML. Dasatinib (Sprycel®) is a potent inhibitor of the bcr-abl kinase as well as the SRC family of kinases, c-kit, and PDGFR-β. It binds to both the active and inactive conformations of the abl kinase domain, thereby overcoming imatinib resistance resulting from bcr-abl mutations (Chu and DeVita, 2009). Common side-effects include fluid retention, rash, hypocalcemia, and hypophosphatemia, diarrhea, nausea and vomiting, headache, dyspnea, and fatigue. Serious side-effects include myelosuppression, pleural effusions, QT prolongation, and hemorrhage (gastrointestinal and cerebral) secondary to platelet dysfunction.

Nilotinib (Tasigna®) is another second-generation bcr-abl kinase inhibitor, which also inhibits c-kit and PDGFR-β kinases. Nilotinib has a higher binding affinity and selectivity for the abl kinase domain when compared to imatinib, and is able to overcome imatinib resistance resulting from bcr-abl mutations (Chu and DeVita, 2009). Common side-effects include edema, pruritis, rash, constipation or diarrhea, myelosuppression, headache, nausea, fatigue, electrolyte disturbances, and elevations in serum lipase. QT prolongation and sudden death have been reported.

Imatinib is predominantly metabolized in the liver by the cytochrome P450 enzymes CYP3A4 and CYP3A5, while dasatinib and nilotinib are primarily metabolized in the liver by CYP3A4. Drug interactions are common and should be considered when caring for a patient on these medications.

Myelodysplasia

DNA METHYLTRANSFERASE INHIBITORS AND NUCLEOSIDE ANALOGS

5-azacitidine (Vidaza®) and 5-aza-2′-deoxycitidine (decitabine) are hypomethylating agents that inhibit DNA meythltransferase by incorporation of either azacitidine triphosphate or decitabine triphosphate into DNA. This leads to a loss of DNA methylation and reactivation of aberrantly silenced genes. They are cell cycle-specific with activity in the S phase. Azacitidine triphosphate is also incorporated into RNA, resulting in inhibition of RNA processing and function. A phase III trial demonstrated a survival advantage for azacitidine over conventional care, and established it as the preferred therapy for patients with high-risk myelodysplasia (MDS) (Fenaux et al., 2009). A similar trial conducted with decitabine did not demonstrate a survival advantage (WijerMans et al., 2008), though many feel the drugs are clinically equivalent and biologically similar.

Common side-effects of these agents include myelosuppression, fatigue and anorexia, nausea, vomiting, constipation and abdominal pain, and peripheral edema. Azacitidine can cause renal toxicity with elevations in serum creatinine, renal tubular acidosis and hypokalemia, while decitabine can cause hyperbilirubinemia. Both medications can also cause dizziness and headache (Chu and DeVita, 2009). CNS toxicity including coma was reported in a small number of patients on a clinical trial who were treated with doses of azacitidine that are higher than those used in current clinical practice (Saiki et al., 1981). Similarly, acute CNS toxicity with severe myalgias and altered mental status was reported in a child receiving high doses of azacitidine (Weisman et al., 1985).

Leukemias, lymphomas, and multiple myeloma

CHEMOTHERAPEUTIC AGENTS

Chemotherapeutic agents are classified according to their mechanism of action. Broad categories include alkylating agents, platinum agents, antimetabolites, topoisomerase inhibitors, antimicrotubule agents, and antibiotics.

Alkylating agents form covalent bonds with DNA bases. Bifunctional alkylators interact with two strands of DNA and form a "cross-link" that covalently links the two strands of the DNA double helix. This prevents the cell from replicating effectively. Common side-effects of alkylating agents include myelosuppression, nausea and vomiting, and alopecia. They are teratogenic and leukemogenic, with secondary myelodysplasia and acute leukemia occurring 7–10 years after therapy (Colvin and Friedman, 2005). Examples of alkylating agents used in hematologic malignancies include cyclophosphamide, ifosfamide, melphalan, and chlorambucil. Ifosfamide can cause CNS toxicity including confusion, somnolence and hallucinations, as well as encephalopathy and seizures.

Platinum agents interact with guanine and adenine residues to form DNA adducts and cross-link DNA strands. If the DNA damage is not repaired or tolerated, apoptosis occurs (Johnson and O'Dwyer, 2005). Examples of platinum agents include cisplatin, carboplatin, and oxaliplatin. Carboplatin is used for second-line treatment of leukemia and lymphoma. Cisplatin can cause peripheral neuropathy and ototoxicity. Oxaliplatin commonly causes both acute and delayed sensory neuropathy. Less commonly, it can cause pharyngolaryngeal dysesthesia and Lhermitte's sign.

Antimetabolites can be subclassified as purine analogs, pyrimidine analogs, and antifolates. They are cell cycle-specific and are therefore active on replicating cells. Antimetabolites interfere with DNA production and replication, causing apoptosis. Purine analogs include the 6-thiopurines 6-mercaptopurine and 6-thioguanine, fludarabine, 2-chlorodeoxyadenosine (2-CdA or cladribine) and pentostatin. Their toxicity profile includes dose-limiting myelosuppression, immunosuppression, pulmonary toxicity, and severe neurotoxicity, although this complication has occurred primarily at significantly greater doses than currently recommended for clinical use. Cladribine can cause a dose-dependent delayed sensorimotor peripheral neuropathy characterized by axonal degeneration and secondary demyelination (Vahdat et al., 1994). Irreversible paraparesis and quadraparesis were reported in patients with refractory acute leukemia and non-Hodgkin lymphoma who were treated with high doses of cladribine (Beutler et al., 1991). High doses of fludarabine and pentostatin are also neurotoxic (Cheson et al., 1994). At standard doses of fludarabine, somnolence and peripheral neuropathy have been reported (Cheson et al., 1994).

The 6-thiopurines are primarily used in treatment of acute leukemia, while fludarabine, cladribine and pentostatin are active in both leukemias and lymphomas.

Pyrimidine analogs include cytarabine, gemcitabine, 5-fluorouracil and capecitabine. Cytarabine is critical in the treatment of acute myeloid leukemia (AML). It is also used in treatment of acute lymphoblastic leukemia (ALL) and lymphomas, including primary central nervous system lymphoma. At high doses, cytarabine crosses the blood–brain barrier and can be effective as prophylaxis for CNS leukemia. High-dose cytarabine is neurotoxic and can cause seizures, cerebral and cerebellar dysfunction, peripheral neuropathy, bilateral rectus muscle palsy, optic neuritis, aphasia, and parkinsonian symptoms. Cerebral dysfunction manifests as generalized encephalopathy, with somnolence, confusion, disorientation, memory loss, cognitive dysfunction, psychosis, and frontal lobe release signs. Rapid infusion of high doses of cytarabine increases the risk of cerebral toxicity (Baker et al., 1991). Clinical signs of cerebellar dysfunction occur in up to 15% of patients within 8 days of treatment and include dysarthria, dysdiadochokinesia, dysmetria, and ataxia. EEG will often demonstrate diffuse slow wave activity. Even when therapy is discontinued, up to 30% of patients with cerebellar toxicity do not fully recover. Peripheral neuropathy is a rare complication of cytarabine therapy, occurring in < 1% of patients. The severity of symptoms increases with higher cumulative doses of cytarabine and can range from a pure sensory neuropathy to a rapidly progressive ascending polyneuropathy (Baker et al., 1991). Neurotoxicity can be reduced by increasing the duration of the infusion to more than 3 hours. Patients older than age 50 and those with elevated serum creatinine are particularly susceptible to neurologic toxicity from high-dose cytarabine (Kummar et al., 2005). Prior to each dose, patients are evaluated for neurotoxicity and doses are held or adjusted as necessary to minimize toxicity.

Cytarabine is also given intrathecally for prophylaxis of CNS leukemia in patients with acute lymphoblastic leukemia (ALL), and to treat leptomeningeal disease in both leukemias and solid tumors. A depot formulation, in which the cytarabine is encapsulated in multivesicular liposomes for sustained release in the CSF, is also available. Doses can be administered through an Ommaya reservoir or via lumbar puncture. For treatment of CNS leukemia, doses are typically given twice weekly until the leukemia is no longer detectable in the CSF. This is followed by weekly doses for 4 weeks, and monthly doses for up to 1 year. The depot formulation is typically given every 2 weeks. Dose-limiting toxicities include headache and arachnoiditis and are more common with the depot formulation. Myelopathy, paraplegia, papilledema, and seizures can also occur (Baker et al., 1991). Occasionally systemic toxicities such as nausea and myelosuppression, are seen with intrathecal cytarabine (Kummar et al., 2005).

Antifolate analogs include methotrexate, raltitrexed and pemetrexed. Methotrexate inhibits dihydrofolate reductase and prevents *de novo* thymidylate and purine nucleotide biosynthesis (Kummar et al., 2005). High dose methotrexate, often used in CNS lymphoma, is occasionally associated with an acute, transient cerebral dysfunction manifesting as paresis, aphasia, and behavioral abnormalities. Seizures have been described in 4–15% of patients who receive high-dose methotrexate. Symptoms generally occur within 6 days of treatment and completely resolve within 48–72 hours. Chronic neurotoxicity with encephalopathy, dementia and motor paresis can occur 2–3 months after administration of high-dose methotrexate (Kummar et al., 2005).

Intrathecal methotrexate is used for CNS prophylaxis in ALL, as well as treatment of CNS leukemia and leptomeningeal involvement by solid tumors. There are three distinct neurotoxic syndromes associated with intrathecal methotrexate (Walker et al., 1984). Acute chemical arachnoiditis can occur immediately after administration and is the most common toxicity. This syndrome is characterized by severe headaches, nuchal rigidity, vomiting, fever, and an inflammatory cell infiltrate in the CSF. A subacute form of neurotoxicity is seen in approximately 10% of patients and usually occurs after the third or fourth course of intrathecal therapy. This most commonly occurs in patients with active meningeal leukemia and consists of motor paralysis, cranial nerve palsies, seizures, and/or coma. Continued intrathecal therapy with methotrexate can result in death, therefore a change in therapy is mandatory. The third syndrome is a chronic demyelinating encephalopathy, which typically occurs in children several months to years after treatment. Patients present with dementia, limb spasticity, and in advanced cases, coma. Ventricular

enlargement, cortical thinning, and diffuse intracerebral calcifications are noted on computed tomographic (CT) scan (Kummar et al., 2005).

Inhibitors of topoisomerase I and II include irinotecan, topotecan, etoposide, and anthracyclines. DNA topoisomerases modify the tertiary structure of DNA without altering the primary nucleotide sequence. Topoisomerase inhibitors generate single and double strand breaks in DNA, resulting in apoptosis and cell death. They are cell cycle-specific. Etoposide and anthracyclines are used in treatment of acute leukemia and lymphomas.

Antimicrotubule agents include the vinca alkaloids (vincristine, vinblastine, vindesine) and the taxanes (paclitaxel and docetaxel). These agents interfere with microtubule function, particularly within the mitotic spindle apparatus. Vinca alkaloids are used in the treatment of ALL and lymphomas. Vincristine is particularly known for causing neurotoxicity, which is characterized by a symmetric, mixed sensorimotor and autonomic polyneuropathy. Pathologically, vincristine interferes with axonal microtubule function and causes axonal degeneration and decreased axonal transport. Symptoms start with a distal symmetric sensory impairment. With continued treatment, neuritic pain and loss of deep tendon reflexes can develop. This may be followed by foot drop, wrist drop, motor dysfunction, ataxia, and paralysis. Cranial nerves are rarely affected, but can manifest as hoarseness, diplopia, jaw pain, and facial palsies. Central toxicity from vincristine is also very rare because of minimal uptake in the CNS. Central effects can include confusion, mental status changes, hallucinations, insomnia, seizures, and coma. Acute, severe autonomic toxicity may be seen with high doses (greater than $2 \, mg/m^2$) or in patients with altered hepatic function. Autonomic toxicities can include constipation and abdominal cramps, ileus, urinary retention, and orthostatic hypotension. In adults, neurotoxicity can occur after treatment with cumulative doses of 5–6 mg, and toxicity can become severe after 15–20 mg. In routine treatment for lymphoma, adult patients receive 2 mg per treatment, with cumulative doses of 12–16 mg being given over 4–6 months. Children appear to be less sensitive, and older patients are particularly susceptible. Patients with preexisting neurologic disorders and hepatic dysfunction are at especially increased risk. The only treatment for vincristine neurotoxicity is discontinuation of the drug. Vinblastine and vindesine rarely cause neurotoxicity (Rowinsky and Tolcher, 2005).

Taxanes, particularly paclitaxel, can also cause neurotoxicity. This is most commonly a peripheral sensory neuropathy in a symmetric stocking-glove distribution. Neurologic examination reveals sensory loss and loss of deep tendon reflexes. Most patients experience mild to moderate effects, but patients with pre-existing neuropathy are more prone to development of taxane-induced neuropathy. Symptoms usually begin after several courses of standard-dose therapy, but can occur as early as 24–72 hours after the first treatment. Motor and autonomic neuropathy has also been reported with paclitaxel. Transient myalgia and arthralgia are also observed and most commonly occur within 24–48 hours after treatment. Treatment with prednisone can reduce myalgia and arthralgia. Taxanes are commonly used in the treatment of solid tumors.

TARGETED THERAPIES

Monoclonal antibodies

Rituximab (Rituxan®) is a chimeric (murine/human) monoclonal antibody against CD20, which is expressed on B lymphocytes. It is used in combination with chemotherapy to treat chronic lymphocytic leukemia, and can be given as a single agent or with chemotherapy to treat CD20 expressing non-Hodgkin's lymphomas. Rituxan is also approved for use in rheumatoid arthritis, and is sometimes used off label to treat autoimmune cytopenias and other autoimmune diseases. Rituxan causes cell lysis through complement-dependent cytotoxicity (CDC) and antibody-dependent cellular cytotoxicity (ADCC). Common side-effects include infusion reactions (hypotension, bronchospasm, rigors, angioedema), fatigue, and myelosuppression. Tumor lysis syndrome can occur in patients with significant tumor burden. Patients with prior hepatitis B infection can have reactivation of the virus, and should be screened for prior infection before the drug is administered. Similarly, reactivation of the JC virus can cause progressive multifocal leukoencephalopathy (PML) in patients who receive Rituxan in combination with chemotherapy, immunosuppression, or stem cell transplant. The largest series reported 57 HIV-negative patients with hematologic malignancies and autoimmune disorders (Carson et al., 2009). Patients commonly presented with confusion/disorientation, motor weakness or hemiparesis, poor motor coordination, and changes in speech or vision. Symptoms progressed over weeks to months. The diagnosis was primarily confirmed by magnetic resonance imaging and JC virus detection in the CSF, or by brain biopsy or autopsy. Mortality was very high: all patients diagnosed with PML within 3 months of the last rituximab dose died, compared with 84% of patients who were diagnosed more than 3 months after the last rituximab dose. There is no standard effective therapy for this condition.

Gemtuzumab ozogamicin (GO or Mylotarg®) is a recombinant humanized IgG4 κ antibody that is conjugated with calicheamicin, a cytotoxic antitumor antibiotic. The antibody portion of GO targets CD33, which is commonly expressed on leukemic blasts. After the antibody binds, a complex is formed and internalized, calicheamicin is released within the myeloid cell lysosomes, and the cell dies. GO is approved for treatment of relapsed leukemia. Common side-effects include infusion reactions, myelosuppression, and hepatotoxicity.

Radioimmunotherapy

Radioimmunotherapy allows the targeted delivery of ionizing radiation to the tumor site, while minimizing toxicity on normal tissue. This is accomplished by conjugating radioactive isotopes to monoclonal antibodies that target tumor cells. Currently, two products are approved for treatment of relapsed and refractory non-Hodgkin lymphoma.

Tositumomab (Bexxar®) and ibritumomab (Zevalin®) are monoclonal antibodies to CD20 that are conjugated with the radionuclides iodine-131 (I-131) and yttrium-90 (Y-90), respectively. Side-effects include infusion reactions, asthenia and fatigue, and myelosuppression. There is also a risk of myelodysplasia and/or acute leukemia (Davies, 2007).

Immunomodulatory drugs

Thalidomide and lenalidomide are immunomodulatory drugs (IMiDs) primarily used in the treatment of multiple myeloma. Lenalidomide is also being studied for treatment of relapsed lymphomas. They have direct cytotoxic effects and induce apoptosis or growth arrest of myeloma cells. They also have potent antiangiogenic and anti-inflammatory effects that appear to inhibit cell growth (Kumar and Rajkumar, 2006). In the 1950s thalidomide was used to treat morning sickness in pregnant women. Several years later it was identified as a teratogen and was not used again until the 1990s, when it was investigated in cancer patients. Common side-effects include constipation, drowsiness and somnolence, neutropenia, and VTE when used in combination with steroids or chemotherapy. Thalidomide also causes a debilitating peripheral neuropathy as well as orthostatic hypotension and dizziness. Lenalidomide, a second-generation IMiD, is much better tolerated, with myelosuppression being the most common side-effect. Lenalidomide can also cause VTE when used in combination with steroids or chemotherapy, but it is not associated with peripheral neuropathy.

Proteosome inhibitors

Bortezomib (Velcade®) is a small molecule that inhibits the activity of the 26S proteasome, which degrades ubiquitinated proteins. The ubiquitin-proteasome pathway is critical for regulating concentrations of intracellular proteins and maintaining intracellular homeostasis. Inhibition of the proteasome prevents this targeted proteolysis and can affect multiple signaling cascades within the cell. Disruption of the normal homeostatic mechanisms can lead to cell death. Bortezomib is active in multiple myeloma as well as non-Hodgkin lymphomas. Common side-effects include constipation or diarrhea, nausea and vomiting, myelosuppression, dyspnea and cough, and peripheral neuropathy. The neuropathy is predominantly sensory, but motor neuropathy has also been reported.

REFERENCES

Abshire T, Kenet G (2004). Recombinant factor VIIa: review of efficacy, dosing regimens and safety in patients with congenital and acquired factor VIII or IX inhibitors. J Thromb Haemost 2: 899–909.

Aguilar MI, Hart RG, Kase CS et al. (2007). Treatment of warfarin-associated intracerebral hemorrhage: literature review and expert opinion. Mayo Clin Proc 82: 82–92.

Albers GW, Amarenco P, Easton JD et al. (2008). Antithrombotic and thrombolytic therapy for ischemic stroke: American College of Chest Physicians evidence-based clinical practice guidelines (8th edition). Chest 133: 630S–669S.

APASS Writing Committee (2004). Antiphospholipid antibodies and subsequent thrombo-occlusive events in patients with ischemic stroke. JAMA 291: 576–584.

Babior BM (2006). Folate, cobalamin and megaloblastic anemias. In: E Beutler, K Kaushansky, TJ Kipps et al. (Eds.), Williams Hematology, McGraw-Hill, United States, pp. 477–509.

Baker JW, Royer GL, Weiss RB (1991). Cytarabine and neurologic toxicity. J Clin Oncol 9: 679–693.

Bauer KA (2006). New anticoagulants. Hematology Am Soc Hematol Educ Program 2006: 450–456.

Bennett CL, Weinberg PD, Rozenberg-Ben-Dror K et al. (1998). Thrombotic thrombocytopenic purpura associated with ticlopidine: a review of 60 cases. Ann Intern Med 128: 541–544.

Bennett CL, Connors JM, Carwile JM et al. (2000). Thrombotic thrombocytopenic purpura associated with clopidogrel. N Engl J Med 342: 1773–1777.

Beutler E, Piro LD, Saven A et al. (1991). 2-Chlorodeoxyadenosine (2-CdA): a potent chemotherapeutic and immunosuppressive nucleoside. Leuk Lymphoma 5: 1–8.

Brandjes DP, Heijboer H, Buller HR et al. (1992). Acenocoumarol and heparin compared with acenocoumarol alone in the initial management of proximal vein thrombosis. N Engl J Med 327: 1485–1489.

Buller HR, Davidson BL, Decousus H et al. (2003). Subcutaneous fondaparinux versus intravenous unfractionated heparin in the initial treatment of pulmonary embolism. N Engl J Med 349: 1695–1702.

Buller HR, Davidson BL, Decousus H et al. (2004). Fondaparinux or enoxaparin for the initial treatment of symptomatic deep venous thrombosis: a randomized trial. Ann Intern Med 140: 867–873.

Butterfield WC, Neviaser RJ, Roberts MP (1972). Femoral neuropathy and anticoagulants. Ann Surg 176: 58–61.

Carson KR, Evens AM, Richey EA et al. (2009). Progressive multifocal leukoencephalopathy after rituximab therapy in HIV-negative patients: a report of 57 cases from the Research on Adverse Drug Events and Reports project. Blood 113: 4834–4840.

Cheson BD, Vena DA, Foss FM et al. (1994). Neurotoxicity of purine analogs: a review. J Clin Oncol 10: 2216–2228.

Chew DP, Bhatt DL, Sapp S et al. (2001). Increased mortality with oral platelet glycoprotein IIb/IIIa antagonists: a metaanalysis of phase II multicenter trials. Circulation 103: 201–206.

Chu E, DeVita VT (2009). Physicians' Cancer Chemotherapy Drug Manual, Jones and Bartlett, Sudbury, MA.

Colvin MO, Friedman HS (2005). Alkylating agents. In: VT DeVita, S Hellman, SA Rosenberg (Eds.), Cancer: Principles and Practice of Oncology, Lipincott Williams and Wilkins, Philadelphia, PA.

Connolly SJ, Ezekowitz MD, Yusuf S et al. (2009). Dabigatran versus warfarin in patients with atrial fibrillation. N Engl J Med 361: 1–11.

Cook JD (2005). Diagnosis and management of iron deficiency anemia. Best Pract Res Clin Haematol 18: 319–332.

Copelan EA, Strohm PL, Kennedy MS et al. (1986). Hemolysis following intravenous immune globulin. Transfusion 26: 410–412.

Cortelazzo S, Finazzi G, Ruggeri M et al. (1995). Hydroxyurea for patients with essential thrombocythemia and a high risk of thrombosis. N Engl J Med 332: 1132–1136.

Davies AJ (2007). Radioimmunotherapy for B-cell lymphoma: Y90 ibritumomab tiuxetan and I(131) tositumomab. Oncogene 26: 3614–3628.

Diener HC, Cunha L, Forbes C (1996). European Stroke Study II Dypiridamole and acetylsalicylic acid in the secondary prevention of stroke. J Neurol Sci 143: 1–13.

Fenaux P, Mufti GJ, Hellstrom-Lindberg E et al. (2009). Efficacy of azacitidine compared with that of conventional care regimens in the treatment of higher-risk myelodysplastic syndromes: a randomised, open-label, phase III study. Lancet Oncol 10: 223–232.

Forristal T, Witt M (1968). Pleocytosis after iron dextran injection. Lancet 1: 1428.

Francis CW (2008). New issues in oral anticoagulants. Hematology Am Soc Hematol Educ Program 2008: 259–265.

Freeman WD, Brott TG, Barrett KM et al. (2004). Recombinant factor IVVa for rapid reversal of warfarin anticoagulation in acute intracranial hemorrhage. Mayo Clin Proc 79: 1495–1500.

Fruchtman SM, Mack K, Kaplan ME et al. (1997). From efficacy to safety: a Polycythemia Vera Study Group report on hydroxyurea in patients with polycythemia vera. Semin Hematol 34: 17–23.

Gorelick PB, Weisman SM (2005). Risk of hemorrhagic stroke with aspirin use – an update. Stroke 36: 1801–1807.

Guidolin L, Vignoli A, Canger R (1998). Worsening in seizure frequency and severity in relation to folic acid administration. Eur J Neurol 5: 301–303.

Harrison CN, Campbell PJ, Buck G et al. (2005). Hydroxyurea compared with anagrelide in high-risk essential thrombocythemia. N Engl J Med 353: 33–45.

Hellstern P (1999). Production and composition of prothrombin complex concentrates: correlation between composition and therapeutic efficiency. Thromb Res 95 (4 Suppl 1): S3–S6.

Hirsh J, Warkentin TE, Shaughnessy SG et al. (2001). Heparin and low-molecular-weight heparin mechanisms of action, pharmacokinetics, dosing, monitoring, efficacy, and safety. Chest 119: 64S–94S.

Hunter R, Barnes J, Oakeley HF et al. (1970). Toxicity of folic acid given in pharmacological doses to healthy volunteers. Lancet 1: 61–63.

Johnson SW, O'Dwyer PJ (2005). Cisplatin and its analogues. In: VT DeVita, S Hellman, SA Rosenberg (Eds.), Cancer: Principles and Practice of Oncology. Lipincott Williams and Wilkins, Philadelphia, PA.

Kelton JG, Hirsh J (1980). Bleeding associated with antithrombotic therapy. Semin Hematol 17: 259–291.

Killip S, Bennett JM, Chambers MD (2007). Iron deficiency anemia. Am Fam Physician 75: 671–678.

Knezevic-Maramica I, Druskall MS (2003). Intravenous immune globulines: an update for clinicians. Transfusion 43: 1460–1480.

Krishnaswamy K, Nair KM (2001). Importance of folate in human nutrition. Br J Nutr 85 (Suppl 2): S115–S124.

Kumar S, Rajkumar SV (2006). Thalidomide and lenalidomide in the treatment of multiple myeloma. Eur J Cancer 42: 1612–1622.

Kummar S, Noronha V, Chu E (2005). Antimetabolites. In: VT DeVita, S Hellman, SA Rosenberg (Eds.), Cancer: Principles and Practice of Oncology. Lipincott Williams and Wilkins, Philadelphia, PA.

Kutteh WH (1996). Antiphospholipid antibody-associated recurrent pregnancy loss: treatment with heparin and low-dose aspirin is superior to low-dose aspirin alone. Am J Obstet Gynecol 174: 1584–1589.

MacLennan S, Barbara JA (2006). Risks and side effects of therapy with plasma and plasma fractions. Best Pract Res Clin Haematol 19: 169–189.

Marie I, Maurey G, Hervé F et al. (2006). Intravenous immunoglobulin-related thrombotic complications. Br J Dermatol 155: 714–721.

Mayer SA, Brun NC, Begtrup K et al. (2008). Efficacy and safety of recombinant activated factor VII for acute intracerebral hemorrhage. N Engl J Med 358: 2127–2137.

McCarthy L, Eichelberger L, Skipworth E et al. (2002). Erythromelalgia due to essential thrombocythemia. Transfusion 42: 1245.

Moore RD, Wong WE, Keruly JC et al. (2000). Incidence of neuropathy in HIV-infected patients on monotherapy versus those on combination therapy with didanosine, stavudine and hydroxyurea. AIDS 14: 273–278.

Stroke Prevention in Reversible Ischemia Trial (SPIRIT) Study Group: a randomized trial of anticoagulants versus aspirin after cerebral ischemia of presumed arterial origin (1997). Ann Neurol 42: 857–865.

Oh RC, Brown DL (2003). Vitamin B_{12} deficiency. Am Fam Physician 67: 979–986.

Orbach H, Katz U, Sherer Y et al. (2005). Intravenous immunoglobulin: adverse effects and safe administration. Clin Rev Allergy Immunol 29: 173–184.

Paran D, Herishanu Y, Elkayam O et al. (2005). Venous and arterial thrombosis following administration of intravenous immunoglobulins. Blood Coagul Fibrinolysis 16: 313–318.

Rai R, Cohen H, Dave M et al. (1997). Randomised controlled trial of aspirin and aspirin plus heparin in pregnant women with recurrent miscarriage associated with phospholipid antibodies (or antiphospholipid antibodies). BMJ 314: 257.

Redman RC, Miller JB, Hood M et al. (2002). Trimethoprim-induced aseptic meningitis in an adolescent male. Pediatrics 110: 1–2.

Reutter A, Luger TA (2004). Efficacy and safety of intravenous immunoglobulin for immune-mediated skin disease: current view. Am J Clin Dermatol 5: 153–160.

Rincon F, Fernandez A, Mayer SA (2007). Hematology interventions for acute central nervous system disease. In: CS Kitchens, BM Alving, CM Kessler (Eds.), Consultative Hemostasis and Thrombosis, Saunders Elsevier, Philadelphia, PA.

Roberts HR, Monroe DM, White GC (2004). The use of recombinant factor VIIa in the treatment of bleeding disorders. Blood 104: 3858–3864.

Rosenberg RD (2001). Redesigning heparin. N Engl J Med 344: 673.

Rowinsky EK, Tolcher AW (2005). Antimicrotubule agents. In: VT DeVita, S Hellman, SA Rosenberg (Eds.), Cancer: Principles and Practice of Oncology, Lipincott Williams and Wilkins, Philadelphia, PA.

Saiki JH, Bodey GP, Hewlett JS et al. (1981). Effect of schedule on activity and toxicity of 5-azacytidine in acute leukemia. Cancer 47: 1739–1742.

Schomig A (2009). Ticagrelor – is there need for a new player in the antiplatelet therapy field? N Engl J Med 361: 1108–1110.

Schulman S, Kearon C, Kakkar AK et al. (2009). Dabigatran versus warfarin in the treatment of acute venous thromboembolism. N Engl J Med 361: 2342–2352.

Silverstein SB (2004). Parenteral iron therapy options. Am J Hematol 76: 74–78.

Stanworth SJ (2007). The evidence-based use of FFP and cryoprecipitate for abnormalities of coagulation tests and clinical coagulopathy. Hematology Am Soc Hematol Educ Program 2007: 179–186.

Tefferi A (2003). Polycythemia vera: a comprehensive review and clinical recommendations. Mayo Clin Proc 78: 174–194.

Triulzi DJ (2006). Transfusion-related acute lung injury: an update. Hematology Am Soc Hematol Educ Program 2006: 497–501.

Umbreit J (2005). Iron deficiency: a concise review. Am J Hematol 78: 225–231.

Vahdat L, Wong ET, Wile MJ et al. (1994). Therapeutic and neurotoxic effects of 2-chlorodeoxyadenosine in adults with acute myeloid leukemia. Blood 84: 3429–3434.

Varon D, Spectre G (2009). Antiplatelet agents. Hematology Am Soc Hematol Educ Program 2009: 267–262.

Verstraete M (1985). Clinical application of inhibitors of fibrinolysis. Drugs 29: 236–261.

Walker RW, Allen JC, Rosen G et al. (1984). Transient cerebral dysfunction secondary to high dose methotrexate. Cancer 53: 1849.

Wallentin L, Varenhorst C, James S (2008). Prasugrel achieves greater and faster P2Y12 receptor mediated platelet inhibition than clopidogrel due to more efficient generation of its active metabolite in aspirin treated patients with coronary artery disease. Eur Heart J 29: 21–30.

Wallentin L, Becker RC, Budaj A et al. (2009). Ticagrelor versus clopidogrel in patients with acute coronary syndromes. N Engl J Med 361: 1045–1057.

Wallerstein RO (1968). Intravenous iron-dextran complex. Blood 32: 690.

Warkentin TE, Maurer BT, Aster RH et al. (2007). Heparin-induced thrombocytopenia associated with fondaparinux. N Engl J Med 356: 2653–2655.

Weisman SJ, Berkow RL, Weetman RM et al. (1985). 5-Azacytidine: acute central nervous system toxicity. Am J Pediatr Hematol Oncol 7: 86–88.

Weitz JI, Hirsh J, Samama MM (2008). New antithrombotic drugs: American College of Chest Physicians evidence-based clinical practice guidelines (8th edition). Chest 133: 234S–256S.

WijerMans P, Suciu S, Baila L et al. (2008). Low dose decitabine versus best supportive care in elderly patients with intermediate or high risk MDS not eligible for intensive chemotherapy: final results of the randomized phase III study (06011) of the EORTC Leukemia and German MDS Study Groups. Blood (ASH Annual Meeting Abstracts) 112: 226.

Wiviott SD, Braunwald E, McCabe CH et al. (2007). Prasugrel versus clopidogrel in patients with acute coronary syndrome. N Engl J Med 361: 1045–1057.

Wysowski DK, Talarico L, Bacsanyi J et al. (1998). Spinal and epidural hematoma and low molecular weight heparin. N Engl J Med 338: 1774.

Index

NB: Page numbers in *italics* refer to figures and tables.